Management of
**Common
Musculoskeletal
Disorders**

Darlene Hertling, B.S., R.P.T.

Lecturer, Division of Physical Therapy
Department of Rehabilitation Medicine
University of Washington School of Medicine
Seattle, Washington

Randolph M. Kessler, M.D.

with 5 additional contributors

Illustrations by Elisabeth Kessler

Management of
Common Musculoskeletal Disorders

Physical Therapy Principles and Methods

THIRD EDITION

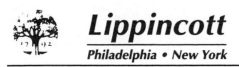
Lippincott
Philadelphia • New York

Sponsoring Editor: **Andrew Allen**
Development Editor: **Laura Dover**
Project Editor: **Tom Gibbons**
Indexer: **Victoria Boyle**
Design Coordinator: **Doug Smock**
Interior Designer: **Maria Karkucinski**
Cover Designer: **Ilene Griff**
Production Manager: **Helen Ewan**
Production Coordinator: **Patricia McCloskey**
Compositor: **Pine Tree Composition, Inc.**
Printer/Binder: **Courier Book Company/ Kendallville**
Cover Printer: **Lehigh**

Third Edition

Library of Congress Cataloging-in-Publication Data

Hertling, Darlene.
    Management of common musculoskeletal disorders : physical
therapy principles and methods / Darlene Hertling, Randolph M.
Kessler; with 5 additional contributors : illustrations by Elizabeth
Kessler. —3rd ed.
        p.   cm.
    A Lippincott physical therapy title.
    Includes bibliographical references and index.
    ISBN 0–397–55150–9
    1. Physical therapy.   2. Musculoskeletal system—Diseases—
Patients—Rehabilitation.   I. Kessler, Randolph M.   II. Kessler,
Randolph M.   III. Title.
    [DNLM: 1. Bone Diseases—therapy.   2. Bone Diseases—
therapy.   3. Physical Therapy.   4. Muscular Diseases—ther-
apy.   5. Physical Therapy.   WE 140 H574m 1996]
RM700.H48   1996
616.7′062—dc20
DNLM/DLC   95–4483
for Library of Congress   CIP

9   8   7   6   5

To Max, Tess, Tera
Gunter, Sonja, and Dieter

Contributors

MITCHELL G. BLAKNEY, B.S., P.T.

Practicing Physical Therapist
Gig Harbor, Washington

NEIL P. CHASAN, B.S., P.T.

Practicing Physical Therapist
Seattle, Washington

DANIEL JONES, B.S., PT

Practicing Physical Therapist
Portland, Oregon

MAUREEN K. LYNCH, M.D., P.T.

Practicing Physician
Seattle, Washington

LARRY J. TILLMAN, PH.D.

Department of Physical Therapy
University of Tennessee
Chattanooga, Tennessee

Preface

In the decade that has elapsed since the first edition of Management of Common Musculoskeletal Disorders, a number of therapeutic advances have either been newly introduced or been made generally available. This book was conceived at a time when the lack of proper textbooks on impaired function and management of common musculoskeletal disorders was a major obstacle to teaching. Now there are numerous texts dealing with the teaching of soft tissue and joint mobilization, stabilization techniques, exercises, and so forth.

This third edition has again been expanded. Three entirely new chapters have been added. The techniques formerly described in the chapters on peripheral joint mobilization techniques and automobilization for the extremities have been absorbed into their respective peripheral joint chapters.

The book comprises three parts: Basic Concepts and Techniques, and Clinical Applications of the Peripheral Joints and the Spine. Part One, dealing with background material, is not meant to be a comprehensive discussion of the musculoskeletal system, which is well covered in other studies. A new Chapter 2, Properties of Dense Connective Tissue and Wound Healing, was authored by Larry Tillman and Neil Chasan. The overview of important concepts concerning connective tissue properties, behavior, injury, and repair is long overdue. The material vital for further discussion of a variety of topics is presented later in this text. We thank these authors for their work, cooperation, and patience.

Chapter 6, Introduction to Manual Therapy, includes a history of mobilization techniques (from the first edition) and a broad overview of manual therapy. This chapter addresses a number of new techniques that sometimes do not enjoy support in the literature but are being used by an ever-increasing number of therapists. It can be disastrous to confine one's interest to one area of specialty and to remain unaware of both the broader context of treatment and the possible alternatives.

The key chapter in this first section, from a clinical standpoint, is Chapter 5, Assessment of Musculoskeletal Disorders. A comprehensive system of patient evaluation is a crucial component of the clinician's overall approach to management. Ways to elicit subjective and objective data are presented, along with guides to the interpretation of findings.

Parts Two and Three encompass the clinical applications of the preceding materials as they relate to selected conditions affecting the peripheral joints and the spine. Each of the regional chapters in these sections is organized to include functional anatomy and biomechanics, specific regional evaluation, and common lesions and their management. Most of the chapters have been expanded, including Chapter 14, which formerly covered only the ankle and hindfoot and now includes the lower leg and forefoot. Chapters on the thoracic spine and the sacroiliac joint have been added for completeness.

Identification of the treatment most likely to succeed continues to improve, emphasizing either "hands on" procedures (Grieves 1986; Maitland 1987) or the "hands off" approach (McKenzie 1979; Holten 1984). Active mobility rather then passive mobility continues to be emphasized. Significant clinical contributions have been made by Robin McKenzie, a New Zealand physiotherapist of international renown who has expanded on an original contribution with his lateral shift treatment technique for patients with lumbar discogenic disorders, and by Brian Edwards of Australia, who has formalized combined movements in examination and treatment.

The works of Lewit, Fryett, Mitchell, Grieves, Janda and others have resulted in new methods of post-isometric relaxation techniques. Lewit (1985), having worked for about 30 years in the field of painful disorders stemming from impaired locomotor function, has observed that movement restrictions are not necessarily due to an articular lesion. Post-isometric relaxation techniques (which employ the patient's active participation during manual therapy techniques) are based on the prime importance of soft tissues, particularly the muscles, as opposed to the skeletal elements of joint structures, in producing various abnormal states of joint pain and movement limitations.

This book was originally written for the student in the advanced stages of training and for the practicing clinician. Originally it was directed toward physical therapists, but we soon recognized that its cross-sectional interest should be much broader. Patients with musculoskeletal disorders are likely to consult any one of a wide variety of practitioners. We trust that orthopaedists, osteopaths, physiatrists, rheumatologists, family practitioners, chiropractors, orthopaedic assistants, occupational therapists, physical therapy assistants, athletic trainers, massage therapists, orthopaedic nurses, and alternative somatic practitioners will also find it useful.

It is our hope that this third edition will continue to provide a foundation for designing creative and appropriate therapeutic programs. Occasionally we have chosen to introduce complex materials at a somewhat superficial level with the intent of exposing the reader to advanced concepts. Readers who wish to pursue topics in depth are encouraged to continue reading in the reference lists at the end of each chapter. Most of the techniques described here are widely accepted. No claim is made for original methods of treatment.

We thank the readers who have been so responsive to our efforts to develop a readable and comprehensive text on management of common musculoskeletal conditions and would like to encourage colleagues in the field to continue their dialogue with us. We acknowledge Professor Jo Ann McMillian, Head of Physical Therapy, Rehabilitation Medicine, University of Washington Medical Center, for her support and continuous encouragement for the research and writing of this edition. Thanks are also due to various people—some students, some colleagues, patients, and a family member who allowed us to use them as pictorial models. Our thanks to the physical therapy students and the staff at the University of Washington for their contributions to the development of this edition. Furthermore, we acknowledge the contributions of the following individuals who reviewed this edition: Laura Robinson, Jenny Cole, Anita Sterling, Beth Mortimer, Kelly Fitzgerald, and Robert Reif.

We particularly recognize the important role Elizabeth Kessler played in providing the art work as well as Bruce Terami in providing the photography. Finally, I am especially appreciative of the invaluable assistance and encouragement provided me by the following members of the editoral staff of Lippincott-Raven Publishers: Andrew Allen, Laura Dover, and Tom Gibbons.

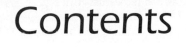

Contents

PART THREE
CLINICAL APPLICATIONS—THE SPINE

Management of
**Common
Musculoskeletal
Disorders**

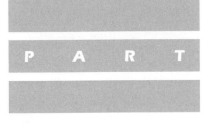

Basic Concepts
and Techniques

CHAPTER 1

Embryology of the Musculoskeletal System

RANDOLPH M. KESSLER

■ Axial Components
■ Limbs
■ Terminology

Knowledge of the development of the musculoskeletal tissues is of particular value to clinicians, whether they deal mainly with patients with developmental disabilities, long-term rehabilitation problems, or common musculoskeletal disorders, because it yields insight into the phenomenon of pain perception, segmental innervation, repair processes, and general body organization. Surely every clinician at some time has wondered, Why does my patient with a neck problem feel pain in the scapula? Why do my patients with shoulder problems feel pain not in the shoulder but in the upper arm? Why do some muscles receive innervation from all of the segments that they cross, whereas some muscles crossing many segments, such as the latissimus dorsi, receive innervation from relatively few segments? What is the explanation for the "spiraling" nature of the dermatomes, especially in the lower limb? The answers to some of these questions are not essential for competent clinical performance. However, some concepts, such as patterns of pain referral, are of the utmost importance in patient evaluation and treatment and should be pursued in depth. The study of embryology adds to our understanding of these concepts and deserves consideration here.

■ AXIAL COMPONENTS

The early developing embryo is composed of three primary, or germinal, layers: ectoderm, endoderm, and mesoderm. By the fourth week of development, the neural plate lying centrally in the ectoderm begins to invaginate into the underlying mesoderm. As this occurs, the peripheral margins of the neural plate gradually become more prominent and begin to approximate one another. Eventually they meet, forming the neural tube, which pinches off from the ectoderm and ends up lying within the mesoderm (Fig. 1-1). A similar phenomenon occurs ventrally; the notochordal process migrates and pinches off to form the notochord, which lies free in the ventral mesodermal layer.

The intrusion of the notochord and neural tube results in compaction of the mesodermal cells lying lateral to them. The compaction of the paraxial mesoderm forms the somites, of which there are originally 42 to 44 pairs: 4 occipital, 8 cervical, 12 thoracic, 5 lumbar, 5 sacral, and 8 to 10 coccygeal. These roughly coincide with what are to become the craniovertebral segments. The ventromedial cells of the vertebral somites, the sclerotomes, migrate medially to surround the notochord and neural tube (Fig. 1-2). In a

Darlene Hertling and Randolph M. Kessler: MANAGEMENT OF COMMON MUSCULOSKELETAL DISORDERS: Physical Therapy Principles and Methods, 3rd ed.
© 1996 Lippincott-Raven Publishers.

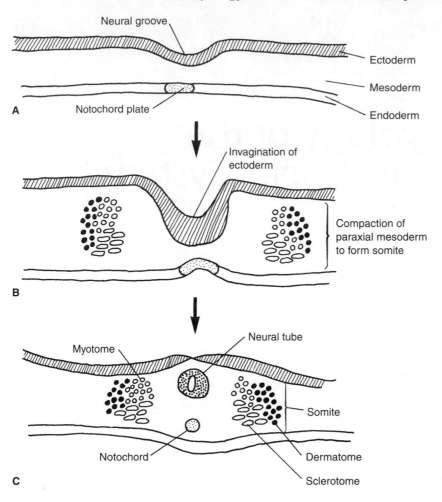

FIG. 1-1. Germinal layers of the early embryo. Invagination of the ectoderm forms the neural tube.

longitudinal cross-section (Fig. 1-3), each sclerotome is divided by a layer of cells called the *perichordal disk.* The cranial half of one sclerotome then unites with the caudal half of the adjacent sclerotome, causing a shift in the relationship between sclerotomes and the remaining somites. The sclerotomes eventually chondrify, or become cartilaginous, and then ossify to become the vertebrae. They also form cartilage, capsules, ligaments, and blood vessels. The peri-

chordal disk becomes the annulus fibrosis, while the notochord becomes the original nucleus pulposus. The neural tube gradually differentiates into nerve tissue, becoming the spinal cord and sending out peripheral nerves to the adjacent mesoderm.

The more dorsomedial somite cells are the myotomes. These cells divide into the hypomere, which migrates around to form the ventrolateral trunk muscles, and the epimere, which forms the segmental muscles of the back. As this occurs, the spinal nerve divides to form the anterior primary ramus, which invades the hypomere, and the posterior primary ramus, which innervates the segmental back muscles. Because of the segmental shift in relationship between the sclerotomes and myotomes, the segmental back muscles each cross at least one segment.

The remaining somatic cells are the dermatomes. These cells migrate out around the body wall, beneath the ectoderm, to form the dermal layer of skin. The dermis becomes innervated by sensory branches of the division (ramus) of the spinal nerve that innervates the muscles underlying it. The epidermal layer of skin is derived from the ectoderm.

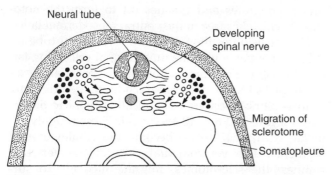

FIG. 1-2. Ventromedial migration of sclerotomic cells.

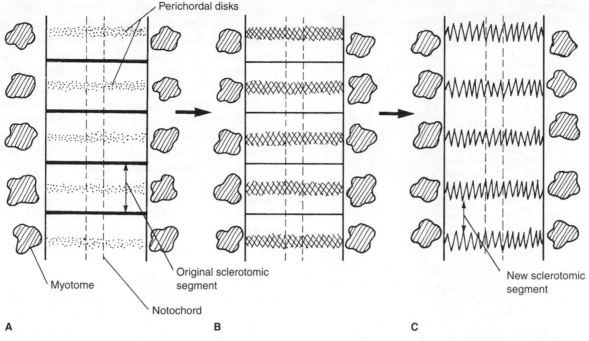

Perichordal disks

Myotome

Original sclerotomic
segment

Notochord

New sclerotomic
segment

A   B   C

FIG. 1-3. *Diagram of the shift in relationship between a sclerotome and remaining somatic segments.*

LIMBS

The limb buds appear during the fourth week in the developing embryo. A few days before the hindlimb appears, the forelimb develops at the lateral body wall level with the C4–T2 segments. The hindlimb appears at an area level with the L1–S2 segments (Fig. 1-4). The early limb bud is a mass of mesenchymal cells arising from the laterally located somatopleure and covered by an ectodermal layer. The mesenchymal cells are pluripotential, in that some will develop into osteoblasts, some into fibroblasts, some into myoblasts, and some into chondroblasts. The muscles of the limb buds develop *in situ* rather than from an invasion of cells from the myotome of the somite; this occurs as a result of differentiation of primitive mesenchymal cells into myoblasts, which become multinucleated muscle cells or fibers. The anterior primary divisions of the spinal nerve invade the developing limb buds to innervate the early muscle masses. Because of the intertwining of segmental nerves throughout the regional plexus and because the early muscle masses tend to divide or fuse with one another, each muscle typically receives innervation from more than one segment, and each segmental nerve tends to innervate more than one muscle. The intertwining of segments through the plexus also explains the overlapping, somewhat unpatterned skin innervation of the limbs.

The original orientation of the limb buds is such that the upper limb is positioned laterally, lying in the frontal plane at about 90° abduction, with the palm facing forward. The lower limb is positioned similarly, with the hip externally rotated, the patella facing posteriorly, and the sole facing forward. Gradually the limbs rotate down into the fetal position. This rotation and adduction of the limb buds explains the spiraling nature of the limb segments (dermatomes, myotomes, and sclerotomes), especially in the lower limbs, which undergo more rotation. It also explains the anteversion and varus angle of the normal femoral neck in relation to the shaft of the femur and the external torsion of the tibial shaft, which compensates for the internal torsion of the femur.

A guide to determining approximate segmental innervation of a limb is to imagine the limb in the original embryological position. In this position, the more cranial aspects of the limb are innervated by cranial segments, and the more caudal aspects by caudal segments. Thus the inner thigh, which was originally located cranially, is innervated by L2, whereas the outer lower leg, which was positioned caudally, is innervated by S1. Also worth noting is the fact that the scapula originates as part of the developing limb bud. As the limb develops, the scapula migrates to become "folded back" on the posterior body wall. This explains why the scapula, although it lies level with thoracic segments, is innervated primarily by cervical segments. Thus, pain of cervical origin is often referred to the scapulae as well as to the arms. Although

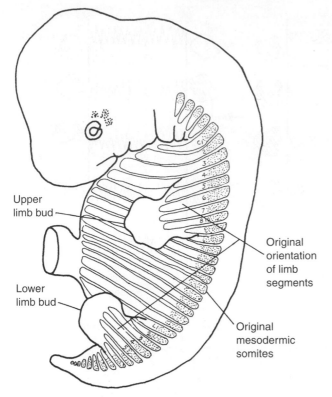

FIG. 1-4. Diagram of embryo at about 5 weeks' gestation.

Labels on figure:
Upper limb bud
Lower limb bud
Original orientation of limb segments
Original mesodermic somites

most limb muscles split or fuse as they develop, some migrate. The latissimus is the most obvious example; it migrates so far that it attains a pelvic attachment. However, like other limb muscles, it is innervated by the anterior primary divisions of mostly cervical segments, in spite of the fact that it lies over the back and extends over thoracic and lumbar segments.

The bones of the limbs also develop *in situ*. A condensation of mesenchymal cells first appears in the axial region of the limb bud. These differentiate into chondrocytes that form a "cartilage model" of the developing bone (Fig. 1-5). Through the process of endochondral ossification, the cartilage model is gradually replaced by bone tissue. This occurs first in the diaphyseal regions of the long bones, extending toward both ends. Secondary centers of ossification appear at both ends, or epiphyses, and are separated from the primary area of ossification by the epiphyseal plates. The epiphyseal plate of cartilage tissue continues to develop cartilage cells that continue to undergo ossification, adding to the bone formed by the primary ossification site. In this way, the bone continues to grow in length until the epiphyseal plate closes in response to hormonal influence during the second decade of postpartum life. The outer layer of the cartilage model remains as mesenchymal tissue, which continually produces chondroblasts and osteoblasts that form bone tissue. This perichondrium, which later becomes the periosteum, is responsible for the growth in width of the bones. It becomes highly innervated and highly vascularized, whereas the underlying layers of bone receive blood supply but little if any innervation.

The axial regions of the developing limb bud, which later become the joints, remain as condensations of mesenchymal tissue. In the case of synovial joints, the layers of "interzonal" mesenchyma adjacent to the developing bone ends differentiate into chondrocytes that secrete cartilage matrix, thus forming articular cartilage. The intervening middle zone undergoes cavitation to form the joint cavities, or discongruities, between joint surfaces. The surrounding layers of cells, which are continuous with the perichondrium, differentiate into fibrous capsule and synovium. The innervation of synovial joints is discussed in Chapter 3, Arthrology.

The development of the cartilage models and joint spaces and the subsequent rotation and adduction of the limb buds occurs by the seventh to eighth week of fetal life. By 8 weeks, often before the mother realizes she is pregnant, the status and form of the fetal musculoskeletal system has largely been determined and any significant teratogenic influences will have taken effect. The development of the musculoskeletal system may be summarized as follows:

1. The musculoskeletal system is largely derived from the mesoderm.
2. The ectoderm forms the epidermal layer of skin and, through its invagination into the mesoderm, the nervous system.
3. Somites form in the paraxial mesoderm. They consist of sclerotomes, which form bones, capsules, ligaments, cartilage, and blood vessels; myotomes, which form muscles; and dermatomes, which form the dermal layer of skin.
4. Because of the division of sclerotomes and subsequent fusion of caudal and cranial divisions of adjacent segments, a shift occurs that offsets the relationship between axial sclerotomes and myotomes.
5. The limbs are not formed from somatic myotomes, sclerotomes, or dermatomes but from the lateral somatic mesoderm, the somatopleure. The musculoskeletal structures of the limbs develop *in situ* from differentiation of primitive mesenchymal cells.

■ TERMINOLOGY

Although the limbs do not form from an invasion of cells from the somatic myotomes, dermatomes, and sclerotomes, these segments are often referred to as existing in the limbs. Clinicians speak of pain being referred to a particular sclerotome, weakness occur-

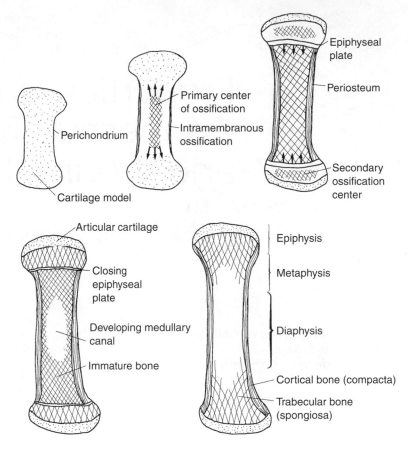

FIG. 1-5. Development of bone.

ring within a particular myotome, or sensory changes in a dermatome. It is important to understand that these terms are useful in clinical description but that they refer only to the source of innervation for a particular type of tissue and not the embryologic origin of the tissue, unless the terms are applied to the axial tissues. Thus, for example, the C5 myotome refers to those muscles in the limb receiving a significant innervation from the C5 anterior primary division or those muscles of the trunk innervated by the posterior primary division of C5. The C5 sclerotome in the limb refers to those structures (*e.g.,* capsules, ligaments, periosteum) receiving innervation from C5. A particular joint is often said to be largely derived from a particular segment. In this manner it is implied that innervation to the structures forming the joint has its source in that spinal segment. More discussion concerning the clinical importance of segmental innervation is found in Chapter 4, Pain.

RECOMMENDED READINGS

Arey LB: Developmental Anatomy, 7th ed. Philadelphia, WB Saunders, 1974

Baume LJ, Holz J: Ontogenesis of the temporomandibular joint: II. Development of the temporal components. J Dent Res 49:864–875, 1970

Christian EL: Embryology and evolution of movement and function. In Scully RM, Barnes MR (eds): Physical Therapy, pp 48–62. Philadelphia, JB Lippincott, 1989

Falkner F: Human Development. Philadelphia, WB Sanders, 1966

Fitzgerald MJT: Human Embryology, A Regional Approach. New York, Harper & Row, 1978

Hamilton WJ, Mossman HW: Human Embryology: Prenatal Development of Form and Function, 4th ed. Baltimore, Williams & Wilkins, 1972

Hollinshead H: Anatomy for Surgeons: Back and Limbs, 3rd ed. New York, Harper & Row, 1982

Lee D: Embryology, development and aging. In Lee D (ed): The Pelvic Girdle, pp 8–16. Edinburgh, Churchill Livingstone, 1989

Lewis WH: The development of the arm in man. Am J Anat 1:145–183, 1902

Lewis WH, Bardeen CR: The development of the limbs, body wall and back in man. Am J Anat 1:1–35, 1901

Moore KL: Before We Are Born, 2nd ed. Philadelphia, WB Saunders, 1983

Moore KL: The Developing Human: Clinically Oriented Embryology, 4th ed. Philadelphia, WB Saunders, 1988

Netter FH, Crelin ES: Embryology. In Netter FH (ed): The Ciba Collection of Medical Illustrations: Vol 8. Musculoskeletal System. Summit, NJ, Ciba-Geigy Co, 1987

O'Rahilly R: Developmental Stage of Human Embryos. Publication No 631. Washington, DC, Carnegie Institute, 1973

O'Rahilly R, Gardner E: The embryology of the movable joints. In Sokoloff L (ed): The Joints and Synovial Fluid, vol 1. San Francisco, Academic Press, 1978

Sarnat HB, Netsky MG: Evolution of the Nervous System, 2nd ed. New York, Oxford Press, 1981

Snell RS: Clinical Embryology for Medical Students, 3rd ed. Boston, Little, Brown & Co, 1983

Taylor JR, Twomey LT: The role of the notochord and blood vessels in vertebral column development and in the aetiology of Schmorl's nodes. In Grieve GP (ed): Modern Manual Therapy of the Vertebral Column, pp 21–29. Edinburgh, Churchill Livingstone, 1986

Thorogood P, Tickel C (eds): Craniofacial development. Development (Suppl) 103:1–254, 1988

Verboat AJ: The development of the vertebral column. Adv Anat Embryol Cell Biol 90:1–118, 1985

Warwick R, Williams P: Gray's Anatomy, 36th ed. Philadelphia, WB Saunders, 1980

Wendall Smith CP, Williams PL: Basic Human Embryology, 3rd ed. London, Pitman, 1984

Properties of Dense Connective Tissue and Wound Healing

LARRY J. TILLMAN AND NEIL P. CHASAN

Manual physical therapy has primary effects on dense connective tissue (DCT) structures. In order for the reader to gain an up-to-date understanding of soft tissue response to injury, a firm grasp of the physical properties of DCT is necessary.

Through the application of scientific principles, the manual therapy clinician can predict a level of success in management of musculoskeletal patients. After the history taking and physical examination, the clinician should have some knowledge about the specific tissue(s) in a lesion. But what then? By development and implementation of a treatment plan that is specific both to the tissue(s) in a lesion and the state of wound healing, the manual therapist will be able to apply the "optimal stimulus for protein synthesis," which lends a high probability to success in the clinic.[23] As the chapter unfolds, the reader will realize that different stimuli are necessary at different phases of the repair cycle in order to achieve an ideal result. Also, collagen has specific physical properties that can be taken advantage of during therapy. Further, manual therapy joint articulation techniques, described later in Chapter 3, Arthrology, have effects both on the mechanoreceptors and the DCT structures in which the receptors reside.

A rationale of treatment applied to a specific lesion or dysfunction gives the manual therapist a basis for evaluating the efficacy of their care. "Clinical Consideration" sections are used throughout the chapter to correlate basic science information with applicable clinical examples.

■ PHYSICAL PROPERTIES OF COLLAGEN

DCT consists of cells and protein fibers surrounded by ground substance. The predominant fiber is collagen.[20] A review of the physical and mechanical properties of collagen is an important starting point to understanding (DCT) healing.

Synthesis of Collagen

Collagen synthesis begins in the rough endoplasmic reticulum (ER) of connective tissue fibroblasts. In the ER, a repeating sequence of specific amino acids is assembled into long polypeptide chains of uniform length. Every third amino acid residue is glycine.

Darlene Hertling and Randolph M. Kessler: MANAGEMENT OF COMMON MUSCULOSKELETAL DISORDERS: Physical Therapy Principles and Methods, 3rd ed. © 1996 Lippincott-Raven Publishers.

Three polypeptide chains attach in a right-handed triple helix formation to form the *procollagen* molecule. Because of the three-dimensional shape of each chain and the relative placement of radicals that react with each other through hydrophobic, hydrophilic, hydrogen, and covalent interactions, the chains fit together in specific configurations of fixed dimensions with uniform length and width (Fig. 2-1). Procollagen is, therefore, an organic crystal. Once the procollagen molecule is extruded from the fibroblast cell membrane into the interstitial space, cleavage at terminal sites of the molecule occurs, and the slightly shortened molecule is now called *tropocollagen*. The tropocollagen molecule is the basic building block of collagen.

Intercellularly, five tropocollagen molecules rapidly aggregate in an overlapping array to form a collagen *microfibril*. The microfibril has been termed a "crystallite" structure, owing to the consistent spatial relationship of its molecules.[51] Groups of microfibrils organize into the *subfibril*, and subfibrils combine to form *fibrils*. It is at the level of the collagen fibril that the characteristic cross-banding or periodicity observed in x-ray diffraction and electron microscopic studies is demonstrated (Fig. 2-2). This cross-banding is the result of the specific overlapping and stacking of the tropocollagen molecules within the larger units, emphasizing the highly structured molecular organization of collagen. The physical and mechanical properties of collagen, therefore, are directly governed by this hierarchy of organization.

Bundles of collagen fibrils combine to form connec-

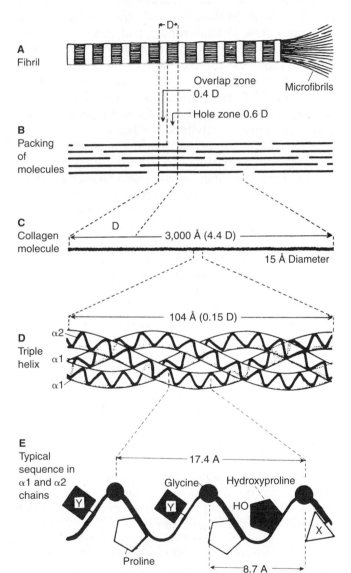

FIG. 2-1. Collagen fibril formation: (**A**) fibril with cross-banding due to overlapping tropocollagen units, (**B**) extracellular stacking of tropocollagen molecules, (**C**) one tropocollagen molecule of fixed 300-nm dimension, (**D**) the right-handed triple helix, and (**E**) the left-handed alpha helix illustrating the regularity of primary sequence. (Illustration by Tagawa B. From Prockop DJ, Guzman NA: Collagen diseases and biosynthesis of collagen. Hosp Pract 12(12):61–68, 1977)

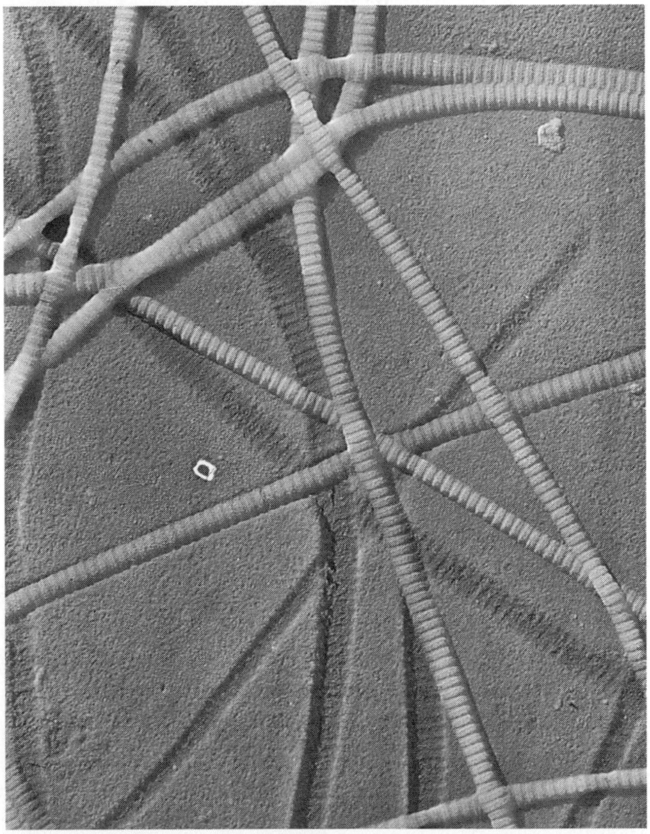

FIG. 2-2. Electron micrograph of metal-shadowed replica of collagen fibers from human skin, demonstrating cross-banding periodicity. (de Duve, C: A Guided Tour of the Living Cell, vol 1, p 38. New York, Scientific American Books, WH Freeman, 1984; and Jerome Gross, Harvard Medical School, Boston, MA 02114)

tive tissue *fascicles.* Whenever subjected to stress during formation, these fascicles form with distinct waveforms or *crimps.* The angle of crimping of collagen at this level of connective tissue development is both predictable and measurable. Collagen fascicles together make up the gross structure of tendon, ligament, and joint capsule (Fig. 2-3). It is at the level of the DCT collagenous fascicle that a tendon or ligament can first be mechanically tested. The compliance of DCT is primarily, therefore, a function of the removal of the crimp. In other words, when working within physiological limits, collagen can become temporarily elongated by straightening out the crimped fascicle. As a result of the dimensions set by the molecular attachments, native collagen cannot shrink or be stretched with permanent elongation. Clinically speaking, any "permanent" elongation signifies tearing or denaturation of the collagen with irreversible damage.

As yet, five classes and numerous subclasses of collagen have been identified. Of these classes, the larger structural, interstitial fibers of tendon and ligament contain mostly type I collagen, and in smaller quantities type II collagen. Articular cartilage is typically made up of type II collagen.

☐ Ground Substance Composition

Ground substance is the amorphous, gel-like material occupying the interstitial space between the collagen fibers, and it is composed of a mixture of water and organic molecules, namely *glycosaminoglycans (GAGs),*

proteoglycans, and *glycoproteins.* Ground substance has enormous water-binding properties, and acts as both a lubricant for movement of adjacent fibers over one another, as well as a source of nourishment for fibroblasts.[1,3]

GAGs (acid mucopolysaccharides), like tropocollagen, are a product of fibroblast metabolism. GAGs interact electrostatically with collagen fibers, binding them together, thus contributing to their aggregation and strength.[7] The distinctive crimping in collagen fascicles is thought to be the result of the attachment of GAGs to the collagen fibers.[28,29,35] Examples of GAGs include hyaluronic acid, chondroitin sulfate, heparan sulfate, keratan sulfate, and dermatan sulfate. Hyaluronic acid is common in cartilage and is thought to be responsible for cohesion within the fibril, enabling the tissue to bear mechanical stresses without distortion.[9,40] Dermatan sulfate is found in dermis, tendons, ligaments, and fibrous cartilage—all structures containing mostly type I collagen.

When GAGs covalently bind to protein chains in the extracellular matrix of DCT, they are called *proteoglycans.* Each type of connective tissue has characteristic proteoglycans present in various proportions. Proteoglycans regulate collagen fibrillogenesis and accelerate polymerization of collagen monomers.[35] Structural *glycoproteins* are organic molecules containing a protein core to which carbohydrates attach. Unlike proteoglycans, the protein core predominates. Glycoproteins, such as fibronectin, chondronectin, and laminin, play an important role in the interaction between DCT cells and their adhesion to collagen.

CLINICAL CONSIDERATION

Ground substance viability depends on motion. GAGs have a half-life of 1.7 to 7 days, and motion is required for ground substance production.[70] Early on, motion at the level of the DCT might imply gentle isometric contractions rather than gross osteokinematic movements. The forces generated by gentle isometric contractions are often sufficient to keep the DCT lubricated during the phase of recovery in which pain-induced splinting occurs.

☐ Maturation Changes in Collagen

There are progressive changes in bonding as the collagen ages and matures. Once the tropocollagen molecules aggregate into microfibrils, gradual chemical changes occur that result in the conversion of unstable hydrogen bonds into stable covalent bonds. Simultaneously, new attachments are formed by the organic

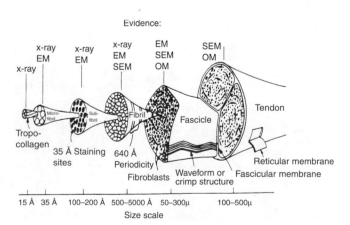

FIG. 2-3. Hierarchical organization of tendon. Note the cross-banding periodicity at the level of the collagen fibril, and the specific crimp formation in the collagen fiber fascicle. (Kastelic J, Galeski A, Baer E: The multicomposite structure of tendon. Connect Tissue Res 6:11–23, 1978)

molecules (GAGs) of the ground substance, which result in additional stability. The end result is that the maturing collagen becomes progressively rigid and strong. In addition to the increase in covalent bonding, two other factors thought to affect collagen strength during maturation include the continuous increase in size of the collagen fibers and the alignment of fibers along lines of stress.[41] Stress as a physical stimulus is a significant factor in the formation and maintenance of collagen in DCT. Deprivation of physical stress results in actual loss of collagen fibers and progressive weakening of the DCT.

MECHANICAL PROPERTIES OF COLLAGEN

The mechanical behavior of tendon and other DCT can be studied by elongating collagen fibers to the point of rupture. The resulting changes in length and tension during stretch can be plotted to produce a *stress/strain curve. Stress* is the amount of load or tension per unit of cross-sectional area placed on the specimen, whereas *strain* refers to the temporary elongation that occurs when stress is applied within physiologic limits.

The Stress/Strain Curve

A stress/strain curve characteristic for tendon that is mechanically strained to the point of rupture, as demonstrated in Figure 2-4, includes five distinct regions:

1. *Toe region*: In the toe region, there is little increase in load with lengthening. This region represents a 1.2 to 1.5 percent strain, and occurs during loading for 1 hour or less. The load stays within the physiologic limit of the tissue. The crimp is temporarily removed at the level of the DCT fascicle without permanently denaturing or damaging the tendon.
2. *Linear region*: In the linear region, increased elongation requires disproportionately larger amounts of stress. Microfailure of the tendon begins early in this region, and the patient complains of tendon stiffness.
3. *Region of progressive failure*: In this region the slope of the stress/strain curve begins to decrease, indicating microscopic disruption of sufficient

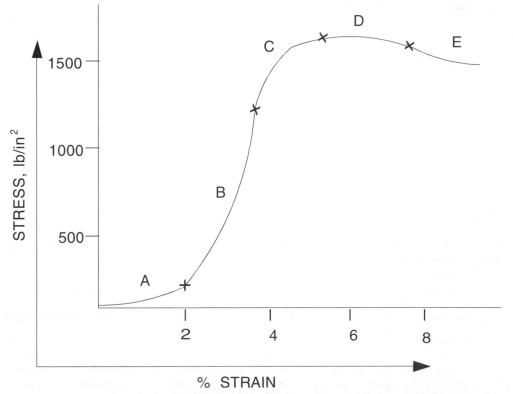

FIG. 2-4. *Stress/strain curve for ruptured Achilles tendon in humans. The five distinct regions are (**A**) toe region, (**B**) linear region, (**C**) progressive failure region, (**D**) major failure region, and (**E**) complete rupture region.*

amounts of DCT structure. The gross tendon, nonetheless, appears to be normal and intact. A decrease in the slope angle on the curve is called *yield* and occurs around 6 percent strain.

4. *Region of major failure*: The slope of the curve now flattens dramatically. Although the gross tendon is intact, there is visible narrowing at numerous points of shear and rupture. This narrowing at points of tear is known as *necking*.

5. *Region of complete rupture*: The slope of the stress/strain curve falls off, indicating a total break in the gross tendon. Tendon failure occurs with 12 to 15 percent strain.

When a load is removed from a tendon prior to incomplete rupture, the tendon returns to its original starting length after a period of rest. The return of the temporarily elongated tendon to its original length is called *recovery*. Being a crystalline structure, collagen can be temporarily deformed by stress, but with the removal of the load, the collagen recovers to its original length.

CLINICAL CONSIDERATION

Manual therapy receptor techniques generally occur in the toe region (prior to any microtrauma). Type I, type II, and type III receptors are active in the beginning range, mid range, and end range of tension of the DCT structure in which they are located (Table 2-1). Type IV receptors are stimulated once the DCT suffers irreversible damage—in the linear region. Trauma might bring the DCT into the region of progressive failure or the region of major failure. If DCT injury occurs, it is likely that there is also injury to the receptors typically residing within the traumatized structures. Early rehabilitation must therefore focus on joint proprioception.

☐ Viscoelastic Properties of Dense Connective Tissue

The viscoelastic properties of tendon and other DCT can be demonstrated when stress/strain studies plot the recovery of tendon following the removal of stress. Interrupted cyclical stress, in which a load is applied to and quickly removed from tendon, produces a stress/strain curve illustrated in Figure 2-5A. The tendon temporarily elongates (*compliance*) but quickly recovers to its original length (*elasticity*). The end result is an initial 1.5 percent strain with recovery. This example demonstrates the elastic behavior of DCT to cyclical (on/off) stress.[52]

When stress is applied to a tendon in a sustained fashion and recovery is allowed to occur, the constant (or uninterrupted cyclical) loading produces a 2.6 percent strain (see Fig. 2-5B). This additional and gradual lengthening of the tendon with sustained stress is called *creep*. The phenomenon of creep describes the viscous or plastic behavior of tendon and DCT.

A tendon stressed 1 percent for 60 minutes recovers. It has been shown that all DCT creep found within physiological limits at 25°C is transitory.[50] In contrast, a 1 percent stress sustained over 1 hour results in irreversible damage to tendon structure and function. Creep in tendons, therefore, occurs at two levels: a temporary elongation that shows recovery when treatment is within physiologic limits, and a permanent elongation that progresses to irreversible damage and rupture.

CLINICAL CONSIDERATION

On occasion, the clinician might choose to perform a manipulation or stretching technique that results in permanent elongation or even rupture of a DCT struc-

TABLE 2-1   MECHANORECEPTORS OF THE DENSE CONNECTIVE TISSUES

RECEPTOR TYPE	WHERE ACTIVE	WHERE FOUND	ACTION/EFFECTS
Type I	Beginning and end range of tension	Superficial layers of joint capsules	Slow adapting, low threshold tension postural reflexogenic effects
Type II	Mid range of tension	Deep layers of joint capsules	Rapidly adapting, low threshold dynamic receptor
Type III	End range of tension	Intrinsic and extrinsic joint ligaments	Slow acting, high threshold dynamic mechanoreceptor
Type IV	Inactive normally; activated by noxious mechanical or chemical stimulation	Fibrous capsules, intrinsic and extrinsic ligaments, fat pads, and periosteum	Nonadapting, high threshold pain receptors

(Wyke B: The neurology of joints. Ann R Coll Surg Engl 41:25, 1967)

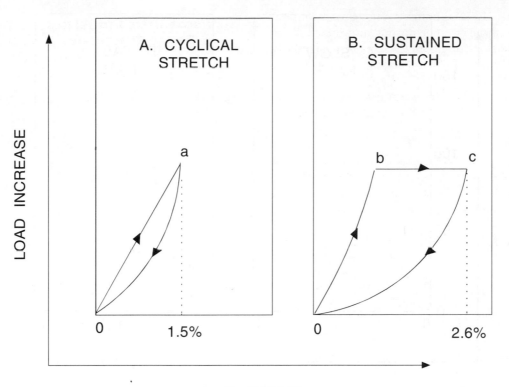

FIG. 2-5. Graphs illustrate the recovery of cyclical stretch (**A**) and sustained stretch (**B**). Increased strain occurs in a sustained stretch owing to the removal of crimp (indicated as b → c). (Modified from Warren CG, Lehman JF, Koblanski JN: Elongation of rat tail tendon: Effect of load and temperature. Arch Phys Med Rehabil 52:466, 1971)

ture, such as a small scar or an adhesion. In the event that the manual therapist performs a technique causing rupture of DCT, the *injury* caused by the technique should be managed as if it is an *acute* trauma that will eventually result in fibrosis. Caution must be taken to prevent further adhesions requiring additional aggressive care.

☐ Rate of Stress

In addition to whether the applied stress to tendon is cyclical or sustained, the *rate* of stretch has been shown to be important.[52] Figure 2-6 illustrates that "slow" stretch allows creep to occur, and thus less force is required to provide more temporary elongation. In contrast, "fast" stretch provides more resistance and results in less elongation. With fast stretch, an increase of tendon resistance to stretch requires greater load to achieve elongation.[64] Although this higher stress might lead to more structural damage of the DCT, high-velocity techniques used to articulate joints benefit from the protection afforded the DCT by the increase in viscoelasticity with higher rates of

stretch. In general, high-velocity techniques are performed at low amplitudes, which implies that the margin for error for the high-velocity thrust is greater at higher speed than for the same stretch applied at a slower rate. If such a technique were to be applied at high amplitudes, the likelihood that the DCT would be damaged is increased. Clinically, caution must be applied during the application of all techniques that stretch DCT so as to avoid permanent damage.

If the physiologic limit of strain is only 1.5 to 2.6 percent with recovery,[51] what is the impetus for physical therapists to temporarily elongate tendon and other collagenous structures? Why bother to do it at all? Stressing collagen within physiological limits provides the effective stimulus for the remodeling of DCT. It has been demonstrated that collagen forms along lines of stress. Tension controls the direction of collagen fiber alignment as well as the formation of collagen into large fascicles. The manual therapist, therefore, can control how the newly synthesized collagen is laid down by providing the proper stimulus for remodeling. This concept is important to remember when dealing with scar tissue formation and wound healing.

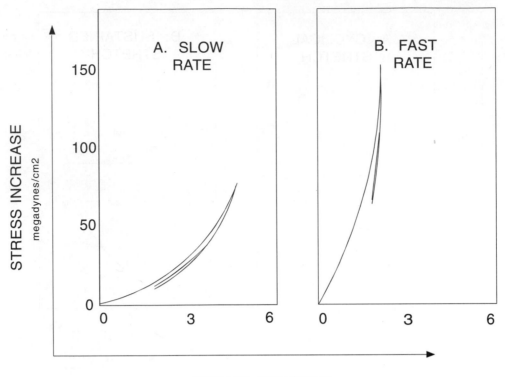

FIG. 2-6. Stress–strain data from extensor digitorum tendon: (**A**) slow rate and (**B**) fast rate. Slower rate of stretch produces greater strain with less stress. (Modified from Van Brocklin JD, Ellis DG: A study of mechanical behavior of toe extensor tendons under applied stress. Arch Phys Med Rehabil 46:371, 1965)

CLINICAL CONSIDERATION

Rehabilitation of the musculoskeletal system requires that the patient exercise the injured joint(s). In order to appropriately stimulate the collagen structures with the "optimal stimulus for regeneration," the exercise must be dosed correctly. Early in the acute phase, the exercise dose must be sufficiently low so as to stress the collagen fibers without overloading them, and as the fibers mature, the dose can be gradually increased. An important clinical consideration, therefore, is to think in terms of the collagen formation, as well as the DCT in general, when designing a rehabilitation program for your patient.

◼ WOUND HEALING: INJURY AND REPAIR OF DENSE CONNECTIVE TISSUE

An *injury* may be defined as an interruption in the continuity of a tissue. Repair begins immediately following injury by attempting to reestablish that continuity. With the exception of teeth, all tissue within the body are capable of repairing injuries.[43,46] Generally speaking, mammals do not regenerate tissue; they re-

pair it with DCT scarring. This quick process reduces the chances of infection. The prompt development of granulation tissue forecasts the repair of the interrupted DCT to produce a scar. It is important for the manual therapist to understand and apply basic biologic principles of wound repair and scar formation in order to predict the outcome of clinical wound management.

The body produces a similar cellular response to tissue irritation, mechanical injury, surgical and other forms of trauma, and bacterial or viral invasion. In wound healing, this cellular response contributes to three broad phases of scar tissue formation: inflammatory, fibroplastic, and remodeling phases.[24]

☐ Inflammatory Phase

Inflammation is a series of reactions by vascularized tissue in response to an injury. The purpose of the inflammatory reaction is to remove all foreign debris along with the dead and dying tissue, thereby reducing the likelihood of infection, so that optimal wound healing can occur. The inflammatory reaction attempts to control the effects of the injurious agent and return the tissue to a normal state.

Vascular and cellular responses play a major role during the inflammatory phase. The clinical signs of pain, heat, redness, swelling, and loss of function relate directly to the acute events of the inflammatory phase.

VASCULAR RESPONSE

Capillary injury results in whole blood flowing into the wound. Coagulation seals off the injured blood vessels and temporarily closes the wound space. Simultaneously, noninjured blood vessels in the vicinity of the wound dilate in response to various vasoactive chemicals released into the wound.[65]

Three interrelated plasma-derived systems mediate the inflammatory response: the kinin system, the complement system, and the clotting system.[37] Kinins, which are plasma polypeptides found in the exudate, contribute to the arteriolar dilation and increased venule permeability. *Bradykinin* becomes activated by Hageman factor XII of the clotting system, to participate in the early period of vascular permeability.

The complement system, known for its role in enhancing antibody–antigen immune complexes, also plays an important role in inflammation. In this capacity, complement (as a series of plasma proteins) acts directly on DCT mast cells. Mast cells, located adjacent to the vessels, respond to specific complement proteins by releasing *histamine.* Histamine produces the initial, short-acting dilation of the noninjured arterioles and increases the vascular permeability of the venules. Increased blood flow to the microvascular beds, as a result of the vasodilation, causes the heat and redness observed during the early hemodynamic changes in inflammation. The dilated noninjured vessels initially release a *transudate,* composed mainly of water and electrolytes, into the interstitium. Increased vascular permeability allows plasma proteins and a few white blood cells to escape into the wound area, and the serous transudate becomes a more viscous *exudate* (Fig. 2-7). This exudation leads to the edematous swelling observed during the inflammatory phase.[12]

The clotting system is a series of plasma proteins that can be activated by Hageman factor XII. Hageman factor XII initiates clotting by converting prothrombin to thrombin. Thrombin acts to convert fibrinogen to fibrin, in the final step of the clotting cascade. Fibrinopeptides are formed during this conversion, which cause increased vascular permeability.[37] Fibrin plugs the capillaries and lymphatics around the wound to seal off the area, effectively preventing infection. Additionally, the water-binding properties of hyaluronic acid released from mast cells result in a "wound gel,"[12] which fills all space in the

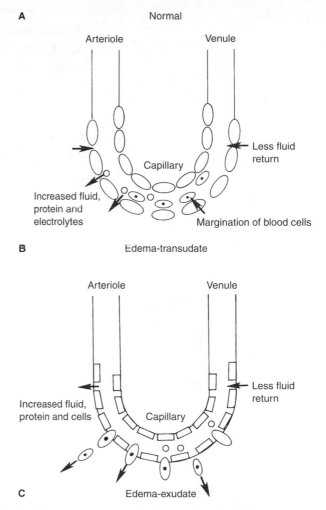

FIG. 2-7. Production of edema during inflammation. Initially a transudate consisting of water, electrolytes, and some plasma proteins is formed (**A**), followed by an exudate made up of increased plasma proteins and white blood cells (**B**). (Modified from Zarro V: Thermal Agents in Rehabilitation, vol 1, p 12. New York, FA Davis, © Holden and Publisher, 1986)

wound. This process results in loss of dermal fat, leading to a thinning of the skin over the wound area.[30]

Arachidonic acid (AA), a polyunsaturated fatty acid product of phospholipid breakdown in ruptured cell membranes, releases metabolites into the exudate, which play an important role in inflammation. *Prostaglandins* (PGs) and leukotrienes, products derived from AA metabolism, can mediate virtually every step of acute inflammation (Fig. 2-8).[37] PGs are long-acting vasodilators, and leukotrienes are a family of compounds that cause increased vascular permeability. These chemical mediators synthesized by injured cell membranes prolong the edematous reaction.

Pain is produced by both the engorgement of tissue spaces from the pressure and swelling, and by chemical irritation of pain-producing nerve endings. Bradykinin, enhanced by prostaglandins, stimulates

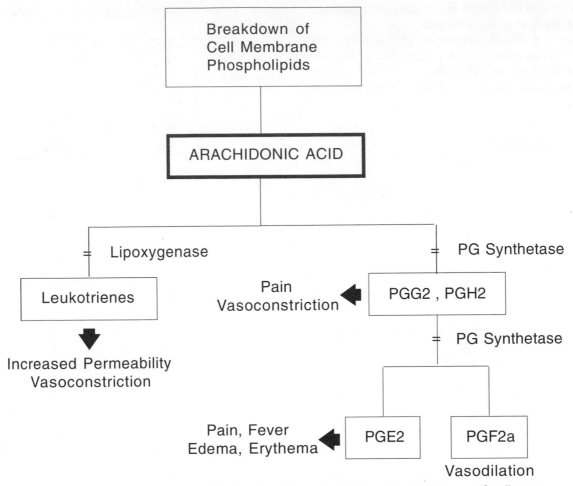

FIG. 2-8. Prostaglandin and leukotriene biosynthesis from the breakdown of cell membrane phospholipids.

the nociceptor receptors in the skin. The increased pain causes the patient to guard the affected wound area, and loss of function results.

Many of the chemical substances in the exudate are chemoattractants for white blood cells (WBCs).[31,32] The arrival of leukocytes at the site of injury is a critical part of the inflammatory process, since phagocytosis of cellular debris and foreign antigens is necessary to ensure proper wound healing.[24]

CELLULAR RESPONSE

Bacterial products, complement and fibrin fractions, histamine, and kinin components are chemotactic mediators of the WBC response that occurs during the inflammatory phase of wound healing.[8,21,49,56,65] Polymorphonuclear leukocytes (PMNs), also known as neutrophils, are chemotactically attracted to the site of injury. The process of cell migration along a chemically mediated concentration gradient is called *chemotaxis*. PMNs act as the first line of WBC phagocytic defense against foreign antigens and bacterial debris.

With increased vascular permeability and escape of plasma proteins, the viscosity of the blood increases, causing sludging of red blood cells and increased frictional resistance to blood flow. During this process, short-lived PMNs follow a specific sequence of events known as margination, pavementing, emigration, chemotaxis, and phagocytosis.

Initially the PMNs *marginate* to the inner walls of the capillaries and post-capillary venules, and there they adhere to the walls, a process called *pavementing*. Next, these neutrophils *emigrate* through the permeable endothelial cells lining the vessels, into the surrounding interstitial space. Through *chemotaxis* they are drawn to the wound area where the bacteria are located. Blood monocytes, lymphocytes, eosinophils, and basophils all use this same pathway.[37] The primary goal of the PMNs is *phagocytosis* of bacterial products and other foreign antigens to prevent or eliminate infection in the wound. PMNs attach to and engulf the foreign particles, release proteolytic enzymes from lysosomal organelles, and, hopefully, degrade and digest the microorganisms. When large numbers of PMNs die and are lysed, the exudate forms pus.

As the inflammatory phase progresses, the number of PMNs declines and DCT macrophages predominate. Neutrophilic, bacterial, and complement factors are chemoattractants for macrophages. These phagocytes are the scavenger cells that dispose of the remaining bacteria and necrotic tissue. Hydrogen peroxide, ascorbic acid, and lactic acid are by-products of phagocytosis.[67] Hydrogen peroxide controls anaerobic bacterial growth, whereas ascorbic and lactic acids increase macrophage activity. This increased activity results in a more intense and prolonged inflammatory response.

The exudative, acute inflammatory phase usually lasts 24 to 48 hours and is completed in 2 weeks. Although the patient's chief complaint is pain, the other clinical signs of heat, redness, swelling, and loss of function relate directly to the sequence of acute hemodynamic changes. Chronic inflammation, on the other hand, lasts months to years and results from either unresolved acute inflammation, repeated episodes of microtrauma, or persistent chronic irritation. Chronic inflammation leads mostly to a DCT cell proliferation response, and the patient complains predominantly of stiffness associated with some minor pain. Assuming, however, that the macrophages resolve the acute inflammation, the resultant clean wound bed is now ready for the rebuilding or fibroplastic phase of healing.

CLINICAL CONSIDERATION

The presence of a persistent irritant, such as local pressure (as in decubitus ulcers), poor oxygen supply, poor surgical closure, malnutrition, vitamin A and C deficiencies, radiation injury, or immunosuppression can adversely affect wound healing and the prevention of infection.[24] Treatment is directed toward assisting the macrophages in their work through the use of topical antibiotics, debridement, occlusive dressings, whirlpool cleaning, RICE regimen, and proper positioning.[24] Additionally, the manual therapist can minimize some of these factors that prevent or prolong inflammation by application of receptor techniques (described in Chapter 3, Arthrology) for inhibition of pain and guarding, and introduction of carefully dosed (pain-free) exercise for edema reduction.

☐ *Fibroplastic Phase*

The fibroplastic phase of wound healing lasts about 3 weeks and is named for the DCT fibroblast, which is primarily responsible for scar tissue formation by synthesizing new collagen and ground substance. Three major components occur simultaneously in this phase: re-epithelialization, fibroplasia with neovascularization, and wound contraction.

RE-EPITHELIALIZATION

Within hours of an injury, superficial wounds initiate the *re-epithelialization* process in skin.[47,67] This process involves the reestablishment of the epidermis across the surface of the wound by mitotically active basal cells of the noninjured epidermal margin. Epidermal growth factor is thought to stimulate the basal cell proliferation.[13] With a viable wound bed, these epithelial cells traverse the wound surface guided by matrix fibrin, fibronectin, and newly formed type IV collagen.[11,50]

Only 48 hours are required for approximated wound edges to re-epithelialize, well before fibroplasia begins.[10] The re-epithelialization of larger wounds takes longer; several weeks are required for the epithelial cells to differentiate into a functional, stratified epidermis firmly attached to the underlying dermis.

The new epithelium forms deep to any scab, or eschar, in order to maintain contact with the vascular network. Although a scab acts as a temporary surface barrier against bacteria and foreign matter, in deeper wounds it impedes rapid re-epithelialization by retarding basal cell migration.[68]

CLINICAL CONSIDERATION

Scab formation of chronic wounds can be minimized by keeping the surface hydrated with various microenvironmental dressings.[26,55] A clean, moist wound with ample blood supply will facilitate proper tissue repair. Although motion provides the ideal stimulus for collagen regeneration, repeated trauma to the wound surface through excessive skin stretching or multiple dressing changes may interfere with healing.

FIBROPLASIA WITH NEOVASCULARIZATION

Macrophages are not only essential to the inflammatory phase of wound healing but also probably necessary to direct the fibroblasts and angioblasts in the formation of new scar.[5] Macrophages release chemotactic substances, such as fibronectin, platelet-derived growth factor (GF), and other growth factors (epidermal GF, fibroblast GF, transforming GFs α and β),[18,27,34,36,60,61] which attract fibroblasts to the wound and play a role in adhesion of fibroblasts to the fibrin meshwork. Angioblasts contribute to the formation of new blood vessels at the wound edge.

In healthy tissue, fibroblasts are sparse and generally quiescent throughout the connective tissue matrix. After injury, fibroblasts are activated to migrate along the fibrin meshwork to the wound site as a result of the concentration gradients of chemical mediators, O_2, CO_2, lactic acid, and pH.[31] They proliferate and produce new collagen, elastin, GAGs, proteoglycans, and glycoproteins, which are utilized to reconstruct the connective tissue matrix.[44] The process of fibroblast migration and proliferation is called *fibroplasia.*

Healing will not be complete unless new, functioning capillaries develop to provide nourishment and oxygen to the injured tissue. Wound healing ends only when local hypoxia and lactic acid concentrations are reversed by the ingrowth of adequate circulation.[72] The process by which new blood vessels originate from preexisting vessels at the wound margin and grow into the wound space is called *neovascularization* or *angiogenesis.* Within 24 hours and up to 5 days post-injury, as directed by macrophage-released chemotactic substances and ischemia,[55] patent blood vessels "sprout" cells called *angioblasts* into the wound space. When these cells contact each other, new capillary loops are formed. The increased vascular circulation to the new wound, together with immature collagen fibers, gives the surface of the wound a pinkish red granular appearance, hence the term *granulation tissue.* The formation of granulation tissue is the hallmark of tissue healing.

CLINICAL CONSIDERATION

The bulky scar at this stage is very fragile and easily disrupted.[39] The new collagen fibers are laid down randomly along strands of clot fibrin and initially are held together by weak hydrogen bonds. Immobilization is often prescribed to permit vascular regrowth and prevent microhemorrhages.[24] Use of gentle stretch to stress the scar will cause elongation of the scar by cell migration, but the application of excessive force will disrupt cell membranes, causing cellular death.[63] It is clinically important to note that edema may still be present in the newly formed granulation tissue, even after the inflammatory phase has ended. This edema is the result of plasma proteins leaking from the new capillaries into the extravascular space.[38]

WOUND CONTRACTION

Wound contraction is the mechanism by which the edges of a wound are centripetally drawn together by forces generated within that wound. This normal healing process shrinks the defect, resulting in a smaller wound to be repaired by scar formation. Although limited by how much each cell can contract (*i.e.,* the capacity of the extracellular fibers and ground

substance to be compacted) and by the tension in surrounding tissues, this process is progressive over time. Wound contraction begins 4 days post-injury and continues through day 21;[48] in other words, it lasts about as long as the fibroplasia. In certain circumstances, such as large burn scars, contraction remains active for longer periods of time, possibly because of the poor circulation associated with such scars.[32,63]

Wound contraction is predominantly mediated by cells called *myofibroblasts.*[37,42,44,71] Myofibroblasts are specialized fibroblasts containing muscle-like contractile proteins which enable them to extend and contract.[45] The myofibroblasts anchor to each other and to fibrillar structures in the extracellular matrix, so that the contraction of each cell is transmitted to the tissue as a whole. The actual process whereby the scar is made smaller can be compared to a ratchet: as collagen turnover occurs, the myofibroblasts reach out and contract the scar, and the new collagen laid down occupies a smaller space, and so on.[5,6]

CLINICAL CONSIDERATION

It is clinically important to distinguish between wound contraction and scar contracture. Wound contraction is a normal part of the healing process that closes a wound after loss of tissue and protects it from the potentially hostile environment. Scar contracture is the result of a contractile process occurring in a healed scar, and often results in an undesirable fixed, rigid scar that causes functional and/or cosmetic deformity. Scar contracture may be the result of wound contraction, adhesions, fibrosis, or other tissue damage.[2] Whereas wound contraction generally occurs in an incompletely epithelialized defect, scar contracture usually occurs in an epithelialized covered defect.[53,54]

☐ **Remodeling Phase**

At the end of the fibroplastic stage, the myofibroblasts and fibroblasts start to leave the scar. At this point the newly formed scar will undergo remodeling in an effort to strengthen the wound along appropriate lines of stress. By increasing the tensile strength of the scar, the ultimate goal of remodeling is the restoration of function. There are two distinct components of scar tissue remodeling: the consolidation and maturation stages.

CONSOLIDATION STAGE

The consolidation phase lasts from day 21 to day 60. The scar typically stops increasing in size by day 21.[41] The tissue gradually changes from a predominantly cellular tissue to a predominantly fibrous tissue, as first many of the myofibroblasts disappear, followed by the fibroblasts. Four weeks is reported to be the minimum amount of time required for this tissue reorganization to occur.[25] As the cell population declines, the vascularity of the scar slowly diminishes. By day 42 the vascularity of the scar equals that of the adjacent skin.[1] During the consolidation stage, in spite of diminishing cell populations, the remaining fibroblasts remain highly active, bringing about substantial changes in the structure and strength of the scar.[1,28]

MATURATION STAGE

The maturation phase lasts from day 60 to day 360. After day 60 the activity of the connective tissue cells greatly diminishes. Collagen turnover remains high through the fourth month, and then gradually tapers off.[3] Between 180 and 360 days, few cells are seen, and the tissue becomes tendonlike.[17,28] The changes in the scar during these last two stages occur very gradually as the scar, which starts out as an extremely cellular tissue, becomes predominantly fibrous by the end of the maturation stage. The bulk of the scar is formed by large and compact, type I collagen fibers. The fully mature scar is only about 3 percent cellular, and its vascularity is greatly reduced.[28,35] As immature scar is converted to mature scar, intracollagen molecular linkage changes from weak hydrogen bonding to strong covalent bonding, resulting in the gradual increase in scar strength.

EFFECTS OF STRESS ON SCAR REMODELING

Stress has a significant effect on scar remodeling, contributing to the shape, strength, and pliability of the scar.[28,35] The DCT cells, GAGs, proteoglycans, and collagen architecture are all affected by the direction and magnitude of mechanical stress applied to the scar.[35] Figure 2-9 is a schematic representation of the affect of stress on collagen formation. Collagen fibers are often randomly oriented in unstressed wounds, yet aggregate in small, parallel bundles in wounds undergoing stress.

Fibroblasts, including their mitotic bundles, orient parallel to the lines of tension,[4] the long axis of the cells lying along stress lines. Mechanical forces, likewise, influence the metabolic activities of fibroblasts. It has been demonstrated that fibroblast tissue cultures subjected to a cyclic strain respond by increasing production of GAGs and proteoglycans after 24 hours.[58] Fibronectin, which anchors strands of myofibroblasts and provides a scaffold on which collagen fiber aggregation occurs, also lies parallel to the direction of wound contraction.[20] This model offers one explanation of how cellular orientation leads to collagen fiber orientation in the early development of DCT.[63]

Collagen fibers are laid down in response to lines of stress resulting from mechanical loads. Collagen under tension has different properties from collagen under compression, owing to the different distribution of piezo-electric charges on the collagen fibers. Physiologic loads of tension cause increased aggregation of collagen, whereas compression causes decreased fiber aggregation.[18] Collagen fibers laid down along stress lines involve the transduction of physical forces into electrochemical events at the molecular level.[63] As a result, the collagen fibers aggregate into small bundles oriented across the wound space, as dictated by the direction of stress.[19]

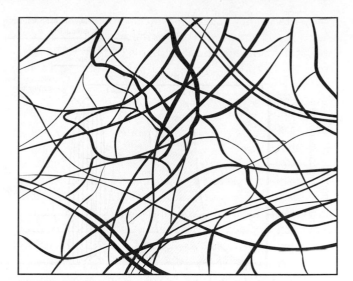

A Wound collagen, unstressed

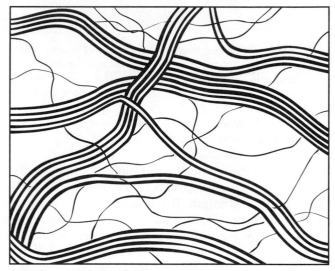

B Wound collagen, stressed

FIG. 2-9. *Unstressed (**A**) and stressed (**B**) wound collagen. In the wound subjected to stress, collagen reorganizes with larger, more parallel aligned fibers.*

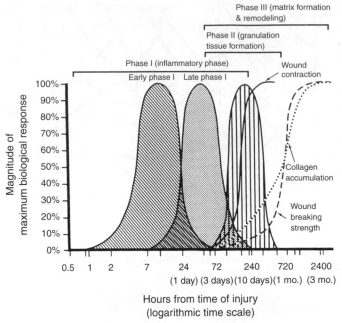

FIG. 2-10. The three overlapping phases of wound repair: phase I, inflammation; phase II, granulation or fibroplastic; and phase III, remodeling. (Daly TJ: The repair phase of wound healing—Re-epithelialization and contraction. In Kolth KC, McCulloch JM, Feedar JA [eds]: Wound Healing: Alternatives in Management, p 15. New York, FA Davis, © Holden and Publisher, 1990)

The magnitude and the duration of stress application also have an effect on collagen deposition and, in turn, on scar strength. If too much stress is applied to newly formed scar, the weakly bonded tissue pulls apart; it is not unusual for excessive strain to increase inflammation and decrease fibroplasia.[22] Scar strength increases with not only the aggregation of collagen fibers along stress lines, but also with the increase of scar collagen volume and the development of stable covalent bonding.[40,63]

The change in shape of scar tissue by remodeling is a slow process. Without the proper amount of stress stimulus, scar can take months to fill in a small space.[31] If remodeling is to occur, there must be a sufficient population of active connective tissue cells to remodel the tissue, and the scar must be malleable enough for therapeutic stress to stimulate remodeling. Additionally, time governs the ability of scar to change shape. For example, a 4-week-old scar significantly remodels shorter to noncyclic strain, whereas a 14-week-old scar is unaffected by the remodeling.[40] This difference may be the result of the reduced number of DCT cells and stronger bonding in the maturing collagen architecture of the older scar.[63] Figure 2-10 summarizes the three overlapping phases of wound healing, providing a post-injury time scale of the events contributing to increased collagen accumulation, wound contraction, and scar strength.

CLINICAL CONSIDERATION

The mission of physical therapy is to restore function. If this implies restoring the ability to perform as well as or better than before injury, then one goal of physical therapy must be to enhance the strength and integrity of the DCT structures. Relative to the richly vascularized contractile tissues, DCT has poor perfusion of nutrients and few active cells. Therefore, the rate of strengthening of DCT is slower than that of muscle. Several studies demonstrate the impact of overloading DCT structures.[57,59] One goal of this chapter has been to alert the reader to the importance of careful dosing of exercise, with DCT structures receiving one's full attention.

■ SUMMARY

The manual physical therapist has several clinical decisions to make during any treatment. Understanding the state of wound healing at the time is critical because the time elapsed since injury modifies the necessary treatment to promote function. Acutely, the manual therapist will perform pain inhibitory receptor techniques and apply light elastic forces to encourage fibroblast alignment along the lines of stress as the tissue repairs. Subacutely, the manual therapist will perform techniques to promote remodeling of dense connective tissues through manual and active stretching of the scar tissue. After 42 days, with less cellular activity, although manual therapy technique will have some effects in the body of the scar, remodeling will primarily occur around the scar periphery, and the emphasis should be on functional restoration. Clearly, the physical and mechanical properties of collagen and wound healing are fundamental principles for the manual therapist.

Further reading is necessary to fully understand the subject matter addressed in this chapter. Each area covered in this chapter is explored in more detail in the chapters and papers suggested for additional reading. Finally, it is suggested that the reader enhance his or her clinical appreciation of exercise dosing in order to maximize the functional outcome.

REFERENCES

1. Akeson WH, Amiel D, Woo S: Immobility effects on synovial joints. The pathomechanics of joint contractures. Biorheology 17:95–110, 1980
2. Alvarez OM, et al: Wound healing. In Fitzpatrick T (ed): Dermatology in General Medicine, 3rd ed, pp 321–336. New York, McGraw-Hill, 1987
3. Amiel D, Akeson WH, Hardwood FL, Frank CB: Stress deprivation effect on metabolic turnover of medial collateral ligament collagen. Clin Orthop 172:25–270, 1983
4. Arem AJ, Madden JW: Effects of stress on healing wounds: 1. Intermittent noncyclical tension. J Surg Res 20:93–102, 1976
5. Baur PS, Larson DL, Stacey TR: The observation of myofibroblasts in hypertrophic scars. Surg Gynecol Obstet 141:22–26, 1975
6. Baur PS, Parks DH: The myofibroblast anchoring strand—the fibronectin connection

in wound healing and the possible loci of collagen fibril assembly. J Trauma 23:853–862, 1983

7. Betch DF, Baer E: Structure and mechanical properties of rat tail tendon. Biorheology 17:83–94, 1980
8. Bevilaquas MP, Pober JS, Wheeler ME, et al: Interleukin 1 acts on cultured human vascular endothelium to increase the adhesion of polymorphonuclear leukocytes, monocytes, and related leukocyte cell lines. J Clin Invest 76:2003–2011, 1984
9. Brody GS, Peng STJ, Landel RE: The etiology of hypertrophic scar contracture: another view. Plas Reconstr Surg 67:673–684, 1977
10. Bryant WM: Wound Healing. Clin Symp 29(3), 1977
11. Clark RAF, et al: Fibronectin and fibrin provide a provisional matrix for epidermal cell migration during wound epithelialization. J Invest Dermatol 70:264–269, 1982
12. Cocke WM, White RR, Lynch DJ, et al: Wound Care. Ann Arbor, MI, Books on Demand, 1986
13. Cohen S: The stimulation of epidermal proliferation by a specific protein (EGF). Dev Biol 12:394–407, 1965
14. Daly TJ: The repair phase of wound healing—Re-epithelialization and contraction. In Kloth KC, McCulloch JM, Feedar JA (eds): Wound Healing: Alternatives in Management, vol 5. Philadelphia, FA Davis, 1990
15. de Duve C: A Guided Tour of the Living Cell, vol 1, p 38. Scientific American Books. New York, WH Freeman, 1984
16. Donaldson DJ, Mahan JT: Fibrinogen and fibronectin as substrates for epidermal cell migration during wound closure. J Cell Sci 62:117–127, 1983
17. Farkas LG, McCain WG, Sweeny P, Wilson W, Hyrs IN, Lindsay WK: An experimental study of the changes following silastic rod preparation of new tendon sheath and subsequent tendon grafting. J Bone Joint Surg 55:149–1158, 1973
18. Flint MH: The basis of the histological demonstration of tension in collagen. In Longacre JJ (ed): The Ultrastructure of Collagen, pp 60–66. Springfield, IL, Charles C Thomas, 1976
19. Forrester JC, Zederfeldt BH, Hayes TUL, Hunt TK: Tape closed and sutured wounds: A comparison by tensiometry and scanning electron microscopy. Br J Surg 57: 729–737, 1970
20. Frank C, Amiel D, Woo Al-Y, Akeson W: Normal ligament properties and ligament healing. Clin Orthop Rel Res 196:15–25, 1985
21. Gamble JR, Harlan JM, Klebanoff SJ, et al: Stimulation of the adherence of neutrophils to umbilical vein endothelium by human recombinant tumor necrosis factor. Proc Natl Acad Sci USA 82:8667–8671, 1985
22. Goldstein WN, Barmada R: Early mobilization of rabbit medial collateral ligament repairs: Biologic and histologic study. Arch Phys Med Rehab 65:239–242, 1984
23. Grimsby O: Medical Exercise Training [Lecture]. Seattle, Ola Grimsby Institute (sponsor), March 1993
24. Hardy MA: The biology of scar formation. Phys Ther 69(12):1014–1024, 1989
25. Hernandez-Jaurequi P, Espereabsa-Garcia C, Gonzales-Angulo A: Morphology of the connective tissue grown in response to implanted silicone rubber: a light and electron microscope study. Surgery 75:631–637, 1974
26. Hinman CC, Maibach HI, Winter GD: Effect of air exposure and occlusion on experimental human skin wounds. Nature 200:377, 1962
27. Hinter H, et al: Expression of basement membrane zone antigens at the dermo-epibolic function in organ culture of human skin. J Invest Dermatol 74:200–205, 1980
28. Hooley CJ, Cohen RE: A model for the creep behavior of tendon. Int J Biol Macromolecules 1:123–132, 1979
29. Hooley CJ, McCrum NG, Cohen RE: The viscoelastic deformation of tendon. J Biomechanics 13:521–528, 1980
30. Houck JC, Jacob RA: The chemistry of local dermal inflammation. J Invest Dermatol 36:451–456, 1961
31. Hunt TK, Banda MJ, Silver IA: Cell Interactions In Post Traumatic Fibrosis. Ciba Foundation Symposium, No. 114, 1985
32. Hunt TK, Van Winkle W: Wound Healing: Normal Repair—Fundamentals of Wound Management in Surgery. South Plainfield, NJ, Chirurgecom, 1976
33. Kastelic J et al: The multicomposite structure of tendon. Connect Tissue Res 6:11–23, 1978.
34. Kariniemi A-L, et al: Cytoskeleton and pericellular matrix organization of pure adult human keratinocytes cultured from suction-blister roof epidermis. J Cell Sci 58:49–61, 1982
35. Kirscher CW, Speer DP: Microvascular changes in Dupuytren's contracture. J Hand Surg 9A:58–62, 1984
36. Kubo M, et al: Human keratinocytes synthesize, secrete, and deposit fibrinectin in the pericellular matrix. J Invest Dermatol 82:580–586, 1984
37. Kumar V, Cotran RS, Robbins SL: Acute and chronic inflammation. In Basic Pathology, 5th ed, pp 25–46. Philadelphia, WB Saunders, 1992
38. Kumar V, Cotran RS, Robbins SL: Wound healing: Repair, cell growth, regeneration, and wound healing. In Basic Pathology, 5th ed, pp 47–60. Philadelphia, WB Saunders Co, 1992
39. Levenson SM, Grever EF, Crowley LV, Oates JF, Rosen H: The healing of rat skin wounds. Ann Surg 161:293–308, 1965
40. Madden JW, De Vore G, Arem AJ: A rational postoperative management program for metacarpophalangeal joint implant arthroplasty. J Hand Surg 2:358–366, 1977
41. Madden JW, Peacock EE: Studies on the biology of collagen during wound healing:

III. Dynamic metabolism of scar collagen and remodeling of dermal wounds. Ann Surg 174:511–520, 1971
42. Majno G, et al: Contraction of granulation tissue in vitro: Similarity to smooth muscle. Science 173:548, 1971
43. McMinn RMH: Tissue Repair. New York, Academic Press, 1969
44. Morgan CJ, Pledger WJ: Fibroblast proliferation. In Cohen et al (eds): Wound Healing, pp 63–75. Philadelphia, WB Saunders Co, 1992
45. Murry JC, Pollack SV, Pinnell SR: Keloids: A review. J Am Acad Dermatol 4:461–470, 1981
46. Needham, AE: Regeneration and Wound Healing. London, Methuen, 1952
47. Odland G, Ross R: Human wound repair. I. Epidermal regeneration. J Cell Biol 39:135–151, 1968
48. Peacock EE, van Winkle W: Structure, synthesis, and interaction of fibrous protein and matrix. In Peacock EE, Van Winkle W (eds): Wound Repair, pp 145–203, Philadelphia, WB Saunders Co, 1976
49. Pohlman TH, Stanness KA, Beatty PG, et al: An endothelial cell surface factior(s) induced in vitro by lipopolysaccharide, interleukin 1, and tumor necrosis factor-α increases neutrophil adherence by a CDα18–dependent mechanism. J Immunol 136:4548–4553, 1986
50. Repesh LA, Fitzgerald TJ, Furcht LT: Fibronectin involvement in granulation tissue and wound healing in rabbits. J Histochem Cytochem 30:351–358, 1982
51. Rigby BJ: The effect of mechanical extension upon the thermal stability of collagen. Biochim Biophys Acta 79:634–636, 1964
52. Rigby BJ, Hirai N, Spikes JD: The mechanical behavior of rat tendon. J Gen Physiol 43:265–283, 1959
53. Rudolph R: Contraction and the control of contraction. World J Surg 4:279–287, 1980
54. Rudolph R, Vande Berg J, Ehrlich HP: Wound contraction and scar contracture. In Cohen et al (eds): Wound Healing, pp 96–114. Philadelphia, WB Saunders Co, 1992
55. Ryan G, Majno G: Inflammation. Kalamazoo, MI, Upjohn Co, 1977
56. Schliemer RP, Rutledge BK: Cultured human vascular endothelial cell surface acquires adhesiveness for neutrophils after stimulation with interluken 1, endotoxin, and tumor-promoting phorbol diesters. J Immunol 136:649–654, 1986
57. Scully TJ, Besterman G: Stress fracture: A preventable training injury. Milit Med 147:285–287, 1982
58. Slack C, Flint MH, Thompson BM: The effect of tensional load on isolated embryonic chick tendons in organ culture. Connective Tissue Research 12:229–247, 1984
59. Stacy RJ, Hungerford RL: A method to reduce work-related injuries during basic recruit training in the New Zealand army. Milit Med 149:318–320, 1984
60. Stanley JR, et al: Detection of basement membrane antigens during epidermal wound healing in pigs. J Invest Dermatol 77:240, 1981
61. Stenn KS, Madri JA, Roll FJ: Migrating epidermis produces AB2 collagen and requires continued collagen synthesis for movement. Nature 277:229–232, 1979
62. Tagawa D: From Prockop DJ, Guzman NA: Collagen diseases and biosynthesis of collagen. Hosp Pract 12:61–68, 1977
63. Tillman LJ, Cummings GS: Biological mechanisms of connective tissue mutability. In Currier DP, Nelson RM (eds): Dynamics of Human Biologic Tissues, vol 8, pp 1–44. Philadelphia, FA Davis Company, 1992
64. Van Brocklin JD, Ellis DG: A study of mechanical behavior of toe extensor tendons under applied stress. Arch Phys Med Rehabil 46:369–371, 1965
65. Wahl CL, Wahl SM: Inflammation. Cohen, et al (eds): Wound Healing, pp 40–62. Philadelphia, WB Saunders, 1992
66. Warren CG, Lehman JF, Koblanski JN: Elongation of rat tail tendon: Effect of load and temperature. Arch Phys Med Rehabil 52:465–484, 1971
67. Werb A, Gordon S: Secretion of a specific collagenase by stimulated macrophages. J Exp Med 142:346–360, 1975
68. Winter GD: Formation of the scab and the rate of epithelialization of superficial wounds in the skin of the young, domestic pig. Nature 193:293, 1962
69. Witte CL, Witte MH, Dummont AE: Significance of protein in edema fluid. Lymphology 4:29–31, 1971
70. Woo SL-Y, Mathews JV, Akeson WH, et al: Connective tissue response to immobility: Correlative study of biomechanical measurements of normal and immobilized rabbit knees. Arthritis Rheum 18:257–264, 1975
71. Wyke B: The neurology of joints. Ann R Coll Surg Engl 41:25, 1967
72. Yannas IV, Huang C: Fracture of tendon collagen. J Polymer Sci 10:577–584, 1972
73. Zarro V: Thermal Agents in Rehabilitation, vol 1, p 12. Philadelphia, FA Davis, 1986.

RECOMMENDED READINGS

Kloth KC, McCulloch JM, Feedar JA (eds): Wound Healing: Alternatives in Management, vol 5, chaps 1–4. Philadelphia, FA Davis, 1990
Currier DP, Nelson RM (eds): Dynamics of Human Biologic Tissues, CPR vol 8, chaps 1, 2. Philadelphia, FA Davis, 1992
Hunt TK, Banda MJ, Silver IA: Cell interactions in post-traumatic fibrosis. In Fibrosis, pp 127–149. London, Pitman (Ciba Foundation Symposium No. 114), 1985

Arthrology

RANDOLPH M. KESSLER AND DARLENE HERTLING

- **Kinematics**
  Classification of Joint Surfaces and Movements
  Arthrokinematics
  Summary of Joint Function
  Clinical Application
- **Neurology**
  Innervation
  Receptors
  Clinical Considerations
- **Joint Nutrition**
  Lubrication

Models of Joint Lubrication
Resolving Problems of Joint-Surface Wear
- **Approach to Management of Joint Dysfunction**
  Pathologic Considerations
  Intervention and Communication
  Arthrosis
  The Degenerative Cycle
  Capsular Tightness
  Clinical Considerations

A complete study of human joints would include synchondroses, syndesmoses, symphyses, gomphoses, sutures, and synovial joints. Each of these classifications includes joints capable of movement. Movement definitely takes place at most syndesmoses, such as the distal tibiofibular joint. The symphysis pubis moves, especially during pregnancy. There is some movement of the teeth in their sockets (gomphoses). In fact, even the sutures of the skull are movable, at least through the third decade of life, and some investigators have claimed that they move spontaneously, with a rhythm independent of heart rate or respiratory rate.[20] Based on this claim, a few practitioners actually apply therapeutic mobilization to the sutures of the cranium.[20,44] However, for the sake of simplicity, and because the emphasis of clinical application is on joint mobilization techniques, the discussion in this chapter will be restricted to the synovial joints, which are the most numerous and most freely movable of the various types of human joints.

The mutual influences of structure and function are emphasized in this discussion because the two cannot

be dealt with adequately or understood when considered independently. The traditional anatomical concept of synovial joints must be expanded to a physiological concept; in addition to those structures that anatomically define a joint, those structures responsible for normal movement at the joint must also be included (Fig. 3-1). With this approach the synovial joint can be considered the basic unit of the musculoskeletal system and used as a reference for discussing normal function and disorders of this system.

KINEMATICS

Classification of Joint Surfaces and Movements

The nature of movement at any joint is largely determined by the joint structure, especially the shapes of the joint surfaces. The traditional classification of synovial joints by structure includes the categories of spheroid, trochoid, condyloid, ginglymoid, ellipsoid,

Darlene Hertling and Randolph M. Kessler: MANAGEMENT OF COMMON MUSCULOSKELETAL DISORDERS: Physical Therapy Principles and Methods, 3rd ed. © 1996 Lippincott-Raven Publishers.

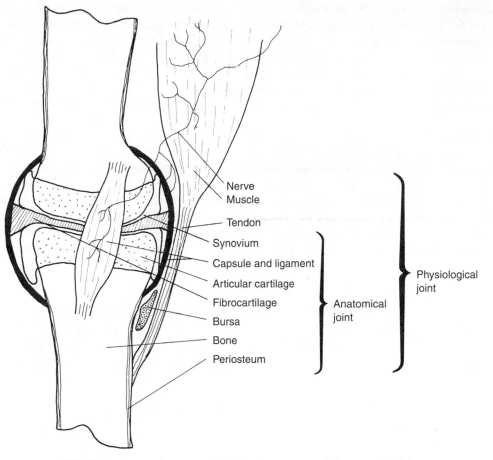

FIG. 3-1. *Anatomic versus physiologic concept of the synovial joint.*

Nerve
Muscle
Tendon
Synovium
Capsule and ligament
Articular cartilage
Fibrocartilage
Bursa
Bone
Periosteum

Anatomical joint

Physiological joint

and planar joints.[58] It should be apparent even to someone with only a basic knowledge of human anatomy and kinesiology that this classification does not accurately define the shapes of joint surfaces or the movements that occur at each type of joint. The heads of the femur and humerus do not form true spheres or even parts of true spheres. A ginglymus, such as the humeroulnar joint, does not allow a true hinge motion on flexion and extension but rather a helical movement involving considerable rotation. The humeroradial joint, which is a trochoid joint, does not move about a single axis, or pivot, because the head of the radius is oval, having a longer diameter anteroposteriorly than mediolaterally. The interphalangeal joints, the carpometacarpal joint of the thumb, the humeroulnar joint, and the calcaneocuboid joints can be considered as sellar. However, the movements occurring at these joints vary greatly, as do the shapes of the joint surfaces. Therefore, although this classification of joint structure may serve a purpose for the anatomist, in itself it is not adequate for the clinician, such as the physical therapist, who must be concerned with the finer details of joint mechanics.

A similar problem exists with classifying joint movement. The traditional classification of joint movement includes the following:[58]

Angular—Indicating an increase or decrease in the angle formed between two bones, for example, flexion-extension at the elbow

Circumduction—Movement of a bone circumscribing a cone, for example, circumduction at the hip or shoulder

Rotation—Movement occurring about the longitudinal axis of a bone, for example, internal-external rotation at the shoulder

Sliding—One bone slides over another with little or no appreciable rotation or angular movement, for example, movement between carpals

There are two problems with this classification system that make it inadequate for those clinicians concerned with joint mechanics. First, it describes movement occurring between bones but ignores movement occurring between joint surfaces. Movement takes place at joints, but often when movement is defined what happens *at the joint* is ignored. An analogy would be to consider the movement of a door but to ignore the hinge. Second, angular movements almost never occur without some rotation; rotation nearly always occurs with some angular movement; gliding usually involves angular and rotary movement, and so on. Again, the classification needs to be expanded to take into consideration the specifics of joint movement.

Movements occurring between bones must be defined in such a way that they can easily be related to movements occurring between respective joint surfaces. Therefore, it is helpful to define the *mechanical axis* of any joint as a line that passes through the moving bone, touching the center of the relatively stationary joint surface and lying perpendicular to it (Fig. 3-2). *Osteokinematic* movement (movement occurring

between two bones) can now be defined according to the mechanical axis rather than according to the long axis of the moving bone, as has been done in the past.[30,58] By relating osteokinematic movement to *arthrokinematic* movement (movement occurring between joint surfaces) the movement of the mechanical axis of the moving bone relative to the stationary joint surface can be considered. In other words, one joint surface can be considered as stationary and its opposing joint surface as moving relative to it. This relative movement is defined according to the path traced by the line representing the mechanical axis of the joint on the stationary surface. The mechanical axis is determined at the starting point of a movement; once movement has begun, it maintains the same relationship to the moving bone while moving relative to the stationary bone.

JOINT SURFACES

Before discussing types of movement, it is necessary to define the shapes of joint surfaces since they largely determine the types of movements that may occur at the joint. No joint surface resembles a true geometric form; joint surfaces are neither spheres, ovals, or ellipses, nor are they true parts of these. However, any joint surface can be thought of as being part of an ovoid surface, that is, resembling the surface of an egg (Fig. 3-3A). If a cross-section of an ovoid surface is examined, it is clear that the radius of the joint surface changes constantly, forming a cardioid curve (Fig. 3-4). A typical example would be a sagittal section of a femoral condyle. Some joint surfaces, rather than representing part of a simple ovoid, might be considered a complex ovoid, or sellar, surface (see Fig. 3-3B). A sellar surface is convex in one cross-sectional plane and concave in the plane perpendicular to it, although the surfaces of each of these cross-sections may be represented by a cardioid curve.

Referring again to a simple ovoid (Fig. 3-5), the shortest distance between any two points on the surface is termed a *chord*, and any other line of continuous concavity toward the chord is an *arc*. A three-sided figure made up of three chords is a *triangle*. A

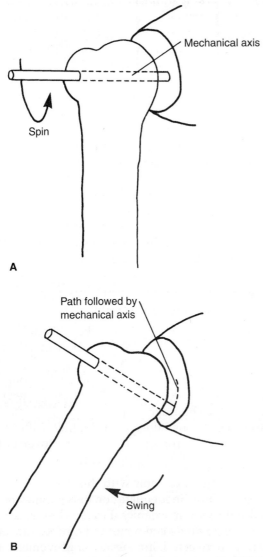

FIG 3-2. Osteokinematic movements may be defined by the mechanical axis. These movements are (**A**) spin and (**B**) swing.

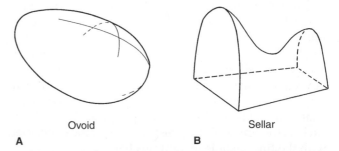

FIG. 3-3. Joint surfaces may be (**A**) ovoid or (**B**) sellar.

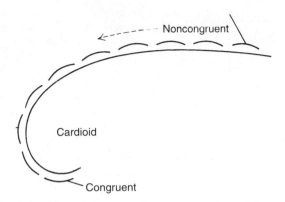

FIG. 3-4. A cardioid curve is representative of the cross-sectional shape of synovial joint surfaces. Because of the constantly changing radius there is one position at which the radius of the opposing joint surface attains maximal congruency.

three-sided figure in which at least one side is formed by an arc is a *trigone*.

JOINT MOVEMENTS

Any movement in which the bone moves but the mechanical axis remains stationary is termed a *spin* (see Fig. 3-2A). True spin of the humerus, then, would be a movement of flexion combined with some abduction, since the glenoid cavity faces slightly forward. The bone, during true spin, would rotate about its mechanical axis. Note that when the mechanical axis of the joint and the long axis of the moving bone coincide, such as at the metacarpophalangeal and the femorotibial joints, the spin is what is traditionally termed *rotation* at the joint. Where axes do not necessarily coincide, such as at the hip and shoulder, spin does not always occur when the joint "rotates." For example, spin occurs during internal and external rotation at the shoulder when the humerus is in a posi-

tion of 90° of abduction; the mechanical axis (defined according to the starting position of movement) coincides with the long axis of the humerus. However, internal and external rotations, performed with the arm to the side, do not involve spin at the joint surfaces; in this position, the mechanical axis does not coincide with the long axis of the humerus. A movement in which the mechanical axis follows the path of a chord is termed a *chordate*, or *pure*, swing. If the end of the mechanical axis should trace the path of an arc during movement of the bone, the bone has undergone an *arcuate*, or *impure*, swing (see Fig. 3-2B).

Note that with flexion or abduction of the humerus, the movement is an impure swing. Pure swing of the humerus occurs during elevation in a plane somewhat midway between the planes of flexion and abduction (because the glenoid cavity faces about 40° forward). Also note that internal and external rotation with the arm at the side is a movement of swing. An impure swing can be thought of as a pure swing with an element of spin, or rotation, about the mechanical axis. This element of rotation, which accompanies every impure swing, is termed *conjunct* rotation. Habitual movements at any joint are usually impure swings. It follows that most habitual movements, or those movements that occur most frequently at any joint, involve some conjunct rotation. It is well known, for example, that the tibia rotates during flexion-extension at the knee. If one carefully watches the ulna flexing and extending on the humerus, a similar rotation is seen; the ulna pronates at the limits of extension and supinates at the extremes of flexion. The interphalangeal joints rotate considerably during flexion and extension. This is easily observed by holding the extended small fingers together, then flexing them simultaneously. The distal phalanges, especially, can be seen to supinate during flexion. Although such conjunct rotation occurs at every joint, it occurs to a much greater degree at joints with sellar surfaces than at those with simple ovoid surfaces. By now it should be evident that most of what have been traditionally considered "angular" movements are actually helical movements because of this element of conjunct rotation that accompanies them. This rotary component is an essential feature of normal joint mechanics.

☐ **Arthrokinematics**

The study of what happens between joint surfaces on joint movement is known as arthrokinematics. When a bone swings relative to another bone, one of two types of movement may occur between joint surfaces.[30,58] If points at certain intervals on the moving surface contact points at the same intervals on the opposing surface, one surface is said to *roll* on the oppos-

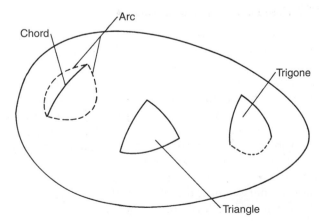

FIG. 3-5. Chords, arcs, a triangle, and a trigone are depicted on an ovoid surface.

ing surface (Fig. 3-6A). This is analogous to a tire on a car contacting the road surface as the car rolls down the street: various points on the tire contact various points on the road, the distance between contact points on the tire and road being the same. If, however, only one point on the moving joint surface contacts various points on the opposing surface, *slide* is taking place (Fig. 3-6B). This is analogous to a tire on a car that is skidding on ice: the tire is not turning but is moving relative to the road surface—it is sliding.

Actually, in most movements at human synovial joints, both slide and roll take place simultaneously. If only roll were to take place, the moving bone would tend to dislocate before much movement could occur; if only slide were to occur, impingement of joint surfaces would prevent full movement (Fig. 3-7). Stated in another way, the moving bone must rotate about a particular center of motion (or centers of motion) in order for normal gliding to occur at the joint surfaces. If the bone should move about any other centroid of movement than what is normal for that joint, abnormal movement will occur between joint surfaces. Conversely, if normal movement does not or cannot occur between joint surfaces, the moving bone cannot move about its normal centroid of movement. This will be discussed later, in the section on analysis of accessory

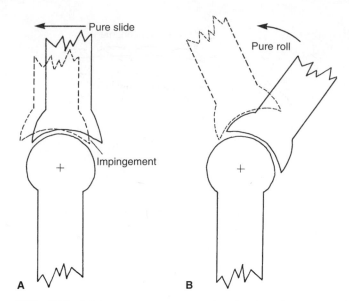

FIG. 3-7. Joint movements occurring in the absence of normal arthrokinematic movement cause (**A**) impingement or (**B**) dislocation.

joint motions. Clinically, a meniscus tear, which causes abnormal movement between joint surfaces, alters the normal centroid of movement at a joint.[15] This often results in abnormal stresses to the joint capsule, which are manifested as pain and muscle guarding. A tight joint capsule, which causes alteration in the normal centroid of movement, will result in abnormal movement between joint surfaces, usually with premature cartilaginous compression before the movement is completed. Physiologically, the fact that slide and roll take place together allows for economy of articular cartilage with respect to the size of the joint surface necessary for movement. It also prevents undue wearing of isolated points on joint surfaces, which would occur if, for example, only slide took place.

THE CONCAVE–CONVEX RULE

Obviously, roll always occurs in the same direction as the swing of the bone. However, the direction of joint slide can be determined only if the shapes of the joint surfaces are known. This is an important rule for anyone concerned with joint mechanics to know and will be referred to as the *concave–convex rule*: If a concave surface moves on a convex surface, roll and slide must occur in the same direction; if a convex surface moves on a concave surface, roll and slide occur in opposite directions (Fig. 3-8). Therefore, if the tibia extends on the stationary femur, the tibial joint surfaces must roll forward and slide forward on the femoral condyles in order for full movement to take place. However, if the

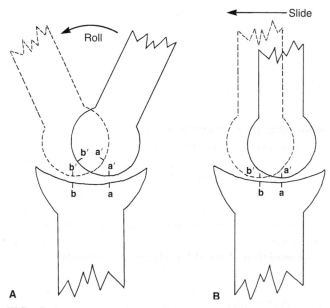

FIG. 3-6. Arthrokinematic movements showing (**A**) roll and (**B**) slide. The letters indicate points on the opposing joint surfaces that come in contact with one another. Points a' and b' are on the moving joint surface; points a and b are on the stationary joint surface. Note that during roll (**A**), points a and b contact various points on the opposing moving joint surface and during slide (**B**), points a and b contact one point on the moving surface.

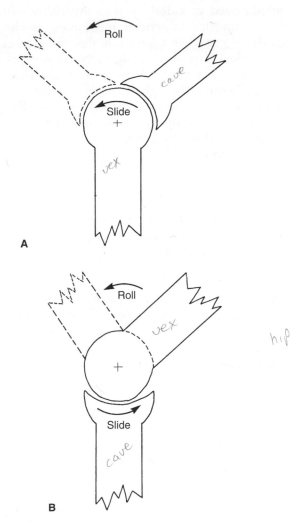

Roll

cave

Slide
+

vex

A

Roll

vex

+

Slide

cave

B

FIG. 3-8. Relationship between arthrokinematic movements and osteokinematic movements for the "concave–convex rule." (**A**) Represents a concave surface moving on a convex surface. (**B**) Represents a convex surface moving on a concave surface.

of the humerus on the glenoid cavity may be restricted as well. The manual therapist may use passive joint mobilization techniques to restore inferior slide in order to facilitate the restoration of upward swing of the humerus. Thus, by knowing the concave–convex rule, the therapist knows in which direction to apply joint slide mobilizations in order to increase any restricted swing of a bone.

The type of joint surface motion that occurs with a spin of a bone about its mechanical axis is actually a form of slide. However, it should be apparent that while slide occurs in one direction at one half of the joint, it occurs in the opposite direction at the other half of the joint surface. This type of slide is referred to as *spin*, as is the osteokinematic movement it accompanies.

Biomechanical analysis demonstrates situations in which the concave–convex rule cannot be applied. These situations include movements at plane joints, movements for which the axis of rotation passes through the articulating surfaces, and movements at joints in which the concave side of the joint forms a deep socket.[28] Joints whose motions are largely dictated by the musculature and tension in the capsule (*i.e.*, joints that are not track-bound), such as the glenohumeral joint, may be controlled more by the tension in the capsular tissue and musculature than by the joint geometry.[22,23,36,46] However, the concave–convex rule is an excellent teaching tool for use with beginning students of manual therapy. This qualitative biomechanical analysis provides a methodical context from which to explain the application of the rule.[28]

THE CLOSE-PACKED POSITION

Separation of joint surfaces is termed *distraction*; approximation of opposing surfaces is *compression*. Whereas some bone movements are accompanied by a relative compression of joint surfaces, other movements involve distraction. By knowing the close-packed position of a joint, one can determine which movements involve compression and which involve distraction.

As mentioned, ovoid surfaces are irregular, in that in any one cross-sectional plane the ovoid surface is of constantly changing radius, defining a cardioid curve. If one imagines an opposing joint surface moving along this curve, it is clear that in most positions the two surfaces do not fit, or are noncongruent. However, one position exists in which the joint surfaces become relatively congruent because their contacting radii are approximately the same (see Fig. 3-4). Thus, while synovial joint surfaces tend to be noncongruent, at least one position exists for each joint in which the

femur extends on the stationary tibia, the femoral condyles must roll forward but slide backward on the tibia. If the humerus is elevated, the humeral head rolls upward but must slide inferiorly. During external rotation, with the arm at the side (a movement of swing), the head of the humerus must slide forward, whereas during internal rotation it must slide backward.

Clinicians must apply these concepts in the approach to restoration of restricted joint motion. Traditionally, in attempts to restore joint movement clinicians have tended to work only on osteokinematic movements. For example, if flexion of the humerus is restricted, active or passive motion into flexion is used in an attempt to increase this movement. However, one must also consider that inferior slide of the head

surfaces become maximally congruent. This position is termed the *close-packed position* of a joint. (See Table 5-4.) At any joint, movement into the close-packed position involves an impure swing and so necessarily involves a conjunct rotation. The rotary component of movement into this position causes the joint capsule and major ligaments supporting the joint to twist, which in turn causes an approximation of joint surfaces. Once the close-packed position is reached, no further movement in that direction is possible.

Therefore, movement toward the close-packed position involves an element of compression, whereas movement out of this position involves distraction. MacConnaill and Basmajian point out that habitual movements at any joint involve movements directed into and out of the close-packed position.[30] It is likely that the resultant intermittent compression of joint surfaces has a bearing on nutrition and lubrication of articular cartilage. The squeezing out of synovial fluid with each compression phase facilitates exchange of nutrients and helps to maintain a lubricant film between surfaces (see sections on joint nutrition and lubrication).

Interestingly, moving the upper extremity in a reciprocating pattern, such that every joint is first moved simultaneously toward its close-packed position and then directly out of the close-packed position, resembles one of the basic patterns used by Knott and Voss in their proprioceptive neuromuscular facilitation techniques.[27] Considering the twisting and untwisting of the capsules and ligaments that occurs, and considering what is known of joint neurology with respect to joint–muscle reflexes (see the section on neurology later in this chapter), it seems likely that the facilitatory effect of the pattern may be related to joint position as well as muscle position.

The close-packed position also has important implications with respect to the pathomechanics of many injuries. For instance, many upper extremity injuries occur from falling on the outstretched hand; Colles' fracture at the wrist, supracondylar elbow fractures, posterior dislocation of the elbow, and anterior dislocation of the shoulder are but a few. This is not surprising if one realizes that falling on the outstretched hand, in such a way that the body rolls away from the arm on impact, throws every major upper extremity joint (except the metacarpophalangeal and acromioclavicular joints) into close-packing. As mentioned, once the close-packed position is reached, the joint becomes locked and no further movement is possible in that direction. If further force is added, a joint must dislocate, a bone must give, or both. The weak link tends to be determined by age; the child is likely to fracture the humerus above the elbow, the adolescent or teenager may dislocate the shoulder, and the middle-aged or elderly person invariably sustains a Colles' fracture. In general, most fractures and dislocations occur when a joint is in the close-packed position. Most capsular or ligamentous sprains occur when the joint is in a loose-packed position. This is simply because the tight fit of the adjoining bones in the close-packed position causes forces applied to the joint to be taken up by the bones rather than by the supporting structures; there is more "intrinsic stability" at the joint.

JOINT PLAY

In a loose-packed position, or in any position of the joint other than the close-packed position, the joint surfaces are incongruent. An obvious example is the knee joint in some position of flexion, although the menisci help to make up for the marked incongruence. In the loose-packed position, the capsule and major supporting ligaments remain relatively lax. This must be so in order to allow a normal range of movement. Thus, in most joint positions a joint has some "play" in it because joint surfaces do not fit tightly and because the capsule and ligaments remain somewhat lax.

This joint play is essential for normal joint function. First, the small spaces that exist because of joint incongruence are necessary to the hydrodynamic component of joint lubrication (see discussion later in this chapter). Second, because the joint surfaces are of varying radii, movement cannot occur around a rigid axis, and so the joint capsule must allow some play in order for full movement to occur. Related to this is the fact that if normal joint distraction (one form of joint play) is lost, then joint surfaces will become prematurely approximated when moving toward the close-packed position, and movement in this direction will, therefore, be restricted. Human synovial joints cannot be compared to a door hinge, except in a limited sense, since a door moves about a single axis at its hinge and requires little or no play. Third, most joint movements are helical, involving movement about more than one axis simultaneously. In order for this type of movement to occur, a certain amount of joint play must exist, unless the movement is track-bound, which is usually not the case. One may, therefore, presume that loss of joint play from some pathology, such as a tight joint capsule, will lead to alteration in joint function, usually involving restriction of motion or pain, or both. Mennell uses the term *joint dysfunction* for loss of joint play.[41] This term is useful in a general discussion of joint mechanics but in clinical use should be avoided in favor of terms that more precisely identify the responsible pathology, since there are many possible causes of loss of joint play.

CONJUNCT ROTATION

Conjunct rotation is the component of spin or rotation that accompanies any impure swing of a bone (Fig. 3-9). It is easily observed when the tibia extends on the femur, the distal phalanges of the fingers flex when held together, or the ulna flexes and extends on the humerus; such movements are helical. This rotation causes the joint capsule to twist when moving toward the close-packed position. At the shoulder, where a particularly large range of movement is possible, some rotation opposite the direction of normal conjunct rotation must occur at the later stages of movement. Thus, pure abduction in the frontal plane involves an impure swing with a medial conjunct rotation at the early phase, the first 90° to 120° of movement. This is because the glenoid cavity faces somewhat forward and the humerus on abduction swings out of the plane of the scapula. If this impure swing were left to continue, at full elevation the joint capsule would be completely twisted on itself. This, however, is impossible, since the twisting of the joint capsule would cause a premature approximation of joint surfaces before full elevation could be attained. To prevent this premature locking of the joint on abduction, the humerus must rotate laterally on its long axis during the final phase of movement, bringing the humeral head back toward the plane of the scapula. Similarly, sagittal flexion involves a lateral conjunct rotation but a medial longitudinal rotation during the

final phase. This is best appreciated by observing it on a skeleton, noting the end position of the humerus on abduction or flexion without rotation and comparing it with elevation in the plane of the scapula, that is, about midway between flexion and abduction.

In addition to accompanying any impure swing, conjunct rotation may occur with a succession of swings, even if each of the swings is a pure swing. In a triangle drawn on a curved surface, such as an ovoid surface, the sum of the interior angles of the triangle may exceed 180° if the surface is convex, or the sum may be less than 180° if the surface is concave. During a succession of movements, in which the mechanical axis follows the path of a triangle or trigone, the amount of conjunct rotation that accompanies the completed cycle will be equal to the difference between the sum of the interior angles of the triangle or trigone and 180° (see Fig. 3-9). This type of conjunct rotation can be visualized by moving the humerus through a succession of movements: starting with the arm at the side, elbow bent, fingers facing forward, flex the humerus 90°, abduct 90° horizontally, then adduct 90°. The fingers are now directed laterally, indicating that the humerus, during this succession of movements, rotated outward 90°. The succession may only be carried out once or twice without derotating the humerus medially because of the twisting of the capsule that results from the lateral conjunct rotation.

☐ **Summary of Joint Function**

The terminology of joint function has been expanded to accommodate the more specific features of joint kinematics, including the relationships between joint structure and function and the types of movements occurring between joint surfaces. In doing so the following osteokinematic terms, or those terms defining movement between two bones, have been defined:

Mechanical axis—Line drawn through the moving bone, at the starting position of a movement, that passes through the center of the opposing joint surface and is perpendicular to it

Spin—Movement of a bone about the mechanical axis

Pure swing—Movement of a bone in which an end of the mechanical axis traces the path of a chord with respect to the ovoid formed by the opposing joint surface; also called *chordate swing*

Impure swing—Movement in which the mechanical axis follows the path of an arc with respect to the opposing ovoid surface

Conjunct rotation—Element of spin that accompanies impure swing; also the rotation that may occur with a succession of swings

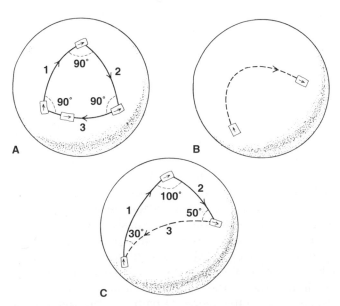

FIG. 3-9. Conjunct rotation occurring (**A**) with a succession of pure swings with return to the starting position (diadochokinetic movement), (**B**) with a single impure swing, and (**C**) with a completed cycle of pure and impure swings (also a diadochokinetic movement).

The following arthrokinematic terms, or those that define the types of movement occurring between joint surfaces, have also been defined:

Roll—Movement in which points at intervals on the moving joint surface contact points at the same intervals on the opposing surface

Slide—Movement in which a single contact point on the moving surface contacts various points on the opposing surface

Spin—Type of slide that accompanies spin of a bone; one half of the joint surface slides in one direction while the other half slides in the opposite direction; that is, the moving joint surface rotates about some point on the opposing joint surface

Distraction—Separation of joint surfaces

Compression—Approximation of joint surfaces; always occurs when moving toward the close-packed position

The *close-packed position* was defined for a joint in which the following three conditions exist:

1. The joint surfaces become maximally congruent.
2. The joint capsule and major ligaments become twisted, causing joint surfaces to approximate.
3. The joint becomes locked so that no further movement is possible in that direction.

☐ Clinical Application

TERMINOLOGY

A rationale for the approach to management of joint dysfunction, including the use of specific joint mobilization techniques, can now be discussed based on the previous analysis of joint movement. However, some additional terms must first be presented. Unfortunately, a jargon has evolved relating to the clinical application of those concepts and is often the source of confusion since the terms are used inconsistently. Therefore, the most common and useful definitions of important terms are presented.

Accessory joint movements are simply those arthrokinematic movements that must occur in order for normal osteokinematic movement to take place. These might include slides, rolls, distractions, compressions, or conjunct rotations. Consider the osteokinematic movement of the humerus moving from the resting position with the arm at the side to the close-packed position. The joint is convex-on-concave. The head of the humerus must roll in the same direction in which the bone swings. It must slide opposite this direction or somewhat inferiorly and inward. Because the close-packed position is being approached, the joint surfaces are becoming approximated. It is a movement of

impure swing, so a conjunct rotation, in this case a lateral rotation, must occur. If any one of these accessory movements does not or cannot occur, then this particular swing of the humerus cannot be performed painlessly or harmlessly through the full range. If full osteokinematic movement does occur, it does so at the expense of the capsule or ligaments, which must be abnormally stretched, or of the articular cartilage, which must be abnormally compressed.

The term *component motions* can be used synonymously with *accessory movements*. For example, lateral rotation of the tibia is referred to as a component of knee extension. Likewise, spreading of the distal tibia and fibula is a component of dorsiflexion at the ankle. The clinician must be aware of the component motions necessary for each osteokinematic movement at a joint. Many of these are listed in Appendix A.

Joint-play movements are those accessory movements that can be produced passively at a joint but cannot be isolated actively. They might include distractions, compressions, slides, rolls, or spins at a joint in a particular position. Joint-play movements are used when applying specific mobilization techniques to restore accessory movements so that full and painless osteokinematic movement may be restored. For example, inferior glide occurs at the shoulder during active elevation. It can be performed passively, but in itself cannot be performed actively by voluntary muscle contraction; inferior glide is a joint-play movement at the glenohumeral joint.

Joint mobilization is a very general term that may be applied to any active or passive attempt to increase movement at a joint. In addition to traditional methods of increasing joint movement, such as active, passive, and active-assisted range-of-motion techniques, joint mobilization includes specific passive mobilization techniques. These techniques are aimed at restoring those component movements that permit pain-free or harmless osteokinematic movement. They are used especially to restore those joint-play movements that cannot be isolated actively.

Specific passive mobilization techniques are graded (Fig. 3-10). Grades 1 through 4 are often referred to as *articulation* techniques, which are passive rhythmic oscillations. Grade 5 is a *manipulation* technique that is a high-velocity, low-amplitude, passive thrust. These grades are relative to the pathologic amplitude of joint-play movement that exists at the joint and *not* to the normal amplitude that should exist. There are two main criteria for the selection of the particular grade to be used: (1) the degree of pain or protective muscle spasm during passive joint-play movement (irritability) and (2) the degree of restriction of joint-play movement. The greater the irritability, the lower the numerical grade of movement used. Pain and spasm

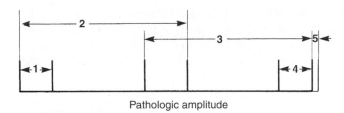

FIG. 3-10. *Grades of joint-play movement.*

must be avoided. Manipulation is used primarily when a very slight, minimally painful restriction exists. A third criterion of selection might apply here, namely the skill and experience of the operator, since manipulative maneuvers should only be attempted after articulation techniques have been mastered and after much practice. The terms of joint movement are presented schematically in Figure 3-11.

Specific accessory joint motions that are limited may be restored by manual oscillations or thrusts. The primary goal of using specific joint mobilization techniques is restoration of normal, pain-free use of the joint. The emphasis is not on forcing a particular anatomic (osteokinematic) movement at a joint, as has been done in the past with traditional methods of mobilization; rather, it is on restoring normal joint mechanics in order to allow full, pain-free osteokinematic movement to occur. In this way, range of motion is restored to the joint with less risk of damaging the joint by compressing isolated portions of articular cartilage, and with less pain and muscle guarding from overstretching isolated capsuloligamentous structures, as may well occur if an osteokinematic movement is forced in the absence of necessary component movements. This is to say that specific passive mobilization, correctly applied, is a safer, more efficient, and less painful method of increasing range of motion at a joint. Mennell, in his lectures, often uses the analogy of a door having lost movement because of a faulty hinge. Efforts to restore motion by pushing hard on the door are likely to result in further damage to the hinge. The logical method to remedy the situation is to direct one's attention to the hinge—to restore nor-

mal mechanics to the hinge, thereby restoring normal movement of the door.[41]

Note that this discussion ignores the physiologic concept of the joint. This is done solely for the sake of simplicity. Obviously when restoring normal joint mechanics is considered, attention must be given to the anatomic joint along with those structures responsible for active movement of the joint. For example, active abduction at the shoulder is often lost because of the absence of inferior glide. Relative to the anatomic joint, the joint-play movement of inferior glide may be limited. However, the problem may also be physiological, in that inferior glide may not be occurring owing to weakness of the supraspinatus muscle. These are very different problems leading to similar results. The nature of the problem must be brought out by a thorough evaluation.

ANALYSIS OF ACCESSORY JOINT MOTIONS

Clinical Assessment. Many of the means of determining which accessory movements are components of specific osteokinematic movements have already been discussed. For instance, the direction of roll is always the same as that for the swing of the bone. If a convex surface moves on a concave surface, slide will occur in the direction opposite to the roll; if a concave surface moves on a convex surface, slide occurs in the same direction as the roll. Distraction occurs when moving out of the close-packed position; compression occurs when moving into the close-packed position. These components can all be determined for any joint moving in any direction. Some of the other component motions, as listed for each joint in Appendix A, must be memorized or deduced anatomically.

One way of assessing the state of a particular accessory movement (its amplitude and irritability) is clinically, by evaluating the joint-play movements. These examination maneuvers are essentially the same as the specific mobilization techniques. Rather than being performed as a graded, therapeutic technique, they are used to determine the amplitude of a joint-play movement and whether the movement causes pain or spasm. The amplitude of movement and possible restriction must be compared with the operator's concept of "normal" for that movement, at that joint, for that body type. This requires experience in evaluating normal as well as pathologic joints. Whenever possible, the pathologic joint must be compared with a healthy contralateral joint. The degree of irritability is determined by the patient's subjective response, as well as by the presence of protective muscle spasm when performing the examination movement. (Refer to regional chapters for the joint-play techniques at each joint.) Proficiency in clinically evaluating joint-

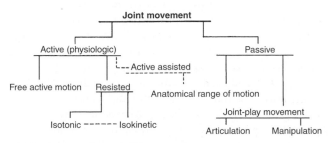

FIG. 3-11. *Terms related to joint movement.*

play movements and correlating findings to knowledge of accessory movements at the joint, as well as other symptoms and signs presenting on examination, is essential to the effective application of joint mobilization techniques and management of musculoskeletal disorders.

Instant Center Analysis. The more scientific method of analyzing arthrokinematic movement has been described by Sammarco and co-workers.[51] This involves a determination of the centroid of movement, or instant center of movement, at various points throughout a joint movement. For any joint, the axis about which motion takes place changes constantly during a particular movement. This is because joint surfaces are irregular. The instant centers of motion can be plotted for a movement through the use of careful roentgenographic studies of a joint that record the relative position of the bones at various points throughout the movement. This is done by choosing two reference points on the moving bone; in Figure 3-12 the points lie on the central axis of the bone, point a on the joint surface, point b 7 cm up on the shaft of the bone. A second roentgenogram taken after the bone has moved is superimposed over the original. In the new position, points a′ and b′ are determined along the central axis; a′ is on the joint surface, b′ is 7 cm up on the shaft. Now lines aa′ and bb′ are constructed, and perpendicular bisectors for each of these lines are drawn. The intersection of these bisectors is the instant center of motion, or the point of zero velocity, for this particular motion of the bone. Using this instant center of motion, point c, a velocity vector can be constructed showing the direction of surface motion that occurred for the particular movement. This is done by drawing a radius from the instant center to the point of contact between bones at the time for which the instant center was determined. In this case, the point of contact—the point at which the center axis of the bone crosses the joint surface—is called point p (Fig. 3-13). A perpendicular line drawn to this radius, at the joint surface, will indicate the direction of surface motion, with the arrow directed toward the movement of the bone.

Once the instant center and surface-velocity vector are determined, an interpretation can be made. An instant center lying on the joint surface at the point of contact between the bones indicates that pure roll is taking place. An instant center lying far from the joint surface point of contact indicates that pure sliding is taking place. A velocity vector pointed away from the opposing (stationary) surface indicates a distraction of the surfaces. A velocity vector aimed into the stationary surface indicates a compression of the surfaces. A velocity vector tangential to the joint surface suggests a smooth gliding motion is occurring.

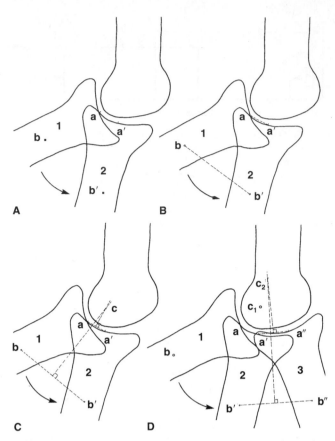

FIG. 3-12. Determination of instant centers of motion (c_1, c_2). (**A**) Two reference points on the moving bone are chosen; point a on the central axis of the joint surface and point b, 7 cm up the shaft of the bone (position 1); the same points, a′ and b′, are chosen in position 2. (**B**) Lines a–a′ and b–b′ are constructed and perpendicular bisections are drawn for these lines (**C,D**). The intersection of the bisectors c_1 and c_2 are the instant centers of motion for movement from position 1 to 2 (**C**) and from position 2 to 3 (**D**).

The above analysis might seem somewhat complex at first but is actually quite simple. The difficult step is obtaining reliable roentgenograms that can be superimposed on each other. Plotting instant centers and surface velocity vectors for a particular movement throughout the range of motion can yield some very specific information about that motion. It reveals the relative amounts of roll and slide for various points throughout the range and how these values change during the complete motion: the closer the instant center comes to the point of contact, the more roll is taking place; the further it moves away, the more slide is occurring. Perhaps more importantly, it reveals possible abnormal compression or distraction of joint surfaces throughout the range (*i.e.*, by comparison to what the operator considers "normal"). This type of scientific analysis of arthrokinematics is not practical

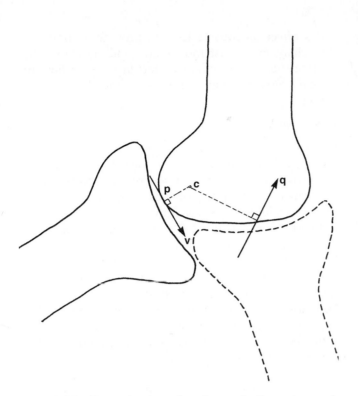

FIG. 3-13. Determination of surface velocity vectors: p is the point of contact during the arc of motion for which c applies; v is the calculated velocity vector indicating tangential surface motion. If q were the vector for the arc of motion for which c applies, one could conclude that joint compression took place during this motion.

for routine diagnostic purposes. However, it offers clinicians an opportunity to demonstrate the value of specific therapeutic interventions in improving abnormal joint mechanics. It has been used already to show the value of certain surgeries, for example, meniscectomy at the knee, in restoring normal joint mechanics.[15]

Because the information is obtained from roentgenograms, which are two-dimensional, arthrokinematic movements can be studied in only two dimensions. This analysis will not yield information concerning the amount of spin or conjunct rotation that is occurring.

NEUROLOGY

The neuroanatomy and, especially, the neurophysiology of joints are subjects not well covered in the current literature. Following the original works of Sherrington on neuromuscular physiology, a vast amount of information was collected concerning the role of muscle and tendon receptors in influencing posture, movement, muscle tone, and various reflex phenomena.[53] Little has been done until recently to identify specific joint receptors, and even less has been done to

determine their clinical significance.[54,62] Since the subject of joint neurology is directly relevant to the management of common musculoskeletal disorders, an overview is presented here.

☐ Innervation

Joints tend to receive innervation from two sources: (1) articular nerves that are branches of adjacent peripheral nerves and (2) branches from nerves that supply muscles controlling the joint. Each joint is usually supplied by several nerves, and their distributions tend to overlap considerably. In general, a particular aspect of a joint capsule is innervated by branches of the nerve supplying the muscle or muscles that would, when contracting, prevent overstretching of that part of the capsule. One notable exception is the anteroinferior aspect of the glenohumeral capsule, which is innervated by a branch from the axillary nerve. The nerve fibers of an articular nerve are purely afferent, with the exception of small vasomotor efferents to the blood vessels. The fiber sizes range from large myelinated fibers to small myelinated and unmyelinated fibers.

☐ Receptors

Joint receptors transmit information about the status of the joint to the central nervous system. The central nervous system interprets the information sent by the joint receptors and responds by coordinating muscle activity around the joint to meet joint mobility and stability requirements.[43,50] Joint receptors function to protect the joint from damage incurred by going into the pathologic range of motion. They are also partly responsible for determining the appropriate balance between synergistic and antagonistic muscular forces and for generating an image of body positioning and movement within the central nervous system. Four types of joint receptors have been identified, each serving a relatively specific role in the sensorimotor integration of joint function.[54,55,58,62]

Type 1: Postural

Description—Encapsulated endings, similar to Ruffini corpuscle

Location—Numerous in the superficial joint capsule; usually found in clusters of six; located primarily in the neck, hip, and shoulder

Related fiber—Small (6–9 μm) myelinated (relatively slow conduction)

Stimulus—Changing mechanical stresses in the joint capsule. May be activated by the presence of positional faults. May be more active with traction techniques than with oscillations

Action—Slowly adapting (acts up to 1 minute following the initial stimulation), low threshold; mechanoreceptor

Function—Provides information concerning the static and dynamic position of the joint; is constantly firing; contributes to regulation of postural muscle tone; contributes to kinesthetic (movement) sense; senses direction and speed of movement; contributes to regulation of muscle tone during movement of the joint; produces increased tone in the muscle being stretched and relaxation in the muscle antagonistic to that being stretched; not active in mid range of motion

Type 2: Dynamic

Description—Thickly encapsulated, similar to pacinian corpuscle

Location—Sparse (relative to type I); found in joint capsule and ligaments (deeper layers and fat pads); primarily located in the lumbar spine, hand, foot, and jaw

Related fiber—Medium (9–12 μm) myelinated

Stimulus—Sudden changes in joint motion; may be more active with oscillation techniques than with traction

Action—Rapidly adapting (acts for ½ second following each motion), low threshold; dynamic mechanoreceptor

Function—Fires only on quick changes in movement; provides information concerning acceleration and deceleration of joint movement; acts at initiation of movement as a "booster" to help overcome inertia of body parts; produces increased tone in the muscle being stretched and relaxation in the muscle antagonistic to the one being stretched when the joint is at end range, not active in mid-range of motion; inhibits pain

Type 3: Inhibitive

Description—Thinly encapsulated, similar to Golgi end organ

Location—Primarily located in intrinsic and extrinsic joint ligaments, superficial layers of the capsule; in the lumbar spine not detected in the longitudinal posterior ligament, longitudinal anterior ligament, or iliolumbar ligament

Related fiber—Large (13–17 μm) myelinated (fast conduction)

Stimulus—Stretch at end range; more active with fast manipulation techniques

Action—Very slowly adapting (acts for several minutes following the initial stimulation), high threshold; dynamic mechanoreceptor

Function—Monitors direction of movement; has reflex effect on muscle tone to provide a "braking" mechanism against movement tending to overdisplace the joint (movement too fast or too far); inhibits muscle tone; responds to stretch at end of range

Type 4: Nociceptive

Description—Free nerve endings and plexus

Location—Located in most tissues: fibrous capsule, intrinsic and extrinsic ligaments, fat pads, periosteum (absent in articular cartilage, intra-articular fibrocartilage, and synovium)

Related fiber—Small (2–5 μm) myelinated and unmyelinated (2 μm) (slow conduction)

Stimulus—Marked mechanical deformation or tension; direct mechanical or chemical irritation

Action—Nonadapting, high threshold; pain receptors

Function—Inactive under normal conditions; active when related tissue is subject to marked deformation or other noxious mechanical or chemical stimulation; produces tonic muscle contraction

☐ Clinical Considerations

It is apparent from the previous descriptions that stimulation of joint receptors contributes to sense of static position (type I), sense of speed of movement (type I), sense of change in speed of movement (type II), sense of direction of movement (types I and III), regulation of postural muscle tone (type I), regulation of muscle tone at the initiation of movement (type II), regulation of muscle tone during movement (coordination) (type II), and regulation of muscle tone during potentially harmful movements (type III). Of course, skin receptors, connective tissue receptors, and muscle receptors also contribute to many of these same functions. The following are some of the clinical problems that remain unresolved, or only partially resolved:

1. How important are these joint receptors, relative to muscle and skin receptors, for example, in the regulation of muscle tone, posture, and movement?
2. Are some of the persistent problems, such as chronic limp, residual incoordination, chronic instability ("giving way"), and chronic muscle atrophy, that are encountered in patients following some joint injuries the result of damage to these receptors?
3. How might treatment techniques, such as joint mobilization, neuromuscular facilitation, and inhibition, be refined to accommodate the functions of these joint receptors?

One particularly interesting study demonstrates a case in which malocclusion of dentures, causing abnormal afferent discharge from the temporomandibular joint capsules, resulted in an almost total reflex inhibition of the temporal muscles during active occlusion by the patient.[26] Restoration of normal joint mechanics, by remodeling of the dentures, restored normal muscular activity. A study by Wyke showed marked postural changes in a boy with apparent alteration of afferent impulses from the ankle capsule following injury to the lateral aspect of the capsule.[62] The postural deficit persisted in spite of an otherwise complete recovery, with restoration of normal strength and range of motion and with no residual pain. The boy's only complaint was that of occasional "giving way" of the ankle. Freeman advocates the use of coordination exercises on a balance board for patients with chronic ankle "instability" in the absence of demonstrable structural instability.[16] He reports good results with such a program, attributing such giving way at the ankle to alteration of normal joint afferent flow following injury to the joint, such as from an ankle sprain. Most physical therapists have encountered the common phenomenon of gross quadriceps atrophy following knee injury in spite of preventive efforts to maintain muscle function. Although there is little current literature on the subject, it seems reasonable to attribute this problem to reflex muscle inhibition by abnormal joint receptor stimulation.[9]

As far as techniques of treatment are concerned, it is interesting to relate what is known about the function of these joint receptors, and what is known of arthrokinematics, to techniques that have already evolved. Consider the diagonal pattern commonly used in proprioceptive neuromuscular facilitation techniques—moving the arm through flexion, abduction, external rotation to extension, adduction, and internal rotation. Part of the explanation of this pattern refers to moving from a position of maximum elongation and unspiraling of functionally related muscles to a position of spiraling and shortening of these same muscles.[57] In addition, this pattern involves moving all joints simultaneously from a close-packed to a loose-packed position. In doing so, the joint capsule of each joint moves from a position of maximum shortening and spiraling to a position of lengthening and unspiraling. Studies thus far on animals have indicated that maximum afferent stimulation occurs when approaching the close-packed position of a joint; this is to be expected since it is the position of maximum tightening of the capsule and ligaments in which the receptors lie. The techniques of proprioceptive neuromuscular facilitation evolved with primary consideration of the neurophysiology of muscles, using movement patterns that combine actions of functionally related muscles to bring about a mutual facilitation of each muscle in the chain. It is now suggested that

these patterns also combine functionally related joint movements that add to the facilitative effect of the patterns on the muscles involved through joint receptor stimulation. It also seems probable that the joint receptors play a significant role in other techniques of facilitation, such as "quick stretch," that tend to stimulate the type II receptor.

It is important to consider the function of joint receptors when using joint mobilization or other treatment techniques involving joint movement. The effectiveness of efforts to increase movement at a joint will naturally be compromised by any muscle contraction tending to restrict joint movement. Emphasis, then, must be made on avoiding reflex muscle contractions that would tend to prevent or restrict a desired joint movement. For this reason—and for other obvious reasons—pain must be avoided during joint mobilization, since it is well known that pain at a joint tends to elicit a reflex muscle response to restrict movement at the joint. Sudden joint movement tends to stimulate firing of the type III receptors, which sets up a reflex muscle contraction to restrict further movement. Gradual initiation of movement tends to stimulate the type II receptor, which effects a small facilitative muscular response. Passive and active mobilization techniques are best performed rhythmically, without sudden changes in speed or direction of movement. A manipulation must be performed so quickly that it is completed before the reflex muscular response produced by stimulation of the type III receptor can act to interfere with the movement. Similarly, it must be performed through a very small amplitude to minimize the number of type III receptors stimulated.

With respect to the type IV pain receptors, it is worth emphasizing that articular cartilage, fibrocartilage (*e.g.*, menisci), synovium, and compact bone are essentially aneural. This is well documented in anatomic studies as well as clinically.[25,54,62] In the anatomic joints the major pain-sensitive structures are the fibrous capsule, ligaments, and periosteum. This carries some important clinical implications. It suggests that pathologic conditions that might alter joint mechanics, such that the articular cartilage undergoes undue compression stress, may go unnoticed by the patient in the initial stages. In fact, the patient may notice nothing until either joint mechanics are altered sufficiently to place an abnormal stress on the joint capsule or until the joint cartilage undergoes sufficient degeneration, causing a low-grade synovitis with resultant pressure on the capsule from effusion. This may explain why persons with "frozen shoulders" or osteoarthrosis of other joints often do not present to a physician until the disease has progressed considerably. It also suggests that clinicians must learn to routinely examine for subtle changes in joint mechanics rather than considering only gross range of motion, strength, and complaints of pain by the patient. Patients presenting with very early symptoms or signs of osteoarthrosis could enjoy complete arrest or reversal of the joint problem if properly managed, rather than resigning themselves to future joint replacement.

As is discussed in more detail in Chapter 4, Pain, small oscillatory articulations may, in themselves, be useful in reducing pain at the joint being moved or at other joints derived from the same segment. The added proprioceptive input may inhibit the perception of pain through modulation at the substantia gelatinosa in the dorsal horn of the spinal cord.

▨ JOINT NUTRITION

In addition to being aneural, articular cartilage is for the most part avascular. This is also true of intra-articular fibrocartilage. Since, in general, body tissues depend on blood supply for nutrition, these structures would seem to be at a disadvantage. It is generally believed that the articular margins do receive some nutrients from the highly vascularized synovium and periosteum adjacent to them.[18] The menisci at the knee also receive nutrients at their peripheral capsular attachments, and it is suggested that the deep layers of articular cartilage are fed by the blood supply to the subchondral bone. However, the problem of nutrition to the more superficial, centrally located portions of the articular cartilage and to the more centrally located parts of the intra-articular fibrocartilage remains. These cartilaginous areas are the primary articulating surfaces, not the more peripheral areas or deeper layers. It is generally agreed that nutrition to these regions occurs by diffusion and imbibition of synovial fluid. This is a unique situation because nutrients must cross at least two barriers in order to reach the chondrocytes embedded within the cartilage. First, they must pass from the capillary bed of the highly vascularized synovium. They must then diffuse through the superficial matrix layers of the cartilaginous surface, before reaching the cell wall of the chondrocyte. Thus, synovial fluid serves a major function as a source of nutrition for articular cartilage and intra-articular fibrocartilage.[18,32,33,35]

Intermittent compression and distraction of joint surfaces must occur in order for an adequate exchange of nutrients and waste products to take place. A joint that is immobilized undergoes atrophy of articular cartilage, just as a joint in which there is prolonged compression of joint surface undergoes similar atrophic changes.[2,12,13,60] The three primary mechanisms by which synovial joints undergo normal compression and distraction are the following: (1) weight-bearing in lower extremity and spinal joints; (2) intermittent contraction of muscles crossing a joint; and (3) twisting and untwisting of the joint capsule as the joint moves toward and away from the close-packed position during habitual movements. With respect to the last mechanism, it is necessary to recall that as the joint approaches the close-packed position, its surfaces not only become compressed but also approach a position of maximal congruency. Thus, compression normally occurs in a position in which greater areas of the opposing joint surfaces are in contact. This ensures that relatively large portions of the joint surfaces undergo adequate exchange of nutrients. From a pathologic standpoint, a joint that has lost movement, such as from a tight joint capsule, does not receive a normal exchange of nutrients over the parts of the joint surfaces that no longer come into contact. This is especially true in the case of a tight joint capsule, since movements toward the close-packed position in which there is maximal joint surface contact are usually the movements that are most restricted.

Attritional changes in articular cartilage related to aging are observed in the relatively noncontacting portions of the joint surfaces.[4,38–40] Several reasons for this may be postulated. First, these are the areas of articular cartilage that undergo less deformation with use of the joint over time; as a result, the rate and degree of exchange of nutrient fluids is less in these areas. Also, with age there is a reduction of the chondroitin sulfate component of cartilaginous tissue. Since the fluid-binding capacity of articular cartilage is largely dependent on its chondroitin sulfate content, a decrease in this constituent might interfere with normal nutrition to the tissue. Furthermore, because loss of joint range of motion occurs with advancing age, the exchange of nutrients to portions of the articular cartilage is reduced.

▢ Lubrication

Synovial fluid, in addition to serving as a nutritional source for articular cartilage, also acts as a lubricant to prevent undue wear of joint surfaces from friction.[11,37,61] In studying lubrication of human joints, however, not just the properties of synovial fluid and how they affect movement and friction between two surfaces are considered. In addition there are the shape and consistency of the joint surfaces as well as the types of movement that occur between joint surfaces. Many models have been proposed for human joint lubrication. Some of the earlier models tend to ignore many of the unique properties of human joints. The more recent models evolved with the sophistication of engineering principles, which are better able to deal with some of the complex factors involved in human joint lubrication. However, it is generally agreed that no one model of joint lubrication applies to all joints under all circumstances. The major mode of lubrication in a particular joint may change, depending on factors such as loading and speed of movement.

Synovial fluid has essentially the same composition as blood plasma, except for the addition of mucin. Mucin is mucopolysaccharide hyaluronic acid, which is a long-chain polymer. The viscous properties of synovial fluid are attributed to hyaluronic acid. The most important property to be considered in this respect is the *thixotropic* or non-newtonian quality of synovial fluid; the viscosity decreases with increased shear rate (increased speed of joint movement).

Models of Joint Lubrication

An analogy cannot accurately be drawn between a machine model of lubrication and the lubrication of synovial joints. One of the major reasons for this is that the physical properties of articular cartilage differ considerably from the physical properties of most machine components. Articular cartilage is porous and relatively spongelike in that it has the capacity to absorb and bind synovial fluid. Articular cartilage is also viscoelastic; the deformation rate is high on initial application of the load and levels off with time. When the load is removed, the initial "reformation" rate is high and decreases over time (Fig. 3-14). Although macroscopically articular cartilage appears quite smooth and shiny, it is, in fact, relatively rough microscopically. Articular cartilage also has the tendency to adsorb large molecules, such as hyaluronic acid in synovial fluid, to its surface. The significance of this is discussed later in this section.

The early model of joint lubrication described a hydrodynamic, or fluid film, situation (Fig. 3-15).[27] In this case, synovial fluid fills in the wedges of space left by the joint surface incongruencies. On movement be-

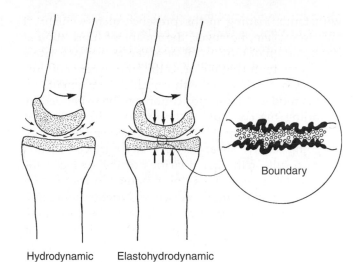

FIG. 3-15. Hydrodynamic, elastohydrodynamic, and boundary models of joint lubrication.

tween surfaces the synovial fluid is attracted to the area of contact between the surfaces. This occurs because of (1) the pressure gradient produced by the movement and (2) the fact that relative movement tends to pull the viscous fluid in the direction of the moving surface. The result of this is the maintenance of a layer of fluids between joint surfaces during movement. Any friction occurring as a result of movement occurs within the fluid rather than between joint surfaces. This meets the requirements of a good lubrication system because it allows free movement and prevents wear to the joint surfaces. This system works well during movement; however, it would tend to fail under very slow velocity or under heavy loading. It would also fail under reciprocal motion, since it would not adapt well to changes in direction of motion, at which time the velocity of movement is zero. Since human joints often move slowly, under heavy loads, and reciprocally, by itself it seems an unsatisfactory model for human joint lubrication.

The hydrodynamic model, however, cannot be completely repudiated because the previous description does not consider the viscoelasticity of joint surfaces. This model can be modified to an elastohydrodynamic system (see Fig. 3-15). Because of the nature of articular cartilage to deform, not all of the energy of heavy loading goes to decreasing the thickness of the layer of film between the surfaces, thus increasing friction between the surfaces. Instead, deformation of the joint surfaces occurs, increasing the effective contact area between surfaces and thus reducing the effective compression stress (force per unit area) to the lubrication fluid. This allows the protective layer of fluid to remain at about the same thickness. Thus, the elastohydrodynamic model describes a system that

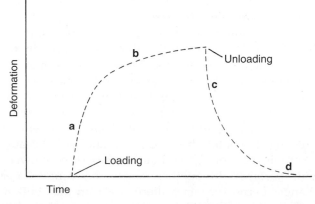

FIG. 3-14. Viscoelastic response of articular cartilage. Parts a and c of the curve are due to elastic properties, while parts b and d show viscous behavior.

withstands loading in the presence of movement. It fails to explain, however, the means of lubrication at the initiation of movement or at the period of relative zero velocity during reciprocating movements or during very heavy loading with very little movement.

This model of joint lubrication can be expanded by including the concepts of boundary lubrication and weeping lubrication.[37,48,56,61] With any materials undergoing relative shear between two surfaces, friction is the result of the irregularities of the surfaces; the greater the irregularities, the greater the friction. Effective lubrication must reduce this friction to a minimum, thus reducing wear of the surfaces to a minimum. In the case of boundary lubrication, the lubricant is adsorbed to the surface of the material, in effect, reducing the roughness of the surfaces by filling in the irregularities. Because articular cartilage is able to adsorb long-chain molecules of hyaluronic acid, these molecules are able to fill in the irregularities as well as to coat the surface. Any friction occurring as the result of shear movement occurs between molecules of the lubricant rather than between the joint surfaces themselves. This probably serves as an adjunct to the elastohydrodynamic system, especially in cases of extreme loading sufficient to decrease significantly the thickness of the layer of fluid maintained by the elastohydrodynamic model under lighter loads. It may also play a role at the initiation of movement or periods of zero velocity, since a layer of fluid would not be present because of its dependence on movement under an elastohydrodynamic system. The concept of weeping lubrication is actually an expansion of the elastohydrodynamic model. Because of the porosity and elastic qualities of articular cartilage, loading sufficient to cause a deformation of the articular surfaces also causes a "squeezing out" of the synovial fluid absorbed by the cartilage. The fluid that is squeezed out further serves to maintain a protective layer of lubricant between joint surfaces.

By the use of this "mixed lubrication" model, which combines elastohydrodynamic concepts with boundary lubrication concepts, the demands of human synovial joints are met.[11,47] The system allows movement, change in direction of movement, loading, and variations in congruencies of joint surfaces. It takes into consideration, at least in general terms, the properties of the lubricant (synovial fluid) and the surface materials. There is still considerable controversy over the relative importance of each of the lubrication models under various conditions, but most authors agree with the general concepts presented previously. Since it is still unknown how each model contributes to normal joint lubrication, very little investigation into the mutual effects of pathologic joint conditions and joint lubrication has taken place. A breakdown in some aspect of the lubrication system is likely to cause or add to the progression of joint disease, such as degenerative joint disease. On the other hand, certain joint diseases result in changes in structure and function of joint constituents. For instance, there is a loss of joint cartilage in degenerative joint disease and changes in synovial fluid viscosity in rheumatoid arthritis. It is probable that in such cases the disease will, in turn, alter the function of the lubrication system, thus contributing to a progressive degenerative cycle.

☐ Resolving Problems of Joint-Surface Wear

It has been emphasized that synovial joint surfaces are incongruent. Because of the incongruency that exists in most positions of movement, a relatively small contact area exists between joint surfaces. The wedges of space that surround this contact area are necessary in order for a hydrodynamic lubrication system to operate effectively; without these spaces the lubricant could not be drawn, or forced, between the contacting surfaces. One may wonder if such a small area of contact might increase the likelihood of wear between joint surfaces, since loading forces from weight-bearing and muscle contraction would be distributed over a small surface area, thus increasing the compressive stress to the joint. This would, in fact, be the case if the area of contact on one or both surfaces was consistently the same throughout habitual movements. In this respect the clinician might be concerned about joints that are relatively track-bound, such as the humeroulnar, patellofemoral, ankle mortise, and interphalangeal joints. In each of these joints movement tends to be restricted to one arc of movement that is determined almost entirely by the shapes of the joint surfaces. It would seem that during movement at these joints, the contacting area on one joint surface would consistently "follow a rut" on the opposing surface, increasing the likelihood of excessive wear in the rut or at the area of the surface contacting the rut. In these joints the problem of excessive wear is resolved in a number of ways. First, these joint surfaces are, relatively speaking, the most congruent in the body, so that forces are distributed over a somewhat larger area. Consider, for example, the close fit between the ulna and the trochlear surface of the humerus. Second, the contact area on each surface is constantly changing throughout an arc of movement. A change in contact areas occurs in one sense because a combination of roll and slide takes place between joint surfaces. In another sense, the contact area changes because contact alternates from the "bottom of the valley to the sides of the slopes" on one surface and correspondingly on the opposing surface. For instance, with the knee in full extension, the articular surface of the patella makes contact with the femur at a strip extending mediolaterally across the middle of the patellar surface. In flexion, however, only the medial and lateral margins of the patella make contact with the femoral condyles while the ridge in the middle of the patellar facets lies freely in the intercondylar notch.[21] A comparable situation occurs at the elbow, ankle, and finger joints throughout their respective movements. Note that at the ankle mortise, which undergoes intermittent heavy loading in habitual use, maximal loading (stance) takes place with the joint closer to its close-packed position, dorsiflexion. This is the position of maximal congruence and, therefore, the position in which the compressive force per unit area would tend to be smallest.

But at joints such as the knee, a more complex situation exists. The knee is markedly incongruent compared with the joints discussed previously; it must be in order to allow some degree of rotation to occur independently of flexion or extension or in conjunction with them. The knee must also withstand heavier loading from weight-bearing in a wide variety of positions. Thus, the knee is often required to undergo heavy loading in positions of flexion, in which the surfaces are very incongruent—a small area of contact withstands relatively large compressive forces. Thus, there might be concern that in a situation of heavy loading, relatively low velocity, and small contact area between surfaces, the lubrication system would not be sufficient to prevent excessive friction (shear) and wear between joint surfaces. This might very well be the case in a joint such as the knee that must undergo such conditions during normal daily activities, such as climbing stairs, squatting, and lifting. There might also be concern about the tendency for the femur to slip forward on the tibia under such conditions, again because of the incongruency of joint surfaces and the lack of intrinsic stability. Are the posterior cruciate, popliteus, and other intrinsic stabilizers sufficient to prevent this problem?

The knee, then, is a joint that must allow movement of spin between the tibia and the femur and swing between the tibia and femur because of the functional demands placed on it. In order for this to be possible, the joint surfaces must be sufficiently incongruent. But because of this incongruence and because of normal heavy loading in a variety of positions, the knee appears susceptible to excessive shear forces between contacting joint surfaces during movement, excessive compressive forces between contacting surfaces on static loading, and intrinsic instability when loaded in flexion. It is probable that the intra-articular menisci serve to compensate for what would otherwise be un-

satisfactory engineering at the knee joint—unsatisfactory in that the joint would not withstand the normal forces applied to it without giving way or undergoing premature wearing of joint surfaces.[29] Under heavy static loading, the menisci act to increase the effective load-bearing surface area at the joint, thus reducing the force per unit area. Being firmly attached to the joint capsule and tibia but mobile enough to conform to the shape of the articulating segments of the femoral condyles, they serve to increase the intrinsic stability of the joint by increasing the effective congruency between joint surfaces. During movement with heavy loading, they again act to increase the load-bearing surface area, but they also maintain a wedge-shaped interval surrounding the area of contact into which the lubricant fluid can be drawn.[29] Since the menisci are semicartilaginous, they can also absorb synovial fluid. With increased loading, fluid can be squeezed out from the menisci as well as the articular load-bearing surface, contributing to a weeping lubrication phenomenon. Also, as the menisci recede before the advancing condyles during movement, they can act to spread a layer of lubricant over the joint surfaces just prior to contact. This, incidentally, may also be a function of the rather large infrapatellar fat pad at the knee.[5] The menisci, because they are semimobile, allow the knee to act as though it were maximally congruent with respect to the requirements of lubrication and intrinsic stability, but to actually function as though it were very incongruent with respect to the types of movement that occur at the joint.

One should also take note of the considerable slide of the femoral condyles along the tibial surface during the complete range of flexion–extension. This feature also reduces the likelihood of excessive wear on the tibial surfaces by distributing the load-bearing surface over a larger area. The degree of slide could not occur normally without the extrinsic control provided by the cruciates, nor without the intrinsic stability provided by the menisci. This type of motion, in which the area of contact of a particular joint surface constantly changes with movement at the joint, is necessary to allow for the intermittent compression of articular cartilage essential to normal nutrition and lubrication. Loss of a constantly changing area of contact during use of a joint is likely to increase the probability of degeneration of articular cartilage by interfering with normal nutrition and normal lubrication, and by increasing the compressive forces over time per unit area per unit time. Unused areas of articular cartilage would not undergo necessary exchanges of nutrients; areas of cartilage in which loading occurs would eventually fail from fatigue (see section on arthrosis later in this chapter).

It is worth mentioning that fibrillation of articular

cartilage in normal hip and shoulder joints occurs first in non–weight-bearing surfaces.[39] Also, a marked acceleration of degenerative changes is shown to occur in weight-bearing animal joints in which a joint is immobilized but full use of the limb is allowed.[12] These are both examples of the effects on articular cartilage of the load-bearing contact area not being distributed over a large area of the opposing surfaces. This is perhaps a partial explanation for the frequency of degenerative arthritis occurring in human hip joints; a relatively small surface area is used for weight-bearing, while much of the articular cartilage receives little or no compression. As will be discussed later in the section on arthrosis, it also contributes to the explanation of how abnormal joint arthrokinematics may lead to joint pathology.

■ APPROACH TO MANAGEMENT OF JOINT DYSFUNCTION

The rationale for specific joint mobilization requires the restoration of normal joint play in order that full, pain-free motion may occur at the joint. The term *joint dysfunction* is used by Mennell to indicate loss of normal joint play.[41] There are many explanations for the causes of joint dysfunction, some of which are specific for certain joints and some of which may be applied to all joints. In the spine, entrapment of "meniscoid inclusions" is postulated by some as a cause of joint dysfunction. Frankel and co-workers have demonstrated through instant center analysis the presence of joint dysfunction at the knee from meniscus tears (confirmed later by surgery) and dysfunction in ankle joints that had been classified as unstable, post-fracture, or having degenerative disease.[15,51] It has also been shown that joint dysfunction in "frozen shoulders" is often caused by adherence of the anteroinferior aspect of the joint capsule to the humeral head.[42] A loose body in a joint may be a cause of dysfunction, as may joint effusion causing some distention of the capsule. The list goes on, the point being that *there is no single cause of joint dysfunction.*

The use of specific mobilization is not indicated in all cases of dysfunction. For this reason, a thorough evaluation performed in an attempt to clarify the nature and extent of the lesion is a necessary step in the management of joint problems. Those cases in which a physical therapist must play a major role in treatment of joint dysfunction are those dysfunctions occurring as a result of isolated or generalized capsular tightness or adhesion. These typically follow traumatic sprains to the capsule or immobilization. In some cases, they occur for no *apparent* reason, for example, "adhesive capsulitis" at the shoulder.

The traditional approach to management of patients presenting with loss of pain-free movement at a joint usually involves various modes of pain relief, active and passive measures to improve osteokinematic movement, and encouragement of normal use of the part. It should be clear that this approach is inadequate and perhaps dangerous. First, it ignores the basic problem, which is often loss of normal arthrokinematics. Second, it involves considerable forcing of osteokinematic movements in the absence of normal arthrokinematic movement, which may only occur at the expense of the articular cartilage. This is to say, the resiliency of the cartilage may allow a certain amount of osteokinematic movement to occur without the normal accompanying arthrokinematic movements. Frankel and co-workers describe the case of a boy who continued to use his knee in the absence of normal external rotation of the tibia on the femur during knee extension.[14] One and a half years later, at surgery, dimpling of the articular cartilage of the medial femoral condyle was observable with the naked eye, presumably due to continued abnormal compression of this portion of the articular surface from loss of normal arthrokinematic movement.

A more logical approach to the management of these patients emphasizes the restoration of joint play to allow free movement between bones. This can be achieved only by (1) evaluating to determine the nature and extent of the lesion, (2) deciding if joint mobilization is indicated based on the evaluation, (3) choosing the appropriate techniques based on the direction and extent of restrictions, and (4) skillfully applying techniques of specific mobilization. Efforts to relieve pain and reduce muscle guarding are, of course, important adjuncts to treatment but do not in themselves constitute a treatment program. Also, some movement should be encouraged in the cardinal planes, but only as normal kinematics are restored. To a certain extent, functional use of the part should be restricted through careful instructions to the patient until normal joint mechanics are restored. This approach minimizes the possible danger of undue stresses to the articular cartilage during attempts to restore movement. It also minimizes the possibility of discharging a patient who has relatively pain-free functional use of the joint, but who may have some residual kinematic disturbance sufficient to cause cartilage fatigue over time and perhaps osteoarthrosis in later years.

□ *Pathologic Considerations*

A high percentage of the chronic musculoskeletal problems seen clinically are fatigue disorders. These are disorders in which abnormal stresses imposed on a structure over a prolonged period result in a tendency toward an increased rate of tissue breakdown. All tissues, including those with low metabolic activity such as articular cartilage, undergo a necessary process of repair to continuously replace the microdamage resulting from normal use. In bone, such microdamage would involve fracturing of bony trabeculae, whereas in other connective tissues there is disruption of individual collagen fibers. As long as the rate of microtrauma does not exceed normal limits, and the rate at which the tissue is able to repair itself is not compromised, the tissue remains "normal." The tendency to maintain an equilibrium against opposing, unbalancing factors is a homeostatic mechanism; a shift in the nature of one factor will cause a compensatory reaction by the body to correspondingly alter the other factor in order to maintain balance.

In general, the nature of the various pathologies affecting the musculoskeletal tissues can be considered according to this homeostatic model. The two factors that the body is attempting to balance are (1) the process of tissue breakdown and (2) the process of tissue production or repair. Thus, in discussing abnormal or pathologic situations, attention must be paid to the causes of and homeostatic responses to a tendency toward increased tissue breakdown and a decreased rate of breakdown. Factors that might disturb the body's ability to maintain an appropriate balance, such as those that might cause an abnormal degree of tissue production and those that might compromise the body's ability to produce enough tissue, must also be considered.

INCREASED RATE OF TISSUE BREAKDOWN

Increased tissue breakdown results when the frequency or magnitude of stresses to the part increases, when the capacity of the tissue to repair itself is reduced, or both. Under conditions of significantly increased stress over time, the body attempts to compensate by laying down more tissue in order to increase the capacity of the tissue to withstand the higher stress levels. The result is tissue hypertrophy. In well-vascularized tissues, this occurs in conjunction with a low-grade inflammatory process incited by the increased rate of tissue damage. A new equilibrium is reached in favor of a more massive structure, better able to withstand higher stress levels without failing. Typical examples include muscle hypertrophy in response to increased loading of a muscle over time; subchondral bony sclerosis in response to increased compressive forces over a joint; and fibrosis of a joint capsule receiving increased stresses from faulty joint movement over a prolonged period of time.

Such tissue hypertrophy, especially when affecting bone and capsuloligamentous structures, causes tissue to gain in strength at the expense of extensibility; the tissue becomes better able to withstand loads without undergoing gross failure but does not deform as readily when loaded. An increase in the ratio of collagen (mineralized collagen in the case of bone) to the remaining extracellular ground substance (mucopolysaccharide) reduces extensibility. This is believed to allow increased interfiber bond formation, with a subsequent reduced mobility, or gliding capacity, of individual elements. The added stiffness reduces the energy-attenuating capacity of the structure. Less of the energy of loading is attenuated as work, and more of the energy must be absorbed internally by the structure or attenuated by increased deformation of other structures that are in series with the hypertrophic tissues. Thus, with sclerosis of subchondral bone, the overlying articular cartilage is made to undergo greater strain per unit of load because of the reduced deformability of the subjacent bone. This is believed to be an important factor in the progressive degeneration of cartilage occurring with degenerative joint disease.[47] With fibrosis of tendon tissue, such as the extensor carpi radialis brevis origin at the elbow, the reduced extensibility of the tendon fibers results in greater strain to the tenoperiosteal junction of the tendon at the lateral humeral epicondyle. The ensuing inflammatory process is responsible for the symptoms and signs of the "tennis elbow" syndrome.

Although in such situations the hypertrophic structure is more massive and less likely to fail when loaded, the rate of microdamage may remain elevated. Although the stress to the structure tends to be reduced because of the increased cross-sectional area resulting from the hypertrophy, the internal energy within the structure may be increased because of the reduced extensibility. An increase in internal energy must be dissipated as heat or microfracturing of individual structural components. Clinically, a painful, low-grade inflammatory reaction may result from the added mechanical and thermal stimulation.

Thus, when a tissue hypertrophies in response to increased stress levels, the rate of microdamage tends to remain elevated—there is simply more tissue present to ensure that the structure, as a whole, does not fail. Pain may arise from the increased internal stresses on the involved tissue or from increased strain on connected tissues.

For any tissue there is a critical point past which the rate of breakdown may exceed the rate at which the tissue is able to repair or strengthen itself. Under normal metabolic conditions, this critical point is reached soonest in tissues with limited capacity for regeneration and repair. These are tissues that are poorly vascularized and have a low metabolic turnover. The typical example of such a tissue is articular cartilage. With increased compressive stress levels to a joint, the well-vascularized bone will tend to hypertrophy, while the cartilage degenerates. Even bone, however, can be stressed at a frequency or magnitude at which it can no longer repair itself fast enough to prevent progressive breakdown. A common clinical disorder in which this occurs is the stress fracture affecting athletes or other persons who habitually engage in high stress–level activities.

REDUCED RATE OF TISSUE BREAKDOWN

Decreased stress levels on tissue over time will reduce the rate of breakdown. Thus, with relative inactivity the rate of microdamage is less and the body takes the opportunity to economize by reducing the rate of tissue production. The tissue no longer needs to be as strong because of the reduction in the everyday stresses it must withstand. The typical condition in which this occurs is disuse atrophy. When a part is immobilized, the bone becomes less dense, and capsules, ligaments, and muscles atrophy. The important clinical consideration in such situations is to gradually increase the stress levels on the tissue in order to promote strengthening of the structure by stimulating increased tissue production, but without causing the weakened structures to fail. This is especially true after healing of a structure such as bone or ligament; not only must new tissue be produced, but it must also mature. Maturation involves reorientation of major structural elements along the lines of stress that the structure will normally undergo. The process of maturation takes time, and the necessary stimulus is the judiciously applied loading of the part in ways that simulate the loads the part will need to withstand with normal use.

INCREASED RATE OF TISSUE PRODUCTION

The rate of tissue production increases in conjunction with any inflammatory process. The reparative phase that follows acute inflammation usually involves a proliferation of collagen tissue. This is especially true in certain virulent inflammatory processes associated with bacterial infections. Chronic, low-grade inflammation, such as that mentioned previously in conjunction with increased stress levels, is also accompanied by increased collagen production. Regardless of the cause, the result is a relatively fibrosed, less extensible structure. Loss of extensibility will be especially marked if the part is immobilized during the period of increased collagen production. The new collagen will not be laid down along the appropriate lines of stress, and abnormal interfiber cross-links develop that do not accommodate normal deformation. If, on the other hand, some movement of the part occurs during the period of increased collagen production, the loss of extensibility will not be so great. Appropriate orienta-

tion of the newly laid fibers is stimulated by the stresses imposed on the tissue by movement. Loss of extensibility in the immobilized part is due to the increased density of the structure, as well as abnormal orientation of the structured elements; whereas in the part in which some movement occurs, reduced extensibility is primarily a result of the change in density.

Clinically, a part that is strictly immobilized during an acute inflammatory process, such as that induced by surgery, trauma, infection, or rheumatoid arthritis, is likely to lose more movement. Further, this loss of movement is likely to be more persistent than in the case of a part in which some movement continues in the presence of a chronic, low-grade inflammation, such as degenerative joint disease.

Restoration of normal extensibility of the tissue requires (1) removing the stimulus of increased tissue production (*e.g.*, stress, infection, trauma); (2) gradually stretching the structure to break down abnormal interfiber cross-links; and (3) restoring normal use of the part to induce normal orientation of structural elements.

REDUCED RATE OF TISSUE PRODUCTION AND REPAIR

Reduced rate of tissue production and repair occurs with reduced stress levels to the tissue, but it may also occur with some change in the metabolic status of the tissue. Examples of the latter include nutritional deficiencies, reduced vascularity, and abnormal hormone levels. When the cause is related to reduced stress levels, amelioration simply involves a gradual return to normal stress conditions. However, when the cause is metabolic, treatment is more complex and will vary with the type of disturbance. In these cases, stress levels must be reduced, since the body is unable to keep up with the normal rate of tissue breakdown. Continued use of the part will result in fatigue failure of the involved tissues.

Typical examples of common musculoskeletal disorders that are related to such an alteration in the metabolic status of the involved tissues include the following:

Supraspinatus tendinitis at the shoulder—The tendon begins to fatigue from reduced vascularity in an area of the tendon close to its insertion. Occasionally the body attempts to compensate for its inability to produce new tendon tissue by laying down calculous deposits. These lesions often progress to complete tendon ruptures because the rate of breakdown continues to exceed the capacity of the tissue to repair itself.

Reflex sympathetic dystrophy—Generalized hypovascularity to a part, caused by increased sympathetic activity, results in atrophy of bone, nails, muscle, and skin—in short, all musculoskeletal components.

Senile and postmenopausal osteoporosis—Bone metabolism is compromised as a result of alteration in hormone levels and other age-related influences. The bone atrophy is most marked in cancellous bone, such as that of the vertebral bodies. Roentgenograms often show collapsed vertebrae, resulting from progressive trabecular buckling.

Age-related tissue changes—Aging, in itself, does not seem to result in changes in the collagen content of musculoskeletal tissues. However, with advancing age, the protein-polysaccharide (glycosaminoglycan) content of most somatic tissues is reduced. There is also an associated reduction in water content, since the protein-polysaccharide component of the tissue matrices is responsible for the fluid-binding capacity of the tissues. The result is a relative fibrosis of the involved tissues, since the ratio of collagen to ground substance is increased. It is postulated that the protein–polysaccharide ground substance normally acts as a lubricating spacer between collagen fibers. As its content is reduced, the collagen fibers approximate one another and form increased numbers of interfiber cross-links (intermolecular bonds), and the fibers no longer glide easily with respect to each other. Thus, the stiffness of the structure increases. Because of the increased stiffness, the tissue as a whole loses its deformability and therefore loses its ability to attenuate the energy of loading. With loading, more stress is imposed on individual structural elements and the rate of tissue breakdown subsequently increases. For many elderly persons this does not pose a problem, since activity levels—and therefore stress levels—decrease with advancing age.

The reduced fluid-binding capacity of the tissue, associated with protein–polysaccharide depletion, may alter the nutritional status of the tissue. This is especially important in structures such as articular cartilage and intervertebral disks that depend on fluid inhibition for normal exchange of nutrients. Thus, the capacity of the tissue to repair itself will also be reduced. This is a likely explanation for the degeneration of intervertebral disks and articular cartilage that occurs with advancing age.

☐ Intervention and Communication

From a clinical standpoint, the clinician should be prepared to estimate the nature of a pathologic process according to this scheme. This is necessary in order to plan a treatment program specific for the type of pathologic process present. Awareness of the various ways the clinician can effectively intervene so as to appropriately alter the pathologic state is also important.

The terms used to refer to common musculoskeletal pathologies usually provide little information relating to the nature of the disorder. The same term may be applied to different conditions in which the cause and nature of the pathologic process are quite distinct. *Tendinitis at the shoulder* is an atrophic, degenerative condition resulting from reduced vascularity to an area of the rotator cuff tendons; *tendinitis at the elbow* is a hypertrophic, fibrotic condition often related to increased stress levels. Also, many terms, such as degenerative joint disease, refer to situations in which a number of tissues may be involved, and the nature of the changes affecting the involved tissues may differ. In the case of degenerative joint disease, for example, the subchondral bone and the joint capsule tend to hypertrophy while the articular cartilage atrophies and degenerates.

Therapeutically, there are many physical agents and procedures that may be used in order to influence various types of pathologic processes. Perhaps the most important form of intervention is well-planned instructions to the patient regarding the performance of specific activities. In order to give appropriate instructions the clinician must gear the patient's activity level to the nature of the disorder. This requires a knowledge of the response of tissues to various loading conditions under normal and abnormal circumstances. A careful examination must be carried out, including a biomechanical assessment. It also requires that the clinician be aware of the types of stresses imposed on a part by various activities. The patient must understand the instructions and be able and willing to carry them out.

☐ Arthrosis

When considering a diseased joint one usually thinks in terms of the physiologic changes that have occurred at the joint. There is much information concerning the histologic and biochemical changes in periarticular tissues, changes in hemodynamics, and synovial fluid changes that accompany some of the more common joint diseases.[3,7,31–34,38] Although mechanical changes also occur, these are usually not dealt with until advanced structural changes have resulted. The treatment then is usually surgical. The earlier, conservative treatment in joint disease typically involves measures to counter the physiologic changes taking place. This seems the logical approach in arthropathies in which the etiology is apparently some physiologic change and in which the primary joint changes are physiologic. Thus, in rheumatoid arthritis, gout, and spondylitis, the primary treatments are those aimed at control of inflammation and metabolic disturbances. The mechanical changes in joint function are generally agreed to be secondary and often left to improve (or degenerate) along with the primary physiologic changes.

Although our knowledge of normal joint mechanics is becoming more sophisticated, little has been written concerning the mechanical changes that occur with, or possibly lead to, joint disease. It is well accepted, however, that joint disease may result from some mechanical disturbance. These cases are usually referred to as *secondary osteoarthritis,* in which some past joint trauma can be cited as a precipitating factor. This is distinguished by many researchers from *primary osteoarthritis,* in which several joints may be involved with no known causative factor. However, the pathologies of primary and secondary osteoarthritis are essentially identical, and since these disorders are for the most part noninflammatory, they are best referred to as *osteoarthroses.* As the probable etiologies of osteoarthroses are investigated, the more it appears that the classifications of primary and secondary are often arbitrary. Although it has been postulated by some that primary osteoarthrosis has a physiologic or metabolic etiology, it appears that in many cases it is due to mechanical changes, of much subtler onset than those causing secondary osteoarthrosis.[17,19,52]

It is generally agreed that changes in the articular cartilage trigger a cycle leading to the progression of degenerative joint disease. Cartilage damage may occur after a single traumatic incident, causing a tension or compression strain sufficient to interfere with the structural integrity of the cartilage. This is relatively rare and usually accompanies a fracture of the adjacent bone. More common is cartilage wearing from fatigue, or the cumulative effects of abnormal stresses, neither of which is sufficient in itself to cause structural damage.[59] Cartilage may be susceptible to fatigue in part because it is aneural; any other musculoskeletal tissue is relatively immune to fatigue because protective reflex inhibition occurs with abnormal stress. This inhibitory response requires, of course, intact innervation. Cartilage is also susceptible to damage because it is avascular. It lacks the normal inflammation and repair response that would replace damaged parts of the tissue. In fact, when cartilage is lacerated without involvement of the vascularized subchondral bone, a brief proliferation of chondrocytes ensues but with no repair of the defect. If the lesion is sufficient to penetrate the subchondral bone, it immediately fills with blood and a clot is formed. This clot is invaded with new blood vessels that apparently bring in undifferentiated mesenchymal cells. These cells proceed to fill the defect with fibrocartilage (not hyaline cartilage).[10,24]

Hyaline cartilage partly makes up for the fact that it is aneural and avascular by its considerable ability to deform when loaded in compression. Much of the substance of articular cartilage is a mucopolysaccharide ground substance, whose chief component is chondroitin sulfate. Chondroitin sulfate is highly hydrophilic with the ability to bind large quantities of water. Cartilage is 70% to 80% water and depends on this water content for its resiliency—its ability to withstand compression stresses without structural damage. The energy of compressive loading is dissipated as cartilage undergoes strain, or deformation. This strain results in tension stresses that are absorbed by the collagen fibers embedded within the ground substance (Fig. 3-16). Thus, the extracellular cartilage matrix normally withstands compression stresses through the mucopolysaccharide gel, and tension stresses through the collagen fibers. Interspersed throughout this matrix are the chondrocytes, or cartilage cells, that are responsible for production of the matrix components. Moreover, a considerable proportion of compressive forces is attenuated by the cancellous subchondral bone that, although stiffer than the articular cartilage, is thicker and has more volume for energy attenuation.[47]

Although cartilage was once believed to be inert metabolically, studies now indicate that turnover of cartilage does occur.[33] Chondrocytes apparently secrete some matrix material continuously to replace that lost by normal attrition. It has also been shown that in response to mild or moderate osteoarthrosis in which cartilage degradation has increased, proliferation and metabolic activity of chondrocytes also increase. At least for a while the chondrocytes are able to keep pace with the disease. For some reason as yet unknown, this process shuts down in later stages of the disease. It is also poorly understood why lacerations of cartilage do not undergo repair, whereas some repair does take place in the earlier stages of osteoarthrosis.

☐ The Degenerative Cycle

The initial changes that occur in the cartilage when abnormal stresses leading to acute damage or chronic fatigue are applied are (1) fibrillation, or fracturing of collagen fibers, and (2) depletion of ground substance, primarily a loss of chondroitin sulfate.[7,31,34,38–40,59] There remains some dispute over which change takes place first; however, it seems to be agreed that once initiated, a cycle of degeneration will follow. This cycle is countered up to a point by the proliferation of chondrocytes and the increased secretion of cartilage

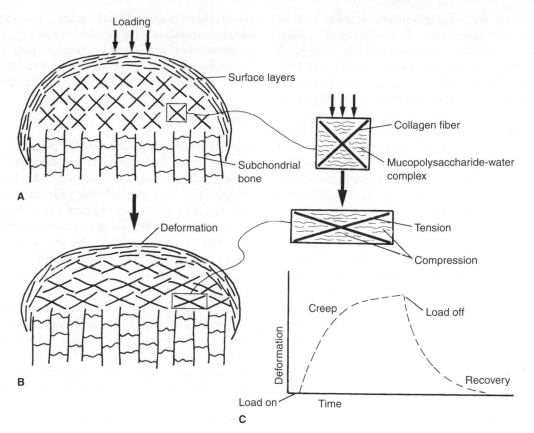

FIG. 3-16. (**A**) Compressive loading of articular cartilage results in (**B**) tension stresses to the collagenous elements and compression stresses to the mucopolysaccharide-water complex. (**C**) The total response is viscoelastic. The viscous creep with sustained loading is largely the result of a time-dependent squeezing out of fluid.

matrix by the chondrocytes. A cycle as shown in Figure 3-17 is likely to develop. Loss of chondroitin sulfate leaves the collagen fibers more susceptible to fracture; fracturing of these fibers causes a "softening" of the surface layers of the cartilage; the cartilage becomes less able to withstand stresses in this region, with the resultant death of local chondrocytes; and the death of chondrocytes is believed to allow the release of proteolytic enzymes that have a further degrada-

tive effect on chondroitin sulfate. The adjacent areas of cartilage, peripheral and deep to this damaged area, must now absorb increased stresses, so the process tends to spread. Added to this mechanical factor in spreading is the chemical factor due to destructive enzyme release.[49]

Because of the absence of pain receptors in articular cartilage, considerable degeneration may take place before symptoms bring the problem to the attention of the patient. Pain or stiffness may not occur until synovial effusion causes sufficient pressure to the joint capsule to fire pain- or pressure-sensitive receptors. The effusion is a result of synovial irritation caused by the release of proteolytic enzymes and other cartilaginous debris. Further irritation may result from abnormal stresses to the joint capsule from altered joint mechanics. In the case of low-grade, chronic inflammation of the synovial lining, the patient may be aware of only transient symptoms. Such a low-grade inflammation, if chronic, will result in capsular fibrosis, or thickening, which will further alter joint mechanics. Fibrosis of the joint capsule may be thought of as a relative increase in the collagen–mucopolysaccharide ratio. The result is that which occurs with any

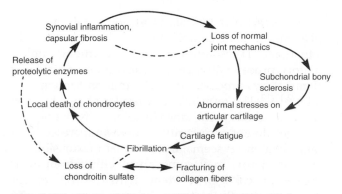

FIG. 3-17. Cycle of degenerative changes in a joint.

scarring process: reduced extensibility from loss of elasticity, gradual contracture, and adherence to adjacent tissues. The loss of capsular mobility often goes unnoticed by the patient until it causes sufficient limitation of motion to interfere with daily activities. In joints such as the shoulder, which in the inactive person may be used only through a small range of motion to perform daily activities, a rather marked limitation of movement may occur before the patient realizes that a problem exists. Such a lack of mobility of the joint capsule will, of course, contribute significantly to the cycle of degeneration shown in Figure 3-17 because of the resultant alteration of normal joint mechanics.

Other reactive joint tissue changes will also occur if the process is allowed to continue, including osteophyte formation, subchondral sclerosis, subchondral sclerosis, subchondral cyst formation, and eburnation of exposed bone. It should be realized that subchondral bone changes are likely to lead to an alteration in the forces that must be absorbed by the articular cartilage, since normally subchondral bone takes up much of the force of compressive loading.[61] In fact, some researchers believe that subchondral bone changes, such as sclerotic changes due to altered blood flow, are often the first changes to take place in the degenerative cycle.[7]

Changes in composition and structure of the articular surface, caused by fibrillation and chondroitin sulfate depletion, are also likely to compromise the lubrication system of the joint. Large irregularities would gradually make boundary lubrication less effective; loss of cartilage resiliency from chondroitin sulfate loss would interfere with weeping lubrication. These potential changes in lubrication efficiency would also seem to contribute further to the progression of degeneration.

☐ **Capsular Tightness**

As indicated in the section on clinical application, specific joint mobilization techniques are primarily used in cases of capsuloligamentous tightness or adherence. There are, of course, cases in which an isolated portion of a joint capsule or supporting ligament is injured and heals in a state of relative shortening or becomes adhered to adjacent tissues during the healing process. Such pathologies are usually of traumatic origin, with a well-defined mechanism of injury and subsequent course. More often, however, the therapist is confronted with cases in which the entire joint capsule is "tight," as suggested by the presence of a capsular pattern of restriction at the joint. Conditions that cause a capsular pattern of restriction at a joint can be classified into two general categories: (1) conditions in which there is considerable joint effusion or synovial inflammation, and (2) conditions in which there is a relative capsular fibrosis. It is important to make this distinction since the implications for management will vary according to the cause of the restriction.

JOINT EFFUSION

Joint effusion causes a capsular pattern of restriction because of the distention of the joint capsule by the excessive intra-articular synovial fluid. Portions of the capsule that are normally lax in order to allow a certain range of movement become taut because of capsular distention. The joint tends to assume a position in which the joint cavity—the space enclosed by the joint capsule—is of maximum volume. The continuous pressure applied to the capsule by the joint fluid may effect abnormal firing of joint receptors, which results in an alteration in function of the muscles controlling the joint.[61] The rapid wasting of the quadriceps in the presence of knee joint effusion is believed to be a result of reflex muscle inhibition from abnormal receptor firing.[9] There may also be reflex facilitation of muscle activity, observed as muscle spasm or guarding, when the joint is moved. Those conditions that cause limited movement because of articular effusion may be broadly classified as inflammatory arthritis. These may, of course, include traumatic arthritis, in which some portion of the joint capsule is torn or stretched, rheumatoid arthritis, in which the synovial layer of the capsule is inflamed, infectious arthritis, gout, and others. In the acute stage of each of these conditions, the capsular restriction is primarily a result of the increased secretion of synovial fluid accompanying the acute stage of the inflammatory process, or it may result from reflex muscle guarding from abnormal firing of joint receptors. The cause of the restriction must be appreciated since, in such cases, clinicians do not wish to stretch the joint capsule to restore movement but rather to assist in the resolution of the acute inflammatory process.

RELATIVE CAPSULAR FIBROSIS

Relative capsular fibrosis most commonly accompanies one, or some combination, of the three following situations: (1) resolution of an acute articular inflammatory process; (2) a chronic, low-grade articular inflammatory process; and (3) immobilization of a joint.[2,12,13] The term *relative capsular fibrosis* has been used, up to this point, since histologically the capsular changes do not necessarily involve an increase in collagen content. It seems, instead, that inextensibility of capsular tissue may come about either from an increase in collagen content with respect to mucopolysaccharide content or from internal changes in the nature of the collagen tissue, such as changes in intermolecular cross-linking. The former might arise from an increased laying down of collagen, such as takes place during the repair phase of any inflammatory process.[1,8] It might also occur from a net loss of mucopolysaccharide content, with the total collagen content remaining constant. This typically occurs with prolonged immobilization of a joint.[12,45,60] One might consider the mucopolysaccharide content of connective tissue as serving as a lubricant for the collagen fibers; loss of the lubricant permits collagen fibers to approximate each other and to form abnormal interfiber cross-links. This inhibits their ability to glide against each other and thus reduces extensibility of the tissue.[1]

Clinically, it seems that conditions in which there is an actual increase in collagen content are more resistant to efforts to restore motion than are those cases of capsular restriction in which there is a net loss of mucopolysaccharide caused simply by immobilization. Also, inflammatory arthritis from infection resolves with a much greater degree of fibrosis (increase in collagen) than the capsular fibrosis that accompanies low-grade, noninfectious joint inflammation such as degenerative joint disease. Thus, the rate of improvement in range of motion might be expected to be more rapid in conditions at the top of the following list and slower when dealing with the capsular fibrosis that follows conditions near the bottom of this list:

Simple immobilization   *improve faster*
Traumatic arthritis
Degenerative arthrosis
Rheumatoid arthritis
Infectious arthritis   ↓ *slower*

Several explanations might be offered to account for the differences in rates of improvement noted above. First, relatively destructive processes, such as infectious arthritis or rheumatoid arthritis, might be met with a more vigorous repair response and, therefore, more collagen production during the resolution of the acute inflammatory process. Second, the period of immobilization, either prescribed or due to pain, is usually greater in acute inflammatory conditions, such as infectious or rheumatoid arthritis, than in relatively chronic conditions such as degenerative joint disease. The tendency, then, is for them to heal with less mobility. Third, during the mobilization period, the tissues may adapt more readily to increased mobility by laying down more mucopolysaccharide ground substance than they could by remodeling collagen. The maturation of the highly collagenous "scar tissue" is a longer, more involved process, involving reabsorption of excess collagen, realignment of collagen fiber orientation, and changes in the intermolecular cross-links within the collagen tissue.[1] In this way, capsular restriction from immobilization only, in which there is no increase in collagen content, is more easily resolved than conditions that lead to an actual increase in the collagen content of the joint capsules. It should be clear from this discussion that in order to accurately set treatment goals, the therapist should understand the nature of the pathologic process and its implications.

☐ Clinical Considerations

Considering what is now known of the pathogenesis of osteoarthrosis, the accompanying biochemical responses, the pathologic tissue changes, and the clinical manifestations, some important conclusions and correlations are worth considering in the management of patients with arthrosis.

Subtle changes in joint kinematics, persisting over a period of time, may cause abnormal stresses sufficient to result in gradual cartilage fatigue, which may, in turn, trigger a progression of changes leading to osteoarthrosis. Perhaps the most convincing evidence of this process is found in studies by Frankel and coworkers that show changes in the normal instant centers of motion in knee joints with minimal clinical signs or symptoms.[14,15] These changes suggested premature compression of joint surfaces accompanying knee extension. On careful clinical testing, loss of longitudinal external rotation of the tibia, with respect to the normal side, was found during extension on the involved side. Subsequent surgery revealed obvious "dimpling" of the cartilaginous joint surface, in the area of the cartilage compressed at full knee extension. In these cases internal derangement of the knee, while not sufficient to cause significant symptoms or signs, was responsible for altering normal knee mechanics enough to cause early cartilaginous changes, observable with the naked eye.

Up to a point in the progression of the disease, the cartilaginous destruction is repaired by increased proliferation and metabolic activity of chondrocytes, with laying down of new cartilage. The suggestion here is that osteoarthrosis is indeed somewhat reversible if managed correctly before severe progression has taken place. It is well known that osteotomy in the case of hip osteoarthrosis will cause the femoral head to become covered with fibrocartilage, with resultant restoration of the joint space on roentgenography. Studies suggest that it is partly a biological phenomenon, perhaps from the hyperemia induced by the surgical procedure, as well as a mechanical phenomenon from the redistribution of stresses over the joint.[6]

If it is accepted that subtle changes in joint kinematics can lead to osteoarthrosis or, taken one step further, if this is the etiology in many of the cases that are considered primary or secondary osteoarthrosis, then evaluation techniques that can detect these changes are valuable. Instant center analysis is probably the best technique for detection of altered joint kinematics. However, because of the extra number of roentgenograms necessary, this technique is not practical for routine evaluation. In view of this, it seems that testing of joint-play movements is the most valuable technique clinically for detecting subtle joint changes that may be causing only minor signs or symptoms but may eventually lead to more serious joint changes in the form of osteoarthrosis. Joint-play techniques are important not only in evaluation of the patient presenting with obscure musculoskeletal complaints but also in evaluating the patient recovering from more serious trauma. Simply because a patient has regained full range of motion and strength does not guarantee that normal joint kinematics have been restored.

If osteoarthrosis may be caused by loss of normal joint mechanics, then primary treatments should be aimed at restoration of normal mechanics. This may entail surgery in cases such as meniscal tears and malalignment of bony structures. In cases of capsular tightness or capsular adhesion, treatment must consist of specific mobilization aimed at restoration of normal accessory movements at the joint. The approach to treatment of joint problems that appear to be mechanical should have a biomechanical basis. At the present time, treatment is too often "supportive" until obvious physiologic changes occur. Currently, treatment tends to be directed at those physiologic changes, including various modalities for pain relief and pharmaceutical agents for controlling inflammation. Efforts to restore joint mechanics too often consist only of range-of-motion exercises and muscle strengthening, carried out without regard for the possible deleterious effects to the joint and without regard for abnormal reflex activity accompanying joint movement in the absence of normal arthrokinematics.

I believe that we, as clinicians, have yet to realize our full potential in the management of patients with mechanical joint disturbances. Knowledge of normal kinematics, ability to detect changes in joint mechanics through joint-play movements, and ability to restore normal component movements to a joint are necessary in successful management of patients with joint problems that are of a mechanical etiology or in which mechanical dysfunction is a prime factor.

REFERENCES

1. Akeson WH: An experimental study of joint stiffness. J Bone Joint Surg 43(A):1022–1034, 1961
2. Akeson WH, Amiel D, LaViolette D: The connective tissue response to immobility. Clin Orthop 51:183–197, 1967
3. Akeson WH, Woo SL, Amiel D: Biomechanical changes in periarticular connective tissues during contracture development in the immobilized rabbit knee. Connect Tissue Res 2:315–323, 1974
4. Barnett CH, Cochrane W, Palfray AJ: Age changes in articular cartilage of rabbits. Ann Rheum Dis 22:389–400, 1963
5. Barnett CH, Davies DV, MacConnaill MA: Synovial Joints: Their Structure and Function. Springfield, IL, Charles C Thomas, 1961
6. Bentley G: Articular cartilage studies and osteoarthrosis. Ann R Coll Surg Engl 57:86–100, 1975
7. Bollett AJ: Connective tissue polysaccharide metabolism and the pathogenesis of osteoarthritis. Adv Intern Med 13:33–60, 1967
8. Clayton ML, James SM, Abdulla M: Experimental investigations of ligamentous healing. Clin Orthop 61:146, 1968
9. de Andrade JR, Grant C, Dixon A: Joint distention and reflex muscle inhibition in the knee. J Bone Joint Surg 47(A):313–322, 1965
10. de Palma A, McKeever LD, Subin DK: Process of repair of articular cartilage demonstrated by histology and autoradiography with tritiated thymidine. Clin Orthop 48:229–242, 1966
11. Dowson D: Modes of lubrication in human joints. In: Lubrication and Wear in Living and Artificial Joints, vol 181. London, Institute of Mechanical Engineers, 1967
12. Ely LW, Mensor MC: Studies on the immobilization of the normal joints. Surg Gynecol Obstet 57:212–215, 1963
13. Evans EB, Eggers GW, Butler JK, Blumel J: Experimental immobilization and remobilization of rat knee joints. J Bone Joint Surg [Am] 42:737–758, 1960
14. Frankel VH: Biomechanics of the knee. In Ingwersen O (ed): The Knee Joint. New York, Elsevier-Dutton, 1973
15. Frankel VH, Burstein AH, Brooks DB: Biomechanics of internal derangement of the knee: Pathomechanics as determined by analysis of the instant centers of motion. J Bone Joint Surg [Am] 53:945–962, 1971
16. Freeman MAR: Treatment of ruptures of the lateral ligament of the ankle. J Bone Joint Surg 47(B):661–668, 1965
17. Freeman MAR: The pathogenesis of primary osteoarthrosis. Mod Trends Orthop 6:40–90, 1972
18. Freeman MAR: Adult Articular Cartilage. London, Pitman & Sons, 1973
19. Freeman MAR: The fatigue of cartilage in the pathogenesis of osteoarthrosis. Acta Orthop Scand 46:323, 1975
20. Frymann VM: A study of the rhythmic motions of the living cranium. J Am Osteopath Assoc 70:928–945, 1971
21. Goodfellow J, Hungerford DS, Woods C: Patellofemoral joint mechanics and pathology: I and II. J Bone Joint Surg 58B:287, 1976
22. Harryman DT, Sides JA, Clark JM, et al: Translation of the humeral head on the glenoid joint with passive glenohumeral motion. J Bone Joint Surg 72A:1334–1343, 1990
23. Howell SM, Galinat BJ, Renzi AJ, et al: Normal and abnormal mechanics of the glenohumeral joint in the horizontal plane. J Bone Joint Surg 70A:227–232, 1988
24. Johnell O, Telhag H: The effect of osteotomy and cartilage damage and mitotic activity: An experimental study in rabbits. Acta Orthop Scand 48:263–265, 1977
25. Kellgren JH: On the distribution of pain arising from deep somatic structures, with charts of segmental pain areas. Clin Sci 4:35, 1939
26. Klineberg IJ, Greenfield BE, Wyke B: Contribution to the reflex control of mastication from mechanoreceptors in the temporomandibular joint capsule. Dent Pract 21:73, 1970
27. Knott M, Voss D: Proprioceptive Neuromuscular Facilitation: Patterns and Techniques. New York, Harper & Row, 1968
28. Loubert PV: A qualitative biomechanical analysis of the concave-convex rule. In Proceedings, 5th International Conference of the International Federation of Orthopaedic Manipulative Therapists, Vail, Colorado, 1992, pp 255–256
29. MacConnaill MA: The function of intra-articular fibrocartilage with special references to the knee and inferior radioulnar joints. J Anat 66:210–227, 1932
30. MacConnaill MA, Basmajian JV: Muscles and Movements: A Basis for Human Kinesiology. Baltimore, Williams & Wilkins, 1969
31. Mankin HJ: Biochemical and metabolic aspects of osteoarthritis. Orthop Clin North Am 2:19–31, 1971
32. Mankin HJ: The reaction of articular cartilage to injury and osteoarthrosis: I. N Engl J Med 291:1284, 1974
33. Mankin HJ: The reaction of articular cartilage to injury and osteoarthrosis: II. N Engl J Med 291:1335, 1974
34. Mankin HJ, Dorfman H, Lipiello L, et al: Biochemical and metabolic abnormalities in articular cartilage from osteoarthritic human hips. J Bone Joint Surg 53A:523–537, 1971
35. Mankin HJ, Thrasher AZ, Hall D: Characteristics of articular cartilage from osteonecrotic femoral heads. J Bone Joint Surg 59A:724–728, 1977
36. McClure PW, Flowers KR: Treatment of limited shoulder motions: A case study based on biomechanical considerations. Phys Ther 72:9229–9236, 1992
37. McCutcheon CW: Lubrication of joints. Br Med J 1:384–385, 1964
38. Meachim G: Articular cartilage lesions in osteoarthritis of the femoral head. J Pathol 107:199–210, 1972
39. Meachim G, Emergy IH: Cartilage fibrillation in shoulder and hip joints in Liverpool necropsies. J Anat 116:161–197, 1973
40. Meachim G, Emergy IH: Quantitative aspects of patellofemoral fibrillation in Liverpool necropsies. Ann Rheum Dis 33:39–47, 1974
41. Mennell J: Joint Pain. Boston, Little, Brown & Co, 1964
42. Nevaiser JS: Adhesive capsulitis of the shoulder: A study of pathologic findings in periarthritis of the shoulder. J Bone Joint Surg 27A:211–222, 1945
43. Norkin CC, Levangie PK: Joint Structure and Function: A Comprehensive Analysis, 2nd ed. Philadelphia, FA Davis, 1992
44. Paris SV: Cranial manipulation. Fysioterapeuten 39:310, 1972
45. Peacock EE: Comparison of collagenous tissue surrounding normal and immobilized joints. Surg Forum 14:440, 1963
46. Poppen NK, Walker PS: Normal and abnormal motion of the shoulder joint. J Bone Joint Surg [Am] 58:195–201, 1976
47. Radin EL, Paul IL: Does cartilage compliance reduce skeletal impact loads? Arthritis Rheum 13:138, 1970
48. Radin EL, Paul IL: A consolidated concept of joint lubrication. J Bone Joint Surg 54A:607–616, 1972
49. Roach JE, Tomblin W, Eyring EJ: Comparison of the effects of aspirin, steroids and sodium salicylate on articular cartilage. Clin Orthop 106:350–356, 1975

50. Rowinski MJ: Afferent neurobiology of the joint. In Gould JA, Davies GJ (eds): Orthopaedic and Sports Physical Therapy, 2nd ed. St Louis, CV Mosby, 1990
51. Sammarco GJ, Curstein AH, Frankel VH: Biomechanics of the ankle: A kinematic study. Orthop Clin North Am 4:75–95, 1973
52. Seileg AJ, Gerath M: An in vivo investigation of wear in animal joints. J Biomech 8:169–172, 1975
53. Sherrington C: The Integrative Action of the Nervous System. New Haven, CT, Yale University Press, 1906
54. Skoglund S. Anatomic and physiologic studies of knee joint innervation in the cat. Acta Physiol Scand (Suppl) 124:1–100, 1956
55. Skolglund S: Joint receptors and kinaesthesis. In Iggo A (ed): Handbook of Sensory Physiology: Vol II. Somatosensory System. New York, Springer-Verlag, 1973
56. Swanson SA: Lubrication of synovial joints. J Physiol 223:22, 1972
57. Voss D, Ionta MK, Myers BJ: Proprioceptive Neuromuscular Facilitation, 3rd ed. Philadelphia, Harper & Row, 1985
58. Warwick R, Williams P (eds): Gray's Anatomy, 36th ed. Philadelphia, WB Saunders, 1980
59. Weightman BO, Freeman MAR, Swanson SAV: Fatigue of articular cartilage. Nature 244:303–304, 1973
60. Woo SL, Matthews JV, Akeson WH, et al: Connective tissue response to immobility. Arthritis Rheum 18:257–264, 1975
61. Wright V (ed): Lubrication and Wear in Joints. Philadelphia, JB Lippincott, 1969
62. Wyke B: The neurology of joints. Ann R Coll Surg Engl 41:25–50, 1967

Pain

MAUREEN K. LYNCH, RANDOLPH M. KESSLER,
AND DARLENE HERTLING

*It is not a fixed response to a noxious stimulus,
its perception is modified by past experiences,
expectations and even by culture. It has a
protective function, warning us that something
biologically harmful is happening, but anyone
who has suffered prolonged severe pain would
regard it as an evil, a punishing affliction that is
harmful in its own right.*

—Ronald Melzack

There are many reasons why the clinician should understand mechanisms of pain perception. Patients are often seen whose primary complaint is pain, which often leads to a loss of function. Usually, a careful assessment of pain behavior is invaluable in determining the nature and extent of the underlying pathologic process. Development of an appropriate treatment program and evaluation of progress may depend largely

on pain assessment. Therefore, it is important for the clinician who sees patients with pain complaints to have a basic understanding of the neurophysiology of pain, including mechanisms of pain perception and the phenomena of referred and projected pain. The clinician should understand how specific treatment modalities influence the nature of pain and how knowledge of pain mechanisms can be applied to its management.

▪ PAIN OF DEEP SOMATIC ORIGIN

When examining a patient with pain of musculoskeletal origin, the clinician often finds that the site that the patient indicates as the most painful does not correspond well with the site of the lesion. The patient often gives a history of proximal or distal radiation of pain and may describe it as moving from one place to another. In addition, cutaneous hyperalgesia or hypalgesia and tenderness to palpation at sites distant from—or at least not directly over—the site of the

Darlene Hertling and Randolph M. Kessler: MANAGEMENT OF COMMON
MUSCULOSKELETAL DISORDERS: Physical Therapy Principles and Methods, 3rd ed.
© 1996 Lippincott-Raven Publishers.

pathologic process are often evident. For example, patients with shoulder problems often describe pain over the lateral brachial region, radiating to the elbow or hand. This type of radiation eliminates muscle spasm as a possible cause of pain, since no muscle traverses the extent of this distribution. Similarly, the patient with a low-back problem often describes more pain in the buttock than in the lumbar region. In the past, a discrepancy between the site of the pathologic process and the site where pain is perceived was often attributed to muscle spasm or sciatic nerve inflammation. These possibilities are unlikely, however, since the pain is often described as traveling distally down the leg and spiraling around the thigh to the front of the lower leg, a distribution that does not correspond to any nerve or muscle. Pain patterns that are associated with deep somatic lesions relate to the embryologic development of the musculoskeletal system (see Chapter 1, Embryology of the Musculoskeletal System). Kellgren and other researchers have clarified and supported this association by mapping areas of pain reference from stimulation of deep somatic structures, by determining the relative sensitivities of the various structures, and by describing the general qualities of pain of somatic origin.[39,43]

☐ Experimental Data

In their series of studies, Kellgren and co-workers injected saline into various joint tissues, including the fibrous capsule, ligaments, tendons, muscle, fascia, menisci, synovia, and articular cartilage.[43,44] They also stimulated the periosteum with a Kirschner wire. These studies revealed several significant findings on the nature of musculoskeletal pain that, unfortunately, are still widely ignored clinically.

> The structures most sensitive to noxious stimulation are the periosteum and joint capsule. Subchondral bone, tendons, and ligaments are moderately pain sensitive, while muscle and cortical bone are somewhat less sensitive. Synovium, articular cartilage, and fibrocartilage are essentially insensitive to nociceptive stimulation.

Thus, cartilaginous erosion accompanying degenerative joint disease, synovitis, or meniscal tears is not painful. Secondary or concomitant involvement of other tissues must occur in order for the patient to be aware of the problem. These, then, are pathologic conditions that can be "silent" for a period, leading to insidious, and often significant, progression before being seen by the clinician.

Tendon and ligament injuries are likely to be most painful when their junction with the periosteum is affected. Too often, muscle is implicated as the source of pain in patients with somatic pain complaints.

> Pain of musculoskeletal origin is usually delocalized; the site at which pain is perceived rarely corresponds exactly with the site of stimulation. Generally, the closer the tissue is to the body surface, the better the site of pain corresponds to the site of stimulation.

This finding deviates markedly from the way we are accustomed to thinking of pain, or sensation in general. Most common sensations affect the skin and are well localized to the site of stimulation. This, however, is not true of subcutaneous sensations, whether somatic or visceral. Thus, for example, pain from lesions about the glenohumeral joint is felt in the lateral brachial region, pain from cervical joints is felt in the scapular area, and pain from the hip joint is felt anywhere from the groin to the knee. These are common cases of deeply situated pathologic processes that cause delocalized sensations. On the other hand, pain from ligament sprains at the knee, ankle, or wrist, all of which are relatively superficial lesions, is well localized to the site of involvement.

Although documented years ago, this characteristic of pain of deep-tissue origin still goes widely unrecognized by clinicians. Patients continue to receive injections, ultrasound, or massage about the scapulae for disorders arising from the neck; the sacroiliac joint or sciatic nerve is often blamed for pain originating in the lumbar spine; and on occasion, an adolescent presenting with slipped capital femoral epiphysis may receive treatment for "knee pain."

> With increased stimulation, pain of deep somatic origin may radiate into a characteristic distribution. The pattern of distribution is always the same for a particular site of stimulation, and tends to follow a segmental, or sclerotomic, pathway. The extent of radiation is dependent upon the intensity of stimulation, and pain tends to radiate distally rather than proximally.

Recall that a sclerotome comprises those deep so-

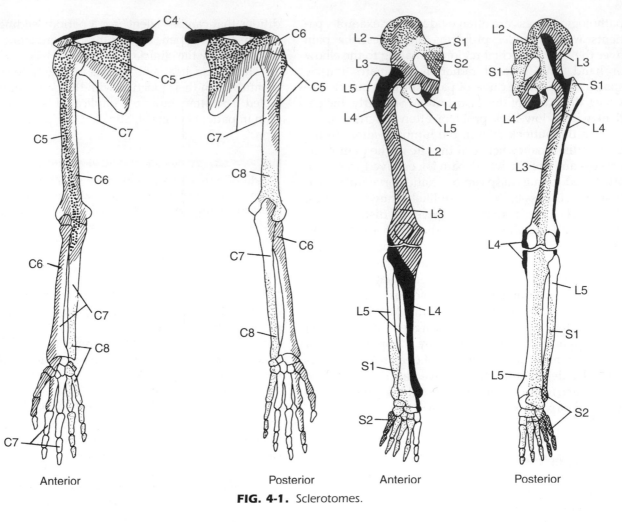

FIG. 4-1. *Sclerotomes.*

matic tissues (fascia, ligaments, capsules, and connective tissue) that are innervated by the same segmental spinal nerve. These areas have been mapped by Inman and Saunders[39] and are shown in Figure 4-1. Note that they do not correspond exactly to dermatomes (Figs. 4-2 and 4-3). When a tissue of a particular sclerotome is irritated, the patient may perceive the resulting pain as arising from any or all of the tissues innervated by the same segmental nerve. This is a result of the lack of precision in central neural connections and is not related to abnormal impulses "spreading down a nerve." In other words, the "problem" is central, not peripheral, and there is nothing wrong with most of the area from which pain seems to arise. Furthermore, it is crucial to realize that *radiating pain does not necessarily imply nerve irritation*.

Thus, patients with supraspinatus tendinitis often have pain referred down the lateral aspect of the arm and forearm to the wrist; disk protrusions may cause pain to radiate into a limb without nerve-root pressure; and trochanteric bursitis is often mistaken for L5 nerve-root irritation or is diagnosed as fasciitis of the iliotibial band. Again, the clinical implications of referred pain cannot be overemphasized and must be appreciated by the clinician seeing patients with musculoskeletal disorders.

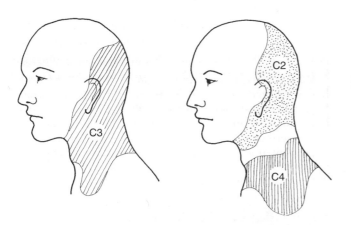

FIG. 4-2. *Dermatomes of the head and neck.*

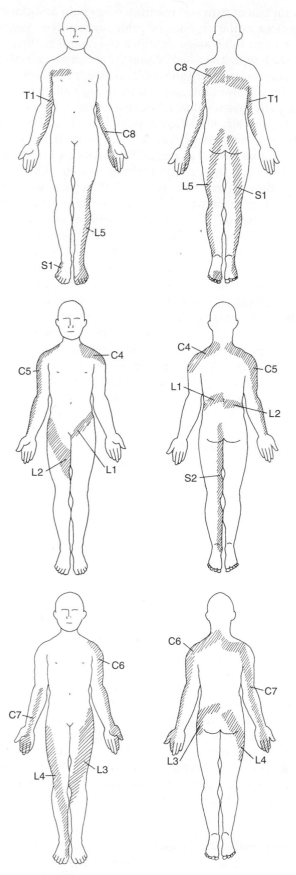

FIG. 4-3. Dermatomes of the body.

Pain of deep somatic origin is of a deep, aching, generalized quality as opposed to the sharp, well-localized pain that may arise from stimulation of the skin. In addition, deep somatic pain is often associated with autonomic phenomena such as increased sweating, pallor, and reduced blood pressure, and is commonly accompanied by a subjective feeling of nausea and faintness.

The terms *sclerotomic* and *dermatomic* are often used to distinguish between pain arising from deep somatic tissues and from the skin. Sclerotomic pain is typically deep, aching, and poorly localized, whereas dermatomic pain is sharp, sometimes shooting, and well localized. In most clinical settings, pain arising from the surface of the skin is not commonly encountered and therefore is insignificant. However, a very important source of both dermatomic and sclerotomic pain is direct irritation of nerve pathways projecting afferent input from a particular area. This is properly referred to as *projected* (or radicular) pain, rather than *referred* (or spondylogenic) pain, and the most common site of irritation is the nerve root. Thus, an intervertebral disk protrusion or bony osteophyte may directly excite nerve fibers subserving sensory or motor functions, producing symptoms or signs confined to the relevant dermatome, myotome, or sclerotome. The symptoms or signs will vary, depending on the fibers affected.

The largest myelinated nerve fibers are most sensitive to pressure, whereas small-diameter, unmyelinated fibers are least sensitive. It is generally agreed that eventual dissociation of the quality of sensation is, in part, related to fiber size, and that sensations may be arranged in order of decreasing fiber size, as follows:

Vibration sense, proprioception—Large, myelinated (A-alpha) fiber
"Fast" (dermatomic) pain, temperature—Small, myelinated (A-delta) fiber
"Slow" (sclerotomic) pain—Unmyelinated (C) fiber

Touch and pressure travel over fibers spanning the entire range of diameters. Consistent with the above scheme is the clinical observation that patients presenting with nerve root irritation may complain of paresthesia (A-alpha stimulation); pain of a sharp, well-localized, dermatomic quality (A-delta irritation); or deep, aching, sclerotomic pain (C-fiber involvement). In any case, the sensation is perceived as arising from any or all of the tissues innervated by the involved nerve.

Differences in central projections between large-fiber afferent input and small-fiber input are responsible for observed differences in associated motor and sensory phenomena. Small-fiber afferent nerves transmitting sclerotomic and visceral pain follow a multisynaptic pathway with diffuse projections to areas such as the hypothalamus, limbic system, and reticular formation. These projections may mediate autonomic changes, such as changes in vasomotor tone, blood pressure, and sweat gland activity, which may accompany the pain experience. They may also be responsible for associated affective phenomena, such as depression, anxiety, fear, and anger. Sensory modalities transmitted over large fibers, such as dermatomic pain and non-noxious sensations, project largely to the thalamus and cortex and skip areas of the brain involved with affective and autonomic mediation. They are thus less likely to be associated with emotional and behavioral changes.

HISTORY AND DEVELOPMENT OF PAIN THEORIES AND MECHANISMS

Inconsistencies in interpreting the experiential and behavioral aspects of pain complicate any discussion of the physiology of a nociceptive system. Although some researchers attempt to discuss pain as a sensory experience, others define pain in terms of associated behavioral responses, both somatic and autonomic. One might argue that extreme pain may affect a person as a sensory experience without being recognized by an observer. Another would counter that even if this were possible, pain is insignificant unless it somehow alters the victim's body functions, behavior, or life-style.

Still another concern of those interested in the phenomenon of pain is the affective component: the suffering, hopelessness, despair, or depression that may accompany pain, especially long-standing pain. On the basis of experience, most would agree that a "painful event" might comprise any combination of sensory, behavioral, or affective components. A person may prick a finger with a pin without significant despair or depression, and in the absence of subsequent shouting, sweating, or shaking of the part. However, smashing the thumb with a hammer is frequently followed by some verbal display of displeasure and significant motor activity, including flailing of the injured part as well as generalized increased sympathetic tone. But this event is not usually associated with depression or sorrow because the person realizes that the swelling will soon subside. On the other hand, loss of a loved one may lead to excruciating "pain" manifested as grieving and sorrow but without a painful sensation. It is often accompanied by diminished motor activity, loss of appetite, and weeping. Interestingly, the sufferer of chronic pain behaves similarly. Although persons in each of the above situations may well complain of pain, psychosocial rewards may condition a person to complain of pain and manifest other pain-associated behaviors in the absence of prior nociceptive events. There seem to be areas in which the neural pathways involved with pain sensation, with certain affective phenomena, and with stereotyped skeletal and smooth muscle activation intersect. Activation of all or part of these pathways results in the experiential or behavioral events generally classified as pain. Which components of the system will be activated depends on the nature of the stimulus as well as central modulation of information reaching the central nervous system (CNS). A given stimulus may or may not result in pain, and pain behavior may occur in the absence of nociception. Everyone has heard stories about soldiers wounded in war who deny pain at the time of severe tissue damage. On the other hand, persons with no demonstrable tissue damage may complain of pain and display disabling pain behaviors. In summary, nociception may occur without pain and pain may occur without nociception. Theories dealing with the neurophysiology of pain must explain these facts in terms of known mechanisms and their anatomical correlates.

Knowledge of the evolution of pain theory is interesting on a historical level and contributes to an appreciation of present pain research. Today's understanding of the nociceptive system is a composite of past and present research, hypotheses, and theories, each of which has emphasized different components of the nociceptive system. Therefore, one approach to understanding pain mechanisms would be to follow the evolution of pain theory and select and combine important contributions.

One of the first recorded pain theories was proposed by Aristotle, who postulated that pain occurs with every kind of stimulation whenever that stimulation becomes excessive. Therefore, anything too hot, too sharp, or abnormally loud causes pain. Excessive stimulation was carried from the periphery by blood vessels to the heart, where it was perceived as a negative passion or absence of pleasure. Aristotle's proposal implied that the pain experience has emotional, psychological, and physiologic dimensions. The proposed anatomic pathway for nociceptive input is, of course, incorrect. Aristotle chose the heart—the center of emotion—as the organ receiving and interpreting painful stimulation, which suggests that he considered the affective or emotional component of pain to be of critical importance. The affective dimension of pain was not emphasized again until the development of modern theories.

☐ Specificity Theory

With the advent of the microscope, scientists became greatly preoccupied with morphologic detail. Investigators in the early 1800s searched for precise anatomic evidence to support hypothesized pain mechanisms. Mueller and others found minute structures in the skin, viscera, and muscles that they believed were receptor end organs for various modalities of sensation.[54,70,71] The primary theory based on microscopic evidence was Von Frey's specificity theory proposed in 1895.[62,87] Von Frey proposed a specific relationship between the type of end organ stimulated and the nature of the resulting sensation. For example, pressure is perceived when the pacinian corpuscles are stimulated, whereas stimulation of free nerve endings causes pain.

It has since been found that such a precise one-to-one relationship between type of receptor and sensation does not exist. Weddell found, for example, that the cornea, which contains only free nerve endings, is sensitive to many types of sensory stimuli.[14,62,80] The specificity theory proponents demonstrated, however, that there are peripheral receptors that must be excited in order for pain sensation to be perceived. Unfortunately, the theory paid little attention to central pain modulation (the influence of spinal cord or brain on input) and considered only the sensory experience of pain. It ignored the associated emotional, psychological, and motor responses.

□ Pattern Theory

Several years later, investigators became interested in peripheral nerves. Head cut a peripheral nerve in his own arm, knowing that smaller nerve fibers regenerate before larger ones. With regeneration of the small nerve fibers, Head noted spontaneous tingling, dysesthesia, and other abnormal nociceptive sensations.[14,24,62] Not until the large nerve fibers regenerated, and sense of light pressure, touch, and vibration returned, were the painful sensations abolished. From this information and from insight gained through their own research (including research on cornea sensation), Weddell and Sinclair proposed a pattern theory of pain.[14,24,62,70,80] The pattern theory emphasized that it is the anatomic variation in fiber size over which afferent impulses travel that leads to temporal and spatial summation of input in central receiving areas. The pattern theory suggested that variation in fiber size was related to both the site of central connections and the pattern of central excitation. For example, input traveling over small fibers ascends multisynaptically in the contralateral anterolateral tract with little cortical input, whereas large-fiber input ascends in the ipsilateral dorsal column to the thalamus, with subsequent projections to the cortex. Weddell also noted that signals traveling over larger fibers reach the spinal cord before small-fiber input. Wed-

dell and Sinclair combined this information in a theory that stated that patterns of input over various fiber sizes are a major determinant of sensation and pain perception. Thus, large-fiber stimulation may be felt as light touch or pressure, whereas small-fiber stimulation tends to cause noxious sensations. A mixture may result in a combination or cancellation of sensory input.

The pattern theory postulates that a specialized system exists that combines and modifies all peripheral sensory input before it ascends to higher brain centers, thus modifying the nature of the resultant sensation. The theory also proposes that all stimulus information from the periphery must summate in the CNS to allow determination and execution of a proper response. Weddell and Sinclair stated that major determinants of intensity and quality of experienced sensations are the discharge characteristics of afferent fibers and the sites of central connections. The weaknesses in the pattern theory are (1) that pain is again considered to be largely a sensory phenomenon, and little reference is made to associated affective phenomena; (2) that knowledge of the role of receptors was ignored or denied; and (3) that the influence of central modulation of input was not considered.

□ Neuroanatomy

Before discussing the gate theory of pain, it is important to compare the pathways taken by large as opposed to small, or nociceptive, afferent nerve fibers. On entering the dorsal horn of the spinal cord, nociceptive afferents from both somatic and visceral tissues travel in the dorsolateral fasciculus (Lissauer's tract) a few segments rostrally and caudally before entering the gray matter of the dorsal horn.[14,48,87] They then relay with cells in the substantia gelatinosa (SG) (laminae II and III) and proceed to synapse ipsilaterally in the dorsal funicular gray matter (lamina V), a nuclear mass that lies at the base of the dorsal horn (Fig. 4-4). The second- or third-order fiber crosses by way of the anterior white commissure to ascend contralaterally in the anterolateral tract. This fiber tract continues rostrally to synapse in the ventroposterolateral and ventroposteromedial nuclei of the thalamus; collaterals also project to the medullary reticular formation, limbic system, and hypothalamus. The nociceptive afferents are small myelinated and unmyelinated, slowly transmitting nerve fibers, and the receptors for this system adapt slowly to the application or removal of the irritating stimulus. The final synapses are in regions where past experience, motivation, and emotion may influence the ultimate response to noxious stimulation.[14,48,87]

Large fiber afferents from proprioceptors and

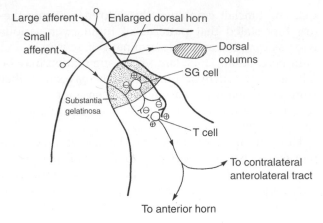

FIG. 4-4. *Modulation of afferent input as proposed by the gate theory. Activation of the T cells results in ascending nociceptive input and reflex motor changes. T cells are inhibited by substantia gelatinosa (SG) cell input, which is, in turn, inhibited by small-fiber input and facilitated by large-fiber input.*

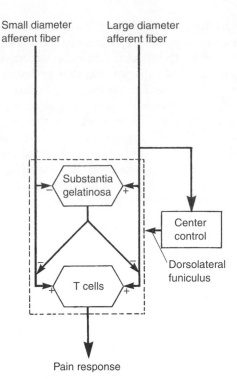

FIG. 4-5. *Scheme of dorsal horn pain-modulating system.*

mechanoreceptors transmitting information concerning light touch, vibration, and joint and muscle position enter the dorsolateral fasciculus and send collaterals to segments several spinal levels above and below the level of entry. The collateral branches enter the dorsal horn and synapse on interneurons in the SG (see Fig. 4-4). The large myelinated fibers then enter the dorsal columns ipsilaterally and ascend to the medulla where they synapse, decussate, and ascend as the medial lemniscus to the ventroposterolateral nuclei of the thalamus. The third-order neuron leaves the thalamus and projects to the postcentral gyrus, the sensory cortex.[14,48,87]

Both large- and small-fiber systems send collaterals to the anterior horn of the spinal cord before entering ascending tracts. These projections mediate reflex motor activity associated with noxious and non-noxious stimulation.

☐ Gate Theory

In 1965 Melzack and Wall proposed the gate theory of pain.[54,57,62,79,87] Several investigators studying the SG measured electrical potentials in some of the interneuron synapses. They found that with small-fiber input (C fibers mediating pain and temperature), hyperpolarization was recorded, and when large fibers were stimulated, depolarization was recorded. Melzack and Wall postulated that interneurons in the SG act as a "gate" to modulate sensory input (Fig. 4-5). They proposed that the SG interneuron projected to the second order neuron of the pain–temperature pathway located in the dorsal funicular gray matter (lamina V),

which they called the *transmission cell* or *T cell*.[54,57] If the SG interneuron were depolarized it would inhibit T-cell firing and thus decrease further transmission of input ascending in the spinothalamic tract. For example, nociceptive fibers enter the dorsal horn and send a collateral fiber into the SG, which hyperpolarizes the interneuron. The nociceptive afferent continues to lamina V where it synapses with the T-cell. On reaching threshold levels of excitation, the T-cell sends nociceptive input rostrally in the anterolateral spinal tract. Large-fiber input (joint movement, pressure, vibration) enters the dorsal horn, sending a collateral into the SG, which depolarizes the SG interneuron. This interneuron projects to lamina V and presynaptically inhibits the T cell, preventing or decreasing ascending nociceptive input.[54,57,62,87] Melzack and Wall thus used concepts presented in the pattern theory and described a specific anatomic pathway by which modulation of peripheral stimuli could occur. Essentially, the theory proposed an analogy to a gate that allows ongoing transmission of painful input when opened. The position of the gate is determined by the balance between large-fiber and small-fiber input to the system and is regulated by interneurons in the SG of the dorsal horn.

The gate theory was, and is, supported by both practical and experimental evidence. When one hits one's shin on a coffee-table corner, the immediate response is to rub the injured area, thus increasing the large-fiber input that decreases the pain. Physical therapists use a large number of modalities to decrease pain by increasing large-fiber input. Hot packs, whirlpools, massage, vibrators, and joint mobilization all act to increase large-fiber input and, therefore, to decrease nociceptive transmission. There are also certain clinical pain states, such as alcoholic neuropathy, in which preferential destruction of large fibers leads to chronic, relatively spontaneous pain.

Melzack and Wall also suggested that the gate could be modified by a descending inhibitory pathway from the brain or brain stem.[54,57,62,87] This was originally proposed largely on the basis of everyday experience. For example, it has been noted that persons injured during stressful, life-threatening, or athletic events often do not realize the seriousness of the injury. Following frontal lobotomy or while on morphine, a patient knows when noxious stimulation is occurring but it is no longer painful or worrisome. Melzack and Wall postulated that these observations could be explained by central inhibitory input descending to the spinal cord to decrease T-cell firing. Sometimes patients experience more pain than expected following a certain amount of noxious input. In these cases it was speculated that learned or affective behavior prevented or decreased inhibition of T-cell activity.

Since the proposal of the gate theory, researchers have identified many clinical pain states that cannot be fully explained by the gate mechanism.[62,87] However, the theory has made several significant contributions to current pain research. First, it directed the attention of researchers to the importance of pain modulation by higher CNS centers. Second, it accommodated most past research findings dealing with receptors, peripheral nerves, the dorsal horn, and ascending sensory pathways. Third, clinical applications of this theory are still useful, and many effective clinical procedures are based on the model provided by the gate theory. Transcutaneous nerve stimulation increases large-fiber input and abolishes or decreases pain to acceptable levels for many patients living with chronic pain. Clinics specializing in treatment for patients with chronic pain use behavior modification techniques to increase a patient's activity level. These techniques may act to increase large-fiber input and decrease pain or they may activate a central descending pathway that inhibits nociceptive input at the spinal cord level.[13,14,21]

Conceptually, the gate control theory[55,58] is still the most comprehensive and relevant to understanding the cognitive aspects of pain. Theories regarding the perpetuation of pain have further extended the gate control theory. The pattern-generating theory proposed by Melzack[55] suggests that the perpetuation of pain is due to sustained activity in the neuron pools, including the dorsal horn and the homologous inter-

acting systems associated with the cranial nerves. With reduction in the inhibitory influences, there is abnormal bursting activity, which continues unchecked and allows recruitment of additional neurons into the abnormally firing pools, leading to the spreading of the pain. Once the pattern-generating mechanisms become capable of producing patterns for pain, any input may act as a trigger. The clinical support for this theory lies in the countless patients who continue to suffer after ablative surgeries such as rhizotomies and cordotomies, or severe phantom limb and back pain after removal of neuromas and removal of nerves and disks.

There remain gaps in the gate control theory, the details of which are being filled in by others. According to the gate control theory, pain phenomena are viewed as consisting of sensory-discriminative, motivational-affective, and cognitive-evaluative components. More than any other theoretical approach, the gate control theory emphasizes the role of psychological variables and how they affect the reaction to pain. (See Weisenberg for a more extensive review of psychological factors in pain control.[81–83])

Recently, other theoretical statements have attempted to fill in the gaps of gate control theory or to introduce new concepts.[33,69,76,77] The functional theory of pain[6] stressed the sensory component of pain, while Dworkin and co-workers[27] presented a theoretical, biobehavioral model designed to show the importance of epidemiological concepts for understanding chronic pain, which involves both extrinsic and intrinsic factors. According to Weisenberg,[84] these theories are not in conflict with gate control but fill in areas not explained in gate control theory.

CENTRAL MODULATION OF NOCICEPTIVE INPUT

During the last decade there has been a wealth of research and discovery related to central pain modulation. Current research continues to explore the relationship between the anatomic and physiologic components of central pain pathways. The spark for this research was provided by technical advancements that have brought a better understanding of biochemical and neurohistological features of the nociceptive system. After years of studying morphine and other opiate derivatives, researchers discovered "endogenous opiates," peptides native to the CNS that are now believed to be involved in nociceptive modulation. More recently the role of other neurotransmitters in the nociceptive system has begun to be elucidated. Additionally, there is much more interest in the affective and behavioral components of the nociceptive system—a return to Aristotle's emphasis. It is becoming generally accepted that any comprehensive pain theory must explain pain as a sensory experience with associated affective and motor (autonomic and somatic) phenomena.

☐ Opiates and Enkephalins

Research leading to the discovery of endogenous opiates, the enkephalins, began with studies of morphine and its mechanism of action. For years researchers and the medical community have searched for a non-addictive opiate agonist. Because morphine exerts analgesic effects with very small doses, researchers generally agreed that morphine might act as a neurotransmitter in the CNS. The subsequent prediction was that receptors for morphine must exist in the CNS.[71,72] Pert and Snyder, using advanced neurohistological and neurochemical techniques, were able to trace morphine receptor sites in the CNS. Kumar, Pert, and Snyder demonstrated the distribution of opiate receptors in many brain regions using direct receptor-binding techniques and autoradiography of brain sections containing radioactive morphine.[38,71] The receptor distribution pathway strikingly parallels the paleospinothalamic pathway (Fig. 4-6), which ascends along the midline of the brain with synapses in the central gray matter of the brain stem, the reticular formation, and the central thalamus. This pathway mediates duller, more chronic, and less localized pain; it is the phylogenetically older pain pathway and contains many synapses and small-diameter, unmyelinated nerves.[14,45,71] Consistent with this is the observation that morphine exerts its analgesic effects on dull pain, whereas sharp, well-localized pain is poorly relieved by opiates.

Other brain areas with opiate receptors are the amygdala, the corpus striatum, and the hypothalamus, all of which are parts of the limbic system—a group of brain regions that largely mediate emotional phenomena.[71,88] These brain regions seem to be concerned with the affective components of pain, such as rage, anger, and depression, and perhaps the euphoric effects of morphine. Hypothalamic connections may mediate associated autonomic activity, such as sweating, pallor, or blood pressure changes. Opiate receptors are also localized in lamina II in the SG of the dorsal horn of the spinal cord—an important synapse area for the upward conduction of nociceptive information—as well as in lamina II of the caudal trigeminal nucleus, which receives nociceptive input from the face.[71,88]

With the discovery of morphine receptors, the search began for an endogenous substance with opiate activity. Several researchers simultaneously identified a morphine-like brain factor consisting of two closely related pentapeptides, which were named *enkephalins*.[38,71,87] It was found that naloxone, a morphine antagonist, also inhibited the analgesic effects of enkephalins.[5,18,20,51,87] Research in morphine addiction revealed that an increase in the presence of morphine is accompanied by a decrease in enkephalin production and release. It was speculated that opiate withdrawal symptoms occur from enkephalin depletion and subside as soon as enkephalin concentrations return to normal.[50,71] Several studies have also described decreased enkephalin levels associated with chronic pain.[6,8,46,47]

The mechanism of enkephalin action as a neurotransmitter is both interesting and speculative. Enkephalin is an excitatory transmitter believed to presynaptically inhibit the dorsal horn T cell of lamina V, and thus modulate input to ascending pain pathways in the spinal cord and the brain.[51,71,87] This has special significance for the gate theory, which 30 years ago suggested that descending inhibition occurred at the level of the dorsal horn in the spinal cord and that perhaps the mechanism was presynaptic inhibition of the T cell in lamina V.[72]

☐ Stimulus-Produced Analgesia

Following the discovery of enkephalins, researchers began to investigate possible mechanisms by which enkephalin-mediated circuits might be activated. Therefore, they have attempted to define the role of enkephalins in the nociceptive system. Opiate receptor sites (and synaptic vesicles of enkephalin) are located in the periventricular, periaqueductal, and mesencephalic central gray matter, in the dorsal horn, and in some limbic regions (*e.g.*, amygdala, corpus striatum) of the CNS.[51,71,87] It was found that electrical stimulation of the periaqueductal gray matter (PAG) in rats, cats, monkeys, and humans produced profound analgesia.[9,11,14,26,45,49–53,64,67,71,87] Subsequently, researchers noted that this stimulus-produced analgesia (SPA) was partially reversed by administering naloxone.[1,4,50,51] Because SPA is only partially reversed by naloxone, it was concluded that SPA was the result of the release of both enkephalin and another unknown neurotransmitter. Investigators have measured in the cerebrospinal fluid a significant increase in enkephalin content following stimulation of the PAG in rats and have found that injections of enkephalin into the central gray matter increase the animal's pain tolerance and produce a long-lasting analgesia to electrically evoked pain.[5,51,67,71,87] It was subsequently postulated that enkephalins were released in the PAG following noxious input. Researchers then administered radioactively labeled amino acids to experimental animals in order to label

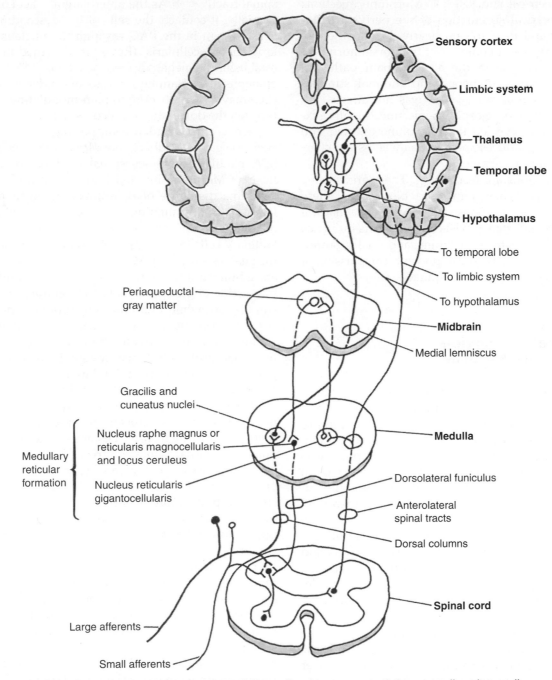

FIG. 4-6. *Scheme of large- and small-fiber afferent systems and the ascending-descending inhibitory loop. The small-fiber system is often referred to as the paleospinothalamic tract and the large-fiber system as the neospinothalamic tract.*

enkephalins, which incorporate the amino acids. Following stimulation of A-delta nerve fibers (which mediate thermal and nociceptive input), the animals' brains were sectioned and analyzed for labeling. It was found that the areas where enkephalins were released overlapped the anatomic substrate for SPA.[71] This area appears to be concentrated in medial brainstem structures extending from the diencephalon (periventricular gray matter and PAG) caudally to the

medullary raphe nuclei, which are part of the midbrain reticular formation.[8,9,26,30,49,51,52,66,88] It was subsequently noted that stimulation of A-delta nerve fibers also caused increased firing of nerve cells located in the medullary raphe nuclei.[8,51]

In humans, stimulation of periventricular structures was effective in relieving diverse pain syndromes.[49,51] Electrical stimulation of the PAG was also shown to increase experimental pain tolerance to both painful heat and electrical shock.[51,87,88] Morphine injections into and electrical stimulation of the periventricular gray matter and PAG in cats clearly depress the discharge of neurons in lamina V of the dorsal horn (site of the first synapse in the afferent pain pathway) evoked by strong cutaneous and thermal stimulation.[26] Non-noxious stimulation was not affected by PAG stimulation or morphine injection. Finally, experiments have revealed that morphine injected into the amygdala produces analgesia as well as the characteristic euphoric behavior.[51,71]

The implications are fascinating. There are specific brain sites that when stimulated block pain; these areas mediate the response to morphine; a natural morphine-like substance exists that exerts its influence in the same brain site as morphine; and finally, stimulation of these brain areas can prevent transmission of nociception at the level of the spinal cord.

☐ Central Descending Inhibitory Pathway

The findings discussed previously strongly suggest that endogenous opiates are neurotransmitters in a nociceptive modulating system.[51,68,72] The physiologic mechanism proposed is an "endogenous pain inhibitory system" or negative feedback loop[21,38] (see Fig. 4-6). Specifically, peripheral nociception leads to activation of the PAG and nuclei of the midbrain and medullary reticular formation. These nuclei then send descending inhibitory signals to the dorsal horn to reduce ongoing transmission of nociceptive input. The descending inhibitory system includes the rostral and caudal PAG, the medullary nuclei of the reticular formation, and connections in the dorsal horn. The descending limb of this feedback loop begins with neurons in the rostral PAG, an important area for SPA that is known to be rich in enkephalins.[9,51,88] The PAG neuron makes an excitatory synapse with the nucleus raphe magnus (NRM) of the medulla, near the caudal PAG, and with the adjacent nucleus reticularis magnocellularis (Rmc), perhaps using dopamine or enkephalin as a neurotransmitter. These two nuclei send fibers to the spinal cord by way of the dorsolateral funiculus that terminate among pain-transmission cells concentrated in laminae II and V of the dorsal horn.[12,13,51] Both the NRM and the nucleus Rmc exert an inhibitory effect specifically on pain-transmission neurons. The NRM uses serotonin as a transmitter; the Rmc transmitter is speculated to be enkephalin. The pain-transmission neurons (activated by substance P following peripheral nociceptive stimulation) cross and project cranially in the anterolateral

spinal tract.[17,37,52] As the anterolateral tract continues cranially, it contacts the cells of the descending analgesia system in the PAG through the nucleus reticularis gigantocellularis (RgC) of the medulla, thus establishing a negative feedback loop.[30,49,51,67] Norepinephrine-containing neurons of the locus ceruleus (LC) may also contribute to pain-modulating systems through the dorsolateral funiculus (DLF).

There is ample evidence supporting the existence of such a negative feedback loop. It has been shown that SPA readily suppresses spinal cord nociceptive reflexes.[51] Morphine injected into PAG can clearly depress the discharge of pain-transmission neurons in lamina V.[87] Stimulation of caudal PAG in the cat markedly inhibits the responses of most dorsal horn lamina V cells to noxious skin stimuli.[26] Furthermore, the analgesia due to PAG stimulation or systemic opiate administration is markedly reduced caudally to transection of the spinal DLF.[12,13] Central gray matter stimulation, while inhibiting nociceptive input, does not affect responses to gentle tactile stimulation.

The critical link provided by NRM in the descending nociceptive inhibitory system is also well supported experimentally. Stimulation of the NRM in cats results in analgesia.[64] Several investigators found that after PAG stimulation or morphine administration, they noted a significant increase in neuronal activity in NRM neurons.[63] Lesions of the NRM block opiate analgesia, while electrical stimulation of the NRM produces a potent analgesia reversed by the opiate antagonist naloxone.[8,66] Studies have demonstrated a population of neurons in the NRM projecting to the spinal cord.[51] It was further found that this population of NRM neurons was excited by electrical stimulation of the PAG as well as by opiates administered systemically or by local injection into midbrain PAG. The PAG and NRM receive a large amount of input from the nucleus RgC, which in turn receives input from spinal cord pain-transmission neurons.[30,51] PAG stimulation in the rat has been shown to suppress the nociceptive responses of neurons in the nucleus RgC.[67] This could have been the result of supraspinal descending inhibition of the nucleus RgC or inhibition of incoming nociceptive input at the spinal cord level.

Bilateral lesions of the DLF in rats reverse the analgesic effects of systemically administered morphine.[12,13,51] Lesions of the DLF also abolish the analgesic effects of morphine injected into the PAG in rats.[12,13,49,51] Other researchers have documented that lesions of the DLF reverse both SPA and morphine-induced analgesia. This evidence implies that a descending pathway inhibits nociceptive input at the level of the spinal cord and that this inhibition functions as part of a negative feedback loop.

☐ Monoaminergic Neurotransmitters

It is interesting that naloxone administration only partially blocks SPA. From recent studies it now appears clear that monoaminergic neurotransmitters also play important roles in SPA and morphine analgesia.[2,29,42,57] These transmitters are serotonin, dopamine, and norepinephrine. Depletion of serotonin with *p*-chlorophenylalanine (*p*-CPA) has been shown to reduce SPA, but the analgesia can be restored by administration of the serotonin precursor 5-hydroxytryptamine.[2,3] *p*-CPA is most effective in reducing SPA when the electrode stimulating sites are in the region of the NRM or dorsal raphe magnus (DRM). Both of these reticular nuclei contain serotoninergic neurons.[17,51] The NRM descends through the DLF to the dorsal horn. The DRM is part of the ascending nociceptive pathway that involves complex multisynaptic pathways first ascending to forebrain structures and then descending to the spinal cord in an as yet unknown circuit.[17] An inhibitor of serotoninergic neurons, LSD-25, has been shown to reduce the inhibitory effect that SPA has on dorsal horn lamina V neurons. Animals treated with *p*-CPA were found to be more reactive to electroshock presentations. Humans with migraine headaches who were treated with *p*-CPA experienced superficial and muscular algesias and pain with facial movement or with clothing friction—in short, fairly spontaneous pain.[51] In animals, injections of a serotonin uptake-blocking drug produces analgesia and will antagonize the hyperalgesia associated with injections of *p*-CPA.[42,60] Lesions of the NRM, DRM, medial forebrain bundle, or the septum produce large reductions in serotonin concentrations, leading to increased pain sensitivity.[51,87] Destruction of the DRM or of the NRM and resultant loss of serotoninergic activity blocks the analgesic effect of systemically administered morphine, while increased serotonin levels potentiates morphine analgesia.[51,60] Another method of disrupting the pain inhibition pathway involves blocking the action of NRM fibers as they synapse in the dorsal horn. Research has documented that morphine-induced analgesia could be antagonized by administration of antiserotonin drugs to the dorsal horn. Other studies have shown that serotonin has an inhibitory effect on those neurons located in the superficial laminae of the dorsal horn that respond to noxious stimuli.[41,42,60] These are also the laminae where NRM fibers terminate. In summary, it has been found that with increased serotonin levels, morphine and stimulus-produced analgesia are potentiated, while depletion of serotonin causes hyperalgesia and spontaneous pain and blocks morphine analgesia and SPA.

Catecholaminergic neurotransmitters (*e.g.*, norepinephrine, dopamine) also appear to be involved in both SPA and morphine analgesia.[2,51,87] Compounds that deplete all monoamines almost completely abolish SPA. When compounds that deplete only catecholamines are used, a smaller reduction in SPA is found.[16] Increasing catecholamine levels with L-dopa, which leads to increased dopamine levels, potentiates SPA.[51] Researchers have found that blocking dopamine receptors inhibits SPA and morphine analgesia, whereas stimulation of dopamine receptors potentiates both. The reverse is true for norepinephrine.[29,51] Depletion of norepinephrine increases the effect of morphine and stimulus-produced analgesia; injections of excess norepinephrine block morphine and SPA.

The evidence for dopaminergic involvement in the nociceptive inhibitory pathway is less extensive than that for serotonin involvement. The only known dopamine systems ascend from the brain stem to forebrain structures, so that dopamine involvement necessitates complex ascending and descending pathways.[29,51,60] Even though the location of the dopamine pathway operating in the descending nociceptive inhibitory pathway is not known, it has been shown that dopamine plays some role. Norepinephrine-containing neurons of the LC in rats and of the subceruleus parabrachialis in cats may contribute to pain modulating systems by sending fibers in the dorsolateral funiculus to lamina V of the dorsal horn.[51]

☐ Central Structures Modulating Descending Inhibition

Other CNS structures may play a role in nociceptive modulation. The PAG region of the midbrain receives diverse inputs from numerous brain areas and is involved in various emotional, motivational, and sensory systems.[51,67] The rostral PAG neurons integrate input from many brain areas, and the resulting output determines the level of nociceptive modulation at the midbrain and spinal cord. The PAG receives nociceptive input from the spinal cord by way of the nucleus RgC while simultaneously receiving thalamic, limbic, and cortical input. In this way, memory, learned responses, and affective components may all contribute to modulation and perception of ascending nociceptive input.

The reticular formation contains the NRM and DRM and a number of other ascending and descending pathways.[17,51] The major descending pathway concerned with nociception is that of the NRM and nucleus Rmc, which both send fibers to the dorsal horn. The ascending pathways include reticular formation (1) to the cortex—a direct pathway; (2) to several thalamic nuclei (posterior, ventral, and intralaminar); and (3) to the hypothalamus, limbic forebrain, and frontal cortex.[17] The pathways also include a catecholamine system that arises in parts of the brain-stem reticular formation and passes through the medial forebrain bundle and septum to reach the neocortex.[17,51] This last pathway may be part of an ascending serotoninergic fiber tract.

These ascending pathways, activated by nociceptive input, excite regions of the brain involved in behavioral, affective, and motor responses to nociception. Output from these higher centers (frontal cortex, limbic regions, and thalamus) may in turn descend to the PAG to modulate ongoing nociception through the previously mentioned descending loop.[10,17,35,51] The higher cortical centers and PAG integration of input appear to determine each person's response to nociceptive input. This explains why some persons perceive intense pain, others a mild discomfort, and some no noxious sensation at all in response to the same nociceptive stimulus.

There are several other brain areas that produce analgesia when electrically stimulated. One well-studied region is the medial forebrain bundle–lateral hypothalamic region.[51] Stimulation of this region in the rat has produced analgesia to pin prick, hot plate, and electric shock. For several reasons it appears that the medial forebrain bundle must produce analgesia by a pathway other than PAG → NRM → dorsal horn. Some evidence indicates that stimulation of the medial forebrain bundle can reduce clinical pain in humans.

Stimulation of the septal region also produces analgesia, again by a seemingly different pathway than the medial brain-stem system. Septal region stimulation has been reported to be effective in relieving clinical pain syndromes in humans.[51]

□ Endorphins

Another class of polypeptides with endogenous opiate activity is the endorphins.[36,67] Beta-endorphin, with a chain of 30 amino acids, is among the most potent endogenous analgesics known. It has been found that a sequence of five amino acids on the amino terminal of the beta-endorphin molecule corresponds to the sequence of enkephalin. This may account for their similar analgesic properties. In fact, beta-endorphins have been shown to bind to some of the same sites in the brain, such as the PAG, as the enkephalins. Endorphins do not appear to bind in the spinal cord, however. There is no evidence that enkephalins are products of endorphins; it is probable that enkephalins are primarily produced within neurons, to be used as neurotransmitters.

Immunochemical studies have demonstrated endorphins in the pituitary, brain, and intestinal tract.

They seem to be released from the pituitary as part of a much larger polypeptide molecule, beta-lipotropin (Fig. 4-7), which may in turn be a product of a still larger "prohormone." Beta-lipotropin is also a precursor of adrenocorticotropic hormone (ACTH), and there is evidence that endorphins are released in response to the same stimuli that trigger ACTH release, for example, stress.[61]

The role of endorphins in pain modulation has not yet been elucidated. Intracerebral injections of endorphins produce profound and prolonged analgesia, but large doses administered into the peripheral bloodstream have no analgesic effects. There is a tendency to want to attribute apparent cases of relative analgesia under stress, as in the case of the war-injured or shark-bite victim, to massive endorphin release. However, there is no experimental evidence to demonstrate analgesia from endorphins released from the pituitary, and it is unlikely that they cross the blood–brain barrier. Although speculation on the role of endorphins in mediating such phenomena as the "runner's high" is interesting, corroboration awaits further study. It is likely, however, that the endorphins do influence the maintenance of behavioral homeostasis, perhaps affecting the central nociceptive modulating system.[36]

□ Summary of Sensory Pathways

Nociceptive stimulation of free nerve endings is usually associated with concomitant stimulation of non-

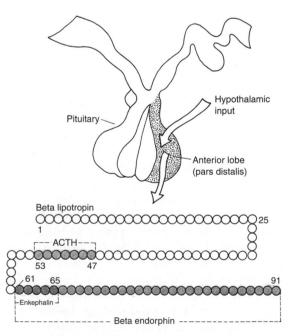

FIG. 4-7. The beta-lipotropin hormone complex released from the anterior pituitary contains amino acid sequences corresponding to ACTH and beta-endorphin. Beta-endorphin, in turn, contains the sequence for enkephalin.

nociceptive receptors, such as mechanoreceptors. Touch and pressure input travels to the cord over large myelinated fibers and to the cortex by a dorsal column–medial lemniscus–thalamus–cortex pathway (see Fig. 4-6). It serves to localize the stimulus, including associated nociceptive input. Nociceptive signals travel by A-delta and unmyelinated C fibers to Lissauer's tract in the apex of the dorsal horn. There they bifurcate into short neurons and ascend or descend one or two segments before synapsing in the SG (lamina II). Cells of laminae I, IV, V, and perhaps VI respond to nociceptive stimulation. Neurons in laminae V and VI project axons to the contralateral cord, which ascend as the anterolateral tract. Some lamina V cells send axons to the ipsilateral anterolateral tract.

Evidence suggests that the spinothalamic system is composed of two divisions, the neospinothalamic tract and the paleospinothalamic tract. The neospinothalamic tract is located laterally and is a more recent evolutionary development. It is composed of myelinated fibers that project directly to the ventrolateral and posterior thalamus, where they synapse. The third-order neuron then projects to the somatosensory cortex. Nociceptive input traveling over this pathway is perceived as sharp, well-localized pain with little or no accompanying affective component and a short latency between stimulus and perception. It travels over larger pain fibers (*e.g.,* A-delta fibers). The paleospinothalamic tract, on the other hand, is located medially and is an evolutionarily older pathway. It is composed of more unmyelinated fibers that make many synapses, so that input travels more slowly than in the neospinothalamic tract. The paleospinothalamic tract projects to the reticular formation (especially the nucleus RgC), to the lateral pons, to the limbic midbrain area, and then to the intralaminar thalamic nuclei. Fibers then continue rostrally and synapse ultimately with neurons in the hypothalamus, in the limbic forebrain structures, and with diffuse projections to many other parts of the brain. Nociceptive input traveling over this pathway is perceived as diffuse, poorly localized pain, with a strong affective component and a long latency between stimulus and perception. The paleospinothalamic tract mediates suprasegmental reflex responses, such as autonomic responses, as well as affective phenomena associated with pain. It is the more important system with respect to clinical pain states.

Nociceptive input to the medullary reticular formation, thalamus, cortex, and limbic regions activates neurons that feed back to the PAG integration center. The PAG in turn provides input to the NRM and the adjacent nucleus Rmc (see Fig. 4-6). Each sends nerve fibers to the dorsal horn through the dorsal lateral funiculus fiber tract. These fibers presynaptically inhibit the nociceptive T cells in laminae I and V of the dorsal horn. As the paleospinothalamic tract ascends rostrally, it synapses and activates the nucleus Rgc in the medulla. The nucleus Rgc sends projections to the PAG and to the NRM. In some manner it also activates the DRM. The DRM (another reticular formation nucleus) forms a portion of the ascending serotoninergic pathway that eventually excites neurons in the hypothalamus, limbic forebrain areas, frontal cortex, and septum. Presumably, the DRM contributes to affective, memory, sensory, autonomic, and somatic motor responses to pain. Descending output from these areas impinges on the PAG, thus modulating nociceptive input originating at spinal cord levels. The nature of modulation depends on the integration of ongoing activity in these areas.

■ CLINICAL APPLICATIONS

Because of the knowledge of the gate theory and the central modulation of pain, clinical applications can be made with variable success. It has been known for centuries that counterirritants such as heat and massage reduce pain. More modern counterirritant techniques, such as transcutaneous nerve stimulation and dorsal column stimulation, may also relieve pain in patients with certain pain problems. All of these techniques stimulate pressure and touch receptors that send information to the dorsal horn through large, myelinated fibers. This large-fiber input leads to partial or complete inhibition of nociceptive T-cell firing, and therefore to less transmission of nociceptive input to higher brain centers by way of segmental modulation.[53]

Some reports suggest that acupuncture-induced analgesia may be reversed by naloxone.[52,86] Generally, it is speculated that the opiate-system activation is involved in acupuncture analgesia, although some studies cast doubt on this.[51,52] It should be noted that acupuncture points, "trigger points," and motor points coincide closely; perhaps they are simply convenient sites for eventual activation of PAG and descending inhibition of nociceptive input by peripheral stimulation.

Behavior modification approaches to management of chronic pain patients often result in decreased pain behavior (fewer complaints, reduced drug dependency), increased activity level, and often a return to a more acceptable life-style.[31,68] Increasing activity, ignoring pain complaints, and replacing old behaviors with new ones may all lead to stimulation of the PAG and, therefore, activate the central descending pathway that inhibits nociceptive input at the spinal cord level. Increasing activity also increases large-fiber input. This may balance small-fiber nociceptive input and lead to inhibition of the nociceptive T cell in lamina V of the dorsal horn. However, many patients with chronic pain have symptoms with apparently minimal somatic contribution but excessive affective components. After behavior modification many patients claim that their pain is the same, even though they are now able to engage in more activities and lead a more normal life. It is likely that more complex pathways are involved than have yet been described.

As more research is done, the evidence becomes highly suggestive that little difference exists between the biological substrate and clinical manifestations of chronic pain and depression. Researchers have measured serotonin levels in severely depressed and suicidal patients and have found them to be markedly reduced. Remember that serotonin inhibitors administered to human subjects lead to hyperalgesia and spontaneous pain syndromes.[3,51] Decreased serotonin levels block morphine effects and SPA in laboratory animals.[29] Patients with chronic pain and depression often behave similarly. Both are generally less active, have altered appetite and sleep patterns, lose motivational and sexual drives, and may become self-abusive.[31] Perhaps the same component of the nociceptive system is involved in both kinds of patients. This may explain why patients with chronic pain exhibit "depressive behaviors," and why depressed patients frequently complain of pain. Interestingly, tricyclic drugs, which inhibit serotonin depletion, have been found to be useful in treating depression as well as chronic pain. This suggests that serotoninergic pathways may be important in both disorders.

Of primary importance clinically is the understanding that pain involves much more than a simple relay of sensory input. Culture, past experience, emotional state, personality, motivation, role expectations, and learned behavior can all contribute to modulation of nociceptive stimuli and can influence the final pain experience. Persons with a strong will to complete a task (*e.g.*, athlete, soldier) undoubtedly receive a barrage of nociceptive input, but pain, suffering, or pain behavior may not accompany nociceptive input, presumably because segmental or central modulation creates a relatively analgesic state. On the other hand, pain can occur without nociceptive input, just as suffering, depression, grief, or other affective phenomena associated with pain can occur without pain or nociception. Many patients exhibit pain behaviors when nociception is no longer present. For clinicians treating patients with pain problems, it is essential to understand the nociceptive process and to consider possible contributing factors affecting nociceptive input. For this purpose, patient history and evaluation are invaluable. The patient with musculoskeletal pain may also be depressed, lonely, have a drug or alcohol problem, or be going through a difficult adjustment period. The clinician must consider these possibilities

when the treatment program is established, as well as provide the appropriate treatment and all other necessary resources to enable the patient to deal with the pain problem most effectively.

◼ GENERAL CONSIDERATIONS OF THE PATIENT IN PAIN

▢ Acute Versus Chronic Pain

Melzack and Wall[59] described three different types of pain based on a time dimension: transient, acute, and chronic pain. Transient pain is typically associated with minimal tissue change. There are two components of transient pain: the sensory and localizing perception followed by the dull, suffering component.

ACUTE PAIN

Acute pain, or pain that persists beyond a few minutes, is a signal of real or impending tissue damage and is the type of pain experienced with a fracture. In an acute pain situation, the perceived stimulus requires either avoidance of the situation or some actual attempt to protect oneself through fight ("fight-or-flee" response).[59] This fight or flight response may actually serve survival needs (see Fig. 8-3).[34]

In addition to the sensory and affective component, acute pain is usually characterized by anxiety. Autonomic changes associated with acute pain include (1) increased systolic and diastolic blood pressure, (2) tachycardia, (3) decrease in gut motility and salivatory flow, (4) increased striated muscle tension, (5) the release of catecholamines, and (6) pupil dilatation.[32,73] These autonomic changes are also consistent with the stress response as described by Cannon.[22] Acute pain appears concurrently with either tissue damage or stress and generally disappears with healing.[16,85]

Acute pain is also a psychological experience that is interpreted in the context of one's experience, cultural background, and environment. Expectations involving the pain typically are positive, since the pain is expected to diminish over time.

CHRONIC PAIN

Chronic benign pain, on the other hand, is pain that persists beyond the expected recovery time. Some clinicians use the arbitrary figure of 6 months to designate pain as chronic.[31,73] The taxonomy of the International Association for the Study of Pain has stipulated an arbitrary time (3 months) beyond which pain is not to be expected and is thus considered chronic.[40]

According to Melzack and Wall,[59] chronic pain is frequently characterized by feelings of depression. It has long been hypothesized that pain and depression are related, although the exact relationship is not understood.[19] Patients with chronic pain display disrupted interpersonal relationships and increased preoccupation with somatic symptoms such as disturbances in sleep, appetite, and libido.

Whereas acute pain indicates tissue damage, chronic pain is less likely to accurately signal ongoing or new tissue damage. Attempts to stabilize chronic pain through rest or the fight-or-flight response are frequently misdirected.[19]

Whereas acute pain encompasses the expected physiologic consequences of nociceptive nervous system activation by an appropriate stimulus, chronic pain becomes disassociated from many of the physiologic evidences of nociception. Thus, the essential criteria of chronic pain are related to the cognitive-behavioral aspects, rather than any nociceptive component.[65,78]

Chronic pain may be caused by chronic pathologic processes in somatic structures or viscera, by prolonged dysfunction of parts of the peripheral or central nervous system, or by both.[15] In contrast to acute pain, chronic pain can also be caused by operant environmental factors and psychopathology. Patients with chronic pain cannot be treated by the modalities and interventions that are appropriate for patients with acute pain. The chronicity of pain itself imposes other components, including psychological, emotional, and sociological impact, which must become part of the treatment.

☐ Characteristics of Chronic Pain

Before proceeding to an outline of the examination of the patient with pain (see Chapter 5, Assessment of Musculoskeletal Disorders and Concepts of Management), it is important to briefly review the general categories of pain, which are often characterized by the location, distribution, and quality of the sensation. It should be noted that these categories overlap.

NOCICEPTIVE (SOMATIC) VERSUS DEAFFERENTATION PAIN

Nociceptive (somatic) pain is sensation referable to ongoing tissue damage detected by thermal receptors and mechanoreceptors leading to A-gamma and C-fiber axons (see earlier text).

It is generally accepted that chronic pain is sustained by central neural pathways that differ significantly from those pathways that signal and provide awareness of acute noxious stimuli.[74] Chronic pain that is secondary to neural trauma is often termed *deafferentation pain*. It is not associated in any consistent fashion with lesions of specific tracts or with lesions at specific levels in the spinal tract.[28] It is believed that deafferentation pain is a consequence of reverberating neuronal circuits set up by hyperactive pools of neurons which, in fact, may be quite remote from the original lesions.[56,75]

The terms patients use to describe their pain are more often variable in cases of deafferentation (*e.g.*, "burning," "crawling," "cold," "gnawing") than in cases of nociception.[28] Deep somatic pain is dull, diffuse, and poorly localized. Both deafferentation and nociceptive pains may be increased by stress and improved with relaxation (see Chapter 8, Relaxation and Related Techniques).

REFERRED PAIN

Referred pain is referred from deep somatic or visceral structures to a distant region within the same neural segment, with or without hyperalgesia and hyperesthesia, deep tenderness, muscle spasms, and autonomic disturbance. No changes are seen in reflexes, and there are no muscle weakness disturbances. Common examples of referred pain include cervical spine disease with referral of sensation to the retro-orbital area and angina referred to the left arm or jaw.

PROJECTED (TRANSMITTED OR TRANSFERRED) PAIN

Projected pain is perceived to be transmitted along the course of a nerve either with a segmental (dermatomal and sclerotomal) or a peripheral distribution, depending on the site of the lesion.[16] Examples of projected pain with segmental distribution are the radiculopathy caused by disease (*i.e.*, herpes zoster) or an intervertebral disk protrusion involving the nerve root or trunk before it divides into its major peripheral branches. Examples of projected pain with peripheral distribution include trigeminal neuralgia, brachial plexus neuralgia, and meralgia paresthetica.

REFLEX PAIN (SYMPATHETIC OR CAUSALGIC PAIN)

Reflex pain is marked by striking hyperalgesia and hyperesthesia as well as vasomotor, sudomotor, and trophic changes. It does not conform to any segmental or peripheral nerve distribution, often involving an entire limb. Major syndromes in this category are reflex sympathetic dystrophies and causalgia. The involved extremity may be so sensitive that it is held immobile, eventually undergoing atrophy and osteoporosis.[28]

☐ Nonorganic Pain
(Psychological Factors
Affecting Pain Sensation)

The location and distribution of pain caused primarily by psychological or psychiatric disorders usually do not fit the normal neuroanatomical patterns. Examples include pain with glove or stocking distribution, pain involving the entire body, and various pains scattered all over the body.[16] Painful sensation in central, segmental, or peripheral distribution may be related to anxiety states, depression, conversion syndromes, and somatization disorders.[28]

These complaints may or may not be associated with somatic or autonomic changes. Such complaints often mimic deafferentation or nociceptive pain and thus greatly complicate the diagnostic process.

☐ Subjective Findings

Subjective findings to help determine the nature and extent of the lesion and the resultant degree of disability include the quality and intensity of pain (*e.g.*, sharp, dull, burning, excruciating). The quality of pain (as emphasized in Chapter 5, Assessment of Musculoskeletal Disorders and Concepts of Management) is a distinguishing characteristic, because it indicates whether the causative factor is superficial or deep. The severity or intensity of pain is another important characteristic. In the usual clinical setting the patient is asked to rate the pain intensity on a numerical scale of 0 to 10 (0 being no pain and 10 being the most severe or intolerable pain imaginable). Verbal descriptor scales and visual analog scales are also used.[23] There are a number of scales that use happy–sad faces to measure pain.[25] The face scale is often used with small children.

Pain is the number one reason people seek physician care. Thirty-three percent of people in industrialized countries suffer from some form of pain.[19] Of these, one half to two thirds are partially or totally disabled for periods of days, weeks, months, or permanently. Despite the frequency of pain and its significant impact on society, controversy remains about its assessment and treatment. A subjective experience, pain eludes precise measurement and successful treatment.

Chronic pain is difficult to treat and is best managed by prevention. It is important to identify patients with chronic pain early and to assist in directing them to a multidisciplinary team for more effective treatment. These patients present with problems both unique and universal. The challenge to the therapist lies in altering a patient's perception of the experience and the enhancing sense of coping with it.

☐ Glossary of Acryonyms

ACTH	Adrenocorticotropin
CNS	Central nervous system
DLF	Dorsolateral funiculus
DRM	Dorsal raphe magnus
LC	Locus ceruleus
NRM	Nucleus raphe magnus
PAG	Periaqueductal gray matter
***p*-CPA**	*p*-chlorophenylalanine
RgC	Nucleus reticularis gigantocellularis
Rmc	Nucleus reticularis magnocellularis
SG	Substantia gelatinosa
SPA	Stimulus produced analgesia

REFERENCES

1. Adams JE: Naloxone reversal of analgesia produced by brain stimulation in the human. Pain 2:161–166, 1976
2. Akil H, Liebeskind JC: Monoaminergic mechanisms of stimulation-produced analgesia. Brain Res 94:279–296, 1975
3. Akil H, Mayer DJ: Antagonisms of stimulation-produced analgesia by p-CPA, a serotonin synthesis inhibitor. Brain Res 44:692–697, 1972
4. Akil H, Mayer DJ, Liebeskind JC: Antagonism of stimulation-produced analgesia by naloxone, a narcotic antagonist. Science 191:961–962, 1976
5. Akil H, Richardson DE, Hughes J, Barchas JD: Enkephalin-like material elevated in ventricular cerebrospinal fluid of pain patients after analgetic focal stimulation. Science 201:463–465, 1978
6. Algom D: Psychophysical analysis of pain: A functional prospective. In Geissler HG, Link SW, Townsend JT (eds): Cognition Information Processing, and Psychophysics: Basic Issues, pp 267–291. Hilldale, NJ, Lawrence Erlbaum, 1992
7. Almay BG, Johansson F, Von Knorring L, Terenius L, Wahlstrom A: Endorphins in chronic pain: Differences in CSF endorphin levels between organic and psychogenic pain syndromes. Pain 5:153–162, 1978
8. Anderson SD, Bausbaum AI, Fields HL: Responses of medullary raphe neurons to peripheral stimulation and to systemic opiates. Brain Res 123:363–368, 1977
9. Balagura S, Ralph T: The analgesic effect of electrical stimulation of the diencephalon and mesencephalon. Brain Res 60:369–381, 1973
10. Barnes DC, Fung SJ, Adams WL: Inhibitory effects of substantia nigra on impulse transmission from nociceptors. Pain 6:207–215, 1979
11. Basbaum AI, Marley N, O'Keefe J: Effects of spinal cord lesions on the analgesic properties of electrical brain stimulation. Presented at a symposium held at the First World Congress on Pain. Advances in Pain Research, p 268, 1975
12. Basbaum AI, Marley N, O'Keefe J, Clanton C: Reversal of morphine and stimulus-produced analgesia by subtotal spinal cord lesions. Pain 3:43–56, 1977
13. Black RG: The chronic pain syndrome. Surg Clin North Am 55:999–1011, 1975
14. Bonica JJ: Neurophysiologic and pathologic aspects of acute and chronic pain. Arch Surg 112:750–761, 1977
15. Bonica JJ: Definitions and taxonomy of pain. In Bonica JJ (ed): The Management of Pain, pp 18–27. Philadelphia, Lea & Febiger, 1990
16. Bonica JJ, Loeser JD: Medical evaluation of the patient with pain. In Bonica JJ (ed): The Management of Pain, 2nd ed, pp 563–579. Philadelphia, Lea & Febiger, 1990
17. Bowsher D: Role of the reticular formation in responses to noxious stimulation. Pain 2:361–378, 1976
18. Buchsbaum MS, Davis GC, Bunney WE: Naloxone alters pain perception and somatosensory evoked potentials in normal subjects. Nature 270:620–622, 1977
19. Buckelew SP, Frank RG: Psychological factors and treatment of pain. In Kaplan PE, Tanner ED: Musculoskeletal Pain and Disability, pp 243–257. Norwalk, CT, Appleton & Lange, 1989
20. Buscher HH, Hill RC, Romer D, Cardinaux F, Closse A, Hauser D, Pless J: Evidence for analgesic activity of enkephalin in the mouse. Nature 261:423–425, 1976
21. Callaghan M, Sternback RA, Nyquist JK, Timmermans G: Changes in somatic sensitivity during transcutaneous electrical analgesia. Pain 5:115–127, 1978
22. Cannon WB: Bodily Changes in Pain, Hunger, Fear and Rage. New York, Appleton, 1929
23. Chapman CR, Syrjala K: Measurement of pain. In Bonica JJ (ed): The Management of Pain, 2nd ed, pp 580–594. Philadelphia, Lea & Febiger, 1990
24. Clark WC, Hunt HF: Pain. In Downey J, Darling R (eds): Physiological Basis of Rehabilitation Medicine, pp 373–401. Philadelphia, WB Saunders, 1971
25. Desparmet-Sheridan JF: Pain in children. In Prithvi Raj P: Practical Management of Pain, 2nd ed, pp 343–366. St Louis, Mosby Year Book, 1992
26. Duggan AW, Griersmith BT: Inhibition of spinal transmission of nociceptive information by supraspinal stimulation in the cat. Pain 6:149–161, 1979
27. Dworkin SF, von Korff MR, Le Resche L: Epidemiologic studies of chronic pain: A dynamic-ecologic perspective. Ann Behav Med 14:3–11, 1992
28. Erickson RK: The physical examination of the patient in pain. In Camic PM, Brown FD; Assessing Chronic Pain: A Multidisciplinary Clinic Handbook, pp 20–46. New York, Springer-Verlag, 1989
29. Fennessy MR, Lee JR: Modification of morphine analgesia by drugs affecting adrenergic and tryptaminergic mechanisms. J Pharm Pharmacol 22:930–935, 1978

30. Fields HL, Anderson SD: Evidence that raphe-spinal neurons mediate opiate and midbrain stimulation-produced analgesias. Pain 5:333–349, 1978
31. Fordyce WE: Behavioral Methods for Chronic Pain and Illness. St Louis, CV Mosby, 1976
32. France RD, Houpt JL: Chronic pain: Update from Duke Medical Center. Gen Hosp Psychiatry 6:37–41, 1984
33. Gamsa A, Vikis-Freibergs V: Psychological events are both risk factors in, and consequences of, chronic pain. Pain 44:271–277, 1991
34. Gellhorn E: Principles of Autonomic-Somatic Interactions. Minneapolis, University of Minnesota Press, 1967
35. Guilbaud G, Peschanski M, Gautron M, Binder D: Neurons responding to noxious stimulation in VB complex and caudal adjacent regions in the thalamus of the rat. Pain 8:303–318, 1980
36. Guillemin R: Beta-lipotropin and endorphins: Implications of current knowledge. Hosp Pract 13(11):53–60, 1978
37. Henry JL, Sessle BJ, Lucier GE, Hu JW: Effects of substance P on nociceptive and nonnociceptive trigeminal brain stem neurons. Pain 8:33–45, 1980
38. Hughes J, Smith TW, Kosterlitz HW, Fothergill LA, Morgan BA, Morris HR: Identification of two related pentapeptides from the brain with potent opiate agonist activity. Nature 258:577–579, 1975
39. Inman VT, Saunders JB: Referred pain from skeletal structures. J Nerv Ment Dis 99:660–667, 1944
40. International Association for the Study of Pain: Classification of chronic pain: Description of chronic pain syndromes and definitions of pain states. In Merskey H (ed): Pain (Suppl 3), S1, 1986
41. Johansson F, Von Knorring L: A double-blind controlled study of a serotonin uptake inhibitor (Zimelidine) versus placebo in chronic pain patients. Pain 7:69–78, 1979
42. Jordan LM, Kenshalo DR, Martin RF, Haber LH, Willis WD: Depression of primate spinothalamic tract neurons by iontophoretic application of 5-hydroxytryptamine. Pain 5:135–142, 1978
43. Kellgren JH: On the distribution of pain arising from deep somatic structures with charts of segmental pain areas. Clin Sci 4:35–46, 1939
44. Kellgren JH, Samuel EP: The sensitivity and innervation of the articular capsule. J Bone Joint Surg 32(B):84–92, 1950
45. Kerr FW, Wilson PR: Pain. Annu Rev Neurosci 1:83–102, 1978
46. Leavitt F, Garron DC: Psychological disturbance and pain report differences in both organic and non-organic low back pain patients. Pain 7:178–195, 1979
47. Lindblom U, Tegner R: Are the endorphins active in clinical pain states? Narcotic antagonism in chronic pain patients. Pain 7:65–68, 1979
48. Loeser JD, Black RG: A taxonomy of pain. Pain 1:81–84, 1975
49. Mayer DJ, Liebeskind JC: Pain reduction by focal electrical stimulation of the brain: An anatomical and behavioral analysis. Brain Res 68:73–93, 1974
50. Mayer DJ, Murphin R: Stimulation-produced analgesia (SPA) and morphine analgesia: Cross tolerance from application at the same brain site. Fed Proc 35:385, 1976
51. Mayer DJ, Price DD: Central nervous system mechanisms of analgesia. Pain 2:379–404, 1976
52. Mayer DJ, Price DD, Rafii A, Barber J: Acupuncture hypalgesia: Evidence for activation of a central control system as a mechanism of action. In Proceedings of the First World Congress in Pain. New York, Raven Press, 1976
53. Mayer DJ, Wolfe TL, Akil H, Carder B, Liebeskind JC: Analgesia from electrical stimulation in the brain stem of the rat. Science 174:1351–1354, 1971
54. Melzack R: The gate theory revisited. In LeRoy PL (ed): Current Concepts in the Management of Chronic Pain. Miami, Symposia Specialists, 1977
55. Melzack R: Neurophysiological foundation of pain. In Sternbach RA (ed): The Psychology of Pain, pp 1–24. New York, Raven Press, 1986
56. Melzack R, Loeser JD: Phantom body pain in paraplegics: Evidence for a central pain generating mechanism for pain. Pain 4:198–210, 1978
57. Melzack R, Wall PD: On the nature of cutaneous sensory mechanisms. Brain 85:331–356, 1962
58. Melzack R, Wall PD: Pain mechanisms: A new theory. Science 150:971–979, 1965
59. Melzack R, Wall PD: The Challenge of Pain. New York, Basic Books, Inc, 1982
60. Messing RB, Lytle LD: Serotonin-containing neurons: Their possible role in pain and analgesia. Pain 4:1–21, 1977
61. Millan MJ, Przewlocki R, Herz A: A non-β-endorphin adenohypophyseal mechanism is essential for an analgesic response to stress. Pain 8:343–353, 1980
62. Nathan PW: The gate-control theory of pain—A critical review. Brain 99:123–158, 1976
63. Oleson TD, Twombly DA, Liebeskind JC: Effects of pain-attenuating brain stimulation and morphine on electrical activity in the raphe nuclei of the awake rat. Pain 4:211–230, 1978
64. Oliveras JL, Woda A, Guilbaud G, Besson JM: Analgesia induced by electrical stimulation of the inferior centralis of the raphe in the cat. Pain 1:139–145, 1975
65. Pilowsky I: Abnormal illness behaviour (dysnosognosia). Psychother Psychosom 46:76–84, 1986
66. Proudfit HK, Anderson ED: Morphine analgesia: Blockade by raphe magnus lesions. Brain Res 98:612–618, 1975
67. Rhodes DL: Periventricular system lesions and stimulation-produced analgesia. Pain 7:51–63, 1979
68. Roberts AH, Reinhardt L: The behavioral management of chronic pain: Long-term follow-up with comparison groups. Pain 8:151–162, 1980
69. Ruby TE, Terns RD, Turk DC: Chronic pain and depression toward a cognitive behavioral mediation model. Pain 35:129–140, 1988
70. Sinclair DC, Weddell G, Feindel WH: Referred pain and associated phenomena. Brain 7:184–211, 1948
71. Snyder SH: Opiate receptors and internal opiates. Sci Am 240(3):44–56, 1977
72. Stacher G, Bauer P, Steinringer A, Schreiber E, Schmierer G: Effects of the synthetic enkephalin analogue FK 33-824 on pain threshold and pain tolerance in man. Pain 7:159–172, 1979
73. Sternbach RA: Pain Patients: Traits and Treatment. New York, Academic Press, 1974
74. Sweet WH: Central mechanisms of chronic pain. In Bonica JJ (ed): Pain, vol 58. New York, Raven Press, 1980
75. Tasker RR, Tsuda T, Hawrylyshyn P: Clinical neurophysiological investigation of deafferentation pain. In Bonica JJ, Linblom U, Iggo A, et al (eds): Advances in Pain Research and Therapy, vol 5, pp 731–738. New York, Raven Press, 1983

76. Turk DC, Flor H: Pain: pain behaviors: the utility and limitations of the behavior construct. Pain 31:277–295, 1987
77. Turk DC, Rudy TE: Cognitive factors and persistent pain: A glimpse into Pandora's box. Cognitive Therapy and Research 16:99–122, 1992
78. Turk DC, Rudy TE: A cognitive-behavioral perspective on chronic pain: Beyond the scalpel and syringe. In Tollison CD (ed): Handbook of Pain Management, 2nd ed, pp 136–151. Baltimore, Williams & Wilkins, 1994
79. Wall PD: The gate control theory of pain mechanisms—A re-examination and restatement. Brain 101:1–18, 1978
80. Weddell G, Palmer E, Pallie W: Nerve endings in mammalian skin. Biol Rev 30:159–193, 1954
81. Weisenberg M: Pain and pain control. Psychol Bull 84:1008–1044, 1977
82. Weisenberg M: Pain and pain control. In Daitzman R (ed): Diagnosis and Intervention in Behavior Therapy and Behavioral Medicine, p 90–149. New York, Springer, 1983
83. Weisenberg M: Psychological intervention for the control of pain. Behav Res Ther 25:301–312, 1987
84. Weisenberg M: Cognitive aspects of pain. In Wall PD, Melzack R (eds): Textbook of Pain, 3rd ed, pp 275–289. Edinburgh, Churchill Livingstone, 1994
85. Wu WH (ed): Pain Management. Assessment and Treatment of Chronic and Acute Syndromes. New York: Human Sciences Press, 1987
86. Wyke B: Neurological mechanisms in the experience of pain. Acupunct Electrother Res Int J 4:27–35, 1979
87. Yaksh TL, Ruby TA: Narcotic analgetics: CNS sites and mechanisms of action as revealed by intracerebral injections techniques. Pain 4:299–359, 1978
88. Yeung JC, Yaksh TL, Ruby TA: Concurrent mapping of brain sites for sensitivity to the direct application of morphine and focal electrical stimulation in the production of antinociception in the rat. Pain 4:23–40, 1977

RECOMMENDED READINGS

Adler M: Endorphins, enkephalins and neurotransmitters. Medical Times 110:32–37, 1982
Aronoff GM (ed): Evaluation and Treatment of Chronic Pain, 3rd ed. Baltimore, Williams & Wilkins, 1992
Basbaum AI, Fields HL: Endogenous pain control systems: Brainstem spinal pathways and endorphin circuitry. Ann Rev Neurosci 7:309–338, 1984
Bond MR: Pain: Its Nature, Analysis and Treatment. New York, Churchill Livingstone, 1984
Bonica JJ (ed): The Management of Pain, vols 1–2. Philadelphia, Lea & Febiger, 1990
Burrows GD, Elton D, Stanley V (eds): Handbook of Chronic Pain Management. Amsterdam, Elsevier, 1987
Caillet R: Pain Mechanisms and Management. Philadelphia, FA Davis, 1993
Camic PM, Brown FD (eds): Assessing Chronic Pain: A Multidisciplinary Clinic Handbook. New York, Springer Verlag, 1989
Chapman CR, Turner JA: Psychological control of acute pain in medical setting. J Pain Symptom Management 1(1):9–20, 1986
Cousins MJ, Bridenbaugh PO: Neural Blockade in Clinical Anesthesia and Management of Pain, 2nd ed. Philadelphia, JB Lippincott, 1988
Dubner R, Bennett GJ: Spinal and trigeminal mechanisms of nociception. Ann Rev Neurosci 6:381–418, 1983
Echtenach JL (ed): Pain. New York, Churchill Livingstone, 1987
Edmeads J: The physiology of pain: A review. Prog Neuropsychopharmacol Biol Psychiatr 7:413–419, 1983
Feinstein B, Langton NJ, Jameson RM, Schiller F: Experiments on pain referred from deep somatic tissues. J Bone Joint Surg 36(A):981–997, 1954
Fields HL: Pain. New York, McGraw-Hill, 1987
Fields HL, Dubner FC, Jones LE (eds): Advances in Pain Research and Therapy, vol 9. New York, Raven Press, 1984
Fields HL, Heinricher MM: Anatomy and physiology of a nociceptive modulatory system. Philos Trans R Soc London [Biol] 13:361–374, 1985
Fordyce WE: Evaluating and managing chronic pain. Geriatrics 33:59–62, 1978
France RD, Krishnam KRR: Chronic Pain. Washington, DC, American Psychiatric Press, 1988
Grieves GP: The autonomic nervous system in vertebral pain syndromes. In Grieves GP (ed): Modern Manual Therapy of the Vertebral Column. New York, Churchill Livingstone, 1986
Grieves GP: Referred pain and other clinical features. In Grieves GP (ed): Modern Manual Therapy of the Vertebral Column, 2nd ed. New York, Churchill Livingstone, 1988
Headley BJ: Chronic pain management. In O'Sullivan SB, Schmitz TJ (eds): Physical Rehabilitation: Assessment and Treatment, 3rd ed, pp 577–602. Philadelphia, FA Davis, 1994
Jensen, TS: Endogenous antinociceptive systems: Studies on spinal and supraspinal modulating mechanism with particular reference to monoaminergic and opioid systems. Acta Neurol Psychol (Suppl) 108: 1–51, 1986
Lewis T, Kellgran JH: Observation relating to referred pain, visceromotor reflexes and other associated phenomena. Clin Sci 49:470–471, 1939
Lundberg TCM: Vibratory stimulation for the alleviation of chronic pain. Acta Physiol Scand (Suppl 523), 1983
Mannheimer JS: Clinical Transcutaneous Electrical Nerve Stimulation. Philadelphia, FA Davis, 1984
McCormack GL: Pain management by occupational therapists. Am J Occup Ther 42:582–590, 1988
Melzack R: Myofascial trigger points: Relation to acupuncture and mechanisms of pain. Arch Phys Med Rehab 62:114–117, 1981
Melzack R: Pain Measurements and Assessment. New York, Raven Press, 1983
Merskey H: Classification of Chronic Pain: Description of Chronic Pain Syndromes and Definitions of Pain Terms. Amsterdam, Elsevier, 1986
Nigl AJ: Biofeedback and Behavioral Strategies in Pain Treatment. New York, SP Medical and Scientific Books, 1984
Paklovitz M: Distributions of neuropeptides in central nervous system: Biochemical mapping studies. Prog Neurobiol 23:151–189, 1984
Prithvi Raj P: Practical Management of Pain. St Louis, Mosby Year Book, 1992

Prithvi Raj P: Practical Management of Pain: With Special Emphasis on Physiology of Pain Management, 2nd ed. Chicago, Year Book Medical Publishers, 1992

Procacci P, Maresca M, Zoppi M: Visceral and deep somatic pain. Acupunct Electrother Res Int J 3:135–160, 1978

Ruda MA, Bennett GJ, Dubner R: Neurochemistry and neural circuitry in the dorsal horn. Prog Brain Res 66:219–268, 1986

Sternbach R (ed): The Psychology of Pain, 2nd ed. New York, Raven Press, 1986

Terman G, Shavit Y, Lewis J, Cannon T, Liebeskind M: Intrinsic mechanisms of pain inhibition: Activated by stress. Science 226:1270–1278, 1984

Tiengo M, et al (eds): Pain and Mobility. Advances in Pain Research and Therapy, vol 10. New York, Raven Press, 1987

Tollison CD, Satterthwaite JR, Tollison JW (eds): Handbook of Pain Management, 2nd ed. Baltimore, Williams & Wilkins, 1994

Turk D, Meichenbaum D, Genest M: Pain and Behavioral Medicine. A Cognitive-Behavioral Perspective. New York, Guilford Press, 1983

Wall PD, Melzack R (eds): The Textbook of Pain, 3rd ed. Edinburgh, Churchill Livingstone, 1994

Warfield RA: Manual of Pain Management. Philadelphia, JB Lippincott, 1991

Watson J: Pain and nociception—mechanism and modulation. In Grieve GP (ed): Modern Manual Therapy of the Vertebral Column. New York, Churchill Livingstone, 1986

Well PE, Frampton V, Bowster D (eds): Pain Management in Physical Therapy. Norwalk, CT, Appleton and Lange, 1988

Willis WD: The pain system: The neural basis of nociceptive transmission in the mammalian nervous system. Pain Headache 8:1–346, 1985

Assessment of Musculoskeletal Disorders and Concepts of Management

DARLENE HERTLING AND RANDOLPH M. KESSLER

■ RATIONALE

A comprehensive examination is, without question, the most important step in the physical therapist's management of patients with common musculoskeletal disorders. The physical therapist's role is to clarify the nature and extent of the lesion, to assess the extent of the resulting disability, and to record significant data in order to establish a basis against which to judge progress. These activities must not be confused with or mistaken for the physician's diagnosis. A diagnosis, in addition to clinical evaluation, often requires the use and interpretation of laboratory tests, roentgenograms, and other data employing skills and knowledge not included in the physical therapist's training. A diagnosis must *differentiate* a particular disease state from other possible causes of the symptoms and signs. The therapist, in performing a *clarifying* examination, is not concerned with such differen-

tiation but with collecting qualitative and quantitative data on the existing lesion.

Diagnosis by a therapist means naming or labeling the movement dysfunction or problem that is the object of therapy treatment.[9,72] Diagnostic labeling is the result of the systematic analysis and grouping of the clinical manifestations of the patient.[5,23,38,70,72] Sahrmann[72] suggests the focus of such classification should be on the primary dysfunction identified in the physical therapy evaluation. Jette[38] suggests that diagnostic categories should include physical impairment and functional disabilities based on the International Classification of Impairments, Disabilities, and Handicaps (ICIDH).[36] Both qualitative and quantitative data on the existing lesion are used so as to judge how best to apply certain treatment procedures and to assess their effectiveness.

Consider the case of a patient referred to a therapist with the diagnosis of "shoulder tendinitis." This is a condition easily managed by physical therapy over a relatively short period of time. However, in order for an effective program to be instituted, several features of the problem must be clarified. The therapist must determine which tendon is at fault in order to know where to direct treatment and at what site on the tendon the lesion exists. Assessment of the lesion's chronicity will influence the choice of treatment procedures and their application. It is important to know whether secondary problems such as stiffness or weakness exist; if so, they must be dealt with as well. The therapist must obtain information concerning the possible behavioral effects of the lesion. Are the conditions accompanying the problem reinforcing in any way to the patient's disease behaviors or is the patient "highly motivated"? Daily activities must be assessed not only to determine the existence of any functional deficit but also to judge whether any present activity will aggravate or prolong the condition. Generally, such information does not accompany the referral, but it is precisely this information that is required in order to institute an effective treatment program. The physical therapist must perform a thorough initial examination on every patient to be treated.

As mentioned, information collected as part of the initial examination is used to set a baseline against which to judge progress and to assess the effectiveness of treatment. Therefore, the therapist not only must perform a complete initial examination but also must assess certain key signs before, during, and after each treatment session. In this way the clinician can determine whether, in fact, a particular procedure is effective and can quantitatively document the patient's progress. Progress must be judged on objective evidence. The patient's subjective report of the degree of pain must be considered but not dwelt on; in itself, it is not a valid measurement of progress. Instead, the therapist should be able to inform the patient as to whether the condition has improved. Treatment sessions should begin less often with, "Hello, Mrs. Jones. How is your back today?" but rather with, "Hello, Mrs. Jones. Let's take a look at your back to see how it's doing." This approach is possible only after complete initial examination and continued assessment of objective signs.

There are, of course, several approaches to patient examination.[14,32,41,42,54,55,58,59,61,62,80] Included in this group are Cyriax,[14] Kaltenborn,[41,42] Maitland,[54,55] McKenzie,[58,59] and Stoddard.[80] Their approaches are frequently used by manual therapists to assess and treat muscle and joint problems. Regardless of which system is selected for assessment, the examiner should establish a sequential method to ensure that no crucial test or step is omitted, which may prevent accurate interpretation. Perhaps no one has contributed more to systematization of soft-tissue examination than James Cyriax.[14] His approach involves observation, subjective examination (patient's history), objective examination (utilization of movements and special tests to elicit signs and symptoms of injury), palpation of soft tissues, and neurological testing.[14]

One of the more common assessment recording methods used today is the problem-oriented medical records method, which uses "S.O.A.P." notes.[45,50,92] S.O.A.P. stands for the four parts of the assessment—Subjective (patient history), Objective, Assessment, and Plan. Progress notes and the discharge summary should also follow the S.O.A.P. format and in combination with the initial examination, assessment, and treatment plan, they become the complete record for most patients. The assessment includes professional judgments about the subjective and/or objective findings formulated into both long-term and short-term goals.

■ HISTORY

To help determine the nature and extent of the lesion and the resultant degree of disability, the clinician must gather data from the patient that cannot be determined by physical examination. These subjective findings are correlated with the findings of the physical examination.

In the case of common musculoskeletal disorders the lesion is usually manifested primarily by pain. Some of the routine questions suggested here as part of every history are directed at obtaining a complete account of the history of the pain and the present status of the pain as perceived by the patient. However, the clinician must also inquire about other symptoms, such as paresthesias, feelings of weakness, feelings of instability, and autonomic disturbances. It is important to keep in mind that the patient's perception of pain and other symptoms offers valuable clues to the nature and extent of the lesion but does not alone serve as an indicator of progress. For that the examiner must rely on assessment of objective signs and examination of the patient's functional status.

Determination of the degree of disability does offer some data by which to legitimately judge progress. It also yields information concerning the nature and extent of the lesion. This is an important part of the history and is too often omitted. To determine the degree of disability the patient's "health-state" behaviors and activity level (occupation, recreation, and other activities of daily life) can be assessed, as well as the patient's "disease-state" behaviors and activity level. Documentation of the disease-state behaviors will set a baseline against which to judge progress; comparison with the patient's health-state behaviors may provide clues to the nature and extent of the problem. For example, the patient with a shoulder problem who has been able to comb her hair all her life but since the onset of the problem is unable to do so, lacks full, pain-free active elevation and external rotation. This is very suggestive of a capsular restriction. In this example there are some data to compare with the physical findings that may help determine the nature and extent of the lesion. One treatment goal will naturally be to restore the patient's ability to comb her hair. A criterion by which to judge progress has also been established. Consequently, when judging progress, the clinician must be less concerned with whether Mrs. Jones had shoulder pain that morning and its extent or duration and more concerned with whether Mrs. Jones was able to comb her hair.

Disability assessment and disease-state behavior assessment become especially important in evaluating patients with a chronic-pain state who have no physical findings or pain that is out of proportion to physical findings and in evaluating patients with a permanent functional deficit from some serious pathologic process. In the first situation, it is often necessary to change from a "medical model," in which treatment is aimed at the lesion in order to change behavior, to an "operant model," in which treatment is aimed at altering the consequences of the disease-state behaviors.[25–27] In the second situation, treatment is no longer directed at the primary lesion (*e.g.,* a spinal cord lesion), but rather at improving residual function. There are some relatively common disorders in which pain complaints and functional disability are out of proportion to the extent of the pathologic process. Some of these abnormal pain states, such as reflex sympathetic dystrophy (see Chapter 11, The Wrist and Hand Complex), have a physiologic basis. Other cases, such as those involving pending litiga-

tion, substantial monetary compensation, or welcomed time away from activities the patient finds undesirable, may have a psychosocial basis. The patient's pain or disability may promise rewards, which may in turn reinforce disease-state behaviors. It is essential that the presence of such abnormal behavior states be determined on examination. In these cases, treatment aimed primarily at some physical pathologic process may only serve to maintain the patient's disability. Primary emphasis must be placed on improved function by altering the consequences of the disabled state (Fig. 5-1).

Although this text emphasizes the assessment and treatment of the lesion itself, clinicians must not lose sight of the fact that they are treating patients and that the ultimate goal in any treatment program is rehabilitation of the patient. Even when treatment is aimed largely at the lesion, care must be taken not to reinforce the disease state or especially pain behavior. Similarly, clinicians must also be concerned with functional deficits associated with the disease state and see that they are resolved, when possible, along with the primary pathologic process. Thus, whether patient management is approached through a "medical model" or through an "operant model," the primary goal is to restore health-state behaviors. When a well-defined lesion exists, and the consequences of the resulting disability appear to have a negative effect on the patient's attitude toward the disability, it can be reasonably expected that resolving the pathologic process will restore health-state behavior. However, when the consequences of disability are rewarding to the patient, treatment of the pathologic process may have little or no effect.

The specific inquiries during the initial history-taking naturally vary according to the site of the lesion, the nature of the lesion, and other factors. Questions

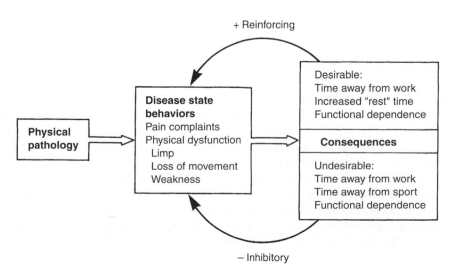

FIG. 5-1. *Disability scheme.*

that are particularly important for specific anatomic regions will be discussed in the respective chapters dealing with those regions. There are, however, certain routine inquiries that should be included in virtually every case.

The most efficient method of obtaining subjective information is to direct a list of specific, predetermined questions to the patient. However, this is not always the *best* method for eliciting certain important pieces of information, and it is certainly not the best method for developing the most effective patient–health care professional relationship. The direct-question approach is *close-ended*; it assumes that the relevant information will fall into predetermined categories, and it does not encourage consideration of factors outside these categories. It leads or directs the line of inquiry to specific categories. The patient often attempts to please the examiner by providing information related to these categories but not necessarily pertinent to the problem at hand.

A close-ended, direct-question method of interviewing creates a patient–therapist relationship in which the therapist assumes the authoritarian role of "healer" while the patient assumes a passive role. Within this relationship the patient need only provide the requested information, after which the examiner will perform the appropriate tests, decide what the problem is, and correct it. Such an approach favors the assumption that there is a specific pathologic process that the therapist will treat while the patient assumes a relatively passive role in the treatment program. This is consistent with a medical model of patient management and excludes from the outset the possibility of an operant disease state or an operant approach to management.

Alternatively, a more *open-ended* approach guides the discussion but does not restrict information to certain categories. Furthermore, it allows the patient the freedom to relate what the patient feels is important, in addition to what the examiner may feel is important. The open-ended patient interview is structured to be a discussion session rather than a question-and-answer period. The examiner structures the discussion carefully, however, to elicit the necessary information. In an open-ended interview, the therapist and patient discuss the patient's problem on a one-to-one basis. The therapist maintains a position as an expert in the field by virtue of the professional atmosphere in which the interview takes place. The patient is the expert with respect to the particular problem, being more familiar with it than anyone else. The interview serves as a forum in which the patient is encouraged to offer information and insight concerning the problem in return for advice and help in overcoming it. Both patient and therapist maintain distinct roles but

remain equals. They establish an understanding that mutual cooperation and effort are required to execute an effective treatment program.

There are appropriate uses for both the open-ended and closed-ended approaches to history-taking. In all situations, it is important to begin the interview open-endedly to establish an effective professional relationship and to get a feeling for the patient's problem. As the nature of the problem becomes more obvious, however, it is necessary to seek more detailed information by directing specific questions to the patient. However, even during a closed line of questioning, examiners must avoid asking leading questions that may elicit irrelevant or inaccurate information. For example, instead of asking, "Does the pain travel down the arm?" the examiner should ask, "Is the pain felt in any other parts?" Instead of, "Do you have a lot of pain in the morning?" one might ask, "When do you typically feel the pain?" The same is true when inquiring about disability. Rather than asking if a particular activity is painful or difficult, one should ask, "Which activities are particularly painful or difficult to perform?" In this way the patient is responsible for judging what information in a particular category is important and is less likely to provide information primarily for the purpose of satisfying the examiner.

The following list of questions is presented to indicate the type of information one should attempt to elicit. As much of the information as possible should be obtained through an open-ended discussion in an environment in which the patient feels free to discuss his problem and provide related information. The setting should be quiet, private, and free from disturbances. The examiner should be seated, and the patient should still be in street clothes. Following a well-structured discussion, any information that has not come out should be sought through specific questions. The discussion should end with a fairly open-ended question, as indicated below, to reestablish an appropriate working relationship.

1. **Tell me about your problem.**

   The patient referred for a back problem may be more concerned with his prostatic neoplasm; some valuable information may be elicited by letting the patient discuss freely whatever he feels is most important. On the other hand, the patient is likely to go on for as long as the examiner allows. One should be prepared to interrupt politely by saying, for example, "I'm beginning to get an idea of the nature of your problem. Now I would like to obtain some specific information pertaining to it." The patient, having been allowed the opportunity to talk freely, is assured that the examiner is interested in him as a person and has begun to involve him in the therapeutic process by listening to his opinion.

2. **Where, exactly, is your pain?**

   The patient is asked to indicate with one hand or one finger the primary area of pain and then any areas to which it might spread. It is important to determine whether in fact it does or does not spread.

   a. If the patient points to one small, localized area and claims that the pain does not spread from it, the lesion is probably not severe or it is relatively superficial, or both.

   b. If a diffuse area is indicated as the primary site, it suggests that the lesion is more severe or more deeply situated, or both.

   c. If the pain spreads, determine if it is confined to a segment. If so, determine if it follows a well-delineated pathway, as in dermatomic radiation, or if it is more diffuse, as in sclerotomic reference of pain. Well-delineated, radiating pain suggests pressure on a nerve root in which the A-delta fibers are irritated but still transmitting. Diffuse, segmental referred pain may have its origin in the viscera, a deep somatic structure, or a nerve root in which the large myelinated fibers are no longer conducting but the small C fibers are. Cyriax proposes that some structures such as the dura mater and viscera will refer pain extrasegmentally.[14]

   d. In general, reference of pain is favored by a strong stimulus (a severe lesion), a lesion of deep somatic structures or nerve tissues, and a lesion lying fairly proximally (since pain is more often referred distally than proximally).

3. **When did the present pain arise? Was the onset gradual or sudden? Was an injury or unusual activity involved?**

   An insidious onset unrelated to injury or unusual activity should always be viewed with suspicion, since this history is typical of a neoplasm. However, degenerative lesions or lesions due to tissue fatigue are common and may also arise in this manner. If the patient blames some injury or activity, keep in mind that she may or may not be correct. The exact nature of the event or mechanism of injury should be determined so that correlation can be made to symptoms and signs for interpretation. Determining the direction and nature of forces producing the injury may give some clues as to which tissues may have been stressed.

4. **What is the quality of the pain (sharp, dull, burning, tingling, aching, constant, boring, excruciating)? Has it changed at all in quality or intensity since its onset?**

   a. Sharp, well-localized pain suggests a superficial lesion.

   b. Sharp, lancinating, shooting pain suggests a nerve lesion, usually at a nerve root, presumably affecting the A-delta fibers.

   c. Tingling suggests stimulation of nerve tissue affecting A-alpha fibers. A segmental distribution suggests a nerve root; a peripheral nerve distribution implicates that nerve. Tingling in both hands, both feet, or all four extremities suggests spinal cord involvement or some other more serious pathologic process.

   d. Dull, aching pain is typical of pain of deep somatic origin.

   e. Excruciating pain, unrelenting pain, intolerable pain, and deep, boring pain all suggest a serious lesion.

   f. Change in intensity of the pain may offer some clue as to the progression of the problem. This must be considered when treatment begins. If the patient's condition was getting worse prior to treatment and continues to worsen once treatment has begun, then the treatment has probably not been effective. However, it is probably not the cause of the worsening following initiation of treatment. On the other hand, if the patient's condition had been improving but stops getting better or gets worse once treatment has begun, the treatment is probably at fault.

   g. Change in quality of the pain may offer many clues as to the nature and extent of the lesion. Progression of nerve-root pressure, such as from a disk protrusion, typically leads to rather marked changes in symptoms (see Chapter 4, Pain).

5. **What aggravates the pain? What relieves it? Is it any better or worse in the morning or evening? When do you typically feel pain?**

   a. Pain not aggravated by activity or relieved by rest should be suspected as arising from some pathologic process other than a common musculoskeletal disorder. The exception is a disk problem that may be aggravated by sitting and relieved by getting up and walking.

   b. Morning pain is suggestive of arthritis, especially the inflammatory varieties. Morning stiffness is suggestive of degenerative joint disease or chronic arthritis.

   c. Pain awakening the patient at night is typical of shoulder or hip problems that may be aggravated by lying on the affected side. Otherwise, a more serious problem should be suspected, particularly if the patient is kept awake and especially if he must get up and walk about.

d. Arthritis in weight-bearing joints leads to pain on fatigue (long walks, etc.) in its early stages. In later stages, the pain is felt when beginning a walk, somewhat relieved once going, and returns after walking too far.

6. **Have you had this problem in the past? If so, how was it resolved? Did you seek help? Was there any treatment? Is the pain the same this time?**

If the examiner should elicit a history of recurrence, the patient might be asked in depth about the first episode and the most recent episode, with an estimate of the number of intervening episodes. Recurrences are typical of spinal cord lesions, but many common extremity lesions such as ankle sprains, minor meniscus lesions or other internal derangements, minor degenerative joint problems, tendinitis, and frozen shoulder also may tend to recur.

By inquiring about previous management, some helpful information may also be obtained for treatment planning. However, the patient's judgment of the effectiveness or value of previous treatment must not be weighed too heavily. If an injection helped before, for example, in the case of supraspinatus tendinitis, it does not necessarily follow that another injection is necessary or indicated. If physical therapy (perhaps inadequately instituted) was unsuccessful in the past, do not assume that it will not be helpful on this occasion.

7. **Are there any other symptoms that you have or have had that you associate with the problem, such as grinding, popping, giving way, numbness, tingling, weakness, dizziness, or nausea?**

By concentrating on the patient's account of pain, the examiner may well overlook some other important symptoms. A wide variety of responses may be elicited with this question, each of which must be carefully weighed and considered. A patient's description of "numbness" is very often not true hypesthesia but is actually referred pain. In most cases, considerable weakness must be present before the patient can accurately perceive it as such, and very often what the patient describes as "weakness" is actually instability or giving way. Symptoms inconsistent with musculoskeletal dysfunction must be viewed with some suspicion and medical consultation sought for interpretation.

8. **How has this problem affected your dressing, grooming, or other daily activities? Has it affected your ability to work at your job or around the house? Has it affected or altered your recreational activities? Is there anything that is diffi-**

cult or impossible for you to do since the onset of this problem?

The patient's normal occupation and daily activity level is determined. The existence of a functional deficit often contributes to interpretation of the problem by considering the demands placed on various musculoskeletal structures in performing the task. Later, quantification of the deficit or residual function during physical examination will set a baseline against which to assess progress.

Any functional deficit must be correlated later with the apparent nature of the lesion, and any inconsistencies must be considered. In cases involving compensation or litigation, the disease state may be reinforced in such a way that a functional deficit is no longer the result of the problem but rather its cause.

9. **What treatment are you having or have you had for the present problem? Are you taking any medications for this problem or for any other reason?**

Here again, it may or may not be helpful to determine whether certain attempts at treatment have had any good or bad effects, especially treatments involving physical agents.

The examiner must determine whether pain medications, anti-inflammatory agents, or muscle relaxants are being taken. Symptoms or signs may be masked accordingly. Certain medications may produce rather marked musculoskeletal changes (in addition to effects on other tissues and functions). Most important, perhaps, is the long-term use of corticosteroids, which produces osteoporosis; proximal muscle weakness; generalized tissue edema; thin, fragile skin; collagen tissue weakening; and increased pain threshold. These factors, of course, will affect findings on examination. More importantly, however, they must be considered when planning treatment.

10. **How is your general health?**

It is necessary to determine whether the patient has or has had any disease process or health problem that may have contributed to the present problem or that may influence the choice of treatment procedures.

11. **Do you have any opinions of your own as to what the problem is?**

Some useful information may be elicited concerning what the patient has learned from others, what his insight is into the problem, and so on. If nothing else, the patient can be reassured that the examiner is interested in her and her opinions and that she is to be involved in the therapeutic program.

■ PHYSICAL EXAMINATION

A complete history performed by the experienced clinician will often be sufficient to determine the extent and nature of the lesion. Even so, the physical examination must not be excluded or cut short. Objective data are needed to facilitate or confirm the interpretation of subjective findings. It is equally important that every effort be made to quantify objective data to allow documentation of a baseline and, therefore, accurate assessment of progress.

Specific tests and measurements will vary, of course, depending on the area to be examined and to a certain extent on the information obtained from the history. In this chapter we present a systematic approach that can be applied to any region to be evaluated; tests specific to particular regions will be discussed in the chapters on those regions. This discussion will include general guidelines and statements meant to assist in interpretation of findings. It should be noted that the order of testing procedures presented here is for the sake of conceptual organization. Clinically, tests must be organized according to patient positioning. This point will be elaborated in the chapters on specific regions.

Having discussed the phenomenon of referred pain, it should be apparent that at times clinicians may be at a loss as to which region should be singled out as the primary area to be examined. For example, elbow pain may have its origin locally or at the neck or shoulder, but surely it is not necessary that each of these areas be examined in depth. The physician's referral or the history, or both, will often implicate the involved area. However, this is not always the case. When such a difficulty arises, it is often helpful to perform a brief *scan examination.* This is done by asking the patient to actively move each joint within the suspected areas and by applying some passive overpressure to the extremes of each motion. If pain or dysfunction is noted at a particular area, it may be examined in depth. In general, every structure derived embryologically from the same segment must be considered as the segment or portion of a segment in which the patient indicates the pain exists.

The physical examination, briefly presented in this chapter, will be described in detail in later chapters. The basic aims of the physical examination are (1) to reproduce the patient's symptoms and (2) to detect the level of dysfunction by provocation of the affected joint or tissues. The main components of the physical examination are as follows:

- Observation
- Inspection
- Selective tissue tension

- Active movements
- Passive movements
  - Passive physiologic movements
  - Joint play
  - Resisted isometric movements
- Neuromuscular tests
- Palpation
- Provocation tests
- Functional assessment
- Special tests
- Testing of related areas
- Other investigations

☐ Observation

The patient's general appearance and functional status can be observed when he walks in, during dressing activities, during the examination and treatment session, and as he leaves. If specific functional disabilities are related during the history, the examiner may ask the patient to attempt to perform the involved activity in order to assess the exact degree and nature of the disability.

The patient's general appearance and body build—slim, obese, muscular, emaciated, short, tall—are noted and recorded. Obvious postural deviations as well as abnormalities in positionings of body parts are reported.

All functional abnormalities or deficits noted during the patient's visit are described as precisely as possible. These might typically include observations relating to gait, guarding of particular movements, use of compensatory or substitution movements, or use of certain aids or assistive devices.

☐ Inspection

The inspection part of the examination entails a closer assessment of the patient's physical status. It is usually performed in conjunction with palpation, which is discussed later in this section. To avoid excluding crucial assessments, it is convenient and helpful to organize inspection of body parts according to the following three layers: bony structure and alignment, subcutaneous soft tissue, and skin.

BONY STRUCTURE AND ALIGNMENT

Inspection of the bony structure and alignment is a critical component of the biomechanical examination, especially when correlated with specific functional abnormalities such as gait deviances and altered range of motion. For example, a person with increased femoral anteversion is likely to present with a loss of external rotation at the hip, but with respect to his structure, a decrease in average external rotation is normal. If a careful assessment of static alignment were not made, one might make the mistake of attempting to restore external rotation in this case. Similarly, a common gait abnormality seen clinically is increased pronation of the hindfoot during stance phase. This often occurs secondary to structural malalignments elsewhere in the extremity, such as increased internal tibial torsion, increased femoral antetorsion, or adduction of the first metatarsal. The ultimate cause of the pronation can only be determined through a careful structural examination. Assessment of structural alignment is likewise of utmost importance following the healing of fractures. A person who has sustained a Colles' fracture invariably ends up with some residual angulation dorsally and radially; restoration of full wrist flexion and ulnar deviation should never be expected. Thus, structural assessment becomes important in planning treatment as well as in setting treatment goals.

Assessment of a particular part in which some pathologic lesion may exist should often include structural assessment of biomechanically related parts. In the case of a patient with a low back disorder, the clinician should examine the alignment of the lower extremities and vice versa. The same is true for the cervical spine and upper extremities. Each part should be assessed with respect to frontal, sagittal, and transverse planes. Key bony landmarks are identified, and their relationships to fixed points of reference (*e.g.,* the ground, wall, or a plumb-line) as well as their relationships to each other are determined. In judging whether malalignments exist, clinicians must often rely on their experience of what is normal, as well as on comparison to a normal side in cases of unilateral problems. Malalignments should be documented through careful measurements when possible.

Specific assessments related to particular regions of the body will be discussed in the chapters on those body regions. The following list includes some key bony landmarks that must often be identified when testing structural alignment and with which the clinician must become familiar:

Navicular tubercles
Talar heads
Malleoli
Fibular heads
Patellar borders
Adductor tubercles
Greater trochanters
Ischial tuberosities
Posterior and anterior iliac spines
Iliac crests

Spinous processes
Scapular borders
Mastoid processes
Clavicles
Acromial processes
Greater tubercles
Olecranons
Humeral epicondyles
Radial and ulnar styloid processes
Lister's tubercles
Carpal bones

SUBCUTANEOUS SOFT TISSUES

The soft tissue is inspected and palpated for abnormalities. The examiner should look for swelling or increase in the size of an area, wasting or atrophy of the part, and alterations in the general contours of the region. When an increase in size is noted, an attempt should be made to distinguish the cause, whether generalized edema, articular effusion, muscle hypertrophy, or hypertrophic changes in other tissues. The area is examined for localized cysts, nodules, or ganglia. In the presence of wasting, the examiner should determine whether localized or generalized muscle atrophy exists or whether there is perhaps some loss of continuity of soft tissues.

Measurements should be taken to carefully document soft-tissue changes and to use as baseline measurements. Volumetric measurements of small parts, such as fingers, hands, and feet, can be made by measuring the displacement of water in a tub. Swelling or wasting elsewhere in an extremity can often be documented with circumferential measurements using a tape measure.

SKIN AND NAILS

Local or generalized changes in the status of the skin are noted and recorded. These changes might include:

- Changes in color either from vascular changes accompanying inflammation (erythema) or vascular deficiency (pallor or cyanosis)
- Changes in texture and moisture. These commonly accompany reflex sympathetic dystrophies, in which the sympathetic activity of the part becomes altered. Increased activity results in hyperhidrosis; smooth, glossy skin; cyanosis; atrophy of skin; and splitting of the nails. Decreased sympathetic activity may result in pink, dry, scaly skin.
- Local scars, distinct blemishes, abnormal hair patterns, calluses, blisters, open wounds, and other localized skin abnormalities. When a scar exists, whether surgical or traumatic, the type of surgery or injury should be determined because it may

have some bearing on the present problem. Blemishes such as large, brownish, pigmented areas (*café au lait* spots) and localized hairy regions often accompany underlying bony defects, such as spina bifida. Calluses develop with increased shear or compressive stresses; blisters occur with increased shear between the skin and subcutaneous tissue. When an open wound is observed, the clinician should determine whether it is of traumatic origin or of insidious origin, as often accompanies diabetes.

Local skin changes are described according to size and location. Size can be most precisely documented by outlining the borders of the defect on a piece of acetate, such as old x-ray film.

☐ Selective Tissue Tension Tests

This portion of the examination consists of specific active, passive, and resisted movement tests designed to assess the status of each of the component tissues of the physiologic joint. When properly interpreted, findings from these tests can yield very specific information relating to both the nature and extent of the pathologic process. The organization and interpretation of these tests is largely the work of Cyriax and is certainly a significant contribution to the field.[14]

I. **Active movements.** These yield very general information, relating primarily to the patient's functional status. They provide information concerning the patient's general willingness and ability to use the part. They offer no true indication of the range of motion or strength of a part. If a patient is asked to lift an arm overhead and only lifts it to horizontal, it cannot be determined at that point whether the loss of function is due to pain, weakness, or stiffness.

Therefore, active movement tests are used primarily to assess the patient's ability to perform common functional activities related to the part being evaluated. For lower extremity and spinal regions, then, active movements should be performed while bearing weight. Upper extremity parts should be moved in functional directions. At the shoulder, for example, internal and external rotation are performed by asking the patient to reach behind and to touch the back of the neck rather than rotating the humerus with the arm to the side.

The following should be noted and documented for the active movements tested:

A. *The patient's account of the onset of, or increase in, pain associated with the movement, and at what point or points in the range of movement the pain occurs.* The existence of a painful arc of movement is best detected on active, weight-bearing, or antigravity movements. A painful arc of movement, in which pain is felt throughout a small arc of movement in the mid range of motion, suggests an irritable structure being (1) pulled across a protuberance or (2) pinched between two structures. An example of the former is a nerve root pulled across a disk protrusion during straight-leg raises. An example of the latter is an inflamed supraspinatus tendon squeezed between the greater tubercle and the acromial arch during abduction of the arm.

B. *The range of motion through which the patient is able to move the part.* This should be measured by some easily reproducible method.

C. *The presence of crepitus.* This can usually be best detected on active movement, with the forces of weight-bearing or muscle contraction maintaining compression of joint surfaces. Crepitus usually indicates roughening of joint surfaces or increased friction between a tendon and its sheath due to swelling or roughening of either the tendon or the sheath. Fine crepitus at a joint suggests early wearing of articular cartilage or tendinous problems, whereas more coarse crepitus implies considerable cartilaginous degeneration. A creaking sound, not unlike that which a large tree makes when swaying in the wind, often occurs when bones articulate in the late stages of joint-surface degeneration.

II. **Passive movements**

A. *Passive range-of-motion testing.* The part is passively put through the major motions in the frontal, sagittal, and transverse planes that normally occur at the joint being moved. Very specific information concerning both the nature and extent of a disorder may be obtained by making the following assessments:

1. Range of movement. The examiner should determine whether movement is normal, restricted, or hypermobile. The degree of any abnormal movements is measured carefully. If there is restriction of movement at a joint, the first and foremost determination that should be made is whether the restriction is in a capsular or noncapsular pattern. Tables 5-1 and 5-2 list the common capsular patterns present in the sequence of most to least restricted.

a. Capsular patterns of restriction indicate loss of mobility of the entire joint capsule from fibrosis, effusion, or inflammation. Differentiation can be made by assessing the "end feel" at the

TABLE 5-1 COMMON CAPSULAR PATTERNS FOR THE UPPER QUADRANT JOINTS

JOINT(S)	PROPORTIONAL LIMITATIONS
Temporomandibular Upper cervical spine (occiput–C2)	Limitation of mouth opening
OA joint	Forward bending more limited than backward bending
AA joint	Restriction with rotation
Lower cervical spine (C3–T2)	Limitation of all motions except flexion (sidebending = rotation > backward bending)
Sternoclavicular	Full elevation limited; pain at extreme range of motion
Acromioclavicular	Full elevation limited; pain at extreme range of motion
Glenohumeral	Greater limitation of external rotation, followed by abduction and internal rotation
Humeroulnar	Loss of flexion > extension
Humeroradial	Loss of flexion > extension
Forearm	Equally restricted in pronation and supination in presence of elbow restriction
Proximal radioulnar	Limitation; pronation = supination
Distal radioulnar	Limitation; pronation = supination
Wrist	Limitation; flexion = extension
Midcarpal	Limitation equal all directions
Trapeziometacarpal	Limitation abduction > extension
Carpometacarpals II–V	Equally restricted all directions
Upper extremity digits	Limitation flexion > extension

OA, occipitoatlantal joint; *AA*, atlantoaxial joint.
(Adapted from references 14, 22, and 41)

TABLE 5-2 COMMON CAPSULAR PATTERNS FOR THE LOWER QUADRANT JOINTS

JOINT(S)	PROPORTIONAL LIMITATIONS
Thoracic spine	Limitation of sidebending and rotation > loss of extension > flexion
Lumbar spine	Marked and equal limitation of sidebending and rotation; loss of extension > flexion
Sacroiliac, symphysis pubis, sacrococcygeal	Pain when joints are stressed
Hip	Limited flexion/internal rotation; some limitation of abduction; no or little limitation of adduction and external rotation
Tibiofemoral (knee)	Flexion grossly limited; slight limitation of extension
Tibiofibular	Pain when joint is stressed
Talocrural (ankle)	Loss of plantarflexion > dorsiflexion
Talocalcaneal (subtalar)	Increasing limitations of varus; joint fixed in valgus (inversion > eversion)
Midtarsal	Supination > pronation (limited dorsiflexion, plantar flexion, adduction, and medial rotation)
First metatarsalphalangeal	Marked limitation of extension; slight limitation of flexion
Metatarsophalangeal (II–V)	Variable; tend toward flexion restrictions
Interphalangeal	Tend toward extension restrictions

(Adapted from references 14, 19, 37, 41, and 50)

extremes of movement (see following). Capsular restrictions typically accompany arthritis or degenerative joint disease (fibrosis, inflammation, or effusion), prolonged immobilization of a joint (fibrosis), or acute trauma to a joint (effusion).

Only joints that are controlled by muscles have a capsular pattern. Thus, joints such as the tibiofibular and sacroiliac do not exhibit a capsular pattern.

b. Noncapsular patterns of joint restrictions typically occur with intra-articular mechanical blockage or extra-articular lesions. Common causes include

i. Isolated ligamentous or capsular adhesion. A common example of isolated ligamentous adhesion is that of adherence of the medial collateral ligament at the knee to the medial femoral condyle during healing of a sprain. This results in restriction of knee flexion to about 90°, with extension being of full range. Isolated anterior capsular tightness at the shoulder often occurs following an anterior dislocation, resulting in a disproportionate loss of external rotation.

ii. Internal derangements, such as displacement of pieces of torn menisci and cartilaginous loose bodies. These typically produce a mechanical block to movement in a noncapsular pattern. The most common example is a "bucket handle" medial meniscus tear, resulting in blockage of knee extension, with flexion remaining relatively free in the absence of significant effusion.

iii. Extra-articular tissue tightness,

such as reduced lengthening of muscles from contracture (fibrosis) or myositis ossificans.

iv. Extra-articular inflammation or swellings, such as those accompanying acute bursitis and neoplasms.

2. *End feel* at extremes of painful or restricted movements. This is the quality of the resistance to movement that the examiner feels when coming to the end point of a particular movement. Some end feels may be normal or pathological, depending on the movement they accompany at a particular joint and the point in the range of movement at which they are felt. Other end feels are strictly pathological. The testing of end feel can be performed on both classical (osteokinematic) and accessory motions.

a. End feels that may be normal or pathologic include:

i. Capsular end feel. This is a firm, "leathery" feeling felt with a slight creep, for example, when forcing the normal shoulder into full external rotation. When felt in conjunction with a capsular pattern of restriction, and in the absence of significant inflammation or effusion, it indicates capsular fibrosis.

ii. Ligamentous end feel. This is a firm end feel with no give or creep. An example of normal ligamentous end feel would be abduction of the extended knee.

iii. Bony end feel. This feels abrupt, as when moving the normal elbow into full extension. When accompanying a restriction of movement, it may suggest hypertrophic bony changes, such as those that occur with degenerative joint disease, or possible malunion of bony segments following healing of a fracture.

iv. Soft-tissue–approximation end feel. This is a soft end feel, as when fully flexing the normal elbow or knee. It may accompany joint restriction in the presence of significant muscular hypertrophy.

v. Muscular end feel. This more rubbery feel resembles what is felt at the extremes of straight-leg raising from tension on the hamstrings. It is less abrupt than a capsular end feel.

b. End feels that are strictly pathologic include:

i. Muscle-spasm end feel. Movement is stopped fairly abruptly, perhaps with some "rebound," owing to muscles contracting reflexively to prevent further movement. It usually accompanies pain felt at the point of restriction. When occurring with a capsular restriction, it indicates some degree of synovial inflammation of the portion of the joint capsule being stretched during the movement.

ii. Capsular (abnormal) end feel. The range of motion is obviously reduced, in a movement pattern characteristic for each joint. Some authors divide abnormal capsular end feel into *hard capsular end feel,* when the feel has a tight resistance to creep or thick quality to it, and *soft capsular end feel,* when it is similar to normal but is painful with induced muscle guarding. A hard end feel is seen in chronic inflammatory conditions. The soft capsular end feel is more often seen in acute inflammatory conditions, with stiffness occurring early in the range and increasing until the end range is reached. Maitland[53] calls this "resistance through range." Many authors also describe a boggy end feel that typically accompanies joint effusion in the absence of significant synovial inflammation.[11]

iii. Boggy end feel. This is a very soft, mushy end feel that typically accompanies joint effusion in the absence of significant synovial inflammation. It will usually occur together with a capsular pattern of restriction.

iv. Internal derangement end feel. This is often a pronounced, springy rebound at the end point of movement. It typically accompanies a noncapsular restriction from a mechanical block produced by a loose body or displaced meniscus.

v. Empty end feel. The examiner feels no restriction to movement, but movement is stopped at the insistence of the patient because of severe pain. This end feel is relatively rare except with acute bursitis at the shoulder or a few other painful extra-articular lesions such as neoplasms. The muscles do not contract to prevent movement since this would cause compression at the painful site and further pain.

c. Additional abnormal end feels described by Paris[67] include:

   i. Adhesions and scarring with a sudden sharp arrest in one direction, commonly seen at the knee

   ii. Bony block. This is a sudden hard stop short of normal range. Examples of abnormal bony blocks are callus formation, myositis ossificans, or fracture within a joint.

   iii. Bony grate. The end feel is rough and grating as occurs in the presence of advanced chondromalacia.

   iv. Pannus. This abnormal end feel is described as a soft, crunchy squelch. The exact nature is unknown but may include synovial infold or trapped fat pad.

   v. Loose. Ligamentous laxity as seen in a ligamentous injury or rheumatoid arthritis.

     The importance of the end feel is that it gives some indication of what is likely to be the most efficient treatment.

3. Another useful way to consider restricted motion is known as the barrier concept.[6,31,37] Barriers exist at the end of normal active range of motion, when the soft tissues about the joint have reached a degree of tension beyond which the person cannot voluntarily move. This is known as the *physiologic barrier.* Other barriers include:

a. Within the total range of motion there is a range of passive movement available which the examiner can introduce (Fig. 5-2*A*). The limits to this barrier have been described by some as the *elastic barrier.*[31] At this point all the tension has been taken up within the joint and its surrounding tissues.

b. Passively, the joint may be taken beyond its elastic barrier to the *anatomic barrier.* Here the soft tissues are on maximum stretch, and going farther will either cause failure of the soft tis-

sues or fracture. According to Sandoz[73] there is a small amount of potential space between the elastic barrier and anatomic barrier described as the *paraphysiologic* space (Fig. 5-2*A*). It is within this area that the high-velocity, low-amplitude thrust appears to generate the popping which is sometimes elicited from this maneuver.[31]

c. In a state of dysfunction, when motion is lost within the range, it can be described as a major or minor loss of mobility (see Fig. 5-2*B*). The barrier which prevents movement in the direction of motion lost is defined as the *restrictive barrier.* The barrier may be described according to the abnormal end feel previously discussed.

d. The loose packed or resting position is often described as the *point of ease* (see Fig. 5-2*A*).[31] Conversely, as one moves away from neutral or the point of maximum ease, in either direction, the soft tissue becomes more tense, where one begins to sense a certain amount of "bind" (see Fig. 5-2*A*). In the normal joint the point of ease is usually near the mid point of range. When there is a restrictive barrier, the point of ease will be found to have moved, usually to about the mid point of the remaining range (actual resting position). When there is a major restriction, the point of ease may be closer to the physiologic barrier at the normal end (see Fig. 5-2*B*).

4. Pain on movement and the point in the range in which it is felt.

a. Pain at the extremes of a movement indicates

   i. A painful structure is being stretched. In this case, one should consider first, a lesion of the joint capsule or a ligament and second, a lesion of a muscle or tendon. For biarticular muscles, the constant-length phenomenon can be used to differentiate the location. Otherwise one must correlate this finding with findings of resisted movement tests (see III, following) in order to differentiate between capsuloligamentous and musculotendinous lesions. If the lesion lies in a muscle or tendon, resistance to

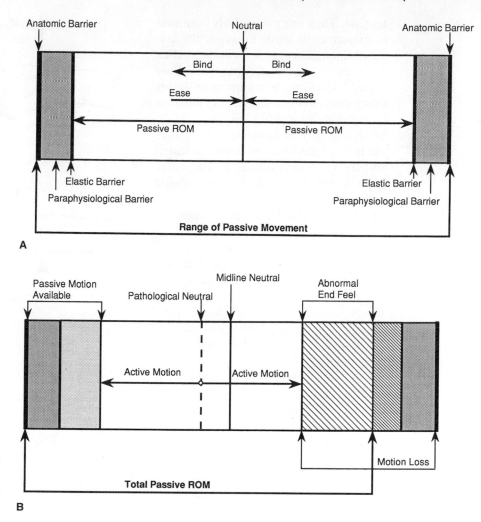

FIG. 5-2. Soft tissue tension development during examination procedures. (**A**) Normal mobility and associated barriers. (**B**) Dysfunction and associated restrictive barriers.

the movement opposite the direction of the painful passive movement will be painful, whereas with capsuloligamentous lesions resisted movements are painless.

ii. A painful structure is being squeezed. This usually occurs with extra-articular lesions such as tendinitis and bursitis. An inflamed subdeltoid bursa is susceptible to impingement beneath the acromial arch; the trochanteric bursa is squeezed on abduction of the hip; the semimembranosus bursa, when swollen, is squeezed on full knee flexion. With supraspinatus tendinitis, pain will be felt on elevation of the arm from squeezing of the involved part of the tendon between the greater tuberosity and the posterior rim of the glenoid cavity.

b. A painful arc may occur with passive movement tests. (See section on active movements for a discussion of its significance.)

5. Joint sound on movement. When moving peripheral joints, the examiner will often feel or hear unusual joint sounds which may or may not indicate pathology.

a. Crepitus on movement. This is best detected by active movement testing but may be noted on passive movement as well. (See section on active movements for discussion.) A creaking, leathery (snowball) crepitus (soft-tissue crepitus) is sometimes perceived in pathologies involving the tendons.[50] Soft tissue crepitus may be palpable in patients with degeneration of the rotator cuff and a bony crepitus will be evident in patients with osteoarthritis.

b. Clicks, such as the normal vacuum click, may be felt in the joint and are usually of no significance. In the normal knee, there is often a click on extension. They are particularly common in hypermobile joints in which the laxity of ligaments enables a bone to click as it moves in relation to its fellow bone.[13] Clicking is common in joints unsupported by muscles or when a loose body lies inside a joint.

   c. Snapping may be heard or felt around joints as ligaments or tendons catch and then slip over a bony prominence. Less common causes of a pathologic nature are

      i. A coarse clunking type of noise accompanying joint subluxation or instability (*e.g.,* rotatory instability of the knee due to ligamentous damage or degenerative changes in the joint).[13]

      ii. A semimembranosus bursa may snap as it jumps from one side of the tendon to the other, as the knee extends.[14]

      iii. A trigger finger is often released into extension with a snap.[14]

   d. Cracks may occur when traction is applied to a joint. Synovial fluid found in a joint cavity contains 15 percent gas, and the crack is thought to be caused by a bubble of gas collapsing.[14,87]

B. *Passive joint-play movement tests (capsuloligamentous stress tests)* are designed to stress various portions of the joint capsule and major ligaments to detect the presence of painful lesions affecting these structures or loss of continuity of these structures. (For the method of performing the movements and the various movements performed at each joint, see the mobilization techniques included in the specific joint chapters in Part II.)

Joint play is assessed by moving one of the articular surfaces of the joint in a direction that is either perpendicular or parallel to the joint (Fig. 5-3). The treatment plane is at right angles to a line drawn from the axis of rotation to the center of the concave articulating surface and lies in the concave surface. Passively moving either bone in a direction perpendicular to the treatment plane constitutes a *traction* or distraction joint-play assessment, and moving either bone in a direction parallel to the treatment plane constitutes a *gliding* or oscillation joint-play assessment. Traction joint-play assessments directed along the axis of the long bone are called *long axis extension* or *distractions* to distinguish them from tractions administered perpendicular to the treatment plane.

Joint-play movement should be assessed in the

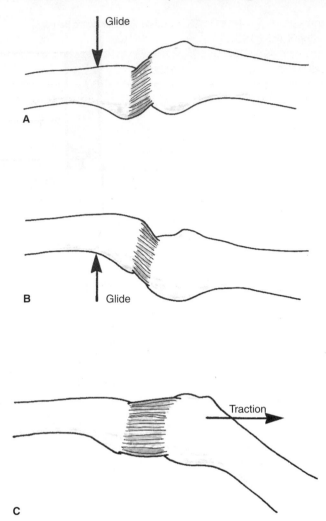

FIG. 5-3. *Glides and traction. Traction is applied perpendicular, and glides are applied parallel to the treatment plane.*

loose (resting) position in which laxity of capsule and ligaments is greatest and there is the least bone contact (minimal congruency between the articular surfaces).[41] The greatest amount of joint play is available in the resting position that is usually considered in the mid range, or it may be just outside the range of pain and spasm (position of most comfort). If limitations in range of motion or pain prevent the examiner from placing the joint in the resting position, then the position most closely approximating the resting position should be used. This is called the *actual resting position.*[22] Examples of resting positions (loose-packed) are shown in Table 5-3.

Joint-play assessment and treatment should not be performed or attempted in the maximal close-packed position (see Chapter 3, Arthrology). The close-packed configuration usually occurs at a position that is the extreme of the most habitual position of the joint, whereas the mid range of a joint movement will be closer to the loose-packed or resting position.[76] For

TABLE 5-3 RESTING (LOOSE-PACKED) JOINT POSITIONS

JOINT(S)	POSITION
Vertebral	Midway between flexion and extension
Temporomandibular	Jaw slightly open (freeway space)
Sternoclavicular	Arm resting by side
Acromioclavicular	Arm resting by side
Glenohumeral	55–70° abduction; 30° horizontal adduction; neutral rotation
Elbow	
Humeroulnar	70° flexion and 10° supination
Humeroradial	Full extension and supination
Forearm	
Proximal radioulnar	70° flexion and 35° supination
Distal radioulnar	10° supination
Radio/ulnocarpal	Neutral with slight ulnar deviation
Hand	
Midcarpal	Neutral with slight flexion and ulnar deviation
Carpometacarpal (2 through 5)	Midway between flexion/extension, mid flexion, and mid extension
Trapeziometacarpal	Midway between flexion/extension and between abduction/adduction
Metacarpophalangeal (MCP)	First MCP joint: slight flexion MCP joints 2–5: Slight flexion with ulnar deviation
Interphalangeal (IP)	Proximal IP joints: 10° flexion Distal IP joints: 30° flexion
Hip	30° flexion, 30° abduction, and slight lateral rotation
Knee	25° flexion
Ankle/Foot	
Talocrural	Mid inversion/eversion and 10° plantar flexion
Subtalar and mid-tarsal	Midway between extremes of range of motion with 10° plantar flexion
Tarsometatarsal	Midway between supination and pronation
Toes	
Metatarsophalangeal	Neutral (extension 10°)
Interphalangeal	Slight flexion

(Adapted from references 22, 41, and 49)

TABLE 5-4 CLOSE-PACKED POSITIONS OF THE JOINTS

JOINT(S)	POSITION
Vertebral	Maximal extension
Temporomandibular	Maximal retrusion (mouth closed with teeth clenched) or maximal anterior position (mouth maximally opened)
Glenohumeral	Maximum abduction and external rotation
Sternoclavicular	Arm maximally elevated
Acromioclavicular	Arm abducted 90°
Elbow	
Humeroulnar	Full extension and supination
Humeroradial	90° flexion, 5° supination
Forearm	
Proximal radioulnar	5° supination, full extension
Distal radioulnar	5° supination
Radiocarpal	Full extension with radial deviation
Hand	
Midcarpal	Full extension
Carpometacarpal	Full opposition
Trapeziometacarpal	Full opposition
Metacarpophalangeal (MCP)	First MCP: Full extension MCP joints 2–5: Full flexion
Interphalangeal	Full extension
Hip	Ligamentous: Full extension, abduction, and internal rotation Bony: 90° flexion, slight abduction, and slight external rotation
Knee	Full extension and external rotation
Ankle/Foot	
Talocrural	Full dorsiflexion
Subtalar	Full inversion
Midtarsal	Full supination
Tarsometatarsal	Full supination
Toes	
Metatarsphalangeal	Full extension
Interphalangeal	Full extension

(Adapted from references 22, 41, 49)

example, the close-packed position for the wrist joint is full extension. The other extreme position of the joint that is less commonly assumed is also very congruent and is called the *potential close-packed position*.[3,49,89] Examples of the close-packed positions of most synovial joints are shown in Table 5-4.

If joint motion is to be avoided, the close-packed position can be used. For example, the spinal segments above and below a segment to be mobilized may be "locked" into a close-packed position in order to isolate the mobilizing force to a particular level.

Generally speaking, rotation will cause a close-packed position.

Joint-play assessment entails determination of the type of resistance felt at the end of range of motion (end feel), the type of pain, and the amount of excursion present in a particular direction. Excursion is determined by comparing the joint with the same joint on the opposite side, assuming that it is not in dysfunction. Joint excursion is evaluated by performing either a glide or traction mobilization and by moving the bone up to and slightly through the first tissue stop. This corresponds to a grade 3 treatment glide or grade 2 to 3 treatment traction (see joint treatment techniques in Chapter 6, Introduction to Manual Therapy). The first tissue stop felt by the clinician corresponds with the end of the elastic phase and the beginning of the plastic phase on the stress–strain curve. Following this scheme one can assess:

1. The degree of mobility (amplitude). The possibilities include:
   a. Hypermobility, suggesting a loss of continuity (partial tear or complete rupture) of the structure being tested
   b. Hypomobility, suggesting fibrosis, as from increased laying down of collagen in the presence of chronic stresses and low-grade inflammation, or suggesting adhesion to adjacent structures, as may occur during healing of a sprain. Hypomobility may be due to protective muscle spasm, in which case some degree of inflammation of the structure or synovial lining is implied.
   c. Normal mobility, implying normal status of the structure being tested
2. Presence of pain or muscle guarding (irritability) at extremes of movement. Pain on joint-play movement testing suggests the presence of a sprain or actual tear of the structure being stressed.
3. One must consider, then, six possible findings on joint-play movement testing and their probable interpretations:
   a. Normal mobility—painless. There is no lesion of the structure tested.
   b. Normal mobility—painful. There is a minor sprain of the structure tested.
   c. Hypomobility—painless. A contracture or adhesion involves the tested structure.
   d. Hypomobility—painful. A more acute sprain of the structure may be accompanied by guarding. If the hypomobility is due to muscle guarding, one cannot, at this point, know whether an actual tear or rupture exists.
   e. Hypermobility—painless. A complete rupture of the structure is suggested; there are no longer intact fibers from which pain can be elicited.
   f. Hypermobility—painful. A partial tear is present in which some fibers of the structure are still intact and being stressed.
4. Accessory movements are usually graded on a scale of 0 to 6, as listed in Table 5-5.[88] Such grading has the following treatment implications:[22]

TABLE 5-5   GRADING ACCESSORY JOINT MOVEMENT

GRADE	JOINT STATUS
0	Ankylosed
1	Considerable hypomobility
2	Slight hypomobility
3	Normal
4	Slight hypermobility
5	Considerable hypermobility
6	Unstable

   a. Grades 0 and 6: Mobilization is not indicated. Surgery should be considered.
   b. Grade 1 and 2: Mobilization is indicated.
   c. Grade 3: Mobilization is not indicated to increase joint extensibility.
   d. Grades 4 and 5: Mobilization is not indicated to increase joint extensibility. Taping, bracing, stabilization through exercises, and education regarding posture and positions to be avoided should be considered.

III. Resisted Isometric Tests

These are tests designed to assess the status of musculotendinous tissue. Traditional muscle testing procedures that are included in the following section on neuromuscular tests are used primarily to evaluate neurologic function, whereas the intention of these tests is to determine whether there is some lesion, or loss of continuity, of the musculotendinous tissue itself. In order to do so, ideally the clinician needs to stress the muscle and tendon that is to be tested without stressing other joint tissues. These tests are performed, then, as maximal isometric contractions, disallowing any movement of the joint. Realistically, in most cases other tissues are going to be squeezed or compressed by the contracting muscles, but this seldom poses a problem when the test is done correctly. A particular muscle and tendon are tested in the position that best isolates them, and in a position in which they are at an optimal length for maximal contraction (usually a mid position). Maximal stabilization is required to prevent substitution and to minimize joint movement.

When performing resisted isometric tests, one must determine whether the contraction is strong or weak and whether it is painful or painless. Weakness may be due to a neurologic deficit or to actual loss of continuity of muscle or tendon tissue;

appropriate neurologic testing may be performed to determine which is the case. Few neurologic disorders result in isolated weakness of a single muscle. A painful contraction signifies the presence of some painful lesion involving the muscle or tendon tissues being tested. In the majority of cases the problem will be in the tendon, since muscle strains are rare except in sports-related injuries. Very often the patient feels the most pain as the contraction is released rather than during maximal contraction. When this occurs, it should be considered a positive test; the lengthening that occurs as a muscle relaxes apparently stresses the involved fibers sufficiently to cause more pain than does the shortening that occurs during contraction. Practically speaking, these resisted tests are often performed in conjunction with standard neuromuscular strength tests.

There are four possible findings on resisted movement tests:

A. *Strong and painless*—There is no lesion or neurologic deficit involving the muscle or tendon tested.

B. *Strong and painful*—A minor lesion of the tested tendon or muscle exists; usually the tendon is at fault. Occasionally auxiliary resisted tests must be performed to differentiate the involved structure from synergists.

C. *Weak and painless*

   1. There may be some interruption of the nerve supply to the muscle tested. The findings must be correlated with those of other muscle tests and neurologic tests.

   2. There may be a complete rupture of tendon or muscle; there are no longer fibers intact from which pain can be elicited.

D. *Weak and painful*

   1. There may be a partial rupture of muscle or tendon in which there are still some intact fibers that are being stressed.

   2. This may be the result of painful inhibition in association with some serious pathologic condition, such as a fracture or neoplasm or an acute inflammatory process.

☐ **Neuromuscular Tests**

If, at this point in the examination, one suspects that there may be a lesion interfering with neural conduction, the appropriate clinical tests should be performed in an attempt to detect loss of neurologic function. The common nerve lesions are extrinsic. Loss of conduction usually results from pressure on a nerve

from some adjacent structure or structures. In the common nerve disorders, the pressure is usually minor or intermittent, or both, and usually involves a single nerve or segment. For this reason, the manifestations of the disorder are often quite subtle; findings on evaluation are largely subjective, and some objective signs may be detected only with more sophisticated electrotesting procedures.

When neurologic function is assessed clinically and a deficit is detected, the approximate site of the lesion can be estimated by correlating the extent of the deficit with peripheral nerve and segmental distributions. More central or serious lesions must be suspected when the extent of the deficit exceeds the distribution of a single segment or a single peripheral nerve. Peripheral nerve and segmental innervations are indicated in Table 5-6 and Figure 5-4. Key segmental distributions, both myotomal and dermatomal, are listed in Table 5-7. These are the muscles and skin areas that are most likely to be affected by involvement of a particular segment. These are important to know, since segmental deficits, such as those that occur with disk protrusions, are very common neural disorders seen clinically. Because of the overlapping of dermatomes and myotomes in the extremities, lesions involving a single segment, even when conduction is completely interrupted, result in only subtle deficits.

The tests described below may be used when performing clinical neurologic assessment.

STRENGTH TESTS

Traditional muscle testing procedures should be employed. It is often necessary to repeat a test, comparing the strength carefully to the normal side if possible, since weaknesses resulting from common nerve lesions are usually subtle. Weaknesses and asymmetries in strength are noted.

SENSORY TESTS

A pin, wisp of cotton, and tuning fork may be used to assess conduction along sensory pathways. Pressure on a nerve will usually result in loss of conduction along the large myelinated fibers first and the small unmyelinated fibers last. Therefore, minor deficits will often be manifested first by loss of vibration sense, with sensation to touch and noxious stimulation being reduced with more severe or long-lasting pressure.

When performing sensory tests, a particular area on the normal side is tested and the patient is asked if the sensation is perceived. Then the involved side

(text continues on page 88)

TABLE 5-6 PERIPHERAL NERVES AND SEGMENTAL INNERVATION

ACTION TO BE TESTED	MUSCLES	CORD SEGMENT	NERVES	PLEXUS
Shoulder Girdle and Upper Extremity				
Flexion of neck Extension of neck Rotation of neck Lateral bending of neck	Deep neck muscles (sternomastoid and trapezius also participate)	C1–C4	Cervical	Cervical
Elevation of upper thorax	Scaleni	C3–C5	Phrenic	
Inspiration	Diaphragm	C3–C5		
Adduction of arm from behind to front	Pectoralis major and minor	C5–C8 T1	Medial and lateral pectoral (from medial and lateral cords of plexus)	Brachial
Forward thrust of shoulder	Serratus anterior	C5–C7	Long thoracic	
Elevation of scapula	Levator scapulae	C5 (C3–C4)	Dorsal scapular	
Medial adduction and elevation of scapula	Rhomboids	C4–C5		
Abduction of arm	Supraspinatus	C4–C6	Suprascapular	
Lateral rotation of arm	Infraspinatus	C4–C6		
Medial rotation of arm Adduction of arm front to back	Latissimus dorsi, teres major, and subscapularis	C5–C8	Subscapular (from posterior cord of plexus)	
Adbuction of arm	Deltoid	C5–C6	Axillary (from posterior cord of plexus)	Brachial
Lateral rotation of arm	Teres minor	C4–C5		
Flexion of forearm Supination of forearm	Biceps brachii	C5–C6	Musculocutaneous (from lateral cord of plexus)	
Adduction of arm Flexion of forearm	Coracobrachialis	C5–C7		
Flexion of forearm	Brachialis	C5–C6		Brachial
Ulnar flexion of hand	Flexor carpi ulnaris	C7–T1	Ulnar (from medial cord of plexus)	
Flexion of terminal phalanx of ring finger and little finger Flexion of hand	Flexor digitorum profundus (ulnar portion)	C7–T1		
Adduction of metacarpal of thumb	Adductor pollicis	C8–T1	Ulnar	Brachial
Abduction of little finger	Abductor digiti quinti	C8–T1		
Opposition of little finger	Opponens digiti quinti	C7–T1		
Flexion of little finger	Flexor digiti quinti brevis	C7–T1		
Flexion of proximal phalanx; extension of two distal phalanges; adduction and abduction of fingers	Interossei	C8–T1		
Pronation of forearm	Pronator teres	C6–C7	Median (C6,C7 from lateral cord of plexus; C8, T1 from medial cord of plexus)	Brachial
Radial flexion of hand	Flexor carpi radialis	C6–C7		
Flexion of hand	Palmaris longus	C7–T1		
Flexion of middle phalanx of index, middle, ring, little fingers	Flexor digitorum sublimis	C7–T1		
Flexion of hand Flexion of terminal phalanx of thumb	Flexor pollicis longus	C7–T1	Median	Brachial
Flexion of terminal phalanx of index finger, and middle finger Flexion of hand	Flexor digitorum profundus (radial portion)	C7–T1		

(continued)

TABLE 5-6   Continued

ACTION TO BE TESTED	MUSCLES	CORD SEGMENT	NERVES	PLEXUS
Shoulder Girdle and Upper Extremity				
Abduction of metacarpal of thumb	Abductor pollicis brevis	C7–T1	Median	Brachial
Flexion of proximal phalanx of thumb	Flexor pollicis brevis	C7–T1		
Opposition of metacarpal of thumb	Opponens pollicis	C8–T1		
Flexion of proximal phalanx and extension of 2 distal phalanges of all fingers	Lumbricales (the two lateral) Lumbricales (the two medial)	C8–T1	Median Ulnar	Brachial
Extension of forearm	Triceps brachii and anconeus	C6–C8	Radial (from posterior cord of plexus)	Brachial
Flexion of forearm	Brachioradialis	C5–C6		
Radial extension of hand	Extensor carpi radialis	C6–C8		
Extension of phalanges of fingers Extension of hand	Extensor digitorum communis	C6–C8		
Extension of phalanges of little finger Extension of hand	Extensor digiti quinti proprius	C6–C8		
Ulnar extension of hand	Extensor carpi ulnaris	C6–C8	Radial	Brachial
Supination of forearm	Supinator	C5–C7		
Abduction of metacarpal of thumb Radial extension of hand	Abductor pollicis longus	C7–C8		
Extension of thumb	Extensor pollicis brevis and longus	C6–C8		
Radial extension of hand Extension of index finger Extension of hand	Extensor indicis proprius	C6–C8		
Trunk and Thorax				
Elevation of ribs Depression of ribs Contraction of abdomen Anteroflexion of trunk Lateral flexion of trunk	Thoracic, abdominal, and back		Thoracic and posterior lumbosacral branches	
Hip Girdle and Lower Extremity				
Flexion of hip	Iliopsoas	L1–L3	Femoral	Lumbar
Flexion of hip and eversion of thigh	Sartorius	L2–L3		
Extension of leg	Quadriceps femoris	L2–L4		
Adduction of thigh	Pectineus	L2–L3	Obturator	Lumbar
	Adductor longus	L2–L3		
	Adductor brevis	L2–L4		
	Adductor magnus	L3–L4		
	Gracilis	L2–L4		
Adduction of thigh Lateral rotation of thigh	Obturator externus	L3–L4		
Abduction of thigh Medial rotation of thigh	Gluteus medius and minimus	L4–S1	Superior gluteal	Sacral
Flexion of thigh	Tensor fasciae latae	L4–L5		
Lateral rotation of thigh	Piriformis	L5–S1		
Abduction of thigh	Gluteus maximus	L4–S2	Inferior gluteal	

(continued)

TABLE 5-6   CONTINUED

ACTION TO BE TESTED	MUSCLES	CORD SEGMENT	NERVES	PLEXUS
Hip Girdle and Lower Extremity				
Lateral rotation of thigh	Obturator internus	L5–S1	Muscular branches from sacral plexus	
	Gemelli	L4–S1		
	Quadratus femoris	L4–S1		
Flexion of leg (assist in extension of thigh)	Biceps femoris	L4–S2	Sciatic (trunk)	Sacral
	Semitendinosus	L4–S1		
	Semimembranosus	L4–S1		
Dorsiflexion of foot Supination of foot	Tibialis anterior	L4–L5	Deep peroneal	Sacral
Extension of toes II–V Dorsiflexion of foot	Extensor digitorum longus	L4–S1		
Extension of great toe Dorsiflexion of foot	Extensor hallucis longus	L4–S1		
Extension of great toe and the three medial toes	Extensor digitorum brevis	L4–S1		
Plantar flexion of foot in pronation	Peronei	L5–S1	Superficial peroneal	Sacral
Plantar flexion of foot in supination	Tibialis posterior and triceps surae	L5–S2	Tibial	Sacral
Plantar flexion of foot in supination Flexion of terminal phalanx of toes II–V	Flexor digitorum longus	L5–S2		
Plantar flexion of foot in supination Flexion of terminal phalanx of great toe	Flexor hallucis longus	L5–S2		
Flexion of middle phalanx of toes II–V	Flexor digitorum brevis	L5–S1		
Flexion of proximal phalanx of great toe	Flexor hallucis brevis	L5–S2		
Spreading and closing of toes Flexion of proximal phalanx of toes	Small muscles of foot	S1–S2		
Voluntary control of pelvic floor	Perineal and sphincters	S2–S4	Pudendal	Sacral

(Chusid JG: Correlative Neuroanatomy and Functional Neurology. Los Altos, CA, Lange Medical Publications, 1970)

is retested and the patient again asked if the sensation is felt. If sensation is intact on both sides, the patient is asked if it felt the same on both sides. This procedure is followed when testing each key segmental sensory area and each peripheral nerve distribution. Sensory deficits and asymmetries in perception are noted.

DEEP TENDON REFLEXES

Lower motor neuron lesions, such as segmental or peripheral nerve disorders, may result in diminution of certain deep-tendon reflexes, while more central, upper motor neuron lesions may cause hyperreflexia. The important assessments to make when testing deep tendon reflexes are whether the responses at homologous tendons are symmetrical and whether any responses are clonic. The presence of hyporeflexia is difficult to judge, since some persons normally have reflexes that are difficult to elicit. In general, if it is equally difficult to elicit responses at corresponding tendons, no significance can be attributed. However, if upper extremity responses are difficult to elicit but lower extremity responses are strong, a myelopathy

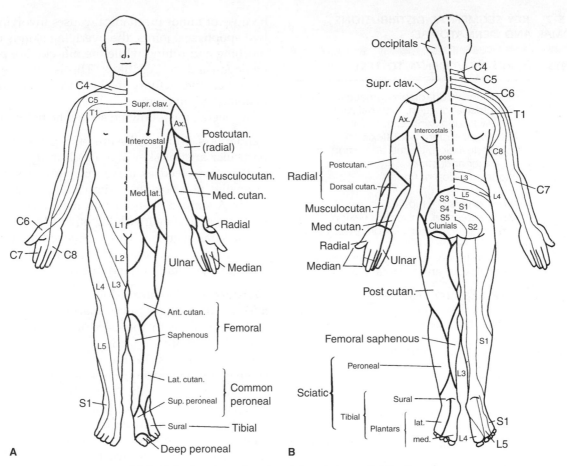

FIG. 5-4. Segmental and peripheral nerve distribution.

or some other more serious pathologic process should be considered.

COORDINATION, TONE, AND PATHOLOGIC REFLEXES

Coordination, tone, and pathologic reflexes should be assessed if myelopathy or other upper motor neuron disturbances are suspected. For example, myelopathy resulting from cervical spondylosis may result in a mildly spastic gait, increased lower extremity tone, lower extremity hyperreflexia, and perhaps a positive Babinski response (dorsiflexion of big toe in response to noxious stimulation along the sole of the foot).

☐ Palpation

Palpation tests are usually conveniently performed at the same time as the inspection tests discussed previously. As in inspection, palpation tests should be organized according to layers, assessing the status of the skin, subcutaneous soft tissues, and bony structures (including tendon and ligament attachments). Significant findings are documented.

Palpation of all tissues associated with the area of symptoms discloses both physiologic and structural changes. The uninvolved side should be palpated first so that the patient has some idea of what to expect. The palpatory examination includes, but is not necessarily limited to, palpation of the myofascial structures in the form of layer palpation and palpation of the bony structures. The tissues that can be palpated include the skin, subcutaneous fascia, blood vessels, nerves, muscle sheaths, muscle bellies, musculotendinous junctions, tendons, deep fascia, ligaments, bones, and joint spaces.

For practical purposes, layer palpation may be categorized into superficial and deep palpation. Superficial palpatory examination includes assessment of tissue temperature and moisture as well as light touch to determine the extensibility and integrity of the superficial connective tissue.

SKIN

The examiner uses the back of the hand to initially discern variations in skin temperature and sweating between symptomatic and nonsymptomatic areas.

The movement of the skin over the underlying but superficial structures is checked next. Depending on

TABLE 5-7 KEY SEGMENTAL DISTRIBUTIONS (MYOTOMAL AND DERMATOMAL)

SEGMENTS	KEY MOVEMENTS TO TEST
C4	Shoulder shrug, diaphragmatic function
C5	Shoulder abduction, external rotation
C6	Elbow flexion, wrist extension
C7	Elbow extension, wrist flexion
C8	Ulnar deviation, thumb abduction, small finger abduction
T1	Approximation of fingers
L2	Hip flexion
L3	Knee extension, hip flexion
L4	Knee extension, ankle dorsiflexion
L5	Ankle/large toe dorsiflexion, eversion of ankle
S1	Plantar flexion, eversion, knee flexion
S2	Knee flexion, ankle plantar flexion
	REFLEXES TO TEST
Cranial nerve V	Jaw jerk[29,66]
C5,C6	Biceps, brachioradialis
(C7),C8	Triceps
(L3–L4)	Patellar tendon (quadriceps)
L5	Great toe jerk[32,83]
S1–S2	Achilles tendon
	KEY SEGMENTAL SENSORY AREAS TO TEST (distal part of segment)
C6	Thumb and index finger, radial border of hand
C7	Middle three fingers
C8	Ring and small finger, ulnar border of hand
L2	Medial thigh
L3	Anteromedial, distal thigh
L4	Medial aspect of large toe
L5	Web space between large and second toes
S1	Below lateral malleolus
S2	Back of heel
S3–S4	Saddle, anal region

Note: Others (*e.g.*, upper cervical, thoracic, and lumbar) are less definite due to overlapping.

(Chusid JG: Correlative Neuroanatomy and Functional Neurology. Los Altos, CA, Lange Medical Publications, 1970)

the body part being tested, either the palm or the fingertips are used to detect restrictions. On broad body surfaces, the palm is firmly but lightly placed on the skin and then displaced in all directions to identify tension and resistance to gentle displacement.

More vigorous displacement in the form of skin rolling (if tolerated and indicated) is often an important part of layer palpation; it gives additional information about the extensibility of the subcutaneous tissues and possible infiltration of the skin and subcutaneous tissue by cellulitis.[51,52] According to the minor intervertebral derangement theory of Maigne,

because of minor mechanical causes involving one or two apophyseal joints, the overlying skin is tender to pinching and rolling while the muscles are painful to palpation and feel cordlike.[44] This is felt to be initiated by nociceptive activity in the posterior primary dermatome and myotome.

In general, the following should be noted:

Tenderness. Minor pressure on a nerve supplying a particular area of skin may result in dysesthesia that may be perceived as a painful burning sensation to normally non-noxious stimulation, such as light touch. A similar phenomenon may also occur in the presence of lesions involving other tissues innervated by the same segment. This is believed to be the result of summation of otherwise subthreshold afferent input to a segment of the spinal cord.

Moisture and Texture. Moisture and texture may be altered with changes in vascularity or changes in sympathetic activity to the part. In the presence of increased sympathetic activity, such as that which commonly occurs in the chronic stages of reflex sympathetic dystrophy, the skin will be abnormally moist and very smooth. With reduced sympathetic activity, sometimes preceding a reflex sympathetic dystrophy, the skin may be dry and scaly. Sudomotor studies have utilized an electrical skin resistance method for measuring sweat gland activity.[46,47,48]

Temperature. Skin temperature will be elevated in the presence of an underlying inflammatory process or with reduced sympathetic activity.[1,18,35] A reduction in skin temperature may accompany vascular deficiency, increased sympathetic activity, or fibro-fatty infiltration.[39] Thermocouples and infrared thermography are sometimes used for differential diagnosis of certain conditions.[64]

Mobility. The skin should be moved relative to the underlying tissues to examine for the presence of skin adhesions. This is especially important following healing of surgical and other traumatic wounds.

SUBCUTANEOUS SOFT TISSUES

The soft tissues are palpated deep to the skin—fat, fascia, muscles, tendons, joint capsules and ligaments, nerves, and blood vessels. No more pressure than what is necessary is used. A common mistake is to press harder and harder in an attempt to distinguish deep structures. This only serves to desensitize the palpating fingertips and does not assist in determining the nature of the tissues being palpated.

The deep palpatory examination includes *compression*, which is palpation through layers of tissue perpendicular to the tissue, and shear. *Shear* is movement of the myofascial tissues between layers, moving parallel to the tissue.[8] Translational muscle play is an effective assessment tool for assessing the mobility of a muscle or muscle group within the fascial sheath. Palpation may progress to probing, to grasping, or displacing muscle bellies and tendons. Resistance to displacement or stretch and crepitus or "catching" should be noted. It is most revealing to palpate the entire extent of a tendon sheath during contraction of its respective muscle. A characteristic vibration, as if the tendon needs lubrication, represents tenosynovitis.[88] Soft tissue palpation may offer information concerning the following:

Tenderness. Tenderness to deep palpation is a very unreliable finding. In itself it is never indicative of the site of a pathologic process because of the prevalence of referred tenderness with lesions of deep somatic tissues. The phenomenon is similar in all respects to that of referred pain. In many common lesions, the area of primary tenderness does not correspond well to the site of the lesion. Patients with low back disorders are often most tender in the buttock, those with supraspinatus tendinitis are most tender over the lateral brachial region, and persons with trochanteric bursitis are most tender over the lateral aspect of the thigh. These "trigger points," or referred areas of tenderness, are found in some area of the segment corresponding to the segment in which the lesion exists. Generally, tenderness associated with more superficial lesions, such as medial ligament sprains at the knee, corresponds more closely with the site of the lesion than does tenderness occurring with more deeply situated pathologic processes.

Edema and Swelling. The size and location of localized soft-tissue swellings are noted. Abnormal fluid accumulations should be differentiated as intra- or extra-articular. Articular effusion will be restricted to the confines of the joint capsule; pressure applied over one side of the joint may, therefore, cause increased distention observed over the opposite side. This type of *ballottement* test can be used with more superficial joints. Often articular effusion is distinguished by its characteristic distribution at a particular joint; these distributions are discussed in the chapters on specific regions. Extra-articular swelling may accompany acute inflammatory processes, such as abscesses and those following acute trauma, because of protein and plasma leaking from capillary walls. Generalized tissue edema may accompany vascular disorders, lymphatic obstructions, and electrolyte imbalances.

Consistency, Continuity, and Mobility. Normal soft tissue is supple and easily moved against underlying tissue. Palpation for abnormalities such as indurated areas, loss of mobility, stringiness, doughiness, nodules, and gaps is done and results noted.

Pulse. Palpating for the pulse of various major arteries can assist in assessing the status of blood supply to the part. Heart rate may also be determined.

BONY STRUCTURES

Bony structures also include ligaments and tendon attachments. When palpating bony structures, the following should be noted:

Tenderness. As with deep, soft-tissue tenderness, tenderness at various bony sites may be referred and is therefore often misleading. Lesions involving both ligaments and tendons commonly occur at the site where these structures join the periosteum. Typically, these are highly innervated regions and may be tender to palpation in the presence of tenoperiosteal or periosteoligamentous strains and sprains. Periosteal tenderness will also accompany specific bony lesions, such as stress fractures or other fractures.

Enlargements. Bony hypertrophy often accompanies healing of a fracture and degenerative joint disease. In the latter, the bony changes will be noted at the joint margins in more superficial joints.

Bony Relationships. Structural malalignments, as discussed in the section on inspection, may be detected clinically by assessing the relationships, in the various planes of reference, of one bony structure to another. This is especially important following healing of fractures and in cases of vague, subtle, insidious disorders that may have a pathomechanical basis.

☐ Provocation Tests

Provocation tests (auxiliary tests) are employed only when no symptoms have been produced by full active movements and other selective tissue tension tests. Additional strategies may be required to reproduce symptoms.

Initial provocation tests may be undertaken in which gentle passive overpressure is applied at the end range of active or passive movement. Sometimes the symptoms are only at the end range, which the patient tends to avoid by moving just short of this point. Additional tests may include repeated active motions and repeated motions at various speeds and sustained pressures.

Should gentle overpressure, sustained pressure, or repeated motions fail to reproduce the pain, greater stress on the structures can be achieved by combined motions or by coupling movements in two or three directions, for example, quadrant tests (see Chapter 20, The Lumbar Spine). These tests have a considerable capacity to reproduce the patient's pain.

☐ Special Tests

The administration of certain special tests, which pertain to the anatomy and pathologic condition of each peripheral joint or spinal region being examined, may be considered. These tests are structured to uncover a specific type of pathology, condition, or injury and are most helpful when previous portions of the examination have led the examiner to suspect the nature of the pathology or condition. There are usually three types of special tests: joint and ligamentous tests, neuromuscular tests, and neurologic tests. These might include tests for joint instability and muscle/tendon pathology and dysfunction. If the examiner suspects a problem with movement of the spinal cord, nerve root, or nerve, any of the tests that stretch the cord may be performed. These include the straight-leg raising test and well leg test, the slump test (see Chapter 20, The Lumbar Spine), the first thoracic nerve root test (see Chapter 19, The Cervical Spine), and upper limb tension tests (see Chapter 9, The Shoulder and Shoulder Girdle).

Other considerations may include tests for intermittent claudication and tests for malingering or non-organic pain.

☐ Examination of Related Areas

It is often necessary to test other related joints to determine if pain arises from these joints. For example, when assessing the lumbar spine, one may need to consider the sacroiliac or hip joint instead of, or in addition to, the spine. When examining the shoulder, one should consider lesion areas known to refer pain to it, including problems of the neck; for example, a herniated cervical disk may radiate pain to the shoulder or scapula, an elbow or distal humeral pathologies can radiate pain proximally (uncommon), and a myocardial infarction may radiate pain to the left shoulder. Shoulder symptoms may also be related to irritation of the diaphragm, which shares the same root innervation as the dermatome covering the shoulder's summit. A general physical examination including the chest may be necessary.

☐ Functional Assessment

Some aspects of functional assessment should be included during the examination of the joint. This procedure may be as simple as observation of certain patient activities involving the joint or region being examined, or be more complex, such as a more detailed examination involving objective measurement of functional task performance.

After any examination, the patient should always be warned of the possibilities of exacerbation of symptoms as a result of the assessment.

☐ Other Investigations

Plain film radiography is the most common first-order diagnostic screening procedure in the evaluation of musculoskeletal diseases and dysfunction. X-ray films need not be taken routinely in all patients, and a particular radiological lesion does not necessarily prove that it is the source of the patient's pain. They are often of most value in demonstrating that no abnormality is present in the bone or joints. At times, findings simply support a moderately firm clinical diagnosis; in others cases, however, the films may provide the only clue to a clinically obscure situation. If radiographs are available, they should be reviewed. If they are not available but the examiner believes they are needed, he may request them before proceeding with treatment. The manual therapist must recognize the presence of skeletal conditions that contraindicate manual examination and treatment.

It is generally felt that procedural tests such as computed tomography (CT) should be kept in reserve for chronic disorders, especially mechanical disorders, that remain undiagnosed and for situations in which surgical intervention is planned.[44] Depending on availability and merit, such tests may include:

Computed tomography (CT)
Magnetic resonance imaging (MRI)
Myelography or radiculography
Discography
Bone scanning

RADIOGRAPHIC EXAMINATION

X-rays are the very short wavelength representatives on the spectrum of electromagnetic radiation. X-ray film, like photographic film, has a clear celluloid or plastic base coated with a silver bromide emulsion which undergoes alterations in response to radiant energy. Chemical development then renders this visible as differential blackening, and the resultant shadows or negatives are available for interpretation.

As the primary x-ray beam traverses a body part it will be absorbed to varying degrees depending on the density and volume of the tissue elements it encounters. High density bone will absorb more x-rays than the adjacent soft tissues, leaving fewer photons available to expose the film, and the resultant image will have a white area of radiopacity. Fat and gas have lower x-ray absorption, permitting more film blackening or radiolucency.

In conventional x-ray films, the absorption densities of many musculoskeletal tissues—cartilage, tendon, and muscle—are identical. Fortunately, fat is often present along tissue planes and between muscle layers, providing visibility by virtue of its lower absorption density (Fig. 5-5). With experience, the examiner becomes able to detect on x-ray examination many important soft-tissue changes such as effusion in joints, tendinous calcifications, ectopic bone in muscle, and tissue displaced by a tumor. Further, the studies enable the examiner to see fractures, dislocations, foreign bodies, and indication of bone loss (Fig. 5-6). For osteoporosis to be evident on film, approximately 30 to 35 percent of the bone must be lost.

Basic proficiency in film interpretation is generally considered a clinical skill beyond the scope of manual therapy. However, a working knowledge of radiological fundamentals and terminology will greatly facili-

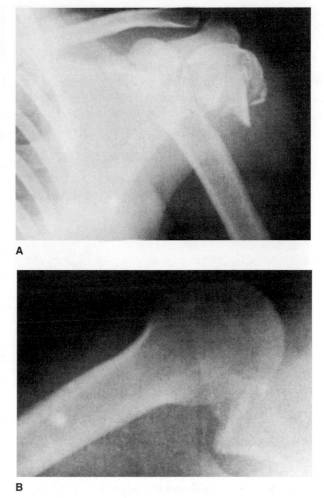

A

B

FIG. 5-6. (**A**) Roentgenogram of a fracture of the proximal humerus, and (**B**) axillary view of an anterior dislocation of the shoulder. A large defect (compression fracture) is present in the posterior position of the humeral head (Hill-Sack lesion). In both situations, the humeral head lies anterior to the glenoid cavity. (D'Ambrosia RD: Musculoskeletal Disorders: Regional Examination and Differential Diagnosis, 2nd ed. Philadelphia, JB Lippincott, 1986)

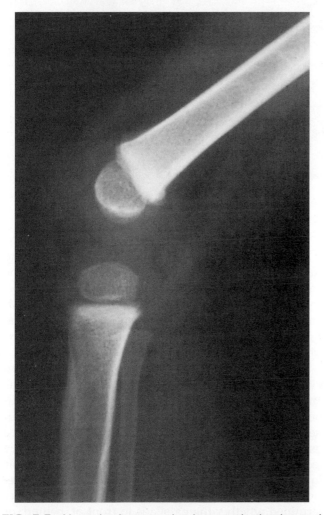

FIG. 5-5. Normal calcareous density, muscle density, and fat density. Fat pads help to outline tendons and articular cartilage at the knee. (D'Ambrosia RD: Musculoskeletal Disorders: Regional Examination and Differential Diagnosis, 2nd ed. Philadelphia, JB Lippincott, 1986)

tate the study of the musculoskeletal system and give access to pertinent information from the radiologist's report to form a more thorough history and physical evaluation of the patient.

The first step is to become familiar with the appearance of normal bones and tissues. They are characterized by clarity, contrast, and transparency of the structures as opposed to the haziness, indistinctness, and translucency associated with diseased tissue.[24] Healthy bone and tissue are further characterized by evenness and regularity of outline, structure, and density. Observation of bone films should include:

I. External observations of bone

    A. Bone shape: Each bone has its own characteristic shape and surface features (Fig. 5-7). The

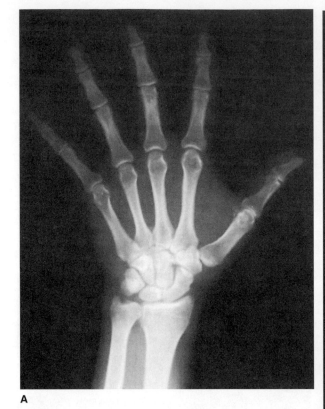

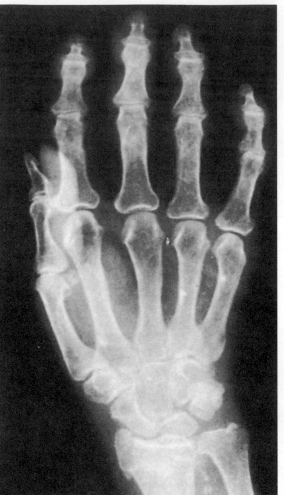

FIG. 5-7. (**A**) Radiograph shows normal shape of the bones of the wrist and hand. (**B**) Radiograph of a hand with senile osteoporosis shows a uniform loss of bone density with a thin, sharply defined cortex. A fracture of the distal radius is present. (**A** from D'Ambrosia RD: *Musculoskeletal Disorders: Regional Examination and Differential Diagnosis*, 2nd ed. Philadelphia, JB Lippincott, 1986; **B** from Greenfield GB: *Radiology of Bone Disease*, 4th ed. Philadelphia, JB Lippincott, 1986)

most frequently encountered example of a deviation from normal shape is a displaced fracture.[86]

B. Bony surfaces: Cortical bone should be smooth, white, and intact, except for cortical roughening normally seen at the site of tendon attachments. Abnormalities of bone surfaces may include periosteal bone formation due to an underlying bone infection and focal erosions in rheumatoid arthritis.

II. **Internal structure of bone**
A. Diffuse changes: Less bone density than normal can be appreciated by comparing normal x-ray films with those which reflect disuse demineralization (see Fig. 5-7).
B. Focal abnormalities: Slowly growing destructive bone lesions will modify the shape of surrounding bones and will often evoke a sclerotic reaction at the margin, which is evident by an increase in density (see Fig. 5-7). More radially growing lesions are characterized by a poorly defined, permeative pattern of destruction.

Spinal radiographs are nearly always included to rule out fracture, dislocation, anomaly, or bone pathology. The radiographs are also used in biomechanical analysis to establish an initial course of treatment for patients. Radiographs of extremity skeletal structures may be included to rule out primary extremity pathologic processes.

Study of any skeletal region requires at least two views, preferably at right angles to each other (such as an anteroposterior [AP] and a lateral view). The patient's history and clinical evaluation are guides that help determine the different views that should be used. At times, modifications and supplementary techniques are required to provide precise diagnosis for effective therapy. For example, in the anteroposterior or frontal projection of the knee, it cannot be determined whether the patella is in front of, behind, or even within the femur (Fig. 5-8*A,B*). A lateral view will obviously localize the patella and give useful information about its configuration (Fig. 5-8*C,D*). However, if there are really concerns about structural integrity of the patella itself, in order to rule out a fracture, a tangential or axial view of it would be necessary (Fig. 5-8E,F).[86]

III. Special examination

Other supplementary techniques and modifications that may be required to provide precise diagnosis for effective therapy and often of particular interest to the manual therapist include:

A. Stress view: Although clinical tests for instability usually subjectively document that laxity is present, standard radiographs should be taken. They will indicate if the laxity is caused by an avulsion of the ligament with its bony attachment or by an epiphyseal separation. In order to determine whether the ligaments are intact after a joint injury, the joint may be x-rayed in a position that would normally tighten or stress the ligament in question; for example, by applying the appropriate varus–valgus or anteroposterior stress to a joint as a standard radiograph is taken. They have proved particularly useful for documenting instabilities at the ankle and epiphyseal injuries of the knee (Fig. 5-9).[43]

B. Dynamic studies: X-ray examinations in both still and cinematic format can be used to assess functional mobility as well as integrity of structure. Examples include cervical spine subluxations (Fig. 5-10) and upper limb motion at the wrist joint.

ARTHROGRAMS

Arthrography is the study of structures in an encapsulated joint using radiographic contrast media. Contrast medium is injected directly into the joint space, distending the capsule and outlining internal structures. When the clinical question is one of a torn meniscus (Fig. 5-11), focal erosion of articular cartilage or a nonopaque intramuscular fragment, arthrography is most informative. Arthrography has been commonly used in evaluating the knee and shoulder joint. Evaluation of the shoulder joint can determine the presence of rotator cuff tears (Fig. 5-12), bicipital tendinitis or tears, and the presence of adhesive capsulitis.

MYELOGRAPHY

Myelography is the study of spinal cord, nerve roots, and dura mater using radiographic contrast media. Myelography is now performed almost exclusively with water-soluble dyes through a spinal puncture. This technique is used to detect nerve root entrapment, spinal stenosis, and tumors of the spinal canal. Extradural techniques can yield supplementary information regarding the state of the disk. Indentation of the dural sac or filling defects indicate abnormality that needs explanation (see Fig. 20-4). In spite of the decreased incidence of spinal headache and discomfort during this procedure, it is still significantly invasive and is usually reserved for chronic disorders that remain undiagnosed and unabated and in situations when surgical intervention is planned.[13,56] Plain films or CT may also be used to visualize more anatomic detail. When CT scanning is used in conjunction with myelography, the image is referred to as a CT myelogram.

DISCOGRAPHY

Discography involves the injection under x-ray control of a contrast medium (a water-soluble radiopaque dye) into the nucleus pulposus. Although rarely indicated, the technique can provide some useful information with respect to disk disease and the level of impingement (see Figs. 20-2A, 20-3A). The test interpretation depends on radiographic abnormalities of degeneration, identification of annular tears, epidural flow, or vertebral flow through vessels transiting the vertebral end-plate.[56]

Other contrast studies include angiography and arteriography (Fig. 5-13), used in evaluating hypervascular tumors and determining vascular anatomy,[7,81] and venography.

COMPUTED TOMOGRAPHY

Computed tomography uses a computerized display to recreate a three-dimensional image. Cuts of film are taken at specific levels of the body. Tomograms may be plain or computer-enhanced. In the latter case, they are referred to as CT scans (computed tomography scans) or CAT scans (computer-assisted or enhanced tomography).[50] Computed tomography has rapidly become the diagnostic procedure of choice for many conditions. Its diagnostic capabilities are based on tissue attenuation of an x-ray beam. Two features render it most useful for musculoskeletal radiology: greater tissue contrast resolution than conventional radiography, and the inherent ability to display cross-sectional anatomy.[30] The CT scan can also be contrast-enhanced (dye injected around the structure) to indicate tumor, bone, or soft-tissue involvement. They are then referred to as CTAs (computed tomoarthrograms).[50] A CAT spinal scan is used to outline structural spinal problems involving both bone and soft tissues. These include spinal stenosis, vertebral diseases, disk prolapse, and abnormalities in the facet joint.

The process begins when an x-ray source rotates around the supine patient and x-rays penetrate the body from numerous angles. Detectors in the surrounding scanner measure tissue x-ray attenuation and transmit this information to the computer. The computer then reconstructs the body image using

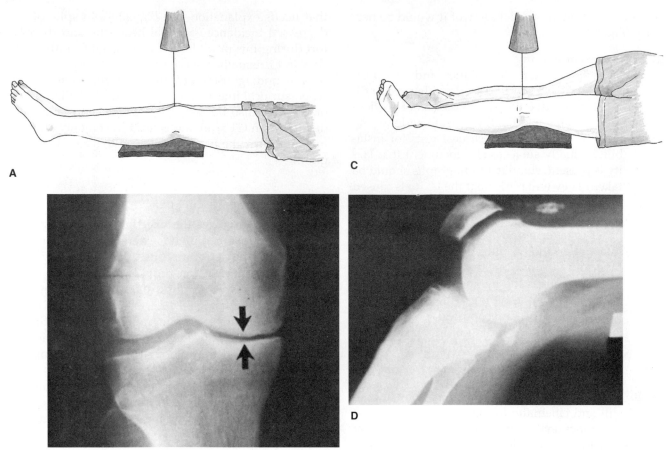

FIG. 5-8. Positioning and resulting x-ray appearance in standard projection for radiography of the knee. (**A,B**) Anterioposterior (AP) projection. (**C,D**) Lateral projection. (**E,F**) Tangential patellar (sunrise) view. (D'Ambrosia RD: Musculoskeletal Disorders: Regional Examination and Differential Diagnosis, 2nd ed. Philadelphia, JB Lippincott, 1986) (*continued*)

these measurements taken at the periphery of the axial slice of the body being scanned (Fig. 5-14).

NUCLEAR MAGNETIC RESONANCE AND MAGNETIC RESONANCE IMAGING

The nuclear magnetic resonance (NMR) scanner is one of the newest tools primarily devised to evaluate vertebral lesions. The development of surface coil technology in the mid-1980s[21] established magnetic resonance imaging (MRI) as a reasonable alternative to myelography and CT in the study of intervertebral disk disease.[2] This technique uses no ionizing radiation to visualize the structures being evaluated and can be used to obtain an image of bone and soft tissue (spinal cord and paravertebral masses). Recently, in orthopedic evaluation, the capabilities of MRI have expanded its role in examination of joints (Fig. 5-15). Excellent soft tissue and bone marrow contrast has led to the early detection of soft tissue and bone tumors.

BONE SCANS

Radioactive isotopes have been developed that will preferentially go to bone, showing increased uptake in portions of the skeleton which are hypervascular or which have an increased rate of bone mineral turnover (Fig. 5-16). Its major role is in identifying pathologic changes, especially infections, tumors, inflammatory diseases, or metabolic bone disease.[10,28,60] It is not specific in differential diagnosis of disease. It is, however, useful in locating a lesion that is symptomatic but not yet visible on roentgenograms. This procedure reveals metastases in 95% of cases.[75]

THERMOGRAPHY

Thermography is a noninvasive procedure that images the temperature distribution of the body surfaces. In contrast to radiography, computed tomogra-

(*text continues on page 98*)

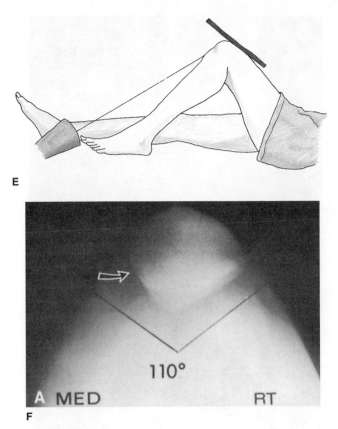

E

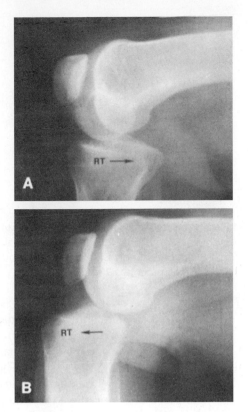

F

FIG. 5-8. (Continued)

FIG. 5-9. Sagittal stress roentgenogram of the knee. (**A**) When a posterior drawer is done, the tibia has a normal relationship to the femoral condyles. (**B**) With an anterior drawer, the tibia subluxes forward, suggesting anteriomedial rotary instability. (D'Ambrosia RD: Musculoskeletal Disorders: Regional Examination and Differential Diagnosis, 2nd ed. Philadelphia, JB Lippincott, 1986)

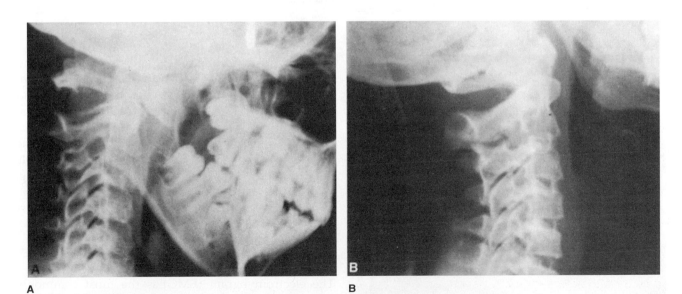

FIG. 5-10. Dynamic study of the cervical spine. (**A**) Flexion view shows marked anterior atlanto-axial subluxation. (**B**) Extension view shows normal atlanto-axial relationships. (Greenfield GB: Radiology of Bone Disease, 4th ed, p 856. Philadelphia, JB Lippincott, 1986)

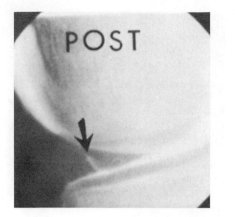

FIG. 5-11. *Arthrogram shows a vertical tear (arrow) in the medial meniscus. (D'Ambrosia RD: Musculoskeletal Disorders: Regional Examination and Differential Diagnosis, 2nd ed. Philadelphia, JB Lippincott, 1986)*

phy, or myelography, which show only anatomic changes, thermography demonstrates functional changes in circulation consequent to damage to nerves, ligaments, muscles, or joints.[68,69,84,94] The procedure allows one to determine the degree of involvement of, for example, a limb in reflex sympathetic dystrophy or peripheral vascular disease. It also permits one to note the activity in stress fractures and diseases such as rheumatoid arthritis and to detect soft tissue tumors such as breast cancer.[12,96]

ULTRASONOGRAPHY

Other technologies such as ultrasound have been suggested as having potential for noninvasive measure-

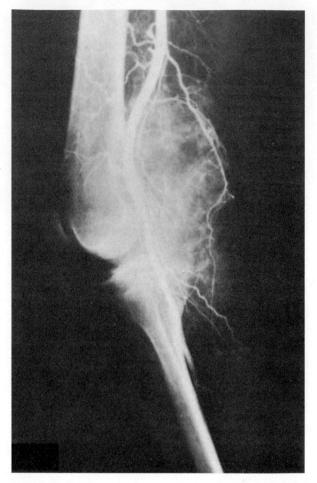

FIG. 5-13. *Angiogram shows anterior displacement of the popliteal artery, and a large soft tissue mass showing tumor vessels. (Greenfield GB: Radiology of Bone Disease, 5th ed. Philadelphia, JB Lippincott, 1990)*

ment of spinal mobility.[57] High frequency sound waves are reflected differently depending on the density of the reflecting tissues. They are received and used to form images of portions of the body. Ultrasonography is also ideally used for evaluating soft tissue masses in the extremities. It has been used in the knee and popliteal space to search for possible popliteal cysts or vascular aneurysms (see Fig. 5-15B).[30]

ELECTRODIAGNOSTIC TESTING

The electromyogram (EMG) is the most commonly done of these tests and is extremely useful in evaluating nerve root denervation, muscular disease, and peripheral neuropathies. It is a helpful tool in the evaluation of herniated disk syndrome. Radicular pain with motor weakness (motor nerve involvement) is well evaluated by EMG.[33] It must be remembered, how-

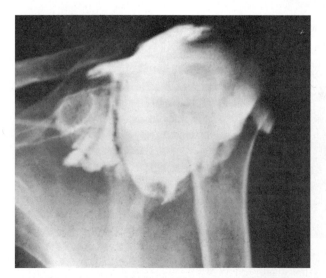

FIG. 5-12. *Arthrogram of the shoulder in a patient with a rotator cuff tear. The dye can be seen to leak into the subdeltoid bursa through the tear. (D'Ambrosia RD: Musculoskeletal Disorders: Regional Examination and Differential Diagnosis, 2nd ed. Philadelphia, JB Lippincott, 1986)*

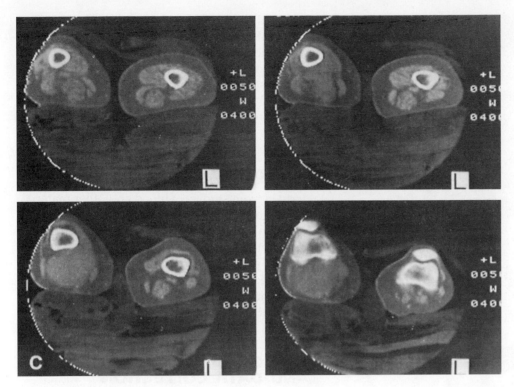

FIG. 5-14. Computed tomography scans show a large soft-tissue mass posterior to the left knee. (Greenfield GB: Radiology of Bone Disease, 5th ed. Philadelphia, JB Lippincott, 1990)

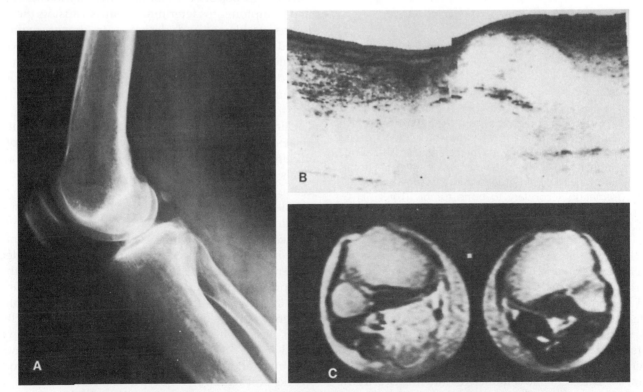

FIG. 5-15. Soft tissue mass in the popliteal region. (**A**) Lateral roentgenogram, (**B**) ultrasound scan, and (**C**) magnetic resonance imaging scan through the popliteal region show extent of the mass. (D'Ambrosia RD: Musculoskeletal Disorders: Regional Examination and Differential Diagnosis, 2nd ed. Philadelphia, JB Lippincott, 1986)

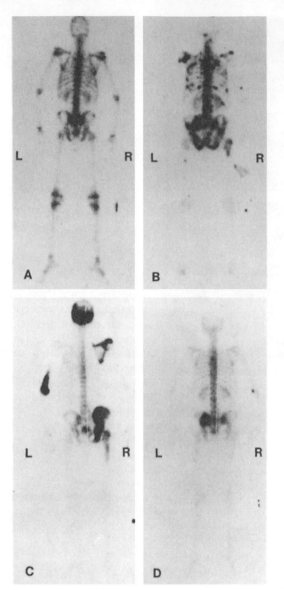

FIG. 5-16. Whole body bone scan. (**A**) Normal adolescent scan. (**B**) Abnormal bone scan showing foci of reactive bone formation consistent with metastatic disease of bone. (**C**) Abnormal bone scan showing patient with metastatic disease of bone. (**D**) Abnormal bone scan showing reactive bone formation secondary to bone tumor. (Turek SL: Orthopaedics: Principles and Their Application, 4th ed. Philadelphia, JB Lippincott, 1984)

ever, that it takes 21 days for the EMG to record denervation potentials.

Electromyography has been used for some time to analyze normal function and pathologic conditions in the spinal musculature. Two distinct patterns of EMG activity have clearly been identified in trunk movements: (1) trunk stabilization and (2) initiation of motion.[4,63] Different movements recruit muscles in different patterns of activity, but most spinal intrinsic musculature is involved in the initiation of most movement and maintenance of posture.[56]

Nerve conduction studies, measuring the velocity of an artificially induced signal through a peripheral nerve, may help to identify the existence and site of peripheral nerve root compression.[82] A current research interest is utilizing somatosensory evoked potentials (SSEP) to assess the afferent system in order to identify lesions of nerves that fail to provoke motor involvement.

LABORATORY INVESTIGATIONS

Data derived from studies of blood and other material in the laboratory are peculiarly disappointing as diagnostic aids in the search for the common causes of musculoskeletal pain.[96] In the differential diagnosis of more serious pathologic conditions some studies may be invaluable. Bone-marrow examination may be indicated for the diagnosis of generalized disorders, especially myeloma and tuberculosis.[79]

■ CLINICAL DECISION-MAKING AND DATA COLLECTION

☐ Treatment Planning

Having completed all parts of the assessment, the examiner is now prepared to look at the pertinent subjective and objective facts, note the significant signs and symptoms to determine what is causing the patient's problems, and design a treatment regimen based on the findings. The reevaluation process should be built into each treatment regimen. Quantified data obtained within the reevaluation phase help to guide future decisions and to promote cost-effective treatment.

Clinical decision-making involves a series of interrelated steps that enable the physical therapist to plan an effective treatment compatible with the needs and goals of the patient and members of the health care team. Various systems and labels for describing the intellectual processes involved in clinical decision-making have been suggested: clinical reasoning,[40] clinical problem solving,[85] and clinical judgment.[17] The intellectual processes involved in clinical decision-making are not addressed in this chapter; rather, the purpose of this presentation is to offer a series of considerations to facilitate effective clinical problem solving. A varied spectrum of models to aid clinicians in their daily decisions has been developed.[9,19,20,34,40,65,71,74,90,91,93,95] Having several models may allow clinicians to identify which model works best with different types of patients.

Often, patients present with a mixture of signs and symptoms that indicates overlapping problems. The novice may recognize the typical feature of an injury yet fail to exclude other potentially coexisting disorders that may share or predispose to the clinical presentation.[40] Only the examiner's knowledge, clinical experience, and diagnosis followed by trial treatment can conclusively delineate the problem. Diagnosis is one of the main decisional acts in clinical reasoning.[23]

☐ Guides to Correlation and Interpretation

Correlation and interpretation of the examination findings is one of the most critical steps in clinical decision-making. This requires that the clinician give meaning and relevance to the data obtained during the examination.

The diagnostician must often make use of abstract relationships such as proximal–distal, deep–superficial, and gradual–sudden and not be centered purely on disjointed lists of signs and symptoms.[40] At times, when faced with an atypical problem, the decision may be an educated guess, since very few problems are textbook perfect. The precise diagnosis of patients with low back pain, for example, is unknown in 80 to 90 percent of patients.[78] Terms such as "disk disease" and "facet joint syndrome" in most instances are ambiguous because it is difficult to measure these phenomena or to clearly define their contribution to pain in a given patient.[15] Instead, terms such as "low back pain with referral into the leg," "low back pain without radiation," and "chronic pain syndrome" are more well-defined and unambiguous.

The Quebec Task Force on Spinal Disorders Classification System (QTFSD) clearly recognized this dilemma of diagnosis. They recommended only 11 classifications of activity-related spinal disorders.[77] DeRosa and Porterfield[15] have proposed a modified version of the QTFSD classification scheme most relevant to physical therapy diagnosis (see Table 20-1).

Judgments relating to the nature and extent of the disorder and the resultant degree of disability can be made by correlating the information obtained during a comprehensive initial patient examination. With respect to the nature of the problem, it is important to judge whether the disease state is a "medical" disorder or if perhaps operant behavior patterns have developed that may account for a significant part of the disability. The clinician should consider whether the degree of disability is consistent with the apparent nature and extent of the physical lesion or whether the patient is exhibiting disability behaviors that are out of proportion to clinical findings. If the latter is the case, the possibility that the disease state is being maintained by external consequences that have a reinforcing effect should be considered. It is essential that such determinations be made, since treatment directed at some physical pathologic process in the presence of an operant disease state will be futile and can further reinforce "learned" disability behaviors.

☐ The Nature of the Lesion

If it appears that some physical pathologic process is primarily responsible for the patient's disorder, the nature of the lesion should be estimated as precisely as possible. To do so, the information obtained on examination must be correlated with knowledge of anatomy, physiology, kinesiology, and pathology in order to identify the involved tissue or tissues. Some estimate should also be made concerning the extent to which these tissues are involved. A few common lesions make up the majority of disorders affecting each musculoskeletal tissue. For each of these lesions, there are also consistent key clinical findings. In developing judgments concerning the nature of common clinical disorders, it is helpful to be aware of the lesions common to each tissue and how they are manifested clinically. The following descriptions are meant to guide the clinician in this respect but are not meant to be all-inclusive.

BONE

Fractures are best identified in the physician's examination through the use of roentgenograms. When examining a patient following healing of a fracture, it is important to determine any malunion of bone on inspection of bone structure and alignment, as this may affect eventual functioning of the part. Dislocations are also best detected through the physician's interpretation of roentgenograms, although dislocations are often obvious on inspection.

ARTICULAR CARTILAGE

Degeneration from wearing due to fatigue is the most common lesion affecting this tissue. It causes roughening of the normally smooth surface layers of cartilage. Clinically this is manifested as crepitus on movements in which opposition of joint surfaces is maintained by weight-bearing or other compressive forces. However, considerable degeneration must usually take place before crepitus is detected clinically.

A loose body is a fragment of articular cartilage that has broken away and lies free in the joint. This may occur in the late stages of cartilage degeneration or as a result of avascular necrosis of an area of subchondral bone (osteochondrosis). A loose body becomes symptomatic when it alters the mechanical functioning of the joint, usually causing a restriction of movement in a noncapsular pattern (joint block).

INTRA-ARTICULAR FIBROCARTILAGE

The common disorder affecting intra-articular fibrocartilaginous disks and menisci is tearing, usually from traumatic injury. Forces sufficient to tear a meniscus or disk in the extremities will usually also cause some strain on the joint capsule to which these structures attach. This causes synovial inflammation in the acute stage. Thus, movement is likely to be restricted in a capsular pattern.

Minor displacement of a torn fragment of fibrocartilage may simply result in "clicking" of the joint on specific movements. Lower extremity joints, namely the knee, may give way when a tag of a torn meniscus is caught between the articular surfaces, suddenly interfering with the normal mechanics of the joint.

A major displacement of a torn fragment may grossly interfere with normal mechanics and block joint movement in a noncapsular pattern. The classic example is a "bucket-handle" tear of a medial meniscus.

When the annular ring of a vertebral disk is torn, secondary neurologic symptoms or signs may result from bulging of the nucleus against adjacent nerve tissue.

JOINT CAPSULE

Fibrosis (see section on capsular tightness) typically occurs with prolonged immobilization of a joint, in association with a chronic, low-grade inflammatory process such as occurs with degenerative joint disease, and with resolution of acute inflammation of the synovium. Joint motion is limited in a capsular pattern, and there is a capsular end feel at the extremes of movement.

Synovial inflammation is commonly caused by rheumatoid arthritis, acute trauma to the joint, joint infection, and arthrotomy. Joint motion is limited in a capsular pattern. There is a painful muscle spasm end feel at the points of restriction of movements.

Inflammation of the synovium results in an increased production of synovial fluid, causing capsular distention and loss of the capsular laxity necessary for full movement. In the more superficial joints, the articular swelling can be observed and palpated. If the effusion persists after resolution of the synovial inflammation, motion will continue to be limited in a capsular fashion, with a boggy end feel to movement.

Patients with capsular pathology typically have some combination of fibrosis, synovial inflammation, and effusion. Therefore, end feels are not always distinct.

Forces sufficient to sprain a ligament usually cause some capsular disruption as well. Occasionally in traumatic injuries, a particular portion of a joint capsule is ruptured, such as the anterior capsule of the shoulder when the humerus dislocates anteriorly. Synovial inflammation and joint effusion usually follow capsular sprains.

In the case of a sprain, the joint-play movement that stresses the involved portion of the capsule will be of normal amplitude. In more severe sprains, the joint may be slightly hypermobile, with a painful muscle-guarding end feel.

LIGAMENTS

The history of a sprain invariably includes a traumatic onset. In the case of a mild sprain, the joint-play movement that stresses the ligament is of normal amplitude and is painful. More severe sprains (partial ruptures) will present as somewhat hypermobile and painful on the associated joint-play test. The synovial lining of the adjacent aspect of the joint capsule will often become inflamed, resulting in capsular effusion in the acute stage. There is usually tenderness over the site of the lesion.

The onset of a rupture is also usually traumatic. The associated joint-play movement test will be *hypermobile* and *painless* in the chronic stages. Even in the acute stage it is usually painless, since there are no fibers intact from which to elicit pain. If adjacent capsular tissue is also sprained, there may be some pain on stress testing in the acute stage. Capsular effusion often does not occur because fluid leaks through the defect. In the chronic stages the patient may give a history of instability. The joint gives way during activities that stress it in the direction that the ruptured ligament is supposed to check.

BURSAE

The common disorder of bursae is inflammation, secondary to chronic irritation, infection, gout, or, rarely, acute trauma. Movement of the nearby joint will cause pain or restriction of motion, or both, in a noncapsular pattern. There may be a painful arc of movement as well.

In acute bursitis, such as at the shoulder, the end feel to movement is often empty and painful; protective muscle spasm would only serve to squeeze the inflamed structure, increasing the pain. There is usually tenderness over the site of the lesion.

TENDONS

Tendinitis is a minor lesion of tendon tissue involving microscopic tearing and a chronic, low-grade inflammatory process. In most cases it is degenerative; the lesion results from tissue fatigue rather than from acute injury. Since progression of the pathologic process will result in a partial tear (macroscopic) or rupture of the tendon, tendinitis should be considered on a continuum with more serious lesions.

The key clinical sign associated with tendinitis is a strong but painful resisted test of the involved musculotendinous structure. There may be pain at the extremes of the passive movement or movements that stretch the tendon. Seldom is there limitation of movement. There may be palpable tenderness at the site of the lesion or referred tenderness into the related segment, or both.

When the involved part of a tendon is that which passes through a sheath, two other terms are often used: tenosynovitis and tenovaginitis. *Tenosynovitis* is an inflammation of the synovial lining of a sheath resulting from friction of a roughened tendon gliding within the sheath. This will present similarly to tendinitis, but there is often pain on activity that produces movement of the tendon within the sheath. Thus, active movement in the direction or opposite the direction of pull of the tendon may be painful. In *tenovaginitis,* a tendon gliding within a swollen, thickened sheath causes pain. The classic example occurs with rheumatoid arthritis. The clinical signs are essentially the same as those for tenosynovitis. There may be palpable and visible swelling of the tendon sheath.

In the case of a partial tendon tear, actual loss of continuity of tendon tissue will cause weak and painful responses to the resisted test for the musculotendinous complex. The passive movement that stretches the tendon may be painful.

When the tendon has torn completely, the findings of the related resisted test will be weak and painless. In some cases, for example, rupture of the Achilles tendon, there may be a palpable gap at the site of the rupture.

MUSCLES

Muscle strains and ruptures are relatively rare. When they do occur they are invariably the result of acute trauma and are therefore most prevalent in sports-medicine settings. Muscles, being well vascularized and resilient, do not commonly undergo fatigue degeneration as do tendons.

In the case of a strain, a minor tear of muscle fibers will result in a strong and painful finding on the resisted test that stresses the involved muscle. There may be pain on full passive stretch of the muscle, as well as palpable tenderness. In the case of a rupture, the associated resisted test results will be weak and painless. A gap may be palpable, or occasionally visible, at the site of the defect.

NERVES

The common conditions affecting nerves are those in which some extrinsic source of pressure results in altered conduction along some or all of the nerve fibers—the so-called *entrapment syndromes.* The most common sites of pressure are the points of exit of the lower cervical and lower lumbar spinal nerves from the intervertebral foramina. Here pressure is usually from a protruding disk or projecting osteophyte. There are other common sites of pressure farther out in the periphery that affect the nerves to the extremities. As indicated in Chapter 4, Pain, pressure tends to alter conduction first along the largest fibers and last along the smallest. Altered nerve conduction is usually manifested subjectively before any objective clinical evidence of neurologic dysfunction can be detected. In fact, in the case of the common entrapment syndromes, objective clinical findings are rare, and when present they are usually quite subtle. Often more sophisticated electrodiagnostic tests are required to objectively detect changes in nerve conduction.

The subjective complaints associated with common entrapment disorders can generally be classified as paresthesia (pins-and-needles), dysesthesia (altered sensation in response to some external stimulus), and pain. Although some patients may describe paresthesia and dysesthesia as painful, pain is usually not a primary complaint when there is pressure on a nerve farther out in the periphery rather than at the nerve-root level. Thus, patients with thoracic outlet syndrome, ulnar nerve palsy, and carpal tunnel syndrome, as well as those who have sat too long with the legs crossed, do not complain of pain but of a pins-and-needles sensation. Pain is a common complaint, however, in cases in which there is pressure on a nerve at nerve-root level. With initial pressure, when the larger, myelinated, "fast pain" fibers are stimulated, patients describe a sharp, shooting dermatomic quality of pain. With prolonged or increased pressure, when the larger fibers cease to conduct and the small, unmyelinated C fibers are stimulated, a dull, aching sclerotomic type of pain will be perceived.

Paresthesia, the primary subjective complaint with pressure farther out in the periphery, may occur with the onset of pressure or when the pressure is released, or both. For example, a person usually feels little or nothing when sitting with legs crossed, with pressure applied to the tibial or peroneal nerve. It is not until the person uncrosses the legs, releasing the pressure, that the pins-and-needles sensation of the foot being "asleep" is felt. A similar situation holds true for pressure on the lower cord of the brachial plexus from depression of the shoulder girdle; the patient invariably describes the onset of pins-and-needles in the early morning hours (1 or 2 AM) some time after the pressure is released. It seems that the interval between the release of pressure and the onset of paresthesia is in some way proportional to the length of time during which the pressure was applied. In other common nerve problems, the onset of symptoms occurs when the pressure is applied. For example, many patients with carpal tunnel syndrome describe paresthesia felt primarily during fine finger movements; the tension on the finger flexor tendons produces pressure on the median nerve sufficient to cause symptoms. Similarly, when a person sits or lies with pressure over the ulnar groove, pins-and-needles are usually felt in the ulnar side of the hand while the pressure is applied, and cease to be felt after the pressure is released.

As mentioned, more objective findings associated with common nerve-pressure disorders are usually very subtle when present. They are more common with nerve-root pressure from a disk protrusion than with more peripheral entrapment syndromes. The earliest evidence of decreased conduction will be related to those functions mediated by the largest myelinated fibers, since these fibers are most sensitive to pressure. Therefore, reduced vibration sense is often the earliest deficit detected by clinical testing. With increased or prolonged pressure, diminished deep-tendon reflexes may be noted, followed by reduced muscle strength. Finally, there is reduced sensation, first to light touch, then to noxious stimulation. Because of overlapping dermatomes and myotomes, and because each muscle and skin area typically receives innervation from more than one segment, even completely severing a nerve root will usually cause only a minor deficit.

Extent of the Lesion

When clinicians speak of acute and chronic lesions, it is often unclear whether they are referring to the length of time that the pathologic process has existed, the severity of the disorder, or the nature of the inflammatory process. There are relatively few consistent clinical findings related to either the duration or the severity of common musculoskeletal problems. However, there are certain symptoms and signs that are consistently present with acute inflammatory processes and others that are pathognomonic of le-

sions in which a more chronic inflammatory state exists. *Acute inflammation* is that stage or type of inflammatory process in which hyperemia, increased capillary permeability with protein and plasma leakage, and an influx of granulocytes and other defense cells take place. *Chronic inflammation* is characterized by an attempt at repair, with increased numbers of fibrocytes and other "tissue-building" cells, and the presence of granulation tissue. An acute lesion is characterized by the following clinical findings:

1. Pain is relatively constant.
2. On passive range of motion of the related joint, there is a muscle spasm end feel or an empty end feel to movement.
3. Pain is likely to be referred over a relatively diffuse area of the related segment.
4. There may be a measurable increase in skin temperature over the site of the lesion.
5. There is often difficulty in falling asleep or difficulty in remaining asleep, or both.

In the presence of chronic lesions, the patient is likely to present with the following symptoms or signs:

1. Pain is increased by specific activities and relieved by rest.
2. On passive movement of the related joint, there is no muscle spasm or empty end feel.
3. Pain is likely to be felt over a relatively localized area, close to the site of the lesion, although often not directly over the site of the lesion.
4. There is little or no temperature elevation over the involved part.
5. Unless the lesion involves the shoulder or hip, there is little or no difficulty in sleeping.

Setting Goals and Priorities

Following the diagnosis, the clinician establishes short-term and long-term goals of treatment. Determining appropriate treatment goals assists the therapist in planning, prioritizing, and measuring the effectiveness of treatment. The goals are derived from the patient's symptom(s), signs, and diagnosis and from the patient's personal, vocational, and social goals. Involvement of the patient is critical in achieving patient compliance.[16] Information obtained from the patient should be integrated with the subjective and objective assessment data. A goal statement should be generated with the patient's full cooperation and understanding.

Long-term goals identify the functional behaviors to be attained by the patient by the end of the treatment program. Once long-term goals have been established, the next step is to determine the component skills that will be needed to attain these goals. Short-term goals identify the progressive functional levels to be attained by the patient at specific intervals within the projected period of treatment.[9] The clinician should determine the appropriate sequence of subskills and prioritize them accordingly. The patient advances through the sequence of short-term goals until he achieves the final end point of long-term goals. The goals and diagnosis direct treatment.

■ CONCEPTS OF MANAGEMENT

Only those procedures that may not be well understood or are new to most professional training programs are discussed in this section. It is assumed that the reader is familiar with many basic therapeutic procedures and modalities, such as therapeutic exercise, use of assistive devices, and electrotherapy. The application of these forms of treatment, in conjunction with traditional therapies, to specific pathologic processes affecting the various extremity regions is discussed in Parts Two and Three.

☐ Rehabilitation

The correlation and interpretation of findings from a comprehensive initial patient examination is the basis for developing a treatment plan. During the initial examination clinicians seek to elicit information that relates to the nature and extent of the pathologic process as well as to the degree of disability. The choice of therapeutic procedures depends on this information.

The primary considerations are the site of the lesion and the type of tissue involved. Once the nature of the lesion has been determined, there is often a tendency to direct treatment primarily at the site of the lesion with the expectation that resolving the pathologic process will alleviate any resultant physical dysfunction, and will in turn restore the patient to a normal health state.

There are many potential fallacies to this approach that make it unsuitable as a reliable treatment model. First, such an approach ignores the secondary effects that a lesion involving a particular structure may have on the normal functioning of other related structures. It calls for treatment of "anatomic structures" rather than "physiologic units." By considering the synovial joints as the basic physiologic—rather than anatomic—unit of the musculoskeletal system, one is better prepared to respect the interactions of the various components of this system under normal and abnormal conditions. This is essential, since an alteration in one component of a functional unit often leads to dys-

function of other components of the same or neighboring units, which may act to maintain the primary pathologic condition, predispose to recurrence, or result in secondary disease. Thus, even in the case of relatively localized lesions, clinicians must respect such interactions and be prepared to deal with them therapeutically.

For example, a painful lesion of the supraspinatus tendon tends to result in reflex inhibition of the supraspinatus and other rotator cuff muscles. This will predispose to subacromial impingement from abnormal movement of the head of the humerus during elevation activities, which may further traumatize the supraspinatus tendon as well as the subdeltoid bursa. Also, muscles such as the deltoid and the trapezius may reflexively contract abnormally during movement of the arm, secondary to abnormal afferent input from the site of the lesion to the lower cervical segments. This may further interfere with normal joint mechanics at the shoulder as well as at the neck, to which the trapezius attaches. It should be clear that effective treatment of this problem involves more than resolution of the pathologic process affecting the tendon. The rotator cuff muscles must, at some time, be strengthened; excessive elevation of the arm must be temporarily avoided; and relaxation of abnormally contracting muscles should be promoted. If one were to treat only the lesion of the tendon, it is likely that treatment would be ineffective or take much longer than necessary to be effective. Continued subacromial impingement would enhance the chance of recurrence. The patient would also be predisposed to the development of a coexistent cervical lesion from increased stresses to the neck due to abnormal muscle activity.

Second, an approach in which treatment is aimed exclusively at some discrete pathologic process tends to ignore etiologic considerations. Temporary amelioration may ensue without true resolution of the problem. Unless underlying causes, such as biomechanical abnormalities, are recognized and dealt with, chronic recurrent problems can be expected. Thus, a patient with chondromalacia patellae resulting from abnormal foot pronation may temporarily do very well on a program of reduced activity and strengthening of the vastus medialis muscle. However, the patient is likely to experience similar problems with the resumption of normal activity levels unless the alignment of the foot and leg is corrected. Similarly, the patient with trochanteric bursitis caused by a tight iliotibial band usually responds well to ultrasound over the site of the lesion, but if extensibility of the iliotibial band is not increased, relief will be short-lived. The clinician should implement the concept that prevention is the ultimate cure by attempting to identify etiologic factors and by employing appropriate measures to deal with them. This should be a major consideration in fatigue disorders that are chronic, since they tend to be self-resolving once the cause of the abnormal stresses is corrected. (See the outlined treatment of chronic disorders that follows.)

Third, and most important, when treatment is directed only at a physical disorder, the psychosocial implications of the problem are not given due respect. Comprehensive rehabilitation requires restoration of an optimal level of function. Although a physical disorder may have been the original cause of physical dysfunction or other "disease behaviors" such as complaints of pain, there are often other factors that may serve to maintain or inhibit the disability behaviors. Such "motivational factors" may eventually assume a greater influence on the disability state than the original pathology (see Fig. 5-1). These factors must be recognized since they often determine whether treatment is successful, whether an optimal level of function is restored, and whether disability behaviors (pain complaints, physical dysfunction, and functional dependence) are resolved. If being disabled carries excessively negative consequences for the patient, such as often occurs in sports-medicine settings, these consequences will strongly inhibit the disability state. As a result, the patient often attempts to do more than is appropriate and imposes deleterious effects on the lesion. This may counteract any beneficial effects of other treatment procedures. On the other hand, if the patient stands to gain in some way from being disabled, such as time away from work, financial compensation, or welcomed dependence, the potential for gain may have a significant reinforcing effect on the disability state. The patient is not likely to improve in spite of otherwise effective treatment of the pathologic condition. In both of these situations, the psychosocial motivational influences are likely to have a greater effect on the disease state than the physical process itself. Unless these influences are dealt with, the patient cannot be truly rehabilitated. To estimate the relative influence of such factors, the clinician must determine whether the degree of disability is consistent with the symptoms and signs manifested by the disease. If there are inconsistencies, significant psychosocial influences affecting the nature of the disability state should be suspected.

☐ Treatment of Patients with Physical Disorders

Although the principle of "treating the patient, not the disease" has become somewhat of a cliché, its application to patients with common musculoskeletal disorders is too often overlooked. The first and foremost

consideration when devising a therapeutic program should always be how the patient's ability to function normally has been compromised. One must ask, what conditions are responsible for the dysfunction and are these conditions reversible? If they are reversible, what would be the most appropriate means of intervening therapeutically so as to affect these conditions? If the conditions at fault appear irreversible, what can be done to optimize residual function? And finally, what can be done to prevent recurrences, secondary problems, and progression of the existing disorder? With such an approach, therapy is disability-oriented rather than pathology-oriented. The primary goal of management becomes restoration of an optimal level of functioning rather than simply resolution of some pathologic process. Resolution of a physical disorder does not necessarily lead to restoration of function, reduction in pain behavior, or other necessary signs of improvement.

In the case of many common musculoskeletal disorders, in which the degree of disability appears to be consistent with the nature and extent of the lesion, physical treatment will constitute a major component of the therapeutic program. When this is the case, clinicians must choose, among the various forms of intervention at their disposal, the procedures and modalities most appropriate for the management of the specific disorder. Treatment must be individualized for each patient and according to the nature and extent of the pathologic process. The tendency to incorporate "standardized" programs of exercises and other treatments, usually for the sake of efficiency, should be avoided. The controversies over and misconceptions about so many forms of treatment (*e.g.,* massage, manipulation, traction, and certain exercises) stem largely from their having been advocated or misconstrued as panaceas for disorders affecting certain regions.

CLASSIFYING PATHOLOGIES: ACUTE VERSUS CHRONIC

As a preface to discussing specific types of treatments and their respective applications, some general concepts that are related to the overall approach to physical treatment are considered. As mentioned previously, approaches to treating a physical disorder should depend on its nature and extent. The two common terms used clinically to classify pathologic processes according to their nature and extent are acute and chronic. These terms should not be used to refer to the severity or duration of a disorder, since when used in these contexts they have little relationship to symptoms and signs. A patient with a relatively severe lesion such as a ligamentous rupture, for example, may present with much less pain and dysfunction than one who has sustained a minor sprain. It is well known, even to those outside the health care professions, that a sprained ankle may be more painful and disabling shortly after injury than a fractured ankle. With respect to duration, disorders of fairly recent onset often present with subtle symptoms and signs when compared with certain long-standing problems. If a clinician has two patients, one with recent onset of aching in the shoulder but no gross loss of function and the other with long-standing severe pain and dysfunction, which condition is acute and which is chronic?

The terms *acute* and *chronic* do have some significance when used to refer to the nature of the symptoms and signs with which a patient presents, as differentiated earlier in this chapter. This is because symptoms and signs reflect the nature of various disorders and, more specifically, they tend to reflect the nature of the inflammation or repair process that accompanies any physical lesion. Because these symptom–sign complexes do relate to the nature of pathologic processes, they are used here as a basis for a discussion of general approaches to management. The following scheme is based on the definitions of acute and chronic.

TREATMENT OF ACUTE AND CHRONIC DISORDERS

I. **General concepts**
  A. *Consider the nature and extent of the disorder, whether* acute *or* chronic.
    1. The terms are sometimes used to refer to duration of the problem and not to symptoms and signs.
    2. They should be used to refer to the nature of the inflammatory process.
      a. Acute hyperemic phase
        i. Pain is felt at rest and aggravated by activity.
        ii. Pain is felt over a relatively diffuse area and may be referred into any or all of the related segments (sclerotome).
        iii. Passive movement of related joints when limited is restricted by pain, muscle guarding, or both.
        iv. The skin temperature over the site of the lesion is often elevated.
      b. Chronic/reparative phase
        i. There is no pain at rest and pain is felt only with specific activities.
        ii. Pain is felt over a fairly localized

area, close to the site of the lesion (often not directly over the site of the lesion, however).
        iii. Movement of related joints, when limited, is restricted by soft-tissue tightness; pain is felt only at the extremes of movement or through a small arc of movement.
    3. The terms are not useful in describing the severity of the lesion. For example, a patient with a complete rupture of a ligament may present with less pain and disability and with fewer cardinal inflammatory signs than a person with only a partial tear of a ligament.
  B. *Assess, control, and monitor the patient's functional status.*
    1. Assess the degree of disability from findings of the history and physical examination. Compare disease (injury) status with health (normal) status, and compare with other symptoms and signs.
      a. Is the degree of disability consistent with the apparent nature and extent of the disorder? This yields important information relating to the patient's motivational status and is a major consideration in treatment planning.
        i. The "well-motivated" patient is one for whom the consequences of injury (disability) are punishing. For example, they imply time away from desirable situations or possibility of financial loss. It can be presumed that resolution of the disease will lead to resolution of the disability state. A medical approach to treatment is appropriate.
        ii. The "poorly motivated" patient is one for whom the consequences of disability are *reinforcing*. For example, they offer time away from undesirable situations or the possibility of financial gain. It cannot be presumed that treatment of the disease will result in resolution of the disability state. Rehabilitation must include attempts to alter the consequences to disability. An operant approach must be incorporated into the treatment program.
      b. Record and use information as a baseline by which to judge progress.
    2. Control functional status (see below under techniques of management).

a. Inappropriate activities must be restricted to prevent prolongation or recurrence of the disorder.

b. Appropriate activities must be resumed as the pathologic process resolves. *This is the ultimate goal of management.*

3. Monitor functional status to judge improvement. The patient is not rehabilitated until an optimal level of function is restored, regardless of the state of the lesion.

II. Treatment of acute inflammatory disorders (traumatic)

The primary goal is to promote progression to a chronic state while minimizing dysfunction.

A. *Physiologic intervention to control the acute inflammatory response*
1. Ice—to reduce blood flow
2. Compression—to prevent and reduce swelling
3. Elevation—to prevent and reduce swelling and hyperemia
4. Relaxation—to reduce pain and muscle spasm

B. *Avoidance and prevention of continued trauma and irritation by reducing loading of the part*
1. Braces, slings, splints, assistive devices, strapping
a. Lower extremity—Crutches or canes to reduce forces of weight-bearing; splints, braces, or strapping to reduce forces of movement
b. Upper extremity—Slings to reduce forces of gravity and, therefore, postural muscle tone; splints, braces, or strapping to reduce the forces imposed by movement
c. Spine—Passive support with collar or corset if indicated
2. Control of activities causing undesirable loading of the part. This requires careful, well-understood instructions to the patient.

C. *Maintaining optimal levels of function and preventing unnecessary dysfunction*
1. Isometric resistive exercises to maintain muscle function, while avoiding undesirable movement of the part
2. In acute nuclear prolapse, isometric activities (*e.g.,* pelvic tilt exercises, straining, and Valsalva maneuvers) must be avoided.
3. With respect to the spine:
a. Rest is interspersed with periods of controlled activity.
b. Positions that increase intradiskal pressure should be avoided (*e.g.,* acute disk protrusions).
4. Gentle active or passive movement (when

appropriate according to the nature of the disorder) to avoid pain and muscle guarding

III. Treatment of chronic disorders

A. Causative factors. The majority of disorders seen in most clinical settings have two primary causes:
1. Abnormal modeling of tissue during resolution of an acute disorder. The following are examples:
a. Malunion of fractures resulting in a change in the direction or magnitude of forces acting on the part during use (increased stress)
b. Abnormalities in collagen maturation or production (scarring, fibrosis, adhesions). An excess amount of collagen may be produced, and that which is produced may not be oriented along the normal lines of stress. Abnormal collagen cross-links are formed, and the tissue may adhere to adjacent structures. The net result is reduced extensibility, and therefore reduced capacity to attenuate energy by deforming when stressed.
2. Fatigue response of tissues. The two types of response are
a. Tissue breakdown—the rate of attrition exceeds the rate of repair (*e.g.,* stress fractures, cartilage degeneration). The tissue becomes "weaker" and begins to yield under loading conditions. It occurs with mild to moderately increased stress levels in tissues with low regenerative capacity (*e.g.,* articular cartilage); with higher stress levels in other tissues (*e.g.,* tendon, bone); under conditions of altered tissue metabolism (*e.g.,* hypovascularity).
b. Tissue hypertrophy (*e.g.,* fibrosis and sclerosis) occurs with mild to moderately increased stress levels in tissues with good regenerative/repair capacity, acting over a prolonged period of time. Tissue becomes stiffer, with reduced energy attenuation capacity. Individual fibers or trabeculae begin to yield under loading conditions, resulting in low-grade inflammation, pain, increased tissue production, and so on.

B. *Treatment planning*
1. Reduce stresses to involved tissue over time.
a. Reduce magnitude of loading (control of activities).

b. Reduce magnitude of stresses by altering direction or magnitude of forces acting on the part through control of activities, use of protective/assistive devices, and use of orthotic devices to control position of the part.

c. Increase surface area of loading (*e.g.,* foot orthosis).

d. Provide for external energy attenuation (*e.g.,* pads, helmets, cushioned heels).

2. Increase energy-attenuating capacity of the part.

a. Increase compensatory muscle strength/activity with strengthening exercises; increase neuromuscular facilitative (afferent) input (*e.g.,* taping, coordination training).

b. Increase tissue extensibility (ability to deform without loss of structural integrity):

i. Active stretching

ii. Passive stretching, using passive range-of-motion stretching for musculotendinous tightness and specific joint mobilization for capsuloligamentous tightness

iii. Use of ultrasound in conjunction with stretch

iv. Use of transverse friction massage to increase interfiber mobility and to prevent or reduce fibrous adhesion without longitudinally stressing the tissue

v. Soft tissue manipulations directed at muscle, ligaments, and fascial layers to restore mobility and extensibility

c. Promote increase in structural integrity of the part (increased "strength"). This requires tissue hypertrophy, without loss of extensibility from overproduction of immature collagenous tissue, and so on, and maturation of collagen fiber orientation along normal lines of stress and development of appropriate cross-links.

The necessary stimulus is stress to the part. This means gradual, controlled return to participation in high-stress-level activities (training).

3. Resumption of optimal activity levels and prevention of recurrence. Judgments are based on:

a. Clinical evidence of having accomplished above objectives

b. Awareness of the nature of stresses imposed by various activities and an estimate of the capacity of the part to withstand those stresses. This requires biomechanical assessment and analysis and familiarity with research related to biomechanical properties of musculoskeletal tissues under various conditions of loading and healing.

c. Extrinsic "motivational" factors—the consequences of disability for the patient

Patients with true chronic pain syndrome should not be treated with the emphasis on pain modulation. Whereas acute pain bears a relatively straightforward relationship to peripheral stimulus, nociception, and tissue damage, chronic pain disability becomes increasingly dissociated from the original physical basis and there may be little if any evidence of any remaining nociceptive stimulus. Emphasis should focus on functional restoration which utilizes sports medicine principles. This approach emphasizes the recognition, through objective quantitative assessment of physical function, of the loss of physical capacity that accompanies disuse (termed the *deconditioning syndrome*).[57] The focus should be on augmenting function and on increasing physical activity, mobility, strength, endurance, and cardiovascular improvement.

☐ Evaluation of Treatment Program

The last step is ongoing and involves continuous reevaluation of the patient and efficacy of treatment. Recognition of the original problems that have been solved and those that need further attention must be made. New short-term goals should be established and appropriate procedures selected. In determining and implementing revised goals and related treatment and criteria, the clinician is again at the problem-solving stages of determining and administering treatment. When long-term goals are reached or are close to being reached, discharge planning and plan for follow-up care (when indicated) can be initiated. The overall success of the treatment plan is dependent on the therapist's clinical decision-making skills and on engaging the patient's cooperation and motivation.[65]

REFERENCES

1. Agarwal A, Lloyd KN, Dovey P: The dermography of the spine and sacroiliac joints in spondylitis. Rheum Phys Med 10:349–355, 1970
2. Aprill C: Radiologic imaging techniques of the spine. In Hochschuler SH, Cotler HB, Guyer RD (eds): Rehabilitation of the Spine, pp 79–111. St Louis, CV Mosby, 1993
3. Barnett C, Davies D, MacConaill MA: Synovial Joints, Their Structure and Mechanics. Springfield, IL, Charles C Thomas, 1961
4. Basmajian J: Muscles Alive: Their Functions Revealed by Electromyography, 4th ed. Baltimore, Williams & Wilkins, 1978
5. Behr D, Katz, Krebs D: Diagnosis enhances, not impedes boundaries of physical therapy practice. Orthop Sports Phys Ther 13:218–219, 1991

6. Bourdillon JG, Day EA, Bookhout MR: Examination: General considerations. In Bourdillon JG, Day EA, Bookhout MR (eds): Spinal Manipulation, 5th ed, pp 46–80. Oxford, Butterworth-Heinemann, 1992
7. Bowers TA, Murray JA: Bone metastases from renal carcinoma. The preoperative use of transcatheter arterial occlusion. J Bone Joint Surg 64(A):749–754, 1982
8. Cantu RI, Grodin AJ: Myofascial Manipulation: Theory and Clinical Application. Gaithersburg, Aspen Pub, 1992
9. Catlin PA: Elements of problem solving. In Greenfield BH (ed): Rehabilitation of the Knee: A Problem-Solving Approach, pp 66–84. Philadelphia, FA Davis, 1993
10. Citrin DL, Bessent RG, Greig WR: A comparison of the sensitivity and accuracy of the Tc-99 phosphate bone scan and skeletal radiographs in the diagnosis of bone metastases. Clin Radiol 28:107–117, 1977
11. Clarkson HM, Gilewich GD: Assessment: Joint Range of Motion and Manual Muscle Strength. Baltimore, Williams & Wilkins, 1989
12. Colodney AK, Raj P: Reflex Sympathetic Dystrophy. In Hochschuler SH, Cotler HB, Guyer RD (eds): Rehabilitation of the Spine: Science and Practice, pp 509–532. St Louis, CV Mosby, 1993
13. Corrigan B, Maitland GD: Examination. In Corrigan B, Maitland GD (eds): Practical Orthopaedic Medicine, pp 9–17. London, Butterworths, 1985
14. Cyriax JH: Textbook of Orthopaedic Medicine, Vol 1. Diagnosis of Soft Tissue Lesions, 8th ed. London, Bailliere Tindall, 1982
15. DeRosa CP, Porterfield JA: A physical therapy model for treatment of low back pain. Phys Ther 72:261–269, 1992
16. DiMatteo M, DiNicola D: Achieving Patient Compliance. Pergamon Press, New York, 1982
17. Downie J, Elstein AS (eds): Professional Judgement: A Reader in Clinical Decision Making. New York, Cambridge University Press, 1988
18. Duensing F, Becker P, Rittmeyer K: Thermographic findings in lumbar disc protrusions. Arch Psychiatr Nervevenkr 217:53–70, 1973
19. Dyrek DA: Assessment and treatment planning strategies for musculoskeletal deficits. In O'Sullivan SB, Schimitz TJ (eds): Physical Rehabilitation and Assessment and Treatment, 3rd ed, pp 61–82. Philadelphia, FA Davis, 1994
20. Echternach JL, Rothstein JM: Hypothesis-oriented algorithms. Phys Ther 69:559–564, 1989
21. Edelman R, Schoukimas G, Stark D, et al: High resolution surface coil imaging of lumbar disc disease. Am J Radiol 144:1123–1129, 1985
22. Edmond SL: Manipulations and Mobilization: Extremity and Spinal Techniques. St Louis, CV Mosby, 1993
23. Feinstein AR: Clinical Judgement. Malabar, FL, Robert E Kreiger, 1967
24. Ferguson AB, D'Ambrosia RD: In D'Ambrosia RD (ed): Musculoskeletal Disorders: Regional Examination and Differential Diagnosis, pp 21–58, 2nd ed. Philadelphia, JB Lippincott, 1986
25. Fordyce WE: Behavioral Methods for Chronic Pain and Illness. St Louis, CV Mosby, 1976
26. Fordyce WE: Evaluating and managing chronic pain. Geriatrics 33:59–62, 1978
27. Fordyce WE, Fowler RS, Lehmann JF, DeLateur BJ, Sands PL, Trieschmann RB: Operant conditioning in the treatment of chronic clinical pain. Arch Phys Med Rehabil 54:399–408, 1973
28. Galasko CSB: The significance of occult skeletal metastases, detected by skeletal scintigraphy, in patients with otherwise apparent "early" mammary carcinoma. Br J Surg 67:694–696, 1975
29. Goldie IF, Reichman S: The biomechanical influence of traction on cervical spine. Scand J Rehab Med 9:31–34, 1977
30. Greenfield GB: Analytical approach to bone radiology. In Greenfield GB (ed): Radiology of Bone Disease, 4th ed, pp 1–30. Philadelphia, JB Lippincott, 1986
31. Greenman PE: Barrier concepts in structural diagnosis. In Greenfield GB (ed): Principles of Manual Therapy, pp 31–38. Baltimore, Williams & Wilkins, 1989
32. Grieve GP: Mobilisation of the Spine: Notes on Examination, Assessment and Clinical Method, 5th ed. Edinburgh, Churchill Livingstone, 1991
33. Handel J, Selby D: Spinal instability. In Hochschuler SH, Cotler HB, Guyer RD (eds): Rehabilitation of the Spine: Science and Practice, pp 153–166. St Louis, CV Mosby, 1993
34. Harris BA, Dyrek DA: A model of orthopaedic dysfunction for clinical decision making in physical therapy. Phys Ther 69:548–553, 1989
35. Huskisson EC, Berry H, Browett J, et al: Measurement of inflammation. Ann Rheum Dis 32:99–102, 1973
36. International Classification of Impairments, Disabilities, and Handicaps. Geneva, Switzerland, World Health Organization, 1980
37. Jensen GM: Musculoskeletal analysis. In Scully RM, Barnes MR (eds): Physical Therapy, pp 326–339. Philadelphia, JB Lippincott, 1989
38. Jette AM: Diagnosis and classification by physical therapist. A special communication. Phys Ther 69:967–969, 1989
39. Jones C: Physical aspects of thermography in relation to clinical techniques. Bibl Radio 6:1–8, 1975
40. Jones MA: Clinical reasoning in manual therapy. Phys Ther 72:875–884, 1992
41. Kaltenborn FM: Mobilization of the Extremities, 3rd ed. Oslo, Norway, Olaf Norlis Bokhandel Universitetsgaten, 1980
42. Kaltenborn FM: The Spine: Basic Evaluation and Mobilization Techniques, 2nd ed. Oslo, Norway, Olaf Norlis Bokhandel Universitetsgaten, 1993
43. Keene JS: Ligament and muscle-tendon-unit injuries. In Gould JA, Davies GJ (eds): Orthopaedic and Sports Physical Therapy, pp 135–165. St Louis, CV Mosby, 1985
44. Kenna C, Murtagh J: Kenna Back Pain and Spinal Manipulation, pp 1–34. Sydney, Butterworth, 1989
45. Kettenbach G: Writing SOAP Notes. Philadelphia, FA Davis, 1990
46. Korr IM, Thomas PE, Wright HM: Patterns of electrical skin resistance in man. Acta Neuroveget 17:77–96, 1958
47. Korr IM, Wright HM, Chase JA: Cutaneous patterns of sympathetic activity in clinical abnormalities of the musculoskeletal system. Acta Neuroveget 4:589–606, 1962
48. Korr IM, Wright HM, Thomas PE: Effect of experimental myofascial insults on cutaneous patterns of sympathetic activity in man. Acta Neuroveget 23:329–355, 1962
49. MacConaill MA, Basmajian JV: Muscles and Movement, pp 13–44. Hunting, NY, Robert E Krieger, 1977
50. Magee DJ: Principles and concepts. In Magee DJ (ed): Orthopedic Physical Assessment, pp 1–32. Philadelphia, WB Saunders, 1992
51. Maigne R: Manipulation of the spine. In Basmajian JV (ed): Manipulation, Traction and Massage, pp 71–96. Baltimore, Williams & Wilkins, 1986
52. Maigne R: Orthopedic Medicine: A New Approach to Vertebral Manipulations. Springfield, IL, Charles C Thomas, 1972
53. Maitland GD: Palpation examination of the posterior cervical spine. The ideal, average and abnormal. Aust J Physiother 28:3–11, 1982
54. Maitland GD: Vertebral Manipulation, 5th ed. Boston, Butterworth, 1986
55. Maitland GD: Peripheral Manipulation, 3rd ed. London, Butterworth-Heinemann, 1991
56. Mayer TG, Gatchel RJ: Quantitative lumbar spine assessment to address the deconditioning syndrome. In Mayer TG, Gatchel RJ (eds): Functional Restoration for Spinal Disorders: The Sports Medicine Approach, pp 115–138. Philadelphia, Lea & Febiger, 1988
57. Mayer TG, Gatchel RJ: The role of the physical therapist: Active sports medicine, not passive modalities. In Mayer TG, Gatchel RJ (eds): In Functional Restoration for Spinal Disorders: The Sports Medicine Approach, pp 218–240. Philadelphia, Lea & Febiger, 1988
58. McKenzie RA: The Lumbar Spine: Mechanical Diagnosis and Therapy. Waikanae, New Zealand, Spinal Publications, 1981
59. McKenzie RA: The Cervical and Thoracic Spine: Mechanical Diagnosis and Therapy. Waikanae, New Zealand, Spinal Publications, 1990
60. McNeil BJ: Value of bone scanning in neoplastic disease. Semin Nucl Med 4:277, 1984
61. Mennell JM: Back Pain: Diagnosis and Treatment Using Manipulative Techniques. Boston, Little, Brown, & Co, 1960
62. Mitchell FL Jr, Moran PS, Pruzzo NA: An Evaluation and Treatment Manual of Osteopathic Muscle Energy Procedures. Valley Park, MO, Mitchell, Moran, and Pruzzo Associates, 1979
63. Morris J, Benner G, Lucas D: An electromyographic study of the intrinsic muscles of the back in man. J Anat 196:509–520, 1962
64. Nyberg R: Clinical assessment of the low back: Active movement and palpation testing. In Basmajian JV, Nyberg R (eds): Rational Manual Therapies, pp 97–140. Baltimore, Williams & Wilkins, 1993
65. O'Sullivan SB: Clinical decision making: Planning effective treatments. In O'Sullivan SB, Schmitz TJ (eds): Physical Rehabilitation Assessment and Treatment, pp 1–8, 3rd ed. Philadelphia, FA Davis, 1994
66. Ongerboer DE, Visser BW, Goor C: Jaw reflexes and masseter electromyograms in mesencephalic and pontine lesions: An electrodiagnostic study. J Neurol Neurosurg Psychiatry 39:90–92, 1976
67. Paris CP: End feel testing: Interrater reliability of end feel testing—Elbow flexion and extension. In: Proceedings of 5th International Conference of the International Federation of Orthopaedic Manipulative Therapists, pp 103–105. Vail, CO, 1992
68. Pochazesky R, Wexler CE, Meyers PH, et al: Liquid crystal thermography of the spine and extremities. J Neurosurg 56:386–395, 1982
69. Pochazesky R: Thermography in skeletal and soft tissue trauma. In Taveras J, Ferrucci J (eds): Radiology. Philadelphia, JB Lippincott, 1987
70. Rose SJ: Physical therapy diagnosis: Role and function. Phys Ther 69:535–537, 1989
71. Rothstein JM, Echternach JL: Hypothesis-oriented algorithm for clinicians: A method for evaluation and treatment planning. Phys Ther 66:1388–1394, 1986
72. Sahrmann SA: Diagnosis by the physical therapist: A prerequisite for treatment. Phys Ther 68:1703–1706, 1988
73. Sandoz R: Some physical mechanisms and effects of spinal adjustments. Ann Swiss Chiro Assoc 6:91–141, 1976
74. Schenkman M, Butler RB: A model for multi-system evaluation, interpretation and treatment of individuals with neurologic dysfunction. Phys Ther 69:538–547, 1989
75. Sim FH: Diagnosis and Management of Metastatic Bone Disease: Multidisciplinary Approach. New York, Raven Press, 1988
76. Simons A, Trossman P: Biomechanical assessment in clinical practice. In Abreu BC (ed): Physical Disabilities Manual, pp 41–56. New York, Raven Press, 1981
77. Spitzer WO: Quebec task force on spinal disorders: Scientific approach to the assessment and management of activity-related spinal disorders. Spine 12:S1–S58, 1987
78. Spratt KF, Lehmann TR, Weinstein JN, et al: A new approach to the low-back physical examination. Spine 15:96–102, 1990
79. Stahl DC, Jacobs B: The diagnosis of obscure lesions of the skeleton. JAMA 201: 229–231, 1967
80. Stoddard A: Manual of Osteopathic Practice. London, Hutchinson & Co, 1969
81. Sunndaresan N, Galicich JH, Lane JM, et al: Surgical treatment of spinal metastases in kidney disease. J Clin Oncol 4:1851–1856, 1985
82. Taylor RG, Fowler WM Jr: Electrodiagnosis of musculoskeletal disorders. In D'Ambrosia RD (ed): Musculoskeletal Disorders: Regional Examination and Differential Diagnosis, 2nd ed, pp 59–94. Philadelphia, JB Lippincott, 1986
83. Taylor TKF, Weinir M: Great-toe extensor reflexes in the diagnosis of lumbar disk disorders. Br Med J 2:487–489, 1969
84. Thomas PS, Zauder HL: Thermography. In Raji PP (ed): The Practical Management of Pain. St Louis, Mosby-Year Book, 1986
85. Thomas-Edding D: Clinical problem solving in physical therapy and its implications for curriculum development. In: Proceedings of the Tenth International Congress of the World Confederation for Physical Therapy, pp 100–104. Sydney, New South Wales, Australia, 1987
86. Troupin RH: Radiologic evaluation of the musculoskeletal system. In Rosse C, Clawson DK (eds): The Musculoskeletal System in Health and Disease, pp 103–118. Philadelphia, Harper and Row, 1980
87. Unsworth A, Doverson D, Wright V: Cracking joints: A bioengineering study of cavitation in the metacarpophalangeal joint. Ann Rheum Dis 30:348–358, 1971
88. Wadsworth CT: Manual Examination and Treatment of the Spine and Extremities, pp 12–27. Baltimore, Williams & Wilkins, 1988
89. Warwick R, Williams P (eds): Gray's Anatomy, 35th ed. Philadelphia, WB Saunders, 1973
90. Watt NT: Decision analysis: A tool for improving physical therapy practice and education. In Wolf SL (ed): Clinical Decision Making in Physical Therapy, pp 7–23. Philadelphia, FA Davis, 1985
91. Watt NT: Clinical decision analysis. Phys Ther 69:569–576, 1989
92. Weed L: Medical records that guide and teach, Part I. New Engl J Med 278:593–600, 1968
93. Weed LL, Zinny NJ: The problem-oriented system, problem-knowledge coupling, and clinical decision making. Phys Ther 69:565–568, 1989
94. Wilson P: Sympathetically maintained pain. In Stanton-Hicks M (ed): Sympathetic Pain. Boston, Kluwer, 1989

95. Zinny NJ, Tandy CJ: Problem-knowledge coupling: A tool for physical therapy clinical practice. Phys Ther 69:155–161, 1989

96. Zohn DA, Mennell J: Ancillary aids in diagnosis. In Zohn DA, Mennell J (eds): Musculoskeletal Pain: Diagnosis and Physical Treatment, pp 65–88. Boston, Little, Brown & Co, 1976

RECOMMENDED READING

PHYSICAL EXAMINATION

Akeson WH, Amiel D, LaViolette D, Secrist D: The connective tissue response to immobility: An accelerated aging response? Exp Gerontol 3:289–300, 1968

Basmajian JV, Nyberg R (eds): Rational Manual Therapies, Baltimore, Williams & Wilkins, 1993

Bourdillon JF, Day EA, Bookhout MR: Spinal Manipulation, 5th ed. Oxford, Butterworh-Heineman, 1992

Cantu R, Grodin AJ: Myofascial Manipulation: Theory and Clinical Application. Gaithersburg, MD, 1992

Clayton ML, James SM, Abdulla M: Experimental investigations of ligamentous healing. Clin Orthop 61:146, 1968

Corrigan B, Maitland GD: Practical Orthopaedic Medicine. Boston, Butterworth, 1985

Cyriax J: Textbook of Orthopaedic Medicine, Vol I. The Diagnosis of Soft Tissue Lesions, 8th ed. London, Bailliere-Tindall, 1982

Cyriax JH, Cyriax PJ: Illustrated Manual of Orthopaedic Medicine, 11th ed. London, Butterworth, 1984

DeLateur BJ, Lehmann JF, Giaconi R: Mechanical work and fatigue: Their roles in the development of muscle work capacity. Arch Phys Med Rehabil 57:321–324, 1976

Dvorak J, Dvorak V: Manual Medicine: Diagnostics, 2nd ed. New York, Thieme Medical, 1990

Dvorak J, Dvorak V, Tritschler T: Manual Medicine: Therapy. New York, Thieme Medical, 1988

Edmond SL: Manipulation & Mobilization: Extremity and Spinal Techniques. St Louis, Mosby–Year Book, 1993

Fordyce WE: Behavioral Methods for Chronic Pain and Illness. St Louis, CV Mosby, 1976

Fordyce WE, Fowler RS, Lehmann JF, et al: Operant conditioning in the treatment of chronic clinical pain. Arch Phys Med Rehabil 54:399–408, 1973

Frankel VH, Hang Y: Recent advances in the biomechanics of sport injuries. Acta Orthop Scand 46:484–497, 1975

Gradosar IA: Fracture stabilization and healing. In Gould JA, Davies GL (eds): Orthopaedic and Sports Physical Therapy. St Louis, CV Mosby, 1990

Greenman PE: Principles of Manual Therapy, Baltimore, Williams & Wilkins, 1989

Grieve G: Modern Manual Therapy of the Vertebral Column. Edinburgh, Churchill Livingstone, 1986

Grieve G: Common Vertebral Joint Problems, 2nd ed. Edinburgh, Churchill Livingstone, 1988

Hammer WI: Functional Soft Tissue Examination and Treatment by Manual Methods: The Extremities. Gaithersburg, MD, Aspen Publications, 1991

Hartley A: Practical Joint Assessment: A Sports Medicine Manual. St Louis, Mosby–Year Book, 1990

Hettinga DL: Inflammatory response of synovial joint structures. In Gould JA, Davies GL (eds): Orthopaedic and Sports Physical Therapy. St Louis, CV Mosby, 1990

Hoppenfeld S: Physical Examination of the Spine and Extremities. New York, Appleton-Century-Crofts, 1976

Kaltenborn FM: The Spine: Basic Evaluation and Mobilization Techniques, 2nd ed. Oslo, Olaf Norlis Bokhandel, 1993

Keene JS: Ligament and muscle-tendon unit injuries. In Gould JA, Davies GL (eds): Orthopaedic and Sports Physical Therapy. St Louis, CV Mosby, 1990

Kenna C, Murtagh J: Back Pain & Spinal Manipulation: A Practical Guide. Sydney, Butterworths, 1989

Kennedy JD, Hawkins RJ, Willis RB, Danylchuk KD: Tension studies in human knee ligaments. J Bone Joint Surg 58(A):350–355, 1976

Knight K: The effects of hypothermia on inflammation and swelling. Athletic Training 11:1, 1976

Lehmann JF, DeLateur BJ, Stonebridge JB, Warren CG: Therapeutic temperature distribution produce by ultrasound as modified by dosage and volume of tissue exposed. Arch Phys Med Rehabil 48:662–666, 1967

Lehmann JF, Warren CF: Therapeutic heat and cold. Clin Orthop 99:207–245, 1974

Lewit K: Manipulative Therapy in Rehabilitation of the Locomotor System, 2nd ed. Oxford, Butterworth-Heinemann, 1991

Magee DJ: Orthopedic Physical Assessment, 2nd ed. Philadelphia, WB Saunders, 1992

Maitland GD: Musculoskeletal Examination and Recording Guide, 3rd ed. Adelaide, Lauderdale Press, 1981

Maitland GD: Vertebral Manipulation, 5th ed. London, Butterworth, 1986

Maitland GD: Peripheral Manipulation, 3rd ed. London, Butterworth-Heinemann, 1991

Mannheimer JS, Lampe GN: Clinical Transcutaneous Electrical Nerve Stimulation. Philadelphia, FA Davis, 1984

McRae R: Clinical Orthopaedic Examination, 2nd ed. Edinburgh, Churchill Livingstone, 1983

Norkin CC, Levangie PK: Joint Structure and Function, 2nd ed. Philadelphia, FA Davis, 1992

Noyes FR, Edward SG: The strength of the anterior cruciate ligament in humans and rhesus monkeys. J Bone Joint Surg 58(A):1074–1082, 1976

Noyes FR, Grood ES, Nussbaum NS, Cooper SM: Effects of intra-articular corticosteroids on ligament properties. Clin Orthop 123:197–209, 1977

Noyes FR, Torvik DJ, Hyde WB, Delucas JL: Biomechanics of ligament failure: An analysis of immobilization, exercise and reconditioning effects in primates. J Bone Joint Surg 56(A):1406–1418, 1974

Radin EL, Paul IL: A comparison of the dynamic force transmitting properties of subchondral bone and articular cartilage. J Bone Joint Surg 52(A):444–456, 1970

Santiesteban JA: Physical agents and musculoskeletal pain. In Gould JA, Davies GL (eds): Orthopaedic and Sports Physical Therapy. St Louis, CV Mosby, 1990

Warren CG, Lehmann JF, Koflanski JN: Heat and stretch procedures: An evaluation using rat tail tendons. Arch Phys Med Rehabil 57:122–126, 1976

White AA, Panjabi MM: Clinical Biomechanics of the Spine, 2nd ed. Philadelphia, JB Lippincott, 1990

CLINICAL DECISION-MAKING AND DATA COLLECTION

Boissonault WG (ed): Examination in Physical Therapy Practice: Screening for Medical Disease. New York, Churchill Livingstone, 1991

Feinstein A: Scientific methodology in clinical medicine, Part I: Introduction, principles and concepts. Ann Intern Med 61:564–579, 1964

Feinstein A: Scientific methodology in clinical medicine, Part IV: Acquisition of clinical data. Ann Intern Med 61:1162–1193, 1964

Feinstein A: An additional basic science for clinical medicine, Part IV: The development of clinimetrics. Ann Inter Med 99:843–848, 1983

Payton O, Nelson C, Ozer M: Patient Participation in Program Planning: A Manual for Therapists. Philadelphia, FA Davis, 1990

Weinstein M, Fineberg H: Clinical Decision Analysis. Philadelphia, WB Saunders, 1980

Wolf S: Clinical Decision Making in Physical Therapy. Philadelphia, FA Davis, 1985

Introduction to Manual Therapy

DARLENE HERTLING AND RANDOLPH M. KESSLER

- **History of Joint Mobilization Techniques**
  Early Practitioners
  Current Schools of Thought
  The Role of the Physical Therapist

- **Hypomobility Treatment**
  Soft Tissue Techniques
  Neural Tissue Mobilization
  Introduction to Joint Mobilization Techniques
  Peripheral Joint Mobilization Techniques

- **Hypermobility Treatment**
  Regional Exercises
  Localized Active Stabilization Techniques (Segmental Strengthening)
  Self-Stabilization Exercises

- **Therapeutic Exercises**

HISTORY OF JOINT MOBILIZATION TECHNIQUES

Although specific mobilization techniques were introduced in physical therapy curricula in this country in the 1980s, their use in the management of patients with musculoskeletal disorders is certainly not new. It seems somewhat odd that physical therapists have been slow in adopting joint mobilization techniques. After all, therapists have been delegated the duty of passive movement for years, and joint mobilization is simply a form of passive movement.

Some time in the past this important method of treatment was lost from medical practice and is just beginning to emerge again. The explanation for its disappearance probably lies in the fact that early users of mobilization techniques based their value on purely empirical evidence of their effectiveness; there was no scientific basis for their use. Later, specific joint mobilization was practiced only by more esoteric "professions" that claimed beneficial effects on all disease processes, usually from manipulations of the spine. This tended to further alienate orthodox medical practitioners, with the result that the use of any and all forms of joint mobilization, other than movement in the cardinal planes, became taboo. The approach to the management of many joint conditions is still largely influenced by the teachings of the early orthopedic surgeons, who advocated strict rest in the management of all joint conditions. Although scientific proof of the effectiveness of specific joint mobilization is still largely lacking, our expanded knowledge of joint kinematics at least provides a scientific *basis* for its use. It is becoming evident that in order to treat mechanical joint dysfunctions effectively and safely, a knowledge of joint kinematics and skill in joint examination and mobilization techniques are required.

☐ Early Practitioners

The use of specific mobilization techniques did not arise with the emergence of osteopathy and chiropractic. Some of the earliest recorded accounts of the use of joint manipulation and spinal traction are from Hippocrates, a physician in the fourth century, B.C. In fact, Hippocrates proposed refinements in some of the techniques used in his time. For example, one traction technique required that the patient be tied to a ladder and dropped 30 feet, upside down, to the ground. Hippocrates suggested that ropes be tied to the ladder so that two people could shake it up and down, thus affecting an "intermittent" traction. Hippocrates also developed many of the methods of reducing dislocations that are still in use today. Accounts of the use of manipulation by Cato, Galen, and other physicians during the time of the Roman Empire also exist.[22]

Little is known of the practice of joint manipulation during the disintegration of the Roman Empire and the beginning of the Middle Ages. During this time most hospitals were attached to monasteries, and treatment was carried out by members of the religious orders. Friar Moulton, of the order of St. Augustine, wrote *The Complete Bonesetter*. The text, which was revised by John Turner in 1656, suggests that manipulation was practiced in medical settings throughout the Middle Ages and early Renaissance. With the reign of Henry VIII in England and the subsequent dissolution of the monasteries, medicine lost its previous "mystic" influences and became the practice of "art and science."

The English orthopedic surgeons of the late 1700s and early 1800s, such as John Hunter and John Hilton, advocated strict rest in the early management of joint trauma.[57] This view was emphasized by Hugh Owen Thomas in the late 1800s. For two centuries this influence prevailed, and joint manipulation remained in the hands of "bonesetters." Bonesetting was practiced by lay people, and the art was passed down over the centuries within bonesetters' families. The bonesetters had no basis for the use of their manipulations other than past experience. The successful bonesetters were those who remembered details of cases in which ill effects had resulted and avoided making the same mistakes over again. Bonesetters tended to guard their techniques, keeping them secret among family members. A few bonesetters, because of their success, became quite famous. One such bonesetter, a Mrs. Mapp, was called upon to treat nobility and royalty.

BONESETTERS VERSUS PHYSICIANS

During this particular period there was extreme rivalry and animosity between physicians and bonesetters. Physicians were well aware of disastrous effects that bonesetting had at times on tuberculous joints or other serious pathologies. It is interesting that Thomas, who was particularly outspoken against bonesetters, was the son and grandson of bonesetters. Thomas, who gave his name to the *Thomas splint*, was the originator of many of the orthopedic principles

concerning immobilization of fractures and joint injuries still adhered to today. It goes without saying that medical opinion of joint manipulation has changed very little since his time.

Despite medical opinion, Sir James Paget, a famous surgeon and contemporary of Thomas in England, recognized the value of judiciously applied bonesetting techniques. His lecture entitled "Cases that Bonesetters Cure," which appeared in the *British Medical Journal* in 1867, spoke of the rivalry between bonesetters and physicians. He described types of lesions for which manipulation may be of value and advised that physicians "imitate what is good and avoid what is bad in the practice of bonesetters." Unfortunately, the medical profession at the time, and for years to come, ignored this advice.

The first medical book on manipulation since Friar Moulton's work was published in the 1870s. It was written by Dr. Wharton Hood, whose father, Dr. Peter Hood, treated a bonesetter, a Mr. Hutton, for a serious illness. Dr. Hood did not charge Hutton since he was aware of Hutton's free services to many poor people. In repayment, however, Hutton offered to teach Hood all he knew of bonesetting. The elder Hood was too busy to accept the offer, but his son Wharton did. In his paper on the subject, published in *Lancet* in 1871, Hood describes Hutton's techniques of spinal and peripheral manipulation.[87] He lists the conditions that Hutton was willing to treat as primarily post-immobilization stiffness, displaced cartilage and tendons, carpal and tarsal subluxations, and ganglionic swellings; he also states that Hutton avoided working on acutely inflamed joints. Hutton usually applied heat before manipulating, especially to the larger joints. Hood describes Hutton's manipulations as being very precise as to the direction and amplitude of motion. They were always of a high-velocity thrust. The illustrated descriptions of some of the common manipulations used by Hutton show them to be essentially identical to the manipulations used by manual therapists and even some orthopedists and physiatrists today. Hutton admitted to knowing nothing of anatomy and felt that in all of his cases a bone was "out." Of his techniques he says that forced pushing and pulling are useless; "the twist is the thing."

OSTEOPATHY AND CHIROPRACTIC

Meanwhile in the United States, Dr. Andrew Taylor Still was practicing medicine in Kansas.[238] It happened that Still's children contracted meningitis and all three died. Still, being frustrated and angered by the failure of current medical practices to save his children, set out to find a solution. For a time he spent his days studying the anatomy of exhumed Indian remains, paying special attention to the relationships among bones, nerves, and arteries. In 1874, through a "divine revelation," Still claimed he had discovered the cause of all bodily disease. His "law of the artery" claimed that all disease processes were a direct result of interference with blood flow through arteries that carried vital nutrients to a part. If normal blood flow to the part could be restored, then the body's natural substances would resolve the disease process. In 1892, Still founded the first school of osteopathy in Kirksville, Missouri, offering a 20-month course. By 1916 the osteopathic course was extended to 3 years, and by 1920 the United States Congress granted equal rights to osteopaths and M.D.s.[176] In the early 1900s, the osteopathic profession gradually became aware that some of Still's original proposals were incorrect. Over the years they incorporated traditional medical thought with the practice of joint manipulation. Especially during the last decade, osteopathic schools have deemphasized the practice of manipulation, and have attained essentially the same standards as medical schools. Osteopaths now qualify for residency programs in all medical and surgical fields.

In 1895 a grocer named D. D. Palmer, who had been a patient of Still, founded the Palmer College of Chiropractics in Davenport, Iowa. No prior education was required, and one of the first graduates was Palmer's 12-year-old son, B. J. Chiropractic theory evolved around the "law of the nerve," which stated that "vital life forces" could be cut off from any body part by small vertebral subluxations placing pressure on nerves. Since this could cause disease in the part to which the nerve ran, most, if not all, disease could be prevented or cured by maintaining proper spinal alignment through manipulation. Chiropractic was a "drugless" remedy that often supplemented manipulative treatment with various herbs, vitamins, and so forth. The chiropractic profession was fraught with internal turmoil from the outset.[216] (B. J. apparently grew up hating his father and later bought him out. When the father died, he stipulated that B. J. was not to attend his funeral.) Unlike osteopaths, most chiropractors adhered to their original concept, the law of the nerve, although the profession has always been divided into two or more schools of thought. They have received bitter opposition from the medical profession, which views them as charlatans and quacks. Today there remains some division in chiropractic philosophy. The "straights" continue to follow the law of the nerve, claiming to treat most disease by manipulating the spine or other body parts. The "mixers" tend to accept the limitations of this practice and use local application of ultrasound, massage, exercises, and so on, to supplement their manipulative treatment. It is significant that due to a strong lobbying force and the realization by chiropractors that, in order to survive, professional standards and education must be upgraded, chiropractors are rapidly gaining acceptance by governing bodies, the public, and even some physicians. It will be interesting to see if the profession of physical therapy keeps abreast of this trend.

□ Current Schools of Thought

In spite of efforts by Paget and Hood to emphasize the value of bonesetting techniques, manipulation was not readopted as a method of treatment by medical doctors until this century. The earliest physicians to practice manipulation were Englishmen. Books on the subject were published by A. G. Timbrell Fisher, an orthopedic surgeon, in 1925, and by James Mennell in 1939.[57,155] Mennell was a doctor of physical medicine at St. Thomas' Hospital. Both he and Fisher often performed their manipulations with the patient anesthetized. In 1934 Mixter and Barr published an article in the *New England Journal of Medicine,* and T. Marlin published *Manipulative Treatment for Medical Practitioners.*[141,162,170] These works have had a powerful effect on medical thought, stimulating much interest and leading to a series of excellent publications since then. Later in the century books advocating manipulative treatment were published by Alan Stoddard and James Cyriax.[35,220] Cyriax was to succeed Mennell at St. Thomas' Hospital. Cyriax advocated manipulations performed without anesthesia. Most of allopathic medicine's knowledge of manipulations can be traced to Mennell and Cyriax; the former made contributions in the field of synovial joints, the latter in the area of the intervertebral disk. Cyriax's examination approach is considered superb and contains a wealth of medical logic.

Currently, a school of thought that has attracted some attention (especially in Europe) is being led by Robert Maigne, who has postulated the "concept of painless and opposite motion."[137] This concept states that a manipulative maneuver should be administered in the direction opposite to the movement that is restricted and causing pain. Maigne, like Cyriax, has worked hard to focus medical attention on manipulative therapy as an effective modality in the relief of pain.

The driving force behind a school of thought that has flourished in Scandinavia is F. M. Kaltenborn.[105] Under his leadership, a systematic post-graduate education program that requires passage of practical and written examinations leads to certification in the specialty of manual therapy. The philosophy behind Kaltenborn's technique is a fusion of what he has considered the best in chiropractic, osteopathy, and physical medicine. He uses Cyriax's methods to evaluate the patient and employs mainly specific osteopathic techniques for treatment. Disk degeneration and facet joint pathologies are the two main spinal pathologies that the Scandinavians theorize are amenable to physical therapy.

Maitland, an Australian physical therapist whose approach is currently being taught in Australia, has a nonpathologic orientation to the treatment of all joints.[33,138] His techniques are fairly similar to the "articulatory" techniques used by osteopaths, involving oscillatory movements performed on a chosen joint. To increase movement of a restricted joint, movement is induced within the patient's available range of movement tolerance. He distinguishes between mobilizations and manipulations but puts heavy emphasis on mobilization. A meticulous examination is essential to this method because examination provides the guideline to treatment.

A prominent figure in the United States has been Dr. John Mennell, the son of the late James Mennell, who came to practice in the U.S. His work on the spine and extremities has been described in several publications and is particularly well known in America. He has made a significant contribution to a better understanding of joint pain and its treatment by placing stress on the function of small involuntary movements within a joint. He refers to these small movements as *joint play*; a disturbance of these movements is termed *joint dysfunction*. He states that full, painless, voluntary range of motion is not possible without restoration of all joint-play motions.[155,156]

In spite of their efforts, Mennell, Cyriax, Stoddard, and Maigne remain among the very few medical physicians to practice joint manipulation. As a result, manipulative treatment was not—and still is not—available to most patients seeking help from the medical profession. The original reasons for avoiding the practice of manipulation stemmed from the teachings of Hilton, Thomas, and Hunter, and the occasional disasters that occurred at the hands of bonesetters and other manipulators. Today many more medical physicians accept the value of judiciously applied manipulative treatment. However, to be effective, this treatment requires considerable evaluative and therapeutic management, and most physicians simply do not have the time to learn or practice manipulative technique.

☐ The Role of the Physical Therapist

Physical therapists are the logical practitioners to assume the responsibility for manipulative treatment. They work closely with physicians, who are capable of ruling out serious pathology. They tend to develop close and ongoing rapport with patients because the nature of their work requires close patient contact. They are taught to evaluate and treat by use of the hands. The advantages of the physician/physical therapist team in orthopedic manual therapy are perhaps best described by Cyriax: "Between them they have every facility: informed selection of cases, a wide range of different types of treatment, alternative approaches when it is clear that manual methods cannot avail."[36]

The United States, which has lagged far behind other countries in the development of orthopedic manual therapy, is gradually catching up. Thanks to the efforts of Mennell and Stanley Paris, a therapist originally from New Zealand, American therapists have at least had the opportunity to take post-graduate courses and to gain some competency in manual therapy and the management of orthopedic patients. It is hoped that the formation of the Orthopaedic Section of the American Physical Therapy Association in 1974 and increased education will improve this situation. Undergraduate courses in the physical therapy schools, clinically oriented long-term courses, postgraduate apprenticeships, and orthopedic specialization in master's degree programs are still needed.

Currently, the techniques therapists use to restore accessory movement are termed *articulations* or *joint mobilizations* and *manipulations*. Generally, manipulation means passive movement of any kind. Many therapists prefer to use the term articulation to denote a passive movement directed at the joint without any high-velocity thrust and within the range of the joint. Articulations or joint mobilizations are passive movements performed at a speed slow enough that the client can stop the movement. The technique may be applied with a sustained stretch or oscillatory motion: a gentle, coaxing, repetitive, rhythmic movement of a joint that can be resisted by the patient. The technique is intended to decrease pain or increase mobility. Unlike manipulation, it can be performed over a wide range and thus involve a series of movements referred to as *stages* (grades of movement). The techniques may use physiologic movements or accessory movements.

Manipulation, in this context, would then denote only passive movement involving a high-velocity, small-amplitude thrust that proceeds quickly enough that the relaxed patient cannot prevent its occurrence. The motion is performed at the end of the pathologic limit of the joint and is intended to alter positional relationships, to stimulate joint receptors, and to snap adhesions.[177] *Pathologic limit* means the end of available range of motion when there is restriction. Thus, the speed of the technique, not necessarily the degree of force, differentiates the two categories of passive movement. Joint manipulation is sometimes referred to as *thrust manipulation* or more recently, in osteopathic manual medicine, as *mobilization with impulse*.[208]

The basic spinal and peripheral joint mobilization techniques presented in this book are only part of the larger scope of manual therapy. In manual therapy we are concerned with the establishment of the normal structural integrity of the body and, to achieve this end, we use a variety of methods. The following is an overview of the practice of manual therapy.

■ HYPOMOBILITY TREATMENT

The term *hypomobility* denotes a decrease in the range of motion in an extremity joint or a spinal segment. In hypomobility there is a subjective stiffness and often pain, particularly when the joint is forcibly moved. Such restrictions often force adjacent joints to become hypermobile to compensate and enable a full range of movement to take place in the area. Treatment methods directed at hypomobility may be classified in four groups.

1. Soft tissue therapies other than joint corrections to normalize activity status, restore extensibility, reduce pain, and relieve abnormal tension in muscles, ligaments, capsules, and fascia.
2. Neural tissue mobilization to increase mobility of dura mater, nerve roots, and peripheral nerves.
3. Techniques of joint mobilization or articulation for the normalization of mobility and position. With hypomobility, the goal of treatment is to mobilize the restricted joint or spinal segment.
4. Other methods which have as their aim the improvement or restoration of normal body mechanics, such as relaxation training, the correction of posture, exercise, and activities which help to maintain the improved normal mechanics, soft tissue length and mobility, and joint mobility.

All of these methods come within the broader aspect of the manual therapy approach.

□ Soft Tissue Therapies

Soft tissue therapies involve manual contacts, pressures, or movements primarily to myofascial tissues. Soft tissue work may be classified into four categories: massage, soft tissue mobilizations or manipulations, acupressure, and stretching techniques ("active" relaxation of muscles, such as proprioceptive neuromuscular facilitation [PNF] and muscle energy techniques, as well as "passive" stretching of shortened muscles and associated connective tissues). *Soft tissue mobilization* is simply defined as the manual manipu-

lation of soft tissues administered for the purpose of producing effects on the nervous, muscular, fascial, lymphatic, and circulatory systems.[249]

CLASSICAL MASSAGE

Classical massage includes the traditional massage techniques that are often taught in the physical therapy curriculum and will not be covered here. The techniques consist of three generally used strokes: effleurage or stroking, petrissage or kneading, and friction. With the exception of tapotement and friction massage, slowly applied sustained pressure is recommended for decreasing soft tissue tone and for improving soft tissue extensibility (see Chapter 8, Relaxation and Related Techniques).

FRICTION MASSAGE

A particular method of friction massage (transverse frictions) was discussed in the 1940s by Mennell[154] and was clinically described later as Cyriax's deep massage and manipulation.[31,36] Although not yet demonstrated by adequately controlled histologic studies, friction massage represents an excellent empirical method of healing that has stood the test of time for the treatment of pathology caused by chronic-overuse soft tissue syndromes (see Chapter 7, Friction Massage).[234]

SOFT TISSUE MANIPULATIONS

Soft tissue manipulations have undoubtedly been performed since the beginning of time and have presently evolved into a variety of formats.* Soft tissue manipulations (including myofascial manipulations and stretching and release treatment methods), as in joint mobilizations, may be used to restore mechanical function of the soft tissue, especially its elasticity and mobility relative to other tissues or tissue layers, to exert a therapeutic effect on the autonomic nervous system by decreasing reflexive holding patterns (connective tissue massage)[12,30,39,43,64,115,174,225] or to change abnormal movement patterns through movement, posture, and body awareness.[9,28]

Mechanical approaches differ from autonomic approaches in that they seek to make mechanical or histologic changes in the myofascial structures.[9,28] *Myofascial manipulations* have been defined as the forceful passive movement of the musculofascial elements through their restrictive direction(s), beginning with the most superficial layers and progressing in depth while taking into account their relationship to the

---

*See references 7–9, 28, 30, 70, 75, 97, 126, 131, 137, 140, 165, 192, and 225.

joints concerned.[28] The technique is characteristically uniform, which distinguishes it from the more usual massage techniques. According to Lewit,[131] the difference between classical massage and myofascial-release types of soft tissue manipulations or mobilizations is that massage ignores the barrier-and-release phenomenon and with its moderate to rapid movements fails to achieve myofascial release. In the movement of shifting or stretching, one first takes up the slack (engages a barrier), after which a release occurs. Release is hypothesized as following reflex neural efferent inhibition and biomechanical hysteresis within the tissues.[70] The resistant barrier may be engaged directly or the tissue may be stretched in a direction away from the barrier in an indirect fashion. There are many combinations, and different authors and teachers of myofascial manipulations show similarities and differences.[9,28,70,75,140,207]

Substantial research has been performed by Akeson, Amiel, Woo, and others to determine the biomechanical characteristics of normal and immobilized connective tissues.[2-6,248] Since the literature is inconsistent at present and available research does not clearly explain how connective tissue is changed with soft tissue mobilization, practitioners must rely on clinical experience until further research is published.[68,75,223,224]

ACUPRESSURE

Acupressure is a method of point massage to acupuncture points or along meridians for the purpose of analgesia. It acts particularly on reflex changes in the soft tissue. Typically, fingertip pressure is used over a finite acupuncture point of highly discernible tenderness according to anatomy or traditional acupuncture, trigger points, or spontaneously tender points (Ah Shi points).[20,77,131,151,195,230] Pressure may also be applied by the thumbs, knuckles, palms, elbows, or even the feet for specific techniques. The stimulus applied may be either deep pressure on trigger points or Ah Shi points that are in muscle, circular or transverse frictions over acupuncture points, or kneading or palm pressure along the course of the meridian. Different systems suggest sustaining pressure from 3 to 90 seconds when a number of points are treated; however, one point can be treated as long as 3 to 4 minutes.[194] It has been found most effective to sustain pressure for as long as it takes to feel a softening of the tissue.[14] Although acupuncture and the various methods of acupuncture point stimulation have gained some acceptance in Western medicine, the theoretical basis for the effects of this type of treatment are viewed with a degree of skepticism. Research into the effects has tied it to the endogenous opiate system.[168]

TRIGGER POINT THERAPY

Trigger point therapy gained prominence as an important modality in treating myofascial pain in the 1960s. Although it had been a recognized type of therapy for many years, it was brought to the forefront by Janet Travell, John Mennell, and David Simons, who supplied much of the needed neurophysiologic information, and trigger point therapy became an accepted therapeutic modality. A *trigger point* is best described as an area of hypersensitivity in a muscle from which impulses travel to the central nervous system, giving rise to referred pain.[231]

Myofascial pain syndrome (MPS) is defined by Travell and Simons as "localized musculoskeletal pain originating from a hyperirritable spot or trigger point with a taut band of skeletal muscle or muscle fascia."[231] Involved muscles may present with a stretch length limitation (muscle tightness) and a local twitch response on palpation.[214,247,250] Physical treatments reported in the literature include transcutaneous nerve stimulation,[66,152] deep massage,[38,213] myofascial manipulations,[9,28,75,140] acupressure or isometric pressure,[20,140] reflex inhibition following minimal or maximal isometric contraction (muscle energy or post-isometric relaxation),[131,160,161,194] laser therapy,[211,218,219,237] ultrasonography,[20,21] trigger point injection or anesthetic blocks,[14,56,59,60,76,152,173] dry needling,[20,77,237] massage with an ice cube, and intense cold and stretching techniques using vapocoolant spray.[14,80,82,83,91,194,210,215,217,229-232] Travell and Simons have stated that "stretch is the action, spray is the distraction."[231] They believe that the cooling effect of the vapocoolant spray blocks pain and reflex muscle spasm, which occurs when a muscle with a trigger point is stretched, thus allowing greater elongation and passive range of motion. Often, a multifaceted approach is needed along with myofascial stretching, exercise, and corrective posture activities.[83,140,145,193]

MUSCLE ENERGY
(POST-ISOMETRIC RELAXATION)

Muscle energy is a form of manipulative treatment using active muscle contraction at varying intensities from a precisely controlled position in a specific direction against a counterforce. The origin of muscle energy is credited to Fred Mitchell, Sr., an osteopathic physician, who described the technique in the 1950s. His work has been documented by Mitchell, Jr., and associates.[160,161] Its other term, *post-isometric relaxation*, indicates the patient's active participation by muscular contraction and inspiration or expiration during manual treatment techniques.[16,49,65,69,74,118,119,131,132,160,161]   These techniques rest on the prime importance of soft tissues, particularly muscles, in producing various, moderately abnormal states of joint pain and movement limitation.

Muscle energy techniques may be used to decrease pain, stretch tight muscles and fascia, reduce muscle tonus, improve local circulation, strengthen weak musculature, and mobilize joint restrictions.[65] This method employs muscle contraction by the patient followed by relaxation and stretch of an antagonist or agonist. It is essentially a mobilization technique using muscular facilitation and inhibition.[132] Moderate to maximal contractions are used to stretch muscles and their fascia while minimal to moderate contractions are used for joint mobilizations.

Lewit[132] has found that muscle energy techniques are as advantageous for muscle relaxation as they have proved to be for joint mobilization, if there is muscle spasm and particularly if there are active trigger points. Lewit recommends the following procedure. The muscle is first brought into a position in which it attains its maximum length without stretching, taking up the slack in the same way as in joint mobilization. In this position, the patient is asked to resist with a minimum of force (isometrically) and to breathe in. This resistance is held for about 10 seconds, after which the patient is told to "let go." With patient relaxation, a greater range is usually obtained. The slack is taken up and the procedure repeated three to five times. If relaxation proves to be unsatisfactory, the isometric phase may be lengthened to as much as half a minute. Wherever possible, the force of gravity is used, as described by Zbojan,[251] for isometric resistance and for relaxation. This method is comparable with the "spray and stretch" method of Travell[228,231,232] but places greater emphasis on relaxation.

THERAPEUTIC MUSCLE STRETCHING

Therapeutic muscle stretching (specific muscle stretching performed, instructed, or supervised by a therapist in a patient with dysfunctions of the musculoskeletal system) has been promoted by Bookhout,[15] Janda,[92] Muhlemann and Cimino,[166] Saal,[200] and Evjenth and Hamberg.[49] The latter investigators have developed highly specific techniques for stretching individual muscles that minimize the risk of injuring the surrounding tissue. Relaxation of incoming neural input is essential for lengthening a contractile unit.[74] This relaxation is best accomplished by a stretch that occurs slowly and evenly and is accompanied by gentle contraction of the antagonist muscle.[118] *Proprioceptive neuromuscular facilitation techniques* (PNF) are methods of promoting or hastening the response of the neuromuscular system through the stimulus of

proprioceptors.[119] PNF is used in the approach of Evjenth and Hamberg. This approach as well as muscle energy is used to bring about relaxation of the antagonist muscle group according to the laws of reciprocal innervation proposed by Sherrington.[74,212] Primary objectives of PNF are also to develop trunk or proximal stability and control as well as to coordinate mobility patterns.

Performing stretching exercises both before and after an exercise period has been demonstrated to result in increased flexibility gains.[163] The ideal length of time for an individual to hold an isolated stretch is probably 15 to 30 seconds.[201] Continuation of the stretch for a period longer than this will not generate any greater flexibility gains, except in the case of pathologic contracture.[123,200,201]

RELAXATION EXERCISES

Relaxation exercises are of particular value in patients with musculoskeletal pain associated with psychogenic or tension states (see Chapter 8, Relaxation and Related Techniques). For example, tension headaches and muscular pain in the region of the cervical spine are often associated with prolonged muscle tension. Relaxation refers to a conscious effort to relieve tension in muscles. These exercises are usually based on the technique described by Jacobson[90] in which minimal contraction of each muscle is followed by a period of maximum relaxation. In addition, as a muscle is contracting, its corresponding antagonistic muscle is inhibited (Sherrington's law of reciprocal innervation).[74,212] Conscious thought can also be used to affect tension in muscle. This has been demonstrated in biofeedback, transcendental meditation, and autogenic training (see Chapter 8, Relaxation and Related Techniques).[135,136,209,235]

☐ **Neural Tissue Mobilization**

Nerve tension tests of the lower limb have been incorporated into mobilization techniques for some time.[138] Both straight leg raising and the slump test position used in testing of the lumbar spine can be employed as a treatment mobilization.[25,138] These methods can be applied when the symptoms or signs indicate pain is arising from the nerve root or its associated investments. Straight leg raising is an example of a direct method of mobilization of the nervous system. It is not considered a method of choice when the limitation is muscular and it should not be used, according to Maitland,[138] until other techniques that do not move the nerve root so much have been found ineffective.

The incorporation of the upper limb tension test (ULTT) into clinical practice was introduced by Robert Elvey (see Chapter 9, The Shoulder and Shoulder Girdle).[46-48] According to Maitland,[138] the ULTT is a most important evaluation tool and should be used by all physical therapists, even at the undergraduate level. The utilization of the ULTT as a treatment technique is just beginning to be developed and there is much more to be learned and many combinations of movements to be explored.[25,48,110] It can be used as an effective treatment technique for both chronic and acute cervical pain and shoulder pain.

When indicated by the examination, Butler[25] gives three related ways of approaching a tension component related to the patient's disorder.

1. Direct mobilization of the nervous system via tension tests and palpation techniques
2. Treatment via interfacing and related tissue such as joints, muscles, and fascia
3. Indirect treatment such as postural advice

☐ Introduction to Joint Mobilization Techniques

GENERAL RULES

The following rules and considerations should guide the therapist when performing joint mobilization techniques.

1. **The patient must be relaxed.** This requires that the patient be properly draped, and that the room be of comfortable temperature without distracting noises, and so on. Joints, other than the joint to be mobilized, must be at rest and well supported.

   The operator's handholds must be firm but comfortable. He must remove watches, jewelry, and so forth, and be sure buttons and belt buckles are not in contact with the patient.

2. **The operator must be relaxed.** This requires good body mechanics, especially with regard to the spine. The operator should attempt to create a situation in which his body and the part to be treated "act as one." This requires close body contact between the operator and patient for optimal control and mobilization.

3. **Do not move into or through the point of pain.** The operator must be able to determine the difference between the discomfort of soft tissue stretch, which is at times desirable, and the pain and muscle guarding that are a signal to ease up lest damage be done.

   The advanced manual therapist at times will move into or through the point of pain, but only

in highly selective circumstances. These techniques are not to be taught, nor are they expected to be learned in a basic-level course.

4. Position of the patient: Ensure that the following criteria are satisfied:
   a. The joint under treatment is accessible and the full range of movement remains unrestricted.
   b. The movement can be localized to the exact area required.

5. The operator should employ good body mechanics. The mobilizing force should be as close to the operator's center of gravity as possible. The force ideally should be directed with gravity assistance, especially when treating larger joints.

6. When performing an assessment mobilization, the joint should be tested in the resting position if the patient is capable of attaining that position. If not, the joint should be tested in the actual resting (present neutral or loose-packed position) position. Maximum joint traction and joint play are available in that position. In some cases, the position to use is the one in which the joint is least painful.

7. Each technique is both an evaluative technique and a treatment technique; therefore, the clinician continually evaluates during treatment. Formal assessments also should be made before and after treatment.

8. In peripheral joints:
   a. The direction of movement during treatment is either perpendicular or parallel to the treatment plane. *Treatment plane* is described by Kaltenborn[105] as a plane perpendicular to a line running from the axis of rotation to the middle of the concave articular surface. The plane is the concave partner, so its position is determined by the position of the concave bone.
      (1) Gliding mobilizations are applied parallel to the treatment plane (see Fig. 5-3).
      (2) Gliding mobilizations are usually performed in the direction in which the mobility test has shown that gliding is actually restricted (direct technique).
      (3) If the mobility test in the desired direction produces pain, gliding mobilization in the other direction should be used (indirect technique).[137] Other indications for the indirect method include joints that are hypermobile or that have little movement (amphiarthrosis).[105]
      (4) Joint traction or distraction techniques are applied perpendicular to the treatment plane.[105] The entire bone is moved so that the joint surfaces are separated (see Fig. 5-3).

b. Treatment force in gliding techniques is applied as close to the opposite joint surface as possible. The larger the contact surface is, the more comfortable the procedure will be.

c. One hand will usually stabilize while the other hand performs the movement. At times the plinth, the patient's body weight, and so on, are used for external stabilization. This allows both hands to assist in the movement. The therapist uses his hand or a belt to fix or stabilize on the joint partner against a firm support. The fixation is maintained close to the joint surface without causing pain. The mobilizing hand grips the joint structure to be moved as close to the joint space as possible.

d. The grip must be firm, yet painless and reassuring, while at the same time allowing the fingertips to be free to palpate the tissues under treatment.

e. The operator must consider:
   (1) Velocity of movement: slow stretching for large capsular restrictions; faster oscillations for minor restrictions
   (2) Amplitude of movement: graded according to pain, guarding, and degree of restriction

f. Accessory joint movement is compared to the opposite side (extremity), if necessary, to determine presence or degree of restriction.

g. One movement is performed at a time, at one joint at a time.

9. In spinal joints:
   a. In the sitting position it is essential that the patient is kept "in balance" so the occiput is in line with the coccyx, thus keeping the apex above the base.
   b. The direction of mobilization is determined by the results obtained from provocation tests. Mobilization initially is in that direction in which the pain and nociceptive reaction are diminished.
   c. Traction may be used to improve pain (levels I–II), prior to applying the specific mobilization technique.

10. Each technique can be used as:
   a. An examination procedure, by taking up the slack only, to determine the existing range of accessory movement and the presence or absence of pain
   b. A therapeutic technique in which a high-velocity, small-amplitude thrust or graded oscillations are applied to regain accessory joint movement and relieve pain

11. Reassessment. This should be done at the beginning of each treatment session, as well as during the treatment session. A selection of a few important "markers" for assessment enables a quick estimate of progress to be made without repeatedly going through the whole examination procedure.

INDICATIONS

Joint mobilization techniques are indicated in cases of joint dysfunction, due to restriction of accessory joint motion causing pain or restriction of motion during normal physiologic movement. However, as discussed in Chapter 3, Arthrology, there may be numerous causes of loss of accessory joint movement. The most common of these include capsuloligamentous tightening or adherence; internal derangement, as from a cartilaginous loose body or meniscus displacement; reflex muscle guarding; and bony blockage, as from hypertrophic degenerative changes. From this it should be clear that the proper indication for using specific mobilization techniques is loss of accessory joint motion (joint-play movement) secondary to capsular or ligamentous tightness or adherence. Other causes of joint dysfunction are relative contraindications. Refer to the section on capsular tightness in Chapter 4, Pain.

CONTRAINDICATIONS

I. **Absolute**
   A. Any undiagnosed lesion
   B. Joint ankylosis
   C. The close-packed position. Close-packed positions produce too much compression force on the articular surfaces.
   D. In the spine:
      1. Malignancy involving the vertebral column
      2. Cauda equina lesions producing disturbance of bladder or bowel function if the lumbar spine is being treated
      3. Where the integrity of ligaments may be affected by the use of steroids, traumatized upper cervical ligaments, Down's syndrome, and rheumatoid collagen necrosis of the vertebral ligaments, particularly if the cervical spine is involved and being treated
      4. Any indication of vertebrobasilar insufficiency in the cervical spine if the cervical spine is being treated
      5. Active inflammatory and infective arthritis

II. **Relative**
   A. Joint effusion from trauma or disease
   B. Arthrosis (*e.g.,* degenerative joint disease) if acute, or if causing a bony block to movement to be restored
   C. Rheumatoid arthritis
   D. Metabolic bone disease, such as osteoporosis, Paget's disease, and tuberculosis
   E. Internal derangement

F. General debilitation (*e.g.,* influenza, chronic disease)

G. Hypermobility. Patients with hypermobility may benefit from gentle joint-play techniques if kept within the limits of motion. Patients with potential necrosis of the ligaments or capsule should not be mobilized.

H. Joints that have yet to ossify. The epithelium is very sensitive in babies owing to the rich blood supply; therefore, in children under 18 to 24 months of age, we work with mobility via muscle elongation and movement.

I. Total joint replacements. The mechanism of the replacement is self-limiting, and therefore mobilizations may be inappropriate.

J. In the spine:

1. Pregnancy, if the lumbar spine or pelvis is being treated
2. Spinal cord involvement or suspected aneurysm in the area being treated
3. Spondylolisthesis or severe scoliosis in the area being treated
4. Where there are symptoms derived from severe radicular involvement

Peripheral Joint Mobilization Techniques

GRADING OF MOVEMENT

Gaining a feel for the appropriate rate, rhythm, and intensity of movement is perhaps the most difficult aspect of learning to administer specific joint mobilization. Generally, rate, rhythm, and intensity must be adjusted according to how the patient presents—whether acute or chronic—and according to the response of the patient to the technique. When significant pain or muscle spasm is elicited, the rate of movement must be adjusted, or the intensity reduced, or both.

The type of movement performed ultimately depends on the immediate effect desired. These techniques, in the majority of cases, are used to provide relief of pain and muscle guarding, to stretch a tight joint capsule or ligament, and, rarely, to reduce an intra-articular derangement that may be blocking movement.

MANUAL TRACTION[105,106]

Traction mobilizations are performed at a right angle to the treatment plane. Treatments are graded according to the amount of excursion imparted to the joint. The distance a joint is passively moved into its total range is its amplitude or grade of mobilization. Traction treatment mobilizations are graded as follows (Fig. 6-1):

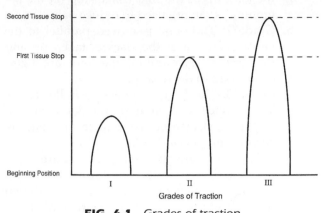
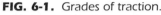

FIG. 6-1. *Grades of traction.*

Grade 1: Traction mobilization is applied by slowly distracting the joint surfaces, then slowly releasing until the joint returns to the starting position. There is little joint separation. Traction grade 1 may be used with all gliding tests and mobilization techniques.

Grade 2: Slow, larger amplitude movement perpendicular to the joint surface is applied, taking up the slack of the joint and the surrounding tissues.

Grade 3: Slow, even larger amplitude movement perpendicular to the joint surface is applied, stretching the tissues crossing the joint.

Grades 1 and 2 are used for pain reduction, whereas grade 3 is used to reduce pain and increase periarticular extensibility.

Other forms of manual traction include oscillatory, inhibitory, progressive, adjustive, and positional traction (see Figs. 17-32 and 20-45). Positional traction may also be applied mechanically. A manual adjustive traction employs a high-velocity thrust.[176]

Kaltenborn[104] advocates the use of *three-dimensional traction,* which describes traction to a joint which has been positioned with respect to the three cardinal planes. For example, a painful joint may be positioned in a pain-free position with a certain amount of abduction, flexion, and rotation before traction is applied to alleviate the pain.

Gliding Mobilizations. Two systems of grading dosages for gliding mobilizations are commonly used: graded oscillation techniques and sustained joint-play techniques.[105–107,139] However, a number of mobilization methods may be considered, such as progressive stretch, continuous stretch, muscle energy techniques, functional techniques, and counterstrain.[18,88,101,172]

1. Sustained translational joint-play or stretch techniques:[105–107]

   a. Grade 1: Small-amplitude glide is applied parallel to the joint surface and does not take the joint up to the first tissue stop (at the beginning of range); used to reduce pain.

b. Grade 2: The bone is moved parallel to the joint surface until the slack is taken up and the tissues surrounding the joint are tightened; used to decrease pain.

c. Grade 3: The bone is moved parallel to the joint surface with an amplitude large enough to place a stretch on the joint capsule and on surrounding periarticular structures.

Traction is always the first procedure. Gliding mobilization is then performed in the direction in which the mobility test has shown that the gliding is actually restricted (direct technique). For restricted joints, apply a minimum of a 6-second stretch force, followed by partial release (to grade 1 or 2), then repeat at 3- to 4-second intervals. When applying stretching techniques, move the bony partner through the available range of motion first (until resistance is felt), and then apply the stretch force against the resistance.

2. Graded oscillation techniques (see Fig. 3-10).[139] Glides are graded along a scale of 1 to 5 as follows:

a. Grade 1: Slow, small-amplitude oscillation parallel to the joint surface at the beginning of range; used to reduce pain.

b. Grade 2: Slow, large-amplitude oscillation parallel to the joint surface within the free range; used to reduce pain (does not move into resistance or limit of range).

c. Grade 3: Slow, large-amplitude oscillation parallel to the joint surface from middle to end of range; used to increase mobility (reaches the limit of range or takes the joint through the first tissue stop).

d. Grade 4: Slow, small-amplitude oscillation parallel to the joint surface at the limit (end) of range; used to increase mobility.

e. Grade 5: Fast, small-amplitude, high-velocity, non-oscillatory movement parallel to the joint surface beyond the pathologic limitation of range (through the first tissue stop), also called a thrust manipulation. Grade V is used when resistance limits movement, in the absence of pain.

Some indications for a thrust manipulation (Grade V) of the peripheral joints may include:[34]

1. Replacement of a joint dislocation, for example, a subluxed cuboid, a dislocated shoulder, or in a child with a pulled elbow

2. Reduction of an internal derangement of a joint in which a torn meniscus (knee) or loose body (elbow) produces blocking of movements

3. Stretching or breaking down adhesions. In chronic adhesive capsulitis of the shoulder, thrust manipulation may be used to break down periarticular adhesions and increase joint mobility.

The oscillatory treatment movements (grades I–III) may be smooth and regular or performed with an irregular rhythm in an attempt to trick muscles when large-amplitude treatment movements are hindered by tension.[34] The oscillatory movements are usually used in one or two methods, either (1) as small- or large-amplitude movements, at a rate of two or three per second, applied anywhere within the range, or (2) combined with sustained stretch as small-amplitude oscillations applied at the limit of the joint range. One may vary the speed of oscillations for different effects such as low-amplitude, high-speed to inhibit pain, or slow speed to relax muscle guarding.[138] If gliding in the restricted direction is too painful, gliding mobilization can be started in the painless direction.

The only consistency between the dosages of the two gliding methods is with grade 1, in which no tension is placed on the joint capsule or surrounding tissue.[115] The choice of using oscillatory or sustained techniques depends on the patient response. When dealing with pain management or high tone, oscillatory techniques are recommended. When dealing with loss of joint play and decreased functional range, sustained techniques are recommended. Traction, grade 1, is used with all gliding tests and gliding mobilizations.

TECHNIQUES FOR THE RELIEF OF PAIN AND MUSCLE GUARDING

Relief of pain and muscle guarding is desirable in relatively acute conditions, as a treatment in and of itself, and in chronic conditions to prepare for more vigorous stretching. The techniques in acute conditions are performed to increase proprioceptive input to the spinal cord so as to inhibit ongoing nociceptive input to anterior horn cells and central receiving areas (see Chapter 4, Pain). They are what Maitland refers to as grades I and II techniques.[138] Movement is performed at the beginning or midpoint of the available joint-play amplitude, avoiding tension to joint capsules and ligaments. A rhythmic oscillation of the joint is produced at a rate of perhaps two to three cycles per second.

In the case of acute joint conditions, these may constitute the only passive mobilization techniques used until the acute manifestations subside. In more chronic cases, these techniques should be used at the initiation of a treatment session, between stretching techniques, and at the end of a session in order to promote relaxation of muscles controlling the joint.

Chronically, they are used on a continuum with stretching techniques, gradually increasing in intensity as the patient relaxes.

Stretching Techniques. Since clinicians use these techniques primarily in cases of capsular tightness or adherence, the goal is ultimately to apply an intermittent stretch to the particular aspect of the capsule that is to be mobilized. In doing so, the clinician must move the joint up to the limit of the pathologic amplitude of a particular joint-play movement and attempt to increase the amplitude of movement. These techniques must be applied rhythmically—no abrupt changes in speed or direction—to prevent reflex contractions of muscles about the joint that might occur from overfiring of joint receptors. They must also be applied slowly in order to allow for the viscous nature—resistance to quick change in length—of connective tissue. The slack that is taken up in the joint-play movement is not released as the movement is performed. In effect, one is applying a prolonged stretch with superimposed rhythmic oscillations of small amplitude. The rationale is twofold. A prolonged stretch is the safest, most effective means of increasing the extensibility of collagenous tissue. In addition, rhythmic oscillations reduce the amount of discomfort and facilitate maximal relaxation during the procedure, presumably by increasing large-fiber input to the "gate."

Stops. When stretching at the limits of a particular osteokinematic movement in the presence of a tight capsule, it is usually helpful to provide a rigid "stop" against which the oscillation is made. It is best for the practitioner to arrange one of his body parts (*e.g.*, thigh, forearm, or trunk) as a stop. In this way the stop is easily moved to allow progressively increased range of movement. Such a stop also gives the patient an indication of exactly how far the therapist is going to move the part during a particular series of oscillations. This will reduce anticipatory muscle guarding to a minimum. If a greater range of movement is desired, the patient is informed where the stop will be made. The therapist rearranges the stop so as to allow a small increase in motion, and the oscillations are resumed. Such a technique seems to be most effective if the patient's body part is brought up rather firmly against the stop with each oscillation. For example, when mobilizing the shoulder, the therapist's thigh is brought up on the plinth to act as a stop for internal (Fig. 6-2) or external rotation (Fig. 6-3).

THE SPINE

There are some specific technical points to be mentioned with respect to the spine. For instance, because it is not possible to move a single segment actively,

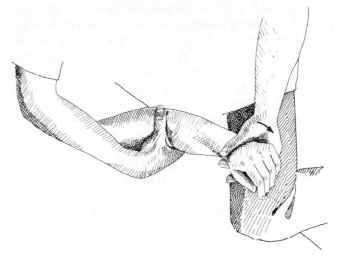

FIG. 6-2. Technique for internal rotation of the shoulder joint (arm close to 90° abduction) using a stop.

passive movement represents, as it were, joint play. Because of this relative difficulty in moving single joints, both specific and nonspecific techniques will be described in the spinal chapters. In the practice of spinal mobilization therapy there are scores of techniques available to the manual therapist. Most of the techniques employed by practitioners have either osteopathic or chiropractic components, although some occasionally make use of Cyriax's and Mennell's techniques.[170] Mobilization can be performed in a physiologic direction (namely, rotation, extension, lateral flexion, or flexion) or in a nonphysiologic direction (*e.g.*, longitudinal traction or anterior-directed posterior-anterior gliding). In practice, rotation, posterior

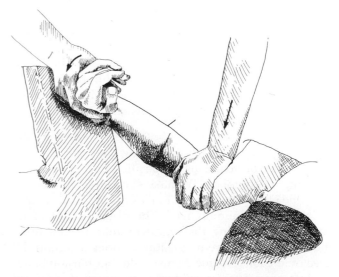

FIG. 6-3. Technique for external rotation of the shoulder joint (posterior glide, arm close to 90° of abduction) with a stop.

gliding, and traction techniques are mainly employed.[109] Spinal mobilization techniques can be classified under the headings of indirect mobilizations, direct mobilizations, specific mobilizations, nonspecific manipulations, oscillatory techniques, progressive loading, and manipulative thrusts.[170] Although there are many mobilization techniques, it is necessary to become proficient with only a few.

INDIRECT MOBILIZATIONS

When using these techniques the operator uses the limbs or pelvic or shoulder girdle as natural levers to influence the spinal column or sacroiliac joint.[170] For example, when a patient is sidelying with the operator applying pressure on the pelvis and the shoulder in opposite directions, the resulting force can cause rotation of the lumbar spine (see Fig. 20-38). Contract–relax or muscle energy techniques may be employed to facilitate maximum range of motion or to correct an anterior sacroiliac dysfunction (see Fig. 20-43). The leg is used as a lever.

DIRECT MOBILIZATIONS

Direct mobilizations involve direct manual pressure on the vertebrae in order to influence the intervertebral joints under treatment. These techniques are sometimes described as pressure techniques. The maneuvers are essentially those of chiropractors.[170] They are executed with the heel or ulnar border of the hand; more exactly, it is the pisiform which constitutes the point of pressure, which is either applied at the level of the transverse process or the spinal process (see Fig. 20-31).

SPECIFIC MOBILIZATIONS

There are specific mobilization techniques intended to influence only one joint at a time. This is achieved in several ways.

Positioning of the Area of Spine Under Treatment

When treating the lumbar spine, for instance, the operator should position the lumbar spine in extension when mobilization of the upper lumbar intervertebral joints is desired, and with a flexed spine for the lower lumbar intervertebral joints (see Figs. 20-30 and 20-32).

Locking

One way of achieving a specific effect is to apply "locking" techniques. To make such a technique specific, the clinician must try to lock all segments except for the one to be mobilized. The principle of locking consists of bringing the segments that are not to be moved into an extreme position, under a certain degree of tension. The mechanism is either tension of ligaments or opposition of bony structures (facet locking).

Ligamentous locking is achieved by moving the joint to the limit of joint range possible and utilizing the resulting capsular tension to lock the joint. The therapist locks the spinal segment by placing it in a movement pattern that constrains movement. When using ligamentous tension locking for localization, it is often desirable to use manual contact to achieve some degree of specificity. For example, a vertebra may be fixed by direct manual contact in a least one direction (*e.g.*, fixation of a spinous process from the side prevents rotation in the opposite direction).

Facet locking is achieved mainly by a careful combination of movement patterns (noncoupled or coupled) that constrains such movement as sidebending and rotation, making use of bony opposition. The therapist positions the patient just short of complete fixation so that a small range of movement is possible in the joint in question but less in the adjacent joints above and below. Usually segments cranial to the treated segment are locked. In some instances, locking may be used both cranial to and caudal to the spinal segment. An in-depth discussion of spinal joint locking is presented in the textbook by Evjenth and Hamberg.[49] To achieve the maximum specific effect, a combination of leverage and locking techniques with direct contact and fixation is commonly used.

Leverage of Movement (Long-Lever Techniques). This is another way to achieve specificity. For example, for treatment of the lower lumbar intervertebral joints, mobilization can be effected by rotating the pelvis or legs on a relatively fixed trunk up to the segment to be mobilized (see Figs. 20-36 and 20-37). Following this principle, the trunk can be rotated on a relatively fixed spine for the treatment of the thoracic spine (see Fig. 19-42).

NONSPECIFIC MANIPULATIONS

There are also nonspecific techniques that can be useful in mobilizing larger sections of the spinal column, such as traction along the long axis of the spine. Whereas traction along the long axis of the spine (see Fig. 20-40) acts on the intervertebral disk, distraction of the apophyseal joints is provided by rotation and side flexion around that same axis (see Fig. 20-45). Other types of nonspecific methods are represented by soft-tissue mobilization, general spinal manipulations, and noncontact manipulations.[81] Nonspecific manipulations are techniques whereby the manipulative force falls on more than one joint. Most of Cyriax's techniques fall under this category in which massive traction is applied to the area of the spine under treatment simultaneously with the manipulative thrust.[35–37] A potential complication of nonspecific techniques (traction and nonspecific manipulations) is the possibility of increasing motion in an unstable joint that was not detected during the evaluation.

OSCILLATORY TECHNIQUES

A variety of oscillatory techniques have evolved. However, more than anyone else, Maitland has successfully developed an excellent system for the application of oscillatory techniques.[138,139] As with the peripheral joints, the operator is guided by the signs and symptoms that the patient brings into the treatment situation. The operator oscillates into the patient's pain but not beyond it. An important feature of these techniques is that the patient is the controller of the treatment, thereby minimizing the possibility of harm. Another component of these techniques is rhythm. The more rhythmic the oscillations, the more tolerable and pleasant the treatment will be for the patient and the more effective.[170] Any diagnostic label is de-emphasized, while the amount of movement in the joint becomes the subject of treatment. This purpose is very much facilitated if the joint is positioned somewhere in mid range in order to move the joint in a chosen direction. (For grading of these techniques, see p. 122.)

PROGRESSIVE LOADING

Progressive loading mobilization involves a successive series of short-amplitude, spring-type pressures.[176] Pressure is imparted at progressive increments of the range on a 1 to 4 scale, as are graded oscillations. The pressures used are transmitted at different ranges; however, the amplitude of each pressure is the same.[172] Grades 1 to 3 occur within the available active range of motion. Grade 4 goes beyond the restrictive barrier and into the passive motion barrier.

MANIPULATIVE THRUSTS

A manipulative thrust (grade V) involves a high-velocity, small-amplitude thrust beyond the pathologic limits of range (through the first tissue stop). Only properly trained and experienced clinicians should apply manipulative thrusts of the spine owing to the skill and judgment necessary to their safe and effective practice. Most therapists have found that they can achieve the same effects by prudent application of other methods of spinal mobilization techniques. The great hallmark of mobilization is its relative safety.

SELF-MOBILIZATION TECHNIQUES OF THE SPINE

Traditionally, home programs have included exercise regimes dealing in a general way with the affected region rather than with the specific segment involved. Many of these home programs for joint dysfunction have, for the most part, stressed active or passive motions that are often poorly controlled by the patient, thus leading to further pain and joint stiffness.[41,185] The logical and most effective approach in the management of capsular restriction is increasing the extensibility through techniques applied directly to the joint. This has lead to the development of special exercises for the joints and muscles involved with vertebral and peripheral joint dysfunction. Self-mobilization techniques of the spine are well known through the works of Kaltenborn,[104] Gustavsen,[78,79] Fisk,[58] Buswell,[23,24] and Lewit.[130,131] In 1975, the first of a series of articles by Rohde on self-mobilization techniques of the extremities appeared in East Germany.[188–191] Among the advantages cited by Rohde are the following:

- Major emphasis is placed on a pain-free position at the end of range, in which mobilization can be most effective with regard to capsular stretch.
- Often the patient can control pain more readily than the therapist can.
- The patient can perform self-mobilization several times a day independently. This reduces the time and expense of formal treatment sessions in a physical therapy department.
- Increased range of motion is possible without excessive force.
- The techniques are simple, easy to apply, and are not time consuming.

Furthermore, it is probable that the oscillatory nature and repetitive motion working within the painful limits reduces pain by increasing proprioceptive input.[29,153] When pain is present, joint irritability is carefully monitored and patients are advised to observe pain behavior and to discontinue the movement if there is an increase in peripheral pain. Self-mobilization must be gentle, slow, and as specific as possible.

In general, self-mobilization is indicated in subacute or chronic painful conditions of the joints, which have resulted in a capsular pattern of restriction and for which restoration of range of motion appears possible. The basic rules and indications are essentially the same as for other mobilization techniques. Precise clinical diagnosis and indication are mandatory. For restricted movement, the patient is advised to gradually work into the painful range in order to stretch tight structures. A particularly effective variation in peripheral joint mobilization is the use of hold–relax techniques applied directly before a specific self-mobilization. All exercises are further enhanced by purposeful breathing.[24] An active altered posture is recommended for all spinal patients.[147,148,181,233]

Self-mobilization exercises are aimed at self-treatment, making the patient the most active member of the rehabilitation team. Selected examples of specific exercise for the relief of pain and increased mobility are described in subsequent chapters.

MUSCLE ENERGY
AND FUNCTIONAL TECHNIQUES

Muscle energy is an extremely valuable technique for correcting positional faults or joint hypomobility, because the technique combines methods to increase extensibility of periarticular tissue with methods to restore a length–tension relationship to the muscles controlling joint motion. The techniques of muscle energy are discussed in a previous section regarding soft tissue mobilization techniques. When muscle energy is used for joint restrictions, the joint is placed in a specific position to facilitate optimal contraction of a particular muscle or muscle group. Isometric muscle contraction against counterpressure provided by the clinician causes the muscle to pull on the bony attachment that is not being stabilized, thus moving one bone in relation to its articulating counterpart. Most isometric contractions are held for 3 to 7 seconds, and techniques are repeated approximately three to five times before reassessment. When isometrics are used for joint mobilization, maximal contractions are not desirable since they tighten, or freeze, the joints.[131] Moderate contractions are much more appropriate for joint mobilization.

An important consideration in this approach is the particular type of three-dimensional movement posture that will best localize the effect to a particular vertebral segment or rib joint. Localization of the force is more important than intensity of force. What is especially welcome about these methods is that they are alternatives to manipulative procedures.[16]

To understand the principles and applications of muscle energy techniques and functional techniques (two forms of post-isometric relaxation techniques), one must be familiar with the concepts of segmental facilitation proposed by Korr and with the work of Patterson and Sherrington on spinal reflexes.[120,121,179,212] According to Korr,[120] when the gamma motoneuron discharge to the muscle spindle is excessive, less external stretch is required to fire the primary annulospiral endings, which reflexly fire the extrafusal muscle fiber via the alpha motoneuron. The exaggerated spindle responses are provoked by motions which tend to lengthen the facilitated muscle and therefore create a restrictive spinal fault. The aim of both muscle energy and functional techniques is to restore the normal neurophysiology of the segment.

The functional method was originated by Harold Hoover, an osteopathic physician.[18,19,88,98,127] The aim of functional techniques is to reduce the exaggerated spindle response from the facilitated segmental muscles and thus restore normal joint mobility.[19,128] Like combined movements[44,45] and strain and counterstrain,[100,101] functional techniques utilize combinations of movements to find the most pain-free starting position, and superimpose on this starting position

gentle, repetitive motions or sustained holding.[19,128] The goal of these approaches is to obtain an antalgic starting position, with subsequent reduction in the input from depolarized nociceptors.[127]

STRAIN–COUNTERSTRAIN
TECHNIQUE[40,71,100,101,125,172]

Strain and counterstrain became popular in the 1970s and the number of practitioners is increasing. The technique was devised by Lawrence Jones, an osteopathic practitioner. It is considered an indirect manipulative technique of extreme gentleness for the treatment of somatic dysfunctions. In *Strain and Counterstrain,* Jones offers two definitions of the technique.[101]

1. "Relieving spinal or other joint pain by passively putting the joint into its position of greatest comfort."
2. "Relieving pain by reduction and arrest of the continuing inappropriate proprioceptor activity." To accomplish this the muscle that contains the malfunctioning muscle spindle is markedly shortened by applying mild strain to its antagonist.

The position of injury is one of strain, which places some muscles in a shortened state and other muscles in a lengthened state. The rationale for strain and counterstrain is based on a neurological model first proposed by Dr. Irvin Korr in 1975.[121,122] According to Korr's muscle spindle theory for neuromuscular disorder, the gamma motor neuron activity to the intrafusal fibers of the shortened muscles is turned up instead of decreased. The resultant tension in the intrafusal mechanism of the shortened muscles causes excitation of the CNS, stimulation of the alpha motor neurons, and the maintenance of extrafusal fiber contraction.

Diagnosis in this method is made by the presence of a specific tender point that overlies the muscle. The tender points may be related to myofascial trigger points and acupuncture points.[40]

The treatment technique is positional. According to Jones, positioning the joint in the exact opposite position to the one that produces the pain will relieve the pain and dysfunction. There are two important aspects of this treatment procedure:[125]

1. Using the tender point as a monitor, the operator is guided into a position of comfort that reduces aberrant afferent flow and returns the muscle to "easy neutral."
2. The position of comfort is held for 90 seconds, the amount of time required for the proprioceptive firing to decrease in frequency and amplitude, and then it is returned to neutral slowly after the positional release.

Strain and counterstrain is considered a gentle, non-traumatic type of mobilization technique especially effective when irregular neuromuscular activities have maintained and perpetuated abnormal mechanical stress to tissue in both acute and chronic conditions. Strain and counterstrain can make a significant contribution when integrated with other manual medicine techniques (*i.e.*, joint mobilization, muscle energy, myofascial release).[125] Although there is limited research data in this area to support the model, the observation of practitioners points to a neural basis through a principle of afferent reduction of abnormal mechanoreceptor and nociceptor stimulation.[71]

HYPERMOBILITY TREATMENT

The term *hypermobility* denotes an increase in the range of motion in an extremity joint or a spinal segment. One can differentiate between minor hypermobility without pain, hypermobility with pain, and complete instability that is considered to be pathologic.[79] Pain may be caused by continued postural imbalances, continued motor performance abnormalities, or delayed stretch pain (tendon pain resulting from overstretching of one or several tendons). According to Gustavsen,[79] this type of tendon pain appears a few seconds after bringing the joint to its barrier and decreases very slowly when the joint is carried to a more normal position.

The two basic types of hypermobility include systematically acquired hypermobility (general constitutional type) and local hypermobility of a peripheral joint or spinal segment. Hypermobility is not a pathologic motion state of a joint but rather one end of the normal mobility spectrum.[67] Hypermobility may be generalized to both spinal and peripheral joints, or it may be a feature of spinal joints alone, peripheral alone, or isolated to one spinal segment. Symptomatic hypermobility occurs when musculoskeletal signs and symptoms may be ascribed to the presence of hypermobility.[42,63] An unstable joint is one with increased range of movement in one (or more) directions in which there is insufficient soft tissue control, be it ligamentous, disk, muscular, or all three.[67]

Many definitions of spinal instability exist without any real consensus.* One consideration is the difference between functional (clinical instability) and mechanical instability. Whereas *mechanical instability* is described as consisting of a measurable abnormal translation of joint opening that is the direct result of disruption of one or more of the mechanical stabilizers of the joint, *functional instability* (which can occur

in the absence of measurable mechanical instability) is manifested by instability of the joint under load.[184] Functional instability is in most cases due to muscular or proprioceptive deficit.

Spinal segment hypermobility may be the result of compensation seen with acquired motion restrictions or congenital motion restrictions. Junctional areas (*i.e.*, C4–5, lumbosacral junction and thoracolumbar junction) of the spinal column tend to become especially hypermobile.[226] Hypermobility in the C4–5 segment is often accompanied by hypomobility in segments C2 and C3 and the cervicothoracic junction as well.[79] Muscular dysfunction is usually present with shortened upper deep neck muscles and weakened long neck and prevertebral muscles. Hypermobility of L4, L5, and S1 is often caused by inappropriate motor activities.[79] Typically these individuals have forgotten how to control their lumbar spine in a position of stability when carrying out activities of daily living. Management of segmental instability should include pain reduction methods. Pain may be caused by continued postural imbalance, continued motor performance abnormalities, or delayed stretch pain. Passive mobilization (grades 1 and 2, posterior–anterior pressures) of the affected segment within its range is particularly effective.[79] Stabilizing and controlling procedures (collars, corsets, taping, *etc.*) when the spinal area is very painful or very unstable, or both, may be helpful.[108,159,167,202,203,206,239,245] These procedures should be temporary while the exercise program is developed.

☐ Regional Exercises

LUMBAR AND THORACIC SPINE

Therapeutic exercises that improve muscle strength, endurance, coordination, and control should be started as soon as possible. Isometric, gravitational exercises, and other forms of exercise should be considered.[72–74,111,157,178] If the spinal extensors (thoracic and lumbar spine) are weak, exercises to strengthen them should avoid inner range hyperextension movements. The starting position should be arranged so that the resisted movement occurs in mid range and the excursion ceases when normal postural length of the muscle is reached.[74] A potent cause of aggravation of low back pain, due to hypermobility, is that of forced extension in the starting position of lying prone. Rotational exercises have been effective in patients who do not respond to other treatments.[182] By increasing muscle control and strength, postural backache and locking will be reduced.

The learning of physiologically correct movement patterns and postural advice is vital and should include avoidance of positions and exercises that lead to

---

*See references 40, 51, 61, 63, 72–74, 89, 112–114, 167, 178, 180, 183, and 201.

strain on joints, such as hyperextension. Exercises need to be selected with care, since those which stress extreme joint positions are liable to exacerbate the condition. In general, one should start with many repetitions at low speed with minimal resistance performed at middle or beginning range. Progression of exercises should focus on increased (isometric) contractions in the inner range of motion and finally on submaximal resistance in any range except the outer range. The purpose is not so much to develop strength but endurance and technique (physiologically correct movement patterns).

Swimming is considered excellent for the lumbar and thoracic spine, because there is little back movement and strong muscle work including co-contractions.[67] Balance exercises using a wobble board, Tumble Form, or Feldenkrais foam roll in standing, sitting, and lying positions are used to improve muscular "speed" reactions and balance reactions. The patient's balance may be challenged also with the use of the Swiss gymnastic ball.[124,129]

The emphasis of long-term management involves the avoidance of excessive load, sustained activities, and especially end-of-range postures.

CERVICAL SPINE

Training follows similar lines as for the thoracic and lumbar spine. Patients will usually benefit from postural retraining of the entire spine. Lumbar exercises offer a properly aligned base of support for the thoracic spine, whereas the position of the thoracic cage is the key to postural control of the balanced cervical spine.[221] As with the thoracic and lumbar spine, the learning of physiologically correct movement patterns, use of relief postures, ergonomic advice, and increased postural awareness are vital to bring about dynamic changes in the musculoskeletal system. Longstanding compulsive patterns need to be modified or removed from the nervous system.[143] Imposing traditional exercise movements on changed or faulty postures and movement patterns will often only perpetuate the existing condition.[55] There are several very effective methods and techniques in current use to facilitate body awareness and movement including the Feldenkrais method,[52–55,142] the Alexander technique,[10,32,62,99] Aston Patterning,[7,8,134,158] ideokinetic facilitation and related body alignment techniques,[222,227] and Kein-Vogelbach's functional kinetics.[117]

There are many methods of strengthening the paravertebral muscles of the neck including proprioceptive facilitation and simple self-administered resistance by hand pressure.[1,23,27,175,187,204,205,252] Exercises for the cervical, upper through mid-thoracic and shoulder girdle region are functionally interre-

lated and need to be addressed. Exercises should not be given arbitrarily as a group but should be judiciously chosen for the treatment program.

☐ Localized Active Stabilization Techniques
(Segmental Strengthening)

Patients with spinal dysfunction need to learn to actively stabilize hypermobile spinal areas. This requires strong and well-functioning muscles. The small extensor and rotator muscles close to the hypermobile joint must become strong enough to be able to fixate a hypermobile segment. Strengthening the segmental musculature is achieved by the principle of stimulating the small but important muscle groups to work isometrically in maintaining the orientation in space of a single segment.[74] Clear evidence exists that degenerative joint conditions are accompanied by changes in the relative population of "fast" and "slow" fibers in the segmental musculature (e.g., multifidus).[102] The deeper intersegmental and polysegmental muscles, particularly the multifidi, are primarily stabilizers controlling posture and assisting in fine adjustments and segmental movement.[11,84,113,236] The multifidi are also believed to protect the facet capsule from being impinged during movement because of its attachment to the joint capsule.[13]

DIRECT METHOD

These stabilization techniques involve direct manual pressure on the spinous process of the hypermobile segment. The thumb pads may be applied to the side of the spinous process in a lateral or oblique direction (lateral technique) or over the spinous process in a posteroanterior direction (sagittal technique) to recruit the small rotators or extensors (see Figs. 20-6C and 20-7A). Moderate but sustained pressure is applied to the bony point while the patient is instructed not to allow the vertebra to be displaced. With encouragement and practice the patient is able to localize the muscular effort. Progression is made by increasing the pressure, both in intensity and duration. Positioning is usually with the spine in a resting position. One can also use ligamentous or facet locking and positioning out of the resting position to influence localization. Progression can also be increased by using an antigravity position (see Fig. 17-37).

INDIRECT METHOD

When using indirect techniques the operator uses the limbs, sacrum, or head to influence the small muscles along the spinal column. For example, when treating the lumbar spine with the patient in a prone position, one hand of the operator is placed on the lumbar region immediately above the segment(s) concerned while moderate but increasing and sustained pressure is applied to the sacrum with the other hand (see Fig. 20-6*A*).

☐ Self-Stabilization Exercises

At home, another person can be taught to give resistance, or pressure can be self-administered by the patient (see Figs. 17-34, 17-35, 20-6*B,C*, 20-7*A,B*). Indirect methods use specific starting positions so that the painful and hypermobile segment does not move during these exercises. Stabilization programs in which the extremities are involved may require a special exercise program to train the muscles so that they can develop the required stabilizing effect (see therapeutic exercises, following). Exercises should emphasize diagonal motion to strengthen the small muscles around the spine.[79]

▮ THERAPEUTIC EXERCISES

Therapeutic exercises have been widely recommended to help prevent the development of spinal and peripheral pathology, to decrease pain, and to increase function. Five types are recognized as necessary to prevent, restore, or maintain a healthy and functional musculoskeletal system: strength training, flexibility training, endurance training, neuromuscular control training, and aerobic training.

Much of our present-day understanding of muscle imbalances and neuromotor training comes from the work of Janda,[93–96] Lewit,[131] Kendall,[108] Bookhout,[15] and Sahrmann.[202] Janda has observed that certain muscle groups respond to dysfunction by tightening and shortening, while other muscle groups react by inhibition, atrophy, and weakness (Table 6-1). Until recently, evaluation of muscle function was concerned primarily with strength testing, with little attention paid to muscle tightness or resting muscle length. According to Janda's clinical experience, to try to strengthen a weakened muscle first is futile, because it will be inhibited by its shortened antagonist.[93,103]

Clinically, injury to one area often affects the functional abilities of the other areas (*e.g.*, the head, neck, and shoulder girdle). Janda describes a muscle imbalance pattern seen typically in the head and shoulder region.[93,96] The proximal or shoulder-crossed syndrome describes a situation in which imbalance exists between the weak lower stabilizers of the scapula and deep neck flexors and the tight and shortened upper trapezius, pectoralis group, and levator scapulae. With a forward head, shortened suboccipital, stern-

TABLE 6-1 FUNCTIONAL DIVISION OF MUSCLE GROUPS

Muscles Prone to Tightness (mainly postural function)

Sternocleidomastoid	Hip flexors
Scalenes	Iliopsoas
Levator scapulae	Tensor fasciae latae
Pectoralis major	Rectus femoris
(clavicular/sternal end)	Lateral hip rotators
Trapezius (upper part)	Piriformis
Flexors of the upper limb	Short hip adductors
Quadratus lumborum	Hamstrings
Back extensors	Plantar flexors
Erector spinae	Gastrocnemius
Longissimus thoracis	Soleus
Rotatores	Tibialis posterior
Multifidus	

Muscles Prone to Weakness (mainly dynamic [phasic] function)

Short cervical flexors	Rectus abdominus
Pectoralis major (abdominal part)	External/internal obliques
	Gluteus maximus
Trapezius (lower part)	Gluteus medius and
Rhomboids	minimus
Serratus anterior	Vastus medialis and lateralis
Subscapularis	Tibialis anterior
Extensors of upper limb	Peronei

(Adapted from Janda V: Muscle Function Testing. London, Butterworth, 1983; and Jull GA, Janda V: Muscles and motor control in low back pain. In Twomey LT, Taylor JR (eds): Physical Therapy of the Low Back, pp 253–278. New York, Churchill Livingstone, 1987)

ocleidomastoid, scalene, and pectoralis minor muscles are often present. When such dysfunctions are present, the shortened muscles must be stretched before the training of the weakened muscles is undertaken.

In the last 10 years, both therapists and patients have shown increasing support for the concept of active self-treatment.[146–150] Training programs such as medical exercise training (MET),[85,86] medical training therapy (MTT),[78,79] aerobic training,[17,144,169,246] back and neck schools,[50,51,133,221,240–244] and dynamic stabilization programs (particularly for the lumbar spine),* have increased our knowledge of how to carry out a patient-oriented training program to provide optimal stimulation of the functional qualities of muscle strength, flexibility, endurance, coordination, and cardiovascular fitness for retraining and improving function.

REFERENCES

1. Adler SS, Beckers D, Buck M: The neck. In Adler SS, Beckers D, Buck M (eds): PNF in Practice: An Illustrated Guide, pp 141–151. Berlin, Springer-Verlag, 1993
2. Akeson WH, Amiel D: The connective tissue response to immobility: A study of the

*See references 144, 164, 175, 186, 196–199, 201, 204, 205, 221, and 243.

chondroitin 4 and 6 sulfate and dermatan sulfate changes in periarticular connective of control and immobilized knees of the dog. Clin Orthop 51:190–197, 1967

3. Akeson WH, Amiel D: Immobility effects of synovial joints: The pathomechanics of joint contracture. Biorheology 17:95–110, 1980

4. Akeson WH, Amiel D, LaViolette D: The connective tissue response to immobility: An accelerated aging response? Exp Gerontol 3:289–301, 1968

5. Akeson WH, Amiel D, Mechanic GL, et al: Collagen cross-linking alteration to joint contractures: Changes in the reducible cross-linking in periarticular connective tissue collagen after nine weeks of immobilization. Connect Tissue Res 5:15–19, 1977

6. Akeson WH, Woo SL-Y, Amiel D, et al: The connective tissue response to immobilization: biomechanical changes in periarticular connective tissue of the rabbit knee. Clin Orthop 93:356–362, 1973

7. Aston J: Movement Dynamics, I. Continuing Education Course. Seattle, The Aston Training Center, 1990

8. Aston J: Movement Dynamics, II. Continuing Education Course. Incline Village, NV, The Aston Training Center, 1992

9. Bajelis D: Hellerwork: The ultimate. Int J Alternative Complementary Med 12:26–39, 1994

10. Barlow W: The Alexander Technique. New York, Warner Books 1973

11. Basmajian JV: Muscles Alive: Their Functions Revealed by Electromyography. Baltimore, Williams & Wilkins, 1978

12. Bischof I, Elminger G: Connective tissue massage. In Licht S (ed): Massage, Manipulation & Traction, pp 57–85. Baltimore, Waverley Press, 1963

13. Bogduk N, Twomey LT: Clinical Anatomy of the Lumbar Spine. New York, Churchill Livingstone, 1987

14. Bonica JJ: Management of myofascial pain syndromes in general practice. JAMA 164:732–738, 1957

15. Bookhout MR: Examination and treatment of muscle imbalances. In Bourdillon JF, Day EA, Bookhout MR (eds): Spinal Manipulation, 5th ed. Oxford, Butterworth-Heinemann Ltd, 1992

16. Bourdillon J, Day EA, Bookhout MR: Spinal Manipulation, 5th ed. Oxford, Butterworth-Heinemann Ltd, 1992

17. Bower KD: The role of exercises in the management of low back pain. In Grieve GP (ed): Modern Manual Therapy of the Vertebral Column, pp 839–848. Edinburgh, Churchill Livingstone, 1986

18. Bowles CH: A functional orientation for technique. Yearbook of the Academy of Applied Osteopathy, pp 177–191, 1955

19. Bowles CH: Functional technique: A modern perspective. J Am Osteopath Assoc 80:326–331, 1981

20. Bradley JA: Acupuncture, acupressure, and trigger point therapy. In Peat M (ed): Current Physical Therapy, pp 228–234. Toronto, BC Decker, 1988

21. Brown BR: Diagnosis and therapy of common myofascial syndromes. JAMA 239:646–648, 1978

22. Burke GL: Backache from Occiput to Coccyx. Vancouver, MacDonald, 1964

23. Buswell JS: A manual of home exercises for the spinal column. Auckland, Pelorus Press, 1977

24. Buswell JS: Exercises in the treatment of vertebral dysfunction. In Grieve G (ed): Modern Manual Therapy of the Vertebral Column, pp 834–838. Edinburgh, Churchill Livingstone, 1986

25. Butler DS: Mobilisation of the Nervous System. Melbourne, Churchill Livingstone, 1991

26. Cailliet R: Soft Tissue Pain and Disability, 2nd ed. Philadelphia, FA Davis, 1988

27. Cailliet R: Subluxations of the cervical spine: The whiplash syndromes. In Cailliet R (ed): Neck and Arm Pain. Philadelphia, FA Davis, 1991

28. Cantu RI, Grodin AJ: Myofascial Manipulation: Theory and Clinical Application. Gaithersburg, MD, Aspen Pub, 1992

29. Casey KL, Melzack R: Neural mechanism of pain: A conceptual model. In Way EL (ed): New Concepts in Pain and Its Clinical Management. Philadelphia, FA Davis, 1967

30. Chaitow L: Neuro-muscular Technique: A Practitioner's Guide to Soft Tissue Manipulation. New York, Thorsons Publishers, 1980

31. Chamberlain GJ: Cyriax's friction massage: A review. J Orthop Sports Phys Ther 4(1):16–22, 1982

32. Chaplan D: Back Trouble: A New Approach to Prevention and Recovery. Gainesville, FL, Triad, 1987

33. Cookson JC, Kent BE: Orthopedic manual therapy—An overview. Phys Ther 59:136–146, 1979

34. Corrigan B, Maitland GD: Practical Orthopaedic Medicine. London, Butterworth, 1985

35. Cyriax J: Textbook of Orthopaedic Medicine, Vol 1. Diagnosis of Soft Tissue Lesions, 8th ed. London, Balliere Tindall, 1982

36. Cyriax J, Coldham M: Textbook of Orthopaedic Medicine. Vol 2, Treatment by Manipulation, Massage and Injection, 11th ed. London, Balliere Tindall, 1984

37. Cyriax JH, Cyriax PJ: Illustrated Manual of Orthopaedic Medicine. London, Butterworth, 1983

38. Danneskiold-Samsoe B, Christiansen E, Anderson RB: Myofascial pain and the role of myoglobin. Scand J Rheumatol 15:174–178, 1986

39. Dicke E, Schliack H, Wolff A: A Manual of Reflexive Therapy of the Connective Tissue. Scarsdale, NY, Simon Publishers, 1978

40. DiGiovanna EL: Counterstrain. In DiGiovanna EL, Schiowitz S (eds): An Osteopathic Approach to Diagnosis and Treatment, pp 85–87. Philadelphia, JB Lippincott Co, 1991

41. Dontigny RL: Passive shoulder exercises. J Phys Ther 50:1707–1709, 1970

42. Dupuis PR, Young-Hing K, Cassidy JD, et al: Radiologic diagnosis of degenerative lumbar spinal instability. Spine 10:662–676, 1985

43. Ebner M: Connective Tissue Manipulations. Malbar, FL, Robert E Kreiger, 1985

44. Edwards BC: Combined movements in the lumbar spine: Examination and significance. Aust J Physiother 25:147–152, 1979

45. Edwards BC: Combined movements in the lumbar spine. Examination and treatment. In Grieve GP (ed): Modern Manual Therapy of the Vertebral Column, pp 561–566. Edinburgh, Churchill Livingstone, 1986

46. Elvey RL: Brachial plexus tension tests and the pathoanatomical origin of arm pain. In: Proceedings of Multidisciplinary International Conference of Manipulative Therapy, pp 105–111. Melbourne, Australia, 1979

47. Elvey RL: Brachial plexus tension test and the pathoanatomical origin of arm pain. In Idczack RM (ed): Aspects of Manipulative Therapy. Carlton, Australia, Lincon Institute of Health Sciences, 1981

48. Elvey RL: Treatment of arm pain associated with abnormal brachial plexus tension. Aust J Physiotherapy 32:225–230, 1986

49. Evjenth O, Hamberg J: Muscle Stretching in Manual Therapy: A Clinical Manual, Vol 1. The Extremities; Vol 2. The Spinal Column and the TMJ. Alfta, Sweden, Alfta Rehab Forlag, 1984

50. Fahrni WH: Back school back then: A personal history. In White AH, Anderson R (eds): Conservative Care of Low Back Pain, pp 37–38. Baltimore, Williams & Wilkins, 1991

51. Farfan HF, Gracovetsky S: The nature of instability of the spine. Spine 9:714–719, 1984

52. Feldenkrais M: Awareness through movement. New York, Schocken Book, 1979

53. Feldenkrais M: The master moves. Cupertino, CA, Meta Publications, 1984

54. Feldenkrais M: Potent self. Cambridge, Harper & Row, 1985

55. Feldenkrais M: Bodily expressions. Somatics 4:52–59, 1988

56. Fine PG, Milano R, Hare BD: The effects of myofascial trigger point injections are naloxone reversible. Pain 32:15–20, 1988

57. Fisher AGT: Treatment by Manipulation, 5th ed. New York, Paul B Hoeber, 1948

58. Fisk JW: The Painful Neck and Back. Diagnosis, Manipulation, Exercise, Prevention, pp 154–205. Springfield, Charles C Thomas, 1977

59. Frost A: Diclofenac versus lidocaine as injection therapy in myofascial pain. Scand J Rheumatol 15:2153–2156, 1986

60. Frost A, Jessen B, Siggaard-Andersen J: A control, double-blind comparison of mepivacaine injection versus saline injection for myofascial pain. Lancet 8:499–500, 1980

61. Frymoyer JW, Krag M: Spinal stability and instability: Definitions, classifications and general principles of management. In Dunsker S, Schmidek H, Frymoyer J, Kahn A (eds): The Unstable Spine, pp 1–16. Orlando, FL, Grune & Stratton, 1986

62. Gelb M: An Introduction to the Alexander Technique: Body Learning. New York, Henry Holt and Co, 1981

63. Gertzbein SD, Seligman J, Holtby R, et al: Centrode patterns and segmental instability in degenerative disc disease. Spine 10:257–261, 1985

64. Gifford J, Gifford L: Connective tissue massage. In Wells PE, Frampton V, Bowsher D: Pain Management in Physical Therapy, pp 218–238. Norwalk, CT, Appleton & Lange, 1988

65. Goodridge JP: Muscle energy technique: Definition, explanation, methods of procedure. J Am Osteopath Assoc 81:249–254, 1981

66. Graff-Radford SB, Reeves JL, Baker RL, et al: Effects of transcutaneous electrical nerve stimulation on myofascial pain and trigger point sensitivity. Pain 37:1–5, 1989

67. Grant ER: Lumbar sagittal mobility in hypermobile individuals and professional dancers. In Grieve GP (ed): Modern Manual Therapy of the Vertebral Column, pp 405–415. Edinburgh, Churchill Livingstone, 1986

68. Gratz CM: Biomechanical studies of fibrous tissues applied to facial surgery. Arch Surg 34:461–495, 1937

69. Greenman PE: Principles of muscle energy techniques. In Greenman PE: Principles of Manual Medicine, pp 88–93. Baltimore, Williams & Wilkins, 1989

70. Greenman PE: Principles of myofascial release technique. In Greenman PE: Principles of Manual Medicine, pp 106–112. Baltimore, Williams & Wilkins, 1989

71. Greenman PE: Osteopathic manipulation of the lumbar spine and pelvis. In White AH, Anderson R (eds): Conservative Care of Low Back Pain, pp. 200–215. Baltimore, Williams & Wilkins, 1991

72. Grieve G: Lumbar instability. Physiotherapy 68:2–9, 1982

73. Grieve G: Lumbar instability. In Grieve G (ed): Modern Manual Therapy of the Vertebral Column, pp 416–441. Edinburgh, Churchill Livingstone, 1986

74. Grieve GP: Mobilisation of the Spine: Notes on Examination, Assessment and Clinical Method, 5th ed. Edinburgh, Churchill Livingstone, 1991

75. Grodin AJ, Cantu RI: Soft tissue mobilization. In Basmajian JV, Nyberg R (eds): Rational Manual Therapies, pp 199–242. Baltimore, Williams & Wilkins, 1993.

76. Grosshandler S, Burney R: The myofascial syndrome. NC Med J 40:562–565, 1979

77. Gunn CC, Ditchburn FG, King MH, et al: Acupuncture loci: A proposal for their classification according to known neural structures. Am J Chin Med 4:183–195, 1976

78. Gustavsen R: Fra Aktiv Avspenning til trening. Oslo, Norlis, 1977

79. Gustavsen R, Streeck R: Training Therapy: Prophylaxis and Rehabilitation. New York, Thieme Medical, 1993

80. Halkovich LR, Personius WJ, Claman HP, et al: Effect of Fluori-Methane spray on passive hip flexion. Phys Ther 61:185–188, 1981

81. Harris JD: History and development of manipulation and mobilization. In Basmajian JV, Nyberg R (eds): Rational Manual Therapies, pp 7–20. Baltimore, Williams & Wilkins, 1993

82. Hey LR, Helewa A: The effects of stretch and spray on women with myofascial pain syndrome: A pilot study [abstract]. Physiother Can 44:4, 1992

83. Hey LR, Helewa A: Myofascial pain syndrome: A critical review of the literature. Physiother Can 46:28–36, 1994

84. Hollinshead WH: Functional Anatomy of the Limbs and Back. Philadelphia, WB Saunders, 1976

85. Holten O: Medical Training Therapy. Continuing education course. Salt Lake City, Holten Institutt for Medisinsk Treningsterapi, 1984

86. Holten O: Norwegian medical exercise therapy. In: Proceedings 5th International Conference of the International Federation of Orthopaedic Manipulative Therapists, pp 58–61. Vail, CO, 1992

87. Hood W: On so-called bone-setting: Its nature and results. Lancet 7:344–349, 1871

88. Hoover HW: Functional technique. Yearbook of the Academy of Applied Osteopathy, 47–51, 1958

89. Ito M, Tadano S, Kaneda K: A biomechanical definition of spinal segmental instability taking personal and disc level differences into account. Spine 18:2295–2304, 1993

90. Jacobson E: Progressive Relaxation, 4th ed. Chicago, University of Chicago Press, 1962

91. Jaeger B, Reeves JL: Quantification of changes in myofascial trigger point sensitivity with the pressure algometer following passive stretch. Pain 27:203–210, 1986

92. Janda V: Die Bedeutung der musklaren Fehlhatung als pathogenetisher Faktor vertebragener Storungen. Arch Phys Ther 20:113–116, 1968

93. Janda V: Muscles, central nervous motor regulation and back problems. In Korr I (ed): The Neurobiologic Mechanisms in Manipulative Therapy, pp 27–41. New York, Plenum Press, 1978

94. Janda V: Muscles as a pathogenic factor in back pain. In: The Treatment of Patients. Proceedings, 4th International Conference of the International Federation of Orthopaedic Manipulative Therapists, pp 1–23. Christchurch, New Zealand, 1980

95. Janda V: Muscle Function Testing. London, Butterworth, 1983

96. Janda V: Muscles and cervicogenic pain syndromes. In Grant R (ed): Physical Therapy of the Cervical and Thoracic Spine, pp 153–166. New York, Churchill Livingstone, 1988
97. Johnson G: Soft tissue mobilizations. In Donatelli R, Wooden MJ (eds): Orthopaedic Physical Therapy, 2nd ed. New York, Churchill Livingstone, 1993
98. Johnston WL: Functional technique. In Basmajian JV, Nyberg R (eds): Rational Manual Therapies, pp 335–346. Baltimore, Williams & Wilkins, 1993
99. Jones F: Body awareness. New York, Schocken Books, 1979
100. Jones LH: Spontaneous release by positioning. Doctor Osteopathy 4:109, 1964
101. Jones LH: Strain and Counterstrain. Colorado Springs, CO, American Academy of Osteopathy, 1981
102. Jowett RL, Fidler MW: Histochemical changes in the multifidus in mechanical derangements of the spine. Orth Clin North Am 6:145–161, 1975
103. Jull GA, Janda V: Muscles and motor control in low back pain. In Twomey LT, Taylor JR (eds): Physical Therapy of the Low Back, pp 253–278. New York, Churchill Livingstone, 1987
104. Kaltenborn FM: Extremity Mobilizations. Vail, CO, Institute of Graduate Health Sciences, 1975
105. Kaltenborn FM: Manual Therapy for the Extremity Joints, 3rd ed. Oslo, Olaf Norlis Bokhandel, 1980
106. Kaltenborn FM: The Spine: Basic Evaluation and Mobilization Techniques, 2nd ed. Oslo, Olaf Norlis Bokhandel, 1993
107. Kaltenborn FM, Evejenth O: Manual Mobilization of the Extremity Joints. Vol II: Advanced Treatment Techniques. Oslo, Olaf Norlis Bokhandel, 1986
108. Kendall FP, McCreary EK, Provance PG: Muscles: Testing and Function, 4th ed. Baltimore, Williams & Wilkins, 1993
109. Kenna C, Murtagh J: Back Pain and Spinal Manipulation. Sydney, Butterworth, 1989
110. Kenneally M, Rubenach H, Elvey R: The upper limb tension test: The SLR test of the arm. In Grant R (ed): Physical Therapy of the Cervical and Thoracic Spine, pp 167–197. New York, Churchill Livingstone, 1988
111. Kennedy B: An Australian programme for management of back problems. Physiotherapy 66:108–111, 1980
112. Kirkaldy-Willis WH: Presidential symposium on instability of the lumbar spine: Introduction. Spine 10:25, 1985
113. Kirkaldy-Willis WH, Burton CV: Managing Low Back Pain, 3rd ed. New York, Churchill Livingstone, 1993
114. Kirkaldy-Willis WH, Farfan WH: Instability of the lumbar spine. Clin Orthop 165:110–123, 1982
115. Kisler CD, Taslitz N: Connective tissue massage: influence of the introductory treatment on autonomic functions. Phys Ther 48:107–119, 1968
116. Kisner C, Colby LA: Therapeutic Exercise: Foundations and Techniques, 2nd ed. Philadelphia, FA Davis, 1990
117. Klein-Vogelbach S: Therapeutic Exercises in Functional Kinetics. Analysis and Instruction of Individually Adaptive Exercises. Berlin, Springer-Verlag, 1991
118. Knott M, Voss DE: Proprioceptive Neuromuscular Facilitation: Patterns and Techniques. New York, Hoeber-Harper Books, 1956
119. Knott M, Voss D: Proprioceptive Neuromuscular Facilitation, 2nd ed. New York, Harper and Row, 1968
120. Korr IM: Proprioceptors and somatic dysfunction. J Am Osteopath Assoc 74:638–650, 1975
121. Korr IM: The facilitated segment: A factor in injury to the body framework. In The Collected Papers of Irvin M Korr. Newark, OH, American Academy of Osteopathy, 1979
122. Korr IM: The neural basis of the osteopathic lesion. In: The Collected Papers of Irvin M Korr. Newark, OH, American Academy of Osteopathy, 1979
123. Kottke F, Pauley D, Ptak R: The rationale for prolonged stretching for correction of shortening of connective tissue. Arch Phys Med Rehab 47:345–352, 1966
124. Kucera M: Exercise on the Gymball. Stuttgart, Gustav Fischer Verlag, 1993
125. Kusunose RS: Strain and counterstrain. In Basmajian JV, Nyberg R (eds): Rational Manual Therapies, pp. 323–333. Baltimore, Williams & Wilkins, 1993
126. LaFreniere JG: LaFreniere Body Techniques: A Therapeutic Approach by Physical Therapy. Chicago, Year Book Medical Publishers, 1984
127. Lamb DW: A review of manual therapy for spinal pain with reference to the lumbar spine. In Grieve GP (ed): Modern Manual Therapy of the Vertebral Column, pp 605–621. Edinburgh, Churchill Livingstone, 1986
128. Lee D: Principles and practice of muscle energy and functional techniques. In Grieve (ed): Modern Manual Therapy of the Vertebral Column, pp 640–655. Edinburgh, Churchill Livingstone, 1986
129. Lester MN: Spinal stabilization and compliance utilizing the therapeutic ball. In: Proceedings, 5th International Conference of the International Federation of Orthopaedic Manipulative Therapists, p 159. Vail, CO, 1992
130. Lewit K: Manuelle Therapie (im Rahmen der artlichen Rehabilitation). Leipzig, JA Barth, 1973
131. Lewit K: Manipulative Therapy in Rehabilitation of the Locomotor System, 2nd ed. Oxford, Butterworth-Heinemann Ltd, 1991
132. Lewit K, Simons DG: Myofascial pain: Relief by post-isometric relaxation. Arch Phys Med Rehabil 64:452–456, 1984
133. Liston CB: Back schools and ergonomics. In Twomey LT, Taylor JR (eds): Physical Therapy of the Low Back, pp 279–301. New York, Churchill Livingstone, 1987
134. Low J: The modern body therapies: A first hand look at leading bodywork therapies, part four. Aston Patterning. Massage Magazine 16:48–56, 1988
135. Luthe W (ed): Autogenic Therapy, Vols 1–6. New York, Grune & Stratton, 1969–1972
136. Maharishi MY: The Science of Being and Art of Living. London, International SRM Publications, 1966
137. Maigne R: Orthopedic Medicine. Springfield, IL, Charles C Thomas, 1972
138. Maitland GD: Vertebral Manipulations, 5th ed. London, Butterworth, 1986
139. Maitland GD: Peripheral Manipulations, 3rd ed. London, Butterworth-Heinemann, 1991
140. Manheim CJ, Lavett DK: The Myofascial Release Manual. Thorofare, NJ, Slack, 1989
141. Marlin T: Manipulative Treatment for the General Practitioner. London, Edward Arnold & Co, 1934
142. Masters R, Houston J: Listening to the Body: The Psychophysical Way to Health and Awareness. New York, Delta Books, 1978
143. May P: Exercise and training for spinal patients: Movement awareness and stabilization training. In Basmajian JV, Nyberg R (eds): Rational Manual Therapies, pp 347–359. Baltimore, Williams & Wilkins, 1993
144. Mayer TG, Gatchel RJ: Functional Restoration for Spinal Disorders: The Sports Medicine Approach. Philadelphia, Lea & Febiger, 1988
145. McCain GA: Role of physical fitness training in fibrositis/fibromyalgia syndrome. Am J Med 81(Suppl 3A):73–77, 1986
146. McKenzie RA: The Lumbar Spine. Waikanae, New Zealand, Spinal Publications, 1980
147. McKenzie RA: Treat Your Own Back. Waikanae, New Zealand, Spinal Publications, 1981
148. McKenzie RA: Care of the Neck. Waikanae, New Zealand, Spinal Publications, 1983
149. McKenzie RA: Mechanical diagnosis and theory for low back Pain: Toward a better understanding. In Twomey LT, Taylor JR (eds): Physical Therapy of the Low Back, pp 157–174. New York, Churchill Livingstone, 1987
150. McKenzie RA: The Cervical and Thoracic Spine: Mechanical Diagnosis and Therapy. Waikanae, New Zealand, Spinal Publications, 1990
151. Melzack R: Prolonged relief of pain by brief intense transcutaneous somatic stimulation. Pain 1:357–373, 1975
152. Melzack R, Stillwell DM, Fox EJ: Trigger points and acupuncture points for pain: Correlations and implications. Pain 3:3–23, 1977
153. Melzack R, Wall PD: Pain mechanisms: A new theory. Science 150:971–979, 1965
154. Mennell JB: Physical Treatment by Movement, Manipulation and Massage, 5th ed. Philadelphia, The Blakiston Co, 1947
155. Mennell JB: The Science and Art of Joint Manipulation. London, J & A Churchill, 1949
156. Mennell J McM: Joint Pain. Boston, Little, Brown & Co, 1964
157. Milanowska K: Conservative treatment. In Weistein JN, Wiesel SW (eds): The Lumbar Spine, pp 500–515. Philadelphia, WB Saunders, 1990
158. Miller B: Alternative somatic therapies. In White A, Anderson R (eds): Conservative Care of Low Back Pain, pp 120–133. Baltimore, Williams & Wilkins, 1991
159. Million R, Nilson KH, Jayson MV, et al: Evaluation of low back pain and assessment of lumbar corsets with and without back supports. Ann Rheum Dis 40:449–454, 1981
160. Mitchell FL Jr: Elements of muscle energy technique. In Basmajian JV, Nyberg R (eds): Rational Manual Therapies, pp 285–321. Baltimore, Williams & Wilkins, 1993
161. Mitchell FL Jr, Moran PS, Pruzzo NA: An evaluation and treatment manual of osteopathic muscle energy procedures. Valley Park, MO, Mitchell, Moran, and Pruzzo, 1979
162. Mixter WJ, Barr JS: Rupture of the intervertebral disc with involvement of the spinal canal. N Engl J Med 211:210–215, 1934
163. Moller M, Oberg B, Gilquist J: Stretching exercise and soccer: Effect of stretching on range of motion in the lower extremity in connection with soccer training. Intern J Sports Med 6:50–52, 1985
164. Morgan D: Concepts in functional training and postural stabilization for the low-back-injured. Top Acute Care Trauma Rehabil 2(4):8–17, 1988
165. Mottice M, Goldberg D, Benner EK, et al: Soft Tissue Mobilization Techniques. Monroe Falls, OH, JEMD Publications, 1986
166. Muhlemann D, Cimino JA: Therapeutic muscle stretching. In Hammer WI (ed): Functional Soft Tissue Examination and Treatment by Manual Methods. Gaithersburg, MD, Aspen Publishers, 1991
167. Nachemson A: Lumbar spine instability: A critical update and symposium summary. Spine 10:290–291, 1985
168. Nicholson GG, Clendaniel RA: Manual techniques. In Scully RM, Barnes MR (eds): Physical Therapy, pp 926–985. Philadelphia, JB Lippincott, 1989
169. Nutter P: Aerobic exercise in the treatment and prevention of low back pain. Occup Med 3:137–145, 1988
170. Nwuga VC: Techniques of spinal manipulation. In Nwuga VC (ed): Manipulation of the Spine, pp 47–81. Baltimore, Williams & Wilkins, 1976
171. Nyberg R: Clinical decision making in orthopaedic physical therapy: The low back. In Wolf SL (ed): Clinical Decision Making in Physical Therapy, pp 255–293. Philadelphia, FA Davis, 1985
172. Nyberg R: Manipulation: Definition, types, application. In Basmajian JV, Nyberg R (eds): Rational Manual Therapies. Baltimore, Williams & Wilkins, 1993
173. Pace JB: Commonly overlooked pain syndromes responsive to simple therapy. Postgrad Med 58:107–113, 1975
174. Palastanga N: Connective tissue massage. In Grieve G (ed): Modern Manual Therapy of the Vertebral Column, pp 827–833. Edinburgh, Churchill Livingstone, 1986
175. Pardy W: Exercise and training for spinal patients: Strength training. In Basmajian JV, Nyberg R (eds): Rational Manual Therapies, pp 387–425. Baltimore, Williams & Wilkins, 1993
176. Paris S: The Spinal Lesion. Christchurch, New Zealand, Pegasus Press, 1965
177. Paris S: Mobilization of the spine. Phys Ther 59:988–995, 1979
178. Paris S: Physical signs of instability. Spine 10:277–279, 1985
179. Patterson MM: A model mechanism for spinal segmental facilitation. J Am Osteopath Assoc 76:121–131, 1976
180. Pettman E: Hypermobility/instability. In: Proceedings, Fifth International Conference of the International Federation of Orthopaedic Manipulative Therapists, pp 40–41. Vail, CO, 1992
181. Pickering SG: Exercises for the Autonomic Nervous System. Springfield, Charles C Thomas, 1981
182. Polermo F, Panjabi MM: Role of trunk rotation endurance exercise in failed back treatment. Arch Phys Med Rehab 67:620, 1986
183. Pope M, Punjabi M: Biomechanical definitions of spinal instability. Spine 10:255–256, 1985
184. Porter-Hoke A: Lumbar instability: Manual therapy evaluation and management. Continuing education course. Seattle, WA, 1993
185. Robins V: Should patients with hemiplegia wear a sling? J Phys Ther 49:1029, 1970
186. Robinson R: The new back school prescription: Stabilization training, Part I. Spine: State of the Art Reviews 5(3):341–355, 1991
187. Rocabado M, Iglarsh ZN: Physical modalities and manual techniques used in the treatment of maxillofacial pain. In Rocabado M, Iglarsh ZN (eds): Musculoskeletal Approach to Maxillofacial Pain, pp 174–193. Philadelphia, JB Lippincott, 1991
188. Rohde J: Die Automobilisation der Extremitatengelenke(I). Zeitschrift fur Physiotherapie 27:57, 1975
189. Rohde J: Die Automobilisation der Extremitatengelenke (II). Zeitschrift fur Physiotherapie 28:51, 1976
190. Rohde J: Die Automobilisation der Extremitatengelenke (III). Zeitschrift fur Physiotherapie 28:121, 1976
191. Rohde J: Die Automobilisation der Extremitatengelenke (IV). Zietschrift fur Physiotherapie 28:427, 1976

192. Rolf I: Rolfing: The Integration of Human Structures. Santa Monica, CA, Dennis-Landman Publishers, 1977

193. Rosomoff HL, Fishbain DA, Goldberg M, et al: Physical findings in patients with chronic intractable benign pain of the neck and/or back. Pain 37:279–287, 1989

194. Rubin D: Myofascial trigger point syndromes: An approach to management. Arch Phys Med Rehabil 62:107–110, 1981

195. Rumsey J: Guidelines for acupuncture massage—Neck pain. Sports Medicine Section, Bulletin of the APTA 4:8–9, 1977

196. Saal JA: Rehabilitation of sports-related lumbar spine injuries. Phys Med Rehabil: State of the Art Reviews 1:613–638, 1987

197. Saal JA: Dynamic muscular stabilization in the nonoperative treatment of lumbar pain syndromes. Orthop Rev 19:691–700, 1990

198. Saal JA: The new back school prescription: Stabilization training, Part II. Spine: State of the Art Reviews 5(3):357–366, 1991

199. Saal JA, Saal JS: Nonoperative treatment of herniated lumbar intervertebral disk with radiculopathy: An outcome study. Spine 14:431–437, 1989

200. Saal JS: Flexibility training. In Saal JS (ed): Rehabilitation of Sports Injuries. Philadelphia, Hanley & Belfus, 1987

201. Saal JS, Saal JA: Strength training and flexibility. In White AH, Anderson R (eds): Conservative Care of Low Back Pain, pp 65–77. Baltimore, Williams & Wilkins, 1991

202. Sahrmann S: A program for correction of muscular imbalance and mechanical imbalance. Clinical Management in PT 3:21–28, 1983

203. Sahrmann S: Diagnosis and treatment of muscle imbalances and associated regional pain. Continuing education course. Seattle, WA, 1993

204. Saliba VL, Johnson GS: Lumbar protective mechanisms. In White AH, Anderson R (eds): Conservative Care of Low Back Pain. Baltimore, Williams & Wilkins, 1991

205. Saliba VL, Johnson GS, Wardlaw CF: Proprioceptive Neuromuscular facilitation. In Basmajian JV, Nyberg R (eds): Rational Manual Therapies, pp 243–284. Baltimore, Williams & Wilkins, 1993

206. Saunders DH: Spinal orthotics. In Saunders DH (ed): Evaluation, Treatment and Prevention of Musculoskeletal Disorders, pp 285–296. Minneapolis, Viking Press, 1985

207. Scariati PD: Myofascial release concepts. In DiGiovanna EL, Schiowitz S (Eds): An Osteopathic Approach to Diagnosis and Treatment, pp 363–368. Philadelphia, JP Lippincott, 1991

208. Schneider W, Dvorak J, Dvorak V, et al: Manual Medicine Therapy. New York, Thieme Medical Pub, 1988

209. Schultz JH, Luthe W: Autogenic Training: A Psychophysiologic Approach in Psychotherapy. New York, Grune & Stratton, 1959

210. Schwartz RG, Gall NG, Grant AE: Abdominal pain in quadriparesis: Myofascial syndrome as unsuspected cause. Arch Phys Med Rehabil, 65:44–46, 1984

211. Scudds RA, Ewart NK, Trachsel L: The treatment of myofascial trigger points with Helim-Neon and Gallium-Arsenide LASER: A blinded, crossover trial (abstract). Pain Suppl 5:768, 1990

212. Sherrington C: The Integrative Action of the Nervous System. New Haven, Yale University Press, 1961

213. Sihvonen T, Hanninen G, Kankkunin P, et al: The relief of static work loading to shoulder musculature (abstract). Scand J Rheum (Suppl) 60:51, 1986

214. Simons DG: Fibrositis/fibromyalgia: A form of myofascial trigger points? Am J Med 81:93–98, 1986

215. Skootsky SA, Jaeger B, Oye RK: Prevalence of myofascial pain in general internal medicine practice. Western J Med 151:157–160, 1989

216. Smith RL: At Your Own Risk: The Case Against Chiropractics. New York, Trident Press, 1969

217. Snow CJ, Aves Wood R, Dowhopoluk V, et al: Randomized controlled clinical trial of stretch and spray for relief of back and neck myofascial pain (abstract). Physiother Can 44:8, 1992

218. Snyder-Mackler L, Barry AJ, Perkins AL, et al: Effects of helium-neon laser irradiation on skin resistance and pain in patients with trigger points in the neck or back. Phys Ther 69:336–341, 1989

219. Snyder-Mackler L, Bork C, Bourbon B, et al: Effect of helium-neon laser on musculoskeletal trigger points. Phys Ther 66:1087–1090, 1986

220. Stoddard A: Manual of Osteopathic Technique. London, Hutchinson, 1978

221. Sweeney T: Neck school: Cervicothoricic stabilization training. Occup Med: State of the Art Review 7:43–54, 1992

222. Sweigard L: Human Movement Potential: Its Ideokinetic Facilitation. New York, Harper and Row, 1974

223. Tabery JC, Tabery C, Tardieu C, et al: physiologic and structural changes in the cat's soleus muscle due to immobilization at different lengths in plaster casts. Am J Physiol 224:231–244, 1972

224. Tabery JC, Tardieu C: Experimental rapid sarcomere loss with concomitant hypoextensibility. Muscle Nerve May/June:198–203, 1981

225. Tappan FM: The bindegewebsmassage system. In Tappan FM: Healing Massage Techniques, 2nd ed. Norwalk, CT, Appleton Lange, 1988

226. Tilscher H: Die Rehabilitation von Wirbelsaulengestorten. Schriftenreihe Manuelle Medizin. Heidlberg, Verlag fur Medizin, 1975

227. Todd ME: The Thinking Body. New York, Dance Horizons, 1937

228. Travell J: Myofascial trigger points: Clinical view. In Bonica JJ, Albe-Fessard A (eds): Advances in Pain Research and Therapy, vol 1, pp 919–926. New York, Raven Press, 1976

229. Travell J: Identification of myofascial trigger point syndromes: A case of atypical facial neuralgia. Arch Phys Med Rehabil 62:100–106, 1981

230. Travell J, Rinzler SH: Myofascial genesis of pain. Post Grad Med 11:425–434, 1952

231. Travell JG, Simons DG: Myofascial Pain and Dysfunction: The Trigger Point Manual, vol 1. Baltimore, Williams & Wilkins, 1983

232. Travell JG, Simons DG: Myofascial Pain and Dysfunction: The Trigger Point Manual, vol 2. Baltimore, Williams & Wilkins, 1992

233. Tucker WE: Home Treatment and Posture. London, E & S Livingstone, 1969

234. Walker JM: Deep transverse friction in ligamentous healing. J Orthop Sports Phys Ther 6:89–94, 1984

235. Wallace RK: Physiological effects of transcendental meditation. Science 167:1751–1754, 1970

236. Warwick R, Williams PL (eds): Gray's Anatomy, 35th Br ed. Philadelphia, WB Saunders Co, 1973

237. Waylonis GW, Wilke S, O'Toole D, et al: Chronic myofascial pain: Management by low-output helium-neon laser therapy. Arch Phys Med Rehabil 69:1017–1020, 1988

238. Webster, GV: Concerning Osteopathy. Norwood, MA, Plimpton Press, 1921

239. Wells PE: Manipulative procedures. In Wells PE, Frampton V, Bower D (eds): Pain Management in Physical Therapy, pp 181–217. Norwald, CO, Appleton & Lange, 1988

240. White AA, Punjabi MM: Clinical Biomechanics of the Spine, pp 106–115. Philadelphia, JB Lippincott, 1990

241. White AH: Back School and Other Conservative Approaches to Low Back Pain. St Louis, CV Mosby, 1983

242. White AH: Back school: State of the art. In Weinstein JN, Wiesel SW (eds): The Lumbar Spine. Philadelphia, WB Saunders Co, 1990

243. White AH: Stabilization of the lumbar spine. In White AH, Anderson R (eds): Conservative Care of the Low Back. pp 106–111. Baltimore, Williams & Wilkins, 1991

244. White AH (ed): Back school. Spine: State of the Art Reviews, 5(3):325–506, 1991

245. Willner S: Effect of a rigid brace on back pain. Acta Orthop Scand 56:40–42, 1985

246. Wolf LB: Exercise and training for spinal patients: Aerobic exercise. In Basmajian JV, Nyberg R (eds): Rational Manual Therapies, pp 425–440. Baltimore, Williams & Wilkins, 1993

247. Wolfe F: Fibrositis, fibromyalgia and musculoskeletal disease: The current status of the fibrositis syndrome. Arch Phys Med Rehabil 69:527–531, 1988

248. Woo S, Matthews JV, Akeson WH, et al: Connective tissue response to immobility. Arthritis Rheum 18:257–264, 1975

249. Wood EC, Becker PD: Beard's Massage, 3rd ed. Philadelphia, WB Saunders, 1981

250. Yunus MB, Kalyan-Raman UP, Kalyan-Raman K: Primary—fibromyalgia syndrome and myofascial pain syndrome: Clinical features and muscle pathology. Arch Phys Med Rehabil 69:451–454, 1988

251. Zbojan L: Antigravitáčna relaxacia, jej podstata a použtie. (Gravity induced relaxation, its principles and practical application). Praktický Lekař 68:147, 1988

252. Zohn DA, Mennell J McM: Musculoskeletal pain conditions. In Zohn DA, Mennell JM (eds): Musculoskeletal Pain: Diagnosis and Physical Treatment, pp 171–198. Boston, Little, Brown and Co, 1976

Friction Massage

RANDOLPH M. KESSLER AND DARLENE HERTLING

- **Principles of Deep Transverse Friction Massage**

- **Clinical Application**
  Indications
  Techniques

Massage, as is true of most forms of manual therapy, is a method of treatment that has been viewed with considerable controversy by the medical community. The "laying on of hands" of any sort tends to be associated with charlatanism. Its value, if any, is frequently felt to be of a psychological nature or the result of the placebo phenomenon. This attitude is not necessarily unfounded, for several reasons. First, those who have advocated the use of massage have often done so on the basis of nonscientific or nonphysiologic mechanisms that the medically oriented professional cannot always accept. Reflex zones, trigger points, fibrositic nodules, and meridians have all been identified as areas to which massage may be directed but have never been identified as true anatomic or physiologic entities. Secondly, there is little empiric or direct scientific evidence for the efficacy of massage. It tends to be used on the basis that it "seems to work"; it makes the patient feel better. So, while there is little question among clinicians who employ massage as a therapeutic measure that it has some value, its value is not well documented. This is primarily because massage is often used for the relief of painful conditions in which there are few associated pathologic signs. This makes reliable measurement of the possible effects of treatment a difficult problem in research design and technology. Finally, the use of massage by lay practitioners, especially in situations of questionable moral

standards, has contributed to the adverse connotations often associated with its use.

The result of the prevailing attitudes toward massage is that it is often not used in the treatment of some conditions for which it might have a significant therapeutic effect. Furthermore, massage is time-consuming, occasionally strenuous, often boring, and relatively costly. Therefore, the clinician as well as the patient may at times avoid it. On the other hand, massage is often employed in circumstances in which it is unnecessary or its therapeutic effect is questionable.

In order to avoid the inappropriate use of any treatment, the clinician should consider not only the objectives but how these objectives fit into the overall plan of management. Although for many conditions seen clinically our primary goal is long-term relief of pain, we cannot necessarily justify the use of massage solely on the basis that it helps relieve pain. Whereas massage may certainly provide *temporary* pain relief in many conditions, it does not necessarily contribute to the *long-term* relief of pain, which requires resolution of the pathologic state. Massage should not be used unless the clinician can rationalize that its use contributes to resolving the physical pathologic process. Such a rationale should have a well-accepted physiologic basis. Otherwise, not only will massage not help the patient to feel better, but because of its often pleasurable effects, it may actually reinforce the disease

Darlene Hertling and Randolph M. Kessler: MANAGEMENT OF COMMON
MUSCULOSKELETAL DISORDERS: Physical Therapy Principles and Methods, 3rd ed.
© 1996 Lippincott-Raven Publishers.

state. The therapist can better expect that treatment of the pathologic process will relieve pain, rather than that relief of pain will improve the patient's condition.

There are several types of conditions for which a particular form of massage, when appropriately administered, may have a direct or indirect effect on the pathologic state. Deep stroking in the presence of certain edematous conditions may assist in the resolution of fluid accumulations. A variety of massage techniques can be used to reflexively promote muscle relaxation for more effective mobilization of a part. This may certainly be useful when abnormal muscle tension is an important factor in the perpetuation of the pathologic process (see Chapter 8, Relaxation and Related Techniques). Deep frictions and kneading types of massage may assist in restoring mobility between tissue interfaces or may increase extensibility of individual structures. Deep massage also tends to increase circulation to the area treated, which may be desirable in certain cases. These effects are generally well described in traditional massage textbooks, along with descriptions of related massage techniques.[12,15,18]

PRINCIPLES OF DEEP TRANSVERSE FRICTION MASSAGE

A particularly important massage technique in the management of many common musculoskeletal disorders is deep transverse friction massage. Its importance and the rationale and technique of application have not been well described in the traditional literature.

As discussed under pathologic considerations in Chapter 3, Arthrology, many of the chronic musculoskeletal disorders seen clinically are manifestations of the body's response to fatigue stresses. Tissues tend to respond to fatigue stresses by increasing the rate of tissue production. Thus, prolonged abnormal stresses to a tissue will lead to tissue hypertrophy, provided that the nutritional status of the tissue is not compromised and that the stress rate (the rate of tissue breakdown) does not exceed the rate at which the tissue can repair the microdamage. Under continuing stress, if nutrition to the tissue is affected or if the rate of tissue breakdown is excessive, the tissue will gradually atrophy and weaken to the point of eventual failure. Tissues that normally have a low metabolic rate (usually those that are relatively poorly vascularized) are most susceptible to such degeneration. Such tissues include articular cartilage, intra-articular fibrocartilage, tendons, and some ligaments. On the other hand, those tissues with good vascularity and a normally high rate of turnover, such as cancellous bone, muscle, capsular tissue, and some ligaments, are more likely to respond

by undergoing hypertrophy. This results in increased density of the structural elements. Of course, even these structures may not be able to keep up with the rate of tissue breakdown under conditions of great stress or reduced nutrition (*e.g.*, hypovascularity).

Under conditions of mildly increased stress rates, the body has the ability to adapt adequately, and no pathologic state (*i.e.*, pain, inflammation, or dysfunction) results. Such conditions might even include situations of high-magnitude stresses if the high stress levels are induced gradually and the stresses are intermittent enough to allow an interval for adequate repair to take place. A typical example is the individual engaging in vigorous athletic activities who goes through a period of gradual training. The training period allows for adequate maturation of new tissue so that structural elements become oriented in ways that best attenuate energy without yielding. Such energy attenuation requires that there be a sufficient mass of tissue to provide some resistance to deformation, but it also requires that the structure be adequately extensible to minimize the strain on individual structural elements. To increase the ability of a structure to attenuate the energy of work done on it (a force tending to deform the structure), new collagen is produced to increase the tissues' total ability to resist the force. However, this new collagen must be sufficiently mobile to permit some deformation. The less it deforms, the greater the resistance the tissue must offer. The greater the resistance it must offer, the greater will be the internal strain on individual collagen fibers or bony trabeculae. The greater the strain on individual structural elements, the greater the rate of microdamage. As the rate of microdamage increases, so does the likelihood of pain and inflammation. As you can see, a more massive tissue is not necessarily one that will permit normal functioning under increased stress. It must also be deformable, and deformability requires time for the new structural elements (collagen fibers and bony trabeculae) to assume the proper "weave."

The effect of the weave, or orientation, of structural elements in contributing to the extensibility of a structure as a whole can be appreciated by examining a Chinese "finger trap" (Fig. 7-1). You can lengthen and shorten the finger trap without changing the length of any of the individual fibers composing it. Its extensibility is due entirely to the weave of the fibers and interfiber mobility. Thus, you can apply an extending force to the structure without inducing internal strain on any of the individual fibers. If the fibers were not in the proper weave or if they were to stick to one another, the deforming force would be met with greater resistance by the structure and greater internal strain to individual fibers. The body adapts to mildly increased stress rates by laying down collagen precursors which, in response to imposed stresses, polymer-

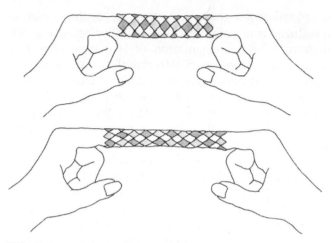

FIG. 7-1. A Chinese finger trap before and after being extended illustrates the extensibility of structural elements.

ize into collagen fibers. The fibers become oriented in the proper weave to allow deformability of the tissue.

Under abnormally high stress levels or altered nutritional conditions, the body's attempt to adapt may be inadequate. The particular structure may not be able to produce new tissue fast enough, or the new tissue that is produced may not have sufficient time or proper inducement to mature. In the former situation, the tissue will degenerate, whereas in the latter, pain and inflammation are likely to result if stresses continue. Tissue degeneration must be treated by reducing stress levels or increasing nutrition to the tissue, depending on the underlying cause. Typical examples of such tissue degeneration include the degradation of articular cartilage in degenerative joint disease and the lesions that commonly affect the soft tissues of the diabetic foot. Articular cartilage, being avascular and having a normally low metabolic turnover, does not adapt well to increased stress levels and is thus susceptible to fatigue degradation. The diabetic foot may have a nutritional deficit because of vascular changes and possibly increased stresses secondary to reduced sensory feedback, leaving it abnormally susceptible to tissue breakdown.

Situations in which the new tissue does not mature adequately are typically those in which the stress levels are not sufficient to cause degeneration but are too excessive to allow time for normal tissue modeling. In bone, the condition is referred to as *sclerosis;* in capsules, ligaments, and tendons, it may be referred to as *fibrosis.* In both situations there is often a normal or increased amount of tissue, but the tissue is not sufficiently deformable to attenuate the energy of loading from use of the part. This can cause pain, inflammation, and increased stresses to adjacent tissues. Correction of such conditions requires that stress levels be reduced while stresses sufficient to stimulate normal tissue modeling are maintained. In addition, normal

extensibility of the structure must be restored. This requires that interfiber mobility be increased. The nutritional status of the tissue must also be considered.

There are many common musculoskeletal disorders that may be related to abnormal or inadequate tissue modeling. Bony sclerosis typically occurs in degenerative joint disease when there are abnormal compressive stresses to a joint. Most tendinitis can be attributed to the tendon having received continuous abnormal stresses, which preclude adequate tissue modeling and create a structure that is not sufficiently deformable. This is especially true of the condition often referred to as *tennis elbow,* in which the origin of the extensor carpi radialis brevis becomes fibrosed, and a chronic inflammatory process arises. Rotator cuff tendinitis, usually involving the supraspinatus or infraspinatus regions of the tendinous cuff, is a very common disorder in which normal modeling is compromised by hypovascularity to the area of involvement. Often these lesions at the shoulder progress to a stage at which gradual degeneration and eventual failure ensue. It is likely that the capsular fibrosis associated with "frozen shoulder" is a similar disorder of tissue modeling; the joint capsule hypertrophies in response to increased stress levels but, in doing so, loses its extensibility. Abnormal tissue modeling will also result when a tissue is immobilized during the repair phase of an inflammatory process. Thus, a fracture may "heal," but normal modeling of bony trabeculae requires resumption of normal stress levels. Similarly, a joint capsule will become fibrosed when the joint is immobilized following arthrotomy; collagen is laid down in response to the traumatic inflammatory process affecting the synovium, but the lack of movement permits an unorganized network of fibers that forms abnormal interfiber bonds (adhesions) that do not extend normally when the part is moved.

Although clinical evidence has substantiated the benefits of friction massage on chronic tendinitis, previous literature discouraged the use of friction massage in chronic bursitis.[4] However, Hammer[7] has found friction massage clinically effective in chronic bursitis of both the hip and shoulder. It appears that the adhesions in chronic bursal problems which are related to pre-existing tendinitis are positively affected by friction massage in the breakdown of bursal scar tissue. An important similarity in both shoulder and hip bursitis is that, in both areas, the initial pathology occurs in the tendons attached to the greater trochanter of the hip and the greater tuberosity of the shoulder.[7] The bursae are believed to be secondarily involved.[1,9,13,14,16]

The approach to treatment of conditions in which continued stresses have not allowed the structure to mature adequately must include measures to reduce stresses to the part. One must consider means of reducing loading of the part as well as means of preventing excessive internal strain. Reduced loading might be accomplished through control of activities, the use of orthotic devices to control alignment or movement, or the use of assistive devices such as crutches. Also, to reduce loading of a particular tissue, the capacity of other tissues to attenuate more of the energy of loading might be increased. This is often done by increasing the strength and activities of related muscles. Thus, if one wishes to reduce the likelihood of excessive loading of the anterior talofibular ligament, the peroneal muscles should be strengthened. However, one can also strap the ankle to provide additional afferent input to reflexively enhance the ability of the peroneals to contract.

Reduction of stress levels alone, however, will not ensure that adequate maturation will take place. As mentioned earlier, stress to the part is a necessary stimulus for the restoration of normal alignment of structural elements. This apparent paradox is understood when one considers that reducing stress is necessary in order to allow new tissue to be laid down and reconstituted, while at the same time some stress is necessary to optimize the nutritional status of the part and to effect proper orientation and mobility of the new tissue. Consequently, in the case of most chronic musculoskeletal disorders, resolution is not likely to take place with either complete rest of the part or unrestricted use. A judgment must be made, then, as to the appropriate activity level for a particular disorder and the rate at which normal activities can be resumed. This judgment must be based on data gained from an examination that reflects the nature and extent of the pathologic process as well as etiological considerations. Knowledge of the healing responses of musculoskeletal tissues and of their responses to various stress conditions must also be applied.

In situations in which significant reduction of activities is necessary in order to allow healing to occur, there are measures that the therapist can, and should, take. The therapist must help prevent undue dysfunction that may result from a mass of tissue being laid down as an unorganized, adherent cicatrix, and from the atrophy of related muscle groups that is likely to take place. There are few conditions, even of an acute inflammatory nature, in which some gentle range of motion and isometric muscle exercises cannot be performed during the healing process without detrimental effects.

Some of the chronic disorders that tend to be the most persistent are minor lesions of tendons and ligaments. These are often refractory to treatments such as rest and anti-inflammation therapy because they are not chronic inflammatory lesions *per se*, but pathologic processes resulting from abnormal modeling of tissue in response to fatigue stresses. Therefore, although rest allows new tissue to be produced, that which is produced is not of normal extensibility because of the lack of a proper orientation of structural elements, abnormal adherence of structural elements to one another, and adherence to adjacent tissues. In some situations, most notably rotator cuff tendinitis, inadequate tissue nutrition is also a factor. Because of the lack of extensibility that accompanies "healing" of these lesions, the structure becomes more susceptible to internal strain when stresses are resumed and less able to attenuate the energy of loads applied to it. The result is recurrence of a low-grade inflammatory process each time use of the part is resumed. The most common of these disorders are supraspinatus tendinitis at the shoulder, tendinitis of the origin of the extensor carpi radialis brevis (tennis elbow), tendinitis of the abductor pollicis longus or extensor pollicis brevis tendons at the wrist (de Quervain's disease), coronary ligament sprain at the knee, and anterior talofibular ligament sprain.

In such chronic, persistent lesions of tendons and ligaments—and occasionally muscle—procedures to promote normal mobility and extensibility of the involved structure are important components of the treatment program. Passive or active exercises that impose a longitudinal strain on the involved structure may be incorporated. However, this creates the risk of maintaining the weakened or unresolved state of healing by contributing to the rate of tissue microdamage. That is probably why these disorders tend not to resolve spontaneously with varying degrees of activity. Too little activity results in loss of extensibility; too much activity does not allow for adequate healing. The appropriate compromise is difficult to judge.

Another method of promoting increased extensibility and mobility of the structure, while reducing stress levels and allowing healing to take place, is the use of deep transverse friction massage.

Friction massage on muscles, ligaments, tendons, and tendon sheaths for the prevention and treatment of inflammatory scar tissue has been used and recommended by numerous authors[2–8,11,17] and was discussed in the 1940s by Mennell (1947).[10] This is a form of treatment advocated primarily by Cyriax, but unfortunately not widely adopted to date. It involves applying a deep massage directly to the site of the lesion in a direction perpendicular to the normal orientation of fibrous elements. This maintains mobility of the structure with respect to adjacent tissues and probably helps to promote increased interfiber mobility of the structure itself without longitudinally stressing it. It may also promote normal orientation of fibers as they are produced. This effect might be likened to the effect of rolling your hand over an unorganized pile of toothpicks; eventually the toothpicks will all become oriented perpendicular to the direction in which the hand moves. In some pathologic processes, such as rotator cuff tendinitis, in which the etiology may be related to a nutritional deficit arising from hypovascularity, the hyperemia induced by the deep friction massage may also contribute to the healing response.

Although highly conjectural, the effects of friction massage are based on sound physiologic and pathologic concepts. Further support is provided by the often dramatically favorable results obtained clinically when friction massage is appropriately incorporated in a treatment program. Studies are needed, however, to substantiate the physiologic effects and the clinical efficacy of friction massage in chronic disorders. Designing a legitimate clinical study would be difficult, because most of the disorders for which friction massage seems to be effective do not present with measurable objective signs, and documentation of subjective improvement is usually unreliable. Basic studies of the effects of friction massage, however, may be fashioned after previous investigations into the effects of exercise, immobility, and other variables on the healing and maturation of collagen tissue. Until there is more concrete evidence of the value of friction massage, its use must be justified on the above considerations combined with "educated empiricism."

CLINICAL APPLICATION

☐ Indications

Friction massage is indicated for chronic conditions of soft tissues—usually tendons, ligaments, or muscles—arising from abnormal modeling of fibrous elements in response to fatigue stresses or accompanying resolution of an acute inflammatory disorder. The intent is to restore or maintain the mobility of the structure with respect to adjacent tissues and to increase the extensibility of the structure under normal loading conditions. The approach is to allow for increased energy-attenuating capacity of the part with reduced strain to individual structural elements. Typical conditions in which friction massage is often indicated include the following:

Tendinitis

Supraspinatus or infraspinatus (shoulder) (tendinitis)
Subscapularis (tendinitis)
Tennis elbow (medial and lateral tendinitis)
Biceps tendon at the bicipital groove (bicipital tendinitis)
de Quervain's (wrist) (tenovaginitis)
Pes anserinus (tendinitis/chronic bursitis)
Patellar tendinitis (knee)
Peroneal tendinitis (ankle or foot)
Achilles tendinitis

Subacute or chronic ligamentous sprains

Acromioclavicular ligament
Intercarpal ligament sprains (wrist)
Coronary ligament sprains (knee)
Minor medial collateral ligament sprains (knee)
Minor anterior talofibular or calcaneocuboid ligament sprains (ankle)

Others

Plica syndrome (knee)
Plantar fascia (foot)

Acute signs and symptoms should be resolved at the time at which friction massage is used (see criteria for acute versus chronic conditions in Chapter 5, Assessment of Musculoskeletal Disorders and Concepts of Management).

☐ Techniques

The part should be well exposed and supported so as to reduce postural muscle tone. The structure to be treated is usually put in a position of neutral tension. It should be positioned so that the site of the lesion is easily accessible to the fingertips. If adherence between a tendon and its sheath is suspected, then the tendon should be kept taut to stabilize it while the sheath is mobilized during the massage.

The therapist should be seated, if possible, with the elbow supported to reduce muscle tension of more proximal parts. The pad of the index finger, middle finger, or thumb is placed directly over the involved site (Figs. 7-2 and 7-3). The remaining fingers should be used to provide further stabilization of the therapist's hand and arm. *No lubricant is used*; the patient's skin must move along with the therapist's fingers.

Beginning with light pressure, the therapist moves the skin over the site of the lesion back and forth, in a direction perpendicular to the normal orientation of the fibers of the involved part. The amplitude of movement is such that tension against the skin at the extremes of each stroke is minimal. This is necessary to avoid friction between the massaging fingers and the skin, which might well produce a blister. Friction may be further avoided by using the thumb and finger of the opposite hand to gather the skin in and somewhat toward the area being massaged. The rate of movement should be about two or three cycles per second and should be rhythmical.

At the beginning of the massage, the patient may feel mild to moderate tenderness. This should not be a deterrent; after 1 or 2 minutes of treatment with light pressure, the tenderness should subside considerably. If it does not, or if tenderness increases, treatment is

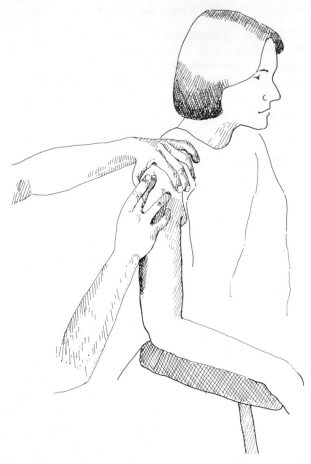

FIG. 7-2. Transverse friction massage to the supraspinatous tendon.

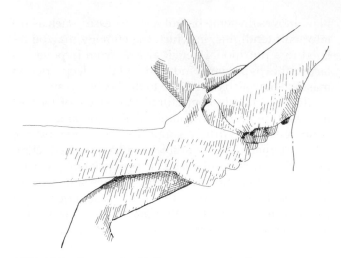

FIG. 7-3. Transverse friction massage to the common extensor tendon at the lateral humeral epicondyle.

stopped. At that point the therapist should consider whether pressure used at the initiation of the massage was excessive. Continuing or increasing tenderness is very rare; more often, the massage has an anesthetic effect. As the tenderness subsides after 1 or 2 minutes, the pressure should be increased somewhat. The patient may feel some tenderness again. After about 2 more minutes, the therapist should again determine if the tenderness has subsided. If it has not, he should discontinue for that session; if it has subsided, he again increases the pressure and massages for about 2 more minutes. During the final 2 minutes of massage, the therapist should feel that the depth of massage is sufficient to affect the involved structure.

During the first treatment, the massage should be stopped after 5 or 6 minutes and the key signs reassessed. If it is a muscular or tendinous lesion, the painful resisted movement is checked; if it is a ligamentous lesion, the painful joint-play movement is retested. The patient should feel some immediate improvement. If he does not, the therapist should consider whether the technique of treatment was appropriate, assuming that the disorder is one for which friction massage is indicated.

With successive treatments, the depth of massage is always gradually increased, as described above, and the length of treatment is gradually increased by about 3 minutes in each session, working up to 12 or 15 minutes each session. However, treatment should not be continued during a particular session nor should the depth of massage be increased if the tenderness to massage increases or does not subside during treatment. Responses will vary, of course, with the patient and with the nature of the disorder. In some cases the duration of treatment must be increased more slowly than in others. There are few conditions that do not resolve after six to ten sessions over 2 or 3 weeks, provided that other components of the treatment program are appropriately carried out and provided that friction massage is indicated.

It is not unusual for a patient to feel some increased "soreness" after the first or second session, but this must be distinguished from exacerbation of symptoms. Some skin or soft-tissue tenderness and soreness are to be expected. This would occur whether the patient did or did not have an underlying problem and should not be misconstrued by the therapist or patient as worsening of the condition, so long as key symptoms and signs related to the patient's condition are no worse.

A common mistake during treatment by friction massage is the development of skin blisters or abrasions. These result either from fingernails that are too long or from poor technique that causes friction between the massaging finger and skin. Another common mistake is for the therapist to apply the massage to the area of pain rather than to the site of the lesion. The two areas do not necessarily coincide.

In addition, the therapist must avoid overstressing the more distal joints of his thumb and fingers when performing the massage. This is especially important if friction massage is being used frequently. Such stresses can be reduced by stabilizing the distal interphalangeal joint of the massaging finger with a free finger, as shown in Figure 7-3, and by alternating fingers during a particular treatment session.

Friction massage should be avoided when the nutritional status of the skin is compromised and in cases of impaired vascular response. These would typically include patients on long-term, high-dose, steroid drug therapy and patients with known peripheral vascular disease.

Specific techniques for friction massage of the supraspinatus tendon and extensor carpi radialis brevis are described below.

SUPRASPINATUS TENDON

Light to deep transverse friction massage is given over the tendon. The patient sits comfortably on a chair, and the arm is put in a neutral or somewhat extended position with the lower arm supported. The therapist sits at the patient's side. A position of neutral or slight humeral extension brings the tendon forward into a position in which the site of the lesion is easily accessible to the fingertips. (see Fig. 7-2). The therapist identifies the site of the supraspinatus tendon lying between the greater tubercle of the humerus and the acromion process. It is essential that the tendon be accurately located by knowledge of anatomy; it cannot be distinguished by palpation. The pad of the therapist's middle finger, reinforced by the index finger (or vice versa), is placed directly over the site of the lesion, which is always just proximal to the tendon insertion on the greater tubercle. The thumb is used to stabilize the arm. The therapist applies friction in a direction perpendicular to the normal orientation of the tendon, using the thumb both as fulcrum and to maintain pressure. The thumb and fingers of the opposite hand support and gather the skin over the shoulder to avoid friction between the massaging finger and skin.

This is the most valuable treatment in the management of supraspinatus tendinitis and is a key component of the treatment program (see Chapter 9, The Shoulder and Shoulder Girdle). A similar technique is used for the other tendons of the rotator cuff.

"TENNIS ELBOW"

Light to deep friction massage is given to the affected fibers of the extensor carpi radialis brevis at the anterior aspect of the lateral humeral epicondyle. The patient sits with the lower arm supported; the elbow is flexed and the forearm is supinated to allow easy access of the massaging finger or thumb. The therapist sits at the side, facing the patient. One hand supports at the elbow. The massaging hand is placed so that the thumb is over the affected fibers (see Fig. 7-3). Counterpressure is applied by the fingers lying against the medial proximal aspect of the forearm. The thumb is drawn across the site of the lesion in a direction perpendicular to the fibers by alternate supination and pronation of the forearm, using the fingers as a fulcrum. The therapist may also use the index or long fingers for massage, as described for friction massage to the supraspinatus tendon.

REFERENCES

1. Booth RE, Marvel JP: Differential diagnosis of shoulder pain. Orthop Clin North Am 6:353–379, 1975
2. Chamberlain GJ: Cyriax's friction massage. A review. J Orthop Sports Phys Ther 4:16–22, 1982
3. Cyriax J: Deep friction. Physiotherapy 63:60–61, 1977
4. Cyriax J, Coldham M: Textbook of Orthopaedic Medicine, Vol 2. Treatment by Manipulation, Massage, and Injections, 11th ed. London, Bailliere Tindall, 1984
5. Gersten JW: Effect of ultrasound on tendon extensibility. Am J Phys Med 34:662, 1955
6. Hammer WI: Friction massage. In Hammer WI: Functional Soft Tissue Examination and Treatment by Manual Methods: The Extremities. Gaithersburg, MD, Aspen Pub, 1991
7. Hammer WI: The use of transverse friction massage in the management of chronic bursitis of the hip and shoulder. J Manipulative Physiol Ther 16:107–111, 1993
8. Hunter SC, Poole RM: The chronically inflamed tendon. Clin Sports Med 6:371–388, 1987
9. Little H: Trochanteric bursitis: A common clinical problem: Orthop Clin North Am 120:456–458, 1979
10. Mennell JB: Physical Treatment by Movement, Manipulation and Massage, 5th ed. Philadelphia, Blakiston, 1947
11. Palastanga N: Connective tissue massage. In Grieve GP (ed): Modern Manual Therapy for the Vertebral Column. New York, Churchill Livingstone, 1986
12. Rogoff JB (ed): Manipulation, Traction and Massage, 2nd ed. Baltimore, Williams & Wilkins, 1980
13. Schapira D, Nahir M, Scharf Y: Trochanteric bursitis: A common clinical problem. Arch Phys Med Rehabil 67:815–817, 1986
14. Swezey RL: Pseudo-radiculopathy in subacute trochanteric bursitis of subgluteus maximus bursa. Arch Phys Med Rehabil 57:387–390, 1976
15. Tappin FM: Healing Massage Techniques: Holistic, Classic, and Emerging Methods, 2nd ed. Norwalk, CT, Appleton & Lange, 1988
16. Uhthoff HK, Sarkar K, Hammond DI: The subacromial bursa: a clincopathological study in surgery of the shoulder. In Bateman JE, Welch RP (eds): Surgery of the Shoulder, pp 121–125. St Louis, CV Mosby, 1984
17. Walker JM: Deep transverse frictions in ligament healing. J Orthop Sports Phys Ther 6:89–94, 1984
18. Wood EC: Beard's Massage: Principles and Techniques, 3rd ed. Philadelphia, WB Saunders, 1981

Relaxation and Related Techniques

DARLENE HERTLING AND DANIEL JONES

Relaxation techniques are being used more than ever before by physical therapists and other health professionals. The concept of relaxation has had a long and varied history. In the early part of this century, Jacobson introduced a form of therapy based on muscular quiescence known as *progressive relaxation*.[59] American interest in the topic of relaxation waned during the 1940s and 1950s. It was not until the introduction of systematic desensitization by Wolpe in 1958, in which progressive relaxation played an important role, that American interest in this topic was once again renewed.[154]

Systematic desensitization is one of the most widely used behavioral therapy techniques to employ relaxation. It is a method used for breaking down neurotic anxiety-response habits in a step-by-step fashion.[155] Relaxation is used as a physiologic anxiety-inhibiting state. The subject is first exposed to a weak anxiety-arousing stimulus, which is repeated until the stimulus progressively loses its ability to evoke anxiety.

Successively stronger stimuli are applied and similarly treated until the habit is overcome, or until the trainee gains some control over it. Relaxation training has since become an integral part of many behavioral procedures; the principles of behavioristic psychology, behavior modification, stress management, and related techniques often employ relaxation training.

Relaxation techniques and related techniques have also found their way into the newly established pain clinics. The prototype, and now probably the largest and best-organized clinic, was begun in 1961 by Bonica and White of the University of Washington Medical School.[101] Other pain clinics have been formed at other hospitals and clinics both here and abroad. Many psychological approaches have been proven to produce some measure of pain relief. According to Sternbach, these include desensitization techniques, hypnotic suggestion techniques, and progressive relaxation.[139]

Interest in relaxation and related techniques has

Darlene Hertling and Randolph M. Kessler: MANAGEMENT OF COMMON MUSCULOSKELETAL DISORDERS: Physical Therapy Principles and Methods, 3rd ed. © 1996 Lippincott-Raven Publishers.

been further augmented by increased self-awareness and by what has been called the "body boom" of the 1960s and 1970s.[79] It has led to increased concern with relaxation, posture, and getting in touch with one's body and thereby one's emotions. Ultimately, it has to do with healing the body and, hopefully, the mind as well. According to Kruger, "The body boom has begot a widely assorted, though in many ways a cohesive family of both medical and nonmedical therapists who do body work—the father of the breed, Reich, the mother, Yoga, and the family estate Esalen, California, which is considered the mecca of the American Human Potential Movement."[79]

Recent research demonstrates that we are more capable of controlling our bodily and psychological processes than was previously believed.[8,60,89,124,128,129,155] The defining mark of the "new body therapies" is their attention to exercise, relaxation, massage, and body and human potential. Theoretical principles include an understanding of the relationship between the body and character structure (first developed by psychoanalyst Wilhelm Reich) and existentialist, physiological, behavioral, and sociological theories. Therapeutic practices include a variety of psychophysiological methods for making use of bodily processes to reduce tension and anxiety. Among them are the following methods:

- The revival of ancient Asian disciplines such as yoga, T'ai Chi, and Zen awareness training, and their Western modifications
- Principles of behavioristic psychology and behavior modification
- Sophisticated instrumentation of Western technology, such as biofeedback
- The neo-Reichian approach of bioenergetics, best known through the work of Lowen.[87,88] Body movements and verbalization are used to release blocked or repressed energy and to reintegrate body and mind.
- The Alexander technique, which changes body alignment by increasing awareness of posture and by the use of suggestion and gentle repositioning of the limbs[1,4]
- The rediscovery of dance therapy. An example is the Feher School of Dance and Relaxation, which works extensively with back problems. It is considered a form of dynamic or active distraction used for relaxation purposes.[79]
- A variety of massage techniques, including massages for different parts of the body to promote relaxation and well-being, and more recently, acupressure massage and acupuncture.[5,33,34,142,152] Chapman of the University of Washington Pain Clinic has experimented with acupuncture. He be-

lieves that one of its effects is to bring about relaxation very quickly, and that it may tend to reduce physiologic stress reactions.[101]
- The revival of the Jacobson relaxation technique, including newer techniques such as the Lamaze technique (associated with natural childbirth), autogenic training (a medical therapy based on sensory awareness devised by J. H. Schultz, a German neurologist), and the relaxation response or Benson's technique (meditation on a single word or color)[6,78,89,124,140]
- Differential relaxation techniques of body parts and systems through respiration exercises, such as Fuchs's functional relaxation and Jencks's respiration exercises for use in daily life activities and coping with stress[66,67]

COMPONENTS OF THE STRESS RESPONSE

Research during the past decade in the management of stress and the application of relaxation and related techniques has received an increasing amount of attention. The existing literature on relaxation and related states is extremely diverse. The foundations on which this body of research rests range from age-old meditative disciplines of Asia to contemporary research on behavior modification, to the newest approach, biofeedback, which is often combined with relaxation techniques.

Components of the stress response identified by theorists include physiologic, psychosomatic, psychological, and sociologic aspects. Selye has spent almost four decades of laboratory research on the physiologic mechanism of adaptation to the stress of life.[128,129] From his studies on overstressed animals, he observed nonspecific changes, which he called the *general adaptation syndrome,* and specific responses that depend on the kind of stressor and on the part of the organism involved. He established a stress index that comprises some major pathologic results of overstress, including enlargement of the adrenal cortex, atrophy of lymphatic tissues, and bleeding ulcers. He has further defined certain pathologic consequences of long-term stress as *diseases of adaptation.* Among these he classified stomach ulcers, cardiovascular disease, high blood pressure, connective tissue disease, and headaches.

Mason, one of the most distinguished investigators of the psychological and psychiatric aspects of biological stress, suggests that emotional stimuli are the most common stressors.[94] They are reflected in the endocrine, autonomic, and musculoskeletal systems (Fig. 8-1). We know that every individual will not

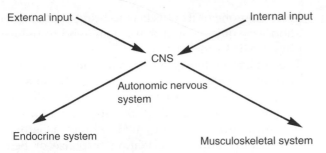

FIG. 8-1. Common stresses.

elicit the same syndrome even with the same degree of stress. Likewise, it is known that the same stressor can cause different lesions in different individuals, which can selectively enhance or inhibit one of the stress effects. Conditioning may be internal (*i.e.,* genetic predisposition, past experience, age, sex) or external (*i.e.,* treatment with certain hormones, drugs, dietary factors). Under the influence of such conditioning factors a normally well-tolerated degree of stress may be pathogenic and may cause diseases of adaptation that selectively affect predisposed areas of the body. Any kind of activity sets our stress mechanism in motion. However, whether the heart, gastrointestinal tract, or musculoskeletal system will suffer most depends largely on accidental conditioning factors. Although all parts of the system are exposed equally to stress, it is the weakest link that breaks down first.

Sternbach has described a scheme for the onset of stress-related disorders and the resultant failure in the homeostatic mechanism to prevent the body from returning to a baseline level of function in many cases.[138] For example, frequent stressors cause an increase in blood pressure. Often, as the result of failure in the homeostatic mechanism, the system readjusts to a new level of increased blood pressure (Fig. 8-2). Similarly, Brown has pointed out that muscle behavior under stress is translated into muscle holding or tension.[13] If stressors are frequent, the following two muscle events occur: (1) muscle tension becomes sustained at higher levels, and (2) the tightness of the muscles causes them to be hyperactive. Under normal conditions, an appropriate adjustment is made by the central muscle control system. Special nerve cells in the muscle tissue sense when a fiber is contracting, how fast it is tensing, and other complex aspects of muscle contraction. The system seems to become inefficient, however, with continued stress or rumination about the stress, since the length of time muscle fibers have been tense does not seem to be relayed to the central muscle control system. As a result, the muscles have little chance to recover from increased tension. Tension becomes sustained at higher levels and may continue to increase. If muscles are not given relief from tension by relaxation or a change of activity, the muscle fibers physiologically "adapt" to states of increased tension.

Hess produced the changes associated with the fight-or-flight response by stimulating a part of the cat's brain within the hypothalamus.[42,55] By stimulating another area within the hypothalamus, he demonstrated a response whose physiologic changes were similar to those measured during the practice of relaxation, that is, a response opposite to the fight-or-flight (ergotropic) response. He described this as a protective mechanism against overstress that belongs to the trophotropic system and promotes a restorative process (Fig. 8-3).

Benson believes the trophotropic response described by Hess in cats is the relaxation response in humans.[7,8] Both of these opposing responses are associated with physiologic changes, and each appears to be controlled by the hypothalamus. Because the fight-or-flight response and the relaxation response are in opposition, one counteracts the effects of the other. This is why Benson and Wallace feel the relaxation response is so important; through its use the harmful effects of inappropriate elicitation of the fight-or-flight response are counteracted. They indicate that most of the relaxation therapies evoke the same physiologic changes as the relaxation response.

■ ROLE OF PHYSICAL THERAPY

One of the common symptoms physical therapists see in many of their patients today is tension pain related to neuromuscular hypertension. Many feel that muscle tension or stress is actually a partial or complete cause of heart attack, cerebrovascular accident, peripheral and neurovascular syndromes, chronic musculoskeletal problems, and the common headache.

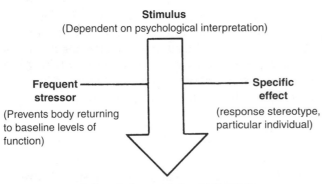

FIG. 8-2. Scheme illustrating onset of stress-related disorders.

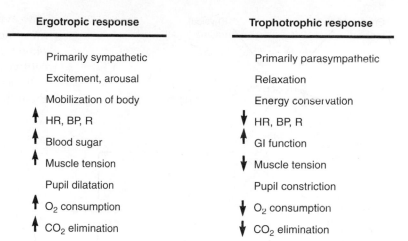

Ergotropic response	Trophotrophic response
Primarily sympathetic	Primarily parasympathetic
Excitement, arousal	Relaxation
Mobilization of body	Energy conservation
↑ HR, BP, R	↓ HR, BP, R
↑ Blood sugar	↑ GI function
↑ Muscle tension	↓ Muscle tension
Pupil dilatation	Pupil constriction
↑ O_2 consumption	↓ O_2 consumption
↑ CO_2 elimination	↓ CO_2 elimination

FIG. 8-3. Effects of the ergotropic and trophotropic responses. *BP,* blood pressure; *HR,* heart rate; *R,* respiration, *GI,* gastrointestinal.

Most physical therapists would agree that a chronic pain patient who is tense will invariably take much longer to treat and need more time to recover. Experience seems to indicate that many musculoskeletal disorders have more severe and more prolonged symptoms when muscular tension is a factor. Since this appears to be true, then certainly one should be aware of tension symptoms in the evaluation process and should develop skills to treat the tension factor in these patients.

Tension may not only prolong a condition but may be the primary factor in the causation of dysfunction. Tension tends not only to aggravate the condition, thus compounding the pathology, but it may actually bring to light what would otherwise have been a subclinical pathologic process. Holmes and Wolff believe that in many instances the primary local cause of backache is minimal, but the muscle tension produced by anxiety and emotional stress causes secondary pain in the back that may outlast and exceed the primary pain.[122] In any event, both the cause of the habitual holding—the tension itself—and the subclinical pathologic process will require treatment.

Relief of Neuromuscular Hypertension

What is neuromuscular hypertension? Certainly we contract muscles isotonically and isometrically all day long, be it small muscle movement of the eyes, or the action of the quadricep, hamstring, and gastrocnemius muscles when running, or some normal activity that requires muscle contraction between the two extremes. This involves normal muscular effort or normal energy expenditure. We also seem to have a remarkable ability to recruit muscular effort when faced with an emergency situation. Humans, however, are creatures of habit and can become accustomed to contracting these muscles subconsciously. This is when problems occur. One gets used to bracing or holding or continuous movement and then carries that muscular effort over into activities that should require a small amount of effort. This is learned behavior. Excess tension may even carry over into periods in which there should be minimal effort, such as lying down or sleeping.

Should some medical condition develop, this tension factor immediately prohibits the natural healing process. According to Jacobson, "Acute conditions may occur after intense or prolonged pain or distress from whatever source, whether physical, as a trauma, angina or colic, or mental, as a fright, bereavement, quarrel or loss."[60] Our society probably perpetuates this holding or contracting habit. The pressures of occupation, family, church, and friends contribute to the overuse of muscle tissue and increased neuromuscular excitability. Whatmore and Kohli describe this as a pathophysiological state made up of errors in energy expenditure.[151] The chronic musculoskeletal problems that therapists are confronted with are seldom found to be associated with only one factor, but with a number of factors. Emotional tension, physical trauma, infection, immobilization, or various combinations may lead to joint dysfunction resulting in a sustaining cycle of pain, muscle guarding, retained metabolites, and restricted motion (Fig. 8-4).

Physical therapy plays an important role in the local relief of tension pain associated with neuromuscular hypertension. Often localized tension may be relieved by heat and massage. Joint mobilization of the involved part is often the most effective treatment for breaking up this sustaining cycle. But physical therapy can also act at a deeper level to relieve underlying muscle holding or tension by teaching the tense individual to relax the body and mind through conscious relaxation during normal daily activities.

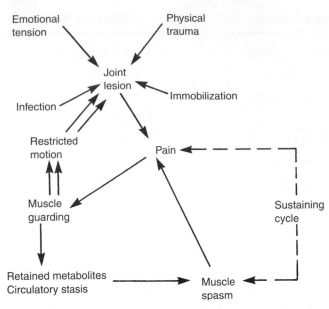

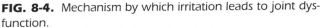

FIG. 8-4. *Mechanism by which irritation leads to joint dysfunction.*

☐ Health Problem Prevention

Another major use of relaxation training is in the prevention of health problems. This use of relaxation training is supported by experimental evidence that stress affects the immune system and can increase the susceptibility to experimental infections or implanted tumors. Animal studies have shown that corticosteroids are released during stress, and these adrenal hormones can suppress immune function by reducing the number of circulating T lymphocytes.[98] Research has also shown that emotional stress can reduce immunocompetence in humans.[76,100,158]

▨ TYPES OF RELAXATION AND RELATED TECHNIQUES

Jacobson's approach has been used in physical therapy almost since its beginning to manage habitual holding. Jacobson's approach to instructing relaxation has been found to be very suitable in our work and certainly is the most well known in the United States. However, a large number and variety of techniques and combinations of techniques are now being used by physical therapists, as well as other medical practitioners. These include Benson's relaxation response, transcendental mediation, and Schultz and Luthe's autogenic training, among others. It is generally felt that individual differences and the diversity of needs require a wide choice of techniques. A review of clinical reports suggests that a judicious mix of techniques may obtain the best results.[13] Of the many techniques

now available to us, most carry similar requirements, most notably the need for practice, a quiet atmosphere, a comfortable position, and a passive and receptive attitude.

Indications are numerous. Jacobson cites some of the following:[60]

- Acute neuromuscular hypertension
- Chronic neuromuscular hypertension
- States of fatigue and exhaustion
- States of debility
- Various preoperative and postoperative conditions
- Sleep disturbances
- Alimentary spasm and peptic ulcers

Some of the most common stress-related conditions treated by physical therapists include

- Tension headaches
- Migraine headaches
- High blood pressure
- Pulmonary disease (asthma and emphysema)[130]
- Muscle guarding
- Spasticity
- Arthritis and related disorders
- Bell's palsy
- Cerebral palsy
- Burns (before treatment with debridement and range-of-motion exercises)
- Various chronic pain conditions associated with muscle tension (*e.g.,* cervical strain, adhesive capsulitis)

Relaxation and related techniques are difficult to categorize, but basically there are two types: the somatic or physical approach and the cognitive or mental approach. Many techniques employ a combination of both approaches. Such a great variety of psychophysiological methods are available to us that only a general survey will be made here, with detail given to some of the more familiar ones. Physical approaches may primarily emphasize passive distraction (*e.g.,* Jacobson's technique, Praskauer massage, and respiratory techniques) or active or dynamic distraction (*e.g.,* Feldenkrais's awareness through movement, T'ai chi, or the Alexander technique). Those that stress the mental or cognitive approach include meditation, sensory awareness techniques, autogenic training, and sentic cycles.

☐ Overview of Psychophysiologic Techniques

The following list of psychophysiologic methods of relaxation and related techniques contains only the more commonly used methods of relaxation and related techniques that are practiced in the United States and Europe today. Many excellent techniques have been omitted.

Active Tonus Regulation (Stokvis, Netherlands)

Ideomotor movements are used to prove the influence of mind over body. Suggestions for relaxation of muscles, respiration, and mind are used to induce an altered state of consciousness.[67]

Alexander Technique (Alexander, England)

Kinesthetics is the key word in the Alexander lexicon. The core of this technique is helping people to become aware of when and where their bodies are tense. Proper alignment of head on spine is used to correct physical misalignments, attitudes, and behavior.[1,4]

Autoanalysis (Bezzola, Switzerland)

This is a simple technique in which the body serves as its own excellent biofeedback instrument through attention to and verbalization of successive internal sensations to induce deep mental and physical relaxation.[67]

Autogenic Training (Schultz, Germany)

Autogenic training is one of the four major relaxation techniques now being used that developed directly from the therapeutic practice of hypnosis for relaxation. The complete program is divided into three categories of exercises: auto-suggestion about relaxation; single-focus meditation (as in yoga); and meditation on abstract qualities. Physical therapists primarily use the first series of exercises, and occasionally the second.[89,124]

Awareness Through Movement (Feldenkrais, Israel)

Sensory awareness involving movements of limbs, breathing, facial expressions, and self-massage is used for balance of tension and postural alignment.[33,34] The late Moshe Feldenkrais (1904–1984) is world renowned for the system of body awareness and exercises he developed over the course of his career.[33–35]

Functional Relaxation (Fuchs, Germany)

Slow, relaxed exhalations and breathing rhythms are used for differential relaxation of the body parts and systems. Gentle hand contact by the therapist and later by the patient is used to detect inhibiting tension. It is considered a medical therapy requiring a therapist's guidance.[67]

Hatha Yoga (India)

Hatha yoga exercises require both physical manipulation and concentration on awareness of body activities. Assumption of certain postures and controlled breathing are used to induce altered states of consciousness.[27,146]

Meditation Techniques

Whether of Hindu, Zen, Buddhist, or other origin, meditation behavior usually entails concentration of attention and awareness on a single idea, object, or point inside or outside the body. Many Western modifications have been developed for their usefulness as antidotes to the stress of ordinary living. Although meditative practices were not originally designed to be relaxation techniques, the experience of relaxation is a by-product of most such techniques.[24,149,152]

Muscular Therapy (Benjamin, U.S.)

This approach to tension relief combines deep massage, tension-release exercises, body-care techniques, and postural re-education. The tension-release exercises make use of the neo-Reichian approach of bioenergetics.[5]

Nyingma System (India)

A system of physical exercises, posture, breathing, and massage forms a basis for sensory awareness and relief of emotional tension. The Nyingma Institute is located in Berkeley, California, and workshops are offered for psychotherapists, physical therapists, and other health professionals.[152]

Passive Movements (Michaux, France)

Passive movement of relaxed body parts, without the active participation of the subject, is used to induce both physical and mental relaxation.[67]

Progressive Relaxation (Jacobson, U.S.)

This is the most widely known of the four major relaxation techniques. Alternate tensing and relaxing of skeletal, respiratory, and facial muscles is used to induce physical and mental relaxation.[59–64]

Proskauer Massage (Proskauer, U.S.)

Also called *breath therapy*, this method couples exhalation and inhalation with an extremely light and delicate massage to different muscle groups, timing the massage with the rhythm of the breathing exercise. Meditation and imagery are used to enhance physical and mental relaxation.[79,152]

Relaxation Response (Benson, U.S.)

From the collected writings of the East (meditation) and the West (autogenic training), Benson has devised a simplified method of eliciting the relaxation response. It consists of two basic categories of exercises: autosuggestion about relaxation and single-focus meditation usually on the mantra "one."[8]

Respiration of Special Accomplishment (Jencks, U.S.)

Self-suggesting technique is coupled with breathing rhythm to enhance relaxation or invigoration, warmth or coolness, for use in daily-life activities and in coping with stress. Jencks's exercises can easily be adapted for use in physical therapy and psychotherapy.[66,67]

Self-Hypnosis (Pierce, U.S.)

Attention is given, with closed eyes, to tensing the skeletal muscles of the body part to a point of fatigue. Attention is then shifted to another body part to bring about automatic complete relaxation. This is followed by a series of eye exercises. Finally, imagery is used as a method of distracting attention to further enhance relaxation.[115,152]

Sensory Awareness Training (Grindler, Germany)

Sensory awareness training originated about 100 years ago in Europe as a training method for performing artists. Several of the teachers later emigrated to the United States. The earliest and perhaps most significant work with sensory awareness training was done by Elsa Grindler (1885–1961).[67] A large number and variety of exercises have evolved, including autogenic training. Most of the therapeutic techniques are used for inducing physical relaxation through sensory awareness of muscle tension and inhibited breathing.

Sentic Cycles (Clynes, U.S.)

This is a behavioral therapy technique composed of eight sentic states or self-induced emotional states. Clynes, a psychophysiologic researcher, has demonstrated the close relationship between emotional states and predictable physiologic change.[18]

Systematic Desensitization (Wolpe, U.S.)

This behavioral therapy technique uses progressive relaxation (following Jacobson) in conjunction with behavioral management techniques. The client develops a series of "scenes" or "visualizations" that are called forth in a hierarchical order based on their fear-evoking ability while attempting to remain relaxed.[154,155]

Transcendental Meditation (T.M.) (Maharishi Mahesh Yogi, U.S.)

This form of meditation has been adapted to Western concepts and philosophical background and most often is used as an adjunct to therapeutic relaxation techniques, including EMG biofeedback.[90,148] Graduates are required to meditate for 20 minutes per day using a mantra that has been assigned to them. Credited courses in T.M. have been given in dozens of colleges and universities in the United States and abroad.

The two major techniques used by physical therapists in the United States are progressive relaxation and autogenic training. Various types of meditation, massage, breathing, and sensory awareness techniques are also employed and are often combined with other techniques. With the exception of self-hypnosis, hypnosis is used primarily by other health professionals in the management of painful conditions of the musculoskeletal system as well as cancer, alcohol and drug abuse, and natural childbirth.

☐ Relaxation and Massage

An invaluable tool in the management of common musculoskeletal disorders is massage. However, since World War II, there seems to have been a general decrease in the use of massage for these conditions, perhaps because massage is time consuming, sometimes strenuous, and demands skill on the part of the person giving the treatment. It is also possible that increased knowledge and sophistication of equipment has made basic massage too simple to use. Another reason is, unfortunately, that the basis for its use has been empirical rather than scientific. However, many therapists, including these authors, believe that experience has shown massage to be an extremely important and beneficial tool. Surely it is not the total answer, but as with heat or cold, exercise, relaxation, mobilization, and electrical stimulation, massage as part of our repertoire helps us treat our patients more effectively.

Our discussion of massage could focus on stroking and effleurage, pétrissage and kneading, friction, percussion, ice, mechanical vibration, or connective tissue massage. It could cover direction (centrifugal *versus* centripetal or proximal *versus* distal), pressure, rate and rhythm, media, positions of patient and clinician, duration, and frequency. However, this basic material and its history can be reviewed in the literature, what little there seems to be. Two of the better sources are *Massage: Principles and Techniques*, by Wood and Becker,[156] and *Healing Massage Techniques: Holistic, Classic, and Emerging Methods*, by Tappin.[142]

As mentioned earlier, much has been written about massage, although little scientific study has been done on the physiologic effects massage has on various body tissues. In one study of injured muscle, animal muscle tissue was subjected to a crushing injury and later examined microscopically. One group of animals was left untreated, while another group received massage. The untreated group showed the following results:

1. Dissociation into fibrillae of muscular fibers as shown by well-marked longitudinal striation
2. Hyperplasia (sometimes simple thickening of the connective tissue)
3. Increase, in places, of the number of nuclei in the connective tissue
4. Interstitial hemorrhages
5. Enlargement of blood vessels, with hyperplasia of their adventitious coats
6. Sarcolemma usually intact, but in one section, a multiplication of nuclei reported, resembling somewhat an interstitial myositis

The treated group, on the other hand, showed the following results:

1. Normal appearance of muscle
2. No secondary fibrous bands separating the muscle fibers

3. No fibrous thickening around the vessels
4. Greater general bulk of the muscle
5. No signs of hemorrhage

It has been concluded from this study and others that massage may lessen the amount of fibrosis that inevitably develops in immobilized, injured, or denervated muscle. Even when there has not been injury, there are innumerable situations that will cause a metabolic imbalance within the soft tissue. Observation, and particularly palpation, will reveal abnormal muscle tissue that is often hard, well defined, stringy, and painful. Massage will benefit this uninjured but abnormal tissue as well.

The discovery of endorphins may soon lead to an explanation of some of the neurophysiological mechanisms involved in the pain relief provided by acupuncture and massage given to specific areas, such as connective tissue.[44] In addition, relaxation instructions and autogenic phrases may be used during massage to assist patients to relax even further.[142]

Sensorimotor stimulation by massage facilitates the development of premature infants and decreases the possibility of emotional disturbance.[114,117,118] The use of deep finger pressure over painful trigger points[116] and the use of acupuncture and acupressure massage have been found to relieve infants' headaches, tummy aches, and other minor problems.

CLINICAL APPLICATION

Massage should usually follow application of heat or cold and should be done in a relaxing rhythm, with media of the therapist's choice. One should have good hand contact, but most importantly, the massage should be deep. That means the therapist must feel for abnormal tissue (hard and tender) during the palpation portion of massage and gradually restore that tissue to its normal soft, elongated, nontender state. This appears to increase circulation, decrease pain sensitivity, and promote relaxation; it certainly reduces tension or stress to the tissues with which the muscle comes in contact.

Because muscle is the only tissue in the body that contracts, it follows that excessive or continuous contraction, especially for prolonged periods of time, can only lead to abnormality. It is interesting to note that over the years many patients, after a few treatments of vigorous deep massage, experience considerable relief from arthritis, adhesive capsulitis, tension headaches, and so forth. Patients also tend to become unhappy if there is a change in personnel to someone who gives a gentler massage. From a practical standpoint, we must realize that acute conditions cannot tolerate deep massage immediately. Occasionally, there will be patients who never tolerate deep massage. Usually

the extremely tense individual who is unwilling to change his daily habits is in this category. However, it is important to realize that some muscles become so tense that the patient has a very difficult time relaxing the tissue without some massage. If mobilization is used, it is common sense that the least amount of force used will add to the safety of patient treatment. Therefore, massage prior to mobilization can be extremely useful. On the other hand, a joint restriction can sometimes cause localized protective spasm, which will be relieved by using mobilization to restore normal joint mobility.

A variety of theories and soft tissue manipulations and techniques have evolved over the last 10 years (see Chapter 6, Introduction to Manual Therapy). Techniques have been categorized under the headings of muscle energy, myofascial release, strain and counterstrain, neuromuscular techniques, trigger point release, and acupressure (including Shiatsu acupressure[95,108,125]). Restoration of muscle function often begins with soft tissue work directed at muscle, ligaments, and fascial layers. Such work must then be followed by muscle re-education and movement training.

☐ Muscle Re-education

Although massage is a valuable tool in relieving tension in muscle, it is imperative that the patient be taught how to relax his muscles in order to achieve prolonged good results. This requires a learning process like that for any other skill we have learned—riding a bike, tying our shoes, reading, playing a sport, or driving a car. It is essentially muscle re-education, a skill physical therapists have used in their practice for years. To teach relaxation, we must develop a muscle awareness in the student. This means practice on the part of the patient.

One way for the patient to develop muscle awareness is to lie down in a comfortable position in a quiet place and practice, in an easy way, three things—the "basic three." The first is belly or abdominal breathing. Explain to the patient that chest breathing requires contraction of various muscles from neck to chest. Since relaxation of muscle tissue is the desired result, and not contraction, abdominal breathing is the method of choice. As the lungs expand with inspiration, their normal space is taken up in the chest cavity. More space can be given to the expanding lungs by allowing the diaphragm, which separates the chest from the abdominal cavity, to be pushed down into the abdominal cavity. Consequently, the external appearance and feel is that the abdomen rises. With exhalation the pressure is reversed; the air is expelled easily, and the diaphragm returns to its normal position. The normal habit of tension is rapid, shallow, chest breathing or sighing types of patterns. Abdominal breathing with a slow, rhythmical, average amount of air is extremely important for relaxation.

Secondly, the patient should "let all the muscles go." Explain that this means no movement and no holding or bracing. Instruct the patient that it is best to have a couple of pillows under the knees to protect the low back. The legs must roll outward, that is, be externally rotated, in order to relax the various hip muscles. One or two pillows may be placed under the head to support the mid-cervical area. The arms may be flexed with the hands resting on the abdomen but not touching or interlocked, or the muscles will tend to contract. Or they may be extended and externally rotated if the bed or plinth allows complete support of the arms.

Several key areas should be pointed out for the patient to "let go." For example, the eyes should not be closed quickly, since this is a contraction, but gradually after a few minutes have passed. Muscle relaxation can never be forced or done with determined effort because relaxation is a negative effort rather than a positive effort of contraction. Point out the various forms of muscle that contract or relax for facial expression and the contraction of the tongue with speech. The neck, upper back, arms, legs, and low back can all be pointed out again as areas where the patient "lets go" or "turns the power off."

The third aspect of the "basic three" is thinking about letting go without hard concentration. Learning, of course, requires some mental energy, and relaxation as a means of combating tension is definitely a learning process. So, by having the patient think—not concentrate hard—about letting go of that residual tension in the various areas of the body mentioned above, he can learn to relax. As Jacobson states, "The mind and body are one operating unit, not two, and this operating unit is based on muscle contractions."[62] Thus, letting the muscle go in itself will help to put the mind at ease.

☐ **Progressive Relaxation**

One of the most widely accepted tools used in learning relaxation is the contract–relax method commonly known as *Jacobson's progressive relaxation*. By teaching the patient to contract a muscle and develop recognition of the tension signals, or effort, she can begin to recognize tension as it occurs in daily life. This is followed by a period of "letting go," "turning the power off," "going negative," or whatever term is most meaningful to a particular patient. In other words, effort is discontinued, and the fibers of that muscle lengthen as relaxation takes place.

The patient is asked to practice 60 minutes each day in a quiet room free from intruders and phone calls. The following eight instructions for steps to be followed consecutively during the first period are adapted in part from Jacobson's *Self-Operations Control Manual.*[62]

Arm Practice

1. Lying on your back with arms at sides, leave eyes open 3 to 4 minutes.
2. Gradually close eyes and keep them closed during the entire hour.
3. After 3 to 4 minutes with eyes closed, bend left hand back. Observe the control sensation 1 to 2 minutes, and how it differs from the strains in the wrist and in the lower portion of the forearm.
4. Go negative for 3 to 4 minutes.
5. Again bend left hand back and observe as described in step 3.
6. Go negative once more for 3 to 4 minutes.
7. Bend left hand back a third and last time, observing the control sensation 1 to 2 minutes.
8. Finally, go negative for the remainder of the hour.

Eight similar steps are taken in the second period, except that the left wrist is flexed instead of extended. The same eight instructions apply during every period of the entire course, except that the motion performed will vary with the number of the period. The motion indicated for a period is usually performed three times at intervals of several minutes.

It should be noted that this does not apply to every third period of practice. During these sessions all motion is omitted, and the patient simply relaxes for the entire hour ("zero period"). In this way, the person avoids forming the bad habit of tensing a part before relaxing it.

The sequence of the movements performed each day and the periods for relaxation of the left arm are as follows:

Period	Left Arm
1	Bend hand back (wrist extension)
2	Bend hand forward (wrist flexion)
3	Relax only (no contraction)
4	Bend at elbow (elbow flexion)
5	Straighten arm (elbow extension)
6	Relax only
7	Progressive tension and relaxation of whole arm

Day 7, and each subsequent period of progressive tension and relaxation of the entire part, involves slowly tightening the entire part—a gradual and continuous increase in the amount of muscle contraction.

When the part has become moderately tense, the patient gradually and slowly relaxes, contracting less and less for the remainder of the 60 minutes.

Periods 8 through 14 follow exactly the same procedures as periods 1 through 7, except with the right arm. The periods then continue to other areas of the body as follows:

Period	Left Leg
15	Bend foot up (dorsiflexion)
16	Bend foot down (plantar flexion)
17	Relax only
18	Raise foot (knee extension)
19	Bend at knee (knee flexion)
20	Relax only
21	Raise knee (hip flexion)
22	Press lower thigh down (hip extension)
23	Relax entire leg
24	Progressive tension and relaxation of entire leg

Following the pattern described above, periods 15 through 24 are focused on the left leg, and periods 25 through 34 are focused on the right leg.

Period	Trunk
35	Pull in abdomen (contraction of abdominals)
36	Arch back slightly (spinal extension)
37	Relax abdomen, back, and legs
38	Observe a deeper breathing pattern
39	Bend shoulders back (contraction of interscapular muscles)
40	Relax only
41	Lift left arm forward and inward (pectorals)
42	Lift right arm forward and inward
43	Relax only
44	Elevate shoulder (upper trapezius and levator scapulae)

Periods 45 through 50 are focused on neck practice.

Period	Neck
45	Bend head back
46	Bend chin toward chest (neck flexion)
47	Relax only
48	Bend head left (left side flexion)
49	Bend head right
50	Relax only

Finally, Periods 51 through 62 are eye-region practice.

Period	Eye Region Practice
51	Wrinkle forehead
52	Frown
53	Relax only
54	Close eyelids tightly
55	Look left with lids closed
56	Relax only
57	Look right with lids closed
58	Look up
59	Relax only
60	Look down with lids closed
61	Look forward with lids closed
62	Relax only

This progressive relaxation can continue into visualization practice, speech-region practice, and practice in other positions, such as sitting, and in activities of daily living as explained in Jacobson's *Self-Operations Control Manual.*[62]

Another variation of Jacobson's progressive relaxation is a tool that has been used for years called the "relaxation lesson." The instructions given to the patient are as follows:

Begin with diaphragmatic breathing; then do some combination breathing with the chest and diaphragm. Settle into a nice rhythmic breathing pattern, with the abdominal muscles relaxed, and the diaphragm doing all the work. Do this lying on your back with the proper supports so that you relax best. Coordinate the following exercises with the breathing rhythm. All exercises should be done with minimal effort; the relaxation period is most important. Concentrate so that you may establish new habits for your muscles.

- Bend fingers, wrist, and elbow (flexion pattern). Relax.
- Straighten fingers, pull back wrist, and stiffen elbow (extension). Let go.
- Roll arm inward (inward rotation). Let go.
- Roll arm outward (outward rotation). Relax.
- Bend hip, knee, push foot down, curl toes (flexion). Let go.
- Pull toes and foot up, stiffen knee, push straight leg into bed (extension). Relax.
- Roll leg inward (rotation). Relax.
- Roll leg outward (outward rotation). Let go.
- Check breathing pattern and rhythm, thinking back to each arm and each leg. They should feel heavy and relaxed. As a muscle relaxes, it softens and lengthens. Concentrate; the exercise is not more important than the rest period.
- Squeeze buttocks together (attempt to use gluteals and sphincters). Relax.
- Arch back (erector spinae group). Let go.

- Pinch shoulder blades back toward spine (rhomboids). Let go.
- Pull shoulders forward (pectorals). Relax.
- Pull shoulder to ears (upper trapezius). Let go.
- Push shoulders toward knees (depressors). Relax.
- Pull abdominals in and relax. This alters breathing rhythm, so once again check your breathing. It should be belly breathing.
- Turn chin to right, left, and straight ahead. Release all the neck muscles.
- Push back of head into bed (neck extensors). Let go.
- Lift head (neck flexors). Relax.
- Pull corners of mouth downward. Let go (platysma fish breathing).
- Raise eyebrows and wiggle scalp. Let go.
- Frown. Relax.
- Squeeze eyelids tightly together. Let go.
- With eyes lightly closed and without moving head, turn eyes right, left, up, down, and straight ahead. Relax.
- Squeeze jaws together. Relax jaw muscles so mouth drops almost open.
- Push tongue against roof of mouth. Relax tongue.
- Swallow. Relax.
- Review mentally. Concentrate on feeling relaxed.

Minimum practice on this lesson is 1 hour per day—two 30-minute periods, six 10-minute periods, four 15-minute periods, or three 20-minute periods. Check your breathing hourly and practice diaphragmatic breathing 5 minutes out of every hour. You must establish new habits to break the pain–tension cycle.

The two contract–relax tools explained above are slight variations of methods of teaching relaxation. The important point is to determine, after evaluating the patient, which method of practice will best suit the patient so that he may learn to relax his muscles. As the patient progresses in his ability to relax, the method will also certainly change and progress. Sometimes isolation of contract–relax is effective. With adhesive capsulitis, learning to relax the rotator cuff muscles can be effective. Learning to extend the neck can relieve tension headaches. Relaxation of the fingers and wrist extensors is valuable in treating tennis elbow.

The patient must develop some understanding of what relaxation is, which means that those of us doing the teaching must have a greater understanding of the muscle relaxation process. However, the key to success is practice and repetition on the part of the patient. Because muscle relaxation is learned, the patient must practice. As mentioned before, 60 minutes is the recommended time period for daily practice. Frequently, the patient is so tense that she finds it ex-

tremely difficult to practice 60 continuous minutes, and shorter periods must be used. In very difficult cases, 5 minutes of practice out of each waking hour can be done. With contract–relax methods the emphasis must always be on the "letting go" phase. Patients will tend to emphasize the contraction phase of the exercises. You must carefully explain and repeat and re-emphasize that the "going negative" or "power off" phase is what is important. It is often helpful to tell the patient that even if she does every movement correctly but does not spend time "letting go" after the movement, the program will not be worth the paper it is printed on. Conversely, even if half the movements are incorrect but the patient really relaxes those muscles following the contraction, then muscle relaxation will be achieved.

BIOFEEDBACK

A comment about biofeedback or electromyography (EMG) equipment is appropriate at this time. As noted in Jacobson's *Progressive Relaxation*, these methods have been used for years.[60] EMG equipment can reveal baseline data regarding the amount of muscle tension initially present and can indicate progress at a later date. Biofeedback equipment used a few times can help the patient to understand through sight and sound what muscle relaxation is. However, like muscle relaxant medications that do not seem to have solved tension conditions, biofeedback appears to be just another crutch for the patient if used as the relaxation method. The key to relaxation appears to be learning and practice on the part of the patient. The patient must accept the major responsibility in combating neuromuscular hypertension problems. The therapist is present to help, to teach, to clarify, to encourage, and to explain.

PRACTICAL APPLICATION

Learning to sense muscle relaxation is only the first step in the progressive relaxation process. In reading, learning the alphabet and the phonetic sounds are the basic steps; the learning is valuable when the letters and sounds are put into words—words with meaning. The same applies to relaxation. Until we begin to adapt our ability to relax to our daily lives, we have nothing more than a tool of no practical value. Practicality comes with continuing periods of awareness of what our muscles are doing throughout the waking hours. By checking ourselves for muscle tension during various activities (*e.g.*, working, driving, walking, eating, participating in recreational activities) we begin to realize how much we contract muscles excessively. Thus, we can begin to let go. Over time, the relaxation of muscle rather than the contraction becomes the habit pattern; relaxation acquires practical value in our lives. Reminders to help us become aware of muscle habits can be helpful. For example, we might use time to develop a mental connotation with relaxation. Every time we look at our watch, or the radio mentions the time, or someone says it is time for lunch or asks what time it is, we can check ourselves. However, reminders must be changed every few days, or the mental connotation will itself become a habit, and the needed awareness of muscle activity will not develop.

☐ Autogenic Training

Autogenic training was developed by Schultz, a German neurologist, from investigations of hypnosis begun around 1900.[89,124] Two basic mental exercises are used: (1) the standard exercises, and (2) the meditative exercises. The six standard exercises are physiologically oriented. The verbal content of the standard formula is focused on the neuromuscular system (heaviness of the limbs), the vasomotor system (warmth of the limbs and coolness of the forehead), the cardiovascular system, and respiratory mechanism. These exercises are practiced several times a day until the patient is able to shift to a less stressful state or the trophotropic state described by Hess.

A reduction of afferent stimuli requires observation of the following points:

- The exercises should take place in a quiet room with moderate temperature and reduced illumination.
- Restrictive clothing should be loosened or removed.
- The body should be as relaxed as possible, and the eyes closed. Three distinctive postures have been found adequate: a horizontal posture; a reclining arm-chair posture; and a simple, relaxed, sitting position.
- The subject's attitude toward the exercises should not be tense or compulsive but of a "let it happen" nature, referred to as *passive concentration.*

The first exercise of the autogenic standard series aims at muscular relaxation. Right-handed individuals should start out with passive concentration on the right arm and heaviness, for example, "My right arm is comfortably heavy." Once the patient achieves the feeling of heaviness in the right arm, and the feeling spreads to the other extremities regularly, the formula is extended to include the other limbs (left arm, both arms, right leg, left leg, both legs, arms and legs). Concentration on heaviness continues until heaviness can be experienced more or less regularly in all four extremities. This may be achieved in 2 to 8 weeks.

Subsequently, passive concentration on warmth is added, starting with the right arm and warmth: "My right arm is comfortably warm." The warmth formula follows the same progressive procedures used for heaviness until all the extremities become regularly heavy and warm. This training on peripheral vasodilation may require another period of 2 to 8 weeks.

After having learned to establish the feeling of heaviness and warmth, the trainee continues with passive concentration on cardiac activity by using the formula, "Heartbeat calm and regular," or just passively observing the heart beat. This is followed by the respiration formula, "Respiration regular—it breathes me," or passively observing the breathing rhythm.

The last two, or final, exercises of the physiologically oriented standard exercises concern the abdominal region ("Solar plexus comfortably warm") and the cranial region, which should be cooler than the rest of the body ("My forehead is cool" or "Forehead pleasantly cool").

After the standard formulas have been repeated four to seven times in the sequence described, the altered state of consciousness is ended in a manner similar to awakening from a deep sleep by stretching, inhaling, or yawning, and gradually opening the eyes. Activation phrases are used, such as "I feel life and energy flowing through my legs, hips, solar plexus, chest, and arms. The energy makes me feel light and alive."

As training progresses, and after all six formulas have been added successively and mastered, they may be shortened. The time needed to establish these exercises effectively may require several months (4 to 6 months according to Schultz). In modern practice, however, Schultz and Luthe's autogenic training techniques have been modified to reduce training to a minimum of 6 weeks, so that a whole "round" can be practiced in 1 hour.[13] After several months of practice, the subject should be able to achieve the induced altered state of consciousness by simply thinking "heaviness—warmth—heartbeat and respiration—solar plexus—forehead."

The meditative exercises are reserved for the trainee who has mastered the standard exercises. They focus primarily on certain mental functions, single-focus mental concentration (as in yogic meditation), and finally meditation on abstract qualities of universal consciousness, much as in yogic or Zen meditation. The standard series of exercises and the single-focus meditation are primarily used in meditation or psychological treatment.

Certainly, the autogenic standard exercises concentrate on somatic attention and have an effect similar to that of progressive relaxation. According to Benson the first five standard exercises have been found to be the most effective in producing the relaxation response.[8] The meditative exercises that give an important role to single-focus concentration or to imagery are more cognitive in nature. They elicit subjective and physiologic changes that are different from those that follow the practice of somatic procedures.

CLINICAL APPLICATION

The clinical usefulness of autogenic training in the treatment of muscular disorders, according to Luthe and Schultz, is largely based on the following factors:[89]

- Muscular relaxation
- Improved local circulation
- Decreased stimulation of pain
- Reduction of unfavorable reactivity to emotional stress
- Possible favorable effects on deviation of certain metabolic and endocrine functions
- Reduction or elimination of relevant medications
- Promotion of the patient's active participation in treatment

Regular practice of autogenic training has been found particularly helpful in relieving complaints associated with arthritis and related disorders (rheumatoid arthritis, osteoarthritis), nonarticular rheumatism (fibromyositis, myalgia), and cervical-root and low-back syndromes (particularly when associated with nerve-root pressure, such as lumbagosciatic syndrome).

When musculoskeletal disorders involve the spine in conditions such as ankylosing spondylitis, degenerative joint disease, or herniation of a vertebral disk, autogenic training may prove to be very helpful when used in combination with other forms of treatment. In such cases, the patient should be encouraged to learn all the standard exercises, with particular emphasis on the heavy and warm formulas. In addition, topographically adapted special formulas are used. Topographically specific heaviness and warmth formulas may cover the entire length of the spine or may be used with passive concentration on a particular area (*e.g.*, "The lower part of my spine is heavy" or "My pelvis is warm"). When used to cover the entire length of the spine, dynamic mental contact has a better effect. This implies that the mental contact does not remain fixed on a given topographical area but shifts progressively over different sections of the spine starting with the cervical section and moving to the coccygeal area, while the mental process of passive concentration (*e.g.*, "My spine is very warm") continues. The mental control travels repeatedly down the spine and is followed by concentration on the arms and legs.

Similarly, in musculoskeletal disorders affecting the joints of the extremities, the emphasis is on frequent practice of the first two standard exercises (heavy and warm formulas) with relatively prolonged passive concentration on the affected area (*e.g.*, "My right knee is warm" or "My right shoulder is warm").

VARIATIONS

Benson and Wallace have devised a simplified method incorporating a modification of the standard autogenic exercises and single-focus attention.[6] Deep relaxation of the muscles, concentrating on heaviness and warmth, begins with the feet and progresses proximally to the calves, thighs, back, neck, arms, and shoulders. This method uses the word *one* as a mantra, while the patient breathes in and out for 10 to 20 minutes during the program. Benson and Wallace suggest that there is not a single method that is unique in eliciting the relaxation response, and that any one of the age-old or newly developed techniques may produce the same physiologic results, regardless of the mental device used.

Jencks has designed an interesting variation of autogenic training for children. Her variation includes all aspects of Schultz's standard formula but works through imagery instead of Schultz's precise meditative exercises.[66] Sensory awareness is aroused through images, for which suggestions are made in the form of Erickson's therapeutic double binds.[29] Jencks refers to this approach as the "autogenic rag doll."

Autogenic training has been found to be a useful adjunct to massage. Frances M. Tappin, a physical therapist and foremost authority on massage, states, "Since one purpose of massage is relaxation and relief of stress, it will be doubly effective if the one doing the massage can provide autogenic phrases to increase the effectiveness of massage."[142] She feels this is particularly true in situations in which tension is a major part of the patient's problem. She suggests a series of autogenic phrases developed by Alyce and Elmer Green of the Menninger Clinic that tend to bring the patient closer to the alpha brain rhythm, which is associated with feelings of calm.[46]

Alpha waves (slow brain waves) increase during the practice of relaxation but are not commonly found in sleep. Although we still do not know the significance of alpha waves, we do know that they are present when people feel relaxed.[8,13]

☐ An Integrated Relaxation Approach

Many physical therapists now use a combination of techniques or an integrated system using a sequential approach. Such an approach is best exemplified in a training program developed by Budzynski, Director of the Biofeedback Institute in Denver.[14,15] A gross awareness of muscle tension is acquired by moving from one form of relaxation to another in order of difficulty. The trainee progresses only after he has mastered a less difficult technique. His training program consists of three major components: progressive relaxation, autogenic training, and finally, a form of stress management combining autogenic training with systematic desensitization. There are six exercise elements that build on each other to produce simultaneous mind–body relaxation. The approach may be used independently or as an adjunct to biofeedback or related clinical procedures.

The first set of exercises is used to develop a gross awareness of muscle tension using a modification of progressive relaxation. Once the trainee can perform the exercises to the therapist's satisfaction, he moves on to differential relaxation (also developed by Jacobson). This allows the trainee to integrate his ability to relax into everyday living situations.[64] Along with practice twice a day, the patient is encouraged to become aware of specific tension areas in his body throughout the day.

The third set of exercises uses the autogenic formulas designed to develop further "muscle sense" with useful cognitive responses. The emphasis is on limb heaviness.

The fourth set moves on to limb heaviness and warmth, and the fifth to the forehead and the face. The fifth set is intended to bring together all of the components learned in the first five.

The final set employs systematic desensitization, a behavioral therapy approach combined with the relaxation techniques. The therapist typically assists the client in developing a series of scenes or visualizations. These are then listed in a hierarchical order, based on their fear-evoking quality. The client begins by visualizing the scene that has the fewest anxiety- or fear-provoking properties. This scene is repeated until the trainee can visualize it while remaining relaxed. He then moves to the next scene.

■ CHRONIC PAIN MANAGEMENT: RELAXATION AND MOVEMENT TRAINING

☐ Relaxation

As with biofeedback, there are numerous reports attesting to the efficacy of various relaxation training procedures in the reduction of chronic pain. Examples of these reports include the successful application of such procedures to low back pain,[106,107,110,120,123,135,141,145] temporomandibular joint pain,[16,40,104,136,137] myofascial pain,[2,20,43,48,126,127] muscle tension headaches,* migraine headache,[37,56,69,119,132–134] and chronic pain of mixed etiology.[57,70–72,82–84,105]

The central pain model presented by Melzack[97] in his pattern-generating theory suggests several methods of intervention with respect to the chronic pain patient. This theory describes the alteration of the central, self-perpetuating feedback loop with either hyperstimulation or hypostimulation. Hyperstimulation can be achieved by rapid changes in the environment such as the use of spray-and-stretch techniques, or acupuncture. Hypostimulation can be achieved during deep states of relaxation, which provides an environment for physiologic elements in which homeostasis can be more readily established.

Central pain management may also address the condition of low endorphin levels. Deep relaxation and imagery may be used to assist in reversing endorphin depletion caused by chronic stress.[12,121] Relaxation training and imagery have been used successfully even with patients having long-standing (15 years) chronic pain.[54] The rationale for this treatment is based on the increased muscle tension and anxiety seen in chronic pain patients and the need to reduce the sympathetic arousal level.[53]

Another method of increasing endorphin levels is exercise.[30,49] McCain[96] has reported that true modulation of pain sensitivity may depend on tissue levels of endogenous opioids, especially on the levels of beta-endorphin and adrenocorticotropic hormone (ACTH) released during exercise. Other researchers[28,31,73,102,103] whose studies have focused on pain and movement have shown that exercise programs can be instrumental in pain relief.

Therapeutic interventions designed to alleviate and control pain may be targeted at a number of components of the response. Approaches such as the operant behavioral approach[38,85] and the cognitive-behavioral approach[144] can be expected to have an impact on the affective mechanism. The cognitive-behavioral approach, which helps patients understand the relationship of their pain to cognitive, affective, and physiologic variables and instructs them in skills to cope more effectively, has an impact on affective distress.[19]

Phillips[112] reported that a cognitive-behavioral treatment package (relaxation, exercise, activity pacing, and cognitive intervention) had a substantial impact on mood, affective reactions to pain, drug intake, exercise capacity, self-efficacy, and avoidance behavior, which continued to improve a full year later. Fordyce and co-workers[39] have shown systematically that exercise helps to reduce pain or the behaviors re-

---

*See references 3, 9–11, 26, 41, 50, 58, 65, 80, 111, 131, 143, 147, 153.

lated to it. Relaxation training reduces both the sensory and affective dimensions of pain and relieves pain intensity.[113] Instructions in imagery, distraction strategies, and biofeedback disrupt the pain–anxiety–tension cycle and enhance perceived self-efficacy.[74,75]

Movement Awareness and Exercise

Research has shown that the body begins to compensate for the changes imposed by an injury within 3 to 5 days post injury.[51,53] These adaptive changes are the result of the body's attempt to attain pain-free postures and movements. Compensatory responses to pain, such as antalgic gait or guarded stance, may become contributing factors to the chronicity of pain.[52] These initial altered patterns of movement and posture are similar to those seen in patients with chronic pain evaluated 1 to 5 years post injury.

According to a study by Headley,[51,52] the difference between acute and chronic pain patients was in awareness. Acute patients are usually aware of postural changes and muscle activity compensations. Headley found that chronic patients were unaware of muscle and postural changes, stating their muscles were relaxed despite EMG findings to the contrary.[52] This dysfunctional movement adaptation results in abnormal shortening or lengthening of muscles, fascia, and ligaments, in addition to altered recruitment or movement strategies. These patients often make extraordinary progress with symptom reduction and increased function when the movement patterns are normalized.

In dealing with chronic pain patients, faulty posture and inefficient movement patterns must be recognized. Failure to correct the dysfunctional movement pattern may contribute to the eventual development of a true central pain phenomenon.[53] These patients often cannot produce slow, smooth controlled movements. The misuse of muscles is significant and is often more of a problem than actual loss of strength. Helping such patients increase awareness can be accomplished in many ways. Various types of relaxation exercises and movement therapies that can facilitate body awareness include Aston Patterning,[86,99] Trager (Psychophysical Integration),[99] the Feldenkrais Method (Functional Integration and Awareness Through Movement),[32–36] the Alexander technique,[1,4,17,68] and T'ai Chi.[21,22,77]

Once muscle recruitment has been normalized and efficiency of the muscle restored, functional strengthening is necessary with monitoring of muscle activity to ensure that the muscle is working as expected during the functional task.[53,93]

In the last 5 years there has been considerable interest in the value of intensive progressive exercises, particularly for patients with chronic low back pain.[25,45,82,92,157] Manniche and colleagues[92] have given an extensive review of the evidence indicating the value of such an exercise program. They concluded that while intensive exercise training can effect a lasting improvement of pain, continued training is essential to avoid relapse. Further studies on the affects of exercise will no doubt enhance the development of movement therapy and exercise programs for the reduction of pain.

GUIDELINES FOR ADMINISTERING RELAXATION TECHNIQUES IN MUSCULOSKELETAL DISORDERS

Evaluation

The most obvious candidates for relaxation techniques that physical therapists see are patients with chronic back and neck problems. These conditions are often the result of many varying factors. The role of our urbanized, overstressed, under-exercised life in the etiology of premorbid states—of which neck and back pain are often the first symptoms—needs special consideration. Today, the initial attack of back pain is frequently precipitated by emotional problems, tension, or unaccustomed work or athletic activities. These causes are often masked by or combined with true mechanical factors, but rarely are they entirely missing. Therefore, when taking the case history, the therapist must not overlook physical signs of emotional stress and muscle tension. The overall picture of the patient needs to be emphasized rather than concentration on the local mechanical problems.

SUBJECTIVE EXAMINATION FOR TENSION

An examination should always be conducted (see Chapter 5, Assessment of Musculoskeletal Disorders and Concepts of Management) for the extremities and for mechanical problems of the spine, which has been discussed and described by authors such as Cyriax, Grieve, and Maitland.[23,47,91] In addition, it may be necessary to further develop the history as it relates to tension and stress factors. The results of stress are often expressed as secondary manifestations, such as irregular sleeping habits, gastrointestinal problems, headaches, and so forth. People under stress experience a wide variety of physical responses, anxiety or restlessness, and emotional symptoms.

The nature of the patient's work and the manner in which the predominant activities of daily life are performed are important clues to whether the patient is under stress. The following are some areas that may need to be explored:

Nature of work—Does the patient like his or her work, superiors, and co-workers? Is the job competitive and stressful?

Way the work is performed—Do the daily activities require repetitive movements of the body? Does the activity allow free movement, or does the patient maintain a fixed position for prolonged periods?

Driving—Commuting for long periods of time is often a source of tension not only from the standpoint of maintaining a fixed position but also as a source of constant daily irritation from heavy traffic.

Physical activities—Does the type of work provide much exercise? If not, what, if anything, does the patient do to compensate for lack of exercise? What is the nature of such activity, and how often is it performed?

Home and family—Is there illness in the family? If married, is the marriage relationship satisfactory? Are there children? The home situation is often an important source of tension.

People under stress may experience a wide variety of physical symptoms. These may include

Cardiovascular and respiratory symptoms—Does the patient experience chest pain, a rapid or racing heart beat, difficult breathing, or shortness of breath? Does he have a problem with high blood pressure?

Eye, ear, nose, and throat symptoms, headaches or head pain—A special cause or starting point of neck pain may be related to grinding and clenching of the teeth. Does the patient frequently experience nasal stuffiness, hoarseness, or difficulty swallowing? Are there frequent migraine or tension headaches? Does the patient experience transient somatic effects such as dizziness or fainting?

Digestive disorders—Does the patient experience frequent stomach problems, a peptic ulcer syndrome, or a "nervous" stomach? Is he or she frequently bothered by indigestion, constipation, or nausea?

Endocrine imbalances—The most frequent endocrine disorders causing muscle pain are hypothyroidism and estrogen deficiency.[78] Does the patient tire easily, require a lot of sleep, or have a weight problem? Is there increased or decreased perspiration? Are there problems with dysmenorrhea or an irregular menstrual cycle?

Muscle-tension pain—Patients often describe only the leading, most severe symptoms and forget a multitude of others that momentarily seem unimportant. Has there been excessive muscle tension or pain in other parts of the body (jaw, forehead, legs, shoulders)? Has the patient been bothered by stiff, sore, or cramping muscles? If so, where?

There must be close observation of whether the pain is primary or secondary. For example, did pain cause the stress or *vice versa?*

Stress is often accompanied by symptoms of anxiety or restlessness. Inquiry or observation during the interview may be useful in determining if some of the following manifestations are present:

- Chewing the lips, grinding and clenching the teeth, and biting fingernails
- Pacing
- Increased eating, smoking, or drinking
- Difficulty falling asleep, waking up feeling exhausted, and being keyed up and jittery during the day

Stress is also accompanied by a variety of emotions. Possibly the most important question concerns the emotional stability of the patient. This aspect is often hard to obtain by direct questioning, but is frequently revealed in the course of the interview and treatment program. The patient's medical chart is also a useful source of information.

And finally, we will want to know

- In what type of situation does the patient become aware of unwanted tension? What is the environment, what is he or she doing at the time, and how?
- Is there any warning signal that tension may be coming on? Any thoughts or behaviors that are an indication of tension?
- When does the patient experience the most tension during a day?
- How does the patient experience tension? If the patient states that he or she feels "nervous," what does this actually mean?
- How does the patient deal with anxiety or unwanted tension?
- What does the patient feel is the source of the tension?

Closer inquiry in these areas and others may pinpoint the source of tension and thereby make it possible to influence it.

Many times the history will indicate that tension is a factor, especially under the following circumstances:

- Symptoms have an insidious onset, with a number of general symptoms of a vague and aching quality.
- Symptoms are related to a specific injury or particular activity and have taken a long time to improve or have actually become worse.
- The patient tires easily and has general symptoms of fatigue.
- There is morning pain and stiffness, aggravated by activity—at times only a minor amount of activity—and relieved by rest. (These patients many

times have difficulty sleeping. They may tell you, "I never have been able to relax.")

- Particular problems have become recurrent. For example, the patient may have experienced a third or fourth episode of shoulder pain, or problems in the other shoulder as well. When muscle tension is involved, problems tend to recur.

- When questioned about medications, the patient indicates she has taken muscle relaxants in the past.

- The patient has gone from doctor to doctor without a specific diagnosis, or has been told he has a "functional illness."

- A specific condition has been identified which is known to be related to muscle tension (*e.g.*, adhesive capsulitis of the shoulder or various types of tendinitis).

- There are general health problems related to tension and fatigue.

A useful tool for measuring the client's stress profile is the "Symptoms of Stress Checklist," a questionnaire that measures the ways people respond to stressful situations.[81] Sets of questions dealing with physical, psychological, or behavioral responses are included. The questionnaire is filled out by the patient during the first week, or it may be filled out prior to the examination. Many other such evaluation forms are now available. They are not only a useful source of information, but many can also be used to assess the patient's progress during the training session and at its end.

PHYSICAL EXAMINATION FOR TENSION

The physical part of evaluation may reveal many signs that point to tension. The first time you see the patient you will see that she is not resting or is constantly moving. For instance, the patient may prefer to stand rather than sit in the waiting room. Once you begin the examination you may observe constant shifting of position in the chair, shifting and movement of arms or legs, use of arms in talking, constant movement of eyes, actual tremors, restlessness, rapid and short breathing patterns or constant sighing, diminished concentration, irritability, and other signs of apparent overactivity of the skeletal muscles.

Inspection can be a relevant part of the examination for tension problems. Bony structure and alignment may be unremarkable, although subcutaneous soft tissues and the skin are affected (*i.e.*, hard, stringy muscle fiber, and adherent skin). You may determine this during palpation. Atrophy from tension fatigue, muscles that are well defined because of contraction in the muscle tissue, or poor general posture may be observed on inspection.

Selective tissue tension tests may elicit some positive signs as well. The patient may hesitate to move actively. There may be hypersensitivity to pain or general anxiety. Or she may move quickly rather than in the requested slow and deliberate pattern.

Passive testing is a key test for tension-related conditions, since it may be impossible to do a pure passive motion—the patient will actually assist you in moving the part. Even after you carefully explain to the patient that you would like her to completely let go, she will continue to assist. Patients often state that they are not aware of using their muscles. It thus becomes important in the remaining examination and treatment to stop frequently to point out that you want the patient to let go, and to explain relaxation. The patient quickly learns that by stopping movement or touching a particular muscle you can feel assistance or resistance, and therefore, she must "let go."

Be aware that although assistance is the most prevalent sign with passive movements, tense patients may actually resist movements. A hypersensitivity to pain and a muscle spasm or muscle tension end feel will occur. Apparent involvement of joint-play movements are more apt to be encountered because of resistance on the part of the patient. There will be involuntary, hyperactive muscle contractions that tend to prohibit testing of various joint-play movements. Many joint-play movements will appear painful, again because of the hyperactive muscle activity. Resistive testing will demonstrate a quick contraction on the part of the patient, and there will usually be several areas that have a pain response, rather than one or two specific movements. A general weakness may be prevalent. Neuromuscular tests may demonstrate hypersensitive responses to various stimuli and will usually produce hyperactive responses when deep-tendon reflexes are tested.

Palpation will elicit distinct signs when tension is present. The skin is often tender and dry, has an elevated temperature, and is adherent to underlying tissue. Palpation of subcutaneous tissue, in a particular muscle, is a key test. The muscle will feel hard and stringy and will be tender to palpation. It is difficult to distinguish between muscle tissue that is tense and that which is in spasm. Both are hard, but it is safe to assume that if several muscle groups are hard and tender, as well as numerous anatomic areas, there is a tension factor involved rather than pure protective spasm. Muscle tissue in a relaxed state is soft, pliable, and not tender to palpation, and the various fibers are elongated. With tension (muscle is the only tissue in the body that contracts) there is just the opposite effect of the relaxed state, and this can be readily palpated.

Clearly, before initiating a program of relaxation training, the therapist must decide if it is realistic to expect that increasing relaxation skills will be a significant factor in alleviating the patient's problems. If the tension occurs in response to a serious problem in the patient's life, it must be dealt with differently (even though relaxation can be beneficial here as well). However, relaxation training can be helpful as a means of eliminating or reducing physical complaints, such as a headache or low-back pain, when there are no strictly organic bases for the complaint that can be treated more directly by other means.

☐ Management

A thorough knowledge of and experience with relaxation procedures, as well as the use of other clinical skills, are essential to effective relaxation training. Relaxation techniques are seldom used alone, because in most cases the patient's problem is combined with true mechanical factors, muscle imbalances and pain, emotional or behavioral problems, and so on. Relaxation training is an integral part of many behavioral procedures. Principles of behavioristic psychology, behavior modification, and biofeedback are often employed in conjunction with relaxation training but are beyond the scope of this chapter. These methods are discussed and described in many excellent books and articles in the literature.

The first session of relaxation training is perhaps the most important. The therapist should

1. Explain and justify the procedures so that the patient can understand and accept the rationale underlying relaxation training.
2. Instill a feeling of confidence in the technique as well as enthusiasm for carrying out necessary "homework." Success at learning relaxation skills requires regular practice once they have been learned in the training session.
3. Explain and set up long-term and short-term goals. An intermediate goal is for the patient to be able to relax at any time using any or all of the techniques that work best for that individual. The ultimate goal is to produce relaxation independent of conditioned responses.

THE PHYSICAL SETTING

A suitable setting for training should be provided. Eliminate all sources of extraneous stimulation. Relaxation should take place in a quiet, dimly lit, attractive room. An important consideration is the chair or couch that the patient uses during relaxation training. Recliner chairs are considered ideal. A treatment table may be used as long as the basic requirement of complete support and comfort are met.

The client should wear loose-fitting, comfortable clothing. Glasses, contact lenses, watches, and shoes should be removed to reduce extraneous stimulation and to allow free movement.

The therapist must be aware of self, touch, and tone of voice. The voice should be used as an instrument to facilitate the relaxation process. How the therapist speaks is just as important as what is actually said. You should speak softly, and the pace of speech should gradually be reduced as the session progresses.

DIRECTING THE PROCEDURE

The therapist directs the sequence of events, which will vary with the training technique employed. The clinical training should generally be continued until the therapist is convinced that the patient is performing a set of exercises correctly and that deep relaxation has, in fact, been achieved. This can usually be determined through questioning after the session and by nonverbal clues that are observed during the treatment session (*e.g.,* fidgeting in the chair).

Post-relaxation questioning should follow each session in order to determine if problems exist, and whether an alternative strategy should be employed. The patient's report usually is a sufficiently reliable guide to his ability to relax and is most helpful as an aid in modifying the approach to that patient. Ask the patient to describe what relaxation feels like, as well as more specific questions regarding any problems that occurred during the session. It is important to ask if anything that was said or done during the session made it more difficult to relax, and what statements or techniques seemed to facilitate relaxation so that they can either be eliminated or emphasized in subsequent sessions.

ASSIGNED HOME PROGRAMS

A home program of relaxation may be started from the very beginning or as soon as the therapist is convinced that the patient is performing a set of exercises correctly. Self-administered relaxation is ideally suited for problems in which tension is a major component and easily lends itself for use in "homework" assignments between therapy sessions. In general, self-administered relaxation can provide benefits as a treatment in itself, or it can be used in conjunction with additional therapeutic techniques.

The importance of practicing cannot be overemphasized to the patient. Relaxation is a skill that improves with practice. The trainee is usually required to practice once or twice a day (varying with the training technique employed, *e.g.,* anywhere from two 10-minute sessions to a single 1-hour session). In many cases, frequent, shorter sessions will be more effective for some patients. Advise the patient to practice at times when she is under minimal or no pressure. For example, just before bedtime is often recommended, although the best times will vary from patient to patient. It is not advisable to practice on a full stomach.

As the patient becomes more and more proficient in relaxation skills, the number of daily practice sessions as well as the time spent can gradually be reduced. Gradually the patient should be weaned away from both therapist and any instrumentation used. The patient must learn to rely on the learned awareness and control, along with other self-generating aids, so that tension can be reduced at any time in day-to-day stressful situations.

Devices may be used to foster home practice and to incorporate these habits into routine activities of daily living. Some clinicians have used small parking-meter timers that can be set to buzz at hourly intervals to remind the patient to practice for anywhere from 30 seconds to 3 minutes. Patel uses an interesting reminder system, instructing patients to use everyday sounds such as ringing telephones or church bells.[109] Others use visual reminders, such as stop lights, so that each time the patient comes to a lengthy stop in traffic, he practices his techniques. Others have patients replace their coffee breaks at work with relaxation breaks. Obviously, it is best if the patient will also allot long periods every day for serious practice in a conducive environment.

Standard relaxation tapes made from Jacobson's and Schultz and Luthe's relaxation techniques, which have been modified to reduce training time, are readily available commercially and are often used in home practice. Budzynski's relaxation approach described earlier is also available on tape. Tape practice, according to Brown, should be used with a bit of caution, however, and should be considered on an individual patient basis. Recent research indicates that recorded relaxation instruction may actually result in increased EMG tension levels in some patients.[13] Tape recorders offer far more flexibility than prerecorded tapes. Each relaxation session can be recorded during the clinical session on a tape recorder provided by the patient, which he can then take home for practice between sessions. This has several advantages. The relaxation technique can be modified to meet the patient's own needs and can become progressively shorter as the patient becomes more skilled in his learning techniques.

Tapes used for home practice have also been found to be useful for patients who have difficulty relaxing in the presence of a therapist. Patients may be started on relaxation learning in this way, and then at a later date start clinical practice with the therapist.

It is usually advisable for patients to do other homework as well. Patients may be requested to chart their painful activities during the day or to record situations that make them tense. This type of record keeping is useful in documenting the patient's progress as well as in helping to pinpoint sources of tension. Encourage the patient to make frequent body checks for muscle tension during the day in order to become more aware of the environment and of tension-causing factors.

Invariably, the patient will need activities of daily living (ADL) training to improve gait, posture, body mechanics, and ways of conserving energy and reducing tension. The most difficult step of all is transferring this learning to the patient's day to day living.

☐ Assessing the Patient's Progress

To assess the success of relaxation training, the therapist can employ several kinds of information about the patient: clinical observation, a subjective stress profile or anxiety-scale evaluation, and objective indicators of relaxation. Important indicators of progress that may be gained by observing the patient during the clinical session include physical signs, such as less observable movement, a reduction in the breathing pattern during the course of the session, and a peaceful, relaxed appearance (a relaxed open jaw or a sleepy-eyed appearance after successful relaxation). The patient's ability to gain deep relaxation in shorter and shorter periods of time is also an indicator.

There should be signs of symptomatic improvement. Furthermore, stimuli that once called forth muscle tension or "fibrositis" (backache) no longer do so under the same condition. By deconditioning the muscle-tension habit or anxiety response that has been partly responsible for her problem, she brings about a proportionate reduction of the symptoms.

Secondary manifestations should decline. Stress-dependent reactions, whether migraines, intestinal cramps, grinding and clenching the teeth, or difficulty falling asleep, can also be used as measures of improvement. A reduction or termination of drugs to reduce pain or encourage muscle relaxation is also a useful indicator of improvement.

It is often an advantage to have objective indicators of relaxation. Jacobson has used EMG.[61] Recently, more convenient equipment such as EMG biofeedback has become available. The equipment can be used as methods of evaluation and as treatment to facilitate relaxation by translating muscle potential into auditory or visual feedback to the patient. Other physiologic measurements might include cardiovascular measurements (heart rate, blood pressure, skin temperature) and the use of brain wave biofeedback (electroencephalogram). Fortunately, the patient's report of changes in symptoms usually serves as a sufficiently reliable guide that relaxation skills have been a significant factor in alleviating the problem.

RESEARCH

To date, quantitative research in this area of relaxation and related techniques has been relatively scant. However, caution should be used in applying these techniques, because there may be side-effects. Symptoms ranging from insomnia to hallucinatory behavior and withdrawal have been reported when relaxation techniques have been practiced for long periods or to excess.[152] Clearly, additional research is needed to test and clarify the numerous hypotheses presented in the current literature. Therapists can help by documenting the claims made for relaxation and for specific treatment strategies that seem to be most effective. And, finally, therapists should review the current studies involving relaxation for possible areas of clinical research as they apply to physical therapy and musculoskeletal disorders.

Relaxation has been found to be a successful alternative to drugs and numerous types of back surgery. Major advantages include cost effectiveness and the fact that the patient is making a contribution to treatment. Relaxation is not a "magic bullet" and will not cure joint dysfunction or other musculoskeletal disorders. It is, however, a key to reducing the muscle tension, anxiety, nervousness, and stress that may lead to a variety of physical and psychological disabilities.

REFERENCES

1. Alexander FM: The Use of Self. London, Re-Education Publications, 1910
2. Amen DV, Mostofsky DI: Behavioral management of myofascial pain syndrome. J R Soc Health 108:81–82, 1991
3. Attanasso V, Andrasik F, Blanchard EB: Cognitive therapy and relaxation training in muscle contraction headache: Efficacy and cost-effectiveness. Headache 27:254–260, 1987
4. Barlow W: The Alexander Technique. New York, Alfred A Knopf, 1973
5. Benjamin BE: Are You Tense? The Benjamin System of Muscular Therapy: Tension Relief Through Deep Massage and Body Care. New York, Pantheon Books, 1978
6. Benson H: The Relaxation Response. New York, Avon Books, 1976
7. Benson H: The Mind/Body Effect. New York, Simon & Schuster, 1979
8. Benson H: Beyond the Relaxation Response. New York, Times Books, 1984
9. Bhargava SC: Progressive muscular relaxation and assertive training in tension headache. Ind J Clin Psychol 10:23–25, 1983
10. Blanchard EB, Andrasik F, Appelbaum BA, et al: Three studies of the psychologic changes in chronic headache patients associated with biofeedback and relaxation therapies. Psychosom Medicine 48:73–83, 1986
11. Blanchard EB, Nicholson NL, Taylor AE, et al: The role of regular home practice in the relaxation treatment of tension headaches. J Consult Clin Psychol 59:467–470, 1991
12. Bonica JJ: General considerations of chronic pain. In Bonica JJ (ed): The Management of Pain, pp 180–196. Philadelphia, Lea & Febiger, 1990
13. Brown BB: Stress and the Art of Biofeedback. New York, Harper & Row, 1977
14. Budzynski TH: Relaxation Training Program. New York, Bio Monitoring Audio Cassette Publications, 1977
15. Budzynski TH, Stoyva J, Adler C: Feedback-induced muscle re-education: Application to tension headaches, Behav Ther Exp Psychiatry 1:205–211, 1970
16. Burdette BH, Gale EN: The effects of treatment on masticatory muscle activity and mandibular posture in myofascial pain dysfunction patients. J Dent Res 67:1126–1130, 1988
17. Caplan D: Back Trouble. Gainesville, FL: Triad Publishing, 1987
18. Clynes M: Toward a view of man. In Clynes M, Milsum J (eds): Biomedical Engineering Systems. New York, McGraw-Hill, 1970
19. Craig KD: Emotional aspects of pain. In Wall DP, Melzack R (eds): Textbook of Pain, 3rd ed, pp 261–274. Edinburgh, Churchill Livingstone, 1994
20. Crockett DJ, Foreman ME, Alden L, et al: A comparison of treatment modes in the management of myofascial pain dysfunction syndrome. Biofeedback Self Regul 11:279–291, 1986
21. Crompton P: The Elements of Tai Chi. Shaftesbury, Dorset, Element, 1990
22. Crompton P: The Art of Tai Chi. Shaftesbury, Dorset, Element, 1993
23. Cyriax J, Coldham M: Textbook of Orthopaedic Medicine, vol 1, 11th ed. London, Bailliäre Tindall, 1984
24. Davis M, Eshelman ER, McKay M: The Relaxation and Stress Reduction Workbook, 2nd ed. Oakland, CA, New Harbinger, 1982
25. Deardorff WW, Rubin MS, Scott DW: Comprehensive multidisciplinary treatment of chronic pain—a follow up study of treated and non-treated groups. Pain 45:35–43, 1991
26. DeBerry S: An evaluation of progressive muscle relaxation on stress related symptoms in a geriatric population. Int J Aging Hum Dev 14:225–269, 1981–1982
27. Devi I: Yoga for Americans. Englewood Cliffs, NJ, Prentice-Hall, 1959
28. Donelson R, Grant W, Kamps L, et al: Pain response to sagittal end-range spinal motion. Spine 72:210–211, 1991
29. Erickson MH, Ross EL: Varieties of double bind. Am J Clin Hypn 17:143–157, 1975
30. Farrell PA: Exercise and endorphins—male response. Med Sci Sports Exerc 17:89–93, 1985
31. Feine JS, Chapman CE, Lund JP, et al: The perception of painful and nonpainful stimuli during voluntary motor activity in man. Somatosens Mot Res 7:113–124, 1990
32. Feldenkrais M: The master moves. Cupertino, CA, Meta, 1984
33. Feldenkrais M: Body and Mature Behavior. New York, International University Press, 1949
34. Feldenkrais M: Awareness Through Movement. New York, Harper & Ross, 1972
35. Feldenkrais M: The Potent Self. Cambridge, Harper & Row, 1985
36. Feldenkrais M: Bodily expressions. Somatics 4:52–59, 1988
37. Fentress DW, Masek BJ, Mehegan JF, et al: Biofeedback and relaxation-response training in the treatment of pediatric migraine. Dev Med Child Neurol 28:139–146, 1986
38. Fordyce WE: Behavioural methods for chronic pain and illness. St Louis, CV Mosby, 1976
39. Fordyce WE, McMahon R, Rainwater G, et al: Pain complaint–exercise performance relationship in chronic pain. Pain 10:311–321, 1981
40. Funch DP, Gale EN: Biofeedback and relaxation therapy for chronic temporomandibular joint pain: predicting successful outcomes. J Consult Clin Psychol 52:928–935, 1984
41. Gada MT: A comparative study of efficacy of EMG biofeedback and progressive muscular relaxation in tension headache. Ind J Psychiatr 26:121–127, 1984
42. Gellhorn E: Principles of Autonomic-Somatic Interactions. Minneapolis, University of Minnesota Press, 1967
43. Gessel AH, Alderman M: Management of myofascial pain dysfunction syndrome of the temporomandibular joint by tension and control training. Psychosomatics 12:302–309, 1971
44. Gifford J, Gifford L: Connective tissue massage. In Wells P, Frampton V, Bowsher D (eds): Pain Management in Physical Therapy, pp 218–238. Norwalk, CT, Appleton & Lange, 1988
45. Godges JJ, Holden MR, Longdon C, et al: The effects of two stretching procedures on hip range of motion and gait economy. J Orthop Sports Phys Ther 10:350–357, 1989
46. Green E, Green A: The ins and outs of mind body energy. In: Science Year 1974: World Book Science Annual. Chicago, Field Enterprises Corporation, 1973
47. Grieve GP: Mobilisation of the Spine: A Primary Handbook of Clinical Methods, 5th ed. Edinburgh, Churchill Livingstone, 1991
48. Graff-Radford SB, Reeves JL, Jaeger B: Management of chronic head and neck pain: Effectiveness of altering factors perpetuating myofascial pain. Headache 27:180–185, 1987
49. Grossman A, Sutton JR: Endorphins: What are they? How are the measured? What is their role in exercise? Med Sci Sports 17:74–81, 1985
50. Hart JD: Predicting differential response to EMG biofeedback and relaxation training: The role of cognitive structure. J Clin Psychol 40:453–457,1984
51. Headley BJ: Postural homeostasis: PT Forum 9:1–4, 1990
52. Headley BJ: EMG and postural dysfunction. Clinical Management 10:14–17, 1990
53. Headley BJ: Chronic pain management. In Sullivan SB, Schmitz TJ: Physical Rehabilitation: Assessment and Treatment, 3rd ed, pp 577–602. Philadelphia, FA Davis, 1994
54. Hendler N, Derogatis L, Avella J: EMG biofeedback in patients with chronic pain. Dis Nervous System 7:505–509, 1977
55. Hess WR: Functional Organization of Diencephalon. New York, Grune & Stratton, 1957
56. Houts AC: Relaxation and thermal feedback treatment of child migraine headache: A case study. Am J Clin Biofeedback 5:154–157, 1982
57. Hyman RB, Feldman HR, Harris RB, et al: The effects of relaxation training on clinical symptoms: a meta-analysis. Nursing Res 38:216–220, 1989
58. Jacob RG, Turner SM, Szelkelv BC, et al: Predicting outcome of relaxation therapy in headaches. The role of "depression." Behav Ther 14:457–465, 1983
59. Jacobson E: Progressive Relaxation. Chicago, University of Chicago Press, 1929
60. Jacobson E: Progressive Relaxation, 4th ed. Chicago, University of Chicago Press, 1962
61. Jacobson E: Anxiety and Tension Control. Philadelphia, JB Lippincott, 1964
62. Jacobson E: Self-Operations Control Manual. Chicago, National Foundation for Progressive Relaxation, 1964
63. Jacobson E: Tension in Medicine. Springfield, IL, Charles C Thomas, 1967
64. Jacobson E: You Must Relax. New York, McGraw-Hill, 1970
65. Janssen K, Neutgens J: Autogenic training and progressive relaxation in the treatment of three kinds of headache. Behav Res Ther 24:199–208, 1986
66. Jencks B: Respiration for Relaxation, Invigoration and Special Accomplishment. Salt Lake City, Jencks, 1974
67. Jencks B: Your Body: Biofeedback at Its Best. Chicago, Nelson Hall, 1977
68. Jones F: Body Awareness. New York, Schocken Books, 1979

69. Jurish SE, Blanchard EB, Andrasik F, et al: Home versus clinic-based treatment of vascular headache. J Consult Clin Psychol 51:743–751, 1983
70. Kabat ZL: An outpatient program in behavioral medicine for chronic pain patients based on the practice of mindfulness meditation: Theoretical considerations and preliminary results. Gen Hosp Psychiatry 4:33–47, 1982
71. Kabat ZL, Lipworth L, Burney R: The clinical use of mindfulness meditation for the self-regulation of chronic pain. J Behav Med 8:163–190, 1985
72. Kabat-Zinn J, Lipworth L, Burney R, et al: Four-year follow up of a meditation-based program for the self regulation of chronic pain: treatment outcomes and compliance. Clin J Pain 2:159–173, 1987
73. Kakigi R, Shibasaki H: Mechanism of pain relief by vibration and movement. J Neurol Neurosurg Psychiatry 55:282–286,1992
74. Keefe FJ, Gil KM: Behavioral concepts in the analysis of chronic pain syndromes. J Consult Clin Psychol 54:776–783, 1986
75. Keefe FJ, Lefevre JC: Behaviour therapy. In Wall PD, Melzack (eds): Textbook of Pain, 3rd ed, pp 1367–1380, 1994
76. Kiecolt-Glaser JK, Williger D, et al: Psychosocial enhancement of immunocompetence in a geriatric population. Health Psychol 4:24–41, 1985
77. Kotsias J: The Essential Movements of Tai Chi. Brookline, MA, Paradigm Publications, 1989
78. Kraus H: Clinical Treatment of Back and Neck Pain. New York, McGraw-Hill, 1970
79. Kruger H: Other Healers, Other Cures. New York, Bobbs-Merrill, 1974
80. Lacroix JM, Clarke MA, Bock JC, et al: Muscle-contraction headaches in multiple pain patients. Treatment under worsening baseline conditions. Arch Phys Med Rehabil 67:14–18, 1986
81. Leckie M, Thompson E: Symptoms of Stress Checklist. Seattle, University of Washington, 1977
82. Linton SJ, Bradley LA, Jenson I: The secondary prevention of low back pain—a controlled study with follow up. Pain 36:197–207, 1989
83. Linton SJ, Gotestam KG: A controlled study of the effects of applied relaxation and applied relaxation plus operant procedures in the regulation of pain. Br J Clin Psychol 23:291–299, 1984
84. Linton SJ, Melin L: Applied relaxation in the management of chronic pain. Behav Psychother 11:337–350, 1983
85. Linton SJ, Melin L, St Jernlof N: The effects of applied relaxation and operant activity training on chronic pain. Behav Psychother 13:87–100, 1985
86. Low J: The modern body therapies. Part four: Aston patterning. Massage Magazine 16:48–52, 1988
87. Lowen A: Physical Dynamics of Character Structure. New York, Grune & Stratton, 1958
88. Lowen A: Breathing, Movement, and Feeling. New York, Institute for Bioenergetics Analysis, 1965
89. Luthe W (ed): Autogenic Therapy, vols. 1–6, New York, Grune & Stratton, 1969–1972
90. Maharishi MY: The Science of Being and Art of Living. London, International SRM Publications, 1966
91. Maitland GD: Vertebral Manipulations, 5th ed. London, Butterworth, 1987
92. Manniche C, Lundberg E, Christensen I, et al: Intensive dynamic back exercises for chronic low back pain. A clinical trial. Pain 47:53–60, 1991
93. May P: Movement awareness and stabilization training. In Basmajian JV, Nyberg R (eds): Rational Manual Therapies. Baltimore, Williams & Wilkins, 1993
94. Mason JW: A re-evaluation of the concept of nonspecificity in stress theory. Psychol Res 8:323–333, 1971
95. Masunaga S, Ohashi W: Zen Shiatsu: How to Harmonize Yin and Yang for Better Health. Tokyo, Japan Publications 1977
96. McCain GA: Role of physical fitness training in the fibrositis/fibromyalgia syndrome. Am J Med 81(Suppl 3A):73–77, 1986
97. Melzack R: Neurophysiological foundation of pain. In Sternbach R (ed): The Psychology of Pain, pp 1–24. Raven Press, New York, 1986
98. Middaugh SJ: Biobehavioral techniques. In Scully R, Barnes MR (eds): Physical Therapy, pp 975–997. Philadelphia, JB Lippincott, 1989
99. Miller B: Alternative somatic therapies. In White AH, Anderson R: Conservative Care of Low Back Pain. Baltimore, Williams & Wilkins, 1991
100. Miller NE: Effects of emotional stress on the immune system. Pavlov J Biol Sci 20:47–52, 1985
101. Mines S: The Concept of Pain. New York, Grosset & Dunlap, 1974
102. Mitchell RI, Carmen GM: Results of a multicenter trial using an active exercise program for treatment of acute soft tissue and back injuries. Spine 15:514–521, 1990
103. Murry PB: Case study: Rehabilitation of a collegiate football placekicker with patellofemoral arthritis. J Orthop Sports Phys Ther 10:224–227, 1988
104. Newbury CR: Tension and relaxation in the individual. Int Dent J 29:173–182, 1979
105. Newshan G, Balamuth R: Use of imagery in a chronic pain outpatient group. Imagination, Cognition and Personality 10:25–38, 1990
106. Nicholas MK, Wilson PH, Goyen J: Operant-behavioral and cognitive-behavioural treatment for chronic low back pain. Behav Res Ther 29:225–238, 1991
107. Nicholas MK, Wilson PH, Goyen J: Comparison of cognitive-behavioral group treatment and an alternative non-psychological treatment for chronic low back pain . Pain 48:339–347, 1992
108. Nicholson GG, Clendaniel RA: Manual techniques. In Scully RM, Barnes MR: Physical Therapy, pp 975–985. Philadelphia, JB Lippincott, 1989
109. Patel C: Randomized controlled trial of yoga and biofeedback in management of hypertension. Lancet 2:93–95, 1975
110. Petty NE, Mastria MA: Management of compliance to progressive relaxation and orthopedic exercises in treatment of chronic back pain. Psychol Rep 52:35–38, 1983
111. Phillips C, Hunter M: The treatment of tension headache: II. EMG "normality" and relaxation. Behav Res Ther 19:499–507, 1981
112. Phillips HC: The effects of behavioural treatment on chronic pain behaviour. Res Therapy 25:365–377, 1987
113. Phillips HC: Changing chronic pain experience. Pain 32:165–172, 1988
114. Portela A: Massage as a stimulation technique for premature infants: An annotated bibliography. Pediatr Phys Ther 2:80–85, 1990
115. Pierce F: Mobilizing the Midbrain. New York, GP Putnam's Sons, 1924
116. Prudden B: Pain Erasure. New York, Evans, 1984
117. Rice R: Neurophysiological development in premature infants following stimulation. Dev Psychology 13:7–26,1977
118. Rice R: Effects of the Rice infant sensorimotor stimulation treatment on the development of high-risk infants. Birth Defects 15:7–26, 1979
119. Richter IL, McGrath PJ, Humphreys PJ, et al: Cognitive and relaxation treatment of paediatric migraine. Pain 25:195–203, 1986
120. Rosomoff HL, Rosomoff RS: Comprehensive multidisciplinary pain center approach to the treatment of low back pain. Neurosurg Clin North Am 2:877–890, 1991
121. Rossi EL: The Psychobiology of Mind-Body Healing. New Concepts of Therapeutic Hypnosis New York, WW Norton, 1986
122. Ruch TC: The nervous system: Sensory function. In Fulton JF (ed): Textbook of Physiology. Philadelphia, WB Saunders, 1955
123. Sanders SH: Component analysis of a behavioral treatment program for chronic low-back pain. Behav Ther 14:697–705, 1983
124. Schultz JH, Luthe W: Autogenic Training: A Psychophysiologic Approach in Psychotherapy. New York, Grune & Stratton, 1959
125. Schultz W: Shiatsu: Japanese Finger Pressure Therapy. New York, Bell, 1976
126. Scott DS: Treatment of the myofascial pain-dysfunction syndrome: Psychological aspects. J Am Dent Assoc 101:611–616, 1981
127. Scott DS: Myofascial pain-dysfunction: A psycho-biological perspective. J Behav Med 4:451–465, 1980
128. Selye H: The Stress of Life. New York, McGraw-Hill, 1956
129. Selye H: Stress Without Distress. Philadelphia, JB Lippincott, 1974
130. Sinclair JD: Exercise in pulmonary disease. In Basmajian JV (ed): Therapeutic Exercise, 3rd ed. Baltimore, Williams & Wilkins, 1976
131. Smith LS: Evaluation and management of muscle contraction headache. Nurs Prac 13:20–23, 26–27, 1988
132. Sorbi MA, Tellegen B: Differential effects of training in relaxation and stress-coping in patients with migraine. Headaches 26:473–481, 1986
133. Sorbi M, Tellegen B: Stress-coping in migraine. Soc Sci Med 26:351–358, 1988
134. Sorbi M, Tellegen B, Dulong A: Long-term effects of training in relaxation and stress-coping in patients with migraine: A 3-year follow-up. Headache 29:111–121, 1989
135. Spinhoven P, Linssen ACG: Behavioral treatment of chronic low back pain. I. Relation of coping strategy to outcome. Pain 45:29–34. 1991
136. Stam HJ, Mcgrath PA, Brooke RI: The effects of cognitive-behavioural treatment program on temporo-mandibular pain and dysfunction syndrome. Psychosom Med 46:534–545, 1984
137. Stam HJ, McGrath PA, Brooke RI: The treatment of temporo-mandibular pain joint syndrome through control of anxiety. J Behav Ther Exp Psychiatry 15:41–45, 1984
138. Sternbach RA: Psychophysiological bases of psychosomatic phenomena. Psychosomatics 7:81–84, 1966
139. Sternbach RA: Strategies and tactics in the treatment of patients with pain. In Crue BL (ed): Pain and Suffering: Selected Aspects. Springfield, IL, Charles C Thomas, 1970
140. Stewart E: To lessen pain: Relaxation and rhythmic breathing. Am J Nurs 76:958–959, 1976
141. Stuckey SJ, Jacobs A, Goldfarb J: EMG biofeedback training, relaxation training and placebo for the relief of chronic back pain. Precept Mot Skills 63:1023–1036, 1986
142. Tappin FM: Healing Massage Techniques: Holistic, Classic, and Emerging Methods, 2nd ed, Norwalk, CT, Appleton & Lange, 1988
143. Tobin DL, Holroyd KA, Baker A, et al: Development and clinical trial of a minimal contact, cognitive-behavioral treatment for tension headaches. Cognitive Ther Res 12:325–339, 1988
144. Turk DC, Meichenbaum DH, Genest M: Pain and behavioural medicine: Theory, research and clinical guide. New York, Guilford, 1983
145. Turner JA: Comparison of group progressive-relaxation training and cognitive-behavioral group therapy for chronic low back pain. J Consult Clin Psychol 50:757–765, 1982
146. Vishnudevananda S: The Complete Illustrated Book of Yoga. New York, Julian Press, 1960
147. Walbaum ABC, Pzewnicki R, Steele H, et al: Progressive muscle relaxation and restructured environmental stimulation therapy for chronic tension headache: A pilot study. Int J Psychosom 38:33–39, 1991
148. Wallace RK: Physiological effects of transcendental meditation. Science 167:1751–1754, 1970
149. Wallace RK, Benson H: The physiology of meditation. Sci Am 226:84–90, 1972
150. Warner G, Lance J: Relaxation therapy in migraine and chronic tension headache. Med J Aust 1:298–301, 1975
151. Whatmore GB, Kohli DR: Dysponesis: A neurophysiologic factor in functional disorders. Behav Sci 13:102–124, 1968
152. White J, Fadiman J (eds): Relax: How You Can Feel Better, Reduce Stress and Overcome Tension. The Confucian Press, 1976
153. Williamson DA, Monguilot JE, Jarrell MP, et al: Relaxation for the treatment of headache: controlled evaluation of two group programs. Behav Mod 8:407–424, 1984
154. Wolpe J: Psychotherapy by Reciprocal Inhibition. Stanford, Stanford University Press, 1958
155. Wolpe J: The Practice of Behavior Therapy, 2nd ed. New York, Pergamon Press, 1973
156. Wood EC, Becker PD: Beard's Massage, 3rd ed. Philadelphia, WB Saunders, 1981
157. Wynn Parry CB: The failed back. In Wall PD, Melzack R (eds): Textbook of Pain, 3rd ed, pp 1075–1094. Edinburgh, Churchill Livingstone, 1994
158. Zachariae R, Kirsten JS, Hokland P, et al: Effect of psychology intervention in the form of relaxation and guided imagery on cellular immune function in normal healthy subjects. Psychother Psychosom 54:32–39, 1990

RECOMMENDED READINGS

GENERAL REFERENCE

Achterberg J: Imagery in Healing: Shamanism and Modern Medicine. Boston, New Science Library, 1985
Bohachick P: Progressive relaxation training in cardiac rehabilitation: Effect on psychologic variables. Nurs Res 22:283, 1984

Gellhorn E: Autonomic Imbalances and the Hypothalamus. Minneapolis, University of Minnesota Press, 1957

Green K, Webster J, Beiman I, et al: Progress and self-induced relaxation training: Their relative effects on subjective and autonomic arousal of fearful stimuli. J Clin Psychol 37:309–315, 1981

Lazarus RS: Psychological Stress and Coping Process. New York, McGraw-Hill, 1966

Lazarus RS: Psychological stress and coping in adaptation and illness. Int J Psychiatry Med 5(4):321–333, 1974

Lynn SJ, Rhue JW: Hypnosis, imagination and fantasy. J Mental Imagery 11:101–113, 1987

Marks DF: Theories of Image Formation. New York, Brandon House, 1986

McKay M, Davis M, Fanning P: Thoughts and Feelings: The Art of Cognitive Stress Intervention. Richmond, CA, New Harbinger Publications, 1981

Rubin R: Mind–brain–body interaction: Elucidation of psychosomatic intervening variables. In Pasnau RO (ed): Consultation-Liaison Psychiatry, pp 73–85. New York, Grune & Stratton, 1975

Selye H: Forty years of stress research: Principal remaining problems and misconceptions. Can Med Assoc J 115:53–56, 1976

Selye H: History and present status of the stress concept. In Goldberger L, Breznits S (eds): Handbook of Stress: Theoretical and Clinical Aspects. New York, The Free Press, 1982

Sheikh A: Imagery: Current Theory, Research, and Application. New York, John Wiley & Sons, 1983

Squires S: The power of positive imagery: Visions to boost immunity. American Health 6:56–61, 1987

Stein M, Schiavi RE, Canerino M: Influence of brain and behavior on the immune system. Science 191:435–440, 1976

Stoyva J, Budzynski TH: Cultivated low arousal—An antistress response? In Dicra LV (ed). Recent Advances in Limbic and Autonomic System Research. New York, Plenum, 1978

Wadden T: Relaxation therapy for essential hypertension: specific or nonspecific effects? J Psychol Res 28:53–61, 1984

RELAXATION AND RELATED TECHNIQUES

Albright GL, Andreassi JL, Brockwell AL: Effects of stress management on blood pressure and other cardiovascular variables. Int J Psychophysiol 11:213–217, 1991

Bell L, Seyfer E: Gentle Yoga. Berkeley, CA, Celestial Arts, 1987

Benson H, Beary JF, Carol MP: The relaxation response. Psychiatry 37:37–45, 1974

Benson H, Kotch JB, Crassweler KD: The relaxation response: A bridge between psychiatry; and medicine. Med Clin North Am 61:929–938, 1977

Benson H, Pomeranz B, Kutz I: The relaxation response and pain. In Wall P, Melzack R (eds): Textbook of Pain, pp 817–822. Edinburgh, Churchill Livingstone, 1984

Bernstein D, Borkovic T: Progressive relaxation training: A manual for the helping profession. Champaign, IL, Research Press, 1973

Borysenko J: Minding the Body, Mending the Mind. Reading, MA, Addison-Wesley, 1987

Bry A: Visualization: Directing the Movies of Our Mind. New York, Barnes & Noble, 1979

Carasso, RL: Treatment of cervical headache with hypnosis, suggestive therapy and relaxation techniques. Am J Clin Hypn 27(4):216–218, 1985

Dimotto JW: Relaxation. Am J Nurs 84:754–758, 1984

French AP, Tupin JP: Therapeutic application of a simple relaxation method. Am J Psychother 28:282–287, 1974

Frownfelter DL: Relaxation principles and techniques. In Frownfelter DL (ed): Chest Physical Therapy and Pulmonary Rehabilitation. Chicago, Year Book Medical Publishers, 1978

Galley PM, Forester AL: Human Movement: An Introductory Text for Physiotherapy Students. London, Churchill Livingstone, 1990

Gaupp LA, Flinn DE, Weddige RL: Adjunctive treatment techniques. In Tollison CD, Satterwaite JR, Tollison JW (eds): Handbook of Pain Amendment, 2nd ed, pp 108–135. Baltimore, Williams & Wilkins, 1994

Goleman D, Schwarts GE: Meditation as an intervention in stress reactivity. J Consult Clin Psychol 44(3):456–466, 1976

Graffam S, Johnson A: A comparison of two relaxation strategies for the relief of pain and its distress. J Pain Symptom Management 2:229–231, 1987

Grzesiak RC: Relaxation techniques in treatment of chronic pain. Arch Phys Med Rehabil 58:270–272, 1977

Hayward C, Piscopo J, Santos A: Physiologic effects of Benson's relaxation response during submaximal aerobic exercise in coronary artery disease patients. J Cardiopulmon Rehabil 7:534–539, 1987

Hillenberg JB, Collins FL: The importance of home practice for progressive relaxation training. Behav Res Ther 21:633–642, 1983

Jaeger B: Are "cervicogenic" headaches due to myofascial pain and cervical spine dysfunction? Cephalagia 9:157–164, 1989

Jessup BA, Gallegos X: Relaxation and biofeedback. In Wall PD, Melzack PD (eds): Text Book of Pain, 3rd ed, pp 1321–1336. Edinburgh, Churchill Livingstone, 1994

Kabat-Zinn J: An outpatient program in behavioral medicine for chronic pain based on the practice of mindfulness meditation: Theoretical considerations and preliminary results. General Hospital Psychiatry 4:33–48, 1982

Kutz I, Borysenko J, Benson H: Meditation and psychotherapy: A rationale for the integration of dynamic psychotherapy, the relaxation response, and mindfulness meditation. Am J Psychol 142:1–8, 1985

Lehrer PM, Woolfolk RL, Rooney AJ, et al: Progressive relaxation and meditation: A study of psychophysiological and therapeutic differences between two techniques. Behav Res Ther 21:651–662, 1983

Leshan L: How to Meditate. New York, Bantam, 1974

Levine S: A Gradual Awakening. Garden City, NY, Anchor Books, 1979

Loehr J, Migdow J: Take a Deep Breath. New York, Villard Books, 1986

Lysaght R, Bodenhamer E: The use of relaxation training to enhance functional outcomes in adults with traumatic head injuries. Am J Occup Ther 44:797–802, 1990

Marshall K: Pain relief in labour. Physiotherapy 67:8–11, 1981

Middaugh SJ: Muscle training. In Doleys DM, Meredith RL, Ciminero AR (eds): Behavioral Medicine: Assessment and Treatment Strategies, pp 145–171. New York, Plenum Press, 1982

Miller KM: Deep breathing relaxation. AORN J 45:484–488, 1987

Mitchell L: The Mitchell method of physiological relaxation. In McGuigan FJ, Sime WE, MacDonald Wallace J (eds): Stress and Tension Control, 2nd ed. New York, Plenum Press, 1984

Morse DR, Martin JS, Furst ML, Dublin LL: A physiological and subjective evaluation of meditation, hypnosis and relaxation. Psychosom Med 39(5):304–324, 1977

Neurnberger P: Freedom from Stress: A Holistic Approach. Honesdale, PA, Himalayan International Institute of Yoga Science and Philosophy Publishers, 1983

Peveler RC, Johnston DW: Subjective and cognitive effects of relaxation. Behav Res Ther 24:413–419, 1986

Phillps HC: Changing chronic pain experience. Pain 32:165–172, 1988

Rossman M: Healing Yourself. New York, Pocket Books, 1990

Schatz MP: Relaxation techniques. In Schatz MP (ed): Basic Care Basics: A Doctor's Gentle Yoga Program for Back and Neck Pain Relief, pp 63–85. Berkeley, CA, Rodmell Press, 1991

Schilling D, Poppen R: Behavioral relaxation training and assessment. J Behav Ther Exp Psychiatry 14:99–107, 1983

Shaw G, Srivastava ED, Sadlier M, et al: Stress management for irritable bowel syndrome: A controlled study. Digestion 50:36–42, 1991

Shea DS, Ohnmeiss DO, Stith WJ, et al: The effect of sensory deprivation in the reduction of pain in patients with chronic low-back pain. Spine 16:560–561, 1990

Showers M: Physical therapy and muscle reeducation. In: Tension Control. Chicago, Chicago Physical Biological Sciences, 1975

Van Dixhoorn J, Duivenvoorden HJ, Staal HA, et al: Cardiac events after myocardial infarction: Possible effects of relaxation therapy. Eur Heart J 8:1210–1214, 1987

Van Dixhoorn J, Duivenvoorden HJ, Staal HA, et al: Physical training and relaxation therapy in cardiac rehabilitation assessed through a composite criterion for training outcome. Am Heart J 118:545–552, 1989

Wallace RK, Benson H: The physiology of meditation. Sci Am 226:84–90, 1972

Weinberger R: Teaching the elderly stress reduction. J Gerontol Nurs 17:23–27, 1991

White J: What is Meditation? New York, Doubleday & Co, 1974

Yorkston JF, Sergeant JD: Simple method of relaxation. Lancet 2:1319–1321, 1960

MANAGEMENT OF STRESS

Bandler R, Grinder J: Frogs into Princes. Moab, UT, Real People Press, 1979

Benson H, Stuart EM: The Wellness Book: The Comprehensive Guide to Maintaining Health and Treating Stress Related Illness. New York, Simon & Schuster, 1992

Bonica J, Fordyce WE: Operant Conditioning for Chronic Pain. Springfield, IL, Charles C Thomas, 1974

Coburn J, Manderino MA: Stress inoculation: An illustration of coping skills training. Rehabil Nurs 11:14–17, 1986

Davis M, Robbins, Eshelman ER, McKay M: The Relaxation & Stress Reduction Workbook. Oakland, CA, Hew Harbinger Publications, 1988

Dettmar DM: The effect of stress release in indices of mandibular dysfunction. Aust Den J 32(1)39–41, 1987

Farquhar JW: The American Way of Life Need Not be Hazardous to Your Health. New York, Norton, 1978

Fletcher DJ, Bezanson D: Coping with stress: How to help patients deal with life's pressure. Postgrad Med 77(4):93–96, 99–100, 1985

Fordyce W: Behavioral Methods for Chronic Pain and Illness. St Louis, CV Mosby, 1976

Kabat-Zinn J: Full Catastrophe Living: Using the Wisdom of Your Body and Mind to Face Stress, Pain and Illness. New York, Delacorte Press, 1990

Kannar AD, Coyne JC, Schaefer C, et al: Comparison of two modes of stress management: daily hassles and uplifts versus major life events. J Behav Med 4:1–39, 1981

Lazarus RS, Folkman S: Coping and adaptation. In Gentry DW (ed): Behavioral Medicine. New York, Guilford Press, 1984

Mandel AR, Keller SM: Stress management in rehabilitation. Arch Phy Med Rehabil 67(6):375–379, 1986

McGuighan FJ, Sime WE, McDonald WJ (eds): Stress and Tension Control, 2nd ed. New York, Plenum Press, 1984

Muse M: Stress-related post traumatic chronic pain syndrome: Behavioral treatment approach. Pain 25(3):389–394, 1986

Ost LG: Applied relaxation: Description of a coping technique and review of controlled studies. Behav Res Ther 25:397–409, 1987

Schwartz GE: Self-regulation of response patterning: Implications for psychophysiological research and therapy. Biofeedback Self Regul 1:7–30, 1976

Schwartz GE, Shapiro D (eds): Consciousness and Self-Regulation. New York, Plenum Press, 1976

Steinmetz J, Blankenship J, Brown L, et al: Managing Stress Before It Manages You. Palo Alto, CA, Bull Publishing, 1982

Stoyva J, Anderson C: A coping rest model of relaxation and stress management. In Goldberger L, Breznitz S (eds): Handbook of Stress: Theoretical and Clinical Aspects. New York, The Free Press, 1982

Whatmore G, Kohli K: The Physiopathology and Treatment of Functional Disorders, Including Anxiety States and Depression and the Role of Biofeedback Training. New York, Grune & Stratton, 1974

Woolfolk RL, Lehrer PM: Principles and Practice of Stress Management. New York, Guilford Press, 1984

BIOFEEDBACK

Asfour SS, Khalil TM, Waly SM, et al: Biofeedback in back muscle strengthening. Spine 15:510–515, 1990

Biedermann HJ, Inglis J, Monga TN, Shanks GL: Differential treatment responses on somatic pain indicators after EMG biofeedback training in back pain patients. Int J Psychosom 36:53–57, 1989

Blanchard EB, Ahles TA: Biofeedback therapy. In Bonica JJ, Loeser JD, Chapman CR, et al (eds): The Management of Pain, 2nd ed, pp 1722–1732. Philadelphia, Lea & Febiger, 1990

Blanchard EB, Applebaum KA, Guarnieri P, et al: A controlled evaluation of thermal biofeedback combined with cognitive therapy in the treatment of vascular headaches. J Consult Clin Psychol 58:216–224, 1990

Blanchard EB, Nicholson NL, Radnitz CL, et al: The role of home practice of thermal biofeedback. J Consult Clin Psychol 59:507–512, 1991

Blanchard E, Young L: Clinical applications of biofeedback training: A review of evidence. Arch Gen Psychiatry 30:573–588, 1974

Budzynski T: Biofeedback procedures in the clinic. Seminars in Psychiatry 5(4):537–547, 1973

Budzynski T, Stoyva J, Adler CS, Mullaney DJ: EMG biofeedback and tension headache: A controlled outcome study. Psychosom Med 35:484–496, 1973

Bush C, Ditto B, Feuerstein M: A controlled evaluation of paraspinal EMG biofeedback in the treatment of chronic low back pain. Health Psychol 4:307–321, 1985

Crockett DJ, Foreman ME, Allen L, et al: A comparison of treatment modes in the management of myofascial pain dysfunction syndrome. Biofeedback Self Regul 11:279–291, 1986

Dalen K, Ellertsen B, Expelid I, et al: EMG feedback in the treatment of myofascial pain dysfunction syndrome. Acta Odontol Scand 44:279–284, 1986

Davis M, Eshelman ER, Mckay M: The Relaxation and Stress Reduction Workbook, 2nd ed. Oakland, CA, New Harbinger, 1982

Duchene P: Effects of biofeedback on childbirth pain. J Pain Symptom Management 4:117–123, 1989

Erland PM, Poppen R: Electromyographic biofeedback and rest position training of masticatory muscles in myofascial pain dysfunction patients. J Prosthet Dent 62:335–338, 1989

Feehan M, Marsh N: The reduction of bruxism using contingent EMG audible biofeedback: A case study. J Behav Ther Exp Psychiatry 20:179–183, 1989

Flor H, Haag G, Turk D: Long-term efficacy of EMG biofeedback for chronic rheumatic back pain. Pain 27:195–202, 1986

Funch CP, Gale EN: Biofeedback and relaxation therapy for chronic temporomandibular joint pain. Consult Clin Psychol 52:928–935, 1984

Gaarder K, Montgomery P: Clinical Biofeedback: A Procedural Manual. Baltimore, Williams & Wilkins, 1977

Gauthier J, Carrier S: Long-term effects of biofeedback on migraine headache: A prospective follow-up study. Headache 31:605–612, 1991

Lynch JJ: Biofeedback: Some reflection on modern behavioral science. Semin Psychiatry; 5(4):551–562, 1972

Middaugh S, Kee WG: Advances in electromyographic monitoring and biofeedback in the treatment of chronic cervical and low back pain. Advances in Rehabilitation Technology 1:137–172, 1987

Miller N: Biofeed: Evaluation of new technique. N Engl J Med 290:685, 1974

Peck C, Kraft G: Electromyographic biofeedback for pain related to muscle tension: A study of tension headache, back and jaw pain. Arch Surg 112:889–895, 1977

Schwartz GE, Sharpiro D; Biofeedback and essential hypertension: Current findings and theoretical concerns. Semin Psychiatry 5:591–603, 1973

Sterman L: Clinical biofeedback. Am J Nurs 75:2006–2009, 1975

Stoyva J: Self-regulation: A context for biofeedback. Biofeedback Self Regul 1:1–6, 1976

Stoyva JM: Guidelines in cultivating general relaxation: Biofeedback and autogenic training combined. In Basmajian JV (ed): Biofeedback: Principles and Practice for Clinicians. Baltimore, Williams & Wilkins, 1983

Stuckey SJ, Jacobs A, Goldfarb J: EMG biofeedback training, relaxation training, and placebo for the relief of chronic back pain. Percept Mot Skills 63:1023–1036, 1986

Turin A, Johnson W: Biofeedback therapy for migraine headaches. Arch Gen Psychiatry 33:517–519, 1976

Turner JA, Chapman CR: Psychological interventions for chronic pain: A Critical review: I. Relaxation training and biofeedback. Pain 12:1–21, 1982

Venables PH, Martin I (eds): Manual of Psychophysiological Methods. Amsterdam, North Holland Pub, 1966

Wells N: The effect of relaxation on postoperative muscle tension and pain. Nurs Res 31:236–238, 1982

Wolf SL, Wolf LB, Segal RL: The relationship of extraneous movements to lumbar paraspinal muscle activity: Implications for EMG biofeedback training applications to low back pain patients. Biofeedback Self Regul 14:63–73, 1989

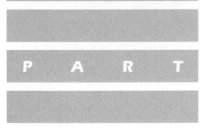

PART TWO

Clinical
Applications—
Peripheral Joints

The Shoulder
and Shoulder Girdle

DARLENE HERTLING AND RANDOLPH M. KESSLER

■ REVIEW OF FUNCTIONAL ANATOMY

Osseous Structures

The osseous components of the functional shoulder girdle include the upper thoracic vertebrae, the first and second ribs, the manubrium, the scapula, the clavicle, and the humerus (Fig. 9-1).[117] For this complex to function adequately, the spine must be stable. To achieve full arm elevation, the upper thoracic vertebrae must be able to extend, rotate, and sidebend to the ipsilateral side, and the bodies of the first and second ribs must be able to descend and move posteriorly (with vertebral rotation). The manubriosternal, costomanubrial, and sternoclavicular joints must permit the manubrium to sidebend and rotate to the ipsilateral side.

The acromioclavicular and sternoclavicular joints provide the mobility of the scapulothoracic mechanism. Movement of the glenohumeral joint provides between 90° (active) and 120° (passive) elevation. For full elevation of the arm, scapular rotation, clavicular elevation, and thoracic extension must accompany humeral elevation. During ipsilateral elevation the upper thoracic vertebrae must be able to extend, rotate, and sidebend to the ipsilateral side, while the lower thoracic vertebrae must sidebend away from the side of motion. For full vertical elevation, exaggeration of lumbar lordosis becomes necessary and is achieved by the action of the spinal muscles.[69]

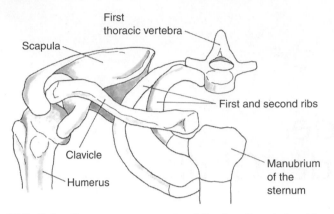

FIG. 9-1. *Osseous components of the functional shoulder girdle.*

Although the joints act interdependently and in concert, we must discuss their structure and movement individually to understand their functions and significance.

☐ Glenohumeral Joint

The humeral head, in the anatomic position, faces medially, slightly posteriorly, and superiorly. The head forms almost half a sphere, with an angular value of about 150°. It forms an angle of about 45° with the humeral shaft (Fig. 9-2).

The glenoid cavity faces laterally, forward, and superiorly. It has an angular value of only 75°. This incongruity between the humeral head and the glenoid cavity is partially compensated for by the fibrous or fi-

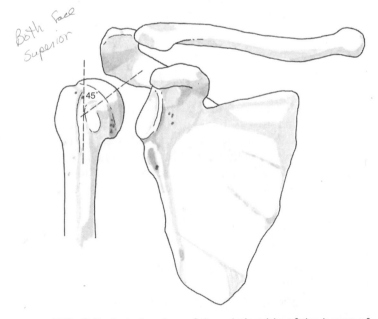

FIG. 9-2. *Anterior view of the relationship of the bones of the glenohumeral joint.*

brocartilaginous glenoid labrum, which serves to deepen the glenoid cavity. The glenoid is pear-shaped—narrow superiorly and wider inferiorly.

☐ Acromioclavicular Joint

The clavicle is S-shaped, the lateral third being concave anteriorly (Fig. 9-3*A*). This provides for extra motion during elevation of the arm (see Biomechanics below). The articular surface of the clavicle is convex. The concave articular surface of the acromion process faces medially and somewhat anterosuperiorly. This joint is oriented in such a way that a strong compression force tends to cause the clavicle to override the acromion. This is what occurs in an acromioclavicular separation, usually caused by a fall on the tip of the acromion.

☐ Sternoclavicular Joint

The sternal end of the clavicle is somewhat bulbous. It is convex in the frontal plane and has a slight concavity anteroposteriorly. It articulates with the upper lateral edge of the manubrium, as well as with the superior surface of the medial aspect of the cartilage of the first rib. It tends to extend above the superior surface of the manubrium by as much as half its width.

☐ Scapulothoracic Mechanism

The scapulothoracic joint complex or mechanism (Fig. 9-4) is not a true anatomic joint, because it has none of the usual joint characteristics. Movements are inescapably associated with the sternoclavicular and acromioclavicular joints. These two anatomic joints and the functional thoracic joint form a closed kinetic chain in which movement in one joint invariably causes motion in the other.

The scapula, viewed from above at rest, makes an angle of about 30° with the frontal plane (see Fig. 9-3*A*). It makes an angle of about 60° with the clavicle, viewed from above.

The medial portion of the scapular spine usually lies level with the T3 spinous process, whereas the inferior angle lies level with the T7 or T8 spinous process. The medial border lies about 6 cm lateral to the thoracic spinous processes.

☐ Ligaments

GLENOHUMERAL JOINT

The articular capsule of the glenohumeral joint (see Fig. 9-4) is quite thin and lax, with redundant folds sit-

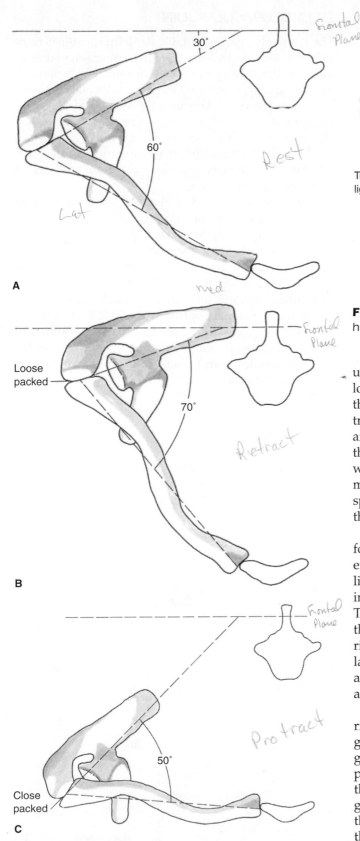

Frontal Plane

30°

60°

Rest

Lat

med

A

Loose packed

Frontal Plane

70°

Retract

B

Frontal Plane

50°

Protract

Close packed

C

FIG. 9-3. Acromioclavicular, sternoclavicular, and scapulothoracic articulations shown (**A**) at rest, (**B**) in retraction, and (**C**) in protraction.

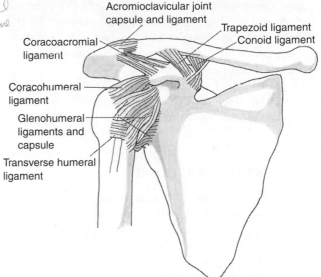

Acromioclavicular joint capsule and ligament

Trapezoid ligament

Conoid ligament

Coracoacromial ligament

Coracohumeral ligament

Glenohumeral ligaments and capsule

Transverse humeral ligament

FIG. 9-4. Anterior view of the ligaments of the glenohumeral and acromioclavicular joints.

uated anteroinferiorly when the arm is at rest. This allows a full range of elevation. Because of the laxity of the joint capsule, the head of the humerus can be distracted laterally about 2 cm in the cadaver, with the arm in a position of slight abduction. With the arm at the side, the superior joint capsule remains taut, whereas the rest of the capsule assumes a forward and medial twist. The tendons of the supraspinatus, infraspinatus, teres minor, and subscapularis blend with the fibers of the joint capsule.

The glenohumeral ligaments provide some reinforcement to the capsule anteriorly, helping to check external rotation. The middle glenohumeral ligament limits lateral rotation up to 90° abduction and is an important anterior stabilizer of the shoulder joint.[134] The inferior glenohumeral ligament is the thickest of the glenohumeral structures and attaches to the anterior, inferior, and posterior margins of the glenoid labrum.[128,143] It strengthens the capsule anteriorly and inferiorly, helping to prevent anterior subluxation and dislocation.[134]

The coracohumeral ligament strengthens the superior capsule and is important in maintaining the glenohumeral relationship. The downward pull of gravity on the arm is counteracted largely by the superior capsule and the coracohumeral ligament. From the root of the coracoid process, it extends to the greater and lesser tubercles of the humerus beneath the supraspinatus tendon. The ligament blends with the rotator cuff and fills in the space between the subscapularis and the supraspinatus muscles.[114] Tension develops mainly in the anterior band during extension and in the posterior band during flexion. The anterior band, running somewhat anteriorly to the vertical axis about which rotation occurs, checks external rotation and perhaps extension. The tension in the posterior band is thought to be a factor in assisting the glenohumeral ligament in medial rotation of the shoulder during flexion.[13,111]

The transverse humeral ligament traverses the intertubercular (bicipital) groove, acting as a retinaculum for the tendon of the long head of the biceps.

ACROMIOCLAVICULAR JOINT

The major ligaments of the acromioclavicular joint (see Fig. 9-4) are the superior and inferior acromioclavicular ligaments and the coracoclavicular ligaments. The superior and inferior ligaments offer some protection to the joint and help prevent overriding of the clavicle on the acromion.

Although situated away from the joint, the coracoclavicular ligaments are of the most importance in providing acromioclavicular joint stability.

The trapezoid ligament lies almost horizontally in the frontal plane and is positioned in such a way that it can check overriding, or lateral, movement of the clavicle on the acromion. It also helps prevent excessive narrowing of the angle between the acromion and clavicle (viewed from above), as occurs with protraction.

The conoid ligament is oriented vertically, medial to the trapezoid ligament, and is twisted on itself. It primarily checks superior movement of the clavicle on the acromion; it also prevents excessive widening of the scapuloclavicular angle. As the arm is abducted, the scapula rotates in such a way that the inferior angle swings laterally and superiorly. This movement increases the distance between the clavicle and the coracoid process, pulling the conoid ligament taut. This tightening causes posterior or external (backward axial) rotation of the clavicle, bringing the acromioclavicular joint back into apposition (because of the S shape of the clavicle). It is necessary for full elevation of the arm (see Biomechanics below).

These ligaments suspend the scapula from the clavicle and transmit the force of the superior fibers of the trapezius to the scapula.[20] Anteriorly, the space between the ligaments is filled with fat and frequently a bursa. In up to 30% of subjects the bony components may be opposed closely and may form a coracoclavicular joint.[20,154]

The coracoacromial ligament, the acromion, and the coracoid process form an important protective arch over the glenohumeral joint (see Fig. 9-4).[96] The arch forms a secondary restraining socket for the humeral head, preventing dislocation of the humeral head superiorly. This arch can be the site of impingement on the greater tubercle, supraspinatus tendon, or subdeltoid bursa in cases of abnormal joint mechanics.

STERNOCLAVICULAR JOINT

The relatively lax sternoclavicular joint capsule is reinforced anteriorly by the anterior sternoclavicular ligament, posteriorly by the posterior sternoclavicular ligaments, and superiorly by the interclavicular ligament (Fig. 9-5). The costoclavicular ligament lies just lateral to the joint. Its anterior fibers run superiorly and laterally, and check elevation and lateral movement of the clavicle. The posterior fibers run superiorly and medially from the first rib, and check elevation and medial movement of the clavicle.

An intra-articular disk is attached above to the clavicle and below to the first costal cartilage and the sternum. It is especially important in helping to prevent medial dislocation of the clavicle, which can occur with a fall on the outstretched arm or on the point of the shoulder. Invariably the clavicle will break or the acromioclavicular joint will dislocate before the sternoclavicular joint dislocates medially. This is true despite the fact that the medial sloping of the joint surfaces and the superior overlap of the clavicle on the sternum would seem to make the joint susceptible to medial dislocation.

☐ **Bursae**

There are usually considered to be eight or nine bursae about the shoulder joint. Practically speaking, only two are worth considering here, because of their clinical significance.

SUBACROMIAL OR SUBDELTOID BURSA

The subacromial or subdeltoid bursa extends over the supraspinatus tendon and distal muscle belly beneath the acromion and deltoid muscle. At times it extends beneath the coracoid process (Fig. 9-6A). It is attached above to the acromial arch and below to the rotator cuff tendons and greater tubercle. It does not normally communicate with the joint capsule but may in

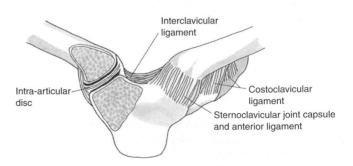

FIG. 9-5. *The sternoclavicular joint.*

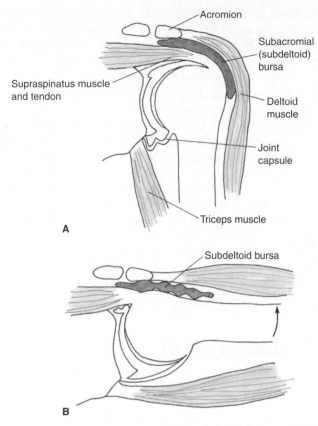

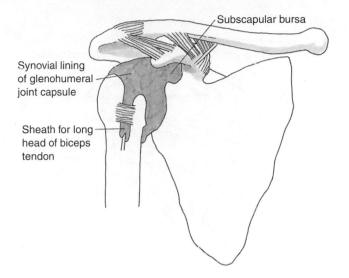

FIG. 9-7. *The subscapular bursa.*

FIG. 9-6. (**A**) *The subacromial (subdeltoid) bursa.* (**B**) *As the humerus elevates, the bursal tissue gathers beneath the acromion.*

the case of a rotator cuff tear. This is seen on arthrography as dye leaking over the top of the supraspinatus tendon. The bursa is susceptible to impingement beneath the acromial arch, especially if it is inflamed and swollen (Fig. 9-6B). Inflammation of the bursa is often attributed to rupture of a supraspinatus calcium deposit superiorly into the underside of the bursa.

SUBSCAPULAR BURSA

The subscapular bursa overlies the anterior joint capsule and lies beneath the subscapularis muscle. It communicates with the joint capsule and fills with dye on arthrography. Articular effusion may be manifested clinically by an anterior swelling, due to distention of the bursa (Fig. 9-7).

☐ Vascular Anatomy of the Rotator Cuff Tendons

The tendons of the rotator cuff include the supraspinatus, infraspinatus, teres minor, and subscapularis. As implied by the term *rotator cuff*, they are not discrete tendons but blend to form a continuous cuff

surrounding the posterior, superior, and anterior aspects of the humeral head. The fibers of the tendinous cuff attach to the articular capsule of the glenohumeral joint by blending with it. This allows the cuff to provide dynamic stabilization of the joint.

The rotator cuff is a frequent site of lesions—usually of a degenerative nature—in response to fatigue stresses. Lesions usually affect the supraspinatus and to a lesser extent the infraspinatus portions of the cuff. Since such degeneration often occurs with normal activity levels, the nutritional status of this frequently involved area of the cuff is of particular interest. Most fatigue or degenerative lesions occur either from increased stress levels or from a nutritional deficit.

The primary blood supply to the rotator cuff tendons is derived from six arteries, three of which contribute in virtually all persons and three of which are sometimes absent (Fig. 9-8).[104] The posterior humeral circumflex and the suprascapular arteries are usually present; they supply primarily the infraspinatus and teres minor areas of the cuff. The subscapularis is supplied by the anterior humeral circumflex artery, which is usually present; the thoracoacromial artery, which is occasionally absent; and the suprahumeral and subscapular arteries, which are often absent. The supraspinatus region receives its supply primarily from the thoracoacromial artery, which as mentioned is not always present. This artery anastomoses with the two circumflex arteries, which also contribute some to the supraspinatus region.

The most significant feature of the blood supply to the rotator cuff is that the supraspinatus and to a lesser extent the infraspinatus regions of the cuff are often considerably hypovascular with respect to the rest of the tendinous cuff. This has been confirmed by injection studies as well as by histological sections.

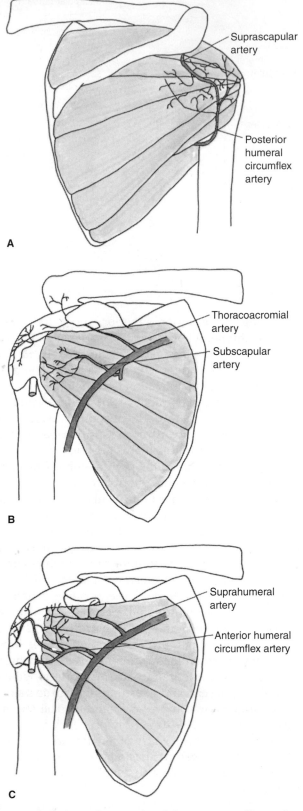

A

B

C

FIG. 9-8. *Vascular supply of the rotator cuff muscles: (**A**) posterior view, (**B**) anterior view, showing the thoracoacromial and subscapular arteries, and (**C**) anterior view, showing the suprahumeral and anterior humeral circumflex arteries.*

Rothman and Parke found that regardless of age, the supraspinatus region was hypovascular in 63% of 72 specimens, and that the infraspinatus region was hypovascular in 37%.[124] When the infraspinatus was undervascularized, so was the supraspinatus. Hypovascularity was demonstrated in the subscapularis region in only 7% of the specimens.

Clinically, the relative incidence of tendinitis in these tendons correlates well with the above relative incidences of hypovascularity. Also, the incidence of shoulder tendinitis tends to increase with advancing age, which is consistent with the findings that tendon hypovascularity in general progresses with age.[104]

It has been proposed that the hypovascularity in the supraspinatus region is at least partly the result of pressure applied to the underside of the tendon by the superior aspect of the humeral head as the tendon passes around and over its insertion on the greater tubercle of the humerus.[87]

■ BIOMECHANICS

□ Joint Stabilization

As mentioned above, the glenohumeral joint capsule is relatively lax. This is somewhat unusual, because most joints rely primarily on their capsules and ligaments to maintain proper orientation of joint surfaces during movement and in response to external forces. The shoulder joint capsule does provide some stabilization of the joint when the arm is at the side, and it does help guide movement of the joint. At the shoulder, however, the muscles also play an essential role in these functions. The shoulder, then, relies on active and passive stabilizing components to maintain joint integrity. This is necessary at the glenohumeral joint because the incongruent bony constituents confer little intrinsic stability, such as that present at the hip joint.

When the arm hangs freely to the side, the superior joint capsule and coracohumeral ligament are normally taut, and the plane of the glenoid cavity faces somewhat upward. A vertical force produced by the weight of the hanging arm is met by a reactive tensile force to the superior joint capsule. The result of these two forces is a force that tends to pull the head of the humerus in against the upward-facing glenoid cavity (Fig. 9-9). In this way the tightness of the superior joint capsule and the orientation of the glenoid stabilize the humerus when the arm hangs freely at the side. Little or no muscle contraction by the deltoid or the rotator cuff muscles is necessary to prevent inferior subluxation of the humerus, even when some weight is held in the hanging hand.[5,6]

Once the arm is elevated from the side in any plane,

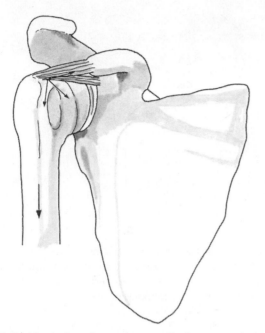

FIG. 9-9. Vertical and reactive tensile forces to the superior joint capsule when the arm is hanging freely at the side.

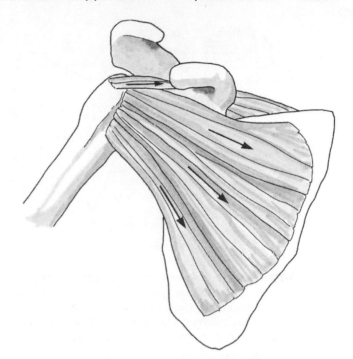

FIG. 9-11. Rotator cuff muscles contract to hold the humerus in proper orientation with respect to the glenoid during movement of the arm.

tension is lost in the superior joint capsule so that it can no longer contribute to the maintenance of joint integrity (Fig. 9-10). Now the rotator cuff muscles, supraspinatus, subscapularis, and teres minor must contract to hold the humerus in a proper orientation with respect to the glenoid cavity during arm move-

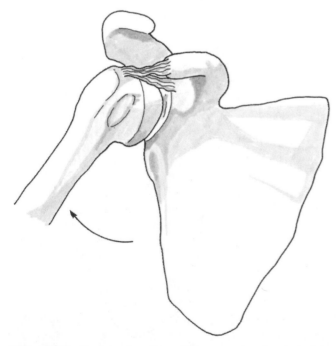

FIG. 9-10. During elevation of the arm, tension is lost in the superior joint capsule.

ment (Fig. 9-11). In this way, the rotator cuff tendons, which blend with the joint capsule, provide for stabilization of the glenohumeral joint when the arm is held away from the side.[5–7,30,64]

Clinically there are some common conditions in which these normal stabilizing mechanisms are compromised. The two common causes are alterations in the normal structural alignment of the bony constituents of the shoulder girdle, and rotator cuff muscle weakness. In a person with a thoracic kyphosis, the scapula follows the contour of the thorax and assumes a downward rotated position; the glenoid cavity no longer faces upward. Also, in this position the freely hanging humerus assumes a position of relative abduction with respect to the scapula, and tension is lost in the superior joint capsule (Fig. 9-12). In this situation, the rotator cuff muscles must contract to maintain joint integrity with the arm at the side, thus preventing inferior subluxation of the humerus. Therefore, the person with a thoracic kyphotic deformity must maintain increased tone in the rotator cuff muscles to compensate for the loss of capsular stabilization. Thoracic kyphosis may be an etiological factor in some cases of frozen shoulder. The increased tone of the rotator cuff muscles results in increased tensile stresses to the joint capsule, with which the rotator cuff tendons blend (Fig. 9-13). The increased stress to the capsule stimulates an increase in collagen production, which leads to a gradual loss of extensibility of the capsule—in other words, capsular fibrosis.

In the patient with shoulder girdle muscle paresis, a

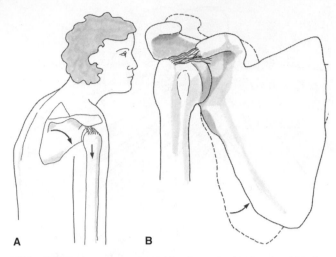

FIG. 9-12. In a person with thoracic kyphosis, (**A**) the scapula assumes a downward, rotated position so that the glenoid fossa no longer faces upward, and (**B**) the freely hanging humerus assumes a position of relative abduction with loss of tension in the superior joint capsule.

similar situation may exist; the weakness of the scapular muscles allows the scapula to assume a downward rotated position on the chest wall (Fig. 9-14A). The common condition in which this occurs is hemiplegia following a stroke. In these patients, rotator cuff muscle activity may also be reduced, and the arm is predisposed to inferior subluxation because of the loss of active and passive stabilizing components (Fig. 9-14B).

☐ Influence of the Glenohumeral Joint Capsule on Movement

The orientation and configuration of the shoulder joint capsule play a major role in determining the degree and type of movement that occur at the joint. When the arm hangs freely to the side, the fibers of the joint capsule are oriented in a forward and medial

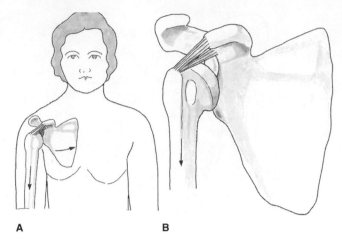

FIG. 9-14. In the person with shoulder-girdle muscle paresis, (**A**) the scapula assumes a downward, rotated position on the chest wall, and (**B**) reduced rotator-cuff tension predisposes to inferior subluxation.

twist (Fig. 9-15).[66] Because the plane of the scapula is oriented midway between the frontal and sagittal planes,[74,118] this capsular twist is increased with abduction (elevation in the frontal plane) and decreased with flexion (elevation in the sagittal plane) (Fig. 9-16).[74,118] Thus, as the arm swings into abduction, the increasing twist in the joint capsule begins to pull the head of the humerus in tightly against the glenoid cavity, and the tension in the capsular fibers gradually increases as the twisting continues. The tension eventually causes the capsule to pull the humerus around

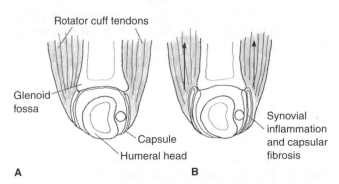

FIG. 9-13. Transverse section of the glenohumeral joint depicting (**A**) normal and (**B**) increased cuff tension.

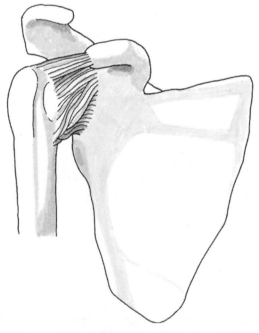

FIG. 9-15. Anterior view of the orientation of the fibers of the joint capsule when the arm hangs freely at the side.

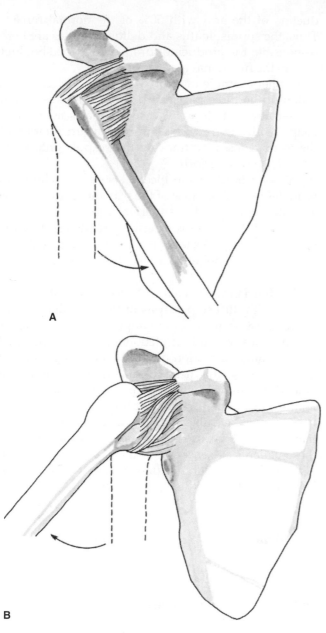

A

B

FIG. 9-16. Capsular twist is (**A**) decreased with flexion and (**B**) increased with abduction.

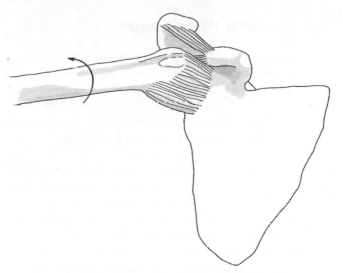

FIG. 9-17. Capsular pull results in external rotation of the humerus and "untwisting" of the capsule during abduction.

tion that tends to increase the twist. If lateral rotation does not occur, full movement is restricted because the joint locks and the greater tubercle impinges on the acromial arch (Fig. 9-18).

A common condition in which external rotation of the humerus becomes restricted is frozen shoulder. With capsular fibrosis at the shoulder, the anterior joint capsule becomes especially tight. The capsule adheres to the anterior aspect of the humeral head, while the redundant folds of the capsule situated anteroinferiorly adhere to one another.[101] In the presence of capsular tightness at the shoulder, abduction is restricted by locking and impingement; this movement should not be forced until external rotation is gained.

into external rotation (Fig. 9-17). This external rotation untwists the joint capsule and allows further movement. If the humerus were not to rotate externally, the joint would lock at the midrange of abduction from the combined effects of abnormal compression of joint surfaces and excessive tension on the capsular fibers. The external rotation that occurs also causes the greater tubercle to clear the coracoacromial arch during abduction.[25,64,84] In this way, the external rotation of the humerus that takes place during abduction is a passive phenomenon, occurring as a result of the twisted configuration of the glenohumeral joint capsule, combined with the fact that abduction involves movement out of the plane of the scapula in a direc-

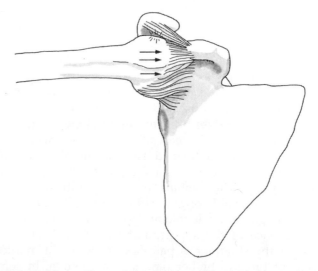

FIG. 9-18 Locking of the joint and impingement of the greater tubercle results if lateral humeral rotation does not occur during abduction.

☐ Muscular Force Couple

The rotator cuff muscles act with the deltoid muscle in a force-couple mechanism during elevation to guide the humerus in its movement on the glenoid cavity.[32,64,84,120,123] The force of elevation, together with active inward and downward pull of the short rotator muscles, establishes the muscle force-couple necessary for limb elevation. When the arm is by the side, the direction of the deltoid muscle force is upward and outward with respect to the humerus, whereas the force of the infraspinatus, teres minor, and subscapularis is inward and downward. The force of the deltoid muscle, acting below the center of rotation, is opposite that of the force of the three rotator muscles applied above the center of rotation and produces a powerful force-couple.[10]

Some anatomists consider the primary function of the supraspinatus muscle to be only the initiation of abduction, thus necessitating contraction of the rotator cuff muscle for the arm to be swung from the side. However, Howell and associates have observed that in the shoulder with a paralyzed supraspinatus muscle, the deltoid can initiate and generate a significant torque from 0° to 30° elevation in the plane of the scapula.[63]

For the glenohumeral joint to be stable and functional within its range, the muscles must generate sufficient force throughout the entire range. The deltoid is well suited in two ways to fulfill this need. First, the muscle fibers are in a multipennate arrangement.[56,117] Functionally, this means there is less change in length of each fiber while providing maximal force during contraction. For a muscle to be powerful, it must develop maximal tension over the range as quickly as possible. This is accomplished better in a multipennate arrangement. Therefore, multipennate muscles are more powerful than muscles with parallel fibers. The second reason why the deltoid is well designed to provide stability to the glenohumeral joint is related to its attachments. Arising from the scapular spine, acromial arch, and clavicle, the deltoid has a broad base and a large muscle mass. More importantly, the origins can be raised during humeral elevation. This scapular rotation decreases the range over which the deltoid must contract during humeral elevation, which in turn increases muscle power throughout the entire range. The combination of the multipennate design and movable origin is of considerable functional advantage for the deltoid and glenohumeral joints.[29]

Absence of the supraspinatus muscle alone, provided the shoulder is pain-free, produces a marked loss of force in higher ranges of abduction. In complete loss of deltoid muscle function, the rotator cuff (including the supraspinatus muscle) can produce abduction of the arm with 50% of the normal force.[10] Thus, the supraspinatus and deltoid muscles are both responsible for producing torque about the shoulder joint in the functional planes of motion.

Another example of a force-couple is the combined action of the three parts of the trapezius muscle and the serratus anterior.[86] The serratus acts as a force-couple with the trapezius during upward rotation of the glenoid fossa by tracking the scapula anteriorly, laterally, and superiorly.[25]

The long head of the biceps also aids in humeral head depression because of the way the tendon acts as a pulley around the superior aspect of the humerus.[64,84] If the arm is externally rotated so that the bicipital groove faces laterally, the long head of the biceps works as a pulley to assist in arm abduction (Fig. 9-19).

The clinician who deals with stroke patients, or any patient with diffuse paralysis of the shoulder musculature, must be aware of the importance of the rotator cuff muscles in guiding glenohumeral movement. If passive range of motion of the shoulder is performed in such cases, the head of the humerus must be guided into inferior glide (depression) passively during flexion and abduction. If it is not, the subacromial tissues may be subjected to repeated trauma. This may explain the onset of shoulder pain in many of these patients as sensation to the shoulder returns. It also emphasizes that "routine" range of motion must be performed by a skilled professional.[100]

☐ Analysis of Shoulder Abduction

When we consider function at the shoulder, we must be concerned with the contribution of several joints in addition to the glenohumeral articulation. These include the acromioclavicular joint, the sternoclavicular joint, the articulation between the scapula and the thorax, the joints of the lower cervical and upper thoracic spine, and the articulation between the coracoacromial arch and the subacromial tissues. An analysis of the function of each of these structures during abduction of the arm emphasizes the importance of a normal interplay between the components of the shoulder complex.

During the first 15° to 30° abduction, much of the movement occurs at the glenohumeral joint, although this varies among people.[44,64,82] During this early phase, the muscles controlling the scapula contract to stabilize the scapula against the chest wall, preparing it for subsequent movement. Because the glenohumeral joint capsule is twisted forward and medially at the starting position, and because abduction is a movement of the humerus out of the plane of the

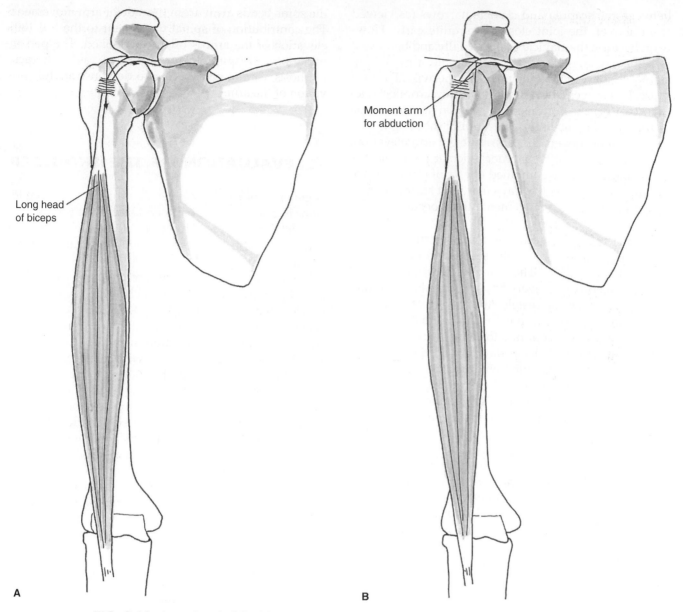

Long head
of biceps

Moment arm
for abduction

A   B

FIG. 9-19. Long head of the biceps acts in the muscular force-couple to create (**A**) vertical and reactive tensile forces and (**B**) moment arm during humeral elevation.

scapula, the medial twist of the capsule begins to increase as abduction proceeds.[66]*

Beginning at 15° to 30° abduction, the scapula begins to move to contribute to arm elevation. In doing so, it moves forward, elevates, and rotates upward on the chest wall. Much of this movement of the scapula can occur because of movement at the sternoclavicular joint; the clavicle protracts about 30°, elevates

about 30°, and rotates backward around its long axis about 50°.[31,64,84] The acromioclavicular joint contributes much less to scapular movement because its planar joint surfaces do not allow much angular movement. The scapula rotates some at the acromioclavicular joint at the beginning of scapular movement. Viewed from above, the angle between the scapula and clavicle narrows as the scapula slides around and forward on the chest wall (see Fig. 9-3C). The rotation that the scapula undergoes in the frontal plane, with respect to the clavicle, causes the conoid ligament to tighten. Since this ligament attaches to the backside of the clavicle, as it pulls tight, it pulls the clavicle into a backward axial rotation. As the angle

*The increasing medial twist is a result of medial conjunct rotation from movement of the humerus around the medial axis as defined at the beginning of movement. This occurs because abduction is an impure swing in which the humerus moves out of the plane of the scapula.

between the scapula and clavicle narrows (as viewed from above), the joint close-packs quite early. However, because the clavicle rotates axially and because it is S-shaped, the joint surfaces maintain a more constant relationship than they would otherwise. Furthermore, less movement is required of the acromioclavicular joint because of this axial rotation and the shape of the clavicle (Fig. 9-20). Thus, out of the roughly 60° that scapular movement contributes to arm elevation, about 30° occurs at the sternoclavicular joint, and the rest occurs from the combined effects of clavicular rotation, which causes the clavicular joint surface to face upward, and the movement that occurs at the acromioclavicular joint.

From 15° or 30° abduction, the humerus continues to elevate with respect to the scapula through a total of 90° to 110°.[9,44,64,84] The humerus contributes about 10° of movement for every 5° contributed by scapular motion. As the humerus elevates, the greater tubercle begins to approximate the coracoacromial arch, and the capsular fibers continue to twist medially. Once a certain amount of tension develops in the joint capsule, the capsule pulls the humerus around into a lateral axial rotation, causing the greater tubercle to be directed behind and beneath the acromion. As this occurs the subdeltoid bursal tissue is gathered proximally beneath the acromion (see Fig. 9-6). If the bursa is distended, or if the tubercle rides too high or does not rotate laterally, subacromial impingement will occur, with either loss of movement or chronic trauma to the subacromial tissues, or both.

The combined glenohumeral and scapular movements contribute about 160° to the full range of abduction. The remaining movement occurs as a result of movement at the lower cervical and upper thoracic spines. If both arms are raised simultaneously, extension occurs at these regions. In unilateral abduction, the spine bends away from the side of arm movement. The contribution of spinal movement to the full 180° elevation of the arm is often overlooked. The person with a fixed spinal deformity, such as a thoracic kyphosis, cannot be expected to demonstrate full elevation of the arm.

■ EVALUATION OF THE SHOULDER

A general approach to the evaluation of soft-tissue lesions is discussed in Chapter 5, Assessment of Musculoskeletal Disorders. However, there are additional concepts and techniques specific to evaluation of the shoulder region.

The shoulder and the arm are common sites of referred pain from other areas, such as the myocardium, cervical region, and diaphragm. Usually the history will suggest the origin of pain. If not, a scan examination consisting of active motion of the neck and all major upper-extremity joints, with passive overpressure at the extremes of each motion, may be useful in reproducing the pain and suggesting the site of the lesion. In discussing examination of the shoulder itself, we assume that the physician's examination, the history, or the scan examination has localized the lesion to the shoulder region. The clinician's in-depth examination clarifies the nature and extent of the lesion so that prescribed treatment modalities may be safely and effectively applied; it also establishes a baseline for judging progress.

I. History
  A. *Specific questions* for shoulder lesions:
    1. Does the pain ever spread to below the elbow?
    2. Can the patient lie on the shoulder at night?
    3. Can the patient use the arm to comb his or her hair?
    4. Can the patient reach into a hip pocket or fasten a bra behind her?
    5. Can the patient eat comfortably with the arm?
    6. Does it hurt to put on or remove a shirt or jacket?
    7. Is it difficult to perform activities that require reaching above shoulder level?
  B. *Site of pain*—Except in acromioclavicular joint sprains, pain is seldom felt at the shoulder itself but rather over the lateral brachial region. It may spread to all or any part of the limb innervated by that spinal segment, from which the glenohumeral joint structures are primarily derived, usually the C5 segment or, in the case

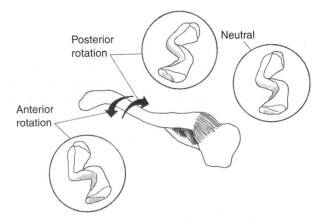

FIG. 9-20. Clavicular rotation in the sagittal plane, as viewed from the proximal end of the clavicle and the frontal plane.

of acromioclavicular problems, the C4 sclerotome (see Figs. 4-1, 4-3, and 5-4).

C. *Nature of pain*—Common lesions at the shoulder tend to be aggravated by use and relieved by rest. Patients with capsular lesions give a history of painful limitation, especially with movements into external rotation and abduction. Patients with noncapsular lesions often present with painful "twinges" during various functions, such as donning a jacket or reaching above shoulder level. In acute bursitis, which is relatively rare, the pain may become quite intense and is often felt even at rest.

D. *Onset of pain*—Except in athletic settings, a history of trauma does not accompany most common shoulder lesions. More often the onset is insidious, as in tendinitis or capsular tightening. In these, the onset is very gradual, whereas in acute bursitis, the patient notes a rapid buildup of pain over 12 to 72 hours.

E. *General health*—The final set of subjective questions should consider the patient's general health, in particular disorders of the cardiac and visceral organs that may cause pain to be referred to the shoulder region (*e.g.*, diaphragmatic irritation, cardiac ischemia, gallbladder problems, pancreatic disease).[14]

II. **Physical Examination**

A. *Observation*
1. Posture of the arm and shoulder girdle
   a. Does the patient hold the arm close to the side or across the chest?
   b. Does the patient tend to support the arm?
2. Function, particularly dressing, and general willingness to use the arm

B. *Inspection*
1. Structure. Observe the patient in a relaxed standing position for
   a. Upper spinal curvatures
   b. Shoulder heights
   c. Bony relationships—acromioclavicular joint; acromion-to-greater-tubercle distance; sternoclavicular joint
   d. Position of scapulae. Note any winging of the scapula. Winging may be due to pseudowinging[43] (*e.g.*, asymmetry of the bony anatomy, as in scoliosis), generalized neuropathy or neuropathy of the long thoracic nerve,[18,43,48,50,90,129,135] muscle injury or muscle disease[79] (*e.g.*, muscular dystrophy), or voluntary winging.[135] This phenomenon, commonly seen in swimmers, is normal.[135] The most common cause of scapular

winging is trauma or overuse injury of the long thoracic nerve.
   e. Rotary position of the humerus hanging freely at the side, as judged by the orientation of the epicondyles and antecubital space
   f. Step deformities over the shoulder. Such a deformity may be caused by an acromioclavicular deformity, with the distal end of the clavicle lying superior to the acromion process. Flattening of the normally round deltoid may indicate an anterior dislocation of the glenohumeral joint or atrophy of the deltoid muscle. If deformity appears when traction is applied to the arm, it may be secondary to multidirectional instability, leading to inferior subluxation. This deformity is referred to as a *sulcus sign*.[89,108]

2. Soft tissues. With the patient sitting, observe for
   a. Atrophy—especially over the shoulder girdles
   b. Swelling
      i. Anteriorly for joint effusion
      ii. Laterally for bursal swelling
      iii. Entire extremity for edema, as from reflex sympathetic dystrophy
   c. General contours—note asymmetries
3. Skin (entire extremity and shoulder girdle)
   a. Color
   b. Moisture
   c. Texture
   d. Scars and blemishes

C. *Selective tissue tension tests*
1. Active movements (sitting). Before observing ipsilateral movements of the shoulder girdle, observe synchrony of motion or identical movements of the shoulder girdle bilaterally.[113] Have the patient simultaneously and sequentially abduct the arms to 90° with the elbows in 90° flexion and neutral glenohumeral rotation; horizontally extend and externally rotate the shoulders. By observing from the rear, one can notice asynchrony in such areas as shoulder elevation, indicating use of the upper trapezius to assist in abducting the arm; oscillating movements of the scapula, indicating the inability to fixate the scapula; muscle fasciculations, indicating local muscle weakness or fatigue; and excessive lateral rotation of the scapula during external rotation, indicating a tight anterior capsule that limits external rotation.

a. Observation

   i. Routine active movements of the shoulder girdle—protraction, retraction, elevation, circumduction, and depression

   ii. Detailed examination with applied passive overpressure at the limits of each active shoulder movement

     —Flexion and extension (observe the scapulohumeral rhythm posteriorly)

     —Abduction (determine whether a painful arc exists)

     —Horizontal adduction

     —External rotation (arm at side with forearm at 90° flexion)

     —Internal rotation with back of hand moving up between scapulae

   iii. Note these factors:

     —Willingness to move

     —Limited range and what appears to limit it

     —Quality of movement

     —Nature of end feel

     —Presence of crepitus

     —Presence and nature of pain

     —Presence of a painful arc

2. Passive movements (supine)

  a. Perform

   i. Flexion and extension

   ii. Internal/external rotation (with elbow bent and arm at 45° abduction)

   iii. Abduction (note painful arc)

   iv. Horizontal adduction

  b. Record

   i. Range of motion

   ii. Pain

   iii. End feel

   iv. Crepitus

3. Resisted isometric movements (supine)

  a. Strong isometric contractions with the arm close to the side (material in parentheses indicates tendons most commonly involved if test is positive)

   i. Internal rotation (subscapularis)

   ii. External rotation with arm close to side (infraspinatus)

   iii. External rotation with arm at 75° abduction (teres minor)

   iv. Abduction with arm close to side (supraspinatus)

   v. Elbow flexion (long head of biceps)

   vi. Forearm supination (biceps)

   vii. Others as necessary for differentiation of the status of the musculotendinous tissue

  b. Record whether strong or weak, painful or painless

4. Joint-play movements

  a. Glenohumeral joint. Tests may be performed either in sitting or supine position. For most of the tests, the open-packed position (resting position) should be used (55° to 70° abduction; 30° horizontal abduction).

   i. Inferior glide (sitting; see Fig. 9-29*A*)

   ii. Inferior glide (supine) (see Fig. 9-28*F*)

   iii. Lateral glide (distraction) with the arm at side (see Fig. 9-32*B*)

   iv. Posterior glide (supine) (see Fig. 9-30*A*)

   v. Anterior glide (prone) (see Fig. 9-31*B*)

  b. Compare to other arm and record

   i. Amplitude of joint play (normal, restricted, hypermobile)

   ii. Presence of pain or muscle guarding

  c. Passive joint-play movements may need to include tests for the cervical and upper thoracic spine and the following related joints:

   i. Sternoclavicular joint (see Fig. 9-34*A-D*)

   ii. Acromioclavicular joint (see Fig. 9-35*A-C*)

   iii. Scapulothoracic mechanism (see Fig. 9-38*A,B*)

D. *Neuromuscular tests*—These tests may be performed if neurological involvement is suspected, such as that following anterior humeral dislocation, or that accompanying a cervical nerve root impingement (see Chap. 5, Assessment of Musculoskeletal Disorders).

1. Included might be upper-extremity muscle testing, sensory testing, and reflex testing (see Tables 5-6, 5-7).

2. Neural tension tests (also known as the brachial tension test and upper limb tension tests).[20,21,38–42,51,68,70,91] Tests of neural tension proposed for the upper limb, upper limb tension tests (ULTTs), have been developed much more recently than those for the lower limb and trunk. Elvey[38] and the Western Australia Institute of Technology are continuing this valuable work. ULTTs are recommended for all patients with symptoms in the arm, head, neck, and thoracic spine.[20,21,91] Since methods of testing for movement of the cervical nerve roots or their sleeves are not yet clear-cut and continue to be developed and modified, the reader should refer to the most current literature. The base test described by Kenneally and associates[70] was based on Elvey's original work.[39] One variation of this test is described below.

a. The patient lies supine, with the examiner facing the patient. The examiner's inner hand maintains constant depressive force over the top of the shoulder girdle with a light and sensitive grasp. With the elbow flexed, the arm is passively abducted (about 110°) and externally rotated at the glenohumeral joint and supported by the operator's thigh (Fig. 9-21A).

b. While continuing to stabilize the shoulder girdle, the elbow is carefully extended and the forearm supinated. In an asymptomatic person the elbow can be fully extended (Fig. 9-21B).

c. Active wrist extension is added depending on the degree of irritability. If indicated, passive overpressure is applied first to wrist extension and then to finger extension (Fig. 9-21C,D). Normal response to this position is a stretch sensation over the anterior shoulder and over the cubital fossa and may be accompanied by slight or definite tingling in the lateral three digits.[51]

d. To impart maximal tension to the neural tissues, in nonirritable conditions contra- and ipsilateral active cervical sideflexion are added while maintaining shoulder girdle depression (Fig. 9-21E).

Symptoms and symptom changes must be identified after each step. This is regarded as the base test of the median nerve; because there are other tests, it is often referred to as the ULTT1 of the median nerve.[20] Additional motions that may be added to the base test include cervical rotation, cervical flexion, bilateral straight leg raising (SLR), and the combination of cervical flexion with double SLR.[91] ULTTs can be directed at any nerve. Butler[20,21] and others[51,68,91] have written extensively on this subject and have encouraged clinicians to use neural sensitizing movements and biases toward particular nerve trunks (the median, radial, and ulnar nerves).

Before neural mobility testing, all joints moved during the tests should be assessed for mobility and symptoms. Muscles should not be placed in stretched positions that could confound the findings. When nerve irritation is present, the patient's response to local palpation or pressure on the nerve will be exaggerated.[68]

Note: When abnormal tension signs are present, treatment should be aimed at the neural tissue rather than capsular or muscle tissue.

E. *Palpation*
   1. Skin
      a. Temperature over joint regions and entire extremity
      b. Moisture, especially distally
      c. Mobility of skin over subcutaneous tissues
      d. Tenderness, especially if neurological involvement is suspected
      e. Texture
   2. Soft tissues
      a. Consistency, tone, and mobility of the shoulder girdle and brachial region
      b. Swelling. Joint effusion may be palpable anteriorly; bursal effusion may be noted laterally.
      c. Pulse. Radial pulse tests (*e.g.,* Adson's maneuver) may be done if thoracic outlet syndrome is suspected. Compare to the opposite side.
      d. Tenderness. Referred tenderness over the lateral brachial region accompanies most common shoulder lesions. Do not be misled.
   3. Bones and soft-tissue attachments
      a. Bony relationships
         i. Acromioclavicular joint
         ii. Sternoclavicular joint
         iii. Acromion-to-greater-tubercle distance
      b. Tenderness
         i. Tenoperiosteal junctions of the supraspinatus, infraspinatus, subscapularis, teres minor, and biceps
         ii. Acromioclavicular joint
         iii. Sternoclavicular joint
      c. Bony contours
F. *Special tests*—Only those special tests that the examiner feels have relevance should be done. If the patient's signs, symptoms, or dysfunction have not been reproduced, additional tests may include:
   1. Locking test.[26,92] The patient lies supine with the arm initially at the side of the

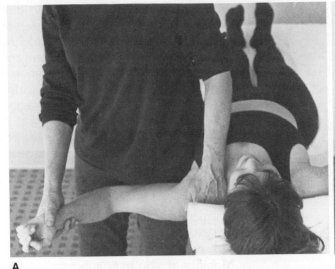

A

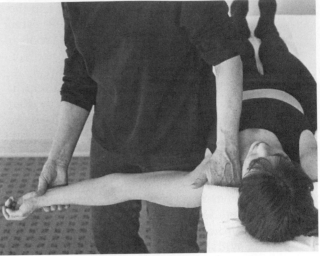

B

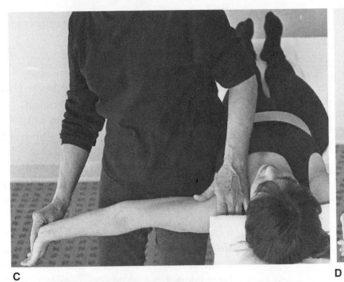

C

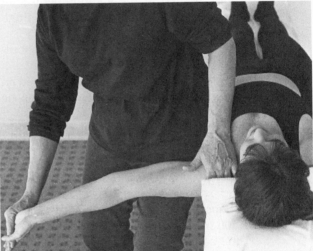

D

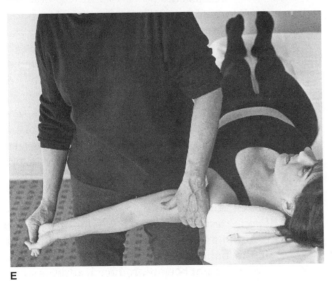

E

FIG. 9-21. Upper limb tension tests. (**A**) With the arm abducted and in about 10° of extension, the arm is supported, on the examiner's thigh, in external rotation, (**B**) the elbow is extended and supinated, (**C**) the wrist is extended, (**D**) and the fingers are extended. (**E**) Cervical sideflexion may be added.

body. The examiner's forearm is used to stabilize the lateral border of the scapula, and the clavicle is stabilized by placing the supinated hand under the shoulder and over the trapezius to prevent shoulder-girdle elevation (Fig. 9-22). With the other hand, the operator flexes the patient's elbow and extends the humerus on the glenohumeral joint with slight internal rotation. The humerus is abducted until it reaches a position where it becomes locked and further movement is impossible, resulting in compression against the inferior surface of the acromion. Normally this maneuver is painless. In some shoulder abnormalities the locking position may not be obtainable and may be painful.

2. Quadrant test.[26,92] The locking position is obtained as described above. The arm is carried forward by first relaxing the pressure on the abducted arm so that it can be moved anteriorly from the coronal plane. The small arc of movement that can be felt during this anterior and rotation movement is known as the *quadrant position*. The humeral head is now unlocked; the arm and forearm are rotated externally and then brought up toward full flexion to a vertical position over the subject's head (Fig. 9-23), producing stress on the anteroinferior joint capsule. The degree and site of pain should be observed.

Overpressure is applied to the arm, moving it backward, which increases the stress on the joint capsule and compresses the acromioclavicular joint. The range of this movement in the sagittal plane should be noted. Patients with joint laxity demon-

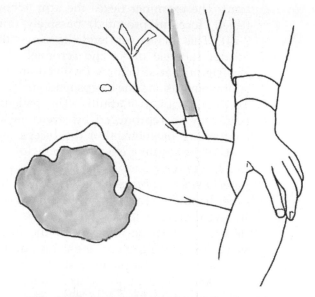

FIG. 9-23. Quadrant position of the shoulder.

strate a pronounced forward movement of the humeral head into the anterosuperior portion of the axilla.

3. Supraspinatus tests
   a. Abduction in the coronal plane is accomplished mainly by the middle portion of the deltoid muscle and the supraspinatus. The patient's arms are abducted to 90° with neutral rotation, and resistance is applied to abduction bilaterally. With the arms abducted to 90°, with the forearm maximally rotated and the arms positioned 30° forward of the coronal plane or in the plane of the scapula, resistance is again given while the examiner looks for weakness or pain, reflecting a positive test result. A positive result may indicate neuropathy of the suprascapular (C5) nerve or a possible tear of the supraspinatus.
   b. Drop-arm test.[98] The drop-arm test is used as an adjunctive test in the assessment of a rotator cuff tear, specifically of the supraspinatus. The examiner abducts the arm to 90° and asks the patient to slowly lower the arm from the abducted position back to the side in the same arc of movement. A positive result is confirmed if the patient cannot return the arm to the side slowly or has severe pain when attempting to do so.

4. Impingement syndrome test. An impingement test is positive when pain is elicited by internal rotation of the humerus in the forward-flexed position (horizontal adduc-

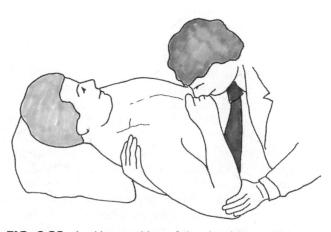

FIG. 9-22. Locking position of the shoulder causing compression of the subacromial physiological joint.

tion). The examiner flexes the arm (elbow flexed, forearm pronated) passively (Fig. 9-24). This maneuver tends to drive the greater tubercle under the acromial arch. The significant structures involved are the supraspinatus and the biceps tendon.[22]

5. Test for bicipital tendinitis. The patient's pain may be reproduced by stretching or contracting (isometrically) the biceps tendon. While resisting elbow flexion with one hand, the examiner simultaneously palpates over the bicipital groove with the other hand. Several tests have been devised to reveal involvement of the biceps muscle or tendon and the integrity of the transverse humeral ligament; these include the Yergason test, Lippman test, Ludington test, and Booth and Marve transverse humeral ligament test.[9,81,85,152]

G. *Miscellaneous.* Because the shoulder and upper extremity articulate with the thorax and spine, they function as a kinetic chain. Involvement of costosternal and costovertebral joints and the upper thoracic and cervical spine can all refer symptoms to the shoulder and may need to be checked. Because thoracic outlet syndrome includes pain in the shoulder, specific tests should be used to rule it out; these include the Adson maneuver, hyperabduction test, and the costoclavicular syndrome test (see Chap. 17, The Cervical Spine).[1,62,83,133] Other conditions that can cause or contribute to thoracic outlet syndrome include fascial fusions of muscles, malunion of old clavicular fractures, the presence of a cervical rib, pseudarthrosis of the clavicle, and exostosis of the first rib.

H. *Ancillary tests*—After completion of the comprehensive physical examination, additional tests may be indicated to provide supplemental information for confirmation of a diagnosis. Evaluation of power and endurance and objective recordings of strength can be valuable. Isokinetic testing is effective in following the progress of rehabilitation.[149]

Nerve-conduction studies have proven beneficial in diagnosing specific neurologic lesions. If it is necessary to further evaluate the intra-articular aspects of the shoulder joint for exact diagnosis, arthrography, arthrotomography, computed tomography, and arthroscopy are available. Shoulder arthrography has been valuable for evaluating rotator cuff pathology.[25]

■ COMMON LESIONS

☐ Impingement Syndrome

The impingement symptom complex primarily involves the coracoacromial arch intruding on the rotator cuff, subacromial bursa, or biceps tendon.[22] There are three theories regarding the factors involved in the development of impingement syndrome: the mechanical-anatomic theory; the vascular compromise theory; and a theory proposed by Perry,[115] which implicates kinesiological factors that limit scapular rotation or promote uncoordinated muscular activity.

Neer, a strong advocate of the mechanical-anatomic theory, recognizes three stages of the syndrome: (1) a benign, self-limiting, overuse syndrome, (2) the development of thickening and fibrosis followed by repeated episodes of the first stage, and (3) development of bony changes, including spurs and eburnation of the humeral tuberosity, leading to possible complications such as rotator cuff tears (Fig. 9-25).[103]

Tendinitis at the shoulder is common. It occurs in young active persons as well as in older persons, and about equally in males and females. In the case of a younger person it may be caused by activities such as tennis, racquetball, or baseball, which increase the stress levels to the rotator cuff tendons. In the older person it is more likely to be a degenerative lesion. Because of the relatively poor blood supply near the insertion of the supraspinatus, nutrition to the area may not meet the metabolic demands of the tendon tissue. The resultant focal cell death sets up an inflammatory response, probably due to the release of irritating enzymes and dead tissue acting as a foreign body.[32,87] The body may react by laying down scar tissue or calcific deposits. Such calcific deposits may be visible on radiographs; however, they are often seen in the absence of symptoms and, conversely, they are not always present in known cases of tendinitis. Superficial

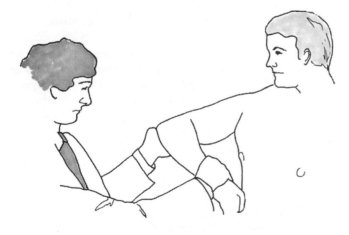

FIG. 9-24. Shoulder impingement syndrome test of possible involvement of the supraspinatus and biceps tendon.

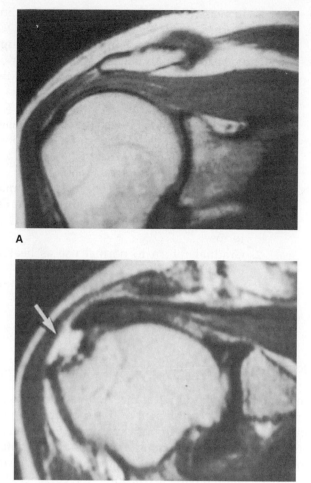

A

B

FIG. 9-25. *Magnetic resonance image of (**A**) normal shoulder rotator cuff and (**B**) a complete rotator cuff tear (arrow). (Esch JC, Baker CL: Arthroscopic Surgery: The Shoulder and Elbow. Philadelphia, JB Lippincott, 1993:31)*

migration of these deposits with rupture into the underside of the subdeltoid bursa is thought to be a major cause of acute bursitis at the shoulder.[88] Because of the poor blood supply to the region, adequate repair may not occur, and the lesion may develop into an actual tear in the tendon.

The degenerative lesions tend to be persistent, with little likelihood of spontaneous resolution. The combined effects of poor blood flow and continued stress to the tendon do not allow for adequate maturation of the healing tissue. It is not unusual for a patient to describe a history of several years of constant or intermittent problems with the shoulder. This by no means should suggest that such patients cannot be helped, since they do respond well, and often dramatically, to the program outlined below.

Transverse friction massage is an essential component of the treatment program in chronic cases. The beneficial effects of friction massage in such cases are not well understood. However, it is proposed that an

increase in the mobility of the developing, or developed, scar tissue occurs without stressing the tendon longitudinally (see Chap. 7, Friction Massage). This prevents the healing tissue from being continually retorn during daily activities.

A factor that may contribute to chronicity and recurrence is weakening of the rotator cuff muscles from reflex inhibition or from actual disuse. Such weakening would predispose to subacromial impingement during elevation of the arm and further mechanical irritation to the site of the lesion. Rotator cuff strengthening is, therefore, an important part of the treatment program. However, if recent or repeated steroid injections to the tendon have been performed, it is necessary to proceed gradually with the strengthening program. Although local steroids do relieve the pain by inhibiting the inflammatory response, they have an antianabolic effect on connective tissue, which may result in structural weakening of the injected tendon.[139]

The differential diagnosis of shoulder pain has been well documented in other publications, and specific conditions afflicting athletes have also been reported.[3,12,55,57,72,113,131]

According to Cahill, the four types of pathologic processes most often neglected are glenohumeral instability, primary acromioclavicular lesions, groove syndrome, and quadrilateral space syndrome. Of these conditions, glenohumeral instability is the one most frequently confused with impingement syndromes.[22] Treatment for impingement syndrome will not benefit the patient with instability.

I. **History**
  A. *Site of pain*—Lateral brachial region, possibly referred below to the elbow in the C5 or C6 sclerotome
  B. *Nature of pain*—Sharp twinges felt on various movements, such as abduction, putting on jacket, or reaching above shoulder level
  C. *Onset of pain*—Usually gradual with no known trauma. May be related to occupational or recreational overuse. May have been present for many months, or even years.
II. **Physical Examination**
  A. *Active movements*—Relatively full range of motion. Often a painful arc is present at midrange of abduction. There is usually slight limitation and pain at full elevation due to pinching of the lesion between the greater tubercle and the posterior rim of the glenoid cavity.
  B. *Passive movements*
    1. Essentially full range of motion
    2. Pain at full elevation, but full range of motion is usually present

3. May be a painful arc on rotation and abduction
4. May be pain on stretch of the involved tendon (*e.g.*, on full internal rotation in the case of supraspinatus or infraspinatus tendinitis)

C. *Resisted movements*—The key test
   1. Maximal isometric contraction of the relevant muscle will reproduce the pain.
   2. In the case of simple tendinitis, the contraction will be fairly strong; if an actual tear exists, it will be weak.
   3. The supraspinatus is the most commonly involved tendon.
   4. Others (biceps, subscapularis, teres minor) are rarely involved.

D. *Palpation*
   1. Tenderness, usually over the involved tendon near its insertion. Soft-tissue crepitus may be palpable in patients with degeneration of the rotator cuff and a bony crepitus in patients with osteoarthritis.[26]
      a. The supraspinatus tendon insertion may be easily palpated as the examiner stands behind the patient and places two fingers of one hand over the greater tuberosity.[26] With the other hand the examiner grasps the forearm above the elbow and passively rotates the arm medially and laterally, while also applying long-axis extension caudally. The normal tendon insertion can be felt to move as a firm cord under the examiner's fingers. At times a gap may be felt if the tendon is disrupted.
      b. The infraspinatus is best palpated near its insertion just below the acromion process and posterior border of the deltoid while the arm is held with the glenohumeral joint at 90° of forward flexion.[26]
      c. The tendinous insertion of the subscapularis may be palpated over the lesser tuberosity just medial to the tendon of the long head of the biceps.
   2. Usually referred tenderness over the lateral brachial region. *Do not be misled.*

E. *Inspection*
   1. Usually negative
   2. Some atrophy may be noted if a chronic tear exists.

III. **Management.** The presence or absence of a calcific deposit, as demonstrated by radiographs, should not affect the treatment plan.
   A. *Ultrasound*
      1. Resolution of inflammatory exudates
      2. Increased blood flow to assist the healing process
      3. May provide some pain relief, although persistent pain is usually not a problem
   B. *Friction massage*—A key component of the treatment program
      1. To form mobile scar
      2. The hyperemia induced by the massage may enhance blood flow to the area to assist the healing response.
   C. *Instruction in appropriate use of the arm*
      1. Strict avoidance of activities that may cause impingement or tension stress at the site of involvement while painless scar forms
      2. Gradual return to normal use as healing progresses
   D. *Restrengthening* of involved muscles and other measures to restore normal joint mechanics

GENERAL GUIDELINES

In most cases of tendinitis at the shoulder, perhaps the only dispensable component of the above program is the use of ultrasound. In our experience, failure to institute any of the remaining measures appropriately increases the likelihood that treatment will be unsuccessful or that the patient will suffer a recurrence. The younger person whose primary complaint is pain during recreational activities such as baseball or racquetball must be advised that temporary abstinence from certain activities is an essential remedial measure. However, restricting activities to "resting" the part is usually not sufficient in itself to effect a resolution of the pathology, although the reduction in pain experienced may often suggest this. Usually, resumption of activities will be accompanied by a recurrence of the previous symptoms, because simply resting the part does not ensure the development of a mature, mobile cicatrix. This is also true for the older person, who may experience pain during normal daily activities. Although appropriate control of activities is usually necessary for resolution of the problem, it alone is usually inadequate. The use of friction massage, passive range of motion (PROM), and, perhaps more importantly, restrengthening exercises should not be excluded.

The therapist must, through a complete history, become aware of the patient's habitual daily activities. This is important because the patient often engages in activities that may contribute to the problem without actually realizing it. Such "fatigue" pathologies typically result from the cumulation of otherwise asymptomatic stresses. Activities that particularly must be avoided are those involving repetitive elevation of the arm to shoulder level or above.

The importance of strengthening exercises can be appreciated by understanding the key role the muscles play in the normal functioning of the shoulder joint. As mentioned earlier, the supraspinatus is largely responsible for maintaining adequate depression of the humeral head during abduction. In the presence of a weak supraspinatus, the head of the humerus will tend to ride high in the glenoid during elevation of the arm because of the disproportionate contraction of the deltoid. This would predispose to impingement of the greater tubercle, along with its tendinous attachments, against the coracoacromial arch. Thus, in cases of tendinitis there is a tendency toward muscle atrophy from reflex inhibition or disuse, and this is often a factor in prolonging the pathologic process.

The muscles of the rotator cuff are tonic and therefore highly dependent on adequate blood supply and oxygen tension. The key to rotator cuff rehabilitation is to provide a pain-free environment for revascularization of the tendons of the rotator cuff. Motion and strengthening exercises that are pain-free stimulate collagen synthesis and collagen fiber organization and neuromodulate pain.[2,148,153]

Remedial strengthening exercises are best performed with the arm close to the side to prevent the possibility of impingement and reflex inhibition during the exercises.

During the early stages of rehabilitation, isometric exercises may be performed with the shoulder in a neutral position following warm-up. *Warm-up* is an increase in body heat by active muscle use for the purposes of lowering soft-tissue viscosity and enhancing body chemical and metabolic functions, to protect and prepare the body for more aggressive physical activity.[9,77] General central muscular body activity (*e.g.,* calisthenics or riding a stationary bicycle) or local exercises (*e.g.,* saw or pendulum exercises) may be used.[12,28] Active muscle activity is likely to be more productive than passive means of heating, because passive heating does not enhance the metabolic and cardiac factors, which are also important.[106]

The position of the shoulder can be altered in several ways to enhance the isometric strengthening of appropriate muscle groups at different angles and lengths in the pain-free range.[45] If pain from joint compression occurs, the use of manual resistance and slight traction to the joint as resistance is given is helpful. Ice is frequently used to reduce postexercise soreness, but the value of ice alone has been questioned, based on experimental data.[151]

A particularly useful rehabilitation approach is that proposed by Grimsby[53], in addition to the regimen for progression of resistive exercises and repetition patterned after Holten's 1-RM (100% resistance maximum) pyramid (Fig. 9-26).[54,60] The initial goal is to facilitate tendon revascularization through isolation and reinforcement of high-repetition, nonresistive tonic cuff musculature activity.[53] The concept of unloading

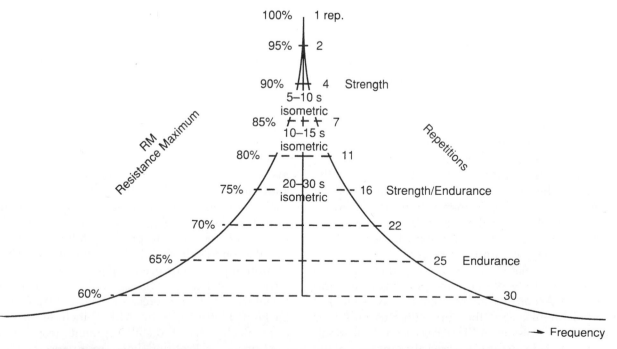

FIG. 9-26. The Odvar Holten pyramid diagram. (Skyhar MJ, Simmons TC: Rehabilitation of the shoulder. In Nickel LV, Botte MJ [eds]: Orthopaedic Rehabilitation. New York, Churchill Livingstone, 1992:758)

is an integral part of this treatment program. During acute inflammation, the weight of the arm alone is enough to aggravate pain.[132] Techniques for performing unweighted axial humeral rotation are initiated, progressing from 50 to 100 repetitions a day of simple pain-free, active internal and external rotation to three sets of 100 repetitions a day. An overhead pulley with forearm support may be used to unweight the limb. Cumulative total repetitions should be 5000 to 6000. Abduction, followed by forward-flexion, begins gradually in an unweighted environment. Axial rotation is again stressed in varying degrees of abduction and forward-flexion. Once satisfactory increases in flexion and abduction have been gained with the arm unweighted, active motions are started in a pain-free environment without irritating the involved muscle(s). This regimen allows the therapist to assess and treat any stage of muscle rehabilitation objectively. Rehabilitation of the scapular stabilizers begins simultaneously with that of the rotator cuff. Finally, sport-specific exercises may begin.

This is a brief overview of this approach. The reader should refer to the works of Holten,[60] Grimsby,[53] and Gustavsen,[54] to adequately plan such a treatment program.

As range of motion improves and healing progresses, the patient is graduated to isotonic exercises for the rotator cuff muscles with manual resistance, free weights, or elastic tension cord resistance (isoflex exercises). Isoflex exercises are convenient, particularly for home programs, and effective, and they allow unlimited arcs of motion with both concentric and eccentric muscle training.[35,45,106]

To strengthen the supraspinatus, the patient should stand with the arm at the side and rotate the shoulder internally to pronate the forearm. Then, moving the arm in a diagonal direction of abduction, the patient should aim to achieve 90° abduction at 30° to 40° in front of the coronal position. This position aligns the muscle parallel to arm movement (in the plane of the scapula); in this position the electromyographic output of the supraspinatus is greatest.[65]

A strong rotator cuff assists in depression of the scapula and the humeral head in the glenoid during overhead activities.[71] It is therefore important to attain a strong rotator cuff before initiating shoulder elevation above 90°. Range of motion can be increased gradually as long as impingement is avoided.

From a functional standpoint, strengthening of the deltoid (particularly the anterior portion) is also important.[15,94] According to Matsen and colleagues,[94] the initial premise that the supraspinatus muscle is the primary depressor and is necessary for full shoulder elevation is incorrect. It primarily functions along with the other rotator cuff muscles as a head concav-ity compressor and stabilizer. *Concavity compression* is a stabilizing mechanism in which compression of the convex humeral head into the concave glenoid fossa stabilizes it against translating forces.[95] Even patients with massive tears of the supraspinatus can still fully elevate their arms. The deltoid plays the major role in elevation of the arm with active flexion and abduction in these conditions.[15,64,116]

Two other exercises important in the prevention of impingement are shoulder shrugs and pushups with the arm abducted to 90°.[16] These exercises strengthen the upper trapezius and serratus anterior, providing normal scapular rotation and thus allowing the acromion to elevate without contracting the rotator cuff.

Shoulder elevation above 90° should be initiated with a D1F (flexion—adduction—external rotation) proprioceptive neuromuscular (PNF) pattern before advancing to a D2F (flexion—abduction—external rotation) pattern.[137] Rotator cuff dysfunction may result in both reduced humeral depression and external rotation.[8,17,23] Neer[102] has reported that the functional arc of shoulder elevation is not lateral, as previously thought, but forward. This results in the suprahumeral structures being impinged against the anterior part of the acromion when the humerus is internally rather than externally rotated.

The advanced phase of rehabilitation concentrates on the progressive return to normal function. In general, the patient continues self-stretching of the rotator cuff and inferior capsule as normal strength and endurance return. During this phase, exercises may be performed on an exercise machine (*e.g.*, Nautilus™, Universal™). Free weights should be used until the patient can safely transfer to the exercise machines for resistive exercise.[16] Pool therapy can be effective for power and endurance training using PNF patterns with hand paddles facilitated by the isokinetic resistance of water,[44] and can also restore range of motion.[27,150]

Closed-chain exercises popular with the lower extremity[112,130,146] are useful in providing joint approximation forces that promote a cocontraction about the joint and provide joint stability.[24,34,110,138,145] Closed-chain training enhances static stability by facilitating compression of the glenohumeral capsule and stimulating joint receptors to provide static control. Traditional closed-chain exercises provide an external fixed motion apparatus or use the patient's body as the external resistance (*i.e.*, basic dips), but the nontraditional closed-chain exercises advocated by Cipriani,[24] Dickhoff-Hoffman,[34] and Wilk[145] include the use of a dynamically fixed distal segment (*e.g.*, dynamic pushups on a Profitter [Fitter International, Calgary, Alberta, Canada] balance board or ball(s), hand gait on a treadmill, and hand stair climber), requiring the shoulder girdle complex to function not only with great stability but also with great mobility.

Although plyometric activity is primarily used for lower-limb training, it has an important place in training the upper limb.[46,107,140,147] Various types of throwing drills and catching activities are examples. Plyometrics are primarily used in late-stage rehabilitation and functional precompetitive testing following the injury of an athlete.

Total body fitness should be initiated no later than the early part of the advanced stage of rehabilitation. This program should consist of exercises to develop cardiovascular fitness, leg strength, and endurance.[97] This is especially important for athletes who engage in sports that predominantly use the muscles of the upper extremity but also require strong lower extremities. It is important to maintain the central cardiovascular system by general aerobic conditioning. A specific aerobic exercise to enhance the endurance of the upper-extremity muscle group consists of sitting behind a stationary bike and pedaling with the hands.

Rehabilitation following surgical repair of the rotator cuff is lengthy and is characterized by slow progress. The surgical techniques are beyond the scope of this text but are well documented in the literature.[9,31,73,100,131,144] Rehabilitation requires an average of 12 to 14 months for an athlete to return to his or her level of activity before the injury.[27] General mobilization to restore accessory motion should be initiated following immobilization. Caudal glides of the humeral head should be emphasized to increase the available space between the acromion and humerus. A program of general shoulder strengthening, capsular stretching, and specific rotator cuff strengthening exercises should be continued as long as the patient uses the shoulder to any great degree in activities of daily living and sports.[16]

Many injuries of the shoulder can be classified as overuse problems resulting from repetitive stresses, with minimal abnormalities.[134] Abnormalities that represent deficits in strength, flexibility, or technique are often easily remedied through appropriate intervention by a skilled therapist.

The successful use of friction massage requires precision with respect to the site of application and the intensity or depth of application (see Chap. 7, Friction Massage). If it is impractical for the patient to be followed regularly for treatment, consider instructing a family member in the technique of application or instructing the patient in self-administration. However, application by a skilled, experienced practitioner is preferred to ensure that the appropriate technique is used and to monitor and document results accurately. As athletic activities or activities involving repetitive

elevation of the arm are resumed, instructing the patient in self-administered friction massage before engaging in the particular function may be an important preventive measure.

☐ Instability

Instabilities may be caused by either static or dynamic factors. Dynamic factors occur primarily as a result of rotator cuff weakness; static factors include damage to the anterior capsule and glenohumeral ligament and glenoid labrum. Several classifications of glenohumeral instabilities are described in the literature. The degree of instability (subluxation or dislocation), the nature (voluntary or involuntary), and the chronicity are all important parameters that must be addressed in the rehabilitation program.[93–95] Shoulder instabilities may be classified as traumatic, atraumatic, or acquired. Matsen and associates[93,94] have provided useful acronyms for this classification. Traumatic patients exhibit Unilateral/Unidirectional instabilities, caused by a Bankart lesion, and usually require Surgery to stabilize the shoulder joint (TUBS). The second type of patient is the Atraumatic, Multidirectional unstable patient, usually Bilaterally involved, in whom Rehabilitation is the first line of defense; if conservative treatment fails, then an Inferior capsular shift procedure is performed, which tightens the inferior capsule and the rotator Interval (AMBRII).

Burkhead and colleagues[19] reported only 15% good to excellent results with conservative treatment in patients with traumatic shoulder dislocations. The success rate was 85% with the atraumatic patient.

I. **History.** The aim is to ascertain the degree (subluxation, dislocation), direction (anterior, posterior), and onset (traumatic, atraumatic, overuse). Considering the two main groups of instability patients (see above) allows us to better appreciate the variations in symptomatic presentation. The AMBRII patient presents with no history of trauma and describes symptoms brought on by certain arm positions or activities. The TUBS patient describes a significant injury causing a dislocation requiring reduction and often subsequent recurrent dislocations. With a subluxation, the patient may describe a feeling of the shoulder "slipping out of the joint" momentarily but going back into place spontaneously. Apprehension is a common feature in patients with recurrent dislocations or subluxation. It is important to determine the nature of the onset of the instability. In traumatic recurrent instability, the shoulder usually displaces anteriorly and rarely posteriorly; in the atraumatic group, multidirectional and posterior displacements are more common.[58]

A. The traumatic patient is asked to re-enact the mechanism of injury to help clarify the body position and the stress placed on the involved tissue. This helps to determine the damaged structure and injury mechanism. The AMBRII patient is asked to demonstrate the positions in which the shoulder feels unstable. Anterior instability is usually associated with the externally rotated and abducted arm position. Posterior instability is manifested with the arm in flexion, internal rotation, and adduction. Inferior laxity is usually noted with axial downward traction on the arm, manifested by a sulcus sign.

B. Patients are asked routinely if they can dislocate the shoulder voluntarily; determine whether voluntary instability is the predominant problem or if it is just a minor facet of the shoulder going out involuntarily. The patient with atraumatic voluntary instability has no history of injury but can remember since childhood the ability to slip one or both shoulders out of place with minimal discomfort.[93] A general appreciation of ligamentous laxity can be observed with bilateral extension of the elbow and thumb to forearm.[11]

II. Physical Examination

A. *Observation*—In the sagittal view, note any anterior displacement of the humeral head. No more than a third of the head of the humerus should be in front of the acromion. Sahrmann's three-finger test may be used.[127] The examiner places the thumb over the head of the humerus anteriorly, the index finger over the acromioclavicular joint, and the ring finger on the posterior aspect of the scapular spine, and notes the relationship of the head of the humerus to the acromion. From the anterior view, note any step deformities suggesting an acromioclavicular dislocation. If the deformity appears when traction is applied to the arm, it may be due to multidirectional instability (sulcus sign).[47,93]

B. *Joint-play movements* are considered key tests for the assessment of instabilities. The amplitude of joint play (hypermobility) and the presence of pain and muscle guarding are noted and compared to the other arm (see Figs. 9-28D, 9-29A, 9-30A, 9-30B).

C. *Tests for instability.* Static instability may be assessed clinically by the anterior and posterior drawer test.[47] Anterior and posterior instability is initially tested with the patient sitting with the forearm resting in the lap and the shoulder relaxed. The examiner grasps the proximal humerus and gently presses the humeral head toward the scapula to center it in the glenoid, ensuring a neutral starting position (Fig. 9-27A). The head is first pushed forward to determine the amount of anterior displacement possible (Fig. 9-27B). The normal shoulder reaches a firm end feel with no pain, apprehension, or clunking. The humerus is returned to the neutral position and then pulled posteriorly to determine the amount of posterior translation relative to the scapula. According to Matsen and associates,[93] the normal shoulder allows posterior translation up to about half of the humeral head diameter. Increased posterior and anterior translation suggests multidirectional instability. A more rigorous test (fulcrum test) is to position the patient in the supine lying position, with the injured shoulder over the edge of the table. The arm is abducted to 90° and externally rotated, and from this position the examiner applies an anterior or posterior force.[93]

Numerous other tests are available to assess multidirectional instability (see Fig. 9-29A),[121,125] anterior instability,[33,47,57,76,119,121,126,141] and posterior instability.[28,93,109] The drawer test, however, has the advantage of eliciting evidence of capsular laxity without threatening the patient with dislocation. Clinical laxity testing has shown that in a few subjects, the magnitude of translation for shoulders with atraumatic instability is essentially the same as that of normal shoulders or shoulders with traumatic instability.[95] Therefore, pay particular attention to the patient's response during the test and determine if the test duplicates his or her symptoms.

III. Management. The strength of the rotator cuff muscles is probably the single most important consideration.[107,136] Whether management is nonoperative or rehabilitative following surgery, strenthening exercises of the rotator cuff (see above) and scapular stabilizing muscles are critical to optimal outcome. According the Sutter,[138] conservative management should be based on immediate motion and strengthening. Several investigators have documented that the incidence of recurrent instability is not affected by the length of glenohumeral immobilization.[37,61,126] The scapulothoracic joint should be strengthened by exercising the muscles that control scapular rota-

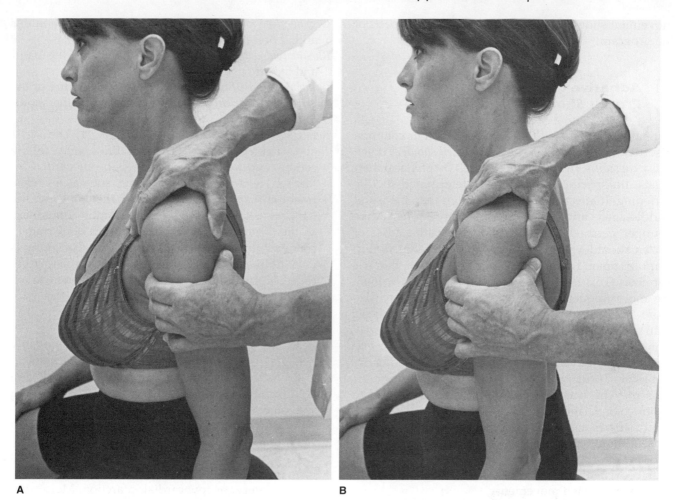

A B

FIG. 9-27. Anterior-posterior drawer test: (**A**) starting position and (**B**) end position.

tion: the levator scapulae and the rhomboids (rowing), the serratus anterior (press-ups), the latissimus dorsi (pull-downs), and the trapezius (shrugging).[107]

Recurrent multidirectional, inferior, and involuntary instability is common in the AMBRII syndrome. The effects of generalized capsular instability can be ameliorated by vigorous rotator cuff strengthening. The goals of instability rehabilitation are to strengthen specific muscle groups and more importantly to increase their sensitivity to stretch. Grimsby's three-stage program is particularly useful.[53,132]

A. *Stage 1* begins with low-speed, high-repetition minimum resistance in the beginning and middle range of motion. This stage is meant to increase muscle endurance and circulation, avoiding overexertion.

B. *Stage 2* involves increasing resistance and adding isometrics in the inner ranges of motion. This is designed to increase strength and sensitivity to stretch.

C. *Stage 3* continues to increase resistance (usually 80% 1-RM) and adds isometrics through a full but not maximal range of motion.

Multidirectional instability requires comprehensive rotator cuff rehabilitation. When treating anterior instability, rehabilitation should concentrate on the internal rotators and adductors (pectorals, subscapularis, latissimus dorsi, anterior deltoid).[132] The external rotators and teres minor and major are emphasized for posterior instability.

The treatment program should also include exercises to enhance neuromuscular control (comprehensive stability and force-couple control), closed-chain (weight-bearing) exercises to facilitate cocontraction, and shoulder stabilization programs (*i.e.,* resisting diagonal PNF patterns with or without the use of equipment).[4] Flexibility training and soft-tissue and joint mobilization are included as necessary. Specificity regarding concentric/eccentric muscle function, aerobic/anaerobic energy pathways, and velocity of movement should be addressed in the final aspects of the program.

☐ Adhesive Capsulitis—Frozen Shoulder

Capsular tightening at the shoulder, another common disorder, is usually referred to as *frozen shoulder* or *adhesive capsulitis*. In most patients seen by physical therapists, no specific cause can be determined for the stiffening. It affects women more often than men, and middle-aged and older persons more often than younger persons. Some so-called idiopathic cases of frozen shoulder probably result from an alteration in scapulohumeral alignment, as occurs with thoracic kyphosis. This is consistent with the fact that women are more frequently affected, since women are also more predisposed to developing thoracic kyphosis than men. Some believe that this problem is a progression of rotator cuff lesions, in which the inflammatory/degenerative process spreads to include the entire joint capsule, resulting in capsular fibrosis.[32,88,99] This may be true in some cases, but there are two major contradictions to this proposal: rotator cuff tendinitis affects men and women fairly equally, whereas frozen shoulder is much more common in women; and persons with a frozen shoulder rarely present with coexistent tendinitis, as evidenced by the absence of pain on resisted movement.

It is commonly thought that these patients stop using the arm because for some reason it is painful, and motion is therefore lost from disuse. In our experience, this is rarely true; instead, the loss of motion is responsible for the pain. The patient continues to use the arm until the restriction of motion progresses to the extent that it interferes with daily activities. Not until this point is reached does the patient feel much pain or is aware of a problem with the arm. The woman first notices that it is difficult to comb her hair and fasten a bra. She may also be awakened at night when rolling onto the affected side. The man notes difficulty reaching into the hip pocket and combing his hair, and may be similarly awakened at night. Because much shoulder motion can be lost before interfering with daily activities of persons in this age group, these patients invariably do not seek medical help until the shoulder has lost about 90° abduction, 60° flexion, 60° external rotation, and 45° internal rotation. In fact, it is rare for a patient to present with significantly more or significantly less than this amount of movement.

Of course, some cases of capsular tightening at the shoulder are associated with particular disease states or conditions. Conditions that might result in capsular tightness at the glenohumeral joint include:

Degenerative joint disease—This is rare at the shoulder and, if present, is relatively asymptomatic.

Rheumatoid arthritis—The smaller joints of the hand and feet are usually affected first.

Immobilization—For example, following fracture of the arm, forearm, or wrist, or dislocation of the shoulder[59]

Reflex sympathetic dystrophy (see Chap. 11, The Wrist and Hand Complex). This condition may follow certain visceral disorders such as a myocardial infarction, or it may follow trauma, such as a Colles' fracture. Capsular stiffening of the joints of the hand, wrist, and shoulder is a common component of this syndrome. A frozen shoulder occurring in conjunction with a reflex sympathetic dystrophy is usually more refractory to treatment, probably because of the abnormal pain state that tends to accompany the disorder.

I. History

    A. *Site of pain*—Lateral brachial region, possibly referred distally into the C5 or C6 segment

    B. *Nature of pain*—Varying from a constant dull ache to pain felt only on activities involving movement into the restricted ranges. The patient is often awakened at night when rolling onto the painful shoulder.

    C. *Onset of pain*—Very gradual. May be related to minor trauma, immobilization, chest surgery, or myocardial infarction. More commonly, no cause can be cited.

II. Physical Examination

    A. *Active movements*—Limitation of motion in a capsular pattern: little glenohumeral movement on abduction, much difficulty and substitution getting the hand behind the neck. Usually there is some limitation when flexing the arm or trying to put the hand behind the back.

    B. *Passive movements*—Limitation in a capsular pattern: external rotation is markedly restricted, abduction is moderately restricted, flexion and internal rotation are somewhat limited.

        1. May be limited by pain with a muscle-guarding end feel (acute)

        2. May be limited by stiffness with a capsular end feel (chronic)

    C. *Joint play*—Restriction of most joint-play movements, especially inferior glide

    D. *Resisted isometric movements*—Strong and painless, unless a tendinitis also is present

    E. *Palpation*—Often referred tenderness over the lateral brachial region. There is often a feeling of increased muscle tone, with induration over the lateral brachial region.

F. *Inspection*—Often negative. Observe for a surgical scar.

III. **Acute vs. Chronic**

A. *Acute*

1. Pain radiates to below the elbow.
2. The patient is awakened by pain at night.
3. On passive movement, limitation is due to pain and muscle guarding, rather than stiffness *per se.*

B. *Chronic*

1. Pain is localized to the lateral brachial region.
2. The patient is not awakened by pain at night.
3. On passive movement, limitation is due to capsular stiffness, and pain is felt only when the capsule is stretched.

C. *Subacute*—Some combination of the above findings

IV. **Management**

A. *Acute stage*

1. Relief of pain and muscle guarding to allow early, gentle mobilization
   a. Ice or superficial heat
   b. Grade I or II joint-play oscillations
2. Maintenance of existing range of motion and efforts to gently begin increasing range of motion
   a. Grade I or II joint-play mobilization. At this stage it is often best to perform these with the patient lying prone and the arm hanging freely at the side of the plinth (see Fig. 9-28*A–C*). Inferior glide is particularly comfortable for most patients and is usually most helpful in relieving muscle spasm. This is an important movement to perform because the spasm, which is usually present in the acute stage, causes the humerus to assume a superior position in the glenoid cavity, further interfering with normal joint mechanics.
   b. Initiation of active assisted range of motion exercises at home, such as auto-mobilization techniques and wand and pendulum exercises.
3. Instruction in isometric strengthening exercises, especially for the rotator cuff muscles. The movements associated with isotonic exercises will usually cause pain and reflex inhibition, thus reducing their effectiveness.
4. Prevention of excessive kyphosis and shoulder-girdle protraction. When appropriate, provide instruction in postural awareness for the upper trunk and shoulder girdles such that the patient learns to differentiate proprioceptively between a kyphotic, protracted posture and a relatively upright, retracted position. A system of regular "postural checks" should be incorporated into the patient's daily activities.
5. Gradual progression of the above program as the condition becomes more chronic (see below)

B. *Chronic stage*—Increase the extensibility of the joint capsule, with special attention to the anteroinferior aspect of the capsule.

1. Ultrasound preceding or accompanying stretching procedures
2. Specific joint mobilizations, with emphasis on the anteroinferior capsular stretch

GENERAL GUIDELINES

When using specific joint mobilization techniques in the presence of a chronically tight joint, the primary objective is to stretch the joint capsule. To do so, the more vigorous grade IV techniques must be used. It is usually best, however, to start with grade I or II oscillations in preparation for more intensive stretching. The lower grades of oscillations promote reduced muscle spasm and pain, probably by increasing large-fiber sensory input. Perhaps the best technique to use when beginning glenohumeral mobilization is the *inferior glide* with the arm to the side (see Fig. 9-28*D–F*); this technique, especially, seems to induce relaxation. These are also good techniques for relieving the cramping sensation a patient may feel during more vigorous movements.

Before or during capsular stretching procedures, ultrasound can be used to help increase the extensibility of the tissue. For example, perform the anteroinferior capsular stretch while an assistant directs ultrasound to the anteroinferior aspect of the joint. Specific joint mobilization techniques are most effective when used in conjunction with the motions they are intended to restore, such as inferior glide performed simultaneously with abduction or flexion, posterior capsular stretch with internal rotation, and anterior capsular stretch with external rotation (see the section on Self Capsular Stretches). Passive stretching can also be combined with appropriate accessory movements (*e.g.,* flexion with inferior glide or abduction with inferior glide).

Instruct the patient in home range of motion exercises. These are necessary to maintain gains made in treatment and to help increase movement. A major goal of the treatment program is to promote independence in mobilization procedures. Once about 120° abduction, 140° flexion, and 60° external rotation are achieved, many patients continue to make satisfactory improvement in range of motion by continuing on a supervised home exercise program. From the outset, though, it is difficult for most patients to make substantial gains in range of motion with home exercises alone; skillfully applied passive movement will significantly accelerate improvement in the early phases of treatment. This is probably because in the relatively acute stage, the reflex muscle spasm that accompanies active movement of the joint prevents patients from exerting an effective stretch to the joint capsule—they simply fight against their own muscles. The therapist skilled in the use of passive joint mobilization procedures can localize the stretch to specific portions of the joint capsule and carefully graduate the intensity of the stretch to avoid eliciting protective muscle contraction. Also, the therapist can combine joint-play movements with certain movements of the arm to reduce cartilaginous or bony impingement at the extremes of movement. For example, when moving the arm into abduction, the therapist can passively move the head of the humerus inferiorly to prevent impingement of the greater tubercle against the acromial arch, which would tend to occur from the loss of external rotation and from a loss of inferior glide of the joint. By doing so, muscle spasm is reduced and a more effective stretch to the inferior capsule is effected. In fact, until significant gains in external rotation are made, patients should not be instructed to stretch into abduction on their own: attempts to do so may traumatize the subacromial tissues more than stretching the inferior aspect of the joint capsule.

The primary goal of treatment is to restore painless functional range of movement; regaining full movement of the arm is not always realistic. This is especially true for persons with some degree of increased thoracic kyphosis, because full elevation of the arm involves extension of the upper thoracic spine. For these patients "normal" elevation is usually about 150° to 160°. Range of motion of the uninvolved shoulder should serve as a guide for setting treatment goals.

In more acute cases of frozen shoulder, the patient's major complaint is often the inability to get a good night's sleep: each time he or she rolls onto the involved side, he or she is awakened by pain. The resultant fatigue adds to the patient's general debilitation. Fortunately, with appropriate management this is usually the first aspect of the problem to resolve. In fact, subjective improvement, in the form of significant reduction in night pain, will usually precede any evidence of objective improvement, such as increased range of motion. In our experience, one or two sessions of gentle joint-play oscillations, especially into inferior glide, preceded by superficial heat or ice, are often enough to alleviate nocturnal symptoms. This leads us to speculate whether the night pain may be related more to the fact that the joint is compressed in a position in which the humerus is held into a cephalad malalignment by muscle spasm, rather than being the result of compression of an inflamed joint capsule. At any rate, relaxation of the associated muscle spasm seems to be one of the more important measures in reducing pain in the acute phase.

In the chronic stage, pain is primarily the result of repeated tensile stresses to the tight joint capsule during daily activities. Treatment is directed primarily at increasing range of motion, although some restriction of activities may be warranted. For the most part, however, in the chronic stage, encourage the patient to use the arm as much as tolerable to minimize habitual disuse, which can be a factor in perpetuating the disorder.

Some authors claim that adhesive capsulitis is a self-limiting disorder, and that spontaneous resolution can be expected in about 12 months.[100,104,139] This has not been consistent with our clinical experience. Even if it were true, this should not be a reason for failing to institute active treatment, because with appropriate therapy satisfactory results can be expected within no longer than 3 to 4 months. The only common exception is when a frozen shoulder is part of a sympathetic reflex dystrophy. These cases are often refractory to conservative management and may require supplementary measures such as sympathetic blocks or manipulation under anesthesia.

Although in most cases of frozen shoulder the prognosis for functional recovery is good, the time frame of recovery is rarely linear. Improvement tends to be characterized by spurts and plateaus. Both the therapist and patient should realize this to avoid undue frustration during periods of limited progress.

☐ Acute Bursitis

Acute bursitis is relatively rare and is thought to occur secondary to calcific tendinitis, in which the deposit migrates superficially into the floor of the subdeltoid bursa.[99]

I. History
  A. *Site of pain*—lateral brachial region, possibly referred distally
  B. *Nature of pain*—intense, constant, dull, sometimes throbbing pain. The patient may present with the arm in a sling, or supporting the arm at the elbow with the uninvolved hand. During this acute period, very little relief is found in any position. All movements are reported to be painful.
  C. *Onset of pain*—History may suggest a chronic tendinitis. The acute pain, however, usually

arises over a period of 12 to 72 hours, with a gradual buildup of pain over this period.

II. Physical Examination

A. *Active movements*—marked restriction in all planes with evidence of severe pain on attempts to elevate the arm

B. *Passive movements*—restricted by pain in a noncapsular pattern with an "empty" end feel; no resistance is felt to movement, but the patient insists that movement be ceased because of intense pain. Rotation with the arm at the side may be fairly free, but abduction past 60° or flexion past 90° is usually not permitted because of complaints of severe pain.

C. *Resisted movements*—There may be some hesitation to perform a maximal contraction, with perhaps some pain on resisted abduction, due to squeezing of the inflamed bursa. When carefully tested, however, most contractions are strong and painless.

D. *Palpation*—possibly some warmth and swelling over the region overlying the subdeltoid bursa; usually considerable tenderness in this area

E. *Inspection*—often unremarkable; possibly some visible swelling laterally at the side of the bursa

III. Management

A. *Early stages*

1. Resolution of the acute inflammatory process
   a. Ice or superficial heat
   b. Support of the arm with a sling to reduce postural tone in the muscles adjacent to the bursa, thereby relieving pressure to the inflamed area
2. Maintaining range of motion—Gentle active-assisted exercises such as wand and pendulum exercises

B. *Chronic stage*

With the above measures, it is rare for the condition to remain "acute" for longer than a few days. Resolution of the acute stage is characterized by the absence of pain at rest and localization of pain to the lateral brachial region. The patient can actively elevate the arm to at least 90° flexion or abduction.

1. Resolution of chronic inflammatory process. Bursitis at the shoulder and of the trochanteric bursa are, in our experience, the two conditions in which the use of ultrasound to provide relief of symptoms, in the presence of a subacute or chronic inflammation, will often have an unequivocally beneficial effect. The increased blood flow induced by the local heat apparently aids in a more rapid resolution of inflammatory irritants and debris.

Unlike tendinitis or frozen shoulder, acute bursitis at the shoulder tends to be self-limiting over a period of several weeks. With appropriate therapy few patients have significant pain or disability 2 weeks after the onset of acute symptoms. However, because calcific rotator cuff tendinitis is often a pre-existing condition, it is important as the acute phase of the bursitis resolves to test for the presence of tendinitis, the clinical signs of which may be obscured by the acute symptoms of bursitis. If tendinitis does exist, appropriate treatment measures should be instituted (see previous discussion on tendinitis).

2. Restoration of full range of motion, joint play, and strength
   a. Instruction in home range of motion procedures
   b. Specific joint mobilization (automobilization or passive movements) if warranted
   c. Instruction in home strengthening exercises

☐ **Other Lesions**

Other, more serious lesions commonly affect the shoulder, such as anterior dislocation and acromioclavicular joint separation. These are usually not seen by the physical therapist until they have been treated by the physician with prolonged immobilization, or perhaps surgery followed by immobilization. At this point, the therapist no longer deals with the original injury so much as with the effects of immobilization. As a result, the goals and techniques of management in such cases are often essentially the same as those for a patient with capsular tightness. There are, however, special considerations with which the therapist should be familiar, depending on the original problem. For example, surgery for recurrent anterior dislocation may be performed with the specific intent of limiting external rotation to help provide anterior stabilization.[23,32] Or, following an anterior dislocation, it may be desirable for the sake of preventing recurrence to allow the anterior capsule to heal in a tightened state. In both cases emphasis on regaining external rotation will be less than what it might be in other cases of capsular tightness. Certain surgical fixations for acromioclavicular separation, such as those involving insertion of a screw from the clavicle to the coracoid, may permanently restrict normal clavicular axial rotation. As long as such a screw is still in place, full elevation of the arm should not be expected; it can occur only if the screw breaks.

Although it is not within the scope of this book to discuss them at length, the therapist must be familiar with these other types of injuries, the current surgical procedures, and such special considerations as those mentioned above.

▮ PASSIVE TREATMENT TECHNIQUES

☐ Joint Mobilization Techniques

(For simplicity, the operator will be referred to as the male, the patient as the female. P—patient; O—operator; M—movement.)

It is always difficult to determine which techniques are likely to be the most effective. Hundreds of techniques are described in the literature. Each technique is either an accessory motion or a particular capsular stretch, and can be applied with any grade of movement. These are also evaluative techniques when performed in the resting position. They should first be used to determine reactivity and the need for mobilization. To reduce the chances of being too aggressive, the operator should try to determine what stage of the healing process the involved joint is in: acute with extravasation, fibroplasia, or chronic with scar formation (see Chap. 2, Properties of Dense Connective Tissue and Wound Healing).

Techniques performed with the arm at the side of the body or in prone with the arm in flexion are primarily used to promote relaxation of the muscles controlling the joint, to relieve pain, and to prepare for more vigorous stretching techniques. In relatively acute cases of adhesive capsulitis, they may constitute the primary techniques used until resolution of the acute state allows more aggressive mobilization. In more chronic cases, they are typically used at the initiation of the mobilization session, between techniques, and at the end of the session to prevent and reduce reflex muscle cramping. As these techniques are performed, the arm may be gradually moved from the side of the body toward positions in which more vigorous techniques may be applied. For chronic conditions, these techniques should be used on a continuing basis in conjunction with the stretching techniques described.

I. **Glenohumeral Joint—General Techniques for Elevation and Relaxation**
   A. *Distraction*—in flexion (Fig. 9-28*A*)
      P—Prone, arm in 90° flexion over the edge of the table
      O—Sitting on a stool, facing the patient's

arm. The hands contact the distal humerus.
      M—The hands apply distraction along the long axis of the arm, applying a caudal force to the glenohumeral joint. This technique may be interspersed with pendulum exercises. While maintaining traction, one may also apply lateral glide (Fig. 9-28B).
   B. *Inferior glide*—in flexion (Fig. 9-28C)
      P—Prone, arm in 90° flexion over the edge of the table
      O—Sitting on a stool. Legs contact the patient's arm and fixate it. The mobilizing hand is positioned with the web space over the cranial surface of the proximal humerus.
      M—The mobilizing hand glides the humerus in a distal direction, while the legs guide and control the position of the arm.
   These are useful techniques for relaxation of spasm, relieving pain, and facilitating flexion, along with inferior glide with the arm at the side (see below). These techniques should be used before and after treatment sessions and between other techniques.
   C. *Inferior glide*—arm at side (Fig. 9-28*D*)
      P—Supine, with arm resting at side of body
      O—Stabilizes the scapula with his foot in the patient's axilla and grasps her distal forearm above the wrist with both hands
      M—By applying gentle traction to the arm and carefully adjusting the angle of his foot, the glenohumeral joint can be distracted. The patient's scapula may also be stabilized using a strap around the axilla as both hands grip the humerus (Fig. 9-28E), or the operator can stabilize the scapula by putting one hand in the axilla against the coracoid process of the scapula and use the other hand to grip the humerus (Fig. 9-28F). The patient's forearm is tucked between the operator's mobilizing arm and trunk, and the operator fixes the patient's arm against his trunk. The mobilizing hand(s) glides the humerus caudally as the operator rotates his trunk away from the joint. Progressive long-axis extension moving toward abduction may be performed by the operator shifting his trunk into outward rotation. As the patient relaxes, the arm may be gradually moved toward abduction. This technique may be

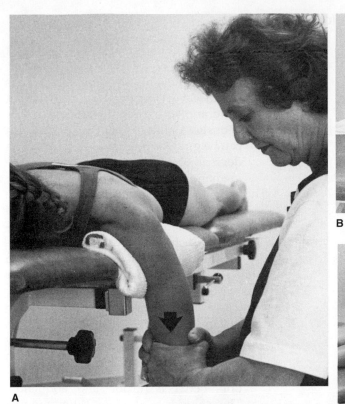

A

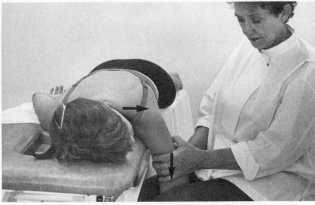

B

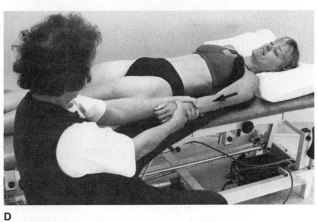

D

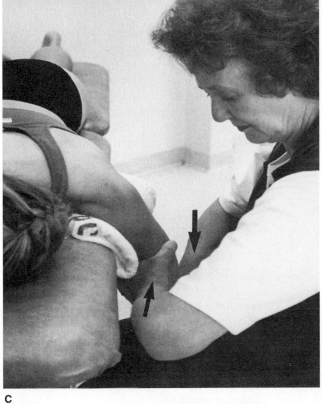

C

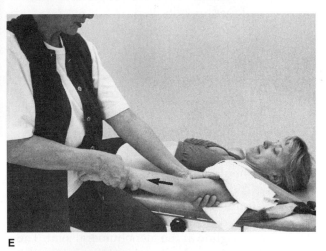

E

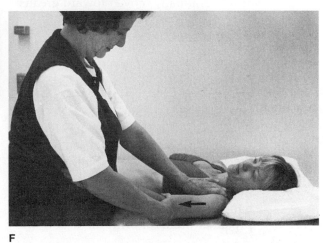

F

FIG. 9-28. General techniques for elevation and relaxation of the shoulder. (**A**) Distraction in flexion, (**B**) distraction with lateral glide, (**C**) distraction with inferior glide, (**D**) inferior glide, arm at side, (**E**) inferior glide, arm at side alternate technique (with a halter), and (**F**) progressive long-axis extension moving toward abduction.

performed up to about 80° abduction. **Note:** This is an important technique for relaxing spasm and relieving pain, to be used before and after a treatment session and between other techniques. For greater ranges of elevation, see Techniques.

II. **Glenohumeral Joint—Inferior Glide Techniques for Elevation**

A. *Inferior glide*—resting position (Fig. 9-29A)

P—Sitting with arms relaxed

O—Patient's arm is supported in resting or neutral position by the operator's forearm and hand. The mobilizing hand is placed on the lateral surface of the upper humerus (just lateral to the acromion process).

M—Mobilizing hand depresses the head of the humerus inferiorly and anteriorly. This technique may be used for assessment of inferior instability (multidirectional) or for loss of joint play, and as a technique to promote flexion and abduction. The limb may be moved out of the resting position and toward 90° of abduction if more aggressive techniques are indicated.

B. *Inferior glide*—moving toward flexion (Fig. 9-29B)

P—Supine, with the humerus flexed 60° to 100° and the elbow bent, with the wrist resting across the clavicular region

O—Grasps the proximal humerus with both hands, the fingers interlaced. The patient's elbow region is contacted with the clavicular region of the operator's shoulder closest to the patient.

M—The operator pulls caudally with his trunk to produce a movement of combined flexion of the humerus and inferior glide at the glenohumeral joint. The arm is gradually moved toward greater ranges of flexion, up to about 110°. For greater degrees of flexion, see Technique IID (below).

C. *Inferior glide*—in abduction (Fig. 9-29C)

P—Supine, elbow bent. The arm is close to the limits of abduction and external rotation, but comfortable.

O—Approaches the arm superiorly. He supports the elbow with the left hand at the distal humerus. The patient's forearm is tucked and supported between the operator's arm and trunk. The right hand contacts the superior aspect of the proximal humerus with the heel of the

hand, with the forearm supinated and the elbow bent.

M—Inferior glide of the humeral head is produced by the right hand as the left hand applies a grade I traction simultaneously. As the patient relaxes, the arm can be guided into gradually increasing degrees of abduction with the stabilizing hand.

This may be performed up to about 90°. The choice of position is guided by the ease with which a relaxed movement can be produced. This technique is used to increase abduction, allowing stretching into abduction while avoiding impingement of the greater tubercle on the acromial arch.

D. *Inferior glide*—in more than 90° elevation (Fig. 9-29D)

P—Supine, with arm elevated comfortably but close to the limits of full elevation in a somewhat horizontally abducted position, between flexion and abduction. The elbow is bent. Note: When moving into ranges past 90°, the patient's forearm may be supported on her forehead or on a pillow above her head, or the operator may support it, as shown.

O—Approaches the arm superiorly. He supports the elbow with the left hand, supporting the patient's arm on his right arm. The operator contacts the superior aspect of the proximal humerus with the right hand, with the thumb positioned ventrally just distal to the acromion.

M—Inferior glide of the humoral head is produced with the right hand. The arm can be guided into gradually increasing degrees of elevation. **Note:** The direction of movement is performed caudally and in a somewhat lateral direction, in keeping with the relationship of the joint surfaces in this position.

Movements in elevation beyond 90° are particularly useful as stretching techniques and may be used even when only a few degrees of elevation are restricted; however, they have no place in the treatment of a very painful shoulder.

III. **Glenohumeral Joint—Internal rotation**

A. *Posterior glide*—arm in various degrees of abduction (10° to 55°) (Fig. 9-30A)

P—Supine, with the arm slightly abducted

O—Standing between the patient's arm and body, supporting the patient's elbow with his right hand. The hand, wrist,

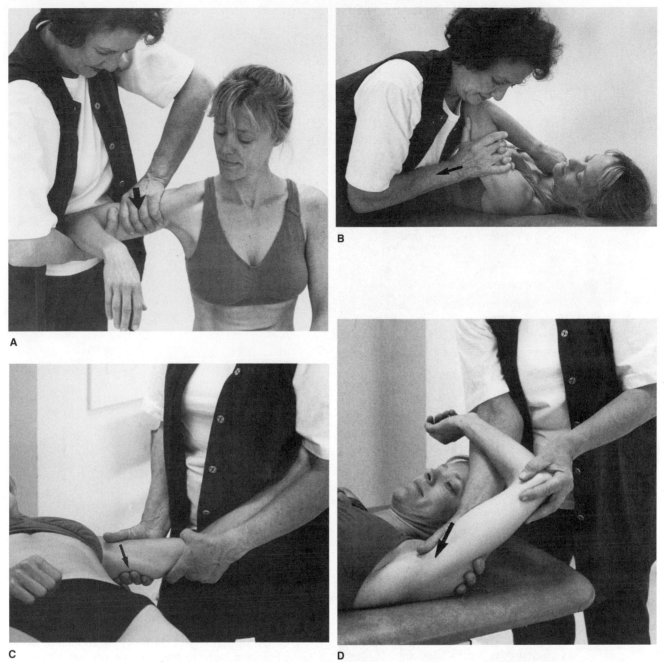

FIG. 9-29. Inferior glides: (**A**) inferior glide in the resting position, sitting, (**B**) inferior glide moving toward flexion, (**C**) inferior glide in abduction, supine, and (**D**) inferior glide in more than 90° elevation.

and forearm are supported by tucking them between his elbow and side. The left hand contacts the anterior aspect of the upper humerus with the heel of the left hand, with the forearm pronated and the elbow straight.

M—A posterior glide is produced by leaning forward slightly and flexing the knees, transmitting the force through the straight arm. This technique is used

to increase joint play necessary for internal rotation and flexion.

B. *Anterior glide*—arm close to the limits of internal rotation (Fig. 9-30*B*)

P—Lying on uninvolved side with the arm behind the back so it rests comfortably, but close to the limits of internal rotation

O—Standing behind the patient with both thumb pads over the posterior humeral

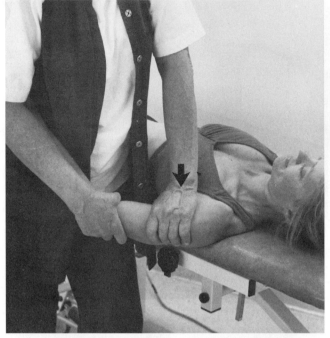

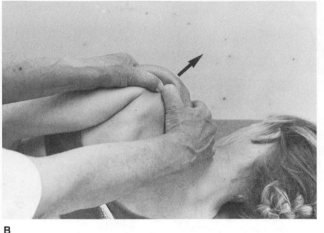

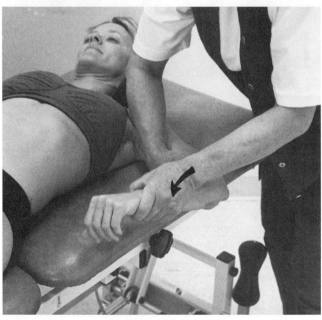

FIG. 9-30. Techniques for internal rotation of the shoulder joint: (**A**) posterior glide, arm slightly abducted, (**B**) anterior glide, arm close to the limits of internal rotation, at side or behind back, (**C**) internal rotation, arm close to 90° abduction.

head. The fingers of the right hand grasp around anteriorly to stabilize at the anterior aspect of the acromion and clavicle. Elbows remain almost fully extended. The left knee may be brought up onto the plinth to support the patient's arm.

M—An anterior glide is produced by leaning forward with the upper trunk, transmitting the force through the thumbs. Internal rotation is gradually increased by progressively moving the patient's hand up the back. This tech-

nique results in a posterior capsular stretch, stretching into internal rotation while avoiding posterior impingement of the humeral head on the glenoid labrum.

C. *Internal rotation technique*—arm close to 90° abduction (Fig. 9-30C)

P—Supine, with the arm resting comfortably but as close to 90° abduction as possible, the elbow bent to 90°, and the forearm pronated

O—Supports the wrist with the left hand; supports under the elbow with the fingers of the right hand from the medial side. He positions the right upper arm in front of and just medial to the shoulder.

M—The right upper arm provides only enough counterpressure to the shoulder to prevent lifting of the shoulder girdle; the hand maintains the arm in abduction. The left hand simultaneously rotates the arm internally. The operator's left thigh may be brought up onto the plinth to act as a stop to internal rotation (see Fig. 6-1). The stop should be close to the limit of movement so as to minimize anticipatory guarding by the patient. The stop is progressively moved as motion increases. This is an oscillatory movement.

Methods for internal rotation are useful for restoring necessary joint-play movements with the arm near the side or in various degrees of abduction (see Technique IIIA), or as a stretching technique in functional position (see Technique IIIB). Internal rotation is accompanied by scapular retraction and associated clavicular movements. Normal internal rotation at the glenohumeral joint, therefore, is not possible without adequate scapular mobility.[114]

IV. Glenohumeral Joint—External rotation

A. *Anterior glide*—arm at side (Fig. 9-31*A*)

P—Supine, arm at the side, elbow bent, forearm supported by operator's arm

O—Stabilizes with the right hand, grasping the distal humerus just proximal to the elbow. He grasps around the posterior aspect of the proximal humerus with the right hand.

M—An anterior glide is effected with the right hand after the slack in the shoulder girdle has been taken up. This is an oscillatory mobilization. This technique is used to increase the joint-play movement necessary for external rotation.

B. *Anterior glide*—prone (Fig. 9-31*B*)

P—Lies prone with the humerus positioned off the edge of the table; a pad supporting the coracoid process provides some stabilization of the scapula

O—Standing, facing the medial side of the upper arm. The glenohumeral joint is positioned in the resting position (if conservative techniques are indicated) or approximating the restricted range (if more aggressive techniques are indicated, such as capsular stretch). He supports the patient's elbow against his

body with the left hand, maintaining the arm in abduction and neutral rotation. The upper limb is lowered slightly into a position in the plane of the scapula (30° to 45° anterior to the coronal plane).[49,66,118] The mobilizing hand is placed over the posterior aspect of the proximal humerus close to the joint.

M—Grade I traction is maintained throughout with the left hand. An anterior glide is produced by leaning forward with the trunk, transmitting the force through the straight arm and flexion of the knees. This technique is used to increase joint play necessary for external rotation, extension, and horizontal abduction.

C. *Anterior glide*—near the limits of external rotation (Fig 9-31*C*)[75]

P—Prone, lying as above

O—Standing, facing the table. The patient's flexed elbow rests on the operator's distal thigh. The outside hand supports the distal forearm above the wrist. The mobilizing hand contacts the proximal dorsal aspect of the humerus.

M—The mobilizing hand glides the humerus in the anterior direction. The amplitude and velocity of this technique is graded according to the patient's symptoms.

D. *Posterior glide*—arm close to 90° abduction (Fig. 9-31*D*)

P—Supine, with the arm resting comfortably but as close to 90° abduction as possible; elbow bent to 90°

O—Supports the wrist with his right hand. He contacts the anterior aspect of the proximal humerus with the heel of the left hand. The thigh may be brought up onto the plinth to act as a stop (Fig. 6-2).

M—Posterior glide is produced with the left hand, while the right hand simultaneously rotates the arm externally. The thigh provides a stop to external rotation close to the limit of movement. This minimizes anticipatory guarding by the patient. The stop is progressively moved as motion increases. This is an oscillatory movement, produced synchronously with posterior glide.

This method results in an anterior capsular stretch, stretching into external rotation while avoiding anterior impingement of the humerus on the glenoid labrum.

V. Glenohumeral   Joint—General   Capsular

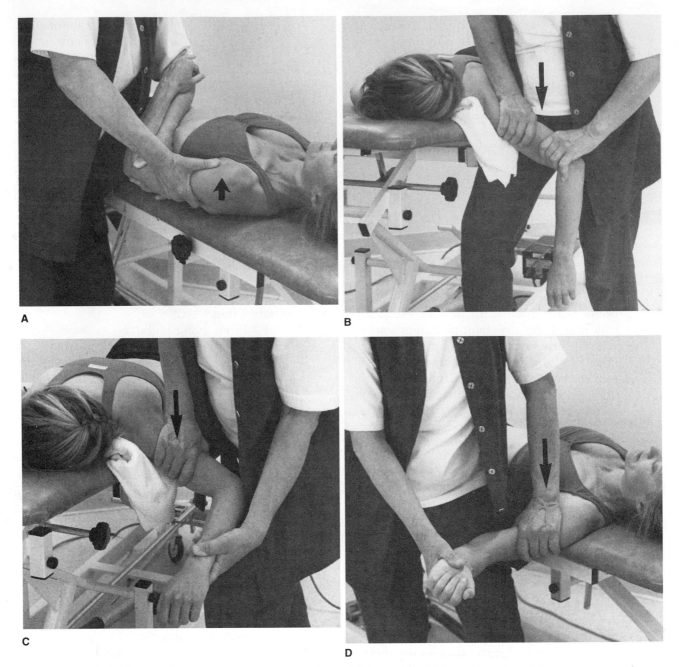

FIG. 9-31. Techniques for external rotation of the shoulder joint: (**A**) anterior glide, arm at side (supine); (**B**) anterior glide (prone); (**C**) anterior glide near the limits of external rotation; (**D**) posterior glide, arm close to 90° of abduction (capsular stretch).

Stretch and Techniques for Horizontal Adduction

A. *Posterior glide or shear* (Fig. 9-32A)

P—Supine, with the arm flexed to 90°. The arm may also be placed in various degrees of horizontal adduction. A pad is placed under the scapula for stabilization.

O—One or both hands are placed over the patient's elbow.

M—Posterior glide is directed through the long axis of the humerus in a slightly lateral direction. This technique is used to increase horizontal adduction, extension, and flexion. Direction of movement may also be directed in a posterior cranial direction.

B. *Lateral glide*—arm at side (glenohumeral distraction) (Fig. 9-32B)

P—Supine, arm at the side, with the elbow bent and the hand resting on her stomach or on the operator's forearm

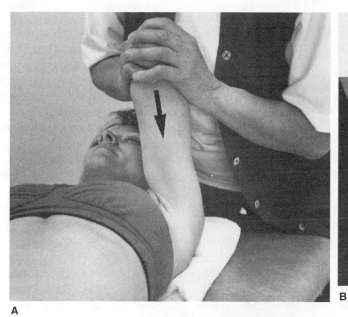

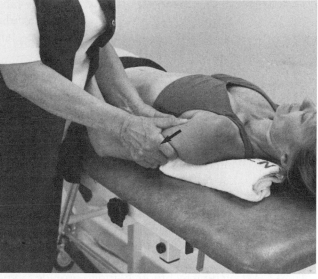

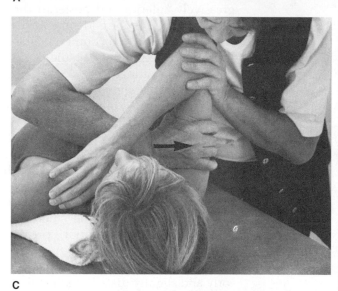

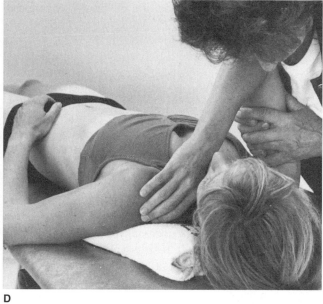

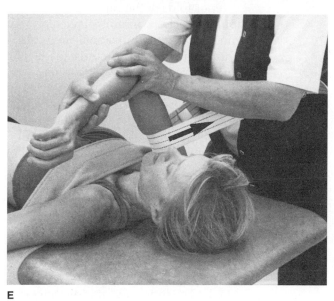

FIG. 9-32. General capsular stretch and techniques for horizontal adduction: (**A**) posterior glide or shear; (**B**) lateral glide, arm at side; (**C**) lateral glide in flexion; (**D**) lateral and backward glide in flexion; (**E**) lateral glide in flexion with a belt.

O—The operator is at the patient's side facing the glenohumeral joint. Both hands grasp the humerus medially, as far proximally as possible.

M—A lateral glide is effected by moving the upper humerus laterally with both hands. The arm should be allowed to move laterally through the same excursion as the humeral head, avoiding a tilting maneuver, unless it is specifically intended to stretch the superior joint capsule. (Anterior, posterior, and inferior glides may also be carried out with this hand placement.)

This technique (performed at the side of the body) is used to promote relaxation, to relieve pain, to prepare for more vigorous stretching techniques, and to provide a general capsular stretch. As the latter, it may be useful in increasing movement toward the close-packed position by helping to prevent premature compression of the joint.

C. *Lateral glide*—in flexion (Fig. 9-32C)

P—Supine, with the arm flexed comfortably to 90° and the elbow bent so that the hand rests on the upper chest

O—Stabilizes the distal humerus with his left hand at the elbow. The right hand is placed against the medial surface of the upper end of the humerus. By bending forward, the arm is placed in a horizontal position in line with the movement.

M—The proximal humerus is moved laterally. This technique is used to restore joint play necessary for horizontal adduction. It results in separation of the joint surfaces (lateral distraction).

D. *Lateral and backward glide*—in flexion (Fig. 9-32D)

P—Supine, with the arm flexed comfortably to 90° and the elbow bent so that the hand rests on the upper chest

O—Stabilizes the distal humerus and elbow by resting them against his trapezial ridge. He grasps the medial aspect of the proximal humerus with both hands, interlacing the fingers.

M—The proximal humerus is moved backward, toward the plinth, and outward simultaneously in a rocking forward and downward movement of the operator's trunk. The arm may be progressively moved toward increased horizontal adduction as the patient relaxes. This technique is used to increase joint play necessary for horizontal adduction

by using lateral glide with a backward glide simultaneously. A belt placed around the patient's proximal humerus and around the operator's pelvis (or waist) may be used to apply lateral glide (traction) by backward leaning of the operator's trunk (Fig. 9-32E).[67]

VI. Glenohumeral Joint—Anteroposterior Glide for the Last Few Degrees of Elevation

A. *Anterior glide*—in supine (Fig. 9-33A)

P—Supine, arm at end range of flexion/abduction

O—Standing, facing the patient's feet. Both hands grip the proximal humerus. The humerus is externally rotated to its limit. The patient's arm is cradled by the operator's arm and body to maintain the plane of scapula position.

M—The hands glide the humerus in a progressively anterior and posterior direction. During anterior glide, the force directs the head of the humerus against the inferior folds of the capsule.

B. *Anterior glide*—in sitting (Fig. 9-33B)

P—Sitting with the shoulder in maximum flexion/abduction and externally rotated

O—Standing next to the patient with the humerus against his chest and arm to maintain plane of scapula position. The stabilizing hand contacts the clavicle and scapular girdle proximal to the glenohumeral joint. The mobilizing hand grips the posterior proximal humerus.

M—The mobilizing force is directed anteriorly and slightly distally against the inferior folds of the capsule.

Scapulothoracic, acromioclavicular, and sternoclavicular mobilizations may also be performed in certain circumstances. However, these are rarely necessary in cases of glenohumeral capsular tightness, because these joints tend to become hypermobile by compensating for the restriction at the glenohumeral joint. They may be useful following immobilization of the entire shoulder complex or in other disorders, such as arthritis or injury in the different joints (*i.e.*, fractures and dislocations) as well as neuromuscular dysfunction.

VII. Sternoclavicular Joint

A. *Distraction* (Fig. 9-34A)[51]

P—Supine

O—Standing on the opposite side of the table. The index and middle fingers rest

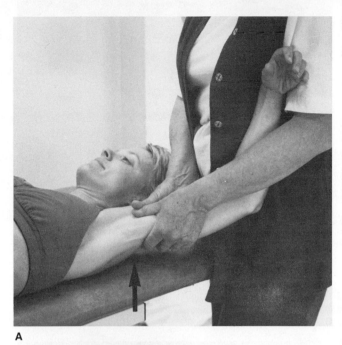

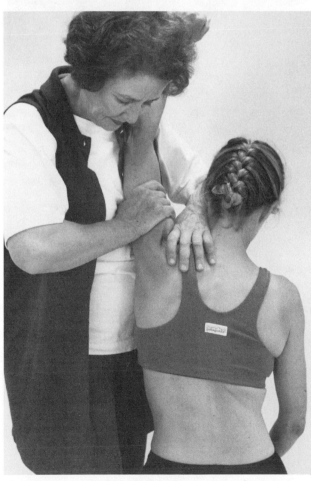

B

FIG. 9-33. Anterior glides for the last few degrees of elevation (flexion, abduction): (**A**) in supine and (**B**) in sitting.

on the first costal cartilage and manubrium sterni to fixate the proximal aspect of the joint. The heel of the mobilizing hand contacts the lateral anterior concavity of the clavicle.

M—Distraction force is applied in the lateral direction. This is considered a test and general technique to restore joint play of the sternoclavicular joint.

B. *Superior glide* (Fig. 9-34B)

P—Supine

O—Standing, facing the patient. Both thumbs contact the inferior aspect of the proximal clavicle. The mobilizing thumb is positioned over the thumb of the guiding hand.

M—The mobilizing hand glides the clavicle in a cephalad, somewhat medial direction in the plane of the joint. This technique is used to increase the joint play of the sternoclavicular joint and increase depression.

C. *Inferior glide* (Fig. 9-34C)

P—Supine

O—Standing at the patient's head. The mobilizing hand is placed over the thumb of the guiding hand.

M—The mobilizing hand glides the clavicle in a caudal, somewhat lateral direction in the plane of the joint. This technique is used to increase joint play and increase elevation.

D. *Posterior glide* (Fig. 9-34D)

P—Supine

O—Standing, facing the patient. Both thumbs contact the proximal end of the clavicle.

M—The thumbs glide in a posterior direction. This technique is used to increase retraction. Gliding anteriorly can be achieved by gripping around the clavicle with the fingers while the stabilizing hand is positioned over the sternum (Fig. 9-34E). The mobilizing hand glides the clavicle in a ventral direction. This technique is used to increase protraction.

VIII. Acromioclavicular Joint—All of the following techniques are considered general techniques to restore joint play of the acromioclavicular joint. The amplitude and velocity of the techniques vary according to the joint's irritability.

A. *Distraction* (Fig. 9-35A)[51]

P—Supine

O—Standing on the opposite side of the table. The clavicle is grasped between the index finger and thumb to provide

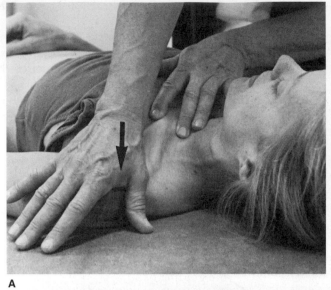

A

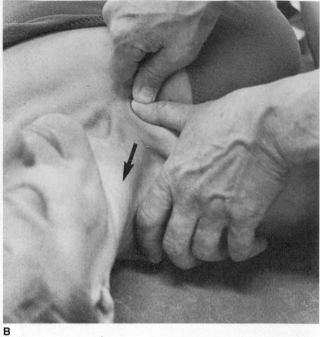

B

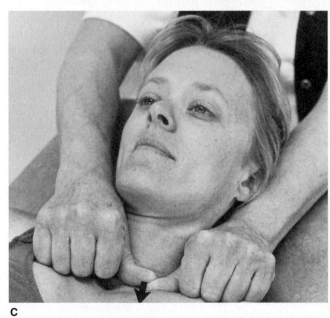

C

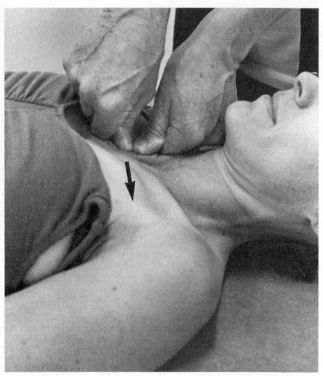

D

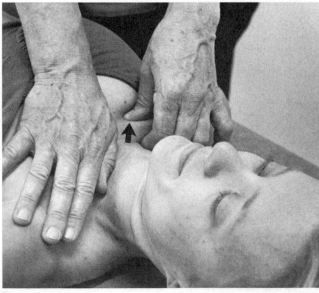

E

FIG. 9-34. Sternoclavicular joint: (**A**) distraction, (**B**) superior glide, (**C**) inferior glide, (**D**) posterior glide, (**E**) anterior glide.

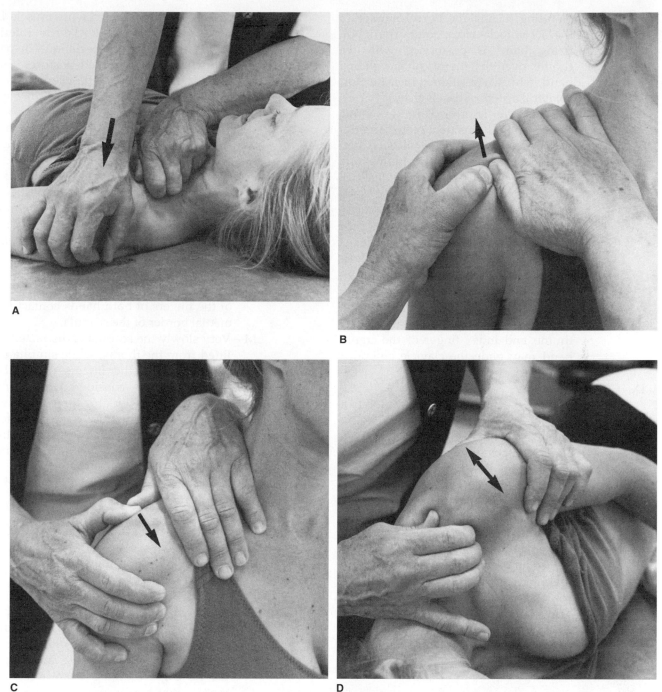

FIG. 9-35. Acromioclavicular joint: (**A**) distraction, (**B**) anteroposterior glide, (**C**) posteroanterior glide, (**D**) anterior and posterior glide in sidelying.

fixation. The mobilizing hand contacts the shoulder, distal to the joint over the acromion.

M—Distraction pressure is applied with the heel of the hand. This technique is considered a test and a general technique to restore joint play of the acromioclavicular joint.

B. *Anteroposterior glide* (Fig. 9-35B)

P—Sitting, the joint in the resting position

O—Facing the ventral surface of the acromion. The thumbs are placed over the anterolateral surface of the clavicle. The medial hand provides stabilization over the dorsal aspect of the scapula.

M—The thumbs glide the clavicle posteriorly.

C. *Posteroanterior glide*

P—Sitting (Fig. 9-35C) or sidelying (Fig. 9-35D), the joint in the resting position

O—Standing, facing the dorsal surface of the acromioclavicular joint. The mobilizing hand is positioned with the thumb over the thumb of the gliding hand, which is positioned over the dorsolateral aspect of the clavicle.

M—The clavicle is glided in a ventral, slightly lateral direction. Note: Anterior and posterior glide may also be performed in sidelying. The thumb and index finger of the stabilizing (cranial) hand contact the distal end of the clavicle with a pincer grasp, while the mobilizing (caudal) hand grasps the acromion process and lateral border of the scapula. The mobilizing hand glides the scapula anteroposterior at the acromioclavicular joint. Alternatively, the caudal hand may stabilize the scapula and proximal humerus and the thumb and index finger of the cranial hand may glide the clavicle anteriorly or posteriorly (see Fig. 9-35D).

IX. Clavicle

A. *Inferior glide*—active physiologic mobilization or isometric technique (Fig. 9-36)[105]

P—Supine

O—Standing, facing the patient. The medial hand grasps the posterior proximal aspect of the humerus and lifts the shoulder girdle into some protraction. The lateral hand holds the distal forearm above the wrist.

M—The patient is instructed to lift the upper limb straight up against the unyielding resistance given by the operator's hand on the forearm. An isometric

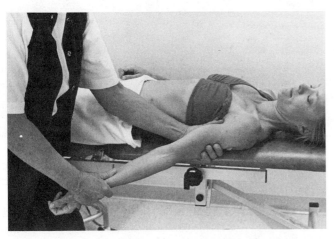

FIG. 9-36. *Inferior glide of the clavicle using isometric technique.*

contraction of the subclavius muscle is produced, moving the clavicle inferiorly. This is a useful technique in patients with forward head postures. Superior subluxation of the clavicle may result from tightness of the sternocleidomastoid.[105] Soft-tissue mobilizations and stretching of the sternocleidomastoid and other restricted soft tissues should be done concurrently.

X. Scapulothoracic Joint—distraction techniques. (This is not a true joint, but the soft tissue is stretched to obtain normal shoulder-girdle mobility.)

A. *Distraction of the medial border of the scapula* (Fig. 9-37A)

P—Prone or sidelying

O—Standing at the patient's side. The pads of the fingers of both hands contact the medial border of the scapula.

M—Very slowly the scapula is distracted or lifted from the thorax, while simultaneously working the fingers under the scapula. This is considered a general technique. The winging or distractive motion is an important movement for reaching behind the back. If there is little mobility, begin in prone and progress to sidelying.

B. *Distraction or inferior glide of the scapula* (Fig. 9-37B)

P—Prone or sidelying

O—The mobilizing hand is placed over the acromion process while the web space of the guiding or stabilizing hand is positioned under the inferior border of the scapula.

M—The mobilizing hand moves the scapula medially and caudally over the guiding or stabilizing hand. The guiding hand assists in lifting the scapula away from the rib cage. Winging is an accessory motion that occurs when a person attempts to place the hand behind the back, accompanying shoulder internal rotation and scapular downward rotation.[73]

C. *Scapulothoracic articulations*—medial-lateral glide, superior-inferior glide, rotation and diagonal patterns (Fig. 9-38)

P—Sidelying, the upper limb supported and draped over the operator's arm

O—Standing, facing the patient. The cranial hand is placed across the acromion process to guide and control the direc-

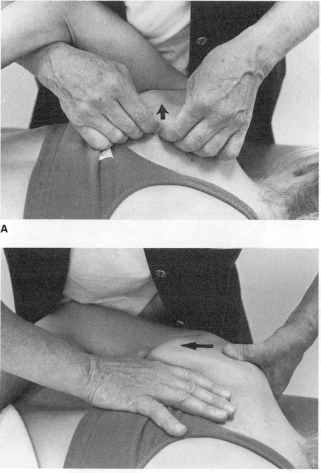

FIG. 9-37. Scapulothoracic joint distractions: (**A**) medial border, (**B**) inferior border.

tion of motion. The caudal hand contacts the inferior angle of the scapula.

M—The scapula is moved in the desired direction by lifting from the inferior angle or by pushing on the acromion process (Fig. 9-38).

☐ **Self-Mobilization Techniques**[122]

(For simplicity, all the techniques described in this section are applied to the patient's *right* extremity, except where indicated. In the self-mobilization techniques, the left hand usually is performing the mobilizations. E—equipment; P—patient; MH—mobilizing hand; M—movement.)

 I. **Inferior Glide**—Long-axis extension (Fig. 9-39)
   E—A high-back chair that is well padded with a blanket or towel on the back of the chair

   P—Sitting, with the right arm over the back of the chair, the axilla firmly fixed over the back of the chair

   MH—Grasps the arm just proximal to the humeral epicondyles so as to gain a purchase on them. An alternate hand-hold would be to grasp the forearm just above the styloid processes.

   M—An inferior glide is produced by pulling directly downward toward the floor while using rhythmic oscillations (Fig. 9-39A). A variation of this technique is to use a weight in the hand (e.g., a bucket of sand) and to perform gentle, pivot-like motions at the end (Fig. 9-39B).

 II. **Inferior Glide**—Shoulder adduction with distraction (Fig. 9-40)
   E—A firm pillow or towel roll placed in the axilla

   P—Standing, with the arm positioned across the chest

   MH—Grasps the forearm just above the styloid processes. MH pulls the arm rhythmically across the chest (into adduction) and downward, resulting in a slight separation of the head of the humerus in the glenoid cavity (Fig. 9-40A). Note: Distraction dorsally may be carried out in a similar fashion if the patient has sufficient internal rotation to place the forearm behind the back. In this case, the elbow is flexed and the MH uses rhythmic oscillations behind the patient's back in a downward direction dorsally (Fig. 9-40B).

 III. **Inferior Glide**—Glenohumeral abduction when the patient has less than 90° abduction (Fig. 9-41A)
   P—Sitting sideways at a table, the right arm is positioned comfortably at the end of painless abduction with the muscles relaxed. The elbow is extended with the hand and the forearm fixed on the table.

   MH—Contacts the anterior-superior aspect of the proximal humerus below the acromion

   M—An inferior glide is produced by pushing directly downward toward the floor, with rhythmic oscillations

 IV. **Inferior Glide**—Glenohumeral abduction when the patient has more than 90° abduction (Fig. 9-41B)
   P—Standing with the right side facing a wall. The arm is positioned comfortably in abduction so that the forearm rests on the wall, with the elbow in 90° flexion.

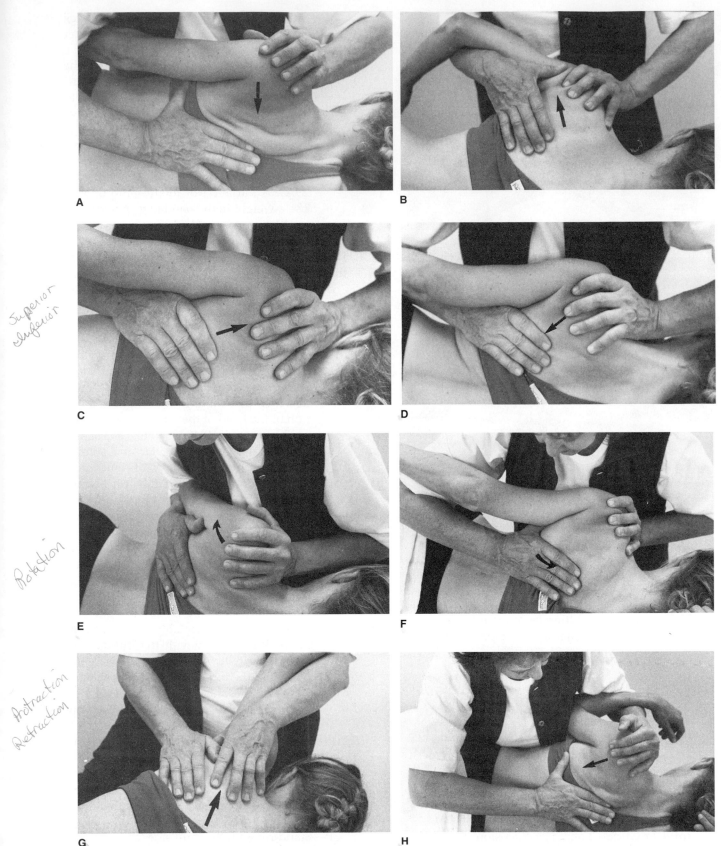

FIG. 9-38. Scapulothoracic joint: (**A**) medial glide, (**B**) lateral glide, (**C**) superior glide, (**D**) inferior glide, (**E**) upward rotation, (**F**) downward rotation, (**G**) elevation and protraction, (**H**) depression and retraction.

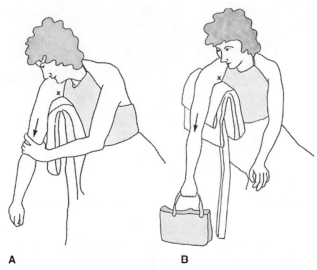

FIG. 9-39. Inferior glide (long-axis extension) of gleno-humeral joint may be performed (**A**) manually or (**B**) by using weights.

MH—Contacts the anterior-superior aspect of the proximal end of the humerus below the acromion

M—An inferior glide is produced by pushing directly downward toward the floor with rhythmic oscillations. A stronger capsular stretch can be performed by bending the knees and using body weight to assist in the movement.

V. **Inferior Glide**—Glenohumeral flexion when the patient has less than 90° flexion (Fig. 9-42*A*)

P—Sitting facing a table. The right forearm is positioned comfortably at the end of painless flexion with the muscles relaxed. A pillow wedge is used under the fore-

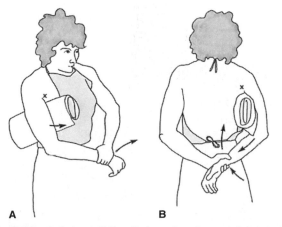

FIG. 9-40. Inferior glide of the glenohumeral joint: (**A**) shoulder adduction with distraction ventrally; (**B**) shoulder adduction with distraction dorsally.

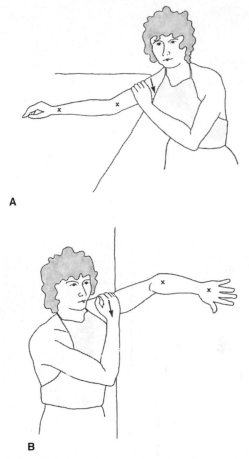

FIG. 9-41. Inferior glide of the glenohumeral joint: (**A**) shoulder abduction for 90° or less; (**B**) shoulder abduction for 90° or more.

arm to provide fixation of the hand and forearm.

MH—Contacts the anterior-superior aspect of the proximal humerus below the acromion

M—An inferior glide is produced by pushing directly downward toward the floor, with rhythmic oscillations

VI. **Inferior Glide**—Glenohumeral flexion when the patient has more than 90° flexion (Fig. 9-42*B*)

P—Standing facing a wall. The right forearm, with the elbow bent to 90° flexion, is positioned at the end of range on the wall for fixation.

MH—Contacts the anterosuperior aspect of the proximal end of the humerus below the acromion

M—An inferior glide is produced by pushing directly downward toward the floor, with rhythmic oscillations. A stronger capsular stretch may be performed by lowering the body weight.

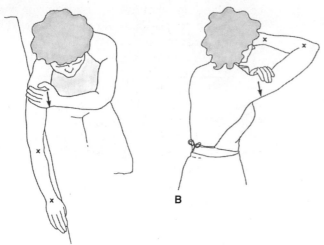

A

FIG. 9-42. Inferior glide of the glenohumeral joint: (**A**) shoulder flexion for 90° or less; (**B**) shoulder flexion for 90° or more flexion.

VII. Anterior Glide—Shoulder extension (Fig. 9-43)

P—Sitting, with the back to a table. The right arm is positioned comfortably at the limits of painless extension with the muscles relaxed. The elbow is extended with the right hand fixed on the table. The trunk is flexed.

MH—Contacts the posterosuperior aspect of the proximal humerus just below the acromion

M—An anterior glide is produced by moving the arm in a ventral-caudal direction, with rhythmic oscillations.

VIII. Shoulder Internal Rotation (Fig. 9-44)

P—Sitting sideways to a table. The right upper arm is positioned so that its entire extent is braced against the table. To do this, the patient bends the trunk to the side toward the upper arm. The elbow is flexed to 90°.

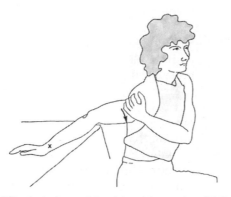

FIG. 9-43. Anterior glide (shoulder extension) of the glenohumeral joint.

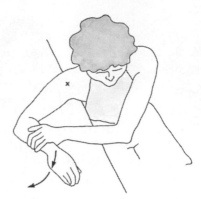

FIG. 9-44. Internal rotation of the glenohumeral joint.

MH—Grasps the dorsal aspect of the wrist with the thumb, and with the fingers wrapped around the ventral aspect

M—The arm is internally rotated as far as possible with rhythmic oscillations performed at the end of the range.

IX. Shoulder External Rotation (Fig. 9-45)

P—Sitting sideways to a table. The right upper arm is positioned so that its entire extent is braced against the table. To do this, the patient bends the trunk to the side toward the upper arm. The elbow is flexed to 90°.

MH—Grasps the ventral aspect of the wrist

M—The forearm is externally rotated, and rhythmic oscillations are performed at the end of the range.

Note: Hold–relax techniques are particularly useful with rotation techniques of the shoulder.

□ **Self Capsular Stretches**

A more aggressive approach to stretching the joint capsule and surrounding musculature usually commences when the patient has attained flexibility of at least 90° abduction. The end feel is firm, and the end

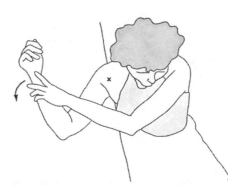

FIG. 9-45. External rotation of the glenohumeral joint.

point is no longer painful. The patient may be instructed to hold at the end range for 10 seconds, with a 5-second rest between consecutive stretches (ten to 15 repetitions), or to apply a longer-duration, low-load stretch. Low-load, long-duration stretches are more efficient in elongating soft tissue than high-load, short-duration stretches.[80,142] Heat in conjunction with low-load, long-duration stretching can be used to facilitate shoulder flexibility.[78] Thus, the patient can be put in a comfortable elongation position with a slight load with heat for 40 seconds or longer.

I. **Anterior Capsule Stretch** (see Fig. 9-46A)

   P—Supine with the involved shoulder over the edge of the table, the elbow flexed to 90° and the shoulder in a comfortable position of abduction, depending on the portion of capsule that is tight. A weight is placed in the hand (starting with 1 or 2 lb or less), or tubing may be used (with tubing securely in the hand and the opposite end attached to the table or

bed). Padding should be used under the upper limb to position the shoulder in the plane of the scapula.

   M—The patient allows the weight or tubing to pull the shoulder into maximum external rotation and some extension. As an exercise to stretch the anterior-inferior capsule, have the patient lie supine with the shoulder over the table edge in a position of about 135° abduction (Fig. 9-46B). Again, padding is used under the upper limb to maintain the plane of scapula position.

II. **Inferior Capsule Stretch** (Fig. 9-46C)

   P—Supine on the table with the shoulder at comfortable end range of flexion. Padding should be used under the upper limb to maintain the plane of scapula position.

   M—A weight or tubing is used to facilitate stretch into fuller flexion.

III. **Posterior Capsule Stretch.** The posterior capsule can be stretched by holding the involved arm in

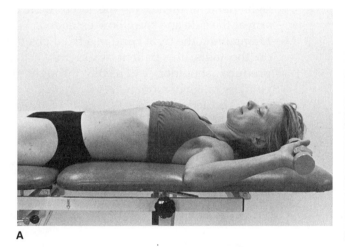

A

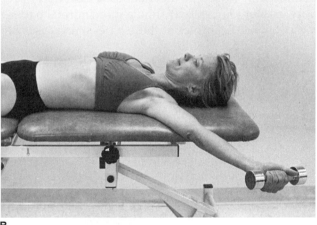

B

C

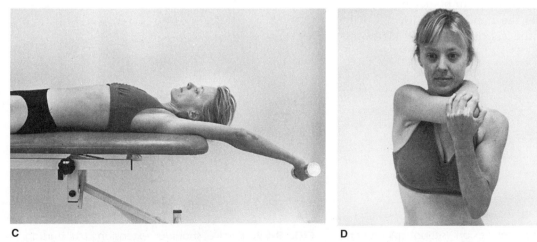

D

FIG. 9-46. Self capsular stretches: (**A**) anterior capsular, (**B**) anterior-inferior capsular, (**C**) inferior capsular, and (**D**) posterior capsular stretch.

horizontal adduction and by placing the hand near the opposite shoulder (Fig. 9-46*D*). A gentle pull is applied with the opposite hand.

☐ Self Range of Motion

Other exercises particularly useful in a home program for painful extremity joints have been advocated by Dontigny[36] and Grimsby.[53] They allow the patient to stretch his or her joints passively by moving the body in relation to the stabilized extremity. This type of movement affords an excellent stretch, minimizes incorrect movements by the patient, and allows a greater degree of pain-free movement. Grimsby maintains that when passive exercise is used for the hip, shoulder, or ankle, the patient uses the concave surface of the joint to mobilize. In so doing, the patient avoids considerable pain and achieves a greater range of motion, because rolling and gliding occur in the same direction.[52] If we compare these exercises to the traditional approach of movement of the extremity in relation to the body, it also appears that using a closed kinetic chain (through the stabilized extremity) provides greater joint stability and a more normal pattern of movement. Examples of these types of exercises are described for the shoulder.

I. **Shoulder Flexion**
 A. *Sitting* (Fig. 9-47)
  P—Sitting at the side of a table with the forearm resting on the table
  M—Patient flexes the trunk and head while sliding the arm forward along the edge of the table, so that the shoulder is moved passively into flexion
 B. *Standing* (Fig. 9-48)
  P—Standing, facing a high countertop (or a high window ledge or bookshelf). The patient rests the hand, palm down, on the edge of the counter with the elbow extended.

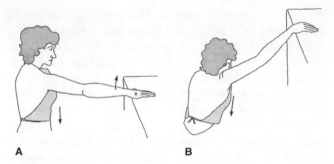

FIG. 9-48. *Passive shoulder flexion (standing):* (**A**) *starting position;* (**B**) *end position.*

  M—The patient lowers the body weight to move the shoulder passively into flexion. Weight-bearing stretches may be done in the all-fours or crawling position. The upper limbs are gradually stretched forward as the body sinks into a prone position (sitting on the heels) to eventually achieve full forward-flexion.
II. **Shoulder Extension** (Fig. 9-49)
 P—Standing with the right side to the table. The right hand is placed on the table, with the arm at the side and the elbow extended.
 M—Maintaining the right hand in a fixed position on the table, the patient walks forward to produce shoulder extension through the painless range of motion.
III. **Shoulder Abduction**
 A. *Sitting* (Fig. 9-50)
  P—Sitting at the side of a table and resting the forearm on the table, with the forearm supinated and the shoulder slightly abducted
  M—The patient sidebends the upper trunk to

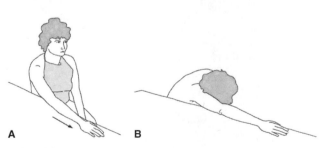

FIG. 9-47. *Passive shoulder flexion (sitting):* (**A**) *starting position;* (**B**) *end position.*

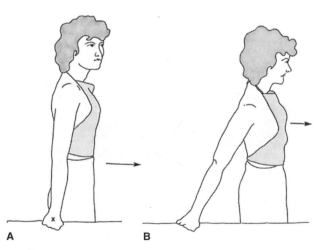

FIG. 9-49. *Passive shoulder extension:* (**A**) *starting position;* (**B**) *end position.*

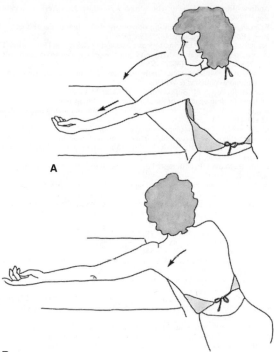

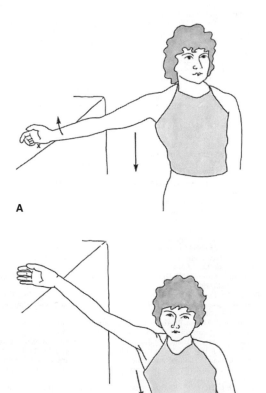

FIG. 9-50. Passive shoulder abduction (sitting): (**A**) starting position; (**B**) end position.

FIG. 9-51. Passive shoulder abduction (standing): (**A**) starting position; (**B**) end position.

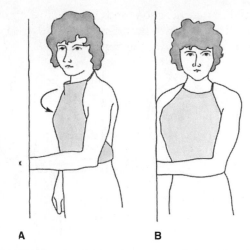

FIG. 9-52. Passive internal rotation of shoulder: (**A**) starting position; (**B**) end position.

the left from the waist while sliding the arm across the table so that the shoulder is moved into abduction as the lower trunk moves away from the table.

   B. *Standing* (Fig. 9-51)
      P—Standing with the right side facing a high countertop (or a high window ledge or bookshelf). The patient rests the hand on the surface with the forearm slightly supinated, elbow extended, and shoulder abducted through partial range.
      M—The patient lowers the body weight, allowing the shoulder to move passively into abduction and external rotation.
IV. Shoulder Internal Rotation (Fig. 9-52)
   P—Standing with the left side toward a door frame. The patient places the back of the hand against the frame so that it will remain fixed with his elbow flexed 90°. The upper arm remains at the side with the elbow held close to the trunk.

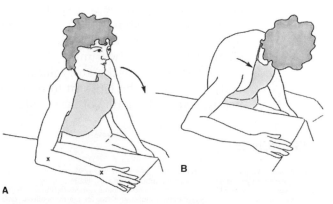

FIG. 9-53. Passive external rotation of shoulder (sitting): (**A**) starting position; (**B**) end position.

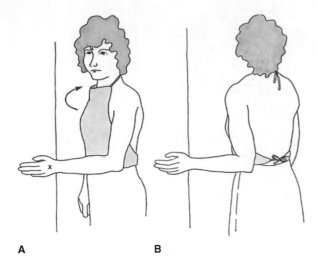

A   **B**

FIG. 9-54. Passive external rotation of shoulder (standing): (**A**) starting position; (**B**) end position.

M—The patient walks forward, rotating toward the left forearm to produce passive internal rotation of the shoulder.

Internal rotation may be done in a standing position, with the patient attempting to reach behind and up the back as far as possible. The opposite limb grasps the involved side at the wrist and attempts to stretch it further. A hand towel can be used behind the back in a similar fashion.

V. Shoulder External Rotation

A. *Sitting* (Fig. 9-53)

    P—Sitting at the side of a table, with the forearm resting on the table, the shoulder abducted, and the elbow flexed

    M—The patient flexes the trunk and head forward toward the table, allowing the shoulder to be moved passively into external rotation.

B. *Standing* (Fig. 9-54)

    P—Standing, facing a door frame. The patient places the palmar surface of the hand against the frame so that it will remain fixed. The elbow is flexed 90°. The upper arm remains at the side with the elbow held close to the trunk.

    M—The patient walks backward, rotating the body away from the left arm to produce passive external rotation of the shoulder.

REFERENCES

1. Adson AW, Coffey JR: Cervical rib: A method of anterior approach for relief of symptoms by division of the scalenus anticus. Ann Surg 85:839–857, 1927
2. Akeson WH, Woo SLY, Amiel D: The connective tissue response to immobility: Biomechanical changes in periarticular connective tissue of the immobilized rabbit knee. Clin Orthop 93:356–362, 1973
3. Andrews JR, Gillogly S: Physical examination of the shoulder in throwing athletes. In Zarins B, Andrews JR, Carson WG (eds): Injuries to the Throwing Arm. Philadelphia, WB Saunders, 1985
4. Andrews JR, Wilk KE (eds): The Athlete's Shoulder. New York, Churchill Livingstone, 1994
5. Basmajian JV: Factors preventing downward dislocation of the abducted shoulder joint. J Bone Joint Surg 41A:1182–1186, 1959
6. Basmajian JV: Weight bearing by ligaments and muscles. Can J Surg 4:166–170, 1961
7. Basmajian JV: Surgical anatomy and function of the arm-trunk mechanism. Surg Clin North Am 43:1471–1482, 1963
8. Basmajian JV: Muscles Alive: Their Functions Revealed by Electromyography, 4th ed. Baltimore, Williams & Wilkins, 1977
9. Bateman JE, Welsh RP. Surgery of the Shoulder. St. Louis, CV Mosby, 1984
10. Bechtol CO: Biomechanics of the shoulder. Clin Orthop 146:37–41, 1980
11. Beighton PH: Articular mobility in an African population. Ann Rheum Dis 32:413–418, 1973
12. Blackburn TA: Throwing injuries to the shoulder. In Donatelli R (ed): Physical Therapy of the Shoulder, 2nd ed. New York, Churchill Livingstone, 1991:239–270
13. Blakely RL, Palmer ML: Analysis of rotation accompanying shoulder flexion. Phys Ther 64:1214–1216, 1984
14. Booth RE, Marvel JP: Differential diagnosis of the shoulder pain. Orthop Clin North Am 6:353–379, 1975
15. Bradley JP, Tibone JE: Electromyographic analysis of muscle action about the shoulder. Clin Sports Med 10:789–805, 1991
16. Brewster CE, Shields CL, Seto JL, Morrissey MC: Rehabilitation of the upper extremity. In Shields CL (ed): Manual of Sports Surgery. New York, Springer-Verlag, 1987:62–90
17. Brunnstrom S: Clinical Kinesiology. Philadelphia, FA Davis, 1962
18. Burdett-Smith P: Experience of scapula winging in an accident and emergency department. Br J Clin Pract 44:643–644, 1990
19. Burkhead WZ, Rockwood CA: Treatment of instability of the shoulder with an exercise program. J Bone Joint Surg 74A:890–896, 1992
20. Butler DS: Mobilization of the Nervous System. Melbourne, Churchill Livingstone, 1991
21. Butler DS: The upper limb tension test revisited. In Grant R: Physical Therapy of the Cervical Spine and Thoracic Spine, 2nd ed. New York, Churchill Livingstone, 1994:217–244
22. Cahill BR: Understanding shoulder pain. In Stauffer ES (ed): Instructional Course Lectures. American Academy of Orthopaedic Surgeons. St. Louis, CV Mosby, 1985
23. Calliet R: Shoulder Pain, 3rd ed. Philadelphia, FA Davis, 1991
24. Cipriani D: Open and closed chain rehabilitation for the shoulder complex. In Andrews JR, Wilk LE (eds): The Athlete's Shoulder. New York, Churchill Livingstone, 1994:577–588
25. Codman EA: The Shoulder. Boston, Thomas Todd, 1934
26. Corrigan B, Maitland GD: Practical Orthopaedic Medicine. Boston, Butterworths, 1985
27. Cunningham J: Applying the Bad Ragaz method to the orthopaedic client. Orthop Phys Ther Clin North Am 3:251–260, 1994
28. Davies GJ, Gould JA, Larson RL: Functional examination of the shoulder girdle. Phys Sports Med 9:82–104, 1981
29. De Luca CJ, Forrest WJ: Force analysis of individual muscles acting simultaneously on the shoulder joint during isometric abduction. J Biomech 6:385–395, 1973
30. Dempster WT: Mechanisms of shoulder movement. Arch Phy Med Rehabil 46:49–67, 1965
31. Deplane AF: Surgical anatomy of the rotator cuff and natural history of degenerative periarthritis. Surg Clin North Am 43:1507–1521, 1963
32. Deplane AF: Surgical anatomy and function of the acromioclavicular and sternoclavicular joints. Surg Clin North Am 43:1541–1521, 1963
33. Deplane AF: Surgery of the Shoulder, 2nd ed. Philadelphia, JB Lippincott, 1973
34. Dickhoff-Hoffman S: Neuromuscular control exercises of shoulder instability. In Andrews JR, Wilk KE (eds): The Athlete's Shoulder. New York, Churchill Livingstone, 1994:435–449
35. Dominguez RH, Gajda R: Total Body Training. New York, Warner Books, 1982
36. Dontigny RL: Passive shoulder exercises. J Phys Ther 50:1707–1709, 1970
37. Ehgartner K: Has the duration of cast fixation after shoulder dislocations had an influence on the frequency of recurrent dislocations? Archi Orthop Unfallchie 89:187–190, 1977
38. Elvey RL: Painful restriction of shoulder movement: A clinical observation study. In Proceedings: Disorders of the knee, ankle and shoulder. Perth, Western Australian Institute of Technology, 1979
39. Elvey RL: Brachial plexus tension test and the pathoanatomical origin of arm pain. In Idczack RM (ed): Aspects of Manipulative Therapy. Lincoln Institute of Health Sciences, Carlton, Australia, 1981
40. Elvey RL: The investigation of arm pain. In Grieves GP (ed): Modern Manual Therapy of the Vertebral Column. New York, Churchill Livingstone, 1986:530–535
41. Elvey RL: Treatment of arm pain associated with abnormal brachial plexus tension. Aust J Physiother 32:224–229, 1986
42. Elvey RL, Quintner JL, Thomas AN: A clinical study of RSI. Aust Fam Physician 15:1314–1322, 1986
43. Fiddian NJ, King RJ: The winged scapula. Clin Orthop 185:228–236, 1984
44. Fish GH: Some observations of motion at the shoulder joint. Can Med Assoc J 50:213–216, 1944
45. Freedman L, Munro R: Abduction of the arm in the scapular plane: Scapular and glenohumeral movements. J Bone Joint Surg 48A:1503–1510, 1966
46. Gamble JN: Strength and conditioning for the competitive athlete. In Kulund DN: The Injured Athlete, 2nd ed. Philadelphia, JB Lippincott, 1988:111–150
47. Gerber C, Ganz R: Clinical assessment of instability of the shoulder, with special reference to the anterior and posterior drawer tests. J Bone Joint Surg 66B:551–556, 1984
48. Gozna ER, Harris WR: Traumatic winging of the scapula. J Bone Joint Surg 61A:1230–1233, 1979
49. Greenfield B: Special considerations in shoulder exercises: Plane of the scapula. In Andrews JR, Wilk KE (eds): The Athlete's Shoulder. New York, Churchill Livingstone, 1994:513–522
50. Gregg JR, Labosky D, Harty M, et al: Serratus anterior paralysis in the young athlete. J Bone Joint Surg 61A:825–832, 1979
51. Grieve GP: Mobilisation of the Spine: A Primary Handbook of Clinical Method, 5th ed. Edinburgh, Churchill Livingstone, 1991

52. Grimsby O: Personal communication, 1977
53. Grimsby O: Fundamentals of Manual Therapy: A Course Workbook. Sorlandets Institute, Everett, WA, 1985
54. Gustavsen R, Streek R: Training Therapy: Prophylaxis and Rehabilitation, 2nd ed. Stuttgart, Georg Thieme Verlag, 1993
55. Halbach JW, Tank RT: The Shoulder. In Gould JA, Davies GJ (eds): Orthopaedic and Sports Physical Therapy. St. Louis, CV Mosby, 1990:483–522
56. Hart DL, Carmichael SW: Biomechanics of the shoulder. J Orthop Sports Phys Ther 6:229–234, 1985
57. Hawkins RJ, Kennedy JC: Impingement syndrome in athletes. Am J Sports Med 8:151–157, 1980
58. Hawkins RJ, Bokor DJ: Clinical evaluation of shoulder problems. In Rockwood CA, Matsen FA III (eds): The Shoulder, vol 1. Philadelphia, WB Saunders, 1990:149–177.
59. Heppenstall RB: Fractures of the proximal humerus. Orthop Clin North Am 9:467–475, 1975
60. Holten O: Medisinsk Trenigsterapi Trykk Fugseth and Lorentzen. Medical Training Course. Salt Lake City, March 1–4, 1984
61. Hovelius L: Recurrence after initial dislocation of the shoulder. J Bone Joint Surg 65A:343–349, 1983
62. Howell JW: Evaluation and management of thoracic outlet syndrome. In Donatelli R (ed): Physical Therapy of the Shoulder, 2nd ed. New York, Churchill Livingstone, 1991:151–190
63. Howell SM, Imobersteg M, Seger DH, Marone DJ: Clarification of the role of the supraspinatus muscle in shoulder function. J Bone Joint Surg 68:398–404, 1986
64. Inman VT, Saunders JB, Abbott LC: Observations of the function of the shoulder joint. J Bone Joint Surg 26A:1–30, 1944
65. Jobe FW, Moynes DR: Delineation of diagnostic criteria and a rehabilitation program for rotator cuff injuries. Am J Sports Med 10:336–339, 1982
66. Johnston TB: Movements of the shoulder joint—plea for use of "plane of the scapula" as the plane of reference for movements occurring at humeroscapular joint. Br J Surg 25:252–260, 1937
67. Kaltenborn FM: Mobilization of the Extremity Joints: Examination and Basic Techniques. Oslo, Olaf Norlis Bokhandel, 1980
68. Kaltenborn FM: The Spine: Basic Evaluation and Mobilization Techniques, 2nd ed. Oslo, Olaf Norlis Bokhandel, 1993
69. Kapandji IA: The Physiology of the Joints: vol 1, Upper Limb. New York, Churchill Livingstone, 1970
70. Kenneally M, Rubenach H, Elvey R: The upper limb tension test: The SLR test of the arm. In Grant R (ed): Physical Therapy of the Cervical and Thoracic Spine. New York, Churchill Livingstone, 1988:167–194
71. Kent BE: Functional anatomy of the shoulder complex: A review. Phys Ther 51:867–888, 1971
72. Kessell L, Walson M: The painful arc syndrome. J Bone Joint Surg 59B:166–172, 1977
73. Kisner C, Colby LA: Therapeutic Exercise: Foundations and Techniques, 2nd ed. Philadelphia, FA Davis, 1993
74. Kondo M, Tazoe S, Yamda M: Changes of the tilting angle of the scapula following elevation of the arm. In Bateman JE, Welsch PR (eds): Surgery of the Shoulder. St. Louis, CV Mosby, 1984:12–16
75. Lee D: A Workbook of Manual Therapy Techniques for the Upper Extremities. Delta BC, Canada, DOPC, 1989
76. Leffert RD, Gumley G: The relationship between dead arm syndrome and thoracic outlet syndrome. Clin Orthop Relat Res 23:20–31, 1987
77. Lehmann F, Warren CG, Scham SM: Therapeutic heat and cold. Clin Orthop 99:207–245, 1974
78. Lentell G, Hetherington T, Eagan J, et al: The use of thermal agents to influence the effectiveness of a low-load prolonged stretch. Orthop Sports Phys Ther 5:200, 1992
79. Letournel E, Fardeau M, Lytle JO, et al: Scapulothoracic arthrodesis for patients who have fascioscapulohumeral muscular dystrophy. J Bone Joint Surg 72A:78–84, 1990
80. Light LE, Nuzik S, Personius W, et al: Low-load prolonged stretch vs. high load in treating knee contractures. Phys Ther 64:330–338, 1984
81. Lippman RK: Frozen shoulder, peri-arthritis, bicipital tenosynovitis. Arch Surg 47:283–296, 1943
82. Lockhart RD: Movements of the normal shoulder joint. J Anat 64:288–302, 1936
83. Lord JW, Rosati LM: Neurovascular compression syndromes of the upper extremity. Clinical Symposia 23:3–23, 1971
84. Lucas DB: Biomechanics of the shoulder joint. Arch Surg 107:425–432, 1973
85. Ludington NA: Rupture of the long head of biceps flexor cubiti muscle. Ann Surg 27:358–363, 1923
86. MacConnaill MH, Basmajian JV: Muscles and Movements: A Basis for Human Kinesiology. Baltimore, Williams & Wilkins, 1969
87. MacNab I: Local steroids in orthopaedic conditions. Scott Med J 17:176–186, 1972
88. MacNab I: Rotator cuff tendinitis. Ann Roy Coll Surg Engl 53:271–287, 1973
89. Magee DJ: The shoulder. In Magee DJ: Orthopedic Physical Assessment, 2nd ed. Philadelphia, WB Saunders, 1992
90. Mahj JY, Otsuka NY: Scapular winging in young athletes. J Pediatr Orthop 12:245–247, 1992
91. Maitland GD: Vertebral Manipulations, 5th ed. Boston, Butterworths, 1986
92. Maitland GD: Peripheral Manipulations, 3rd ed. London, Butterworths, 1991
93. Matsen FA III, Thomas SC, Rockwood CA: Glenohumeral instability. In Rockwood CA, Matsen FA (eds): The Shoulder, vol. 1. Philadelphia, WB Saunders, 1990:526–622
94. Matsen FA III, Harryman DT, Sidles JA: Mechanics of glenohumeral instability. Clin Sports Med 10:783–788, 1991
95. Matsen FA III, Lippitt SB, Sidles JA, et al: Practical Evaluation and Management of the Shoulder. Philadelphia, WB Saunders, 1994
96. Moore KL: Clinically Oriented Anatomy. Baltimore, Williams & Wilkins, 1980
97. Morehouse L, Gross L: Maximum Performance. New York, Simon & Shuster, 1977
98. Moseley HF: Disorders of the shoulder. Clinical Symposia 12:1–30, 1960
99. Moseley HF: The natural history and clinical syndromes produced by calcific deposits in the rotator cuff. Surg Clin North Am 43:1489–1492, 1963
100. Moseley HF: Shoulder Lesions, 3rd ed. Edinburgh, Churchill Livingstone, 1969
101. Najenson T, Yacibovich E, Pikelni S: Rotator cuff injury in shoulder joints of hemiplegic patients. Scand J Rehab Med 3:131–137, 1971
102. Neer OS II. Anterior acromioplasty for chronic impingement syndrome in the shoulder. J Bone Joint Surg 54A:41–50, 1972
103. Neer OS II: Impingement lesions. Clin Orthop 173:70–77, 1983
104. Neviaser JS: Adhesive capsulitis of the shoulder; a study of pathological findings in periarthritis of the shoulder. J Bone Joint Surg 27A:211–222, 1945
105. Nicholson GG, Clendaniel RA: Manual techniques. In Scully RM, Branes MR (eds): Physical Therapy. Philadelphia, JB Lippincott, 1989:926–989
106. Nirschl R: Rehabilitation of the athlete's elbow. In Morrey BR (ed): The Elbow and Its Disorders. Philadelphia, WB Saunders, 1985:524–525
107. Norris CM: Sports Injuries: Diagnosis and Management for Physiotherapists. Oxford, Butterworths-Heinemann, 1993
108. Norris TR: Diagnostic technique for shoulder instability. In Sauffer ES (ed): Instructional Course Lectures. St. Louis, CV Mosby, 1985:239–257
109. Norwood LA, Terry GC: Shoulder posterior subluxation. Am J Sports Med 12:25–30, 1984
110. Paine RM: The role of the scapula in the shoulder. In Andrews JR, Wilk KE: The Athlete's Shoulder. New York, Churchill Livingstone, 1994:495–512
111. Palmer L, Blakely R: Documentation of medial rotation accompanying shoulder flexion: A case report. Phys Ther 68:55–58, 1986
112. Palmittier RA, An KN, Scott SG, et al: Kinetic chain exercise in knee rehabilitation. Sports Med 11:402–413, 1991
113. Pappas AM, Zaacki RM, McCarthy CF: Rehabilitation of the pitching shoulder. Am J Sports Med 13(4):223–235, 1985
114. Peat M: Functional anatomy of the shoulder complex. Phys Ther 66:1855–1865, 1986
115. Perry J. Anatomy and biomechanics of the shoulder in throwing, swimming, gymnastics and tennis. Clin Sports Med 2:247–270, 1983
116. Perry J, Glousman RE: Biomechanics of throwing. In Nicholas JA, Hershman EB (eds): The Upper Extremity in Sports Medicine. St. Louis, CV Mosby, 1990:727–751
117. Pettman E: The "functional" shoulder girdle. International Federation of Orthopaedic Manipulative Therapists, Vancouver, BC, 1984
118. Poppen NK, Walker PS: Normal and abnormal motion of the shoulder. J Bone Joint Surg 58A: 195–201, 1976
119. Protzman RR: Anterior instability of the shoulder. J Bone Joint Surg 62A:908–918, 1980
120. Radin E: Relevant biomechanics in the treatment of musculoskeletal injuries and disorders. Clin Orthop 146:2–3, 1980
121. Rockwood CA: Subluxations and dislocations about the shoulder. In Rockwood CA, Green DP (eds): Fractures in Adults. Philadelphia, JB Lippincott, 1984
122. Rohde J: Die Automobilisation der Extremitatengelenke (III). Zschr Physiother 27:121–134, 1975
123. Rothman RH, Marvel JP, Heppenstall RB: Anatomical considerations in the glenohumeral joint. Orthop Clin North Am 6:341–352, 1975
124. Rothman RH, Parke BB: The vascular anatomy of the rotator cuff. Clin Orthop 41:176–186, 1965
125. Rowe CR: Dislocations of the shoulder. In Rowe CR (ed): The Shoulder. Edinburgh, Churchill Livingstone, 1988:165–292
126. Rowe CR, Sakellarides HT: Factors related to recurrences of anterior dislocations of the shoulder. Clin Orthop 20:40, 1961
127. Sahrmann S: Diagnosis and treatment of muscle imbalances and associated regional pain syndromes. Level I and II continuing education course, Seattle, 1993
128. Sarrafian SK: Gross and functional anatomy of the shoulder. Clin Orthop 173:11–18, 1983
129. Schultz JS, Leonard JA Jr: Long thoracic neuropathy from athletic activity. Arch Phys Med Rehabil 73:87–90, 1992
130. Sheldbourne DK, Nitz PA: Accelerated rehabilitation after anterior cruciate ligament reconstruction. Am J Sports Med 18:292–299, 1990
131. Shields CL: Manual of Sports Surgery. New York, Springer-Verlag, 1987
132. Skyhar MJ, Simmons TC: Rehabilitation of the shoulder. In Nickel VL, Botte MJ (eds): Orthopaedic Rehabilitation, 2nd ed. New York, Churchill Livingstone, 1992:747–763
133. Smith KF: The thoracic outlet syndrome, a protocol of treatment. J Orthop Sports Phys Ther 1:89–97, 1979
134. Spencer J, Turkel MA, Ithaca MC, et al: Stabilizing mechanism preventing anterior dislocation of the glenohumeral joint. J Bone Joint Surg 63A:1208–1217, 1981
135. Steele R, Anthony J, Rice EL, et al: The winged scapula: Diagnosing the atypical case. Phys Sports Med 22:47–54, 1994
136. Stillman JF, Hawkins RJ: Current concepts and recent advances in the athlete's shoulder. Clin Sports Med 10:693–706, 1991
137. Sullivan PE, Markos PD, Minor MA: An Integrated Approach to Therapeutic Exercise: Theory and Clinical Application. Reston, Virginia, Reston Publishing Co., 1982
138. Sutter JS: Conservative treatment of shoulder instability. In Andrews JR, Wilk KE (eds): The Athlete's Shoulder. New York, Churchill Livingstone, 1994:589–604
139. Turek SL: Orthopaedics: Principles and Their Applications, 3rd ed. Philadelphia, JB Lippincott, 1977
140. Voight ML, Dravitch P: Plyometrics. In Albert MA (ed): Eccentric Muscle Training in Sports and Orthopaedics. New York, Churchill Livingstone, 1991:45–73
141. Walsh DA: Shoulder evaluation of the throwing athlete. Sports Med Update 4:24–27, 1989
142. Warren CG, Lehmann JK, Koblanski JN: Elongation of rat-tail tendon: Effect of load and temperature. Arch Phys Med Rehab 52:465–474, 1971
143. Warwick R (ed): Gray's Anatomy, 36th British ed. Philadelphia, WB Saunders, 1980
144. Watson-Jones RR: Fractures and Joint Injuries, vol II, 4th ed. Baltimore, Williams & Wilkins, 1960
145. Wilk KE: Current concepts in the rehabilitation of athletic shoulder injuries. In Andrews JR, Wilk KE (eds): The Athlete's Shoulder. New York, Churchill Livingstone, 1994:335–354
146. Wilk KE, Andrews JR: Current concepts in the treatment of anterior cruciate ligament disruption. J Orthop Sports Phys Ther 15:279–292, 1992
147. Wilk KE, Voight ML: Plyometrics for the shoulder complex. In Andrews JR, Wilk KE (eds): The Athlete's Shoulder. New York, Churchill Livingstone, 1994:543–565
148. Woo SLY, Mathews SV, Akeson WH: Connective tissue response to immobility: Correlative study of biomechanical measurements of normal and immobilized rabbit knees. Arthritis Rheum 18:257–264, 1973
149. Wooden MJ: Isokinetic evaluation and treatment of the shoulder. In Donatelli R (ed): Physical Therapy of the Shoulder. New York, Churchill Livingstone, 1987
150. Woolfenden JT: Aquatic physical therapy approaches for the extremities. Orthop Phys Ther Clin North Am 3:209–230, 1994

151. Yackzan L, Adams C, Francis KT: The effects of ice massage on delayed muscle soreness. Am J Sports Med 12:159, 1984
152. Yergason RM: Supination sign. J Bone Joint Surg 13:160, 1931
153. Wyke BD: The neurology of joints. Ann Roy Coll Surg Engl 41:25–50, 1967
154. Zuckerman JD, Matsen FA III: Biomechanics of the shoulder. In Nordin M, Frankel VH (eds): Basic Biomechanics of the Musculoskeletal System, 2nd ed. Philadelphia, Lea & Febiger, 1989:209–247

RECOMMENDED READINGS

Andrews JR, Wilk KE: The Athlete's Shoulder. New York, Churchill Livingstone, 1994
Aronen JG, Regan K: Decreasing the incidence of recurrence of first-time anterior dislocations with rehabilitation. Am J Sports Med 12:283–291, 1984
Atwater AE: Biomechanics of overarm throwing movements and injuries. Exerc Sport Sci Rev 7:43–85, 1979
Ellman H, Gartsman GM: Arthroscopic Shoulder Surgery and Related Procedures. Philadelphia, Lea & Febiger, 1993
Matsen FA, Lippitt SB, Sidles JA, et al: Practical Evaluation and Management of the Shoulder. Philadelphia, WB Saunders, 1994
McNab I, McCulloch J: Neck Ache and Shoulder Pain. Baltimore, Williams & Wilkins, 1994
Pappas AM, Zawacki RM, Sullivan TJ: Biomechanics of baseball pitching: A preliminary report. Am J Sports Med 13:216–222, 1985
Moynes DR: Prevention of injury to the shoulder through exercise and therapy. Clin Sports Med 2:413–422, 1983
Rockwood CA, Matsen FA: The Shoulder. Philadelphia, WB Saunders, 1990
Zarins B, Rowe CR: Current concepts in the diagnosis and treatment of shoulder instability in athletes. Med Sci Sports Exerc 15:44–448, 1984

10
CHAPTER

The Elbow and Forearm

DARLENE HERTLING AND RANDOLPH M. KESSLER

■ REVIEW OF FUNCTIONAL ANATOMY

□ Osteology

DISTAL HUMERUS

At the distal anterior end of the humerus there are two articular surfaces: the trochlea, which is pulley-shaped, somewhat like an hourglass or spool lying on its side, and the capitellum, which forms most of a sphere mediolaterally and half of a sphere anteroposteriorly. The lateral epicondyle extends laterally above the capitellum for attachment of the extensor muscles. The medial epicondyle is the site of attachment of the flexor–pronator group. The coronoid fossa lies immediately above the trochlea, and the radial fossa is immediately above the capitellum. These fossae receive the coronoid process and the anterior rim of the radial head, respectively, on full elbow flexion (Fig. 10-1).

If one looks laterally or medially, the distal humerus angulates anteriorly such that the longitudinal axis of the trochlea is directed anteriorly, 45° to the

shaft of the humerus. As implied above, the hemisphere of the capitellum faces anteriorly, with the articular surface having an angular value of about 180° (Fig. 10-2).

Posteriorly (Fig. 10-3), the large, deep olecranon fossa accepts the olecranon process on full elbow extension. At times it communicates with the coronoid fossa. The trochlear articular surface, with its median groove, extends posteriorly. The medial half of the trochlea extends farther distally than does the lateral half. The groove usually runs obliquely, distally, and laterally; it dictates the path that the ulna must follow during flexion and extension of the forearm. The asymmetry of the trochlea causes the ulna to angulate laterally on the humerus when the elbow extends. This abduction of the forearm on full extension is referred to as the *carrying angle* of the elbow.

PROXIMAL RADIUS

The proximal end of the radius includes the head, neck, and bicipital tuberosity (see Fig. 10-1). The ra-

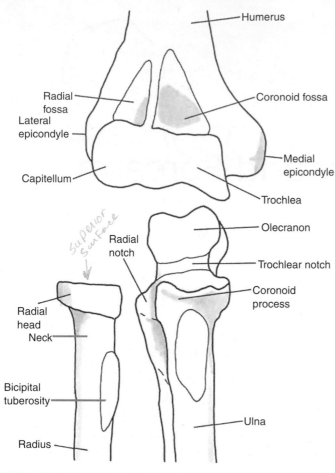

FIG. 10-1. Bones of the right elbow.

dial head is concave on its superior surface for articulation with the convex capitellum. Viewed from above, the radial head is slightly oval, being longer anteroposteriorly, so that with pronation it is displaced slightly laterally (Fig. 10-4).

PROXIMAL ULNA

The proximal ulna consists of the olecranon and the coronoid process, between which is the trochlear notch. With the elbow extended, the trochlear notch faces anteriorly and superiorly, corresponding to the 45° angulation of the distal humerus (see Fig. 10-2A). Lying inferiorly and medially to the trochlear notch is the radial notch, which faces laterally for articulation with the radial head (see Fig. 10-1).

The angulation of the distal humerus and trochlear notch of the proximal ulna allows about 160° elbow flexion and 180° extension. The angulation is necessary to provide room for the anterior muscle groups of the arm and forearm, which approximate on elbow flexion (Fig. 10-5). Any bony malalignment that interferes with these critical angles (*e.g.*, following a supracondylar fracture) will make normal movement impossible.

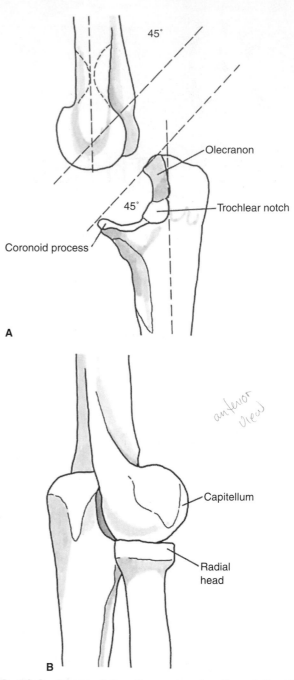

FIG. 10-2. Bones of the elbow, showing the relationship of (**A**) distal humerus and proximal ulna and (**B**) proximal radius (lateral view).

☐ Joint Articulations

The elbow is a compound synovial joint composed of three joints: the humeroulnar, humeroradial, and superior radioulnar. These three joints make up the cubital articulations. The capsule and joint cavity are continuous for all three joints. MacConaill and Basmajian[49] have classified the cubital complex as a paracondylar joint in that one bone (the humerus) articulates with two others (the radius and ulna) by way of

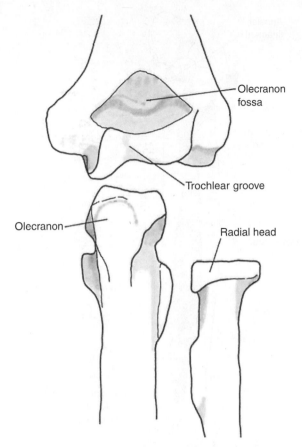

FIG. 10-3. Posterior view of bones of the elbow.

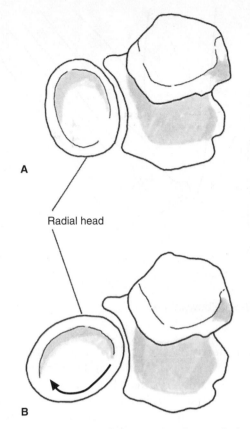

FIG. 10-4. Relationship of proximal radius and ulna in (**A**) pronation and (**B**) supination, as viewed from above.

two facets. This enables one of the latter two bones to undergo movement independent of the other. The middle radioulnar joint should also be considered when examining the elbow.

HUMEROULNAR JOINT

The humeroulnar joint is a uniaxial hinge joint formed between the trochlear notch of the ulna and the trochlea of the humerus (see Figs. 10-2A and 10-3). The ulnar trochlear notch, like the trochlea of the humerus with which it articulates, is a sellar surface. It is concave in the sagittal plane and convex in the frontal plane.[48] The trochlea covers the anterior, inferior, and posterior aspects of the medial humeral condyle.[92] It is a sellar articular surface that is concave in the frontal plane and convex in the sagittal plane. The trochlea of the humerus is asymmetrical. Its axis of motion points superolateral to inferomedial. This causes an angulation of the elbow, the carrying angle. When the arm is at the side, the carrying angle is 10° to 15° in men and 20° to 25° in women. The asymmetry of the trochlea allows for joint play needed for full range of motion. This incongruency produces the following accessory movements: a slight screw action (the ulna is slightly supinated during flexion and

pronated during extension) and abduction and adduction and gliding of the radial head on both the humerus and ulna. On full extension, the medial part of the olecranon process is not in contact with the trochlea; on full flexion, the lateral part of the olecranon process is not in contact with the trochlea. This range allows the side-to-side joint-play movement necessary for supination and pronation. The ulna rotates internally 5° in early elbow flexion and externally 5° at end range of flexion.[10,94]

HUMERORADIAL JOINT

The humeroradial joint allows flexion and extension of the forearm and pronation and supination of the radius. In the humeroradial joint the convex-shaped capitellum articulates with the cup-shaped, concave proximal portion of the radial head (see Fig. 10-2B). It is a triaxial ball-and-socket joint.

PROXIMAL RADIOULNAR JOINT

The articular surfaces of the superior radioulnar joint include the cylindrical rim of the radial head and an osseofibrous ring composed of the radial notch of the ulna and the annular ligament (see Fig. 10-1). The

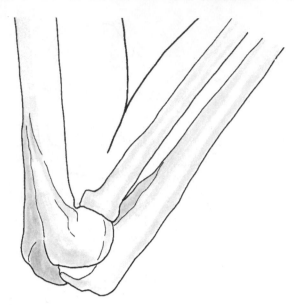

FIG. 10-5. Elbow in flexion.

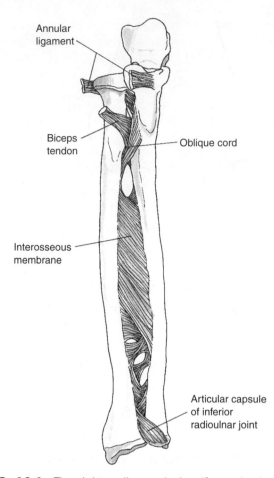

FIG. 10-6. The right radius and ulna (front view), showing structures that reinforce the superior and inferior radioulnar joints.

spherical head of the radius allows the rotation needed for forearm pronation and supination. Movement of the radius on the ulna reaches about 85° of both pronation and supination. Accessory movements include rotation and gliding of the radial head relative to the capitellum, lateral displacement of the radial axis during pronation due to a larger anteroposterior head diameter (allowing room for the radial tuberosity), and distal-lateral tilt of the plane of the proximal surface of the radial head during pronation.[37,38]

INFERIOR RADIOULNAR JOINT

The inferior radioulnar joint is also a critical component in forearm rotation. It anchors the distal radius and ulna, and along with the superior radioulnar joint provides a pivot for radial movement (Fig. 10-6). This joint is discussed further in Chapter 11, The Wrist and Hand Complex.

MIDDLE RADIOULNAR JOINT

The middle radioulnar syndesmosis includes the interosseous membrane and the oblique cord between the shafts of the radius and ulna (see Fig. 10-6). Although this articulation is not really a joint, nor part of the elbow joint complex, it is affected by injury or immobilization of the elbow; conversely, injury to this area can affect the mechanics of the elbow articulation. The oblique cord is a flat cord formed in the fascia overlying the deep head of the supinator and running to the radial tuberosity. It resists distal displacement of the radius during pulling movements. The interosseous membrane (a broad collage-

nous sheet) runs distally and medially from the radius and ulna. It provides stability for both the superior and inferior radioulnar joints. The interosseous membrane not only binds the joints together, but when under tension also provides for transmission of forces from the hand and distal end of the radius to the ulna.[64] The interosseous membrane stabilizes the elbow by resisting proximal displacement of the radius on the ulna during pushing movements. The fibers of the interosseous membrane are tight midway between supination and pronation.

☐ Ligaments

The capsule of the elbow is reinforced by ulnar (medial) and radial (lateral) collateral ligaments. These ligaments serve to restrict medial or lateral angulation of the ulna on the humerus. They also help prevent dislocation of the ulna from the trochlea. Each collateral ligament consists of anterior, intermediate, and posterior fibers. The anterior fibers of both help reinforce the annular ligament of the radioulnar articulation (Fig. 10-7). The capsule is strengthened anteriorly by an anterior oblique ligament (Fig. 10-8).

The annular ligament runs from the anterior margin of the radial notch of the ulna around the radial head to the posterior margin of the radial notch. It is lined with articular cartilage so that with pronation and supination the radial head articulates with the capitellum of the humerus and the radial notch of the ulna, as well as with the annular ligament (see Figs. 10-7 to 10-9).

The joint capsule of the elbow encloses the humeroulnar joint, the radiohumeral joint, and the proximal radioulnar joint (see Figs. 10-7 and 10-8). Some anatomists describe the existence of a quadrate ligament (ligament of Denucé) at the distal border of the annular ligament whose anterior fibers become taut on forearm supination and whose posterior fibers become taut on pronation (see Fig. 10-9).[15,52,76]

The joint capsule of the elbow encloses the humeroulnar joint, the humeroradial joint, and the proximal radioulnar joint (see Figs. 10-7 and 10-8). The anterior and posterior parts of the capsule are broad and thin.

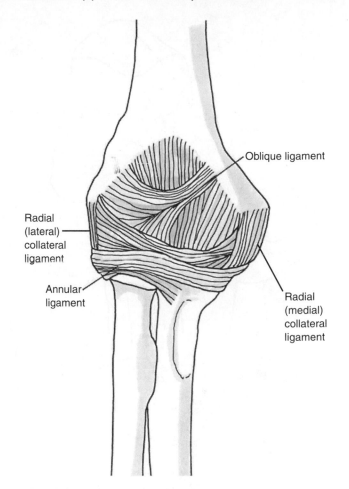

FIG. 10-8. Anterior view of the ligaments of the elbow.

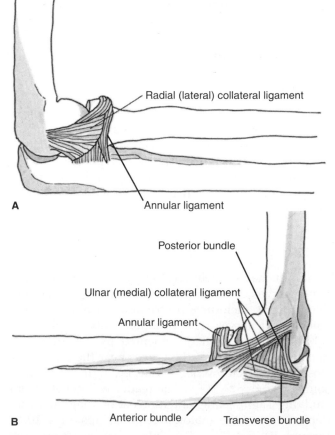

FIG. 10-7. Ligaments of the elbow viewed (**A**) laterally and (**B**) medially.

Forty-five degrees of flexion permits maximum volume of the joint, which is the position a patient assumes to accommodate diffuse swelling secondary to joint trauma or a supracondylar fracture.[33] Fat pads exist between the fibrous capsule and the synovial membrane over the fossae; thus, they are intracapsular but extrasynovial. The classic radiographic "fat pad sign" (used to detect effusion) is often associated with the presence of a fracture and is considered positive when a translucent area appears between the soft tissue and the bone in the area of the fat pad. In any condition leading to joint hemorrhage, effusion, or synovitis, the fat pad may be displaced so that it is visible (Fig. 10-10).

☐ Bursae

The olecranon bursa overlies the olecranon posteriorly, lying between the superior olecranon and the skin. It may become inflamed from trauma, prolonged pressure ("student's elbow"), or other inflammatory afflictions such as infection and gout (Fig. 10-11).

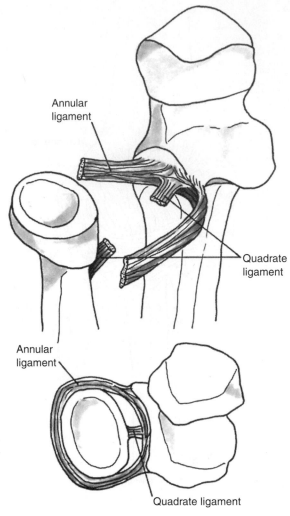

Annular
ligament

Quadrate
ligament

Annular
ligament

Quadrate ligament

FIG. 10-9. The quadrate ligament.

☐ Tendinous Origins

The flexor–pronator muscles of the wrist have their tendinous origins at a common aponeurosis that originates at the medial epicondyle of the humerus. The wrist extensor group has its common aponeurotic origin at the lateral epicondyle. From superior to inferior on the humerus, the brachioradialis inserts first, followed by the extensor carpi radialis longus, the extensor carpi radialis brevis, and the remaining extensor muscles (Fig. 10-12). The extensor carpi radialis brevis is the uppermost muscle to attach to the common extensor tendon. The extensor carpi radialis longus and the brachioradialis do not contribute to the common tendon but rather attach above the epicondyle.

The extensor carpi radialis brevis is important clinically since its tendon is most frequently involved in cases of lateral tennis elbow. Although it originates in part from the common extensor tendon, the extensor brevis also has proximal attachments to the lateral col-

lateral ligament of the elbow, and often to the annular ligament (see Fig. 10-12).

Deep to the tendon of the extensor brevis, and just distal to its insertion at the lateral epicondyle, is a small space normally filled with loose, areolar connective tissue. This is termed the *subaponeurotic space*[24] and is bordered on the ulnar side by the extensor digitorum tendon and distally by the attachment of the brevis to the annular ligament (see Fig. 10-12). Surgical findings commonly reveal granulation tissue in this space in cases of lateral tennis elbow. Histological studies show hypervascularization and the ingrowth of numerous free nerve endings into this space with granulation.[12,24] The granulation probably represents the reactions of adjacent tissues to chronic irritation of the extensor brevis origin, resulting from tension stresses.[24,60]

On full forearm pronation, with the elbow extended, the orientation of the extensor carpi radialis brevis is such that proximally it is stretched over the prominence of the radial head (see Fig. 10-4). This fulcrum effect from the radial head adds to the normal tensile forces transmitted to the origin of this muscle when stretched during combined wrist flexion, forearm pronation, and elbow extension.[60] This may in part explain the susceptibility of this tendon to chronic inflammation at or near its attachment.

☐ Nerves and Arteries

BLOOD SUPPLY

Blood supply to the elbow joint is usually abundant. The medial portion of the elbow is supplied from superior and inferior ulnar collateral arteries and two ulnar recurrent arteries. The lateral portion is supplied by the radial and middle collateral branches of the profunda artery and the radial and interosseous recurrent arteries.[45,55]

INNERVATION

Joint branches are believed to be derived from all the major nerves crossing over this joint (*i.e.*, radial, median, ulnar), including contributions from the musculoskeletal nerves. The variations and relative contributions have been documented by Gardner.[21] A detailed description of the nerves near the level of or close to the elbow joint can be found in other sources.[2,15,21,32,45,65,75,77] The reader will benefit from studying sagittal and anteroposterior diagrams that depict some of the anatomic relationships (Figs. 10-13 through 10-15).

Clinically, the examiner must be aware of potential

(text continues on page 224)

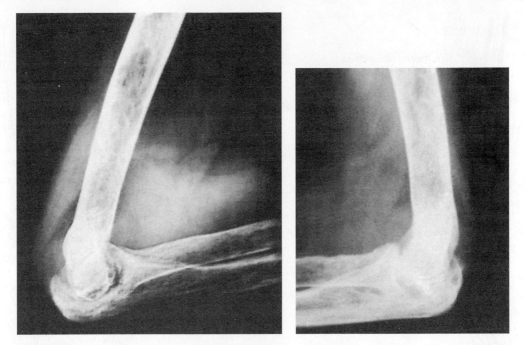

FIG. 10-10. Fat pad sign. Rheumatoid arthritis (elbow). Bilateral positive fat pad signs are seen; erosive changes of rheumatoid arthritis and osteoporosis are also noted. (Greenfield GB: Radiology of Bone Diseases, 5th ed. Philadelphia, JB Lippincott, 1990:782)

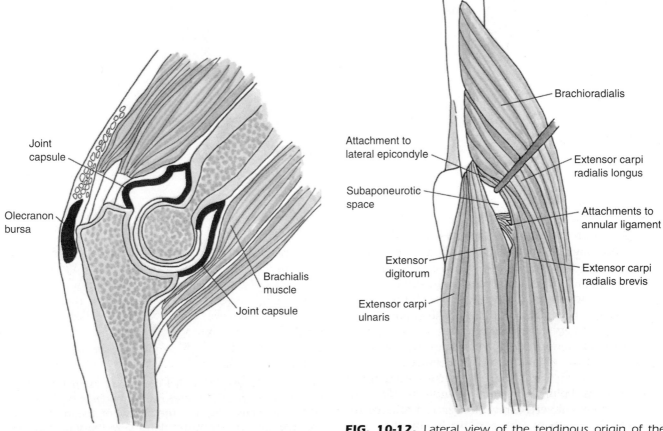

FIG. 10-11. Sagittal section through the elbow.

FIG. 10-12. Lateral view of the tendinous origin of the forearm muscles.

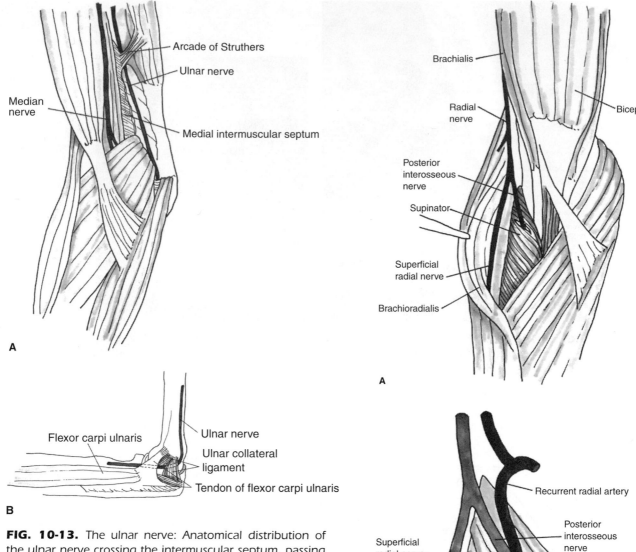

FIG. 10-13. The ulnar nerve: Anatomical distribution of the ulnar nerve crossing the intermuscular septum, passing under the arcade of Struthers (**A**) and the cubital tunnel at the elbow (**B**).

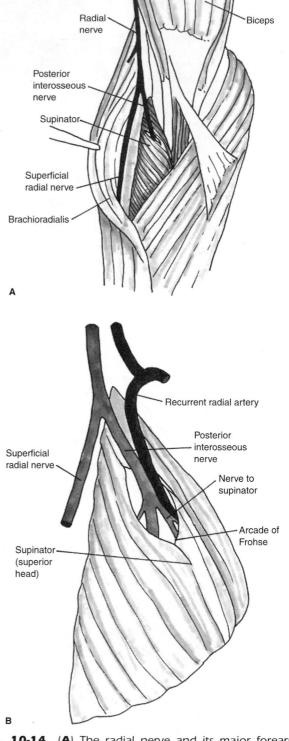

FIG. 10-14. (**A**) The radial nerve and its major forearm branches, the posterior interosseous nerve and the superficial radial nerve. (**B**) Enlarged view of the posterior interosseous nerve and its relationship to the supinator muscle and the arcade of Frohse.

injury or pinching of various nerves near the level of the elbow. For example, for the most part, resistant lateral tennis elbow may be caused by lateral epicondylitis and its associated fascial tears or calcification.[78] On occasion, persistent complaints may be due either to compression of the posterior interosseous nerve or to a combination of persistent localized epicondylitis and nerve compression.[9,67,72]

Of the several entrapment syndromes near the level of the elbow, the ulnar tunnel syndrome is the most common.[14,31,43,75,77–79,86,88–90] The ulnar nerve at the elbow passes behind the medial epicondyle in a groove that is converted into an osseofibrous canal, the cubital tunnel, by the arcuate ligament, which runs from the medial epicondyle to the olecranon

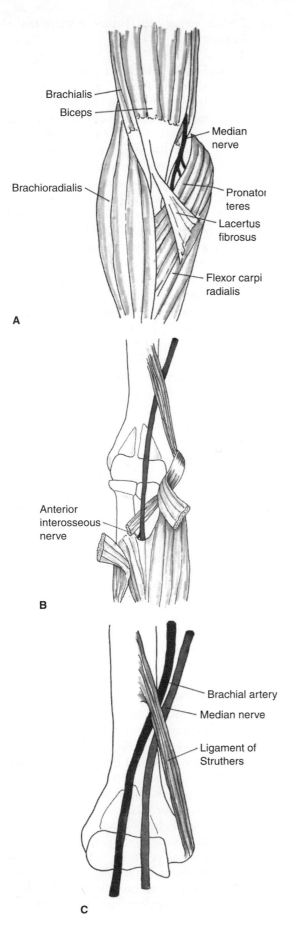

process (see Fig. 10-13*B*).[14,90] The arcuate ligament is taut at 90° flexion and lax in extension. An entrapment neuropathy of the ulnar nerve is common especially after prolonged sitting, overuse of the elbow, or repeated microtrauma from occupations that involve leaning on the elbow.[14]

Next in frequency of occurrence is the posterior interosseous nerve syndrome, or radial tunnel syndrome.[9,18,25,30,47,53,57,59,65,66,70,73,78–80,86,87] The most common compression site of the posterior interosseous nerve is as it passes under the fibrous origin of the extensor carpi radialis and then pierces the supinator muscles (in the region of the arcade of Frohse) to pass along the interosseous membrane, where it supplies the extensor muscles of the forearm, to reach the wrist (see Fig. 10-14).[4,53,59,66,70,73]

The anterior interosseous nerve syndrome and the pronator syndrome, which involves the median nerve, are less common. The median nerve may be compressed just before the anterior interosseous branch on entering the forearm beneath the edge of the lacertus fibrosus of the biceps, resulting in the pronator syndrome (see Fig. 10-15),[43,56,69] while the anterior interosseous nerve is occasionally pinched or entrapped as it passes between the two heads of the pronator teres.[19,41,44,50,68,71,75,78,91]

Other types of entrapment neuropathies are much rarer. Median nerve entrapment is occasionally combined with that of the brachial artery, caused by a supracondylar spur or Struther's ligament (see Fig. 10-15*C*).[22,32,77,80] Ulnar nerve entrapment is caused by Struther's arcade, made up of fibers arising from the medial head of the triceps that interweave to the intermuscular septum (see Fig. 10-13*A*).[36,77,78]

■ EVALUATION OF THE ELBOW

☐ History

Routine questions to be asked while evaluating patients with common musculoskeletal disorders are discussed in Chapter 5, Assessment of Musculoskeletal Disorders. The following questions are of particular concern when evaluating patients with elbow disorders:

1. What activities (*e.g.*, athletic or occupational) do you engage in that involve vigorous or repetitive use of the arm? (Except for the arthritides, most

FIG. 10-15. The median nerve, proximal to the lacertus fibrosus (**A**), the lacertus fibrosus released exposing the anterior interosseous nerve (**B**), and the ligament of Struthers, an anomalous structure (**C**).

elbow conditions are traumatic or degenerative conditions, such as tennis elbow, that become active with certain activities.)

2. Are any other joints involved? (Except for the degenerative or traumatic lesions, rheumatoid arthritis is one of the few remaining causes of elbow pain of local origin.)

The elbow is largely derived from C6 and C7 and may, therefore, be the site of referred pain from other structures of the same segmental derivation; it may also refer pain to other structures in these segments.

☐ Physical Examination

I. **Observation**
   A. *Posture and attitude* in which the arm is held
   B. *Functional use* of the arm during gait, dressing, and other activities
II. **Inspection** (include the entire extremity)
   A. *Structure*—observe the extremities with the patient in a relaxed, standing position.
      1. Shoulder height
      2. Elbow carrying angle (valgus–varus angle)
      3. Elbow flexion–extension angle
      4. Positions of medial and lateral epicondyles, radial head, and olecranon
   B. *Soft tissue*
      1. Atrophy. Observe and measure the girth of the arm or forearm.
      2. Swelling
         a. Marked posterior swelling is usually bursal swelling.
         b. Articular effusion is often visible anteriorly and posteriorly.
      3. General contours
   C. *Skin*
      1. Color changes
      2. Scars or blemishes
      3. Moisture
      4. Texture
III. **Selective Tissue Tension Tests**
   A. *Active movements* (sitting)
      1. Observe
         a. Elbow flexion–extension
         b. Forearm pronation–supination (with elbow at 90°)
         c. Wrist flexion–extension
      2. Apply slight overpressure. Assess effect on pain; assess end feel; feel for crepitus.
      3. Record significant findings relating to range of motion, pain, end feel, and crepitus.

B. *Passive movements* (supine for optimal stabilization)
   1. Tests
      a. Elbow flexion–extension with the shoulder flexed, extended, and in neutral position for constant-length phenomenon in case of muscular pain and tightness. This phenomenon results when the limitation of one joint depends on the position in which another joint is held.
      b. Elbow pronation–supination
      c. Wrist flexion with ulnar deviation (the elbow is held extended and the forearm pronated, stretching the common extensor tendon)
      d. Wrist extension with the forearm supinated and the elbow extended (common flexor–pronator tendon stretched)
   2. Record range of motion, pain, crepitus, and type of end feel. Characteristics of normal end feel are:
      a. Extension: bone-to-bone
      b. Flexion: soft-tissue approximation
      c. Pronation–supination: leathery or elastic
         When motion of the joint is restricted, a pathologic motion barrier impedes movement of the joint before the anatomic barrier is reached. Common pathologic barriers (abnormal end feel) encountered at the elbow are a springy block, suggesting a loose body[17], and muscle guarding, suggesting an acute inflammation of the joint or extra-articular tissues.
C. *Joint-play movements*
   1. Joint-play movements of the elbow are the same as the mobilization techniques (see Treatment Techniques below) except that they are always performed in the resting position. Specific joint-play (accessory) motions to be tested include:
      a. Distraction of the humeroulnar joint (see Fig. 10-18A)
      b. Medial-lateral tilt of the humeroulnar joint (see Fig. 10-19)
      c. Superior (approximation) glide for humeroradial joint (see Fig. 10-21)
      d. Distal glide of radius on ulna for proximal radioulnar joint (see Fig. 10-22)
      e. Dorsal-ventral glide at the proximal radioulnar joint (see Fig. 10-23A)
      f. Dorsal-ventral glide of the distal radioulnar joint (see Fig. 11-30)

2. Record significant findings related to degree of mobility and presence of pain and muscle guarding.

D. *Resisted isometric movements (supine)*
1. Resisted wrist movements. The patient grips the examiner's hand and squeezes strongly. If elbow pain is reproduced, additional isometric contractions of the wrist are examined (*i.e.*, wrist flexion and extension).
2. Resisted elbow movements. The four elbow movements of flexion, extension, supination, and pronation are tested using isometric contractions.
3. If referred pain from more proximal regions is suspected, include resisted isometric contraction tests of the shoulder and cervical spine movements.
4. Record whether the resisted isometric contraction is strong or weak and whether it is painful or painless.

IV. Palpation
A. *Skin*
1. Temperature—especially over brachialis and joint
2. Moisture—especially over hand and forearm
3. Texture
4. Mobility of skin over subcutaneous tissues, especially after immobilization
5. Tenderness—primarily if neurological involvement is suspected (*e.g.*, ulnar nerve lesion)

B. *Subcutaneous soft tissues*
1. Consistency, tone, mobility
2. Swelling. Joint effusion is often palpable anteriorly by ballottement.
3. Tenderness
   a. Common tendon insertions
   b. Soft-tissue attachments

C. *Bones*
1. Bony relationships—especially position of the radial head
2. Tenderness—tenoperiosteal junctions of common flexor and common extensor groups
3. Bony contours

V. Neuromuscular Tests.
The neurological examination includes motor function, light touch sensation, and deep tendon reflexes (DTRs). Motor function may be assessed with resisted isometric movements as performed in the cervical–upper extremity scan examination (see Chapter 18, The Cervical–Upper Limb Scan Examination). Elbow proprioception is also assessed after any injury to the joint or its ligamentous structures.

VI. Special Tests
A. *Joint and ligamentous tests*—to assess the integrity of the medial and lateral collateral ligaments, varus and valgus stress tests may be performed.
1. Valgus stress: To test the integrity of the ulnar collateral ligament (see Fig. 10-7B), the examiner applies a valgus stress to the elbow with the arm slightly flexed (slightly out of the close-packed position), thus attenuating the anterior bundle (Fig. 10-16A). The test is repeated with the

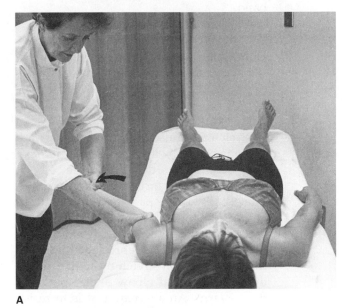

A

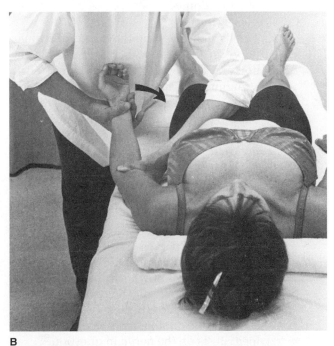

B

FIG. 10-16. Testing the collateral ligaments of the elbow. (**A**) Ulnar collateral ligament. (**B**) Medial collateral ligament.

forearm flexed to 90°, to stress the transverse bundle, and fully flexed, to stress the posterior bundle.[46]

2. Varus stress: To test the integrity of the radial collateral ligament (see Fig. 10-7A), the examiner applies a varus stress to the elbow with the arm slightly flexed (slightly out of the close-packed position), thus stressing the anterior band of the radial collateral ligament (see Fig. 10-16B). The test is repeated with the forearm flexed to 90°, to stress the medial band, and fully flexed, to stress the posterior band.[46]

B. *Musculotendinous tests*

1. Lateral tennis elbow. Pain of lateral tennis elbow may be reproduced at the site of the common extensor tendon. Resistance to wrist extension and radial deviation is applied as the patient attempts to make a fist and pronate the forearm. A key test is to stretch the muscles inserting at the lateral epicondyle, with the wrist in full flexion with ulnar deviation, the elbow straight, and the forearm fully pronated. The examiner may palpate the epicondyle at the same time.

2. Medial tennis elbow. The pain of medial tennis elbow may be reproduced by placing the flexors on stretch by fully extending the wrist and elbow and supinating the forearm. An alternate test is to resist wrist flexion.

C. *Neurologic tests*

1. Tinel's sign. Tapping the area of the ulnar nerve in the groove between the olecranon and the medial epicondyle may elicit a tingling sensation down the forearm if a neuroma or nerve entrapment is present. Tapping at the radial head and radial tunnel (radial nerve) and the carpal tunnel (median) may also reproduce the symptoms in entrapment syndromes of the peripheral nerves.

2. The test of neural tension proposed for the upper limb tension tests (ULTTs) should be conducted for the radial, ulnar, and median nerves (see Chapter 9, The Shoulder and Shoulder Girdle).[7]

3. Nerve conduction velocity. If there is any evidence of peripheral nerve compression, it can be confirmed by performing sensory and motor nerve conduction velocity tests on the nerve in question.[26]

VII. Other Tests. If there is any question about the integrity of the forearm circulation, the brachial pulse may be palpated in the cubital fossa medial to the biceps tendon, as well as the radial pulse lateral to the flexor carpi radialis tendon at the wrist. Results of roentgenograms, laboratory tests, and electromyograms should be reviewed if available.

■ COMMON LESIONS

☐ Elbow Tendinitis

Elbow tendinitis is a common disorder affecting the elbow. The tendon most commonly involved is the extensor carpi radialis brevis, at or near its insertion at the lateral epicondyle.[6,12,17,24,60] At times, other common extensor tendons are also involved concurrently or, rarely, by themselves. Much less frequently, the common flexor tendon is involved at the tenoperiosteal junction. Even more uncommon is tendinitis of the triceps at its attachment to the olecranon.

Confusion about the pathology and treatment of tennis elbow has plagued the medical community since the 19th century. Surgical studies have clearly identified classic tennis elbow as tendinitis, which Nirschl and Pettrone have divided into lateral, medial, and posterior areas and have classified on an anatomic basis:[61,63]

Lateral tennis elbow. Lateral tendinitis (lateral epicondylitis) involves primarily the extensor carpi radialis brevis and occasionally the extensor digitorum, extensor carpi radialis longus, and, more rarely, the extensor carpi ulnaris.[61,63]

Medial tennis elbow. Medial tendinitis (also known as golfer's elbow or medial epicondylitis) involves primarily the pronator teres and flexor carpi radialis and occasionally the palmaris longus, flexor carpi ulnaris, and flexor digitorum superficialis. An additional factor is compression neurapraxia of the ulnar groove.[62]

Posterior tennis elbow. Tendinitis of the triceps at its attachment to the olecranon is rare. It typically follows sudden severe strain to the triceps tendon (*e.g.,* in javelin throwers) as the arm is fully extended.[14]

Tendinitis affecting the elbow is rarely of acute traumatic origin. Except in sports medicine clinics, most patients presenting with tennis elbow do not relate the onset or aggravation of the problem to athletic endeavors such as tennis. Even when the chief complaint is the development of pain during some activity, the onset is usually gradual and pain is felt most *after* the activity. This is because lateral tennis elbow is usually a "degenerative" disorder: it represents tissue response to fatigue stresses. The inflammatory response that characterizes the disorder is an attempt to speed the rate of tissue production to compensate for an increased rate of tissue microdamage (*e.g.*, collagen fiber fracturing). The microdamage rate is increased because of greater internal strain to the tendon fibers over time. This might occur from some increase in use of the tendon—for example, with carpentry, pruning shrubs, or playing tennis. It may also occur with normal activity levels if the tendon's capacity to attenuate tensile loads is reduced. This typically occurs with aging, in which a loss of the mucopolysaccharide chondroitin sulfate makes the tendon less extensible; more of the energy of tensile loading must be absorbed as internal strain to collagen fibers rather than by deformation of the tissue.

The extensor carpi radialis brevis's susceptibility to excessive strain is probably related to the added tensile load imposed on the tendon by the radial head when the tendon is stretched (*e.g.*, wrist flexion, elbow extension, and forearm pronation). In this position the tendon is further stretched over the prominence of the radial head.[60] Because the development of tennis elbow may be due to age-related tissue changes, most patients presenting with this problem are 35 years or older.[6,12,17]

Lateral tennis elbow is classically a persistent disorder that does not tend toward spontaneous resolution. If the patient with tennis elbow continues to perform activities that stress the tendon, the immature collagen produced in an attempt at repair continues to break down before it has the chance to mature adequately, and the chronic inflammatory process continues. If the part is completely immobilized, there may not be adequate stress to the new collagen to stimulate maturation, in which case the scar will again break down on resumption of activities. For treatment to be successful, this dilemma must be resolved.

Medial tennis elbow characteristically occurs with wrist flexor activity and active pronation, as in pitching a baseball and pull-through strokes of swimming.[62] Typically it occurs in middle-aged patients, often those involved in sports or occupational activities that require a strong hand grip and an adduction movement of the elbow.

Posterior tennis elbow consists of intrinsic overload of the triceps attachment in activities that cause a sudden snapping of elbow extension. Pain is reproduced on fully resisting extension of the elbow while the patient stands with the elbow flexed and the forearm fully supinated.

According to Nirschl, the primary overload abuse in tendinitis is caused by intrinsic concentric muscular contraction.[60] Curwin and Standish maintain that decreased flexibility causes the muscles to be overstretched during eccentric contraction and overloading of the extensors.[16] They argue that maximum strengthening of the muscles must necessarily include eccentric work, since this is the nature of the force producing the injury and since eccentric exercise produces greater tensile force on the tendon.

EXAMINATION AND MANAGEMENT

I. **History**
   A. *Site of pain*
      1. Lateral tennis elbow—over the lateral humeral epicondyle, often referred into the C7 segment, down the posterior forearm into the dorsum of the hand, and perhaps into the ring and long fingers
      2. Medial tennis elbow—over the medial epicondyle, rarely referred into the ulnar aspect of the forearm
      3. Posterior tennis elbow—over the posterior compartment of the elbow
   B. *Onset of pain*—usually gradual. May be related to wrist extension activities in lateral tennis elbow, such as grasping, hitting a backhand stroke in tennis, or pruning shrubs, or to wrist flexion and pronation activities in medial tennis elbow. The patient rarely recalls a sudden onset of pain during these activities, however. At times a direct blow to the epicondyle initiates the problem.
   C. *Nature of pain*—varies from a dull ache or no pain at rest to sharp twinges or a straining sensation with activities, as mentioned above. Lateral tennis elbow is particularly aggravated by grasping activities because the wrist extensors must contract to stabilize the wrist during use of the finger flexors. Medial tennis elbow is worsened by repeated wrist flexion and gripping.

II. **Physical Examination**
   A. *Active movements*—usually fairly painless. In more severe cases of lateral tennis elbow, there may be some pain with active wrist flexion with the elbow in extension from the stretch placed on the tendon. Active wrist extension does not usually produce enough tension to reproduce the pain. Similarly, there may be some pain with active wrist extension with the elbow extended in medial tennis elbow, but usually not on active wrist flexion.
   B. *Passive movements*
      1. One of the key tests that should reproduce the pain in lateral tennis elbow is full passive wrist flexion with ulnar deviation, forearm pronation, and elbow extension.

Passive elbow movements alone are painless.

2. Full wrist extension with supination and elbow extension reproduces the pain in medial tennis elbow.

C. *Resisted isometric movements*—The other key test is resisted wrist extension (with the elbow extended), reproducing the pain in lateral tennis elbow; resisted wrist flexion reproduces pain in medial tennis elbow. At times, resisted pronation is painful in medial tennis elbow. Resisted elbow extension with the elbow in flexion and the forearm fully supinated is a key test for posterior tennis elbow.

D. *Joint-play movements*—should be full and painless

E. *Palpation*

1. Exquisite tenderness occurs usually over the epicondyles in medial and lateral tennis elbow. An area of tenderness may be palpated over the insertion of the triceps tendon into the olecranon in posterior tennis elbow.

2. In lateral tennis elbow, the tenderness may often extend down into the muscle belly. Less often, the tenderness is felt superior to the epicondyle at the insertion of the extensor carpi radialis longus.

3. Warmth may be noted over the respective epicondyle and olecranon.

F. *Inspection*—usually no significant findings

G. *Differential diagnoses.* Other entities include De Quervain's tenovaginitis (see Chapter 11, The Wrist and Hand Complex) and extensor carpi ulnaris tendinitis at the wrist; pronator syndrome in the forearm; and radial nerve entrapment accompanying lateral epicondylitis at the elbow.[13,42] Associated problems can appear either independently or in combination with the various forms of tennis elbow tendinitis.[62] These may include ulnar nerve neurapraxia,[62] carpal tunnel syndrome,[60,63] intra-articular abnormalities, joint laxity,[35,58,93] and associated soft-tissue or myofascial trigger point syndromes.[3,5,25,30,34,40,82,84] The multiplicity of conditions and treatments found in the literature is typified by Cyriax's coverage of tennis elbow.[17]

Gunn attributed the tennis elbow symptoms in one group of patients to reflex localization of pain from radiculopathy of the cervical spine.[28,29] Maigne has observed that about 60% of cases with clinical epicondylitis have minor intervertebral derangement at C5–C7 or C6–C7 levels on the side of the tennis elbow.[51] About half of these cases are associated with some degree of periarthritis of the elbow and thus are considered mixed forms.

III. **Management**
  A. *Goals*
    1. To restore normal, painless use of the involved extremity
    2. To restore normal strength and extensibility of the musculotendinous unit
    3. To encourage proper maturation of scar tissue and collagen formation, to allow extensibility and the ability of the tendon to attenuate tensile stresses
  B. *Objectives*
    1. Resolution of the chronic inflammatory process
    2. Maturation of the scar (healed area of the tendon). The new collagen must be sufficiently strong and extensible to withstand the tensile stresses imposed by activity. There must be an appropriate amount of tissue that is oriented to attenuate tensile stresses with a minimum of internal strain.
    3. Restoration of strength and extensibility to the muscle—tendon complex
  C. *Techniques*
    1. Acute cases. Lateral tennis elbow is by nature a chronic disorder, but some patients may present with acute symptoms and signs associated with lateral tennis elbow; pain is referred into the entire forearm and perhaps the hand, and occasionally up the back of the arm. There may be some pain at rest, and some degree of muscle spasm is elicited when the tendon is stressed passively or by resisted movements. In such cases, the immediate goal is to promote progression to a more chronic state, assisting in the resolution of the acute inflammation.
      a. Instruct the patient to apply ice to the site several times a day. The physical therapy modality of high-voltage galvanic stimulation has been helpful in relieving pain and inflammation.[62]
      b. Continued stress to the tendon must be prevented. If the patient presents with acute symptoms and signs as outlined above, this is best achieved by immobilizing the wrist, hand, and fingers (not the elbow) in a resting splint. In some cases a simple wrist cock-up splint will suffice, since this obviates the need for the wrist extensors to contract when the finger flexors are used. Activities involving grasping, pinching, and fine

finger movements must be restricted. This is often the most difficult component of the program to institute but at the same time the most important at this stage. The effectiveness of any other treatment measures will be compromised if the patient continues to engage in activities that stress the lesion site. For example, a carpenter must take some time off from work or temporarily change duties, a tennis player must abstain from playing for a while, and persons who enjoy knitting, sewing, or gardening must temporarily alter their activities.

c. A few times a day, the patient should remove the splint and actively move the wrist into flexion, the forearm into pronation, and the elbow into extension, simultaneously, to minimize loss of extensibility of the muscle and tendon. This should be done *gently*, avoiding significant discomfort, and slowly to prevent high strain-rate loading of the tissue.

If appropriate instructions are given and the patient faithfully follows the outlined program, progression to a more chronic status should occur over a period of a few (3 to 5) days.

2. Chronic cases (lateral tennis elbow). If the pain is fairly localized over the lateral elbow region and there is little or no pain at rest, the disorder should be treated as chronic tendinitis.

a. Advise the patient explicitly as to the appropriate level and type of activity that may be performed. Strong, repetitive, grasping activities, such as hammering, and activities that particularly stress the tendon, such as tennis, must be restricted until there is little pain on resisted isometric wrist extension and little or no pain when the tendon is passively stretched (wrist flexion, forearm pronation, and elbow extension). Such activities must be resumed gradually, with some protection of the part. Protection may be provided by counterforce bracing with an inelastic cuff worn firmly around the proximal forearm (the forearm extensors for lateral tennis elbow and the forearm flexors for medial tennis elbow). The concept of elbow bracing for tennis elbow was initially introduced by Ilfeld and Field

in 1966.[34] Nirschl later introduced a wider device, curved for better fit and support of the conical shape of the forearm.[60]

In theory, constraining full muscle expansion when muscles contract should diminish the potential force generated in the muscle. Cybex testing and biomechanical studies have demonstrated both angular velocity and the sequence of the electromyographic recording of muscular activity, and have confirmed the clinical validity of this concept.[61,62] If such a device is used, the therapist should gradually wean the patient from it as strength, mobility, and painless function increase.

Also, as normal activities are resumed, certain adaptations may be implemented to minimize the stresses imposed on the wrist extensors. For example, the tennis player typically receives high strain-rate loading to the wrist extensor group when using a backhand stroke if the ball strikes the racquet above the center point of the strings. This produces a moment arm about which the force of the ball hitting the racquet can create a high pronatory torque. If the wrist extensors are weak, the wrist might also be forced into flexion. The combined effects of the active and passive tension created in the wrist extensor group result in high loading of the extensor tendons. The passive component can be minimized by hitting the ball on center and by having adequate wrist extensor strength to keep the wrist from flexing. The passive pronatory torque can also be reduced by increasing the diameter of the racquet handle. Other considerations would include the tension of the strings on the racquet and the flexibility of the racquet shaft. High string tension and low racquet flexibility will result in reduced attenuation of forces by the racquet and, therefore, greater transmission of high strain-rate forces to the arm. Also, the larger the racquet head, the greater the potential moment arm about which pronatory forces can act. Thus, a tennis player might benefit from taking lessons to improve the likelihood of hitting the ball on center, from reducing string tension, and from using a relatively flexible racquet with a handle of maximum tolerable diameter and a head of standard size.

Each patient's activities should be similarly assessed for ways to reduce the loads imposed on the wrist extensor group.

b. Ultrasound and friction massage are used to assist in the resolution of the chronic inflammatory process and to promote maturation at the site of healing.

Resolution of inflammatory exudates, such as lysosomal enzymes and other cellular debris, may be enhanced by the increased blood flow stimulated by the heating effects of ultrasound. Ultrasound must often be applied underwater because of the irregular surface contour of the lateral elbow region.

Friction massage is an essential component of the treatment program. Its beneficial effects in cases of tendinitis are not well understood but are probably related to the induced hyperemia and the mechanical influence it may have on tissue maturation (see Chapter 7, Friction Massage). The hyperemic effects are of greatest importance in cases of tendinitis that may be related to hypovascularity, for instance, at the shoulder. Hyperemia does not seem to be a significant factor in the etiology of tennis elbow, however, and this may in part explain why friction massage is effective over a shorter period of time in cases of rotator cuff tendinitis than it is on cases of tennis elbow. The mechanical effects of the deep massage may promote orientation of immature collagen along the lines of stress. This would be an important factor in pathologic disorders, such as tennis elbow, in which some type of mechanical stimulus is necessary for adequate tissue maturation. Use of deep transverse massage may assist in tissue maturation without imposing a longitudinal stress to the healing tendon tissue and, therefore, without continued rupturing of fibers at the site of the lesion. Thus, the defect heals with a maximum degree of tissue extensibility and is less likely to be overstressed as use of the part is resumed. This seems to be a solution to the dilemma mentioned above. If the patient continues to use the part, he or she perpetuates the problem by producing continued damage at the lesion site; if the patient completely immobilizes the part, there is no stimulus for tissue maturation, and as soon as activity is resumed, the healed tissue begins to break down.

c. Strength and mobility must be restored. As symptoms and signs indicate improvement, the patient must resume activities gradually. Excessive internal strain to the tendon can be minimized during stressful activities by optimizing tissue extensibility. No vigorous activities should be allowed until it is determined if the muscle–tendon complex has sufficient extensibility. Following the ultrasound and friction massage, the therapist should gently and slowly stretch the tissue by holding the elbow extended, the forearm pronated, and the wrist ulnarly deviated, while flexing the wrist and fingers. The patient is instructed to perform this stretch at home, emphasizing that it must be performed slowly and gently. The patient should notice a stretching sensation but no pain. As vigorous activities such as tennis, carpentry, and gardening are resumed, the patient can be taught to administer friction massage for a few minutes before engaging in the activity.

Also, before a normal activity level is resumed, it is important to ensure that good forearm strength has been restored. In lateral tennis elbow, wrist extensor strengthening exercises are always necessary, since the muscles invariably undergo atrophy from disuse and reflex inhibition. Good extensor strength is necessary to protect the tendon from high strain-rate passive loading, which may occur with many types of activities. A convenient method of wrist extensor strengthening is to have the patient tie a rope 3 feet long to the center of a 1-inch dowel and a weight to the end of the rope; the patient grasps both ends of the dowel and rotates it toward him or her until the entire rope becomes wrapped around the dowel. This can be repeated as appropriate; the weight may be varied as necessary.

Forearm rehabilitative exercises to increase muscle power, flexibility, and endurance are important. Continued strengthening of uninjured areas and protective exercises for the injured area are necessary. Isometric, isotonic, isokinetic, and isoflex exercises are all used. Isoflex exercises consist of muscle strengthening, employing both concentric and eccentric training, using the resistance of an elasticized tension cord.[62] Maximum strengthening of the muscles must necessarily include eccentric exercise.[16]

    d. Local anti-inflammatory therapy, such as infiltration with a corticosteroid, is commonly used in cases of tendinitis. Although symptomatic improvement is often dramatic, such treatment has only temporary value. It has no lasting beneficial effect on the pathologic process and does not influence etiological factors. At best, it should be considered an adjunct to management in the acute state. Too often other important components of the treatment program are ignored when an apparent "cure" is heralded by dramatic symptomatic improvement.

☐ Postimmobilization Capsular Tightness

Patients with restricted movement at the elbow from capsular tightness are often referred to physical therapists. Since capsular restriction from degenerative joint disease at the elbow is rare, the patients with capsular restriction seen by physical therapists are usually those whose elbows have been immobilized. The only other frequent cause of capsular restriction at this joint is inflammatory arthritis (usually rheumatoid arthritis but occasionally traumatic arthritis).

The common injuries for which management may involve elbow immobilization include fractures of the arm or forearm (humeral shaft fractures, supracondylar fractures, and Colles' fractures are the most common) and elbow dislocations (usually posterior dislocation of the ulna on the humerus).

  I. **History.** Determine the date of injury, dates of subsequent surgery (if any), duration of immobilization, and date of removal of supports or splints. Any suggestion of complications following the injury or immobilization, such as vascular dysfunction, should be noted. Determine whether there have been previous attempts at remobilization, and if so, what these entailed. Assess the patient's functional disability in terms of limitations on dressing or grooming and on occupational and recreational activities. These should be documented and used as a means by which to judge progress.

  II. **Physical Examination.** The key sign is limitation of motion in a capsular pattern. However, note any complication that may have ensued.

    A. *Reflex sympathetic dystrophy* (see Chapter 11, The Wrist and Hand Complex)

      1. Key signs include capsular restriction of all or most upper-extremity joints to varying degrees; generalized edema of the forearm and hand; trophic changes in skin and nails (glossy smooth skin, hyperhidrosis, hypohidrosis, cyanosis, brittle or ridged nails); and dysesthesias, with pain hypersensitivity even to light touch. Roentgenograms often reveal marked osteopenia, especially of the bones of the hand and wrist.

      2. The exact cause of this disorder is unknown. It is especially prevalent in patients who have sustained a Colles'-type fracture. It is believed to be related to nerve trauma (such as trauma to the median nerve in Colles' fracture), the degree of edema, immobilization, and psychological factors. Preventive measures to be taken during immobilization should include frequent active exercise of the free joints (usually the shoulder and fingers) and regular periods of elevation of the involved extremity.

        Development of a true reflex sympathetic dystrophy, often referred to as a shoulder–hand syndrome, can be a significant complicating factor in the rehabilitation program following immobilization. The marked articular restrictions and pain hypersensitivity make efforts at remobilization especially difficult.

    B. *Malalignment of bony fragments.* This is occasionally seen following a supracondylar fracture at the elbow and invariably follows a Colles' fracture (see Chapter 11, The Wrist and Hand Complex).

      Elbow malalignment is easily detected by observing the carrying angle of the arm and by assessing structural alignment. With a supracondylar fracture, the distal fragment tends to displace posteriorly and medially with an angulation medially. Rotational displacement, medial or lateral displacements, and posterior or anterior displacements are not significant in the young person, since these usually resolve with bone remodeling. Angular displacements, however, tend to persist. Typically, the malalignment following a supracondylar fracture presents as a decrease or reversal of the normal carrying angle. The medial epicondyle is positioned higher than the lateral epicondyle, and the olecranon becomes directed medially. Such malalignment usually does not result in a functional deficit but may be cosmetically unacceptable.

C. *Brachialis contusion.* The displacement of bony parts that accompanies supracondylar elbow fractures and elbow dislocations may result in a contusion to the distal brachialis muscle belly, which overlies and is in close contact with the distal end of the humerus (Fig. 10-17). The consequence of such a contusion may be eventual metaplasia of the contused portion of this muscle into osseous tissue, a condition referred to as myositis ossificans.[1,23] Myositis ossificans usually results in permanent restriction of motion at the elbow; extension is restricted more than flexion.

It is questionable whether mobilization of the part (active, passive, prolonged, or otherwise) actually affects the eventual outcome. Some believe that the condition is often the result of overzealous attempts to remobilize the part. This may be the case if the brachialis muscle is stretched. In cases of capsular restriction, however, in which the stretch is applied to the anterior capsule rather than the brachialis muscle, it is doubtful that any form of mobilization would predispose to development of myositis ossificans of the brachialis muscle. Myositis ossificans, after injuries in which the brachialis muscle is traumatized, probably develops as an inevitable event resulting from the original injury.

The therapist must be protected medicolegally in the event that myositis ossificans should occur. This can be done by recognizing the two common conditions (supracondylar fracture and posterior dislocation) that especially predispose to development of myositis ossificans, and by distinguishing between capsular and muscular restriction of motion at the elbow. Fortunately, fractures and dislocations at the elbow occur primarily in children; because of this, remobilization is not a major problem and passive mobilization is seldom required.

However, if mobilization procedures are requested for a patient whose extremity has been immobilized following a supracondylar fracture or elbow dislocation, the therapist must take certain precautions.

First, the cause of the restriction is determined. Limitation of extension more than flexion with an elastic end feel suggests a muscular restriction. The constant length phenomenon is used to determine whether it is the biceps or brachialis. Limitation of motion in a capsular pattern with a capsular end feel suggests a capsular restriction. Stretching a tight elbow flexor muscle in such a case must not be done vigorously, except in cases of persistent restriction of elbow extension, and then only with agreement of the referring physician and with the patient's understanding.

Second, whether the restriction appears capsular or muscular, the therapist must attempt to detect any signs of inflammation of the brachialis muscle. This is done by palpating for a hematoma or excessive tenderness over the distal brachialis muscle belly. Any suggestion of inflammation or hematoma of the distal brachialis muscle belly should preclude vigorous mobilization, barring the stipulations indicated above. Regardless of the intensity of the mobilization program, the therapist would do well to record thermistor readings over the distal brachialis region before and after each treatment session. A rise in temperature that persists over, for example, a 24-hour period might indicate that the intensity of the program should be reduced, especially if a muscular restriction is at fault.

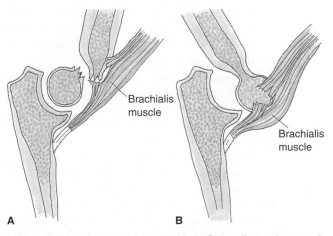

FIG. 10-17. Two common injuries of the elbow that result in displacement of bony parts: (**A**) supracondylar fracture; (**B**) posterior dislocation of ulna on humerus.

III. Management of Capsular Tightness

A. *Acute.* Since most capsular elbow restrictions are those that follow immobilization after injury, they are rarely found in an acute stage, since the acute inflammatory process subsides during immobilization.

1. Provide relief of pain and muscle guarding using ice, superficial heat, and grade I and II joint-play movements.
2. Maintain existing range of motion and increase movement as pain and guarding abate.
   a. Use gentle joint-play movements, grades I and II.
   b. Initiate an active-assisted home range of motion exercise program.
3. Strengthen progressively the muscles controlling the shoulder, elbow, forearm, and wrist as necessary. Use isometrics in the acute stage, since joint movement might cause reflex inhibition of the muscles to be strengthened.

B. *Chronic*
1. Ultrasound to tight capsular tissues along with or followed by capsular stretching, with joint-play mobilization techniques. If the therapist is treating a stiff elbow following a radial head resection, special attention should be given to preventing the development of a valgus contracture at the elbow by use of the "varus tilt" mobilization technique. The radius tends to migrate superiorly since the radial head no longer abuts the capitellum of the humerus. This may also result in problems at the distal radioulnar joint.
2. Progression of home program to include prolonged stretch as tolerated and indicated.
3. Progression of home strengthening program, including exercises to increase flexibility, endurance, and eccentric control.

☐ Cubital Tunnel Syndrome

Entrapment neuropathy in the elbow region is most common at the cubital tunnel because of constriction by the aponeurosis (tendinous insertion) of the flexor carpi ulnaris, located about 2 to 3 cm below the medial epicondyle (see Fig. 10-13B).[39] This is known as the cubital tunnel syndrome.[54] Cubital tunnel is common especially after prolonged flexion of the elbow. Ulnar nerve injuries are common in throwing athletes and manual laborers.[83] The nerve may be damaged by a single traumatic episode as it lies superficially in its grove, by repeated trauma from occupations that involve leaning on the elbow, by previous trauma that has resulted in a cubitus valgus deformity that gradu-

ally stretches the nerve, or by overuse of the elbow, resulting in entrapment as the nerve is tethered in its groove.[14] Ligamentous laxity, hyperflexed elbow posturing, recurrent subluxation or dislocation of the nerve out of the ulnar groove, or restriction of the nerve by adhesions in the cubital tunnel may result in nerve compression.[83,85,86,88–90]

I. **Physical Examination.** Symptoms are mainly sensory, with pain and/or paresthesias in the sensory distribution of the nerve to the medial one and a half fingers.[14] Other symptoms include clumsiness of the hand due to weakness, hyperesthesia or numbness, and complaints of muscle cramping. There may be a dull ache after activity or at rest. Pain may radiate up the forearm to the elbow and as far as the shoulder. Symptoms are aggravated by activity and relieved by rest.

A. On examination, there may be weakness and wasting of the hypothenar eminence and of the adductor muscles of the thumb (clawing of the ring or little finger and grade III paresis).[8] Sensation may be disturbed in the hand.

B. Sensory symptoms may be reproduced by pressure over the ulnar nerve behind the medial epicondyle, where tenderness or thickening of the nerve may be found. The ULTT for an ulnar nerve bias is positive, as is Tinel's sign.[7] Elbow hyperflexion usually elicits symptoms.

C. Diagnosis must be confirmed by nerve conduction studies and appropriate electromyographic tests, since similar symptoms may arise from lesions in the neck, such as thoracic outlet syndrome or cervical nerve root entrapment from discogenic disease.[8]

II. **Management**

A. *Conservative treatment.* Conservative treatment should be tried initially, consisting of relief of symptoms with physical agents, extra rest to the elbow, and education of the patient to avoid aggravating activities or postures (especially repeated or excessive flexion). Soft elbow pads are helpful and should be worn continuously. Exercises to increase flexibility of the forearm muscles and functional activities are introduced slowly.[81] Appropriate neck and shoulder-girdle postures are considered throughout the therapy program.

B. *Surgical management.* In the past surgical management has included translocation of the ulnar nerve, which may be combined with excision of the medial epicondyle. Currently division of the tendinous origin of the flexor carpi ulnaris from the humerus is the procedure of choice in most cases.[11]

■ PASSIVE TREATMENT TECHNIQUES

(For simplicity, the operator is referred to as the male, the patient as the female. All the techniques described apply to the patient's *left* extremity except where indicated. P—patient; O—operator; M—movement; MH—mobilizing hand.)

□ Joint Mobilization Techniques

I. **Humeroulnar Joint—Distraction**
  A. *Joint distraction*—in flexion (ulna moved inferiorly) (Fig. 10-18*A*)
    P—Supine with arm at side, elbow bent, forearm supinated
    O—Stabilizes the wrist with the left hand. He grasps the proximal forearm high up in the antecubital space with the right hand in a pronated position, using the web of the hand for contact.
    M—The proximal ulna is moved inferiorly, affecting a joint distraction, with perhaps some inferior glide. As movement increases, the elbow can be progressively flexed.
  This technique is used as a general capsular stretch, primarily to increase elbow flexion.
  B. *Joint distraction*—in flexion (ulna moved superiorly) (Fig. 10-18*B*)
    P—Supine, with arm at side, forearm supinated, elbow flexed
    O—Stabilizes the upper arm by holding the distal humerus at the elbow down against the plinth with the right hand. With the left hand, he grasps the back of the supinated wrist.
    M—The proximal ulna is moved superiorly (towards the ceiling), producing joint distraction. **Note:** By holding the forearm against his body, the operator can combine distraction with increasing flexion (oscillatory movement) by a rocking motion of his body, while maintaining constant stabilization of the humerus.
  This technique is also used to increase elbow flexion.
  C. *Joint distraction*—moving toward extension (Fig. 10-18*C*)
    P—Supine, with arm at side, elbow bent, forearm in neutral position
    O—Stabilizes the distal humerus against the plinth with the left hand, forearm pronated. He grasps the distal ulna with

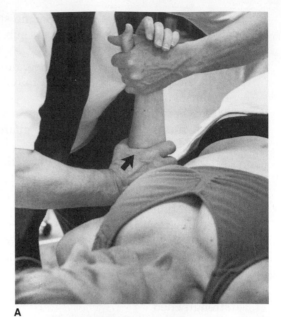

A

B

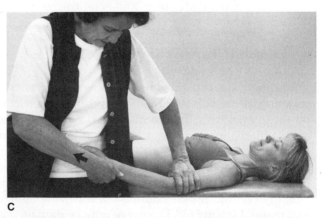

C

FIG. 10-18. Techniques for distraction of the humeroulnar joint: (**A**) joint distraction in flexion (ulna moved inferiorly); (**B**), joint distraction in flexion (ulna moved superiorly); (**C**) joint distraction, moving toward extension.

his right hand, using primarily the thumb and index finger.

M—Ulnar distraction is effected as a distal pull and by a little outward rotation of the operator's entire body. The elbow may be gradually extended as movement increases.

This technique may be considered an inferior glide of the coronoid on the trochlea or, in a sense, a joint distraction. When used at the limit of extension it becomes an anterior capsular stretch.

II. **Humeroulnar Joint—Medial-Lateral Tilt** (Fig. 10-19)

P—Supine, with arm at side, forearm supinated, elbow close to the limit of extension

O—Supports the forearm with the left hand; grasps the humeral epicondyles, supporting the olecranon in the palm of the hand

M—Keeping the patient's forearm stationary, the right hand moves medially or laterally, producing a medial (Fig. 10-19A) or lateral (Fig.

10-19B) (valgus or varus) tilt of the patient's humeroulnar joint. The elbow is gradually extended as movement increases.

These techniques are used only when the elbow lacks a few degrees of extension. It is intended to increase a joint-play movement necessary for full elbow extension.

III. **Humeroulnar Joint—Anterior Glide** (Fig. 10-20A)

P—Prone

O—Standing, facing the head of the table. With the medial hand, stabilize the distal (right) humerus. With the heel of the lateral hand, contact the posterior aspect of the olecranon process. The forearm is supported on the operator's thigh at the limit of the physiologic range of motion.

M—From this position, glide the ulna anteriorly (towards the floor).

This technique is used to increase flexion. This technique may also be performed in supine position, with the head of the treatment table elevated, the upper arm supported on the table, and the forearm over the edge of the table and supported at the wrist (Fig. 10-20B).

IV. **Humeroradial Joint—Approximation** (Fig. 10-21)

P—Supine with the humerus on the table and elbow flexed to 90°

O—The stabilizing hand grips the distal humerus while the mobilizing hand grasps the patient's hand, thenar to thenar and thumb around thumb.

M—The shaft of the radius is moved downward indirectly through the wrist by the operator leaning his shoulder on the interlocking hands, causing the radius to approximate into the humerus. The forearm may be alternately pronated and supinated.

This technique may be used to reduce a distal positional fault of the radius and, when combined with pronation and supination, to increase pronation and supination, respectively.

V. **Proximal Radioulnar Joint—Distal Glide of Radius on Ulna** (Fig. 10-22)

P—Supine, with arm resting at the side, elbow bent, and forearm in neutral position

O—Stabilizes the distal humerus against the plinth with his left hand, forearm pronated. He grasps the distal radius with his right hand, using primarily the thumb, index, and long fingers.

M—The radius is pulled distally with the right hand and by a little outward rotation of the operator's entire body. The elbow may be gradually extended as movement increases.

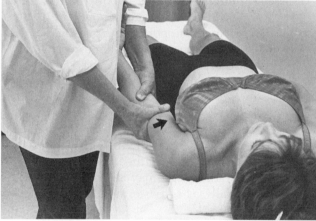

A

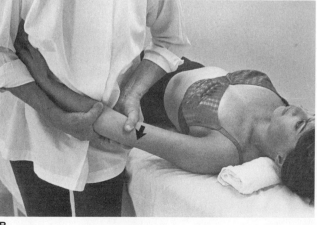

B

FIG. 10-19. Medial-lateral tilt of humeroulnar joint: (**A**) medial tilt (glide); (**B**) lateral tilt (glide).

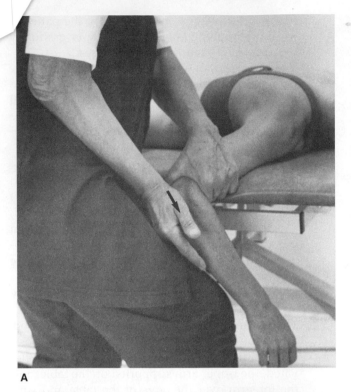

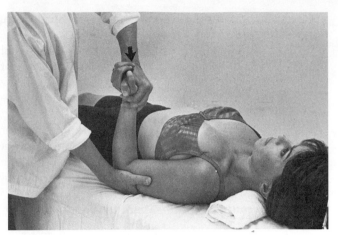

FIG. 10-21. Humeroradial joint: approximation.

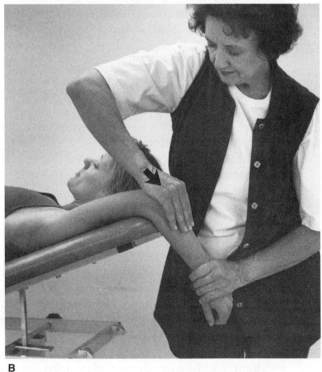

FIG. 10-20. Humeroulnar joint: (**A**) anterior glide in prone; (**B**) anterior glide in supine.

This technique may also be considered distraction at the radiohumeral joint and is intended to increase joint-play movement necessary for full elbow extension.

VI. **Proximal Radioulnar Joint—Dorsal-Ventral Glide** (Fig. 10-23A)

P—Supine, arm at side, elbow slightly flexed, forearm in slight supination. The patient's forearm is supported by placing her hand lightly on the operator's left forearm.

O—Supports the medial aspect of the distal humerus and proximal surface of the upper forearm with his left hand. The right hand holds the ventral surface of the proximal radius with the thumb and the dorsal surface with the crook of the flexed proximal interphalangeal joint of the index finger.

M—The radial head may be moved dorsally or ventrally as separate motions. These move-

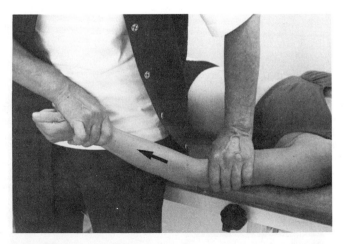

FIG. 10-22. Distal glide of radius on ulna for proximal radioulnar joint.

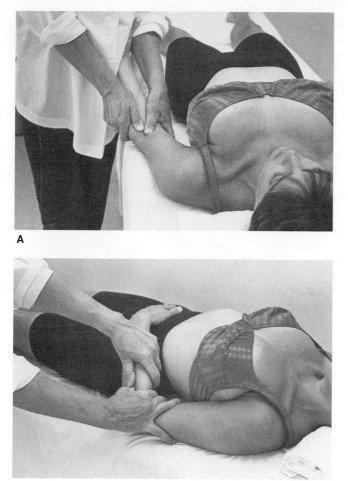

FIG. 10-23. Dorsal-ventral glide of proximal radioulnar joint: (**A**) dorsal glide in resting position; (**B**) ventral glide in restricted range.

the thenar eminence of his right hand over the anterior aspect of the head of the radius and maintains the patient's upper arm on the plinth. The position of the head of the patient's radius is maintained with his thenar eminence.

M—The carrying angle of the patient's elbow is increased by the operator's hand at the wrist while maintaining full supination (Fig. 10-24A). Maintaining both supination and the carrying angle of the forearm, the operator flexes the patient's elbow until the head of the radius is felt to press firmly against his right thenar eminence (Fig. 10-24B). While maintaining the forearm in this position with firm pressure against the radial head, the forearm is moved into pronation (Fig. 10-24C). **Note:** This technique requires considerable practice to be effective. If supination, flexion, and pressure of the thenar eminence are not maintained throughout the technique, the proper movement will not be achieved. The angle of flexion should not be altered while the forearm is moved from supination to pronation.

This is a valuable technique in regaining joint-play movements necessary for pronation and supination. It is particularly helpful with dysfunction of the radial head. This dysfunction usually presents with a history of forceful pronation–supination of the elbow and forearm.[20]

Self-Mobilization Techniques

I. Humeroulnar Joint

  A. *Medial-lateral tilt* (sidebending oscillations) (Fig. 10-25)

    P—Standing in a doorway with the right forearm and hand fixed against the wall. The elbow is in slight flexion or close to the limit of extension.

    MH—Grasps the upper arm near the humeral epicondyles

    M—Keeping the forearm stationary, the MH moves the humerus medially or laterally, effecting a medial or lateral tilt of the humeroulnar joint.

  B. *Distraction in flexion* (Fig. 10-26)

    P—Sitting, with the shoulder abducted 90°. The upper arm is supported on a table. (A kitchen counter is usually a good height.) The elbow is flexed over a firm pillow or towel roll.

ments can be performed in varying degrees of elbow flexion, extension, supination, or pronation.

This technique may also be considered a movement at the radiohumeral joint. It is used to increase joint movement necessary for pronation and supination.

The proximal radioulnar joint is positioned in the resting position (see Fig. 10-23A) if conservative techniques are indicated, or approximating the restricted range if more aggressive range techniques are indicated (see Fig. 10-23B).

VII. Proximal Radioulnar Joint—Technique to Regain Pronation (after Zohn and Mennell[95]) (Fig. 10-24)

  P—Supine, with arm in full supination and slightly abducted

  O—With his left hand, he supports the wrist with his fingers over the ventral aspect and his thumb on the dorsal aspect. He places

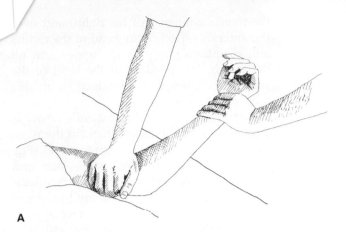

A

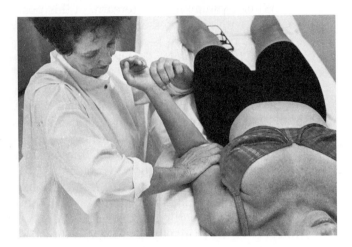

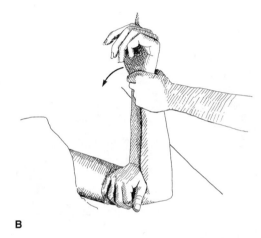

B

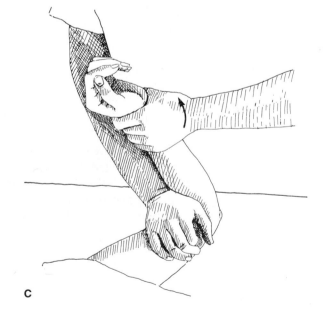

C

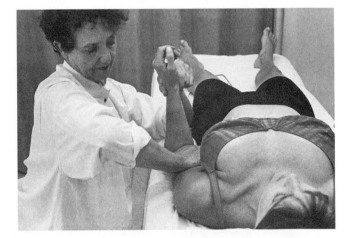

FIG. 10-24. Technique to regain pronation of proximal radiolunar joint (after Zohn and Mennell): (**A**) increasing the carrying angle of the elbow; (**B**) moving the arm toward flexion; (**C**) pronation of arm near the end of motion.

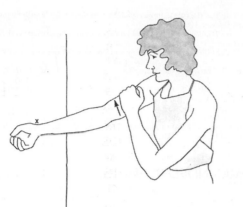

FIG. 10-25. Medial-lateral tilt (sidebending oscillations) of humeroulnar joint.

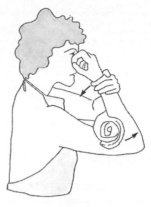

FIG. 10-26. Distraction in flexion of humeroulnar joint.

MH —Placed over the lower arm and dorsum of the hand

M—Slow, gentle, oscillating movements are performed downward in the direction of flexion.

REFERENCES

1. Ackerman LV: Extra-osseous localization non-neoplastic bone and cartilage formation (so-called myositis ossificans). J Bone Joint Surg 40A:279–298, 1958
2. Anson BJ, McVay CB: Surgical Anatomy, vol 2, 5th ed. Philadelphia, WB Saunders, 1971
3. Bernhang AM: The many causes of tennis elbow. NY State J Med 79:1363–1366, 1979
4. Blom S, Hele P, Parkman L: The supinator channel syndrome. Scan J Plast Reconstr Surg 5:71–73, 1971
5. Bowden BW: Tennis elbow. JAOA 78:97–102, 1978
6. Boyd HB: Tennis elbow. J Bone Joint Surg 55A:1183–1187, 1973
7. Butler D: Mobilisation of the Nervous System. Melbourne, Australia, Churchill Livingstone, 1991
8. Cailliet R: Elbow pain. In Cailliet R: Soft Tissue Pain and Disability. Philadelphia, FA Davis, 1988:209–222
9. Capener N: The vulnerability of the posterior interosseous nerve of the forearm. J Bone Joint Surg 48B:7:70–783, 1966
10. Chiao E, Morrey B: Three-dimensional rotation of the elbow. J Biomech 11:57–73, 1978
11. Conway RR, Tanner ED: Elbow pain. In Kaplan PE, Tanner ED: Musculoskeletal Pain and Disability. Norwalk, CT, Appleton & Lange, 1989:133–142
12. Coonard RW: Tennis elbow: Its course, natural history, conservative and surgical management. J Bone Joint Surg 55:1177–1182, 1973
13. Cooney WP III: Bursitis and tendinitis in the hand, wrist and elbow. Minn Med 8:491–494, 1983
14. Corrigan B, Maitland GD: Practical Orthopaedic Medicine. Boston, Butterworths, 1983
15. Cunningham DJ: Myology. In Romanes GJ (ed): Textbook of Anatomy, 12th ed. New York, Oxford University Press, 1981
16. Curwin S, Standish WD: Tendinitis: Its Etiology and Treatment. Lexington, MA, The Collator Press, 1984:115–132
17. Cyriax J: Textbook of Orthopaedic Medicine, vol I: The Diagnosis of Soft Tissue Lesions, 8th ed. Baltimore, Williams & Wilkins, 1982:168–181
18. Dharapak C, Nimberg GA: Posterior interosseous nerve compression: Report of a case caused by traumatic aneurysm. Clin Orthop 101:225–228, 1974
19. Farber JS, Bryan RS: The anterior interosseous nerve syndrome. J Bone Joint Surg 50A:521–523, 1968
20. Gale PA: Joint mobilization. In Hammer WI (ed): Functional Soft Tissue Examination and Treatment by Manual Methods. Gaithersburg, MD, Aspen, 1991
21. Gardner E: The innervation of the elbow joint. Anat Rec 102:161–174, 1948
22. Gessini L, Jandolo B, Pietrangeli A: Entrapment Neuropathies of the median nerve at and above the elbow. Surg Neurol 19:112–116, 1983
23. Gilmer WS, Anderson LD: Reaction of soft somatic tissue which may progress to bone formation: Circumscribed myositis ossificans. South Med J 52:1432–1448, 1959
24. Goldie I: Epicondylitis lateralis humeri. Acta Chir Scand [Suppl] 339:3–119, 1964
25. Goldman S, Honet JC, Sobel R, Goldstein AS: Posterior interosseous nerve palsy in the absence of trauma. Arch Neurol 21:435–441, 1969
26. Goodgold J, Eberstein A: Electrodiagnosis of Neuromuscular Diseases. Baltimore, Williams & Wilkins, 1972
27. Grant JCB: Upper Limb. In Basmajian JV (ed): Grant's Methods of Anatomy, 10th ed. Baltimore, Williams & Wilkins, 1980
28. Gunn CC, Milbrand WE: Tennis elbow and the cervical spine. Can Med Assoc J 114:803–809, 1976
29. Gunn CC, Milbrandt WE: Tennis elbow and acupuncture. Am J Acupuncture 5:61–66, 1977
30. Hagert CG, Lunborg G, Hansen T: Entrapment of the posterior interosseous nerve. Scand J Plast Reconstr Surg 11:205–212, 1977
31. Hayashi Y, Kohimc, Kohno TH: A case of cubital syndrome caused by the snapping of the medial head of the triceps brachii muscle. J Hand Surg 9A:96–99, 1984
32. Hollinshead WH: Anatomy for Surgeons, vol 3: The Back and Limbs, 3rd ed. New York, Harper & Row, 1982
33. Hoppenfeld S: Physical Examination of the Spine and Extremities. New York, Appleton-Century-Crofts, 1976
34. Ilfeld FW, Field SM: Treatment of tennis elbow. Use of special brace. JAMA 195(2):67–70, 1966
35. Indelicato PA, Jobe FW, Kerlan RK, Carter VS, Shields CL, Lomardo S: Correctable elbow lesions in professional baseball players: A review of 25 cases. Am J Sports Med 7(1):72–75, 1979
36. Kane E, Daplan EB, Spinner M: Observation of the course of the ulnar nerve in the arm. Ann Chir 27:487–496, 1973
37. Kapandji IA: The inferior radioulnar joint and pronosupination. In Tubiana R (ed): The Hand, vol. 1. Philadelphia, WB Saunders, 1981
38. Kapandji IA: The Physiology of the Joints, vol 1, 2nd ed. London, E & S Livingstone, 1987
39. Katz RT, Marciniak CA: Electrodiagnosis in musculoskeletal medicine. In Kaplan PE, Tanner ED (eds): Musculoskeletal Pain and Disability. Norwalk, CT, Appleton Lange, 1989:259–289
40. Kelly M: Pain in the forearm and hand due to muscular lesions. Med J Aust 2:185–188, 1947
41. Kiloh LG, Nevin S: Isolated neuritis of the anterior interosseous nerve. Br Med J 1:850–851, 1952
42. Kopell HP, Thompsen WAL: Pronator syndrome. N Engl J Med 259:713–715, 1958
43. Kopell HP, Thompsen WAL: Peripheral Entrapment Neuropathies. Baltimore, Williams & Wilkins, 1963
44. Lake PA: Anterior interosseous nerve syndrome. J Neurosurg 41:306–309, 1974
45. Langman J, Woerdeman MW: Atlas of Medical Anatomy. Philadelphia, WB Saunders, 1976
46. Lee D: A Workbook of Manual Therapy Techniques for the Upper Extremity. Delta, BC, DOPC, 1989
47. Lister GD, Belsole RB, Kleinert HE: The radial tunnel syndrome. J Hand Surg 4:52–60, 1979
48. London JT: Kinematics of the elbow. J Bone Joint Surg 63A:529–535, 1981
49. MacConaill MA, Basmajian JJ: Muscles and Movement: A Basis for Human Kinesiology. Baltimore, Williams & Wilkins, 1969
50. Maeda K, Miura T, Komada T, et al: Anterior interosseous nerve paralysis—Report of 13 cases and review of Japanese literature. Hand 9:165–171, 1977
51. Maigne R: Tennis elbow (epicondylitis). In Liberson WT (ed): Orthopedic Medicine, A New Approach to Vertebral Manipulations. Springfield, Charles C. Thomas, 1972:244–254
52. Martin BF: The annular ligament of the superior radioulnar joint. J Anat 92:473–482, 1958
53. Mayer JH, Mayfield PH: Surgery of the posterior interosseous branch of the radial nerve. Surg Gynecol Obstet 84:979–982, 1947
54. Miller RG: The cubital tunnel syndrome: precise localization and diagnosis. Ann Neurol 6:56–59, 1979
55. Morrey BF: The Elbow and Its Disorders. Philadelphia, WB Saunders, 1985
56. Morris HH, Defers BH: Pronator syndrome: Clinical and electrophysiological features in seven cases. J Neurol Neurosurg Psychiatry 39:461–464, 1976
57. Mulholland RC: Nontraumatic progressive paralysis of the posterior interosseous nerve. J Bone Joint Surg 48B:781–785, 1966
58. Newman JH, Goodfellow JW: Fibrillation of the head of the radius: One cause of tennis elbow. J Bone Joint Surg 57B:115, 1975
59. Nielson HO: Posterior interosseous nerve paralysis caused by a fibrous band compression of the supinator muscle—A report of four cases. Acta Orthop Scand 47:304–307, 1976
60. Nirschl RD: Tennis elbow. Orthop Clin North Am 4:787, 1973
61. Nirschl RD: Medial tennis elbow: The surgical treatment. Annual Meeting of the American Academy of Orthopedic Surgeons. Atlanta, March 1, 1980
62. Nirschl RD: Muscle and tendon trauma: Tennis elbow. In Morrey BF (ed): The Elbow and Its Disorders. Philadelphia, WB Saunders, 1985
63. Nirschl RD, Pettrone F: Tennis elbow: The surgical treatment of lateral epicondylitis. J Bone Joint Surg 61A: 832–839, 1979

64. Norkin CC, Levangie PK: Joint Structure and Function: A Comprehensive Analysis, 2nd ed. Philadelphia, FA Davis, 1992
65. Omer G, Spinner M: Peripheral Nerve Problems. Philadelphia, WB Saunders, 1980
66. Riordan DC: Radial nerve paralysis. Orthop Clin North Am 5:283–287, 1974
67. Roles NC, Maudsley RH: Radial tunnel syndrome, resistant tennis elbow as a nerve entrapment. J Bone Joint Surg 54B:499–508, 1972
68. Rosk MR: Anterior interosseous nerve entrapment: Report of seven cases. Clin Orthop 142:176–181, 1979
69. Seyffarth H: Primary myoses in the m. pronator teres as a cause of lesions of the n. medianus (the pronator syndrome). Acta Psychiatr Scand [Suppl] 74:251–256, 1951
70. Sharrard WJW: Anterior interosseous neuritis—Report of a case. J Bone Joint Surg 50B:804–805, 1968
71. Sharrard WJW: Posterior interosseous neuritis. J Bone Joint Surg 48B:777–780, 1966
72. Somerville EW: Pain in the upper limb. Proceedings of the British Orthopaedic Association. J Bone Joint Surg 45B:620–621, 1963
73. Spinner M: The arcade of Frohse and its relationship to posterior interosseous nerve paralysis. J Bone Joint Surg 50B:809–812, 1968
74. Spinner M: The anterior interosseous nerve syndrome with special attention to its variations. J Bone Joint Surg 52A:84–94, 1970
75. Spinner M. Injuries to the Major Branches of the Peripheral Nerves of the Forearm, 2nd ed. Philadelphia, WB Saunders, 1978
76. Spinner M, Kaplan EB: The quadrate ligament of the elbow: Its relationship to the stability of the proximal radio-ulnar joint. Acta Orthop Scand 41:632–647, 1970
77. Spinner M, Kaplan EB: The relationship of the ulnar nerve to the medial intermuscular septum in the arm and its clinical significance. Hand 8:239–242, 1976
78. Spinner M, Linschied RL: Nerve entrapment syndromes. In Morrey BF (ed): The Elbow and Its Disorders. Philadelphia, WB Saunders, 1985:691–712
79. Spinner M, Spencer PS: Nerve compression lesions of the upper extremity—A clinical and experimental review. Clin Orthop 104:46–67, 1974
80. Tajima T: Functional anatomy of the elbow joint. In Kashiwagi D (ed): Elbow Joint. Amsterdam, Elsevier, 1985
81. Tomberlin JP, Saunders HD: The elbow. In Tomberlin JP, Saunders HD (eds): Evaluation, Treatment and Prevention of Musculoskeletal Disorders, vol 2: Extremities. Chaska, MN, The Saunders Group Inc, 1994:249–274
82. Travel JG, Simons DG: Myofascial Dysfunction—The Trigger Point Manual. Baltimore, Williams & Wilkins, 1983
83. Tullos HS, Bryan WJ: Examination of the throwing elbow. In Zarins JR, Andrews JR (eds): Injuries to the Throwing Athlete. Philadelphia, WB Saunders, 1985
84. Van Rossum J, Buruma OJS, Kamphuisen HAC, et al: Tennis elbow—a radial tunnel syndrome. J Bone Joint Surg 60B:197–198, 1978
85. Vanderpool DW, Edinburg JC, Lamb DW, et al: Peripheral compression lesion of the ulnar nerve. J Bone Joint Surg 50:792–803, 1968
86. Wadsworth TG: The external compression syndrome of the ulnar nerve at the cubital tunnel. Clin Orthop 124:189–204, 1977
87. Wadsworth TG: The Elbow. New York, Churchill Livingstone, 1982
88. Wadsworth TG: Entrapment neuropathy in the upper limb. In Birch R, Brook D (eds): Operative Surgery, The Hand. London, Butterworths, 1984:469–486
89. Wadsworth TG: The cubital tunnel syndrome. In Kashiwagi D (ed): Elbow Joint. Amsterdam, Elsevier, 1985
90. Wadsworth TG, Williams JR: Cubital tunnel external compression syndrome. Br Med J 1:662–666, 1973
91. Wiens E, Lau SCK: The anterior interosseous nerve syndrome. Can J Surg 21:354–357, 1978
92. Williams PL, Warwick R (eds): Gray's Anatomy, 36th ed. Philadelphia, WB Saunders, 1989
93. Woods GW, Tullos HS, King JW: The throwing arm—Elbow joint injuries. J Sports Med [Suppl 1] 4:43–47, 1973
94. Youm Y, Dryer R, Thambyrajan K, et al: Biomechanical analyses of forearm pronation-supination and elbow flexion-extension. J Biomechanics 12:245–255, 1979
95. Zohn DA, Mennell JM: Musculoskeletal pain conditions. In Musculoskeletal Pain: Diagnosis and Physical Treatment. Boston, Little, Brown, 1975

RECOMMENDED READINGS

An KW, Morrey BF: Biomechanics of the elbow. In Morrey BF (ed): The Elbow and Its Disorders. Philadelphia, WB Saunders, 1985:43–61

Bowling RW, Rockar PA: The elbow complex. In Gould JA, Davies GJ: Orthopaedic and Sports Physical Therapy. St. Louis, CV Mosby, 1983

Brewster CI, Shields CL, Seto TL, Morrissey MC: Rehabilitation of the upper extremity. In Shields CL (ed). Manual of Sports Surgery. New York, Springer-Verlag, 1987

Corrigan B, Maitland GD: Practical Orthopedic Medicine. Boston, Butterworths, 1983

Heppenstall RB: Injuries of the elbow. In Heppenstall RB (ed): Fracture Treatment and Healing. Philadelphia, WB Saunders, 1980

Kisner C, Lynn AC: Therapeutic Exercises—Foundations and Techniques, 2nd ed. Philadelphia, FA Davis, 1990:281–296

La Freniere JG: "Tennis elbow": evaluation, treatment and prevention. Phys Ther 59:742–746, 1979

London JT: Kinematics of the elbow. J Bone Joint Surg 63A:529–535, 1981

Murtagn JE: Tennis elbow, description and treatment. Aust Fam Physician 7:1307–1310, 1978

Nirschl R: Rehabilitation of the athlete's elbow. In Morrey BF (ed): The Elbow and Its Disorders. Philadelphia, WB Saunders, 1985:523–529

Nirschl RP, Pettrone FA: Tennis elbow: The surgical treatment of lateral epicondylitis. J Bone Joint Surg 61A:832–839, 1979

Nirschl RP, Sobel J: Conservative treatment of tennis elbow. Phys Sports Med 9:43–54, 1981

Priest JD, Braden V, Gerberich SG: The elbow and tennis, part 1 and 2. Phys Sports Med 8:81–91, 1980

Tucker K: Some aspects of post-traumatic elbow stiffness. Injury 9:216–220, 1978

The Wrist and Hand Complex

DARLENE HERTLING AND RANDOLPH M. KESSLER

FUNCTIONAL ANATOMY

The Wrist Complex

OSTEOLOGY

Distal End of Radius. The radius flares distally, and this end is much larger than the distal end of the ulna. It extends farther laterally than medially. The distal lateral extension of the radius is the radial styloid process. The radial styloid normally extends about 1 cm farther distally than the ulnar styloid (Fig. 11-1).

The medial aspect of the distal radius is a concave surface anteroposteriorly. The medial concavity is the ulnar notch, which articulates with the head of the ulna, allowing pronation and supination to occur. The distal end of the radius is triangular in its transverse cross section. The distal articular surface of the radius is composed of two concave facets, one for articulation with the scaphoid and one for articulation with the lunate (Fig. 11-2). The distal articular surface of the radius faces slightly palmarly (average of 10°) and somewhat ulnarly (average of 20°) (Fig. 11-3).

Distal End of Ulna. The distal end of the ulna flares only mildly compared with the distal end of the radius. The ulnar styloid process is a small conical projection from the dorsomedial aspect of the distal end of the ulna. The radial aspect of the ulnar head is convex anteroposteriorly. It is cartilage-covered for articulation with the ulnar notch of the radius during pronation and supination (see Figs. 11-1 and 11-2).

The distal end of the ulna is somewhat circular on transverse cross section, except for the irregularity

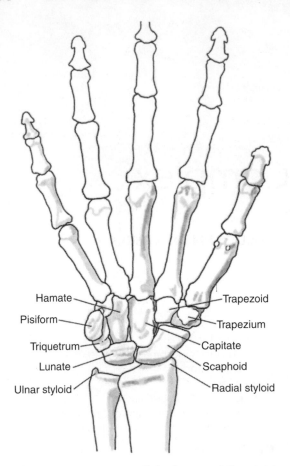

FIG. 11-1. *Palmar aspect of the bones of the right wrist and hand.*

formed by the styloid process dorsomedially. The ulna's distal surface is covered with articular cartilage for articulation with the articular disk (not with the carpals). There is movement between the ulna and disk primarily on pronation and supination, during which the disk must sweep across the distal end of the ulna.

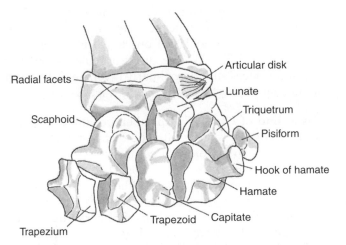

FIG. 11-2. *Inferior aspect of the lower end of the radius and ulna and the carpal bones of the hand.*

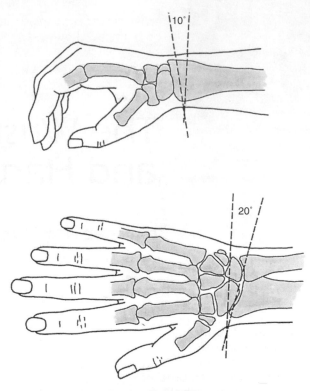

FIG. 11-3. *Normal wrist alignment.*

Carpals. The proximal row of carpals consists of the triquetrum, pisiform, lunate, and scaphoid bones. The scaphoid has a biconvex articular surface proximally for articulation with the lateral facet of the distal end of the radius. The lunate is also convex proximally and articulates with the medial facet of the distal radius and with the articular disk in positions of radial deviation. The triquetrum has a small convex articular surface proximally. This surface is in contact with the ulnar collateral ligament when the wrist is in neutral position and articulates with the articular disk primarily in positions of ulnar deviation. The flexor carpi ulnaris tendon inserts onto the pisiform bone, which lies palmarly over the triquetrum.

The distal end of the scaphoid consists of two distal articular surfaces. The radial surface of the distal scaphoid is convex for articulation with the concave surface formed by the combined proximal ends of the trapezoid and trapezium. The ulnar articulating surface of the distal scaphoid is concave and faces somewhat palmarly and ulnarly. It articulates with the proximal end of the capitate. The distal surface of the lunate is quite concave anteroposteriorly but less so mediolaterally. It grasps the convex proximal end of the capitate and also articulates, to a lesser extent, with the hamate. The distal surface of the triquetrum is concave for articulation with the hamate (see Figs. 11-1 and 11-2).

There is some movement between the bones of the proximal row of carpals. For this reason each of the proximal carpals is lined with articular cartilage on its radial or ulnar surfaces, or both, to allow for such movement.

Ulnarly to radially, the distal carpals are the hamate, capitate, trapezoid, and trapezium (see Fig. 11-1). The combined proximal surfaces of the hamate and capitate form a convex surface that articulates with the concave surface formed by the combined distal surfaces of the triquetrum, lunate, and scaphoid (see Fig. 11-2). The combined proximal surfaces of the trapezoid and trapezium form a concave surface for articulation with the convex distal articular surface of the scaphoid. The distal end of the trapezium is a sellar surface that articulates with the correspondingly sellar surface of the proximal aspect of the first metacarpal. The trapezoid articulates distally with the second metacarpal, the capitate with the third metacarpal, and the hamate with the fourth and fifth metacarpals (see Fig. 11-1).

Because there is a small amount of movement between adjacent bones of the distal row, these are also lined with articular cartilage radially and ulnarly to allow for such intercarpal movement.

The carpals, taken together, form an arch in the transverse plane that is concave palmarly. This arch deepens with wrist flexion and flattens on wrist extension. The "hook" of the hamate, a large prominence on the hamate's palmar aspect, and the pisiform bone, situated on the palmar aspect of the triquetrum, form the ulnar side of this arch. The trapezium, which tends to be oriented about 45° from the plane of the palm, and the radial aspect of the scaphoid, which curves palmarly, form the radial side of the arch. The flexor retinaculum, or transverse carpal ligament, traverses this arch (Fig. 11-4). The flexor ulnaris tendon inserts onto the pisiform. When this muscle contracts it pulls on the pisiform, causing tightening of the flexor retinaculum. This tightening deepens the transverse carpal arch.

LIGAMENTS, CAPSULES, SYNOVIA, AND DISK

The articular cavity of the distal radioulnar joint is usually distinct from the articular cavity of the radiocarpal joint, which is also separate from that of the midcarpal joint. The carpometacarpal joints often share a common joint cavity; in some cases this communicates with the midcarpal joint (Fig. 11-5).

The distal radioulnar joint is bordered proximally by the lax "sacciform recess" in the capsule, which loops proximally between the radius and ulna. Distally this joint is bordered by the triangular articular disk. This fibrocartilaginous disk attaches ulnarly to the ulnar styloid process and radially to the ulnar margin of the distal radial articular surface. It separates the distal ra-

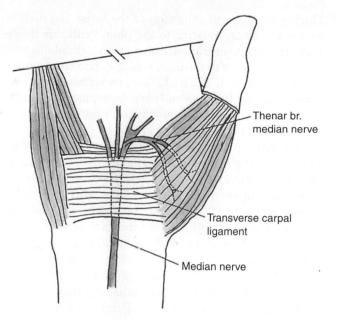

FIG. 11-4. *Transverse carpal ligament and median nerve.*

dioulnar joint from the radiocarpal joint. Anteriorly and posteriorly the margins of the disk attach to the joint capsule. The superior aspect of the disk is a cartilage-lined concave surface for articulation with the distal end of the ulna. The disk moves with the radius on pronation and supination and must therefore sweep across the distal end of the ulna on these movements.

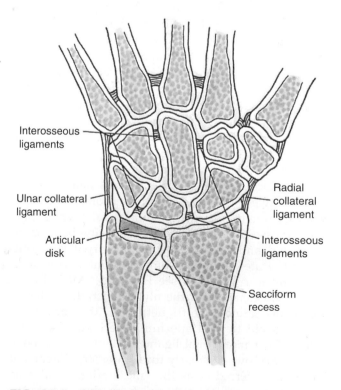

FIG. 11-5. *Cross section through the articulations of the wrist, showing the synovial cavities.*

During flexion and extension of the wrist, the disk remains stationary relative to the ulna. With this movement the lunate or triquetrum, or both, articulates with the distal surface of the disk, which is also concave and cartilage-covered. The disk, then, provides two articular surfaces for the ulna and carpals, separates the adjacent joint cavities, and binds together the distal ends of the ulna and radius (see Fig. 11-5).

The radiocarpal joint is bordered proximally by the radius and the articular disk. Distally it is bordered by the three proximal carpals and their respective interosseous ligaments, which are flush with the continuous convex articular surface formed by the proximal carpals. Medially and laterally the joint is bordered by the strong ulnar and radial collateral ligaments. Both collateral ligaments attach proximally to the styloid processes. Distally, the ulnar ligament attaches to the triquetrum and pisiform; the radial ligament attaches to the scaphoid and trapezium. Palmarly and dorsally the capsule of this joint is reinforced by the palmar and the dorsal radiocarpal ligaments (Fig. 11-6). Palmarly, there is also an ulnocarpal ligament. These ligaments ensure that the carpals follow the radius during pronation and supination. Synovium lines the capsuloligamentous structures mentioned, as well as the interosseous ligaments between the triquetrum and lunate and between the scaphoid and lunate.

The articulations between the proximal and distal carpal bones are enclosed in a common joint cavity. Anatomically, the midcarpal joint is considered the compound joint between the two rows of carpals. However, functionally the distinction is not so simple. Proximally the midcarpal joint is bordered by the scaphoid, lunate, and triquetrum and their interosseous ligaments, which intervene between the proximal ends of these bones. In this way the intercarpal articulations between the proximal carpals are enclosed within the midcarpal joint cavity. Distally the midcarpal joint is bordered by the distal carpals and their interosseous ligaments, which intervene about midway, or further distally, between the distal carpals. Occasionally an interosseous ligament intervenes between the capitate and scaphoid, dividing the midcarpal joint into medial and lateral cavities. Since an interosseous ligament is often missing between the trapezoid and trapezium, the midcarpal joint often communicates with the common joint cavity of the carpometacarpal joints (see Fig. 11-5). Medially and laterally, extensions of the ulnar and radial collateral ligaments connect the triquetrum to the hamate and the scaphoid to the trapezium. There are also dorsal and palmar intercarpal ligaments between the bones of the two rows. Palmarly these intercarpal ligaments are often referred to as the "radiate ligament" since they tend to radiate outward from the capitate (see Fig. 11-6).

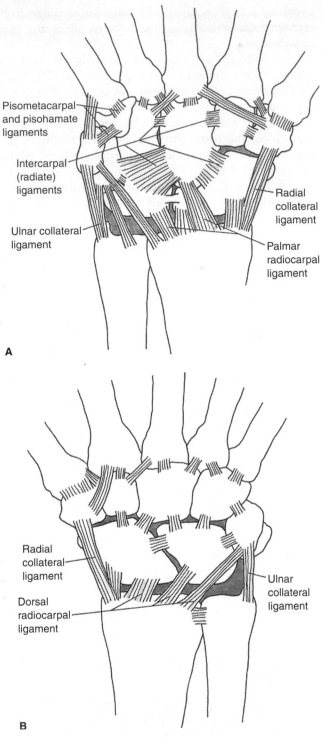

FIG. 11-6. Palmar aspect (**A**) and dorsal aspect (**B**) of the ligaments of the right wrist and metacarpus.

Palmar and dorsal intercarpal ligaments also connect the carpals within a row. The pisohamate ligament (from the pisiform to the hook of the hamate) and the pisometacarpal ligament (to the base of the fifth metacarpal) are believed to be continuations of the flexor carpi ulnaris tendon that attaches to the pisiform (see Fig. 11-6). The joint between the pisiform and triquetrum is usually distinct from the other joints mentioned, having its own joint capsule and synovium-lined cavity.

☐ The Hand Complex

The hand consists of five digits, or four fingers and a thumb. There are 19 long bones distal to the carpals and 19 joints that make up the hand complex. These are divided in five rays, with each ray making up a polyarticulated chain comprising the metacarpals and phalanges. The base of each metacarpal articulates with the distal row of carpals.

CARPOMETACARPAL JOINTS OF THE FINGERS

In the carpometacarpal joint area there are two stable joints that permit little or no motion: the carpometacarpal joints of the index and middle fingers. There are also two very mobile joints: the carpometacarpal joints of the thumb and the little finger.[94] Since thumb function differs significantly from that of the other digits, it will be examined separately. The second metacarpal articulates primarily with the trapezoid and secondarily with the trapezium, capitate, and third metacarpal (see Fig. 11-1). The trapezoid is mortised in the base of the index metacarpal, affording a very secure fixation.

The middle or third metacarpal articulates primarily with the capitate and is also bound to the adjacent second and fourth metacarpal (see Fig. 11-1). Therefore, all the carpals in the distal carpal row and the index and middle metacarpal bases are firmly joined and function together as a single osseoligamentous unit, the fixed stable portion of the hand.[71]

The little finger metacarpal articulates with the hamate and fourth metacarpal (see Fig. 11-1). The hamate is a saddle-like joint, and its articulation with the little metacarpal resembles that of the thumb carpometacarpal joint but is not as mobile.[94] The articular surface of the base of the fifth metacarpal is convex in the volar-dorsal direction and concave in the radioulnar axis.[99]

The ring finger metacarpal base articulates with the hamate primarily in a joint similar to that of the little finger but with even less motion permitted. It also articulates with the capitate, as well as the middle and little finger metacarpals (see Fig. 11-1).

While the little finger carpometacarpal joint is considered a saddle joint with two degrees of freedom, the other finger carpometacarpal joints are plane synovial joints with one degree of freedom: flexion–extension.[54,85] Their proximal surface may be considered concave, the distal end convex.

The capsular pattern of restriction is limitation of motion equally in all directions. All are supported by strong transverse and weaker longitudinal ligaments volarly and dorsally (see Fig. 11-6). This ligamentous structure controls the total range of motion available at each carpometacarpal joint. The function of the carpometacarpal joints of the fingers is primarily to contribute to the hollowing of the palm to allow the hand and digits to conform optimally to the shape of the object being held.[85]

CARPOMETACARPAL JOINT OF THE THUMB

The carpometacarpal joint of the trapezium–thumb metacarpal joint is a very mobile articulation. Although described as a saddle-type joint, it is actually a reciprocally biconcave joint resembling two saddles whose concave surfaces are opposed to each other at right angles or 90° rotation (Fig. 11-7). All motions are possible, including circumduction.[16,94] The carpometacarpal articulation is specialized to produce automatic axial rotation of the first metacarpal during angular movements. Zancolli and associates[124] proposed the concept that the trapezium is formed by two different types of joints. One part, the saddle area, occupies the center of the articular surfaces and takes part in simple angular movements. The other part, located on the palmar side, is an ovoid area that represents a ball-and-socket joint for complex rotatory movements. The saddle part of the joint favors the circumduction motion to the motion of opposition. The trapezium is firmly bound to the trapezoid and indeed to the entire distal carpal row and has virtually no independent motion.

According to Zancolli and colleagues,[124,125] the

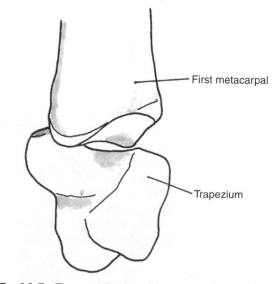

FIG. 11-7. *The saddle-shaped carpometacarpal articulation of the thumb.*

First metacarpal

Trapezium

greatest stability of the first metacarpal is achieved after complete pronation in the position of full opposition when ligamentous tension, muscular contraction, and joint congruence produce the maximal effect in achieving stabilization of pinch. Opposition with simultaneous pronation (or axial rotation) is sequentially abduction, flexion, and adduction of the first metacarpal. Axial rotation occurring in the carpometacarpal joint is made possible because of the laxity of the joint capsule and the joint configuration.[18,85,124,125] The tension in the ligaments combined with muscle activity of opposition and reposition form couples (paired parallel forces) that produce this axial rotation. The function of muscles crossing the joint is essential. According to Kauer,[56] the close structural relationship between the tendon of the abductor pollicis longus and the first carpometacarpal joint influences the restraining and directing function of the ligamentous system. The functional significance of the movement of opposition can be appreciated when one realizes that use of the thumb against a finger occurs in almost all forms of prehension.[85]

The strongest carpometacarpal joint ligament is the deep ulnar or anterior oblique carpometacarpal ligament that unites the tubercle of the trapezium and the volar beak of the metacarpal base (Fig. 11-8).[99] Extrinsic support is provided by the extensor pollicis longus and the origin of the thenar muscles.

METACARPOPHALANGEAL JOINTS OF THE FINGERS

The distal metacarpophalangeal (MCP) joints of the fingers are made of an irregular spheroidal (convex) metacarpal head proximally and the concave base of the first phalanx distally (Fig. 11-9A). They are multiaxial condyloid joints and allow primarily flexion and extension, but also abduction, adduction, and some axial rotation. The most extensive movements are flexion and extension. The average flexion range is 90°

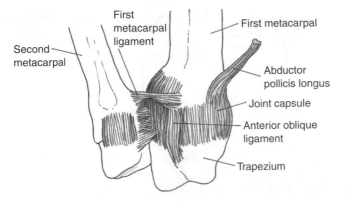

FIG. 11-8. Volar view of the right first carpometacarpal joint and the arrangement of the ligaments.

to 95°, but hyperextension of 20° to 30° and even as much as 45° is common. The articular surface of the metacarpal head is rounded dorsally and is flat volarly (Fig. 11-9B). It has 180° of articular surface in the sagittal plane, with the predominant portion lying volarly. This is apposed to about 20° of articular surface on the phalanx, resulting in poorly mated surfaces.[85]

The joint is surrounded by a capsule that is lax in extension and in conjunction with the poorly mated surfaces allows some passive axial rotation of the proximal phalanx in this position (Fig. 11-10).[85] The primary ligament support of the MCP joint includes two lateral collateral ligaments, two accessory collateral ligaments, and the volar plate (Figs. 11-10 and 11-11). The volar plate or ligament is a thick, tough fibrocartilaginous structure tat firmly inserts into the volar base of the proximal phalanx. Proximally it thins to become nearly membranous at its metacarpal attachment. The volar plate with the two accessory ligaments on the sides enlarges the cavity of the MCP joint, permitting the head of the metacarpal to remain in the articular cavity as the MCP joint flexes (see Fig. 11-10). During flexion, this thin proximal portion folds in like the billows of an accordion or a telephone-booth door.[94] The plate also helps to restrict the hyperextension permitted by the loose capsule. Distally and laterally the volar plate on both sides is attached to a lateral collateral ligament, and in its midposition laterally to an accessory ligament (see Fig. 11-11). The four volar plates of the MCP joints also blend with and are interconnected by the transverse metacarpal ligament, which connects the adjacent lateral borders of the index, middle, ring, and little fingers. While the dorsal surface of the volar plate is in contact with the head of the metacarpal, the volar surface of this ligament is in contact with the flexor tendon. The volar plate and transverse metacarpal ligament form the dorsal wall of the vaginal ligament, which forms a tunnel and completely surrounds the flexor tendons (see Fig. 11-9). The flexible attachment of the volar plate to the phalanx permits the plate to glide distally along the volar surface of the metacarpal head without restricting motion during flexion, and also prevents impingement by the joint of the long flexor tendons (Fig. 11-12).

The MCP joint is the most stable in maximal flexion since the lateral collateral ligaments are stretched tautly in this position and the accessory collateral ligaments offer additional stability by firmly holding the volar plate against the volar surface of the metacarpal head (see Fig. 11-12). The capsule also becomes taut in this close-packed position (see Fig. 11-10). In extension the capsule and lateral collateral ligaments are lax and the MCP joint is relatively mobile, permitting abduction and adduction as well as some axial rotation by the intrinsic muscles. Disparity

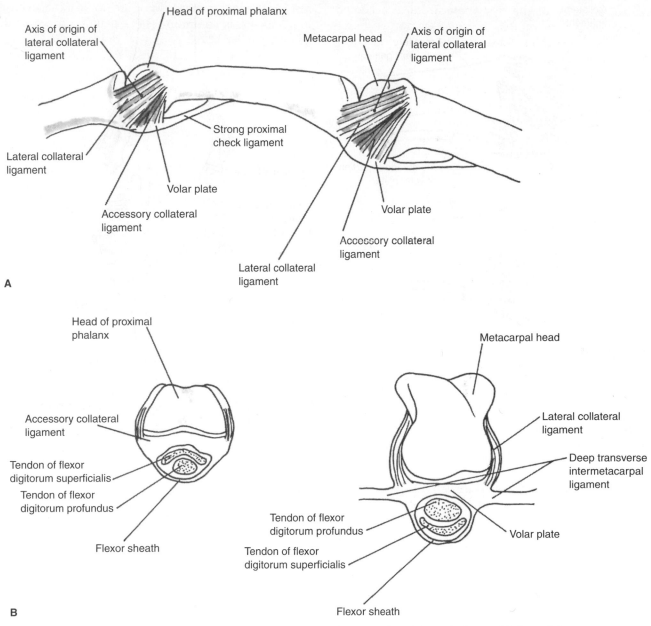

FIG. 11-9. (**A**) *Sagittal view of the metacarpophalangeal and interphalangeal joints of the fingers.* (**B**) *Anterior view of metacarpal and proximal phalanx head.*

of the articular surfaces and laxity of the ligaments at these joints allow for considerable passive range of movement in all positions of these joints except the close-packed position. Together with the transverse metacarpal arch, the passive movements at the MCP joints enhance the plasticity of the hand and facilitate its adaptability to the size and shape of the object being grasped.[92]

The asymmetry of the metacarpal heads, as well as the difference in length and direction of the collateral ligaments, explains why the ulnar inclination of the digits normally is greater than the radial inclination.[109] The normal ulnar inclination of the fingers occurs at the MCP joints and is most marked in the index finger. Inclination is less in the middle and little

fingers and almost nonexistent in the ring finger. Normal ulnar inclination is due to several anatomic factors, which have been the subject of numerous studies in recent years.[33,40,42,98,124]

MCP JOINT OF THE THUMB

The MCP joint of the thumb is a semicondyloid-type articulation between the head of the first metacarpal and the base of its proximal phalanx. Two sesamoid bones are constantly present extracapsularly on its volar surface: a somewhat larger lateral sesamoid and a medial sesamoid (Fig. 11-13).[99] The joint has two degrees of freedom (flexion–extension, abduction–adduction) and limited axial rotation.[55] The capsule is

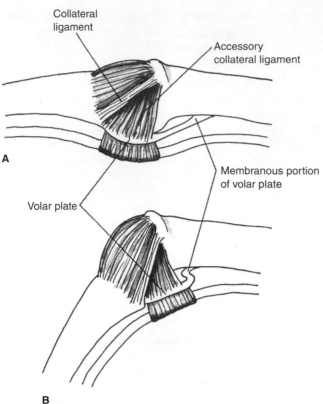

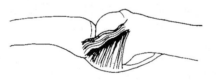

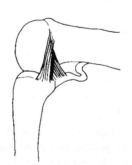

FIG. 11-10. The metacarpophalangeal joint during extension (**A**) and flexion (**B**).

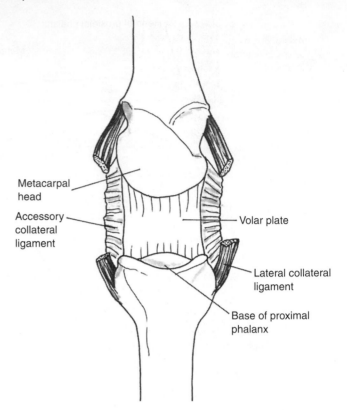

FIG. 11-11. Metacarpophalangeal joint with collateral ligaments divided.

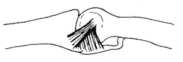

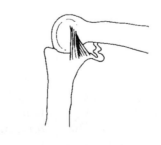

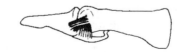

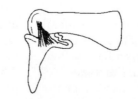

FIG. 11-12. Lateral view showing the volar plate and the two parts of the collateral ligament of the metacarpophalangeal (**A**), proximal interphalangeal (**B**), and distal interphalangeal joints with the joints extended and flexed (**C**).

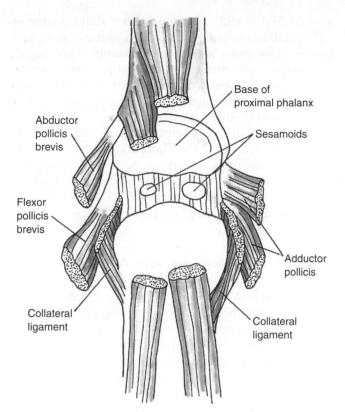

FIG. 11-13. *Inner view of the metacarpophalangeal joint of the right thumb. The capsule and lateral ligaments are excised with the parts attached shown. The volar plate with the sesamoids is shown at the bottom of the joint.*

inserted in the ridge separating the articulation of the proximal phalanx and the metacarpal. The capsule is reinforced on each side by the collateral ligaments, similar to those of the other MCP joints. Each collateral ligament is inserted into a tubercle on the base of the phalanx and into the corresponding sesamoid (Fig. 11-14). The two sesamoids are incorporated into the fibrocartilage of the volar plate.[96] The tunnel of the flexor pollicis longus is intimately connected to the volar plate, so the tunnel is an integral part of the apparatus, connecting the lateral ligaments and the volar plate with the sesamoids. The volar plate is attached firmly to the proximal phalanx but loosely to the metacarpal; it is the proximal attachment that has given way with irreducible dislocation.[16]

There is considerable individual variation in joint ranges, depending on the anatomic configuration of the single broad condyle of the metacarpal.[11] Flexion ranges from 5° to 100°, with an average of about 75°.[94] If the head is round, 90° to 100° flexion is achieved. If it is flat (only 10% to 15% of cases), little flexion is possible. The main functional contribution of the first MCP joint is to provide additional range to the thumb pad in opposition and to allow the thumb to grasp and contour to objects.[85] The literature contains little information on the function of the sesamoids. The most common belief is that they increase the leverage of certain muscles connected with the tendons running to these joints.[99]

INTERPHALANGEAL ARTICULATIONS OF THE FINGERS

The interphalangeal joints of the digits are each composed of the head of a phalanx and the base of the phalanx distal to it (see Fig. 11-9). Each is a true synovial hinge joint that functions uniquely in flexion and extension with one degree of freedom. From a clinical standpoint, each phalanx has a head (caput) or a distal end with a convex surface and a body (corpus) and a base or proximal end with a concave surface.[51] The head of each phalanx, divided into two condyles separated by a cleft, fits the contiguous articular surface of the phalangeal base and articulates in a tongue-and-groove configuration (see Fig. 11-9).[94] Their trochlea-shaped articulations are closely congruent through excursion of the joint.[109]

The proximal interphalangeal (PIP) joint has the greatest range of flexion and extension of any digital joint, with an average of 105°. The intrinsic ligamentous support of the PIP joint resembles that of the MCP joint and includes two lateral collateral ligaments, two accessory collateral ligaments, and a volar plate (see Fig. 11-12*B*). The volar plate, which prevents hyperextension, has a thick distal insertion and two check ligaments proximally inserted on the middle phalanx (Fig. 11-15). Traumatic ruptures of the volar plate occur in the thicker distal insertion rather than the proximal insertion.[109] The fibrous flexor sheath is inserted on the volar plate on the base of the phalanx proximally and

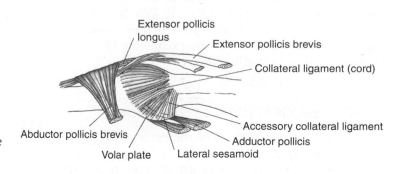

FIG. 11-14. *The metacarpophalangeal joint of the right thumb, radial aspect.*

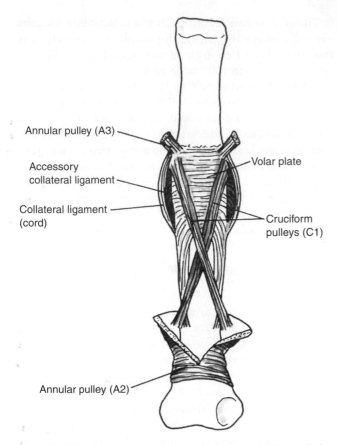

Annular pulley (A3)

Accessory collateral ligament

Collateral ligament (cord)

Volar plate

Cruciform pulleys (C1)

Annular pulley (A2)

FIG. 11-15. The proximal interphalangeal joint and the arrangement of the components of the flexor sheath and volar plate.

distally. This differs from the insertion at the MCP joint, where the flexor sheath inserts on the volar plate and base of the proximal phalanx but not on the metacarpal. This arrangement involving the collateral ligaments, volar plate, and flexor sheath is the key to interphalangeal stability.[26] Little hyperextension of this joint is possible, in contrast to the MCP joint.

The distal interphalangeal (DIP) joint resembles the PIP joint in function and ligamentous structure but has less stability and allows some hyperextension, giving a larger pulp contact (see Fig. 11-12C). DIP flexion rarely exceeds 80°, but hyperextension is greater than at the PIP joint because the DIP joint's volar plate does not have the check ligaments proximally.[94]

The total range of flexion–extension available to the index finger is 100° to 110° at the PIP joint and 80° at the DIP joint. The range at each joint increases ulnarly, with the proximal and distal joints achieving 135° and 90°, respectively, in the little finger.[85]

INTERPHALANGEAL JOINT OF THE THUMB

The interphalangeal joint of the thumb is structurally and functionally similar to the DIP joints of the fingers. It is a trochlear type of articulation, allowing

mainly flexion and extension, with a slight degree of axial rotation toward pronation. Axial rotation, in fact, occurs at all three joints of the thumb: (1) trapezio-metacarpal—automatic longitudinal rotation at a saddle joint; (2) MCP—active longitudinal rotation at a condylar joint through the action of the lateral thenar muscles; and (3) interphalangeal joint.[52,53]

At the end of the extension range, motion is restricted by the volar plate. There is considerable variation in the amount of extension permitted: many normal persons can hyperextend the joint.[16] Lack of extension of this joint, if greater than 15°, is functionally more disabling than lack of flexion.[109]

☐ Tendons, Nerves, and Arteries

These structures are not discussed in detail here, but the reader will benefit from studying cross-sectional diagrams showing the anatomic relationships of these structures (Fig. 11-16). The relationships described below are most important clinically.

The transverse carpal ligament (flexor retinaculum) forms a roof over the palmar arch of the carpal bones (see Figs. 11-4 and 11-16). Through the resulting tunnel pass the tendons of the flexor digitorum profundus and flexor digitorum superficialis. These tendons are all enclosed in a common synovial sheath. The flexor carpi radialis tendon and the flexor pollicis longus tendon also pass through the "carpal tunnel," each enclosed in a separate sheath. Superficial to the common flexor tendon sheath and deep to the flexor retinaculum passes the median nerve. At the distal end of the tunnel the nerve divides into several digital branches, one of which turns rather sharply around the distal border of the flexor retinaculum to innervate the thenar muscle (see Fig. 11-4). "Carpal tunnel syn-

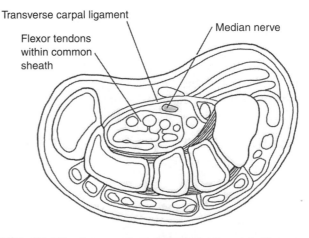

Transverse carpal ligament

Median nerve

Flexor tendons within common sheath

FIG. 11-16. Cross section of the wrist through the carpus, demonstrating the relationship of the median nerve to the flexor tendons and transverse carpal ligaments (flexor retinaculum).

drome" is the result of compression of the median nerve within the tunnel or, occasionally, of just the thenar branch of the nerve as it turns around the distal border of the retinaculum. The palmaris longus tendon and the ulnar nerve and artery pass superficially to the flexor retinaculum. The nerve and artery travel beneath the flexor carpi ulnaris tendon, then radially to the pisiform bone before dividing to enter the hand.

The tendons of the extensor pollicis brevis and the abductor pollicis longus are enclosed in a common sheath as they pass across the lateral aspect of the distal radius. Inflammation of this sheath, or of the tendons within the sheath, is a fairly common disorder known as *De Quervain's disease,* or tenosynovitis. These tendons form the radial side of the "anatomical snuff box." The extensor pollicis longus tendon passes around Lister's tubercle on the dorsal aspect of the distal radius in a pulley-like fashion. It turns obliquely toward the thumb to form the ulnar side of the snuff box. The radial artery travels laterally to the flexor carpi radialis tendon before turning deep beneath the abductor pollicis longus and extensor pollicis brevis tendons. It becomes superficial dorsally and can be palpated in the snuff box.

At the level of the fingers, the long flexor tendons are attached to the volar aspect by three fibrous sheaths: the first lies just proximal to the metacarpal head, the second on the palmar surface of the proximal phalanx, and the third on the same surface of the second phalanx (Fig. 11-17). These form fibrous tunnels or digital pulleys along with the slightly concave osseous palmar surface of the phalanges. Between these three sheaths the tendons are held down by annular oblique and cruciate fibers that cover the MCP and PIP joints in a crosswise position (see Fig. 11-15). The two digital pulleys are the most important elements of the flexor tendon sheaths; the cruciate pulleys play an accessory role.[97] Synovial sheaths allow gliding of the tendons within their tunnels.

The synovial sheaths of the flexor tendons start in the forearm proximal to the flexor retinaculum (see Fig. 11-16). The skin creases on the flexor aspect of the fingers, except for the proximal crease, lie immediately proximal to the corresponding joints. At this level the skin is directly in contact with the synovial sheath, which can be readily infected.[54]

The long extensor muscles of the hand also run along fibro-osseous tunnels, but since their course on the whole is convex these tunnels are less numerous. They are seen only at the wrist, where the tendons become concave outward during extension.[54]

A more detailed description of the anatomy of the hand and wrist complex can be found in other sources.[10,39,43,52,54,56,67,80,105,109]

☐ Surface Anatomy of the Wrist

Because the wrist consists of many small structures in close proximity, the clinician must pay special attention to identifying these structures. The following exercise can help the reader identify the clinically significant structures about the wrist.

The distal end of the radius is easily palpated. Notice how it flares distally. Palpate along its radial border to the styloid process; note the gap between the radial styloid and the carpals when the wrist and thumb are relaxed. Extend the thumb and notice how the abductor pollicis longus and extensor pollicis brevis tendons bridge this gap. The prominence on the dorsal aspect of the distal radius, Lister's tubercle, is easily palpated. Again, extend the thumb and follow the extensor pollicis longus tendon from this tubercle, about which it curves, down to the thumb.

With the thumb extended and the wrist slightly dorsiflexed, once again locate the abductor pollicis longus tendon. Now palpate ulnarly on the palmar aspect of the wrist, level with the radial styloid. The next prominent tendon is the flexor carpi radialis tendon. Palpate the radial pulse just radial to this tendon. Once again palpate in an ulnar direction. The next tendon, just ulnar to the flexor carpi radialis, is the palmaris longus tendon. The median nerve lies deep to this tendon, beneath the flexor retinaculum.

The distal end of the ulna is also easily palpated.

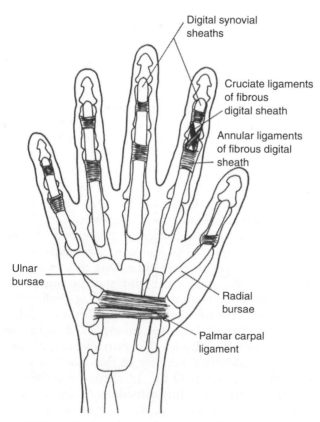

FIG. 11-17. *Bursae and lumbrical sheaths of hand.*

Digital synovial sheaths

Cruciate ligaments of fibrous digital sheath

Annular ligaments of fibrous digital sheath

Ulnar bursae

Radial bursae

Palmar carpal ligament

Feel the interval between it and the distal radius. Notice how much smaller the distal ulna is than the radius. The ulnar styloid process is quite prominent on the dorsoulnar aspect of the distal ulna. Palpate to the end of the ulnar styloid, and notice the gap between it and the carpals, which opens with radial deviation and closes with ulnar deviation. With the wrist in radial deviation, the ulnar collateral ligament can be felt bridging this gap.

From the ulnar styloid process dorsoulnarly, palpate distally to the next large prominence—the dorsal aspect of the triquetrum. From the dorsal aspect of the triquetrum, palpate around palmarly to the prominent pisiform, situated in the palmoulnar corner of the palm. Grasp the pisiform with two fingers and notice how it can be wriggled back and forth with the wrist in flexion, but not with the wrist in extension. This is because of the increased tension on the flexor carpi ulnaris tendon that attaches to the pisiform. Palpate the flexor carpi ulnaris tendon proximal to the pisiform. Feel the pulse from the ulnar artery just radial to this tendon. The ulnar nerve is situated just deep to and between the ulnar artery and the flexor carpi ulnaris tendon. Once again, locate the dorsal aspect of the triquetrum, the large prominence just distal to the prominent ulnar styloid. Slide your palpating finger distally over the dorsal aspect of the triquetrum. Feel the small interval or "joint line" between it and the hamate. With the index finger over the dorsal aspect of the hamate, bring the thumb around palmarly at the same level. With the thumb, palpate the prominent hook of the hamate deep in the hypothenar eminence; it is usually slightly tender to palpation. Between the hook of the hamate and the pisiform, beneath the pisohamate ligament, is the tunnel of Guyon. The ulnar nerve and artery pass through this tunnel.

Now imagine a line running dorsally from the base of the middle finger to Lister's tubercle. At the midpoint of this line, or just radial to it, the base of the third metacarpal can be felt as a prominence. The capitate lies just proximally to this prominence. With the wrist in neutral position, the dorsal concavity of the capitate can be palpated as a depression at the dorsum of the wrist. Just proximal to this depression is the lunate. If a palpating finger is placed over the lunate and capitate while passively flexing and extending the wrist, the distal end of the lunate can be felt to slide into the depression in the capitate on extension and out on flexion.

In the deepest portion of the anatomic snuff box, the dorsoradial aspect of the scaphoid bone can be palpated. It is most easily felt with the wrist in ulnar deviation. Just distal to the scaphoid you can feel the trapezium. You should be able to identify the trapezium–first metacarpal articulation. The trapezoid is easily palpated as a prominence at the base of the second metacarpal.

BIOMECHANICS OF THE WRIST

The wrist is composed of three joints: the distal radioulnar joint, the radiocarpal joint, and the midcarpal joint. With this description it is understood that the radiocarpal joint includes the articulation between the disk and the carpals, since the disk acts as an ulnar extension of the distal radial joint surface. From a functional standpoint, however, it is best to speak of an ulnomeniscotriquetral joint in addition to the three joints listed above. In this way the movements of the ulna and the carpals can be better considered in relation to the disk. (Refer to Appendix A for a description of the movements that occur at these joints and the arthrokinematic motions that accompany these movements.)

The movements among the many bones of the wrist are complex. The clinician must have a basic knowledge of the major interarticular movements to be successful in evaluating painful conditions affecting the wrist and in restoring movement when it is lost.

☐ Flexion–Extension

The primary axis of movement for wrist flexion–extension passes through the capitate. The wrist close-packs in full dorsiflexion, since it must assume a state of maximal intrinsic stability to allow one to transmit pressure from the hand to the forearm. In functional activities, such force transmission usually occurs with the wrist in dorsiflexion—for example, when pushing a heavy object or walking on all fours. As with any synovial joint, the close-packed position at the wrist is achieved by a "screw home" movement—a movement involving a conjunct rotation (see Chapter 3, Arthrology). The carpus, on dorsiflexion, moves in a supinatory rotation. This is easily observed by watching the wrist as it passes from neutral to full extension. The reason for this rotation is that the scaphoid moves in a manner different from that of other proximal carpal bones.[73] As the wrist moves from a position of flexion to neutral, the distal row of carpals remains relatively loose-packed with respect to the proximal row, and the proximal row remains loose-packed with respect to the radius. Disk movement occurs at both the radiocarpal joint and the midcarpal joint. At about the neutral position, or just slightly beyond, as the wrist continues into dorsiflexion, the distal row of carpals becomes close-packed with the scaphoid but not with the other proximal carpals (lunate and triquetrum). Because of this close-packing, the scaphoid moves with the distal row of carpals as the wrist moves into full dorsiflexion. During this final stage of dorsiflexion, then, movement must occur between the scaphoid and lunate as the distal row continues to dorsiflex against the lunate and triquetrum. Looking at it another way, the scaphoid moves more with respect to the radius than do the lunate and triquetrum. This asymmetry of movement results in a supinatory twisting of the carpus that twists capsules and ligaments to close-pack the remaining joints at full dorsiflexion (Fig. 11-18).

As in any joint, the bones forming the wrist are most susceptible to fracture or dislocation when in the close-packed position. Most frequently fractured are the scaphoid and the distal end of the radius. The most common dislocations are a palmar dislocation of the lunate relative to the radius and remaining carpals and a dorsal dislocation of the carpals with respect to the lunate and the radius. The common mechanism of injury for all the above injuries, as would be expected, is a fall on the dorsiflexed hand.

☐ Radial–Ulnar Deviation

The axis of movement for radial–ulnar deviation also passes through the capitate. Ulnar deviation occurs over a much greater range of movement than radial deviation. This is because radial deviation is limited by contact of the scaphoid tubercle against the radial styloid process, whereas the triquetrum easily clears the ulnar styloid process, which is situated more dorsally and is less prominent than the radial styloid process. Both radial and ulnar deviation involve movements at the radiocarpal and midcarpal joints.[121] The associated arthrokinematic movements are not pure, but rather involve rotary movements between the proximal row and the radius, and between the distal row and the proximal row. As described by Kapandji, the proximal row tends to move into pronation, flexion, and ulnar glide during radial deviation with respect to the radius and disk (Fig. 11-19).[53] At the same time, the distal row moves into supination, extension, and ulnar glide with respect to the proximal row. The opposite movements occur during ulnar deviation (Fig. 11-20). This can be easily observed on a cadaver and seems to be due entirely to the shapes of the joint surfaces rather than the capsuloligamentous influences. Radial deviation involves close-packing of primarily the midcarpal joint.

▪ FUNCTION AND ARCHITECTURE OF THE HAND

The hand is a complex machine: it may be used as a means of expression, a tactile organ, and a weapon. The study of the hand is inseparable from that of the wrist and forearm, which function as a single physiologic unit, with the wrist being the key joint. In prona-

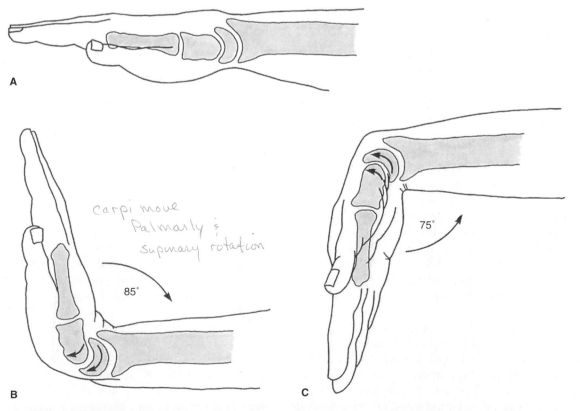

FIG. 11-18. Flexion-extension of the wrist showing neutral position (**A**), dorsiflexion with carpus moving palmarly and in supinatory rotation (**B**), and plamar flexion with carpus moving dorsally (**C**).

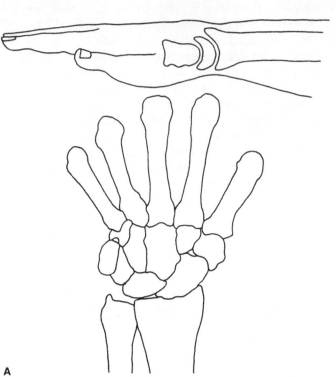

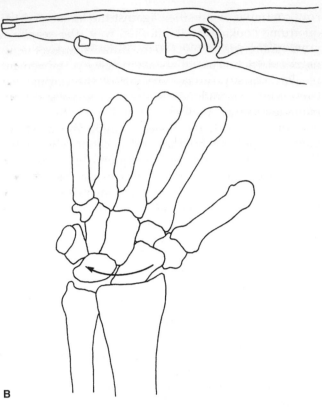

A

B

FIG. 11-19. Radial deviation of the wrist. (**A**) The wrist is shown in neutral position. (**B**) With radial deviation, the proximal row of carpals moves into dorsal and ulnar glide.

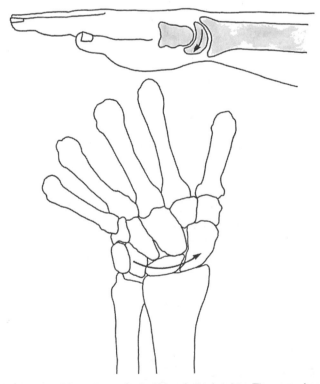

FIG. 11-20. Ulnar deviation of the wrist. The proximal row of carpals moves into palmar and radial glide.

tion–supination the movement of the radius in relation to the ulna is in fact the movement of the hand around its longitudinal axis.[50,109] The entire upper limb is subservient to the hand.

☐ Functional Arches of the Hand

To grasp objects the hand must change its shape. Cupping of the hand occurs with finger flexion, and flattening of the hand occurs with extension. Cupping

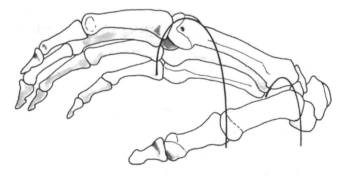

FIG. 11-21. The longitudinal and transverse arches of the hand, side view.

improves the mobility of the hand for functional use, and flattening is used for release of objects. Structurally the hand and wrist conform to three basic physiologic functional arches, which are concave palmarly. Usually three transverse arches (two carpal and one metacarpal arch) and one longitudinal arch are described (Fig. 11-21). To these the oblique arches of opposition between the thumb and each of the fingers may be added.[53,54] These arches allow coordinated synergistic digital flexion and thumb–little finger opposition. Usually the distal phalanges flex toward the scaphoid tubercle or obliquely; only the index ray flexes in a sagittal plane. Full thumb–little finger opposition usually achieves parallel pulp-to-pulp contact of the distal phalanges of these two digits.

The longitudinal arch (or arches, since each ray with its corresponding metacarpal and adjacent carpal forms its own arch) is centered about the MCP articulations, whose thick anterior glenoid capsules and volar plates prevent excessive hyperextension. The long finger ray and the capitate are the focal point.[94]

Two transverse carpal arches may be considered the proximal and distal carpal arch (see Fig. 11-21). The proximal arch is more mobile than the distal carpal row because of its connections to the radius and the distal row. The scaphoid, lunate, and triquetrum, which make up this row, have their own distinct movements.

The transverse arch of the distal row originates basically at the central carpus, specifically at the capitate, which moves with the fixed metacarpals. The trapezium, trapezoid, and hamate also make up this distal row.

The metacarpal arch is formed by the metacarpal heads (see Fig. 11-21). The long axis of the carpal gutter traverses the lunate, the capitate, and the third metacarpal bones. This arch is endowed with a great deal of adaptability because of the mobility of the peripheral metacarpals. It is relatively flat when the hand is at rest but demonstrates considerable curvature with strong clenching of a fist or with thumb–little finger opposition.

Pathological conditions may destroy the arches of the hand and cause severe functional disability by flattening the transverse arches and flattening or reversing the longitudinal arch.

☐ Length–Tension Relationships

Flatt[34] states, "In the normal limb, the placing of the hand is largely controlled by the multi-axial wrist joint." The wrist provides a stable base for the hand, and its position controls the length of the extrinsic muscles to the digits. The muscles that control wrist motion serve two important functions. They provide the fine adjustment of the hand into its functioning position, and once this position is achieved they stabilize the wrist to provide a stable base for the hand.

As the fingers flex, the wrist must be stabilized by the wrist extensor muscles to prevent the long finger flexor muscles from simultaneously flexing the wrist, and allow for optimal length–tension in the long finger muscles. As the wrist position changes, the effective functional length of the finger flexors change, and hypothetically the magnitude of force should also change. As grip becomes stronger, synchronous wrist extension lengthens the extrinsic flexor tendons across the wrist and maintains a favorable length of the musculotendinous unit for a strong contraction.

Hazelton and associates[42] investigated the peak force that could be exerted at the interphalangeal joints of the finger during different wrist positions. They found the greatest interphalangeal flexion force occurred with ulnar deviation of the wrist (neutral flexion–extension). The wrist position in which the least force is generated is volar flexion. For strong finger or thumb extension, the wrist flexor muscles stabilize or flex the wrist so the long finger extensors can function more efficiently.

When the wrist is extended, the pulp (soft cushion on the palmar aspect of the distal phalanges) of the thumb and index finger is passively in contact; when the wrist is in flexion, the pulp of the thumb reaches the level of the PIP joint of the index finger. The position of the wrist has important repercussions on the position of the thumb and finger. Movements of the wrist are usually in reverse of movements of the fingers and reinforce the action of the extrinsic muscles of the fingers.

EXTENSOR MECHANISM

The extensor mechanism, also called the dorsal finger mechanism or extensor apparatus, is a subject of great interest and complexity (Fig. 11-22). The extensor tendons have the advantage of running almost entirely extrasynovially, which facilitates repair, but because they are also thin they tend to become rapidly adherent to the underlying bones and joints. Excursion of the extensor tendons of the hand is considerably less than that of the flexors, and thus it is more difficult to compensate for a loss of length.[109]

The extensor tendons are discrete and obvious at the level of the dorsal forearm, wrist, and hand. At the level of the MCP joint it is proper to speak of the dorsal tendinous structures as the extensor mechanism or apparatus. The extensor mechanism is a broad, flat aponeurotic band composed of extrinsic extensor tendon and the lateral bands formed by the tendons of the interosseous and lumbrical muscles (see Fig.

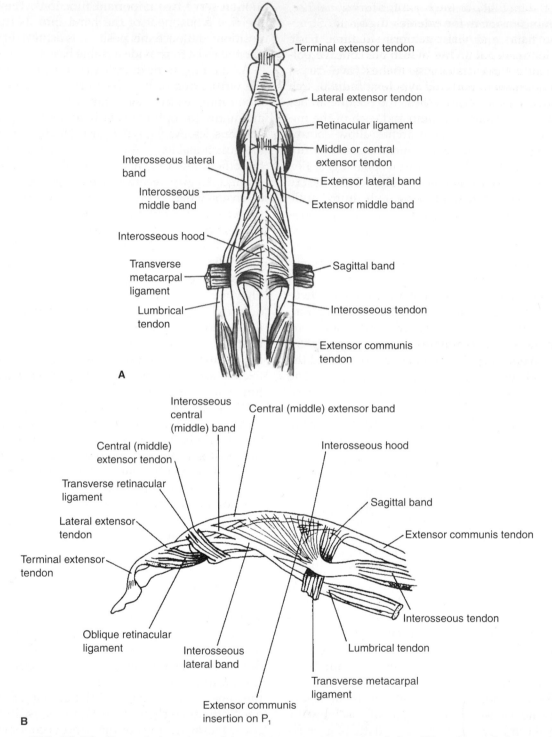

Terminal extensor tendon

Lateral extensor tendon

Retinacular ligament

Middle or central extensor tendon

Interosseous lateral band

Interosseous middle band

Extensor lateral band

Extensor middle band

Interosseous hood

Transverse metacarpal ligament

Sagittal band

Lumbrical tendon

Interosseous tendon

Extensor communis tendon

A

Interosseous central (middle) band

Central (middle) extensor band

Central (middle) extensor tendon

Interosseous hood

Transverse retinacular ligament

Lateral extensor tendon

Sagittal band

Terminal extensor tendon

Extensor communis tendon

Oblique retinacular ligament

Interosseous lateral band

Interosseous tendon

Lumbrical tendon

Transverse metacarpal ligament

Extensor communis insertion on P_1

B

FIG. 11-22. The main insertions of the extensor apparatus: dorsal view (**A**) and lateral view (**B**).

11-22). The extrinsic tendons exert their primary force at the MCP joints. An isolated contraction of the extensor digitorum produces clawing of the fingers (MCP hyperextension with interphalangeal flexion from passive pull of the extrinsic flexor tendons).

The intrinsic tendons are primary extensors of the interphalangeal joints of the fingers. The intrinsic tendons lie volar to the axis of motion of the MCP joints and are actually MCP flexors. They lie dorsal to the axis of motion of the PIP and DIP joints and are, therefore, extensors of those joints.[84] PIP and DIP extension occurs concurrently and can be caused by the lumbrical or interosseous muscles through their pull on the extensor hood (a flattened portion of the communis tendon just distal to the MCP joint; see Fig. 11-22). There must be tension in the extensor digitorum.

The thumb has a similar anatomic situation, with one important exception. The thumb has an extrinsic extensor (extensor pollicis longus) that exerts its force on the distal phalanx. Forceful hyperextension of the interphalangeal joint is prevented and thumb extension is reduced with the loss of this tendon.[84]

PREHENSION

The major musculoskeletal function of the hand lies in its ability to grip objects. Prehension is seen in all forms of the animal world. According to Rabischong,[91] forms of prehension may be divided into four types: organs that pinch (*i.e.*, pincers of the lobster), encircle, push, and adhere. Usually an animal can use only one of these forms of prehension; only in humans has it obtained perfection. This is largely due to opposition of the thumb, which brings it into contact with each finger.[52,53] Since this requires the hand to function as a unit, prehension can never be fully measured in terms of the movement of an individual joint. Many classifications of these movements were used until Napler[83] divided them into two categories: power grip and precision grip.

Power Grip. Power grip is a forceful act resulting in flexion at all fingers: the thumb, when used, acts as a stabilizer to the object held between the fingers and the palm (Fig. 11-23). This typically involves clamping an object with partially flexed fingers against the palm of the hand, with counterpressure from the adducted thumb. The fingers assume a position of sustained (isometric function) flexion that varies with the weight, size, and shape of the object. The ulnar two fingers flex

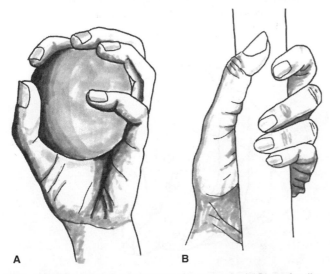

FIG. 11-23. *Modes of power grip: spherical (**A**) and cylindrical (**B**) grip positions.*

across toward the thenar eminence. In the final posture the hypothenar and the thenar eminences are used as buttresses as the fingers flex around the object to be grasped.[19] With all power grips the hand is kept stable and the power movements are produced by either radial or ulnar deviation of the wrist, as in the action of hammering, by supination and pronation of the wrist, and by extension of the elbow. Varieties of power grip include cylindrical grip, spherical grip, hook grip, and lateral prehension.[72]

A crude form of this grip (cylindrical) is used while gripping a heavy object—for example, forcefully driving a nail with a hammer, using the thumb to provide stability and power. A more refined power grip is the ulnar grip, used when a lighter object lying across the palm is gripped mainly by the two ulnar fingers; the thumb is used for control.[19]

Power grip is the result of a sequence of (1) opening the hand, (2) positioning the fingers, (3) approaching the fingers to the object, and (4) maintaining a static phase, which actually constitutes the grip.[64]

Precision Grip. Precision grip shares the first three steps of the power grip sequence but does not have a static phase. The first three steps are followed by dynamic movement rather than a static phase; *precision handling* may be a better term. The muscles primarily function isotonically.[64] The object must be picked up and manipulated by the fingers and thumb (Fig. 11-24). The object is not in contact with the palm of the hand but is manipulated between the opposing thumb and against the fingers—mainly against the next two fingers or the index finger.

The sensory surface of the digits is used for maximum sensory input to influence delicate adjustments. Varieties of precision grip include (1) palmar pinch, in which the pad of the thumb is opposed to the pad of one or more fingers—this is used for picking up and holding an object; (2) lateral pinch or opposition, in which the palmar aspect of the thumb pad presses on the radial surface of the first phalanx of the index finger—for instance, holding a coin or a sheet of paper; and (3) tip prehension, in which the tip of the pad or even the edge of the thumbnail is opposed to the tip of the index finger (or middle finger)—it allows one to hold a thin object or pick up a very fine object such as a pin.[52,53] Tip prehension is the finest and most precise grip and is easily upset by any disease of the hand, since it requires a whole range of movements and fine muscle control.

The functions of the digits can be related to the patterns of the nerve supply. Opening the hand depends on the radial nerve. The muscles of the thumb required for opposition are innervated by both the median and ulnar nerves. Flexion and sensation of the radial digits, important in precision grip, are controlled

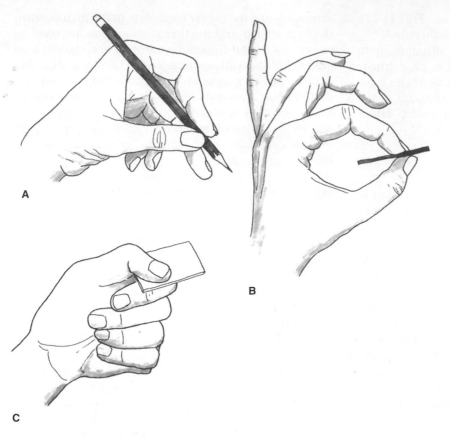

FIG. 11-24. Modes of prehension: palmar (**A**), tip (**B**), and lateral (**C**).

chiefly by the median nerve, whereas flexion and sensation of the ulnar digits depend on the ulnar nerve.

FUNCTIONAL POSITIONS OF THE WRIST AND HAND

The functional position of the wrist and hand is that which is naturally assumed by the hand to grasp an object or the position from which optimal function is most likely to occur.[53,85] From this position it is possible to grasp an object with minimal effort. The functional position is one in which (1) the wrist is slightly extended (20°) and ulnarly deviated (10°); (2) the fingers are slightly flexed at all their joints, with the degree of flexion increasing somewhat from the index to the little finger; and (3) the thumb is in midrange opposition, with the MCP joint moderately flexed and the interphalangeal joints slightly flexed (Fig. 11-25).

This is not necessarily the position in which a hand should be immobilized. The preferred position for immobilization depends on the disability. However, this position is often the position of choice since other positions may result in serious functional sequelae. For example, if a finger is immobilized in extension it may become ankylosed.

The wrist and hand have a fixed and a mobile segment. The fixed segment consists of the distal row of carpal bones (hamate, capitate, trapezoid, and trapezium) and the second and third metacarpals. This is the stabilizing segment of the wrist and hand (see Fig. 11-1), and there is less movement between these bones than between the bones of the mobile segments. The mobile segment is made up of the five phalanges and the first, fourth, and fifth metacarpals. This arrangement allows stability without rigidity.

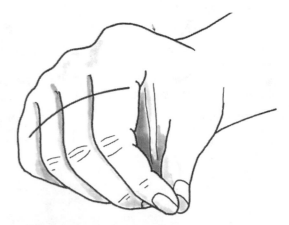

FIG. 11-25. The functional position of a hand.

EXAMINATION

The wrist structures are innervated primarily from C6 through C8. Lesions affecting structures of similar segmental derivation may refer pain to the wrist; conversely, lesions at or about the wrist may refer pain into the relevant segments. Since the wrist is located distally, and pain is more commonly referred in a proximal-to-distal direction than in a retrograde direction, pain from lesions at or about the wrist is fairly well localized. A more proximal origin, however, must always be suspected with symptoms experienced at the wrist or hand. Common lesions that often refer pain to this region include lower cervical pathologic processes (*e.g.,* spondylosis, disk disease), tendinitis or capsulitis at the shoulder, thoracic outlet syndrome, and tennis elbow. If subjective findings do not seem to implicate a local problem, a scan examination of the neck and entire extremity may be warranted before proceeding with an in-depth evaluation of the wrist (see Chapter 18, The Cervical–Upper Limb Scan Examination).

☐ History

A structured line of questioning should be pursued, as set out in Chapter 5, Assessment of Musculoskeletal Disorders.

Common lesions at or about the wrist vary in onset from insidious (carpal tunnel syndrome, De Quervain's tenosynovitis, rheumatoid arthritis) to those in which an incident of trauma is definitely recalled (Colles' fracture, scaphoid fracture, lunate dislocation, or capsuloligamentous sprains). Again, the clinician must be prepared to direct the line of questioning to elicit information concerning more proximal regions, especially if the onset is insidious. If a traumatic event is cited, the examiner should attempt to determine the exact mechanism of injury. Since rheumatoid arthritis is not uncommon at the wrist, questions might be asked about possible bilateral problems and problems with the MCP joints and the joints of the feet.

☐ Physical Examination

I. Observation

   A. *General appearance and body build*

   B. *Functional activities.* Observe the way the person shakes hands, noting the firmness of grasp and temperature and moisture of the hand. Note during dressing activities whether one hand tends to be favored. Observe for fumbling with fasteners or small objects—a problem typical of carpal tunnel syndrome or neurologic dysfunction of more proximal origin. Note whether the patient willingly puts pressure through the wrist, as when standing up from a chair.

   C. *General posture and positioning of body parts.* Note how the arm and hand are carried, and especially whether they swing naturally when walking. The person with a reflex sympathetic dystrophy, not an infrequent complication after healing of a Colles' fracture, invariably walks in with the elbow flexed and the forearm held across the upper abdomen.

   D. *General posture of the hands.* The hands should be observed in their resting position. The dominant hand is usually larger. The posture at rest will often demonstrate common deformities.

   1. An abnormal hand posture may be characteristic and establish the diagnosis, as with a typical ulnar claw, or as with wrist drop and flexion of the wrist and MCP joints, pathognomonic of radial nerve palsy.[109]

   2. Somewhat less typical is the dissociated radial palsy simulating an ulnar claw, in which extension of the thumb and index and middle fingers is preserved.[75]

   3. Dissociated median nerve forearm palsy commonly results from compression of the anterior interosseous nerve supplying the flexor pollicis longus, the radial half of the flexor digitorum profundus, and the pronator quadratus. It also produces a characteristic deformity known as the anterior interosseous nerve syndrome.[57,108] During pinch the distal phalanges of the thumb and index finger cannot flex and stay in extension.

   4. Clawing of the two ulnar digits, caused by paralysis of the interosseous muscle, is variable (ulnar nerve palsy). This deformity is often referred to as "bishop's hand" or "benediction hand" deformity.

   5. Dupuytren's contracture is a contracture of the palmar aponeurosis, which pulls the fingers into flexion.

   6. Mallet finger, which results in flexion of the DIP joint, is caused by an avulsion fracture or a tear of the distal extensor tendon from the distal phalanx.

   7. Swan-neck deformity presents as flexion of the MCP and DIP joints, and is caused by trauma with damage to the volar plate or by rheumatoid arthritis.

   8. Boutonnière deformity—extension of the MCP and DIP joints and flexion of the PIP

joint—is usually the result of a rupture of the central tendinous slip of the extensor hood. It is common following trauma or in rheumatoid arthritis.

II. **Inspection**

A. *Bony structure and alignment.* This is especially important following a fracture of the distal radius. The most common complication following Colles' fracture is healing of the fragments in a malaligned position, resulting in a "dinner fork" deformity (Figs. 11-26 and 11-27). In such a deformity the distal end of the radius is displaced and angulated dorsally, foreshortened, and often rotated into supination. Such a deformity must be considered when determining treatment goals, since normal range of motion can never be obtained in such cases.

   1. Note the structural alignment of the head, neck, shoulder girdle, arm, and forearm.
   2. Note carefully the structural alignment and relationships of the distal end of the radius and ulna, the carpals, and the metacarpals (see section on the surface anatomy).
   3. Note any structural deformities of the hands and fingers, such as boutonnière or swan-neck deformities, ulnar drift, claw hand, or ape hand.

B. *Soft tissue*
   1. Muscle contours
      a. Note especially any atrophy of the

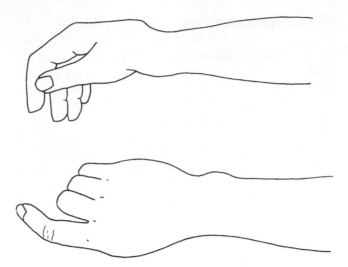

FIG. 11-27. Lateral and dorsal views of the characteristic "dinner fork" deformity resulting from a Colles' fracture.

thenar muscles (this may accompany carpal tunnel syndrome), the hypothenar muscles (suggestive of an ulnar nerve lesion), and intrinsics.
      b. Note any generalized atrophy of the arm or forearm (this invariably occurs with immobilization but may be masked by edema).
      c. Note any localized atrophy about the shoulder girdle and the rest of the limb, which may suggest neuromuscular involvement of related segments.
   2. Joint regions
      a. Inspect for effusion of any upper-extremity joints.
      b. Notice other periarticular swellings: Heberden's nodes about the DIP joints are characteristic of osteoarthrosis of those joints.
      c. Small pea-sized ganglia are commonly found on the dorsal or palmar aspect of the wrist and are usually of little significance.
      d. Large nodules about the wrist, extensor surface of the forearm, and elbow are characteristic of rheumatoid arthritis.
   3. General soft-tissue inspection
      a. Generalized edema of the distal extremity is invariably present following immobilization in all but younger patients.
      b. Localized edema over the dorsum of the hand suggests an infection involving any part of the hand.
      c. If swelling or edema is present, volu-

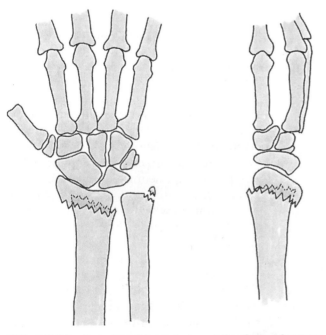

FIG. 11-26. Dorsal and lateral views of a Colles' fracture, showing extension fracture of the lower end of the radius.

metric measurements and girth measurements should be taken to document a baseline.

C. *Skin*
   1. Color
      a. Redness with inflammation
      b. Often cyanotic in reflex sympathetic dystrophy
      c. Colorless with severe neurologic deficit
   2. Texture (see under palpation)
   3. Moisture (see under palpation)
   4. Scars, blemishes
D. *Nails*
   1. Splitting, ridging (typical in reflex sympathetic dystrophy)
   2. Clubbing (may suggest a cardiopulmonary disorder)
   3. Hollowing

III. **Selective Tissue Tension Tests.** Both tendon excursion (active range of motion) and joint motion (passive range of motion) are evaluated by computing total active motion (TAM) and total passive motion (TPM), as recommended by the Clinical Assessment Committee of the American Society for Surgery of the Hand. This method is used to measure and record finger and thumb motions.[3] If joint stiffness is present, closely examine the end feel of each joint before measuring passive range of motion with a goniometer.

A. *Active movements.* Record range of motion, pain, and crepitus.
   1. Wrist flexion–extension and radioulnar deviation and forearm pronation and supination. Active radial and ulnar deviation performed with the thumb held in a fist under the other fingers may be helpful in distinguishing De Quervain's tenovaginitis from osteoarthrosis of the trapezium–first metacarpal joint (both of which are common lesions).
   2. Include shoulder and elbow movements, especially after immobilization and when reflex sympathetic dystrophy is suspected.

B. *Passive movements.* Record range of motion, pain, crepitus, and end feel.
   1. Same movements as above
   2. Also ask the patient to place the hand flat on a table with the wrist dorsiflexed and the elbow extended and to lean forward so as to transmit body weight through the forearm and wrist.

C. *Resisted movements.* Record as strong or weak, painful or painless.
   1. Resist all wrist, forearm, finger, and thumb movements.

2. If referred pain from more proximal regions is suspected, include resisted elbow and shoulder movements.

D. *Joint-play movements.* Joint-play movements of the wrist and hand complex are the same as the mobilization techniques (see Treatment Techniques below) but are performed in the resting position. Record mobility and irritability (pain or muscle guarding).
   1. Specific joint-play (accessory) motions to be tested include:
      a. Distal radioulnar joint: dorsal and ventral glide and distraction (see Figs. 11-30 and 11-32)
      b. Radiocarpal joint: dorsal and palmar glide, ulnar glide, and radial glide (see Figs. 11-33 and 11-34)
      c. Midcarpal joint: traction, dorsal and volar glide
      d. MCP joint: distraction, dorsal and palmar glide, radioulnar glide (or tilt), and rotation (see Figs. 11-41 to 11-44)
      e. Interphalangeal joint: distraction, dorsal–volar glide, side tilt, and rotation
   2. Special intercarpal movements should be performed if an intercarpal ligament sprain is suspected. Kaltenborn[51] has developed a systematic approach to examination of joint play of the individual carpal bones (see Fig. 11-1).
      a. Stabilize the capitate and move the trapezium and trapezoid as a unit.
      b. Stabilize the capitate and move the scaphoid.
      c. Stabilize the capitate and move the lunate.
      d. Stabilize the capitate and move the hamate.
      e. Stabilize the scaphoid and move the trapezium and trapezoid as a unit.
      f. Stabilize the radius and move the scaphoid (see Fig. 11-36).
      g. Stabilize the radius and move the lunate.
      h. Stabilize the ulna with the articular disk and move the triquetrum.
      i. Stabilize the triquetrum and move the hamate.
      j. Stabilize the triquetrum and move the pisiform.

IV. **Neuromuscular Tests** (see Chapter 5, Assessment of Musculoskeletal Disorders, for relevant tests)
   A. Strength, sensation, reflex, and coordination testing should be done at this point if neuromuscular involvement is suggested by find-

ings thus far in the examination. Gross grip strength can be measured by a dynamometer. Force generated by the normal man is about 46 kg, that by the normal woman about 23 kg.[103,123] If the subject cannot grip the dynamometer, a sphygmomanometer may be used—the normal male grip usually exceeds 300 mm Hg, and the female grip is about 300 mm Hg.[111] A pinch-meter is used to test pinch strength.

The status of the motor system can be further described in terms of muscle tone. Coordination can be tested by performing activities such as tracing a diagram or buttoning a button. Standardized tests such as the Jebson Hand Function Test, the Minnesota Rate of Manipulation Test, the Purdue Pegboard Test, the Valpar Work Sample Series, and the O'Conner Dexterity Test are available for more detailed evaluation of manual dexterity and coordination.[6,31,47]

B. A useful test for median nerve pressure at the carpal tunnel is to ask the patient to strongly flex the wrist while maintaining a strong three-jaw-chuck grasp. This position should be held for 1 minute. The onset of paresthesias into the first three or four fingers during this test suggests carpal tunnel syndrome.

C. If carpal tunnel syndrome is suspected, percuss the median nerve where it passes through the carpal tunnel. Reproduction of paresthesias suggests nerve involvement at this level (Tinel's sign).

D. Involvement of the cervical nerve roots and peripheral nerves may affect both muscle strength and sensation of the upper extremity. The level of the cervical nerve root or peripheral nerves may be determined by identifying "key muscles" or joint actions and sensory areas, which are representative (see Chapter 5, Assessment of Musculoskeletal Disorders). Numerous tests have been described to evaluate the various sensory modalities of the hands. Two-point discrimination, vibratory threshold, temperature, and sudomotor activity may assist in lesion identification.[23,32,123]

V. Palpation
  A. *Skin*
    1. Moisture
    2. Texture
    3. Temperature
    4. Mobility
    5. Tenderness. Dysesthesias, such as burning on light palpation, suggest nerve root or peripheral nerve pathology (*e.g.*, pressure).
    6. A common condition following immobi-

lization (especially after Colles' fracture) is a reflex sympathetic dystrophy. The exact cause is unknown. Many believe it to be related to the development of edema during immobilization. Some believe it results from trauma to a nerve from the original injury (*e.g.*, contusion of the median nerve from the displaced distal fragment in Colles' fracture). Others believe psychological factors also play an important role. In early phases of this disorder the skin may be dry, rough, and warm from decreased sympathetic activity. Later, increased sympathetic activity, with hyperhidrosis and vasoconstriction, seems to predominate. Skin palpation reveals several findings in this disorder:
    a. Hyperhidrosis
    b. Smooth, glossy skin
    c. Decreased temperature (cold, clammy hands)
    d. Hypersensitivity to normally nonnoxious sensory stimuli; even light touch may be painful.
    e. Loss of mobility of the skin in relation to subcutaneous tissues from interstitial fibrosis accompanying tissue edema

  B. *Soft tissues*
    1. Tenderness. Palpate tendons and ligaments, especially for local tenderness.
    2. Mobility, consistency. Soft tissues feel indurated and adherent in reflex sympathetic dystrophy from interstitial fibrosis, as well as atrophied, fibrotic muscle.
    3. Edema and swelling (common with reflex sympathetic dystrophy)
    4. Pulse, radial and ulnar arteries. This may be performed in conjunction with various maneuvers of the arm (hyperabduction), shoulder girdle (depression, elevation, and retraction), and neck if thoracic outlet syndrome is suspected. The Allen test is usually performed to determine the patency of the radial, ulnar, and digital arteries: the patient pumps the blood out of the hand and then maintains a fist while the examiner occludes both arteries at the wrist; when the hand is opened it will appear white, and arterial filling on the respective side can be observed as pressure is released from one artery at a time.[44]

  C. *Bones*
    1. Tenderness. The radial styloid process is often the site of referred tenderness from more proximal lesions, usually within the

C5 or C6 segment. It is usually also tender in De Quervain's tenosynovitis.

2. Relationships. Palpate for structural alignment and positioning of the bony components of the wrist.

VI. **Special Tests**

A. A test for intrinsic tightness has been described by Bunnell.[12] This test is performed by holding the patient's MCP joint in extension (stretching the intrinsics) and then passively flexing the PIP joint. The intrinsics are then relaxed by flexing the MCP joint. If the PIP joint can be passively flexed more with the MCP joint in flexion than when it is in extension, there is tightness of the intrinsics. Capsular or collateral ligament tightness of the PIP joint will limit proximal phalangeal motion, regardless of the position of the MCP joint. Loss of flexion at the DIP joint can also be due to a joint contracture or to a contracture of the oblique retinacular ligament.[44,63]

B. Phalen's modified test (three-jaw-chuck test) (see Fig. 17-25). This test aids in the diagnosis of carpal tunnel syndrome. The patient performs a "three-jaw-chuck" pinch with both hands and maintains both wrists in extreme flexion by pressing the dorsum of the hands against one another. This position is held for 30 to 60 seconds. The production of pain or paresthesias is noted.

C. Tinel's sign. Whenever there are neural signs, cervical disk (C6) lesions, brachial plexus, and thoracic outlet must be ruled out. Tap on the volar carpal ligament (carpal tunnels). A positive test causes tingling that spreads into the thumb, index finger, and the lateral half of the ring finger (median nerve distribution). The tingling or paresthesia must be felt distal to the point of pressure for a positive test.

D. Allen test (circulatory problems). This test determines the efficacy of blood flow in the radial and ulnar arteries. The patient makes a fist, then releases it several times. Next the patient makes a fist and holds it so that the venous blood is forced from the palm. The examiner locates the radial artery with his or her thumb and the ulnar artery with the index and middle fingers. Pressure is exerted on these arteries to occlude them, and the patient opens the hand. The examiner releases the pressure on one of the arteries and watches for immediate flushing. If this does not occur, or the response is slow, there is interference with the normal blood supply to the hand. The procedure is repeated for the other artery.

E. Functional assessment of the patient with a hand disability is done most effectively by using a variety of testing methods.[2,3,96]

■ COMMON LESIONS

☐ Carpal Tunnel Syndrome

Carpal tunnel syndrome is very common. It is more common in women than men, and it rarely affects young people. The cause varies. In certain instances it is due to some known disorder involving increased pressure within the carpal tunnel. Such situations include a displaced fracture of the distal radius, a lunar or perilunar dislocation, and swelling of the common flexor tendon sheath. In most cases, the cause is not readily determined. Some believe it to be a vascular deficiency of the median nerve at the carpal tunnel, while others believe direct pressure to the nerve is the cause. Symptoms and signs accompanying this disorder are more suggestive of a pressure phenomenon.[20]

I. **History**

A. *Onset of symptoms*—usually insidious, unless they follow trauma resulting in fracture, dislocation, or swelling of the wrist

B. *Nature of symptoms*—The complaint is most often that of paresthesias (pins and needles) felt into the first three or four fingers. The patient is most troubled by being awakened at night, usually in the early morning, from paresthesias in the hand. The onset of paresthesias often occurs with activities involving prolonged use of the finger flexors, such as writing and sewing. Often the patient complains of clumsiness on activities requiring fine finger movements. At times a burning sensation is felt in the median nerve distribution of the hand as well. Subjective complaints of actual weakness are rare. The problem can be unilateral or bilateral.

C6 or C7 nerve root involvement and thoracic outlet syndrome often present as paresthesias in a similar distribution as that of carpal tunnel syndrome. In the case of nerve root involvement, however, the patient is rarely awakened by paresthesias, and use of the hand does not bring on symptoms. Differentiating carpal tunnel from thoracic outlet syndrome, based on subjective findings, is more difficult, since these patients are usually awakened at night with paresthesias, and paresthesias may occur with certain activities involving use of the upper extremity. In thoracic outlet syndrome, paresthesias are more likely to involve the entire hand—although often the patient is not sure in just how many fingers paresthesias are felt—or perhaps just the more ulnar side of the hand from lower cord involvement only. The objective examination will help differentiate the two conditions in any case.

II. **Physical Examination**

A. *Observation.* There may be some clumsiness with activities requiring fine finger movements, such as handling buttons or other fasteners.

B. *Inspection.* Some thenar atrophy may be noticed, but usually only in chronic cases.

C. *Selective tissue tension tests.* Results are noncontributory, except perhaps some subtle weakness on resisted thumb movements.

D. *Neuromuscular tests.* Only in severe, chronic cases can true weakness of the first two lumbricals of the thumb be noticed. Substitution, overlapping innervation, or subtle involvement make motor testing unreliable.

   1. Careful sensory testing may reveal some deficit in the tips or dorsal ends of the first three or four fingers (usually the second or third). However, mild or early cases sufficient to cause significant symptoms may not present with a detectable sensory deficit.

   2. The special tests mentioned under "Neuromuscular Tests" will usually reproduce the paresthesias.

   3. Tinel's sign (reproduction of paresthesias by tapping the median nerve at the wrist) may be positive.

   4. Nerve conduction studies of the median nerve are the most reliable but are often unnecessary for diagnosis.

E. *Palpation*—usually noncontributory

III. **Management**

These patients often do remarkably well simply by wearing a resting-splint for the wrist at night. The reason why this helps is not entirely clear, except that it maintains the wrist in a neutral position, the position of least pressure within the carpal tunnel. (For this reason it seems more likely that this disorder is a pressure phenomenon rather than a release phenomenon.)

The patient can be shown how to don the splint without impairing venous return from fastening straps or wraps too tightly. The splint may or may not include the fingers. It is usually unnecessary to wear the splint during the day. However, if night use does not provide relief of symptoms, a several-day trial of continuous use of the splint followed by gradual weaning should be instituted. Whether the splint is worn continuously or at night only, after 1 or 2 weeks of relief from symptoms, use of the splint can gradually be decreased and eventually discontinued.

Only in persistent cases is surgery required to divide the flexor retinaculum and relieve the pressure.

☐ **Ligamentous Sprains**

Ligamentous sprains are also common and often lead to chronic wrist pain unless treated appropriately. Most commonly involved are the lunate-capitate ligament, dorsally, and the radiocarpal ligament, palmarly. However, any of the ligaments about the wrist may conceivably be sprained.

I. **History**

A. *Onset of pain.* Ligamentous lesions are invariably of traumatic, not degenerative, onset. The patient usually recalls the traumatic event. A fall on the outstretched hand may rupture one or more of several ligaments about the wrist, but often one of the ligaments attached to the lunate is sprained. This is because of the tendency toward a lunar or perilunar dislocation with such an injury. In fact, at this point in the examination, such a dislocation cannot be ruled out. Because a fall on the outstretched hand tends to force the wrist into hyperextension, the palmar radiolunate and palmar lunocapitate ligaments tend to be sprained. However, if the lunate partially dislocates palmarly with spontaneous reduction, the dorsal radiolunate ligaments may also be sprained (Fig. 11-28).

   Occasionally the fall is such that the person strikes the dorsum of the hand, forcing the wrist into extreme palmar flexion. This usually results in a sprain of one of the ligaments attached dorsally to the capitate. The ulnar collateral ligament is often sprained with a Colles' fracture.

B. *Site of pain.* The pain is usually well localized to a small area that corresponds well to the site of the lesion.

C. *Nature of pain.* The pain is felt with use of the wrist. Often a particular activity is cited as being most aggravating; the activity stresses the involved ligament. In the case of a dorsal radiocarpal sprain, often the activity that tends to reproduce the pain puts pressure down through the hand (as when doing pushups).

II. **Physical Examination**

A. *Observation*—usually noncontributory

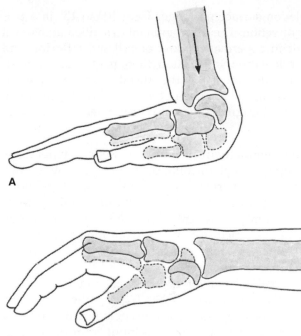

A

B

FIG. 11-28. Lunate dislocation. **(A)** The injury occurs when the radius forces the lunate in a palmar direction, resulting in dislocation **(B)**.

B. *Inspection*—usually noncontributory. Localized swelling following an injury to the wrist almost never accompanies a ligamentous injury only. Fracture or dislocation should be suspected.

C. *Selective tissue tension tests*
  1. Active movements. Some pain may be noted on the extreme of a movement that stresses the ligament.
  2. Passive movements
     a. A ligamentous lesion may exist that is not stressed at the extreme of any passive anatomic movement.
     b. Often the only maneuver that reproduces the pain, other than some specific joint-play movement test, is having the patient lean forward, transmitting the body weight through the arm, forearm, extended wrist, and hand. This is most likely to reproduce pain from a lesion of the palmar radiolunate or dorsal lunocapitate ligaments.
     c. The dorsal radiocarpal ligament may be stressed on full passive pronation (applying the force through the hand and wrist to the forearm), and the palmar radiocarpal ligament may be stressed on full passive supination.
  3. Resisted movements. Strong and painless.
  Note: Resist pronation and supination at

the distal forearm, not at the hand, to avoid stressing the radiocarpal ligaments.
  4. Joint-play movements
     a. The specific intra-articular movement that stresses the involved ligament is likely to reproduce the pain, but again joint-play movement in itself may not be sufficient to reproduce the pain.
     b. The most important movements to perform are dorsal–palmar glide of the capitate on the lunate and the lunate on the radius.
     c. Some hypermobility of the lunate may be detected following partial dislocation and spontaneous reduction of the lunate with a fall on the dorsiflexed hand.
     d. Some hypermobility of the capitate may be detected following a fall on the palmarly flexed hand in which a lunocapitate or capitate–third metacarpal ligament may be ruptured.

D. *Neuromuscular tests*—noncontributory
E. *Palpation.* Localized tenderness usually corresponds well with the site of the lesion.

III. **Management**
  A. Temporary restriction of activities that tend to stress the involved ligament
  B. Friction massage to the site of the lesion to increase mobility of the collagen fibers without longitudinally stressing the ligament. As an adjunct, ultrasound may be used to assist in the resolution of chronic inflammatory exudates.

☐ Colles' Fracture

In most outpatient settings, patients who have sustained a Colles' fracture make up the largest proportion of those with wrist disorders. The term *Colles' fracture* is usually used to refer to fractures of the distal end of the radius, with or without an associated fracture at the distal ulna. This is one of the most common of all fractures. It affects primarily older people. Women are afflicted more often than men because of the prevalence of osteoporosis, especially in older women. These patients are often referred to physical therapists after the period of immobilization because of complications resulting in residual loss of function. The two most common complications following these injuries are malunion (*not* nonunion) of bony fragments, and development of a reflex sympathetic dystrophy. Pain and loss of movement are the major factors limiting function following immobilization of a Colles' fracture.

MECHANISM AND NATURE OF INJURY

Colles' fracture usually results from a fall on the outstretched hand in an older person. The patient lands with the wrist in dorsiflexion and the forearm in pronation. The lunate acts as a wedge to shear the distal 2 cm or so of the radius off in a dorsal direction. The momentum of the body weight causes the distal fragment to displace radially and rotate in a supinatory direction with respect to the proximal bone end (see Fig. 11-26). Because this metaphyseal area of bone is typically osteoporotic, the compression force often results in comminution and impaction of the distal fragment. The major fracture line runs transversely across the distal radius, usually about 2 cm proximal to the radiocarpal joint. The momentum that results in radial displacement may also cause a sprain of the ulnar collateral ligament and an avulsion fracture of the ulnar styloid process.[24]

The characteristic "dinner fork" deformity results from the wrist and hand being displaced dorsally with respect to the forearm (see Fig. 11-27). Often included in the deformity is radial displacement of the wrist and hand.

MANAGEMENT BY THE PHYSICIAN

Closed manipulative reduction is usually performed in an effort to bring the fragments back into anatomic alignment. Reduction is usually not so much of a problem as is maintenance of reduction. In unstable, comminuted fractures the distal fragment tends to slip back into its postinjury position of dorsal, radial, and supinatory displacement. In an attempt to maintain anatomic reduction, the wrist is usually splinted in a position of flexion and ulnar deviation, with pronation. Sometimes external fixation with a Roger Anderson device may be used. The elbow is usually left free. Since the elbow is left free, splinting in a position of excessive pronation may result in a force tending to pull the distal fragment into radial displacement and supination from tension on the brachioradialis with elbow extension. This would defeat the original purpose of positioning the part in pronation and ulnar deviation.

The plaster splint is left on for at least 4 weeks. Nonunion is rare since this fracture occurs in highly vascularized, metaphyseal bone.

COMPLICATIONS

Malunion. A Colles' fracture rarely heals without some residual malalignment. The radius invariably ends up foreshortened such that the radial styloid process no longer extends beyond the ulnar styloid process. The distal end of the radius also tends to be angulated and displaced dorsally; the distal radial articulation surface no longer faces 10° to 15° in a palmar direction. The malalignment described above will result in a permanent loss of full wrist flexion and ulnar deviation. In addition, there may be some residual malalignment of the distal fragment toward supination, resulting in a permanent loss of pronation. The distal fragment may also heal when displaced radially, but this would have little effect on motion.

Reflex Sympathetic Dystrophy. Reflex sympathetic dystrophy is not uncommon following Colles' fracture; in our experience it develops more often following Colles' fracture than after any other injury. Most patients sent to physical therapy after immobilization of a Colles' fracture have this condition to some degree; otherwise they probably would not require ongoing physical therapy.[13,25,82,100,101,120]

The pathophysiology is not well understood. It is generally agreed, however, that sympathetic dysfunction occurs as part of a vicious circle initiated reflexly by some alteration in afferent input from the periphery. Several proposals have been offered as to the precipitating factor, including direct trauma to a peripheral nerve, edema from prolonged immobilization, pain, and psychological predisposition. The characteristic features of the disorder are hyperalgesia, edema, and capsular tightness of the joints of the hand, wrist, and often the shoulder—it is often referred to as shoulder-hand syndrome, although the shoulder is not always involved. The elbow occasionally stiffens as well. In other than the early phases of this condition, there is usually increased sympathetic activity involving the distal part of the extremity, with vasoconstriction and hyperhidrosis. The vasoconstriction causes a cyanotic appearance and atrophy of the musculoskeletal tissues; the skin becomes glossy and thin, the nails brittle, and the bones osteoporotic. (Early osteopenia, seen on roentgenography, is often marked. This early bone atrophy is believed to be a result of the hyperemia often present in the earlier stages; excessive blood flow to bone causes increased resorption.)

Carpal Tunnel Syndrome. The median nerve may be traumatized at the time of injury. Prolonged pressure to the nerve may occur from malalignment of bony fragments, persistent edema involving the carpal tunnel, or both. (See the section on carpal tunnel syndrome above for a discussion of symptoms and signs.)

Late Rupture of the Extensor Pollicis Longus Tendon. The extensor pollicis longus tendon normally takes quite a sharp turn around Lister's tubercle at the dorsum of the distal radius on its way to inserting at the thumb. Malalignment of bony parts following Colles' fracture may cause excessive friction to this tendon, which may result in fraying of the tendon and eventual rupture. Pain on active and passive thumb flexion or opposition, and pain on resisted thumb extension suggest such a problem before actual rupture. Painless weakness of thumb extension, at some time after the injury, is characteristic of rupture of the tendon.

I. **History**
  A. Determine the date of the initial injury, subsequent treatment, the length of time the part was immobilized, and the dates of splint removal. Ask whether exercise and elevation activities were performed while the part was immobilized. A patient whose wrist has been immobilized for 8 weeks with no instruction in shoulder exercises and elevation activities and who has not used the part since removal of the splint 2 weeks ago will present with more dysfunction and disability than the patient who has just come out of the splint after having had the wrist immobilized for 6 weeks, during which time range of motion for the shoulder was performed, along with intermittent periods of elevation and active finger movements.
  B. Ask the standard questions relating to the patient's pain (see Chapter 5, Assessment of Musculoskeletal Disorders). Any acute inflammatory process, initiated at the time of injury, should have resolved during immobilization. Considering this, any residual pain would be expected to be due primarily to stiffness and would be associated with use of the part. Complaints of pain at rest, pain that awakens the patient at night, and inability to use the part because of pain suggest reflex sympathetic dystrophy in this case. Note any complaints of shoulder pain because of the possibility of stiffening of the shoulder from immobilization and perhaps shoulder-hand syndrome. Pain on use of the thumb may suggest involvement of the extensor pollicis longus tendon. Complaints of burning pain or paresthesias into the median nerve distribution of the hand should lead one to suspect carpal tunnel syndrome.
  C. Determine and document the patient's present functional status.
    1. What specific daily activities cannot be performed with the involved hand that could be performed before the injury?
    2. What activities can be performed but with difficulty or pain?
    3. Consider, especially, eating, grooming, dressing, household chores, occupational activities, and recreational activities.

II. **Physical Examination**
  A. *Observation.* Typically these patients walk into the room holding the hand and forearm out in front of them, across the chest or abdomen.
    1. Is the arm used when rising from a chair?
    2. Does the arm hang normally to the side and swing freely and normally when walking?
    3. Does the patient use the hand and arm during dressing activities, or does he or she guard it carefully?
    4. Observe the face for wincing during movement of the part.
  B. *Inspection*
    1. Skin and nails. Note especially trophic changes suggestive of a reflex sympathetic dystrophy: brittle, split nails; smooth, glossy skin; cyanotic appearance to skin in the distal part of the extremity.
    2. Subcutaneous soft tissue. Atrophy of the forearm muscles is invariably found but may be masked by edema, which is usually noticed most in the hand and forearm.
    3. Bony structure and alignment. Some degree of malalignment is likely to be present. In the classic "dinner fork" deformity, the wrist and hand are offset dorsally with respect to the forearm. There is usually some displacement radially also. The radial styloid process may no longer extend further distally than the ulnar styloid process, as it should, because of impaction of the distal fragment.
  C. *Selective tissue tension tests*
    1. Active and passive range of motion
      a. The interphalangeal and MCP joints of the hand are usually restricted in a capsular pattern—the MCP joints are especially restricted in flexion, the interphalangeal joints especially restricted in extension.
      b. Wrist and forearm movements are restricted in all planes. Flexion, ulnar deviation, and pronation are likely to be restricted from bony malalignment; check for bony end feel. Extension, radial deviation, and supination are likely to be limited because the hand is usually immobilized in a position opposite each of these movements (see above).
      c. All movements are likely to be painful at the extremes, especially in the presence of a reflex sympathetic dystrophy.
      d. Check shoulder range of motion for possible capsular tightening.
    2. Resisted movements
      a. Pain on resisted thumb extension may suggest involvement of the extensor

pollicis longus tendon secondary to bony malalignment.

b. Otherwise, resisted movements should be strong and painless.

3. Joint-play movements. Considerable restriction of all joint-play movements of the wrist and hand is likely to be found.

D. *Neuromuscular tests.* Here concern is primarily with the function of the median nerve. The special tests mentioned under carpal tunnel syndrome should be performed.

E. *Palpation*

1. Skin

a. The skin is likely to feel cool, moist, smooth, and tight, especially in the presence of a reflex sympathetic dystrophy.

b. Tenderness to light palpation of the skin is characteristic of a reflex sympathetic dystrophy.

2. Subcutaneous soft tissue. Pitting-type edema is very often present distally. The tissues may feel "tight" and bound down in the hand and forearm because of the fibrosis accompanying prolonged edema.

3. Bones. Careful bony palpation will reveal the extent of residual malalignment.

F. *Other.* A radiologist's report should be ordered so that the therapist can determine the degree of bony malalignment. This is helpful in setting treatment goals. Also, marked osteoporosis usually accompanies a reflex sympathetic dystrophy. As much as 40% of bone resorption may occur before osteopenia shows up on roentgenograms. If roentgenograms suggest considerable osteoporosis, techniques to regain range of motion must not be performed using forces applied over a long lever arm.

MANAGEMENT

Functional use of the part is lost or restricted primarily due to pain and loss of motion. As in any joint in which motion is lost from capsular tightening, much of the pain may be due to joint stiffness; the joint capsule is stretched excessively during use of the part. However, these patients often complain of pain out of proportion to the extent of the dysfunction. Such an abnormal pain state is characteristic of a reflex sympathetic dystrophy. In such situations the patient may complain of severe pain to light touch or another normally nonnoxious stimulation. This complaint may act as a considerable barrier to efforts to regain joint motion.

Pain Management. If such an abnormal pain state is apparent, special care must be taken not to reinforce the patient's pain behavior and not to allow such rein-

forcement by family members, so as to avoid development of an operant pain problem. On the other hand, the patient's very real pain problem cannot be ignored. The patient must be advised that although he or she is not imagining the pain, it does not serve a useful function by signaling potential harm to tissues. Unless the problem is carefully explained to the patient, he or she cannot be expected to follow home instructions that may include exercises and other activities that may be painful. The patient will also doubt the therapist's professional judgment if certain techniques that cause considerable discomfort are used, unless the rationale of their use is carefully explained.

The therapist must also try to make the treatment sessions as painless as possible. This is one disorder in which some modality or procedure might be used solely for its effect to reduce pain, so as to allow the therapist to perform other treatment procedures, such as joint mobilization. A whirlpool bath during or just before mobilization procedures may act as a counterirritant, as well as increasing blood flow to the part. The part may be kept in the water for application of ultrasound in preparation for mobilization procedures.

Restoration of Joint Motion. These patients require an intensive mobilization program. All the joints of the extremity, with the possible exception of the elbow, are likely to be restricted in the case of a reflex sympathetic dystrophy. It is usually desirable to have the patient come in for treatment at least three times a week for passive mobilization. Treatment should include ultrasound to help increase the extensibility of capsular tissue, followed by specific joint mobilization techniques. Such techniques are especially indicated because they are performed with forces applied over very short lever arms.

A home program of active and active-assisted range of motion exercises should be instituted. Take care to show the patient exercises that do not involve forces applied over long lever arms, especially when working on finger flexion and extension. These patients usually have some degree of tissue edema that contributes to the restriction in range of motion. Frequent elevation of the part with activation of the muscle pump should be included in the home program. Encourage use of the part for dressing, grooming, and light activities.

Simple strengthening exercises for finger, wrist, and shoulder muscles should also be instituted. Strengthening the rotator cuff is especially important because of the important role these muscles play biomechanically. Exercises should be kept simple, and the number of exercises should be minimized. The patient who becomes confused or exhausted with a home program is likely to abandon the program completely. This is an important consideration: these patients need to perform range of motion exercises for most of the upper extremity joints, in addition to strengthening exercises and elevation activities. Whenever possible, exercises should be designed that incorporate strengthening, range of motion, and elevation so as to keep the program simple and concise.

If a marked or persistent reflex sympathetic dystrophy presents a major obstruction to rehabilitation, the patient may undergo a series of sympathetic blocks. In such a program the patient may be admitted to the hospital or to ambulatory surgery. The stellate ganglion is injected with an anesthetic in an attempt to reduce sympathetic activity to the part and to break up the cycle. Typically, a series of five injections is given on a daily basis. Such a program in no way precludes continuation of the normal physical therapy program. In fact, the ideal situation is for the patient to be seen in physical therapy each day after the block for mobilization procedures. Obviously, close communication and cooperation among orthopedics, anesthesiology, and physical therapy personnel is important here.

The active phase of a reflex sympathetic dystrophy following a Colles' fracture tends to resolve over several months. However, the patient may be left with some residual disability. Some residual loss of motion is not unlikely because of the often extensive fibrosis of joint capsules as well as extra-articular structures. Goals, in these cases, should be set toward restoring *functional* motion, not necessarily *physiologic* motion. In older persons, the two are less likely to coincide. Of more significance, however, is the tendency for a chronic pain state to develop. Operant management at this point may be indicated over, or in addition to, continued physical treatment. The possibility of psychological consultation should be discussed with the physician.

Too often these patients continue to come in for treatment over a prolonged period without demonstrable improvement in function. While vigorous treatment is indicated in the early phase after immobilization, once improvement plateaus for, say, a 2- or 3-week period, treatment should gradually be discontinued in favor of a progressive home program. However, improvement is rarely linear in such cases, and some fluctuation between spurts of improvement and periods of plateauing can be expected. Until satisfactory, functional use of the part is regained, intermittent follow-up visits should be arranged for reassessment and progression of the home program. As usual, improvement should be based primarily on objective findings and subjective reports of increased function, not on subjective reports of decreased pain.

De Quervain's Tenovaginitis

De Quervain's tenovaginitis is relatively common. It is generally believed to be an inflammation and swelling of the synovial lining of the common sheath of the abductor pollicis longus and the extensor pollicis brevis tendons where they pass along the distal-radial aspect of the radius.

I. **History.** Pain is felt over the distal-radial aspect of the radius, perhaps radiating distally into the thumb or even proximally up the forearm. The onset is usually insidious. The patient notes pain primarily with activities involving thumb movements, such as wringing or grasping activities.

II. **Physical Examination.** This condition must be differentiated from osteoarthrosis of the trapezium–first metacarpal joint, also a fairly common disorder. In osteoarthrosis, **A.** and **B.** below are negative, and joint-play movements at the trapezium–first metacarpal joint are restricted and painful.

   A. Pain on resisted thumb extension and abduction

   B. Pain on ulnar deviation of the wrist with the thumb held fixed in flexion. On this movement the tendons and the sheath are placed on a stretch.

   C. Tenderness to palpation over the tendon sheath in the region of the radial styloid process.

III. **Management**

   A. The physician may elect to inject the sheath with a corticosteroid preparation or a local anesthetic. Surgical incision of the sheath is occasionally performed.

   B. If injection is not contemplated or if it is unsuccessful, a trial of ultrasound and friction massage over a 1- or 2-week period, on a basis of three to five times a week, is warranted. The goal of this program is to maintain and increase mobility of the tendons within the sheath and to help resolve the chronic inflammatory process. In more severe or persistent cases, temporary restriction of thumb movements with a small opponens splint should be considered to prevent continued irritation to the inflamed sheath process.

Scaphoid Fracture and Lunate Dislocation

In an older person, a fall on the outstretched hand results in a Colles' fracture, since the proximal carpals are jammed into the weak osteoporotic radius. However, in a younger person, in whom the radius is strong and healthy, the scaphoid may fracture on impact, or the radius may force the lunate palmarly, resulting in lunate dislocation in a palmar direction (see Fig. 11-28).

A lunate dislocation may be detected on a standard anteroposterior roentgenogram by the lunate's appearing triangular rather than quadrangular and, in a lateral view, by its abnormal position. The therapist should always palpate for lunate positioning in patients referred to physical therapy after a fall on the outstretched hand.

A scaphoid fracture is not always so obvious (Fig. 11-29). Often a fracture here does not show up on standard roentgenograms. A key clinical sign is localized bony tenderness in the anatomic snuff box on palpation. When this is found in a patient referred following a fall on the outstretched hand, the therapist should suspect a scaphoid fracture and should consult the physician. The incidence of avascular necrosis of the proximal fragment of the scaphoid is high with this fracture because the blood supply to the scaphoid often enters only from the distal aspect of the bone. The fracture, then, cuts off the blood supply to the proximal fragment. Strict, prolonged immobilization of the wrist and thumb is necessary to minimize the possibility of avascular necrosis and nonunion.

☐ Secondary Osteoarthritis of the Thumb

The carpometacarpal joint of the thumb is particularly susceptible to osteoarthrosis. Women are more predisposed to this disorder than are men, and it can occur without evidence of osteoarthrosis in any other

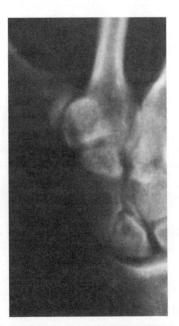

FIG. 11-29. Transverse fracture at the level of the proximal third of the scaphoid. (D'Ambrosia RD [ed]: Musculoskeletal Disorders: Regional Examination and Differential Diagnosis, 2nd ed. Philadelphia, JB Lippincott, 1986:440)

joint.[13,14] Typically it is bilateral, although it can be unilateral and may occur following prolonged overuse or trauma. It is a common finding following Bennett's fracture.[123]

The key structures in the trapeziometacarpal joint are the palmar or ulnar ligaments, which hold the beak of the thumb metacarpal down to the ridge on the trapezium, and the intermetacarpal ligaments, which hold the first to the second metacarpal (see Fig. 11-8).[86] In normal flexion and extension these ligaments undergo very little stress. However, in opposition and power pinch the joint surfaces twist one on the other and are prevented from coming apart by these ligaments.[62] Unequal stresses over time, an incongruency resulting from injured joint surface, or ligamentous disruption can result in osteoarthrosis (as the initial stage) with the ultimate development of osteoarthritis.[69]

Initially, erosion of the joint surfaces causes pain. After a time, the joint commonly subluxates because of degenerative changes, causing a gradual proximal travel of the metacarpal base of the saddle of the trapezium, together with an adduction deformity.[16] A secondary hyperextension deformity of the MCP joint may develop with attempted abduction, resulting in weakness and loss of function.

I. History

The patient's first complaints are usually of pain aggravated by use. Advice is often sought long before destructive changes occur. Typical symptoms include:

  A. Pain on extremes of movement of the thumb or when gripping or holding tools for long periods. The pain is usually localized to the base of the thumb, just anterior and distal to the anatomic snuff box.

  B. Marked instability and weakness of the hand, with a tendency to drop things and difficulty guiding or manipulating tools

  C. Occasional subjective complaints of numbness of the thumb and stiffness

  D. Deep-seated grinding, which is particularly uncomfortable

  E. Occasional swelling

II. Physical Examination

  A. In later stages the patient may present with an adduction deformity and hyperextension of the MCP joint.

  B. Active range of motion will often reveal crepitus and increased motion.

  C. Passive backward stretching of the thumb in abduction brings on the pain.

  D. Joint-play motions, particularly axial rotation, reproduce the pain. Later instability of the joint is evidenced by the prominence of the metacarpal base and hypermobility.[69]

E. Resisted motions are painless. Pinch strength will progressively decrease.

F. Tenderness is well localized over the joint on its anterior aspect. Osteophytes are sometimes palpable anteriorly.

III. Management

A. In the early stages the physician may elect to use corticosteroid injections. In advanced cases intra-articular silicone is often effective, and for this reason arthroplasty and arthrodesis are required less often than formerly.[21] If arthritis clearly involves other trapezial joints, arthrodesis of the trapeziometacarpal joint will give only limited relief of symptoms, as will arthroplasty of that joint. Excision of the trapezium may be necessary, and good results have been reported from this procedure alone.[16,22,37] If the joint remains unstable, replacement of the excised trapezium by rolled tendon[79] or fascia[120] or with a Silastic prosthesis is increasingly practiced.[27,30,68,90,104]

B. In the early stages, osteoarthrosis or traumatic arthritis responds well to friction massage.[21] At any point, relief can be provided by fitting the patient with a splint. Patients often find it useful to continue to use the splint for many months or even years while undertaking heavy work. Mobilization techniques, when indicated, and isometric exercises are useful. Patient education should include emphasis on avoiding positions of stress and activities that provoke the symptoms.

■ THE STIFF HAND

Stiffness and capsular restriction at the wrist and hand proper are common clinical problems seen by physical therapists. Whether due to fracture immobilization, soft-tissue contractures (Dupuytren's disease), burns, reflex sympathetic dystrophy, postoperative reconstructive hand surgery, complications of mastectomy, joint disease, peripheral nerve injury, or constriction by a cast or poorly applied dressing, the stiffness of the fingers and hand proper (metacarpals) that may result can be ruinous. Mobility is essential in normal function, and it can be disastrous when roentgenographic results of a fracture of the hand are normal but the patient is left with a stiff "frozen" hand.[123]

The major contributor to the stiff or frozen hand is edema. Postoperative or posttraumatic edema of the hand has been shown to be a normal physiologic response to injury. Edema is reversible; the degree and rapidity of reversibility determine its deleterious effect. If edema can be controlled early, subsequent scar formation is minimized in comparison with scar that forms if edema is prolonged and brawny. Persistence of edema may lead to joint stiffness and a reflex sympathetic dystrophy.

The measures against persistent posttraumatic or postsurgical edema merit particular attention. Edema is usually the result of an impairment of the microcirculation combined with the release of vasodilatating substances such as histamine and kinins, which also increase the vascular permeability.[81] Vascular dilatation evoked by pain receptors also plays a role. Abnormal autonomic reflexes are believed to be a major contributor in the early and later stages of reflex sympathetic dystrophy, in which edema is the most constant physical finding (see Colles' Fracture above). As time passes, the swelling worsens rather than improves.[65] Later motion is further inhibited by joint stiffness and brawny edema.

The sequence of events following edema has been described by Bunnell:[8,12]

When a hand remains swollen, from whatever cause, the movable parts are bathed in serofibrinous exudate. Fibrin is deposited between the various tissue layers and the folds of the joint capsules, between the tendons and their sheaths, throughout the ligamentous tissue itself and between and within the muscles. While soaked in the exudate, all of these tissues swell with edema and become shorter and thicker. The fibrin seals them in this condition and soon as the fibroblastic growth transforms all to connective tissue, ligaments become shorter and thicker. The folds of synovial membrane, the capsules of the joints, the plicae of tendon sheaths and the tendons and their sheaths become plastered together with organized adhesions.

Typically in the hand proper, edema is localized to the dorsum of the hand, where the tissues are most easily distended. The swelling of the dorsal aspect causes MCP joint extension, which predisposes to stiffness, scar formation, and contractures. Then fibrosis ensues, and a vicious circle begins.

Finger joints may stiffen after injury even though the insult was distant. The tendency toward stiffness of the fingers is greatest in adults and the aged but varies among individuals. Some persons tend to form scar tissue in the periarticular tissues, while others form keloids in the skin.[110] Anatomic factors that can cause limitations of motion include joint or capsular restriction, scar contraction of the skin (burns), contracted muscle, or an adherent tendon and a bony block or exostosis. All tissues can contract or become adherent: subcutaneous tissue, fascia, nerves, vessels, and cartilaginous and bony structures.

Stiffness of the hand resulting from edema, scar formation, muscle contraction, or a combination of these problems renders the hand stiff by interfering with either joint mobility or power gliding of the musculotendinous unit. The effects of edema on tendon gliding result in fluid collection in the layered paratenon, causing increased work to effect tendon gliding and a decrease in longitudinal paratenon gliding. Consequently, edema forming even after a minor injury may restrict gliding even though the joints exhibit a near-normal range of motion.[117] Full passive extension of the joints may be impossible because the swollen paratenon restricts gliding of the flexor tendons. The degree of joint impairment depends more on the anatomy of the joint, its supporting structures, and the position of the joint when the cicatrix was forming and maturing. Scar formation is particularly disabling in regard to tendon gliding because no matter what the position of the tendons, tendon gliding is impaired. Scar forms not only at the site of the lesion but also at many sites far removed. For example, a tendon lacerated in the fibro-osseous tunnel may evoke scar formation in the paratenon of the flexor tendons proximal to the wrist.[117,118]

Involvement of muscle compounds functional loss. Muscles may become involved by internal or external cicatrix formation or by myostatic contracture. Muscle imbalance in nerve palsy can result in contractures combined with the effects of edema and cicatrix reaction to the initial injury.[117,118]

☐ Examination

HISTORY

The patient presents with a primary complaint of loss of hand function due to stiffness following posttraumatic or postsurgical immobilization or lack of immobilization. Stiffness alone is usually not painful; the presence of pain poses a diagnostic problem. Nonunion of a fracture, neuroma, or degenerative arthritis must be considered. Once these causes have been eliminated, the distinction is made between pain that occurs during mobilization, which appears to be due to traction at the gliding planes or irregularities of the articular surfaces, or pain presenting in the absence of mobilization. The latter may be related to sympathetic dystrophy.

INSPECTION

A stiff hand may restrict the normal swinging movement of the arm as the hand is held stiffly by the side. Some swelling may be present; it may be intra-articular or extra-articular. Synovitis of the MCP and PIP joints bulges into the looser tissues on the extensor surface of the hand. Its shape is determined by the synovial attachments around the joints, which tend to spread on either side of the tendon in a proximal direction. Synovitis produces a diffuse swelling and can be easily differentiated from traumatic swelling of the joint structures, which usually forms a localized swelling on one side of the joint.

Extra-articular swelling may be either localized or diffuse. Diffuse swelling of a digit produces a sausage-shaped deformity. Localized swelling may involve the soft tissues around a joint and tendon sheath. In the palm and fingers it usually involves the flexor tendon sheath and may then be associated with nodule formation and triggering of the thumb or finger.[16,19,69]

Localized swelling may be due to ganglia or cystic swellings associated with Heberden's nodes.

SELECTIVE TISSUE TENSION AND NEUROLOGIC TESTS

Assessment of range of motion, strength, sensibility, and ability to perform activities of daily living completes the evaluation. Knowledge of the causes of joint stiffness is essential before evaluating the range of motion of the chronically stiff hand. Testing for skin tightness is routinely done.[2,3,96]

The capsular and extracapsular structures contributing to joint stiffness will be discussed according to the position of stiffness of the joint.

MCP JOINT

The initial response following trauma to a hand is an increase in tissue fluid (lymph, hemorrhage, or both). Fluid increases in the tissues of the joints. The fluid in the tissue of the capsule and collateral ligaments tends to produce an effective shortening of the structures. Fluid in the joint distends the capsule, and the joint assumes a position of maximum capacity. The anatomic positions are greatest in the MCP joints, and these joints are the key to the resultant negative hand: MCP extension, interphalangeal flexion, and wrist flexion.[116] Left in this attitude, certain periarticular changes occur and contractures develop.

STIFFNESS IN EXTENSION

Stiffness in extension can be due to contraction of the dorsal skin, extensor apparatus, capsular restriction (dorsal aspect), contraction of the collateral ligaments, or lesions of the joint structures. The joint factors that contribute to stiffness of the joint include capsular restriction, pannus formation in the volar synovial pouch, and articular surface erosions with or without pannus invasion. Extracapsular factors that can contribute to stiffness of the MCP joint in extension include skin contractures, extensor tendon adhesions at the dorsum of the wrist, unopposed extension (loss of active MCP flexion), and forearm extensor muscle contractures.

STIFFNESS IN FLEXION

Capsular factors that can contribute to stiffness of the MCP joints in flexion include deformities of the MCP joints, contractures or binding of the proximal sinus of the volar plate, contraction of the collateral or accessory collateral ligaments, and erosion of the articular surfaces with or without fusion.[110,117] Extracapsular factors contributing to MCP joint stiffness in flexion include contractures of the palmar skin and fascia, adhesions or contractures of the flexor tendons, and intrinsic muscle contractures.

PIP JOINT

At the PIP joint, the flexor superficialis comes into contact with the distal portion of the volar plate and may become adherent to it. The same is true of the flexor profundus at the DIP joint. The fibrous sheath of the flexor tendon extends from the PIP joint to the MCP joint. It inserts on the volar plate and on the phalanges but not on the metacarpal. This explains the important role it may play in stiffness in flexion of the PIP joint but not in stiffness of the MCP joint.[110] Other problems limiting extension of the PIP joints include adherence of the retinacular ligament to the collateral ligaments, adherence of the collateral ligaments, a bony block or exostosis, scarring of the skin on the volar surface of the finger and contraction of the superficial fascia or forearm musculature, and contraction of the fibrous portion of the fibro-osseous tunnel.

Abnormalities limiting flexion of the PIP joints include scar contracture of the dorsal skin of the finger, an adherent extensor tendon, capsular restriction, adherence of the collateral ligaments or retinacular ligament to the lateral capsular ligament or of the volar capsular ligament to the proximal phalanx, interosseous or lumbrical tendon adherence, intrinsic muscle contracture exostosis, a bony block, or articular surface erosion or pannus formation.[110]

☐ **Management**

An understanding of the capsular and extracapsular factors responsible for normal joint stability and the factors responsible for the development of stiff joints is required in posttraumatic and postoperative mobilization of stiff joints. It is obviously better to prevent stiffness than to have to treat it. One of the most important aspects is to prevent edema; such action is taken as soon after the injury or elective surgery as possible. Active motion, elevation, massage, anti-inflammatory medications, the use of a continuous passive motion device,[93] intermittent compressive thera-

pics, ice immersions, compressive wrapping or gloves, elastic tape for wrapping of individual fingers, and string wrapping may be considered.[15,17,45,89] Placing the hand in a protective position with a functional resting splint (secured with a figure-of-eight elastic wrap to help distribute pressure over a wide area) should be considered with severe edema.[77]

ACTIVE MOBILIZATION

The mainstay of the therapeutic program is active exercise. Early active mobilization should be started as soon as the lesions allow, but two extremes must be avoided: prolonged immobilization and excessive painful mobilization. The need for active use of the hand in mobilizing stiff joints cannot be overemphasized. Voluntary exercises and the use of the hand by the patient throughout the day produce far better results than does forceful passive range of motion applied for brief periods per day. Daily forcing of the finger joints causes reactive pain and swelling and is equivalent to spraining them daily, according to Bunnel.[8] Correct motions of the fingers and wrist are more important than strength of motion. Cocontraction of the agonist and antagonist should be prevented. Biofeedback often helps prevent unwanted muscle activity. Certain activities such as precision tasks can be done in elevation. Active exercises should include full range of motion to the elbow and shoulder of the involved arm.

MODIFICATION OF SCAR TISSUE

The most accepted clinical method of accelerating the modification of scar tissue is the application of stress to the scar. Treatment by mobilization is based on concepts that were initially empirical but that have more recently been proved in laboratory studies.[9,74,88,119] Slight persistent tension can remodel the collagen within scar tissue. Active mobilization can be profitably combined with massage to increase suppleness and prevent contractures.[105] Direct application of stress to the scar tissue can be accomplished in several ways: (1) direct pressure by massage or bandages, (2) serial or dynamic splints, (3) joint mobilization techniques in the presence of capsuloligamentous tightening or adherence, and (4) passive range of motion or stretching techniques.

MASSAGE

According to Wynn-Parry,[123] massage has no place in hand therapy to reduce muscle spasm, relieve pain, or improve circulation. Ice and active mobilization are the best means of reducing spasm. Pain is more efficiently and less expensively relieved by analgesia or other methods of modulation. Active exercises are infinitely better at increasing circulation than massage. Massage (soft-tissue mobilization) is most effective in breaking down adhesions and fibrosis; mobilizing scar tissue; stretching restricted fasciae, skin, joint capsules, and ligaments; and helping to reduce edema. Massage applies compressive and distractive forces directly to the scar and also helps to alter the fibrotic process and reduce any edema present. Deep friction massage is particularly useful for managing tenosynovitis and for decreasing the adhesions that form at ligaments after a sprain (see Chapter 7, Friction Massage).[21] Joint massage is a valuable adjunct in treating degenerative joints with stiffness or pain.[87]

Connective tissue massage often can provide gentle stretch of the capsule without traumatizing the joint structures.[28,107] A common problem in the management of the hand is overstretching of the capsules in the small joints of the fingers. These joints must be stretched gently—forceful stretching causes reactive pain and swelling, with the joints becoming stiffer than ever. Various soft-tissue mobilization techniques have been used effectively through the years to stretch abnormal fibrous tissue and to increase flexibility and range of motion.[4,49,70]

SPLINTING

Between physical therapy sessions, when retraction is marked, serial splints as advocated by Wynn-Parry and dynamic or static splints can be used to provide a prolonged pull or traction on the scar tissue.[123] In longstanding contractures, elongation by slow traction is necessary. Continuous mild traction provides a light prolonged stretch on the restraining tissues until, by cell multiplication, they actually grow longer, so that lengthening is permanent.[61,95]

Dynamic splints must be well adapted to the patient. If limitation in the range of motion is strictly related to a soft-tissue contracture around a particular joint, a splint must be designed to apply traction to that specific joint. Traction must be perpendicular (at a right angle to the treatment plane) to the involved phalanx.

When restrictions in active range of motion are due to a combination of joint contracture and muscle tightness, a two-stage splinting program is required.[77] Initially a splint is designed to increase the passive range of motion of the involved joint. Later, when normal joint mechanics have been restored, the splinting program is directed at providing stretch to the involved intrinsic or extrinsic musculature.

JOINT MOBILIZATION

Free joint play within a useful or functional range of motion is necessary to avoid joint trauma. If joint play is restricted, joint-mobilizing techniques should be used.[51] When pain is the dominant factor, grade I and II mobilization techniques are appropriate. If these techniques are successful and pain-free active motion increases, treatment is taken further into the range. Chronically, these stretching techniques can be vigorous as long as pain and irritation are avoided. Before initiating stretching techniques to muscle or inert tissue, there should be normal gliding of the joint surfaces to avoid joint damage. Both joint dynamics and muscle strength and flexibility must be balanced as the hand is restored to functional use.

PASSIVE RANGE OF MOTION AND STRETCHING TECHNIQUES

In vitro research has shown that prolonged low-intensity stretching at elevated tissue temperatures maximizes permanent lengthening of connective tissue and minimizes deterioration in tensile strength.[5,7,35,36,38,46,61,66,95,112,114,115] When using this principle of combining heat and stretch to a stiff hand, McEntee suggests applying an elastic tape to the involved finger(s) in the direction in which increased motion is desired to maintain a prolonged stretch.[77] Once the hand is stretched with the tape, it can be dipped in paraffin or placed under a hot pack for the desired time. Active exercises should follow immediately for the best results. As an adjunct to prolonged stretch, manual passive range of motion or stretching techniques may be used.

The complexity of the joints and multijoint muscles of the fingers requires careful evaluation and management. Fingers should always be stretched individually, not grossly. When stretching the extrinsic muscles (which are multijoint muscles), elongation over all the joints, simultaneously, should be avoided. Stretching in this manner can result in joint compression and damage to the smaller or less stable joints. Gently distract the joints to avoid compressing the segments being mobilized. Use short levers whenever possible and apply the stretch force in a gentle, slow, sustained manner. Hold the patient in the stretched position for at least 15 to 30 seconds.

Muscles are more amenable to stretch after some form of warm-up exercise. The best and most specific warm-up exercise is contraction against resistance. Successive techniques of isometric contractions, relaxation, and stretching (contract–relax method), followed by stimulation of the antagonist, help relax the muscles so they are more easily stretched.[29,41,48,59,60,76,106,113,122]

Therapy is more effective if supplemented by frequent self-stretching. In general, the more frequent the stretching, the more moderate the intensity. The principle of moving the body in relationship to the stabilized extremity affords an excellent stretch and allows a greater degree of pain-free movement. For example, to stretch the long finger flexors, have the patient (in a standing position) rest the palm of the involved hand on a table. Using the other hand the patient extends the joints from distal to proximal in succession, or actively extends them, unassisted, when possible. When the joints are extended, the patient fixates or maintains this position with the other hand as he or she actively moves the trunk forward; this brings the arm (with the elbow extended) up over the hand, resulting in wrist extension.[58] Motion is taken to the point of discomfort and maintained. Motion is progressed as the length improves.

Reverse stretching techniques can also be used. For example, to stretch the extensor digitorum communis, the patient maximally flexes the elbow and then actively flexes the fingers to their maximum range, beginning with the most distal joint and progressing proximally until the wrist is simultaneously flexed. Once all the slack is taken up in the hand, the elbow is straightened. As a result, the stretch is primarily directed at the muscle belly rather than the tendons and joint structures of the hand.

RESISTIVE EXERCISE

Joint motion without adequate muscle support can cause additional trauma to the joints as functional activities are resumed. Initially isometric exercises are recommended to increase strength when there is a loss of joint play and when there is significant pain. Once joint play is restored, resistive isotonic exercises are recommended within the available range.[58] This does not imply that normal range of motion needs to be present, but that joint play, within the available range, must be present. Graded resistive activity, progressing from manual resistive exercises using proprioceptive neuromuscular facilitation techniques to progressive resistive exercises using weights, the resistance of an elasticized tension cord (isoflex exercises), or self-resistance, and activities such as woodworking can help increase the strength of the hand. Squeezing activities, such as squeezing a rubber ball or a bit of putty, should be forbidden: they prevent full range of flexion, which is one of the goals of treatment.

Full range of motion is the primary target. Therapeutic and functional activities, as well as early return to work, are preferred to increase strength, endurance, and active motion of the chronically stiff hand. Acceptance of the hand by the patient, motivation, re-education, and preparing the patient to return to a former job and activities are all responsibilities of the hand-care team.

Management of the postsurgical hand is beyond the scope of this book, but details of preoperative and postoperative care are readily available in the literature.[1,8,16,22,27,30,37,68,71,79,90,104]

■ PASSIVE TREATMENT TECHNIQUES

(For simplicity, the patient is referred to as female, the operator as the male. P—patient; O—operator; M—movement)

Underwrap placed between the skin and the operator's mobilizing hand or the use of surgical gloves may allow the operator to obtain a firmer grip by reducing slippage against the patient's skin.

☐ Joint Mobilization Techniques

WRIST AND HAND

I. **Distal Radioulnar Joint—Dorsal-Ventral Glide** (Fig. 11-30)

P—Supine, with the arm somewhat abducted and the elbow bent, so that the forearm may rest on the plinth in a neutral position with respect to pronation and supination

O—Stabilizes the distal radius against the plinth, grasping it between the heel of his hand and the pads of the second through fifth fingers. He grasps the distal ulna dorsally with the thumb pad and ventrally with the pads of the index and long fingers.

M—The distal ulna may be moved dorsally or

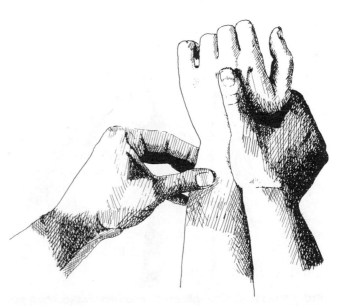

FIG. 11-30. Dorsal-ventral glide of distal radioulnar joint.

ventrally relative to the distal radius. These motions should be performed separately. Note: Alternatively, the distal ulna may be stabilized and the distal radius moved by reversing the hand-holds. The movement may also be performed with the forearm vertical.

These techniques are used to increase joint-play motions necessary for pronation and supination.

II. **Ulnomeniscotriquetral Joint—Dorsal Glide** (Fig. 11-31)

P—Supine or sitting, with the elbow resting on the plinth or table and the forearm vertical

O—Stabilizes the radial side of the wrist and hand with his left hand. The right hand contacts the dorsal aspect of the head of the ulna with the thumb, and the palmar aspect of the triquetrum and the pisiform with the radial aspect of the crook of the flexed PIP joint of his index finger.

M—A dorsal glide of the pisiform and triquetrum on the ulna is produced by a squeezing action between the thumb and the crook of the index finger.

This technique is used to increase joint-play movements necessary for pronation and supination.

III. **Radiocarpal Joint (and Ulnomeniscotriquetral Joint)—Joint Distraction** (Fig. 11-32)

P—Sitting or supine, with the elbow bent and resting on the plinth, and the forearm in neutral pronation and supination

O—Stabilizes the distal humerus and elbow

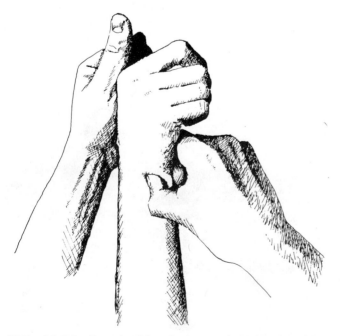

FIG. 11-31. *Dorsal glide of ulnomeniscotriquetral joint (right hand).*

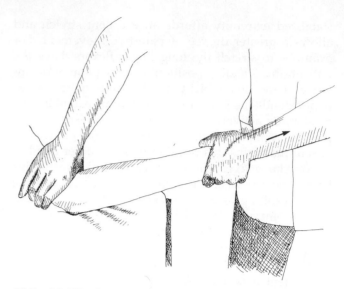

FIG. 11-32. *Distraction of radiocarpal joint (and ulnomeniscotriquetral joint) (right hand).*

against the plinth with his right hand at the antecubital space. The left hand grasps around the proximal row of carpals, just distal to the styloid processes.

M—A distraction is produced with the left hand, paying particular attention to the radiocarpal joint.

This technique is used as a general mobilization procedure to increase joint play at the radiocarpal joint. Distraction tends to occur with palmar flexion of the wrist. By increasing the amount of joint distraction, movement toward the close-packed position, dorsiflexion, may be increased. This prevents premature compression of joint surfaces.

IV. **Radiocarpal Joint—Dorsal-Palmar Glide** (Fig. 11-33)

P—Sitting with the arm somewhat abducted, the elbow bent, and the forearm resting on the plinth in pronation. The hand extends over the edge of the table or plinth.

O—Stabilizes the distal end of the forearm with his right hand, just proximal to the styloid processes. He grasps the proximal row of carpals with his left hand using the styloid processes and pisiform for landmarks.

M—The proximal row of carpals may be moved dorsally or palmarly, paying particular attention to the radiocarpal joint. Dorsal glide and palmar glide should be performed as separate techniques. Note: Dorsal glide may be performed more effectively with the arm in full supination and the hand extended over the edge of the plinth or table.

Palmar glide is used to increase joint-play

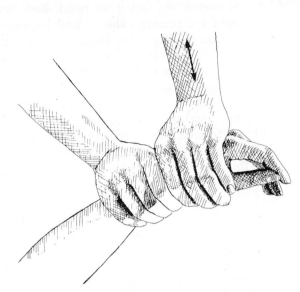

FIG. 11-33. Dorsal-palmar glide of radiocarpal joint.

movements necessary for dorsal flexion. Dorsal glide is used to increase joint-play movements necessary for palmar flexion.

V. **Radiocarpal Joint (and Ulnomeniscotriquetral Joint)—Radial-Ulnar Glide (or Tilt)** (Fig. 11-34)

   P—Sitting, with the arm near the side, the elbow bent, and the forearm resting on the plinth in neutral pronation and supination. The radial aspect of the forearm faces superiorly.

   O—Stabilizes the distal end of the forearm with the left hand, just proximal to the styloid processes. He grasps the proximal row of carpals with his right hand.

   M—The proximal row of carpals may be glided

radially or ulnarly on the distal ends of the radius and ulna (articular disk). Alternatively, a radial tilt or ulnar tilt may be produced.

Radial glide and ulnar tilt are joint-play movements necessary for ulnar deviation. Ulnar glide and radial tilt are joint-play movements necessary for radial deviation.

VI. **Midcarpal Joint—Joint Distraction**

This technique is produced in exactly the same way as that for the radiocarpal joint, except that the left hand-hold moves distally to grasp the distal row of carpals. This technique is used for general mobilization to increase joint play at the midcarpal joint.

VII. **Midcarpal Joint—Dorsal-Palmar Glide**

This technique is produced in exactly the same way as that for the radiocarpal joint, except that the left hand-hold moves distally to grasp the distal row of carpals. Palmar glide is used to increase the joint-play movements necessary for dorsal flexion. Dorsal glide is used to increase the joint-play movements necessary for palmar flexion.

VIII. **Midcarpal Joint—Palmar Glide of the Distal Row of Carpals on the Proximal Row of Carpals** (Fig. 11-35)

   P—Sitting or supine, with the elbow resting on the plinth and the forearm vertical

   O—Approaches from the ulnar aspect. The thenar eminence of his left hand contacts the distal row of carpals dorsally. The thenar eminence of his right hand contacts the proximal row of carpals palmarly. The fingers are interlaced over the radial aspect of the wrist. The forearms are directed outward, perpendicular to the plane of the palm.

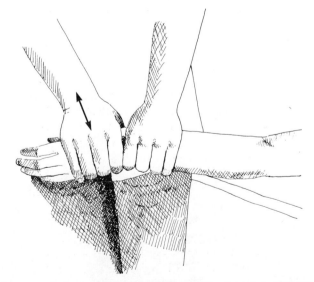

FIG. 11-34. Radial-ulnar glide (or tilt) of radiocarpal joint (and ulnomeniscotriquetral joint).

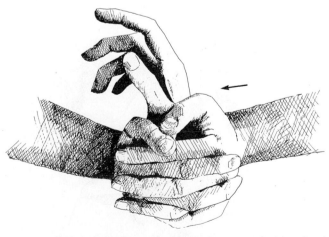

FIG. 11-35. Palmar glide of the distal row on the proximal row for midcarpal joint (right hand).

M—A palmar glide of the distal row of carpals on the proximal row is produced by a squeezing motion between the thenar eminences.

Note: This is a more effective method of palmar glide than that described for dorsal-palmar glide. The performance of this movement depends on the accurate placement of the operator's thenar eminences over the correct bones. Extension and spreading of the patient's fingers should occur when this movement is done correctly.[12] This technique is used to increase joint-play motion necessary for dorsal flexion of the wrist.

Specific movements between adjacent bones of the wrist and carpal joints may be indicated. Mobility between the triquetrum and lunate, the lunate and radius, or the capitate and lunate, for example, can be tested and mobilized. In general, one joint partner is always fixated while the other is moved. The individual carpal bones can be mobilized by placing the thumb and index finger on the volar and dorsal sides of two adjacent carpal bones (*e.g.,* the lunate and capitate), respectively. The thumbs may mobilize one carpal while the index fingers stabilize the other carpal bone, or vice versa. The reader is referred to detailed descriptions of these advanced techniques by Kaltenborn and others.[51,78,102] Only one example will be described.

IX. **Intercarpal Joints—Palmar Glide of the Scaphoid on the Radius** (Fig. 11-36)

P—Sitting or supine, with the forearm resting on the table, or with the arm held forward by the operator

O—Stands or sits facing the hand. Both hands hold the patient's thenar and hypothenar eminence. The index fingers are placed on the proximal palmar surface of the radius, stabilizing it in this position. The thumbs contact the scaphoid dorsally.

M—The scaphoid is moved palmarly relative to the distal end of the radius.

This technique is used to increase joint-play motion necessary for dorsal glide of the scaphoid on the radius.

X. **Trapeziometacarpal Joint—Distraction** (Fig. 11-37)

P—Sitting or supine with the ulnar aspect of the forearm resting on the table

O—The stabilizing hand grips the trapezium with the thumb on the dorsal surface and the index finger on the volar surface. The mobilizing hand grips the proximal metacarpal, with the thumb on the dorsal surface and the index finger on the volar surface.

M—A long-axis distraction is produced by the mobilizing hand moving the metacarpal distally.

Note: The metacarpal may be moved dorsally or ventrally relative to the trapezium using the same hand grips. These techniques are used to decrease pain and increase joint play of the trapeziometacarpal joint. Dorsal-volar glides are used to increase range of motion into trapeziometacarpal abduction and adduction. The trapeziometacarpal joint is in the resting position if conservative techniques are indicated or approximates the restricted range if more aggressive techniques are indicated.

XI. **Trapeziometacarpal Joint—Radial and Ulnar Glide** (Fig. 11-38)

P—Sitting or supine with the ulnar aspect of the forearm resting on the table

O—The stabilizing hand grips the trapezium with the thumb on the radial surface and the index finger on the ulnar surface. The mobilizing hand grips the proximal metacarpal on the radial and ulnar surfaces.

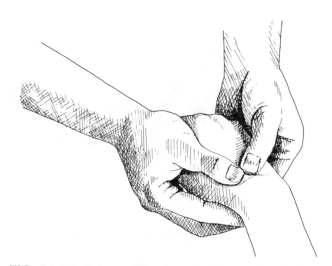

FIG. 11-36. *Palmar glide of scaphoid on radius for intercarpal joints.*

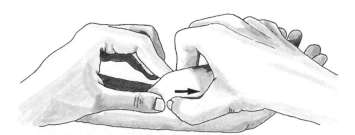

FIG. 11-37. *Distraction of the trapeziometacarpal joint.*

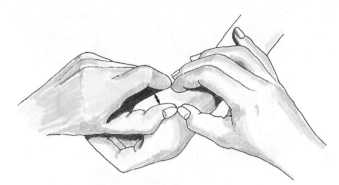

FIG. 11-38. *Radial-ulnar glide of the trapeziometacarpal joint.*

M—Radial or ulnar glide or tilt may be produced with the thumb pad in one direction and the index finger in the other.
Radial glide (ulnar tilt) is necessary for trapeziometacarpal extension. Ulnar glide (radial tilt) is necessary for trapeziometacarpal flexion.

XII. Carpometacarpal–Intermetacarpal Joints (II Through V)—Distraction (Fig. 11-39)
P—Sitting with the forearm resting on the table, palm down
O—Stabilizes the respective carpal with one hand, grasping with the thumb on the dorsal aspect and the index finger on the volar aspect. The mobilizing hand grips the base of the metacarpal of the joint being mobilized, with the thumb on the dorsal surface and the index finger on the volar surface.
M—Long-axis distraction is applied to the metacarpal; the second metacarpal is moved distal on the trapezoid, the third metacarpal distal on the capitate, the fourth metacarpal distal on the hamate, and the fifth metacarpal on the hamate.
Note: Volar glide may also be performed using the same stabilization and hand placement. Movement in these joints is minimal, especially in the second and third carpometacarpal joints. These techniques are used to increase joint play in the carpometacarpal joints and increase mobility of the arch of the hand.

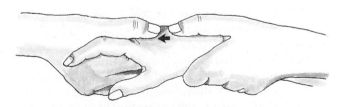

FIG. 11-39. *Distraction of the carpometacarpal intermetacarpal joints, II through V.*

XIII. Intermetacarpal Joints—Dorsal-Palmar Glide (Fig. 11-40) (These joints between the metacarpal heads are not true synovial joints, but movement must occur here during grasp and release, as described in Appendix A.)
P—Sitting or supine, with the elbow resting on the plinth, the forearm pronated
O—Approaches from the dorsal aspect. The left hand stabilizes the head and neck of the third metacarpal. The thumb pad contacts dorsally, the pads of the index and long fingers palmarly. The left hand grasps the head and neck of the fourth metacarpal in similar fashion.
M—The head of the fourth metacarpal can be moved palmarly or dorsally with respect to the third metacarpal. Similarly, the right hand can stabilize the third metacarpal, while the left hand moves the second metacarpal. The third metacarpal is the "center of movement" as the hand flattens and arches during release and grasp. It is always stabilized, while the other metacarpals are moved relative to it.
These techniques are used to increase joint-play movements necessary for the arching and flattening of the hand that occur with grasp and release.

FINGERS

Note: Traction grade 1 should be used with most gliding and mobilizing techniques of the fingers.

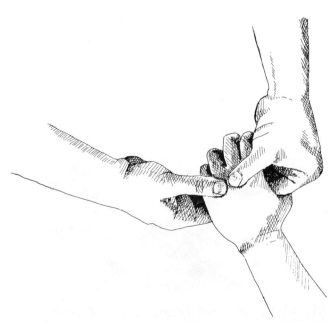

FIG. 11-40. *Dorsal-palmar glide of intermetacarpal joints.*

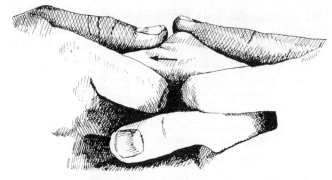

FIG. 11-41. *Distraction of metacarpophalangeal or interphalangeal joints (right hand).*

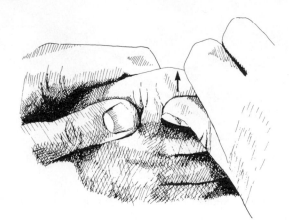

FIG. 11-43. *Radial-ulnar glide of metacarpophalangeal or interphalangeal joints (right hand).*

I. **MCP or Interphalangeal Joints—Distraction** (Fig. 11-41)

P—Sitting or supine

O—Supports the forearm and elbow by tucking them between his forearm and side. To treat the more radial joints, the operator approaches from the ulnar side for the thumb, index, and long fingers, and from the radial side for the ring and small fingers. He grasps the head of the proximal bone dorsally with the thumb pad and palmarly with the crook of the index finger. He grasps the base of the distal bone in a similar manner.

M—Keeping the joint in slight flexion (avoiding the close-packed position), a long-axis distraction is produced with the operator's more distal hand.

These techniques are used for general joint mobilization to increase joint play. Distraction is necessary, especially during flexion at the MP joints and extension at the interphalangeal joints, since these are movements toward the close-packed position. Premature compression of joint surfaces will result if sufficient joint play into distraction cannot occur.

II. **MCP or Interphalangeal Joints—Dorsal-Palmar Glide** (Fig. 11-42)

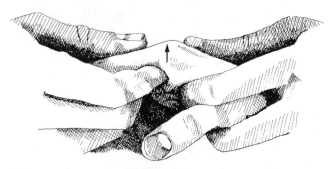

FIG. 11-42. *Dorsal-palmar glide of metacarpophalangeal or interphalangeal joints (right hand).*

P—Supine or sitting

O—The hand-holds are essentially the same as those for distraction, except that during dorsal glide the palmar contact of the more distal hand is with the pad of the index finger.

M—The base of the distal bone may be moved palmarly or dorsally.

Palmar glide is necessary for flexion. Dorsal glide is a joint-play movement necessary for extension.

III. **MCP or Interphalangeal Joints—Radioulnar Glide (or Tilt)** (Fig. 11-43)

P—Supine or sitting

O—The hand-holds are similar to those used for distraction, except that the thumbs are brought around to the aspect of the bones closest to the operator, and the crooks or pads of the index fingers are brought around to the aspect of the bone farthest from the operator. The contacts are then made on the radial and ulnar sides of the joint.

M—Radial or ulnar glide or tilt may be produced by the thumb pad in one direction, and by the index pad in the other. While one pad is producing the movement, the other moves to the more distal part of the bone.

Ulnar glide (radial tilt) is necessary for extension at the interphalangeal joints. Radial glide (ulnar tilt) is necessary for flexion at the interphalangeal joints. The same is true, but to a lesser extent, at the MP joints.

IV. **MCP or Interphalangeal Joints—Rotation (Pronation and Supination)** (Fig. 11-44)

P—Supine or sitting

O—The proximal hand-hold is the same as that for distraction. The distal hand-holds are also similar to those used for long-axis distraction, except the operator may gain some leverage by holding the more distal segment

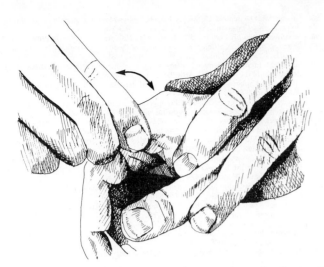

FIG. 11-44. Rotation (pronation and supination) of metacarpophalangeal or interphalangeal joints (right hand).

of the digit, semiflexed, in his remaining fingers. This must be performed with caution.

M—A pronation or supination of the distal end of the bone is produced by the operator's more distal hand.

Supination is a joint-play movement (conjunct rotation) necessary for flexion, especially at the interphalangeal joints. Pronation occurs during extension. **Note:** The same techniques may be used at the carpometacarpal joint of the thumb. As for their specific uses in this case, consider the convex–concave rule and how it applies to this sellar joint.

REFERENCES

1. American Academy of Orthopedic Surgeons: Symposium on Tendon Surgery in the Hand. Philadelphia, CV Mosby, 1975
2. American Society for Surgery of the Hand: The Hand: Examination and diagnosis. Aurora, CO: The Society, 1978
3. American Society for Surgery of the Hand: The Hand: Examination and diagnosis. New York, Churchill Livingstone, 1983
4. Bajelis D: Myofascial release, IV: Management of sports injuries. Presented at a course on physical therapy, management of the extremities, Seattle, July 1986
5. Barcroft H, Edholm OG: The effect of temperature on blood flow and deep temperature in the human forearm. J Physiol 102:5–20, 1943
6. Baxter PL, Ballard MS: Evaluation of the hand by functional tests. In Hunter JM, Schneider LH, Mackin EJ, Bell JA (eds): Rehabilitation of the Hand. St. Louis, CV Mosby, 1984
7. Becker AH: Traction for knee-flexion contractures. Phys Ther 59:1114, 1979
8. Boyes JH (ed): Bunnell's Surgery of the Hand. Philadelphia, JB Lippincott, 1970
9. Brand PW: Clinical Mechanics of the Hand. St. Louis, CV Mosby, 1985
10. Brand PW: Hand rehabilitation management by objectives. In Hunter JM, Schneider LH, Mackin EJ, Bell JA (eds): Rehabilitation of the Hand. St. Louis, CV Mosby, 1978
11. Brown CP, McGrouther DA: The excursion of the tendon of the flexor pollicis longus and its relation to dynamic splintage. J Hand Surg 9A:787–791, 1984
12. Bunnell S: Ischaemic contracture, local, in the hand. J Bone Joint Surg 35A:88–101, 1953
13. Cailliet R: Hand Pain and Impairment, 4th ed. Philadelphia, FA Davis, 1994
14. Cailliet R: Reflex sympathetic referred pain. In Shoulder Pain, 2nd ed. Philadelphia, FA Davis, 1991:108–124
15. Cain HD, Liebgold HB: Compressive centripetal wrapping technique for reduction of edema. Arch Phys Med 48:420–423, 1967
16. Campbell-Reid DA, McGrouther DA: Surgery of the Thumb. Boston, Butterworths, 1986
17. Carter PR: Common Hand Injuries and Infections: A Practical Approach to Early Treatment. Philadelphia, WB Saunders, 1983
18. Cornacchia M: Considerazioni sulla meccanica articolare del pollice. Chir Organi Mov 33:137–153, 1949
19. Corrigan B, Maitland GD: Practical Orthopaedic Medicine. Boston, Butterworths, 1985
20. Cyriax J: Textbook of Orthopaedic Medicine, vol 1, 11th ed. Baltimore, Williams & Wilkins, 1984:136–137
21. Cyriax J: Textbook of Orthopaedic Medicine, vol 2, 5th ed. Baltimore, Williams & Wilkins, 1969:333–338
22. De Palma F: The Management of Fractures and Dislocations: An Atlas, 2nd ed. Philadelphia, WB Saunders, 1970
23. Dell PC, Brushart TM, Smith RT: Treatment of trapeziometacarpal arthritis. Results of resection arthroplasty. J Hand Surg 5:243–249, 1978
24. Dellon AL: Evaluation of Sensibility and Re-Education of Sensation in the Hand. Baltimore, Williams & Wilkins, 1981
25. deTakas G: Nature of painful vasodilatation in causalgic states. Arch Neur Psychiat 50:318–326, 1943
26. Eaton RG: Joint Injuries of the Hand. Springfield, Ill., Charles C. Thomas, 1971
27. Eaton RG: Replacement of the trapezium for arthritis of the basal articulation. A new technique with stabilization by tenodesis. J Bone Joint Surg 61A:76–83, 1979
28. Ebner M: Connective Tissue Manipulation, Therapy and Therapeutic Application. Malabar, FL, Robert Knieger, 1985
29. Evjenth O, Hamberg J: Muscle Stretching in Manual Therapy: A Clinical Manual—The Extremities, vol 1. Alfta, Sweden, Alfta Rehab Forleg, 1984
30. Ferlic DC, Busbee GA, Clayton ML: Degenerative arthritis of the carpometacarpal joint of the thumb. A clinical follow-up of 11 Niebauer prostheses. J Hand Surg 2:212–215, 1977
31. Fess EE, Harmon KS, Strockland JW, et al: Evaluation of the hand by objective measurement. In Hunter JM, Schneider LH, Markin EJ, Bell JA (eds): Rehabilitation of the Hand. St. Louis, CV Mosby, 1978
32. Fess EE, Moran CA: Clinical Assessment Recommendations. Aurora, CO, American Society of Hand Therapists, 1981
33. Flatt AE, Fischer GW: Stability during flexion and extension at the MCP joints. In La Main Rheumatoide, Monographie du GEM. Paris, L'Expansion Scientifique Fran\u00e1aise, 1967:51–61
34. Flatt AE: The Pathomechanics of Ulnar Drift. Final Report. Washington DC, Department of Health, Education, and Welfare, 1971
35. Flax HJ, Miller RV, Horvath SM: Alterations in peripheral circulation and tissue temperature following local application of short-wave diathermy. Arch Phys Med Rehabil 3:630–637, 1949
36. Gersten JW, Wakin KG, Herrick JF, Krusen FH: The effect of microwave diathermy on the peripheral circulation and on tissue temperature in man. Arch Phys Med Rehabil 30:7–25, 1949
37. Gervis WH: A review of excision of the trapezium for osteoarthritis of the trapeziometacarpal joint after 25 years. J Bone Joint Surg 55B:56–57, 1973
38. Glazer RM: Rehabilitation. In Happenstall RB (ed): Fracture Treatment and Healing. Philadelphia, WB Saunders, 1980
39. Grant JCB, Basmajian JV: Grant's Method of Anatomy, 9th ed. Baltimore, Williams & Wilkins, 1991
40. Hakstian RW, Tubiana R: Ulnar deviation of the fingers. The role of joint structure and function. J Bone Joint Surg 49A:299–316, 1967
41. Haugen P, Stern-Knudsen O: The effect of a small stretch on latency relaxation and the short-range elastic stiffness in isolated frog muscle fibres. Acta Physiol Scand 112:121–128, 1981
42. Hazelton FT, Smidt GL, Flatt AE: The influence of wrist position on the force produced by the finger flexors. J Biomech 8:301–306, 1975
43. Hollinshead WH: Anatomy for Surgeons, vol 3: The Back and Limbs, 4th ed. New York, Harper Medical, 1985
44. Hoppenfeld S: Physical Examination of the Spine and Extremities. New York, Appleton-Century-Crofts, 1976
45. Hunter JM, Schneider LH, Mackin EJ, et al (eds): Rehabilitation of the Hand. St. Louis, CV Mosby, 1984
46. Jackman RV: Device to stretch the Achilles tendon. J Am Phys Ther Assoc 43:729, 1963
47. Jebson RH, Taylor N, Trieschman RB, et al: An objective and standardized test of hand function. Arch Phys Med Rehabil 5:311–319, 1969
48. Jenkins RB, Little RW: A constitutive equation for parallel-fibered elastic tissue. J Biomech 7:397–402, 1974
49. Johnson G: Functional orthopedics II: Advanced techniques of soft-tissue mobilization for evaluation and treatment of the extremities and trunk. Presented at a course at the Institute of Physical Arts, San Francisco, 1985
50. Johnson RK, Shrewsbury MM: The pronator quadratus in motions and in stabilization of the radius and ulna at the distal radioulnar joint. J Hand Surg 1:205–209, 1976
51. Kaltenborn FM: Mobilization of the Extremity Joints, 3rd ed. Oslo, Olaf Norlis Bokhandel, 1980
52. Kapandji IA: Biomechanics of the interphalangeal joint of the thumb. In Tubiana R (ed): The Hand, vol I. Philadelphia, WB Saunders, 1981
53. Kapandji IA: The Physiology of the Joints, vol I: Upper Limb. 5th ed. New York, Churchill Livingstone, 1982
54. Kapandji IA: Biomechanics of the thumb. In Tubiana R (ed): The Hand, vol I. Philadelphia, WB Saunders, 1981
55. Kaplan EB: The participation of the MCP joint of the thumb in the act of opposition. Bull Hosp Joint Dis 27:39–45, 1966
56. Kauer JMG: Functional anatomy of the carpometacarpal joint of the thumb. Clin Orthop 220:7–13, 1987
57. Kiloh LG, Nevin S: Isolated neuritis of the anterior interosseous nerve. Br Med J 1:850–851, 1952
58. Kisner C, Colby LA: Therapeutic Exercise: Foundations and Techniques, 2nd ed. Philadelphia, FA Davis, 1990
59. Knott M, Voss DE: Proprioceptive Neuromuscular Facilitation, Patterns and Techniques. New York, Hoeber & Harper, 1956
60. Knutsson E: Proprioceptive neuromuscular facilitation. Scand J Rehab Med [Suppl 7]:106–112, 1980
61. Kottke FJ, Pauley DL, Ptak KA: The rationale for prolonged stretching for correction of shortening of connective tissue. Arch Phys Med Rehabil 47:345–352, 1966
62. Kuckynski K: The thumb and saddle. Hand 7:120–195, 1975

63. Landsmeer JMF: Power grip and precision handling. Ann Rheum Dis 22:164–197, 1962

64. Landsmeer JMF: The anatomy of the dorsal aponeurosis of the human finger and its functional significance. Anat Rec 104:31–453, 1949

65. Lankford LL: Reflex sympathetic dystrophy. In Green LL (ed): Operative Hand Surgery, vol I. New York, Churchill Livingstone, 1982

66. Lehmann JF, DeLateur BJ, Silverman DRT: Selective heating effects of ultrasound in human beings. Arch Phys Med Rehabil 47:331–339, 1966

67. Lewis OJ, Hamshere RJ, Bucknill TM: The anatomy of the wrist joint. J Anat 106:539–552, 1970

68. Lister GD, Kleinert HE, Kutz JE, et al: Arthritis of the trapezial articulations treated by prosthetic replacement. Hand 9:117–129, 1977

69. Lister GD: The Hand. Diagnosis and Indications, 2nd ed. New York, Churchill Livingstone, 1984

70. Little KE: Toward more effective manipulative management of chronic myofascial strain and stress syndromes. JAOA 68:675–685, 1969

71. Littler JW: Principles of reconstructive surgery of the hand. In JM Converse (ed): Reconstructive Plastic Surgery. Philadelphia, JB Lippincott, 1977

72. Long C, Conrad DW, Hall EA: Intrinsic-extrinsic muscle control of the hand in power grip and precision handling. J Bone Joint Surg 52A:853–867, 1970

73. MacConaill MA: Mechanical anatomy of the carpus and its bearing on surgical problems. J Anat 75:166–175, 1941

74. Madden JW, de Vore G, Arem AJ: A rational postoperative management program for MCP joint implant arthroplasty. J Hand Surg 2:358–366, 1977

75. Marie P, Meige H, Patrikious: Paralysie radiale dissociÇe simulant une griffe cubitale. Rev Neurol 24:123–124, 1917

76. Markos P: Ipsilateral and contralateral effects of proprioceptive neuromuscular facilitation techniques on hip motion and electromyographic activity. Phys Ther 59:1366–1373, 1979

77. McEntee PA: Therapist's management of the stiff hand. In Hunter JM, Schneider LH, Mackin EJ, Bell JA (eds): Rehabilitation of the Hand. St. Louis, CV Mosby, 1984

78. Mennell JMCM: Joint Pain. Boston, Little, Brown & Co., 1964

79. Menon J, Schoene H, Hohl J: Trapeziometacarpal arthritis. Results of tendon interpositional arthroplasty. J Hand Surg 6:442–446, 1981

80. Milford LW: Restraining Ligaments of the Digits of the Hand: Gross and Microscopic Anatomic Study. Philadelphia, WB Saunders, 1968

81. Mittelbach HR: The Injured Hand: A Clinical Handbook for General Surgeons. New York, Springer-Verlag, 1979

82. Moberg E: Shoulder–hand–finger syndrome. Surg Clin North Am 40:367–373, 1960

83. Napler JR: The prehensile movements of the human hand. J Bone Joint Surg 38B:902–913, 1956

84. Newmeyer WL: Primary Care of Hand Injuries. Philadelphia, Lea & Febiger, 1979

85. Norkin C, Levangie DK: Joint Structure and Function: A Comprehensive Analysis, 2nd ed. Philadelphia, FA Davis, 1992

86. Pagalidis T, Kuczynski K, Lamb DW: Ligamentous stability of the base of the thumb. Hand 13:29–35, 1981

87. Paris SV: The Spinal Lesion. Christ Church, New Zealand, Pegasus Press, 1965

88. Peacock EE: Some biomechanical and biophysical aspects of joint stiffness; role of collagen synthesis as opposed to altered molecular bonding. Ann Surg 164:1–12, 1966

89. Perry JF: Use of a surgical glove in treatment of edema in hand. J Am Phys Ther Assoc 54:498–499, 1974

90. Poppen N, Niebauer J: "Tie in" trapezium prosthesis: Long-term results. J Hand Surg 3:445–450, 1978

91. Rabischong P: Les problèmes fondamentaux du rétablissement de la préhensime. Ann Chir 25:927–933, 1971

92. Rosse C: The hand. In Rosse C, Clawson DK (eds): The Musculoskeletal System in Health and Disease. Philadelphia, Harper & Row, 1980:227

93. Salter RB: Textbook of Disorders and Injuries of the Musculoskeletal System, 2nd ed. Baltimore, Williams & Wilkins, 1983

94. Sandzen SC: Atlas of Wrist and Hand Fractures. Littleton, Mass., PSG Publishing Co., 1979

95. Sapega AA, Quedenfeld TC, Moyer RA, et al: physiological factors in range-of-motion exercises. Physician in Sports Medicine 9:57–65, 1981

96. Schamber D: Simply Performed Tests of the Hand. New York, Vantage Press, 1984

97. Simmons BP, De La Caffiniere JF: Physiology of flexion of the fingers. In Tubiana R (ed): The Hand, vol I, Philadelphia, WB Saunders, 1981

98. Smith EM, Juvinall R, Bender L, Pearson J: Role of the finger flexors in rheumatoid deformities of the MCP joints. Arthritis Rheum 7:467–480, 1964

99. Spinner M: Kaplan's Functional and Surgical Anatomy of the Hand. Philadelphia, JB Lippincott, 1984

100. Steinbrocker O, Argyros TG: The shoulder–hand syndrome: Present status as a diagnostic and therapeutic entity. Med Clin North Am 42:1533–1553, 1958

101. Steinbrocker O, Spitzer N, Friedman NH: The shoulder–hand syndrome in reflex dystrophy of the upper extremity. Ann Int Med 29:22–52, 1948

102. Svendsen B, Moe K, Merritt R: Joint Mobilization, Laboratory Manual. Loma Linda, CA, Loma Linda University, 1981

103. Swanson AB, Goran-Hagert C, Swanson G: Evaluation of impairment of hand function. In Hunter JM, Schneider LH, Mackin EJ, Bell JA (eds): Rehabilitation of the Hand. St. Louis, CV Mosby, 1978

104. Swanson AB, Swanson G, Watermeier JJ: Trapezium implant arthroplasty—Long-term evaluation of 150 cases. J Hand Surg 6:128–141, 1981

105. Taleisnic J: The ligaments of the wrist. J Hand Surg 1:110–118, 1976

106. Tanigava MC: Comparison of the hold–relax procedure and passive mobilization on increasing muscle length. Phys Ther 52:725–735, 1972

107. Tappan FM: Holistic, Classical Massage and Emerging Methods, 2nd ed. Norwalk, CT, Appleton-Lange, 1988

108. Tinel J: Le signe du "fourmillement" dans les lesions des nerf peripheriques. Presse Med 47:388–389, 1915

109. Tubiana R: Examination of the Hand and Upper Limb. Philadelphia, WB Saunders, 1984

110. Tubiana R: The Hand, vol I. Philadelphia, WB Saunders, 1981

111. Wadsworth CT: Wrist and hand examination and interpretation. J Orthop Sports Phys Ther 5:108–120, 1983

112. Wakim KG, Krusen FH: Influence of physical agents and of certain drugs on intra-articular temperature. Arch Phys Med Rehabil 32:714–721, 1951

113. Wallin D, Ekblom B, Grahn R, Nordenborg T: Improvement of muscle flexibility: A comparison between two techniques. Am J Sports Med 13:263–268, 1985

114. Warren CB, Lehmann JF, Koblanski JN: Heat and stretch procedures: An evaluation using rat tail tendon. Arch Phys Med Rehabil 57:122–126, 1976

115. Warren CG, Lehmann JF, Koblanski JN: Elongation of rat tail tendon: Effect of load and temperature. Arch Phys Med Rehabil 52:465–474, 1971

116. Watson HK: Stiff joints. In Green DP (ed): Operative Hand Surgery, vol I. New York, Churchill Livingstone, 1982

117. Weeks PM, Wray R, Kux M: The results of nonoperative management of stiff joints in the hand. Plast Reconstr Surg 62:58–63, 1978

118. Weeks PM, Wray RC: Management of Acute Hand Injuries. St. Louis, CV Mosby, 1973

119. Wilson J: Arthroplasty of the trapeziometacarpal joint. Plast Reconstr Surg 49:143–148, 1972

120. Woolf D: Shoulder–hand syndrome. Practitioner 213:176–183, 1974

121. Youm Y, McMurtry Ry, Flatt AB, et al: Kinematics of the wrist. I. An experimental study of radioulnar deviation and flexion–extension. J Bone Joint Surg 60A:432–434, 1978

122. Wright V, Johns R: Physical factors concerned with stiffness of normal and diseased joints. Bull Johns Hopkins Hosp 106:215–231, 1960

123. Wynn-Parry CB: Rehabilitation of the Hand. Toronto, Butterworths, 1973

124. Zancolli EA, Ziadenberg C, Zancolli E: Biomechanics of the trapeziometacarpal joint. Clin Orthop 220:14–26, 1987

125. Zancolli EA: Structural and Dynamic Bases of Hand Surgery. Philadelphia, JB Lippincott, 1979

The Hip

DARLENE HERTLING AND RANDOLPH M. KESSLER

REVIEW OF FUNCTIONAL ANATOMY

Osteology

The acetabulum is formed superiorly by the ilium, posteroinferiorly by the ischium, and anteroinferiorly by the pubis. The acetabulum faces laterally, anteriorly, and inferiorly (Fig. 12-1*A*). It is deepened by the fibrocartilaginous acetabular labrum, allowing it to enclose slightly more than half a sphere. The bony, fibrocartilaginous labrum and cartilaginous constituents of the acetabulum are interrupted inferiorly by the acetabular notch (Fig. 12-1*B*). This notch is traversed by the transverse ligament of the acetabulum (Fig. 12-1*C*).

The head of the femur constitutes about two thirds of a sphere. Slightly below and behind the center of

the articular surface of the head is a roughened indentation termed the *fovea*, to which the ligament of the head of the femur attaches (see Fig. 12-1*B*). The neck of the femur connects the head and shaft of the femur. In the frontal plane, the angle formed by the neck and shaft of the femur is about 125° in the adult but closer to 150° in the young child. This is often termed the *angle of inclination* (Fig. 12-2). In the transverse plane, the neck forms an angle of about 15° with the transverse axis of the femoral condyles, such that with the transverse axis of the condyles lying in the frontal plane, the neck of the femur is directed about 15° forward (Fig. 12-3). This is referred to as the *angle of torsion* or *angle of declination* of the hip.

In the anatomic position, both the acetabulum and the neck of the femur are directed anteriorly. Because of this, in the normal standing position, a large area of the articular surface of the head of the femur is ex-

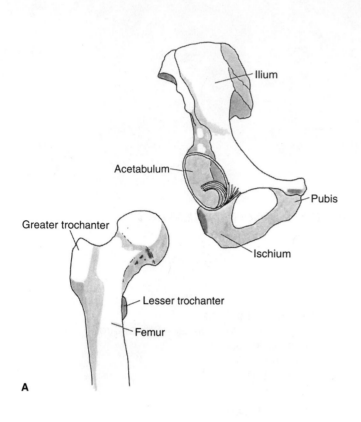

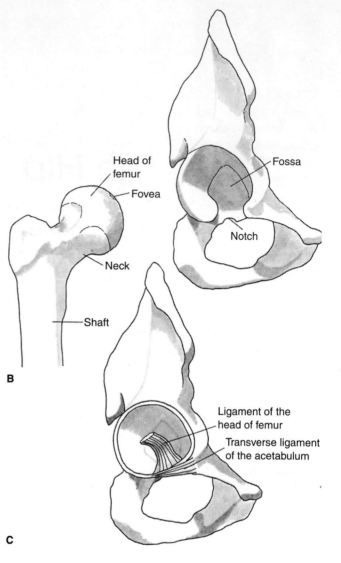

FIG. 12-1. Components of the right hip joint, showing the relationship of the acetabulum to the femur (**A**), the acetabular fossa to the proximal femur (**B**), and the ligaments of the acetabulum (**C**).

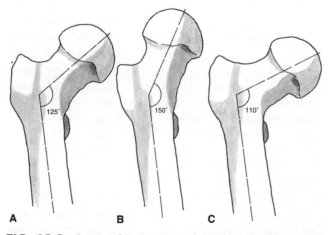

FIG. 12-2. Angle of inclination of the femur: (**A**) normal, (**B**) coxa valgum; (**C**) coxa varum.

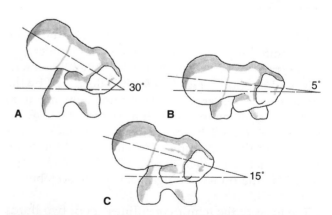

FIG. 12-3. Angle of torsion or declination of the femur in the transverse plane: (**A**) antetorsion; (**B**) retrotorsion; (**C**) normal angle.

posed anteriorly, and the effective weight-bearing surface of the head is confined to a relatively small area on the posterosuperior aspect of the head.

An increase in degrees of the normal inclination angle is referred to as *coxa valgum*; a decrease in the angle is called *coxa varum* (see Fig. 12-2). When an increased torsion angle is present, we speak of antetorsion; when the torsion angle is less than normal, it is called retrotorsion (see Fig. 12-3). The term *antetorsion* should not be confused with *anteversion*. Anteversion is not associated with alignment of any other part of the femur, but is a feature of the hip joint alone.[33,40] Anteversion is a positional change in which either the acetabulum or the head and neck of the femur are directed anteriorly, relative to the frontal plane.[9] Antetorsion is a medial twist of the shaft of the bone, distal on proximal. When the transcondylar axis is aligned on the frontal plane, the femoral head and neck are directed anteriorly, indicating the existence of torsion in the femoral shaft. The result is a medially displaced patella. More distally, the feet are aligned either in a noncompensatory in-toed stance or in a compensatory out-toed stance.[9]

A patient with an anteverted hip will appear to lack external rotation, and a patient with a retroverted hip will appear to lack internal rotation. Also, the person with an anteverted hip will tend to walk with a toe-in gait; with retroversion, a toe-out gait is characteristic.

The greater trochanter is a prominence projecting laterally and superiorly from the junction of the neck and shaft of the femur. It serves as an area for attachment of many of the muscles controlling movement at the hip. Situated posteromedially to the junction of the neck and shaft is a smaller prominence, the lesser trochanter; it also provides an area of insertion for muscles controlling the hip (see Fig. 12-1*A*).

☐ Trabeculae

The trabecular patterns of the upper femur reflect the normal stresses sustained by the hip; they correspond to the normal lines of force in this area (Fig. 12-4). The main system of trabeculae consists of two sets of trabeculae. The arcuate bundle resists a bending moment or a tendency for the weight of the body to shear the head and neck inferiorly with respect to the shaft of the femur; this bending moment is brought about by the lever arm created by the medially projecting neck of the femur. The vertical bundle resists vertical compressive forces through the head of the femur. The arcuate bundle runs from the lateral cortex of the shaft of the femur, just inferior to the greater trochanter, upward and medially to the middle and inferior cortical region of the head of the femur. The vertical bundle is contiguous with the medial cortex of the shaft of the

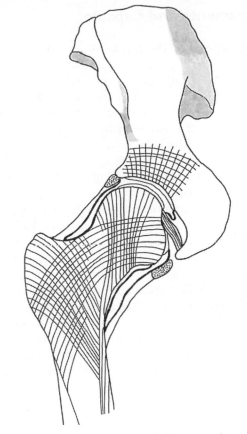

FIG. 12-4. Trabecular patterns of the upper femur.

femur, running straight upward to the superior cortex of the head.

Another trabecular system runs from the medial cortex at the base of the neck, upward laterally through the greater trochanter. These trabeculae resist the tensile forces from the muscles attaching to the trochanter.

The areas where the vertical bundle and the trochanteric bundle intersect the arcuate bundle are areas of particular strength. The intervening region is an area of relative weakness, made weaker by osteoporosis in older people. This region is often the site of femoral neck fractures.

☐ Articular Cartilage

The area of the acetabulum covered by articular cartilage is horseshoe-shaped. The area not covered by articular cartilage corresponds to the total sweep of the ligament of the head of the femur when the hip is moved through a full range of movement in all planes. This nonarticular portion is the acetabular fossa and is lined by a fat pad (see Fig. 12-1*B*). The entire head of the femur is covered by articular cartilage except for the small fovea where the ligament of the head attaches.

Ligaments and Capsule

The joint capsule of the hip joint is thick and strong and is reinforced by strong ligaments. Its fibers run longitudinally, parallel to the neck of the femur (Fig. 12-5). The capsule runs from the rim of the acetabulum and labrum to the intertrochanteric line anteriorly and to about 1 cm proximal to the intertrochanteric crest posteriorly. Much of the neck of the femur, then, is intracapsular. Some deep fibers of the joint capsule run circularly around the neck of the femur, forming the zona orbicularis.

The iliofemoral ligament is one of the strongest ligaments in the body. It is sometimes referred to as the Y ligament of Bigelow, since it resembles an inverted Y. It attaches proximally to the lower portion of the anterior-inferior iliac spine and to an area on the ilium just proximal to the superior and posterosuperior rim of the acetabulum. The ligament, as a whole, spirals around to overlie the anterior aspect of the joint, attaching to the intertrochanteric line. The more lateral fork of the Y attaches to the anterior aspect of the greater trochanter, whereas the more medial fibers twist around to attach just anterior to the lesser trochanter (Fig. 12-5A).

This ligament primarily checks internal rotation and extension. It allows a person to stand with the joint in extension using a minimum of muscle action; by rolling the pelvis backward, a person can "hang" on the ligaments. The ligament prevents excessive movement in the direction toward the close-packed position of the hip joint. Looking at it another way, with movement toward the close-packed position, this ligament becomes taut and twisted on itself, causing an approximation of the joint surfaces and a "locking"

of the joint. Some of the lateral fibers of the iliofemoral ligament probably pull tight on adduction.

The ischiofemoral ligament attaches proximally to an area of the ischium just posterior and posteroinferior to the rim of the acetabulum. Its fibers run upward and laterally to attach to the posterosuperior aspect of the neck of the femur, where the neck meets the greater trochanter (Fig. 12-5B). The ischiofemoral ligament also pulls tight on extension and internal rotation of the hip.

The pubofemoral ligament runs from the pubis, near the acetabulum, to the femur, just anterior to the lesser trochanter. It tightens primarily on abduction but also helps check internal rotation of the hip (see Fig. 12-5A).

The ligament of the head of the femur (ligamentum teres) attaches to the roughened nonarticular area of the acetabulum inferiorly near the acetabular notch, to both sides of the notch, and to the transverse ligament that traverses the notch. It lies in the nonarticular acetabular fossa as it runs up and around the head of the femur to the fovea (see Fig. 12-1C).

Although the ligament of the head of the femur pulls tight on adduction of the hip, its mechanical function is relatively unimportant. Of more significance is its role in providing some vascularization to the head of the femur and perhaps in assisting with lubrication of the joint. The ligament of the head of the femur is lined with synovium. It is believed that this ligament may act somewhat similarly to the meniscus at the knee by spreading a layer of synovial fluid over the articular surface of the head of the femur as it advances to contact the opposing surface of the acetabulum.

As mentioned, the transverse ligament crosses the acetabular notch to fill in the gap. It converts the notch into a foramen through which the acetabular artery (from the obturator artery) runs, eventually becoming the artery of the ligament of the head of the femur (see Fig. 12-1C).

Synovium

The synovial membrane of the hip joint lines the fibrous layer of the capsule. It also lines the acetabular labrum and, inferiorly, continues inward at the acetabular notch to line the fat pad in the floor of the acetabular fossa and to cover the ligament of the head of the femur. From the femoral attachment of the capsule at the base of the neck, the synovium reflects backward proximally to line the neck of the femur.

The synovial "cavity" of the joint often communicates anteriorly with the iliopectineal bursa. It does so through a gap between the pubofemoral ligament and the medial portion of the iliofemoral ligament.

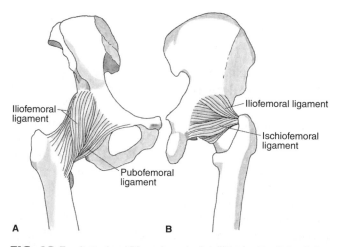

Iliofemoral ligament

Iliofemoral ligament

Ischiofemoral ligament

Pubofemoral ligament

A   **B**

FIG. 12-5. Anterior (**A**) and posterior (**B**) views of the joint capsule of the hip joint.

☐ Bursae

The rather large iliopectineal bursa overlies the anterior aspect of the hip joint and the pubis and lies beneath the iliopsoas muscle as it crosses in front of the hip joint. This bursa often communicates with the hip joint anteriorly through a space between the pubofemoral and iliofemoral ligaments. This may be a factor in the characteristic anterior pain experienced by patients with hip joint disease (Fig. 12-6).

One or more trochanteric bursae overlie the greater trochanter, reducing friction between it and the gluteus maximus, which passes over the trochanter, and the other gluteals, which attach to the trochanter. This bursa is most extensive posterolaterally to the trochanter, where it underlies the gluteus maximus. It is important clinically because of the prevalence of trochanteric bursitis.

☐ Blood Supply
(Fig. 12-7)

The blood supply to the head of the femur is of particular importance because of its significance in common pathologic conditions at the hip, including fractures and osteochondrosis of the femoral head (Legg-Perthes disease). The head of the femur receives its vascularization from two sources, the artery of the ligament of the head of the femur and the arteries that ascend along the neck of the femur. The importance of the artery of the ligament of the head of the femur is variable, but for the most part it supplies only a small area adjacent to the fovea. In as many as 20% of persons it fails to anastomose with the other arteries supplying the head of the femur.

The primary blood supply to the head of the femur,

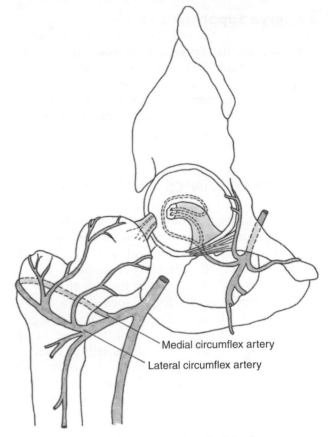

FIG. 12-7. Blood supply to the head of the femur.

Medial circumflex artery
Lateral circumflex artery

then, is derived from the arteries that ascend proximally along the neck of the femur to pierce the head of this bone just distal to the margin of the articular cartilage. These are branches of the medial and lateral femoral circumflex arteries. The medial circumflex artery passes around posteriorly to give off branches that ascend along the posteroinferior and posterosuperior aspects of the neck of the femur. The lateral circumflex artery crosses anteriorly to give off an anterior ascending artery at about the level of the intertrochanteric line. The ascending arteries pierce the joint capsule near its distal attachment to the femur and run proximally along the neck of the femur intracapsularly. They run deep to the synovial lining of the neck. Because of their relationship to the neck, they are subject to interruption in the case of a femoral neck fracture. Also, since they are intracapsular, it is believed that increased intracapsular pressure caused by joint effusion may stop flow. This is believed to be a factor in osteochondrosis and in some cases of idiopathic avascular necrosis of the head of the femur. The circumflex vessels give off extracapsular branches to the trochanteric regions of the femur. This area also receives vascularization from the superior gluteal artery and a perforating branch of the profunda.

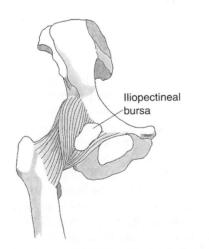

FIG. 12-6. Anterior aspect of the hip joint showing the iliopectineal bursa.

Iliopectineal bursa

☐ Nerve Supply

Innervation to the hip joint is supplied by branches from the obturator nerve, the superior gluteal nerve, and the nerve to the quadratus femoris and by branches from the femoral nerve, both muscular and articular. These nerves represent segments L2 through S1.

■ BIOMECHANICS

The hip joint, being a ball-and-socket joint, exhibits three degrees of freedom of motion. In this respect it is analogous to the glenohumeral joint. Unlike the shoulder, however, the hip is intrinsically a very stable joint. This is due, in part, to the fact that the acetabulum forms a much deeper socket than the glenoid cavity; the head of the femur comes closer to forming a full sphere than does the head of the humerus. The acetabulum, with its labrum, can enclose over half a sphere and can grasp passively the head of the femur to maintain joint integrity; it is difficult to pull the head from the acetabulum without removing or tearing the acetabular labrum.

Coaptation of joint surfaces is also maintained, in part, by atmospheric pressure. Because of the relatively large surface area of contact between joint surfaces, the atmospheric pressures holding the joint surfaces together may be as much as 25 kg. This is sufficient to maintain coaptation of the joint with all soft tissues about the joint removed and the limb hanging freely. Only when the vacuum created between the joint surfaces (by the close fit) is released (by, say, drilling a hole through the acetabulum) will the limb drop free.

Intrinsic stability at the joint is further enhanced by the strong ligamentous support at the hip. Since the major ligaments at the hip pull taut and are twisted on themselves with extension, the hip joint is particularly stable in the standing position. As mentioned, the twisting of the capsule that occurs with movement toward the close-packed position effects a type of "screw home" movement at the hip in which the joint surfaces become tightly approximated. As with any joint, the close-packed position at the hip (extension–abduction–internal rotation) is the position of maximal congruence of joint surfaces.

Because the acetabulum and the neck of the femur are both directed anteriorly, their respective mechanical axes are not coincidental. There are two positions of the hip in which these axes are brought into alignment. One position is attained by flexing the hip to about 90°, abducting slightly, and rotating slightly externally. The other position is one of extension, abduction, and internal rotation. The former position is the one that the hip would assume in a quadruped situation, and the latter is the close-packed position of the joint. As mentioned, in the upright position, a considerable portion of the articular cartilage of the head of the femur is exposed anteriorly. During normal use of the joint, as in walking, there is a relatively small contact area between the acetabulum and the femoral head. This may be a factor in the prevalence of degenerative hip disease in humans; stresses of weight-bearing are borne by a small surface area of cartilage, and a relatively large area of cartilage may not undergo the intermittent compression necessary for adequate nutrition (see Chapter 3, Arthrology).

The smaller the torsion angle at the hip (the less it is anteverted), the greater the stability of the bone, since the axes of the acetabulum and neck of the femur are closer to being in alignment. A smaller torsion angle also favors an increase in the effective contact area between joint surfaces, for the same reason.

Because of its intrinsic stability, the normal hip joint rarely dislocates when compared with, say, the shoulder or elbow. The shoulder, elbow, or any other joint usually dislocates when a force is applied over the joint when it is in its close-packed position. This is not true at the hip, which will usually dislocate only when its capsule and major ligaments are lax and its joint surfaces and bony axes are out of congruence. Thus, the hip is most prone to dislocation when in a position of flexion (ligaments lax), abduction, and internal rotation (noncongruence). Dislocation usually occurs with a force driving the femur backward on the pelvis with the hip in this position—for example, striking the knee on the dashboard of a car in a head-on collision. With such an injury, the head of the femur is driven posteriorly through the relatively weak posterior capsule.

Since the hip is freely movable in all vertical planes, it is not subject to capsuloligamentous strain from horizontal forces applied to it in most positions, even though, due to the length of the leg, these forces acting over a long lever arm are potentially quite large. However, since the hip is a weight-bearing joint, it is subject to vertical loading that must be borne by its bony and cartilaginous components.

In the case of a person bearing equal weight through both legs, the vertical force on each femoral head is equal to half the weight of the body minus the weight of the legs. When standing on one leg, however, the weight-bearing femoral head must support more than the weight of the body. This is because the center of gravity (at about S2) is located some distance medially to the supporting femoral head. This lever arm through which the force is acting causes a rotary moment about the supporting femoral head, with a tendency for the opposite side of the pelvis to drop.

This rotary moment must be countered by the hip abductor muscles, primarily the gluteus medius, gluteus minimus, and tensor fasciae latae, on the weight-bearing side. The point of application of this counterforce provided by the abductor pull is at the greater trochanter, which is considerably closer to the fulcrum (femoral head) than is the center of gravity line that represents the force produced by the body weight. Since the distance from the femoral head to the trochanter is about half the distance from the femoral head to the center of gravity line, the abductors must pull with a force equal to two times the superincumbent body weight to prevent the pelvis from dropping to the non-weight-bearing side. The total force acting vertically at the femoral head is equal to the force produced by the pull of the abductors plus the force produced by the body weight, or up to *three times* the body weight.[28,37,38,63] In this case "body weight" is actually the total body weight minus the weight of the supporting leg.

During stance phase of the normal gait cycle, the vertical forces acting at the femoral head are substantial. If the abductors are not strong enough to counter the forces tending to rotate or tilt the pelvis downward to the opposite side, an abnormal gait pattern results. Either the pelvis will drop noticeably to the opposite side of the weakness, usually resulting in a short swing phase on that side, or the person will lurch toward the side of weakness during stance phase on the weak side. The effect of the lurch is to shift the center of gravity toward the fulcrum (femoral head), reducing the moment arm about which the forces from the body weight may act, thereby reducing the necessary counterpull by the abductors. In fact, a marked lurch may actually shift the center of gravity lateral to the fulcrum, allowing gravity to substitute for the hip abductors, thus preventing the pelvis from dropping to the opposite side. This lurching gait is often referred to as a "compensated gluteus medius gait." It is usually seen in patients with painful hip conditions, such as degenerative joint disease, in which there is some weakness of the abductors and in which it is desirable to reduce compressive forces acting at the joint for relief of pain. It is also seen in patients with abductor paralysis.

The "abductor lurch" may be prevented by providing an external means of preventing the pelvis from dropping toward the uninvolved side during stance phase on the involved side. This external force may be provided by using a cane on the uninvolved side. An upward force is transmitted from the ground through the cane to counter the weight of the body tending to rotate the pelvis downward on that side. The forces acting through the cane do so about a moment arm even longer than that about which the force of gravity on the body weight acts, since the point of contact of the hand on the cane is farther from the supporting femoral head than is the center of gravity line. For this reason, a relatively small force applied through the cane is required to compensate for the abductors and relieve the vertical forces acting at the involved hip. The forces acting upward through the cane must be transmitted to the pelvis through contraction of the lateral trunk muscles, shoulder depressors, elbow extensors, and wrist flexors on the side of the cane.

Clearly, forces of muscle contraction contribute significantly to compressive loading at the hip. This is not only true in a weight-bearing situation. Studies in which strain gauges have been inserted into prosthetic hips suggest that supine straight-leg raising causes a compressive force to the hip that is greater than the body weight.[44] This is an important consideration in the early management of patients who have undergone an internal fixation for a hip fracture.[31]

■ EVALUATION

☐ History

The hip joint is derived from segments L2 through S1. Clinically, however, pain of hip joint origin is primarily perceived as involving the L3 segment. Typically, the patient with hip joint disease complains first of pain in the midinguinal region. As the process progresses, or as the painful stimulus intensifies, pain is likely to be felt into the anterior thigh and knee. At this point pain may also be described in the greater trochanteric region and buttock as well. In some instances (and not uncommonly) pain is felt most in the knee, and the patient may actually believe the knee is at fault. In general, pain in the trochanteric region spreading into the lateral thigh is more suggestive of trochanteric bursitis. Pain in the buttock spreading into the lateral or posterior thigh is more suggestive of pain of lower spinal origin.

Because of its freedom of movement in all planes and its great stability, the hip is seldom afflicted by disorders of acute traumatic origin. The hip is a common site, however, of degenerative joint disease and, to a lesser extent, rheumatoid arthritis. The clinician should ask whether the patient suffered any childhood hip disorders such as congenital dysplasia, osteochondrosis (Legg-Perthes disease), or slipped capital epiphysis, since these may predispose to early hip degeneration. Bursitis, either trochanteric or iliopectineal, is also fairly common at the hip.

The clinician must also determine whether the patient has a history of back problems. Low back disorders may mimic hip disease and vice versa because of the segmental relationships. Also, hip disease often leads to back problems because of the biomechanical relationships. See Chapter 5, Assessment of Musculoskeletal Disorders, for a complete list of questions to be included in the history.

☐ Physical Examination

I. **Observation**
  A. *Gait*
    1. A lurch to one side during stance phase suggests hip pain, abductor weakness, or both on the side to which the lurch occurs.
    2. Dropping of the pelvis on the opposite side of the stance leg suggests abductor weakness (uncompensated) on the side of the stance leg.
    3. Development of an excessive lordosis during stance phase may suggest hip flexion contracture on the side of the stance leg.
    4. A backward lurch of the trunk during stance phase may suggest hip extensor weakness on the side of the stance leg, or hip flexor weakness on the side of the swing leg.
    5. A persistent inclination of the pelvis to one side during all phases of the gait cycle, combined with a lack of heel-strike on the side of inclination, suggests an adduction contracture on the side of the inclination.
  B. *Functional activities*
    1. Loss of hip motion may result in considerable difficulty removing and donning shoes, socks, and slacks.
    2. The patient may "sacral sit" to compensate for a lack of hip flexion.
  C. Note general posture and body build.

II. **Inspection**
  A. *Skin*—usually noncontributory in common hip disorders. Observe for old surgical scars.
  B. *Soft tissue*
    1. Observe for atrophy about the hip and thigh. Document thigh atrophy by girth measurements.
    2. Hip joint effusion is usually not visible due to heavy soft-tissue covering.
  C. *Bony structure and alignment.* Measure and record deviations.
    1. Use plumb bob to assess mediolateral and anteroposterior alignment in the standing position (including the spine).
    2. Assess relative heights of the following structures:
      a. Navicular tubercles
      b. Medial malleoli
      c. Fibular heads
      d. Popliteal folds
      e. Gluteal folds
      f. Greater trochanters
      g. Anterior-superior iliac spines
      h. Posterior-superior iliac spines
      i. Iliac crests

   Note: A vertical structural deviation arising from some abnormality at the hip joint or upper end of the femur is suggested if, from the floor upward, all of the above-mentioned landmarks are level up to the trochanters, but the anterior-superior iliac spines, posterior-superior iliac spines, and iliac crests are not. Note whether the relative levels of the anterior-superior and posterior-superior iliac spines on one side are the same as the levels on the opposite side. If not, the asymmetry may be due to a sacroiliac torsion rather than some abnormality at the hip joint or upper femur. If the trochanters are level and the anterior-superior and posterior-superior iliac spines and iliac crest on one side are lower by the same amount than their counterparts on the opposite side, one may suspect one of several possibilities: coxa varum on the low side, coxa valgum on the high side, a shortened femoral neck on the low side or a lengthened neck on the high side (rare), or cartilaginous narrowing from hip joint degeneration on the low side. The two most common of these are coxa varum and hip joint degeneration. Coxa varum is usually associated with a decreased angle of declination (torsion angle); hip joint degeneration sufficient to cause a clinically detectable vertical asymmetry will be accompanied by other symptoms and signs of degenerative joint disease (see Common Lesions below).

   The extent of coxa varum, hip joint narrowing, or other cause of asymmetry may be documented by assessing the position of the greater trochanter relative to a line drawn from the anterior-superior iliac spine to the ischial tuberosity (Nélaton's line). The "normal" trochanter should lie about on this line. This measurement is primarily useful in unilateral conditions in which it may be compared with the "normal" side. Documentation of total leg-length discrepancy should be made by measuring from the anterior-superior iliac spine to the medial malleolus of the same side.

III. **Selective Tissue Tension Tests**
  A. *Active movements.* The emphasis is on assessing functional activities involving use of the hip. Functional activities (in order of sequence) should include the following:
    1. Gait
    2. Sitting, bending forward to touch the toes, and crossing the legs
    3. Going up and down stairs, one step at a time

4. One-legged standing (observe for dropping of the pelvis to the opposite side—Trendelenburg's sign)
5. Running straight ahead
6. Running and twisting
7. Jumping

In the hip, the active movements commonly tested in standing are flexion and extension, since more information about the other motions of the hip can usually be obtained from tests of passive and combined movements. The normal range of hip flexion (knee bent) is 120°, but there is a wide variation.

B. *Passive movements.* Passive movements should be compared with the uninvolved side. The type of end feel is noted and passive overpressure applied. Although the movement must be gentle, the examiner should apply passive overpressure at end range to find out the type of end feel, whether there is any limitation of motion (hypomobility) or excessive range (hypermobility), and if it is painful.

1. Flexion–extension
   a. Joint motions are best assessed with a Mundale pelvic femoral angle measurement using the standardized sidelying position.[47] Draw a transverse line for the pelvis, connecting the anterior-superior and posterior-superior iliac spines (line *AB* in Figure 12-8A), with the hip in full flexion (with the knee flexed) or extension (with the knee

straight). Construct a perpendicular line *CD* from this line to the most superior point of the greater trochanter; the angle between this line and the long axis of the femur, *DE*, is measured in full flexion and extension. By using the same landmarks the clinician can assess other hip positions, including weight-bearing flexion.

Considering the ease of measurement, reliability, and reproducibility, the use of the prone extension test is recommended to measure hip extension in children with cerebral palsy and those with meningomyelocele. The Thomas test is recommended in the supine position as an alternative for nonspastic patients.[2,70]

   b. Straight-leg raising. Measurement of hamstring flexibility can be determined by using the same sidelying positioning and landmarks as in Mundale's measurement. Between lines *CD* and *DE*, an angle alpha exists in the resting position (see Fig. 12-8A). In maximum flexion an angle beta is obtained between the reference lines (Fig. 12-8B). To obtain the result of isolated coxofemoral flexion, alpha must be subtracted from beta. Once the angle alpha is determined, the subject is asked to perform maximal hip flexion without bending the knee. Abduction of the

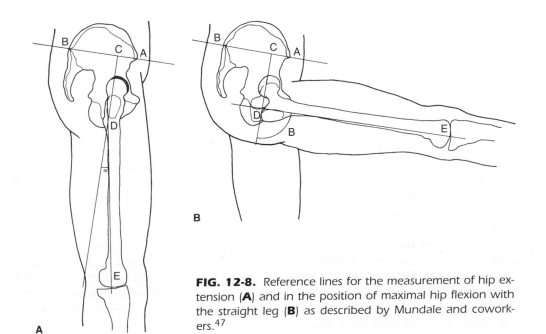

FIG. 12-8. Reference lines for the measurement of hip extension (**A**) and in the position of maximal hip flexion with the straight leg (**B**) as described by Mundale and coworkers.[47]

subject's leg is eliminated by supporting the leg on a powder board table. Instruct the subject not to perform movements of knee flexion, hip rotation, or movements of the ankle joint during hamstring measurement. Finally, the angle beta is determined (see Fig. 12-8B).[72]

2. Abduction–adduction. When measuring, be sure to prevent internal–external hip rotation and lateral tilting of the pelvis. The pelvis must first be fixed by the examiner with one hand while the extended leg is then passively abducted with the other hand. When assessing abduction (supine), the leg to be tested should be close to the edge of the plinth so that when full abduction of the extended leg is reached, the knee can be passively flexed to assess one-joint adduction (mainly pectineus and the adductors) versus two-joint adduction (gracilis, biceps femoris, semimembranosus, and semitendinous).[29]

Adduction of the hip is normally limited by one leg coming into contact with the other. One leg should be held in slight flexion so as to cross over the other leg.

  a. Capsular restriction will result in marked limitation of abduction and mild limitation of adduction.
  b. Full motion with pain at the extremes of adduction, abduction, or both may be present with trochanteric bursitis.

3. Internal–external rotation. Passive hip rotation may be tested by three methods.

  a. Assess while the patient lies supine with the hip and knees extended. The examiner rapidly rotates the leg inward and outward via the ankle. In the early stages of hip disease, before hip deformity develops, a characteristic type of end feel due to loss of normal fluid type is perceived.[8] This test also becomes a useful mobilization technique.
  b. Measure sitting with hips and knees flexed.
  c. Measure prone with the knee flexed (this is a more "functional" measurement since the hip is extended as in walking).
  d. Limited internal rotation and *excessive* external rotation suggest retrotorsion (decreased angle of torsion). Limited external rotation and *excessive* internal rotation suggest increased antetorsion (increased angle of torsion). If internal rotation is considerably limited and external rotation somewhat limited, capsular tightening is likely.

4. Combined hip flexion–adduction–rotation. This test uses the femur as a lever and stretches the posterolateral and inferior capsule and compresses the superior and medial portions of the capsule. With the patient supine, the examiner flexes the patient's knee and hip fully and then adducts the leg. As the knee is moved fully toward the patient's opposite shoulder, the examiner compresses the hip joint.

  a. The examiner should stabilize the pelvis and apply passive overpressure at the end of range. This test will also reveal tightness of the external rotators, particularly the piriformis.[29] If a tight piriformis is present, adduction and internal rotation range are decreased and painful. This test may produce pain in the buttock if a tight piriformis is impinging on the sciatic nerve or if an inflamed bursa is compressed beneath the stretched gluteus maximus. The distance of the knee from the chest is noted.
  b. The range and pain response to the adduction component should also be assessed with the hip in different positions of flexion and rotation.

5. On all passive movements, note the following:

  a. Range of motion. The capsular pattern of restriction is marked limitation of internal rotation and abduction, moderate limitation of flexion and extension, and some limitation of external rotation and adduction.
  b. Pain
  c. Crepitus
  d. End feel

C. *Resisted isometric movements*

1. Resist maximal isometric contraction of muscles controlling all major hip movements, allowing no motion of the joint. Resisted knee flexion and extension should be done as well as the six isometric tests of the hip:

  a. Flexion (supine) with the legs extended or with the hip and knee flexed to 90°. Resistance is applied above the knee. Painful weakness may indicate a psoas tendinitis; a painless weakness may be due to rupture of the psoas or to an L2 nerve root lesion.[8]

b. Extension (supine) with an extended knee. Apply resistance at the heel. Pain in the upper thigh may be due to a lesion of the origin of the hamstrings.

c. Adduction (supine) bilaterally. The knees are squeezed against the examiner's closed fist. Pain on resisted adduction suggests a lesion of the adductors (rider's sprain).[10]

d. Abduction (prone) with the opposite leg well stabilized. The hand around the patient's knee resists the patient's attempt to abduct the thigh. Resisted abduction can compress the gluteal bursa, as may passive abduction. A painful weakness may be due to a gluteus medius tendinitis.[8]

e. Internal and external rotation (prone) with a flexed knee. Resistance is applied at the ankle. Pain, on resisted rotation, is considered an accessory sign in gluteal bursitis.[10]

2. Bursitis about the hip is very rare, but resisted hip flexion may reproduce pain in the presence of iliopectineal bursitis, and resisted hip abduction, or resisted hip extension and external rotation, may reproduce pain in trochanteric bursitis.

D. *Joint-play movement tests*

1. The same movements used for specific joint mobilization techniques are used as examination maneuvers, except when evaluating joint play the femur should be in its resting position (30° of flexion and abduction; slight external rotation).

a. Distraction (Fig. 12-9). With the patient lying supine, the joint is distracted by applying a distolateral force parallel to the neck of the femur. The operator's hands are placed around the subject's thigh.

b. Inferior glide (Fig. 12-10). With the patient lying supine and the femur in its resting position, the examiner's hands are placed around the subject's thigh. An inferolateral force (inferior femoral glide) is applied along the longitudinal axis of the femur by the examiner leaning backward.

c. Posterior glide (Fig. 12-11). With the hip maintained in its resting position, a posterior glide is performed with the examiner's hands by leaning forward with the trunk.

d. Anterior glide. With the subject in the same position as in Figure 12-11, the

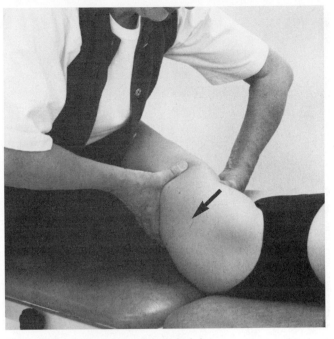

FIG. 12-9. *Distraction of the hip joint.*

slack is taken up, and an anterior glide of the femur is performed with the examiner's hands by leaning backward with the trunk (see Fig. 12-15*A*).

2. Assess:

a. Amplitude of movement: hypomobile, normal, hypermobile

b. Irritability: pain, protective muscle spasm

IV. **Neuromuscular Tests**

A. If a neurologic deficit is suspected at this

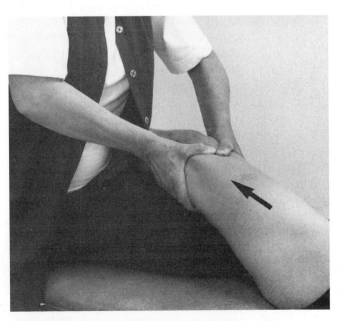

FIG. 12-10. *Inferior glide of the hip joint.*

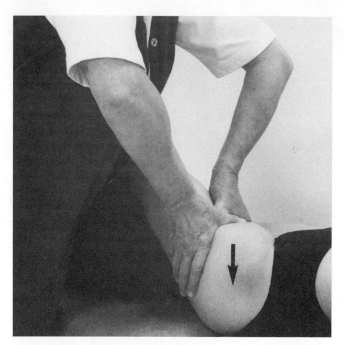

FIG. 12-11. Posterior glide of the hip joint.

point in the examination, it may be appropriate to perform sensory, motor, reflex, and coordination tests (see Chapter 5, Assessment of Musculoskeletal Disorders).

B. Most chronic joint conditions result in some weakness of the muscles controlling the joint because of disuse and reflex inhibition. At the hip some muscle groups are so powerful that mild or even moderate weakness may not be detected by manual muscle testing. Even if detected, manual testing does not permit documentation of the extent of weakness (or strength). For this reason, it is best to test each of the major muscle groups controlling the hip—abductors, adductors, flexors, and extensors—by determining the number of repetitions that can be performed against a constant load—for example, by determining the 10 RM (repetition maximum). This allows for comparison with the "normal" side or predetermined norm, and for documentation of a baseline.

V. Palpation
   A. *Skin.* Palpate hip girdles and lower extremities (usually noncontributory in local lesions at or about the hip because of heavy soft-tissue covering).
      1. Temperature
      2. Moisture
      3. Tenderness
      4. Texture
      5. Mobility

   B. *Soft tissue*
      1. Mobility and consistency
      2. Swelling (joint effusion usually cannot be palpated at the hip)
      3. Tenderness
         a. There may be localized tenderness anteriorly if the iliopectineal bursa is inflamed or distended. It may be distended with joint effusion since it often communicates with the joint.[76]
         b. There may be localized tenderness laterally if the trochanteric bursa is inflamed.
         c. There may be areas of referred tenderness (so-called trigger points) in the related segments (L2–S1) if a lesion is affecting any of the deep somatic tissues at or about the hip.
   C. *Bony structures* (see under Inspection)

VI. Special Tests
   A. *Assessment of common shortened muscle groups*
      1. Hip flexors
         a. The Thomas test detects a fixed hip flexion deformity in patients who have developed a compensatory lumbar lordosis that then masks the hip flexion.[71] With the patient supine, with the coccyx just over the edge of the plinth, the contralateral hip is flexed until the pelvis is tilted backward and the lumbar lordosis is eliminated. A flexed hip position shows shortening of the iliopsoas; a tendency toward simultaneous extension in the knee joint points to shortening of both the iliopsoas and the rectus femoris. Hip adduction of less than 18º to 20º indicates tightness of the tensor fasciae and iliotibial band. Decreased range of hip abduction and compensatory hip flexion (with the knee flexed) are signs of shortness of one-joint thigh adductors (see Fig. 21-29).
         b. Ely's test for the iliopsoas and rectus femoris.[24] The patient lies prone. If the iliopsoas is shortened, the hip remains in flexion. If passive flexion of the knee provokes a compensatory increase of flexion in the hip joint and hyperlordosis of the lumbar spine, the rectus femoris muscle is tight.
         c. Weight-bearing test with the patient assuming normal standing posture, using the pelvic femoral angle to assess the hip flexion angle in relationship to the floor (see Fig. 12-8).[47]

2. Hamstrings (supine)
   a. 90°–90° straight-leg raise.[65] The patient flexes the hip to 90° and grasps behind the knee with both hands. The examiner then extends the knee through the available range. A measurement of 20° from full knee extension is within normal limits.
   b. Straight-leg raising test. The examiner flexes the hip so the knee is kept in extension. To avoid error, the lumbar spine should be monitored and kept flat on the plinth so there is no lordosis or kyphosis of the lumbar spine. When the hip flexors are shortened, the contralateral leg should be flexed at the hip and the knee joint passively or flexed with the sole of the foot on the plinth so the lumbar spine is kept flat.
3. Tensor fasciae latae (iliotibial band)
   a. A positive Ober test indicates a contracture of the iliotibial band.[53] It is performed in the sidelying position with the lower leg flexed at the hip and knee for stability and the pelvis well stabilized by the examiner. The examiner then passively abducts and extends the upper leg with the knee straight or flexed. Maintaining extension and neutral rotation of the hip, the leg is allowed to passively drop toward the plinth. If shortening is present, the leg will remain abducted. With the knee flexed the iliotibial band is slack and the flexibility of the tensor fasciae latae is revealed.[24] The movement may reproduce pain associated with trochanteric bursitis or tendinitis at the tibial insertion of the iliotibial band.

B. *Other tests*
   1. Scouring (quadrant test) (Fig. 12-12) stresses the posterior and lateral hip capsule. It also reveals an abnormal end feel as the hip is rotated.[21,65] Normally the end feel is that of a smooth arc. In early joint changes, a clearly perceived bump in the arch is noted. A grating sensation or sound may be elicited in an osteoarthritic hip.
      a. The subject lies supine with the hip flexed and adducted and the knee fully flexed. The examiner stands on the same side of the table, hands clasped over the patient's anterior knee.
      b. The examiner passively flexes, adducts, medially rotates, and longitudinally

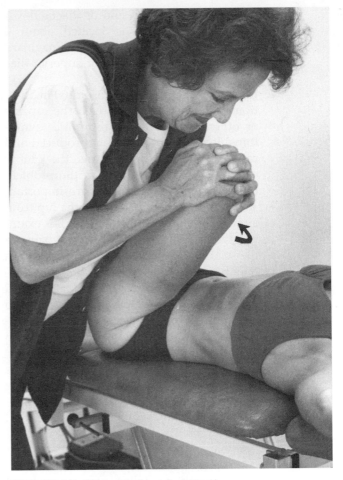

FIG. 12-12. Scouring (quadrant test).

compresses the femur to scour the inner aspect of the joint. The examiner then takes the femur into abduction and lateral rotation. The femur is rotated repetitively in the acetabulum between 90° of hip flexion and 140°.
      c. Compare the movement with that of the contralateral side to determine whether symptoms are reproduced or if there is just routine discomfort. Both the quality of motion and the presence and location of pain are noted.
   2. Noble's compression test[50] is used to reveal a possible iliotibial band friction syndrome near the knee. With the patient supine and the knee and hip flexed to 90°, thumb pressure is applied lateral to the femoral epicondyle (or 1 to 2 cm proximal to it). While maintaining thumb pressure, the patient's knee is slowly extended passively. Severe pain elicited at about 30° flexion indicates a positive test.
   3. Baer's sacroiliac point is tender in the pres-

ence of a sacroiliac lesion or iliacus flexor spasms. This point is located about 2 inches from the umbilicus on an imaginary line drawn from the anterior-superior iliac spine to the umbilicus.[44]

4. Joint-clearing tests take the joint(s) in question to end range and stretch the capsule or other soft tissues to reproduce symptoms. If no symptoms are reproduced and range is within normal limits, the joint is cleared from involvement in the problem being assessed. These tests are important since pain may be referred to the hip from joints above and below the hip. For example, the lumbar spine may project pain via the sciatic or femoral nerve, and knee pain may be projected up to the hip via the obturator nerve. Tests such as squatting and valgus–varus stress tests may be used to clear the knee. Full active flexion, extension, and lateral flexion may be used to clear the lumbar spine.

5. Femoral torsion tests. Various clinical tests (Craig's test or Ryder's method) have been proposed to assess the degree of hip anteversion.[41] Comparative ranges of internal and external hip rotation in the prone position may suggest increased retroversion or anteversion. In weight-bearing, the appearance of the patellae often suggests excessive femoral torsion when the patient stands with the knees in full extension and the feet pointing straight ahead. In excessive anteversion, the patellae face inward (squinting patellae). When the hips are externally rotated until the patellae are facing to the front, the feet and legs will be pointed outward.

6. Assessment of leg-length equality. Several anatomic (a decrease in the vertical dimensions of bony structure) and functional (a right/left asymmetry in joint position) methods have been proposed for assessing true and apparent leg-length discrepancies.[7,13,27,46,49,78] From a clinical standpoint, limb-length assessment should be done with the patient in a weight-bearing position with measurements determined by placing a calibrated block under the sole of the foot to level the pelvis. A gravity goniometer or level placed between the posterior-superior iliac spine can be used to assess when the pelvis is level. Discrepancy is determined by the height of the calibrated blocks needed for correction. Assessment should be accompanied by palpation and additional tests, if indicated, to determine the source of discrepancy (*i.e.*, foot, ankle, knee, sacroiliac, and lumbar spine tests). With the exception of one tape-measure method, clinical tests for determining leg length have been shown to be inaccurate when compared to radiographic measurements.[3] Observer error of up to ±10 mm has been found in clinical methods for assessing leg length.[7,46,49] When using the tape-measure method for determining leg length, an average of two tests may improve validity.[3]

a. Cartilaginous narrowing. Compare clinical to roentgenographic findings.

b. Coxa varum/coxa valgum. Malleoli, fibular heads, and trochanters are level. Posterior-superior and anterior-superior iliac spines and iliac crests are lower on the varus side and higher on the valgus side. Coxa varum is often associated with retroversion; coxa valgum is usually associated with increased anteversion. In coxa varum, the trochanter lies above Nélaton's line; in coxa valgum, it lies below. Compare clinical findings to roentgenograms.

c. Short femoral shaft. Malleoli, fibular heads, and popliteal folds are level. The greater trochanter and pelvic landmarks are lower on the short side.

d. Short tibia. The malleoli are level. The popliteal folds, fibular heads, and tibial tubercles are lower on the short side.

Note: Dynamic evaluation should include a gait analysis and assessment of shoes.

■ COMMON LESIONS

□ Degenerative Joint Disease (Osteoarthrosis)

Degenerative joint disease (DJD) at the hip often progresses to a point at which it results in significant disability. This is true at the hip more so than at any other joint. Clinically, persons with DJD of the hip frequently present to outpatient health-care services because of pain and disability. DJD is the most common disease process affecting the hip. Primary DJD is distinguished from secondary DJD by eliminating predisposing factors and is considered a result of aging alone; *secondary osteoarthritis* is the term used when the condition follows previous damage by disease or mechanical disorders.

The etiology of DJD of the hip varies, and in many patients the etiology is unclear. Age is an important factor, but the pathologic process of DJD is not a result of tissue changes with aging *per se*. In fact, the cartilaginous changes occurring with normal aging are seen first in the "nonarticular" areas of cartilage, whereas changes found in DJD are seen first in areas of cartilage that undergo most frequent contact—for example, during weight-bearing.[1,5,14,17,43,45,61,74] DJD is a disease of older persons, because it takes a long time to cause the fatigue of tissue, such as fibrillation of articular cartilage, characteristic of the disease.[28]

The asymptomatic changes occurring with normal aging of articular cartilage probably result from a nutritional deficiency; the areas of cartilage not undergoing frequent intermittent compression do not undergo the absorption and squeezing out of synovial fluid necessary for adequate nutrition. This is especially true in older persons, because they tend to use their joints less frequently and through smaller ranges of movement.

The degenerative tissue changes that occur with primary DJD are usually reactions to increased stress to the joint over time.[14,17,42,45,48,59] The tissue changes may be of a "compensatory" hypertrophic nature, such as the bony proliferation that typically occurs at the joint margins and subchondral bone or capsular fibrosis. They may also be of an atrophic nature, such as the fatigue of cartilaginous collagen fibers or the degradation of cartilage ground substance (proteoglycan). Perhaps the most disputed issue with respect to pathogenesis is whether the first tissue changes occur in the subchondral bone or in the articular cartilage. It is generally accepted, however, that regardless of which tissue changes occur first, they take place first and foremost in the regions undergoing greatest stress with normal activities, and changes in subchondral bone will, over time, result in changes in articular cartilage, and vice versa.[61,68] Normal attenuation of the forces applied to a joint depends on the elastic properties of subchondral bone as well as those of articular cartilage. If stresses are not normally attenuated in one of these tissues, the other will undergo increased stresses.[58,59] Thus, with subchondral bony sclerosis, the overlying articular cartilage undergoes increased stress as the subchondral bone becomes stiffer and less elastic. With fibrillation and softening of articular cartilage, increased stress is transmitted to the subchondral bone. Such abnormal stresses inevitably lead to progression of the process (see Chapter 3, Arthrology).

It is interesting to note the difference in eventual reaction to increased stress between subchondral bone and articular cartilage: subchondral bone becomes more dense (sclerotic), whereas articular cartilage breaks down. This difference reflects the differences in the vascularity and regenerative capacities of the two tissues.

If one accepts that in many, if not most, cases of DJD the pathogenesis is closely related to increased stress to joint tissues over time (or fatigue), then conditions that may predispose the joint to increased stresses must be considered as possible contributors to the etiology of DJD. Perhaps the most important condition at the hip to consider in this regard is congenital hip dysplasia.[5,19,26,45] A deficient acetabular roof and increased femoral antetorsion angle are common sequelae of this condition. The resultant decrease in effective weight-bearing surface area at the joint predisposes the posterosuperolateral femoral head and superolateral acetabulum to early degenerative changes. Residual structural changes in joint components that may follow osteochondrosis or slipped femoral capital epiphysis—both of which affect younger persons—may have similar effects.

Leg-length disparity may be a factor in predisposing to unilateral DJD of the hip on the side of the longer leg.[18,20] In the standing position, the pelvic obliquity produced by the leg-length discrepancy would cause the long limb to assume a position of relative adduction with respect to the acetabulum. The increased adduction angulation on weight-bearing results in an increased joint incongruence, causing greater stress to the lateral roof of the acetabulum. In addition, the center of gravity is shifted toward the short-leg side, increasing the moment arm about which the force of the superincumbent body weight acts at the supporting femoral head on the long-leg side (see section on Biomechanics). A greater pull by the abductors on the long side then is required to prevent the pelvis from dropping to the short side during stance on the long side. This would increase the vertical compressive force acting at the femoral head during weight-bearing on the long-leg side.

Another condition that may contribute to accelerated hip degeneration is capsular tightness.[5,39,56] Traditionally, capsular tightness has been regarded as more of a *result* than a *cause* of hip degeneration. While this is true, the clinician must consider the role that capsular tightening may play in accelerating the progression of the disease and in some cases in actually initiating the degenerative process. The hip, unlike the shoulder, is a joint that is continually brought close to its close-packed position during normal functional activities, such as walking. With every step, at push-off, the hip is brought into a position of extension, internal rotation, and abduction, taking up most of the slack in the joint capsule by twisting the capsule on itself. The twisting of the capsule effects a compression of the joint surfaces. The compression force is normally in addition to, but acts after, the peak vertical compressive force of weight-bearing. In other words, the peak compressive loading due to capsular twisting is normally not superimposed on that of weight-bearing; rather, these forces are successively applied to the joint during the stance phase.[45,56] This is in accordance with the viscoelastic property of articular cartilage, which favors gradual loading over time as opposed to quick "shock-loading" with respect to its ability to attenuate compressive forces.[58–60] If for whatever reason the hip joint capsule loses extensibility, the slack will be taken up in the joint capsule sooner and the joint surfaces will become *prematurely* approximated during walking. This premature approximation causes the peak compressive loading from capsular twisting to become closer to being superimposed on the peak compressive loading of weight-bearing. It causes a greater magnitude of compressive forces to be applied to the articular cartilage over a shorter period of time, approximating a situation of shock-loading. Certain studies suggest that shock-loading, even more than loss of normal lubrication, is one of the most important factors in fatigue of articular cartilage.[60]

Symptoms of pain on weight-bearing in the presence of hip DJD are not due to compressive forces *per se* but result from strain to the capsuloligamentous structures as they pull prematurely tight with each step (recall that articular cartilage is aneural). Such capsular pain is enhanced by the low-grade capsular inflammation that tends to develop as the disease progresses.[5] Studies in which compressive forces have been calculated in degenerated hips before surgery and then determined after total hip arthroplasty suggest that such surgery does reduce the "flexor moment" acting at the hip from a tight capsule.[56] This may explain the often dramatic symptomatic improvement enjoyed by these patients soon after surgery.

A major goal of conservative management in the earlier stages of hip DJD should be prevention and reduction of capsular tightening of the joint. Such an approach, in addition to providing symptomatic improvement, may help slow the acceleration of the degenerative process; the effective weight-bearing surface area of cartilage is increased, and shock-loading is decreased.

Longstanding obesity may also contribute to accelerated degenerative changes at the hip. Because of the moment arm about which the force of gravity on the body weight acts at the femoral head during stance phase, an additional 3 pounds may act at the supporting femoral head for each added pound of body weight.

I. History

A. *Onset of symptoms.* The patient is usually a middle-aged or older person who describes an insidious onset of groin or trochanteric pain. The pain is first noticed after use of the joint, such as long periods of walking, hiking, or running. The patient may relate some childhood hip problem or an old injury, but more often does not.

B. *Site of pain.* The pain is typically felt first in the groin. As the problem progresses, the pain is more likely to be referred farther into the L2 or L3 segment, to the anterior thigh and knee. Later, other segments may become involved, with pain felt laterally and posteriorly. An occasional patient presents with a primary complaint of knee pain—this is because both the knee and the hip are largely derived embryologically from the same segment. Rarely is pain referred below the knee in a person with only hip joint disease.

C. *Nature of pain.* The pain is noticed first at the end of the day, after considerable use of the joint; relief is obtained by rest. Later, as some low-grade inflammation develops, the patient notices some morning stiffness. At this point, pain and stiffness are noticed when getting up from sitting; the pain largely subsides after several steps (after "getting the joint loosened up"), then returns again after walking a certain distance. As the degeneration becomes more advanced, some constant aching may be noticed. The pain is increased by any amount of walking, and the patient is frequently awakened with pain at night.

With progressive capsular tightness, the patient first notices some difficulty squatting—for instance, when picking up an object from the ground. Gradually, it becomes more difficult to put on stockings and tie shoes. The ability to climb stairs may be lost in the later stages, and the patient may be able to ambulate only with the assistance of canes or crutches. Some discomfort with sitting may develop as hip flexion becomes restricted.

II. Physical Examination

A. *Observation*

1. The patient may hesitate or have difficulty when rising from sitting and initiating ambulation.

2. An abduction or antalgic gait, a swinging type of gait if the hip is stiff, a lurching of the trunk toward the affected side if there is any shortening of the limb, or a Trendelenburg gait if any weakness of the abductors is present may be noted.

3. The patient may have some difficulty removing shoes, socks, and slacks.

4. Note use of aids.

B. *Inspection*
  1. Some localized (abductor or gluteal) or generalized atrophy may be noticed on the involved side. Document thigh girth, if appropriate.
  2. If significant adduction and flexion contractures are present, the patient may tend to stand with the heel raised, the hip laterally rotated, and the pelvis elevated on the involved side.
  3. If a flexion contracture and adduction contracture are present, and the patient stands with both feet flat and knees extended, the lumbar spine will be in some hyperlordosis, the pelvis will be shifted laterally toward the involved side (noticed in plumbbob alignment), and the spine will be functionally scoliotic so as to bring the upper trunk back to the midline.
  4. Assess levels of bony landmarks for leg-length equality. If this is unequal, attempt to determine the source of the discrepancy.
C. *Selective tissue tension tests.* The capsular pattern of restriction of the hip is one in which the greatest loss is that of abduction, flexion, and internal rotation. These motions are always limited, although the order of restriction may vary. The one exception is the medial type of osteoarthritis in which the head of the femur is displaced into the deepened acetabular cavity, so that rotation, in both directions, and abduction tend to be most limited.[8]
  1. Active movements
    a. Assess functional activities
      i. Squatting—usually unable to perform in moderate to advanced cases
      ii. One-legged stance. Pelvis will drop to the opposite side if the abductors are significantly weak (positive Trendelenburg sign).
      iii. Stair climbing—may be restricted in advanced cases
      iv. Sit and bend forward—usually painful or restricted
    b. Note ability to perform, pain, and crepitus.
  2. Passive movements
    a. Limited in a capsular pattern of restriction
      i. May be limited by pain and spasm—acute
      ii. May be limited by soft-tissue restriction and discomfort—chronic
    b. Note pain, crepitus, range of motion, and end feel.
  3. Resisted movements—strong and painless
  4. Joint-play movements
    a. Hypomobility of all joint-play movements
    b. Note whether they are restricted by pain and spasm or by soft-tissue restriction.
D. *Neuromuscular tests*
  1. If at this point a possible coexistent spinal lesion is suspected, motor, sensory, and reflex testing, in addition to other tests, may be warranted.
  2. Assess the patient's "balance" (*e.g.,* one-legged standing with eyes closed); this is often affected due to alteration in afferent input from the joint capsule receptors and controlling muscles.[11]
  3. Mild to even moderate muscle weakness of the large muscle groups controlling the hip must be tested by heavy, repetitive loading. Weakness, especially of the abductors, will be found in all but minor cases.
E. *Palpation*
  1. Often noncontributory
  2. Possibly some warmth anteriorly
  3. Usually some tenderness anteriorly, over the trochanter and buttock; possibly some "trigger points" of referred tenderness elsewhere in the thigh
F. *Other*
  1. Compare roentgenographic findings with clinical findings. However, early DJD can be detected clinically before roentgenograms show positive findings, and rather extensive changes may show on roentgenograms in the absence of significant symptoms. Migration of the femoral head upward in relation to the pelvis, which may be observed on radiographs due to degeneration as seen in osteoarthritis, is referred to as the "teardrop" sign (Fig. 12-13).[24]
  2. Because of the loss of hip extension characteristic of DJD and the compensatory hyperlordosis that develops when standing, these patients are predisposed to the development of back problems. A back evaluation may be warranted.
III. **Management.** Management depends on the stage of the disease as determined by the extent of the lesion and the degree of disability. In early disease, pain is noticed only with fatigue. There is only mild limitation of internal rotation, extension, and abduction associated with pain at the extremes of these movements. The patient walks

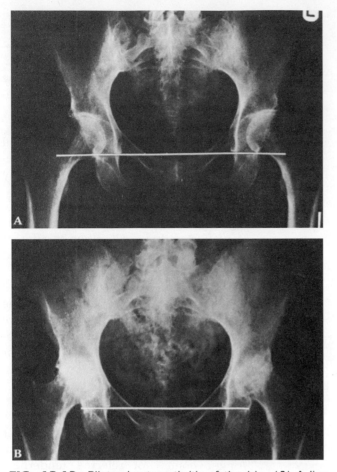

FIG. 12-13. Bilateral osteoarthritis of the hip. (**A**) A line has been drawn between the two "teardrops" and extended into the femoral neck. Note the left hip has migrated more superiorly than the right. (**B**) At a later date, both hips have moved upward as a result of loss of bone at the apex. The left hip is now higher than the right, confirming the original observation that the process of destruction in the left hip was ahead of that in the right. (Bruebel-Lee DM: Disorders of the Hip. Philadelphia, JB Lippincott, 1983:61)

with little or no limp. In advanced disease, there is constant aching, the patient is often awakened at night, and there is considerable morning stiffness. Motion is markedly limited in a capsular pattern. Ambulation is performed with a marked limp or with the use of canes or crutches.

These criteria reflect the two extremes; many patients fall somewhere between these. Information from roentgenograms is not included as a criterion, since it cannot be reliably correlated to symptoms, signs, degree of disability, or prognosis.

The major difficulty facing the physical therapist is that rarely is a patient with *mild* DJD of the hip seen—and this is the patient to whom therapists ultimately have the most to offer. The reason

for this is twofold: (1) considerable progression of the disease may ensue before the patient experiences sufficient pain or disability to warrant seeking medical help, and (2) physicians often do not refer patients with symptoms and signs of early DJD to physical therapists because therapists in the past have not met their potential in managing these patients. Too often the patient is issued a cane and advised to return if the condition worsens, at which time surgical intervention may be indicated.

A. *Early stages*
  1. Goals
     a. Restore normal joint mechanics
     b. Prevent further progression of the disease—capsular tightness or other possible causes of increased stress to the joint
  2. Therapeutic procedures
     a. Restore normal capsular mobility with joint mobilization and active and active-assisted range of motion program. Ultrasound should be helpful in increasing capsular mobility when used during or before mobilization procedures.
     b. Restore normal muscle strength with progressive-resistive exercise program. Emphasize abductor strengthening.
     c. Range of motion exercises to be done indefinitely, instruction in appropriate levels, and other measures to minimize compressive stress to the hip
     d. Attempt to determine if there is an underlying biomechanical or constitutional factor that may predispose the joint to abnormal stresses.
        i. Obesity. For each additional pound of body weight, an additional 3 pounds is applied to each hip joint during stance phase of normal walking. Although few physical therapists are qualified to institute a weight-loss program, the patient can be directed to the appropriate services, on agreement by the physician. A general conditioning program may be supervised by the therapist as an adjunct to a weight-loss program. The patient must be shown simple exercises to help maintain hip range of motion; these are to be done indefinitely on a regular basis.
        ii. Leg-length disparity. Inequality of leg length may be a factor in devel-

opment of DJD on the long-leg side. Gradual, serial elevation of the heel and sole on the uninvolved (short) side, by ¼ inch at a time, may be indicated, along with regular range of motion exercises.

iii. Congenital hip dysplasia and epiphyseolysis (slipped capital epiphysis). Both of these conditions result in permanent structural abnormalities that often lead to increased stress to joint surfaces at the superolateral aspect of the hip joint. Some increased congruity of joint surfaces may be achieved by elevating the heel and sole of the shoe on the uninvolved side in unilateral cases. This places the involved hip in a relative position of abduction, as well as automatically shifting the center of gravity line closer to the involved hip so as to reduce the moment arm about which it acts during stance phase on the involved side.

Since these patients are more or less permanently predisposed to accelerated degenerative changes, they should be encouraged to avoid activities that may be particularly stressful to the hip. Jogging and long-distance walking should be abandoned in favor of swimming and non-weight-bearing exercises. For patients whose regular activities involve considerable walking, alternative modes of travel and perhaps use of a cane should be encouraged.

These patients especially must maintain good strength and motion at their hips for maximal stabilization and maximal distribution of weight-bearing forces over joint surfaces.

B. *Moderate to advanced stages*

Unfortunately, the patient is often given the impression that he or she must simply wait until the disease progresses to a point at which surgery is indicated. Accordingly, the patient is often not referred to rehabilitative services, again because therapists have not demonstrated in the past that they have much to offer these patients. When these patients are referred to physical therapy, it is often simply for instruction in the use of a cane.

Our approach to these patients must be more comprehensive and vigorous. Surgery becomes inevitable unless appropriate measures are taken in the early or moderate stages of the disease. Even so, one may simply be delaying a potentially inevitable event. But one must also consider that these patients are usually middle-aged or older and that if progression of the disease can be retarded and a satisfactory level of function maintained, the patient may very well live out his or her life without undergoing major surgery.

1. Goals
    a. Restore function to optimal level
    b. Restore joint mechanics to optimal level
2. Therapeutic procedures
    a. Instruct the patient in the use of the appropriate walking aid to reduce compressive loading at the hip, to relieve pain on ambulation, and to increase ambulation endurance.
    b. A raised toilet seat may be desirable.
    c. The patient may be made aware of special adaptations in shoe fasteners and devices to help put on and take off shoes and socks. An occupational therapist can be of assistance.
    d. The use of other adaptive aids and devices should be instituted if they may help the patient to perform daily activities with less pain or difficulty.
    e. Primary considerations in regard to improving joint mechanics include increasing capsular extensibility and increasing the strength of the muscles controlling the hip. The basic program is outlined above under management in the early stages. In moderate or advanced stages, however, the joint is likely to be more "irritable," in that motion tends to be limited more by pain and muscle spasm than by a pure capsular restriction. For this reason, progression of the mobilization program must often proceed more slowly. In addition, at some point in more advanced cases, motion in some planes may reach a point at which it is restricted by bony impingement because of the bony hypertrophic changes characteristic of the disease.

    In most respects, the approach to management of these patients should closely resemble that of patients with a frozen shoulder. The primary differences are functional considerations and the concern for reducing compressive forces in patients with hip disease. However, there is no reason not to proceed with an intensive mobilization and strengthening program in cases of capsular hip restriction, as is done routinely with patients with capsular tightness at the shoulder. Remember that it is the tight capsule in cases of DJD at the hip that is a primary source of pain; it is a chief factor in intensifying and localizing compressive forces at the hip joint during walking.

Surgery should be considered in patients with severe pain or disability or who fail to respond to conservative treatment. Total hip replacement is the treatment of choice in older patients, while a femoral osteotomy may still have a role in surgical management.[8]

☐ Trochanteric Bursitis

Trochanteric bursitis is one of the few other common musculoskeletal disorders affecting the hip region for which patients are often referred to physical therapy.[64]

I. **History**
  A. *Onset*—usually insidious. Occasionally an acute onset is described in association with a particular activity, such as getting out of a car, during which a "snap" is felt at the lateral or posterolateral hip region. Presumably such an incident involves a snapping of a portion of the iliotibial band over the trochanter, with mechanical irritation of the intervening bursa.
  B. *Site of pain*—primarily over the lateral hip region. It tends to radiate distally into the L5 segment; the patient describes pain over the lateral aspect of the thigh to the knee and occasionally into the lower leg. Some patients also experience pain referred into the lumbosacral region on the side of involvement. This pain pattern closely resembles that of an L5 spinal lesion, which is a more common disorder than trochanteric bursitis and which must be differentiated by means of careful examination.
  C. *Nature of pain*—aggravated most by ascending stairs (the strongly contracting gluteus maximus compresses the inflamed bursa) and by rolling onto the involved side at night. Indeed, the greatest complaint is often that of

being awakened at night with pain. The pain is a deep, aching, "scleratogenous" pain rather than the sharp, lancinating, dermatomal pain characteristic of L5 nerve root irritation.

II. **Physical Examination**
  A. *Observation*—usually noncontributory. The lesion is not severe enough to cause a limp.
  B. *Inspection*—usually noncontributory. If the iliotibial band is tight, the patient may stand with the pelvis shifted laterally, away from the involved side on mediolateral plumb-bob assessment, with perhaps some increased valgus of the knee on the involved side.
  C. *Selective tissue tension tests*
    1. Active movements—no functional limitations
    2. Passive movements
      a. Full passive abduction may cause pain from squeezing of the bursa between the trochanter and the lateral aspect of the pelvis.
      b. Placement of the hip into full passive flexion combined with adduction and internal rotation compresses the inflamed bursa beneath the stretched gluteus maximus.
      c. An Ober test may reveal iliotibial band tightness.
    3. Resisted movements
      a. Resisted abduction will reproduce the pain by squeezing the bursa beneath the strongly contracting gluteals.
      b. Resisted extension and resisted external rotation may cause pain if the bursa underlying the gluteus maximus is involved.
    4. Joint-play movements—mobility is normal and painless.
  D. *Neuromuscular examination*—noncontributory
  E. *Palpation.* A discrete point of tenderness is found over the site of the lesion, usually over the posterolateral aspect of the greater trochanter. Other areas of referred tenderness are often found elsewhere in the L5 segment, usually over the lateral aspect of the thigh. No increased temperature can be detected.

III. **Management**
  A. *Goals*
    1. Resolve the chronic inflammatory process
    2. Prevent recurrence
  B. *Techniques*
    1. Temporarily avoid continued irritation to the bursa
      a. Arrange pillows so as to avoid rolling onto the painful side

b. Avoid climbing stairs and long walks

c. Ultrasound to the site of the lesion. Ultrasound is often dramatically effective over three to six sessions. The increase in blood flow apparently assists in the resolution of the inflammatory process.

2. A tight iliotibial band may be the cause or the result of the disorder.[64] Full mobility of the iliotibial band should be restored as the condition resolves. Ensure that good muscle strength of the gluteals is restored, since they may weaken in longstanding cases.

☐ Iliopectineal Bursitis

Iliopectineal bursitis is less common than trochanteric bursitis. It presents in a similar manner, but resisted hip flexion and full passive hip extension reproduce the pain. The onset is insidious. The pain is felt most in the groin, with a tendency toward radiation into the L2 or L3 segment. Since this bursa often communicates with the joint, ascertain whether involvement of the bursa is a manifestation of hip joint effusion by checking for a capsular pattern of pain or restriction. Management should follow the same approach as for trochanteric bursitis.

☐ Muscle Strains

Strains may be defined as damage of some part of the contractile unit caused by overuse (chronic strain) or overstress (acute strain). Strains are graded as mild (first degree), moderate (second degree), and severe (third degree).[54] In severe strains, there is a loss of function of the muscle, tendon, or its attachment caused by a complete tear. The strain occurs at the weakest link of the muscle–tendon unit. Under stress, the muscle may tear, the musculotendinous junction may give way, or the tendon or its bony attachment may be damaged.

The most commonly strained muscles of the hip are the hamstrings, adductor longus, iliopsoas, and rectus femoris.[62,64] Resisted isometric muscle contraction will reproduce the pain as well as passive stretch (except in a complete tear). For a definitive diagnosis of the lesion, muscles must be isolated one at a time. The involved structures are tender to palpation.

Perhaps the muscle strain most dreaded by the athlete is that of the hamstring muscle group.[36] Rehabilitation time is from 2 to 3 weeks for mild injuries, 2 to 6 months for severe conditions. The hamstrings may be injured either at their attachment to the ischial tuberosity or within their midbellies, and less commonly at the knee.[52] Garrett and coworkers[16] found that the injuries were primarily proximal and lateral in the hamstring group.

Potential causes of this injury include decreased flexibility, comparative bilateral strength deficits, lack of coordination, poor posture, fatigue, and inappropriate quadriceps/hamstring strength ratios.[12] The optimum value of the hamstrings to that of the quadriceps muscles (HQ ratio) varies from 50% to 80%; the average is about 60%.[34] After knee injury, quadriceps wasting may result in the two muscle groups producing the same power, giving an HQ ratio of 100%.[5] A deficit above 10% between the two sets of hamstrings also has been cited as a predisposing factor in hamstring strain.[4]

With a hamstring injury, pain is apparent on straight-leg raising and resisted knee flexion. Resisted flexion and tibial rotation determine whether the biceps femoris or inner hamstrings are affected. In severe cases, ecchymosis, hemorrhage, and a muscle defect may be visible several days after the injury. Crutches may be necessary for ambulation.[12]

Treatment of muscle strain follows a common pattern. In acute strains rest, anti-inflammatory agents, and physical methods are prescribed. Initially ice and compression may be indicated. Up to 5 to 7 days after the injury, the muscle remains vulnerable to reinjury because of the loss in loading capabilities and the risk of intermuscular hemorrhage.[35] Warm-up, stretch, resistive exercise, and gradual resumption of activity follow. To prevent random alignment of new collagen fibers, deep friction massage should be used. The consequences of inelastic scar tissue formation within the muscle bellies must be minimized. Improper management can lead to recurrent tears and, in the case of the hamstrings, to a condition known as the hamstring syndrome (entrapment of the sciatic nerve).[36,57] Myofascial release forms of massage, gentle stretching, and phonophoresis can be initiated early to reduce the risk of this occurrence.

With chronic strains, prevention is more important than cure. Gradually building up activities so that the muscle–tendon unit can withstand a heavier workload is a key component of rehabilitation. Closed kinetic chain exercises and eccentric and plyometric training[15,51,73,75] in late-stage rehabilitation for the athlete should be considered.

According to Stanton and Purdam,[69] the use of eccentric exercises as part of a general leg-conditioning program may strengthen the elastic components within the hamstrings, making them better equipped to withstand loading at heel-strike. Schwane and Armstrong[66] showed that eccentric training by downhill running can prevent ultrastructural muscle injury in rats. A study by Jensen and DiFabio[31] indicated that training for eccentric strength can be an effective treatment for patellar tendinitis, and Jonhagen and associates[32] found that sprinters with a history of hamstring injury had tight hamstring muscles and were weaker in eccentric contractions at all velocities (30°, 180°, and 230° per second) compared with uninjured sprinters.

Plyometric training consists of rapid eccentric contraction used immediately before an explosive concentric action. This type of training was first used in Eastern bloc countries in the development of power (speed/strength).[73] The aim of plyometric exercise is to train the patient's nervous system to react with maximum speed to the lengthening of muscle and to develop the muscle's ability to shorten rapidly with maximum force. According to Norris,[51] the rapid stretch of the muscle stimulates a stretch reflex, which in turn generates greater tension within the lengthening muscle fibers. In addition to increased tension, the release of stored energy within the elastic components of muscle makes the concentric contraction greater than it would be in isolation.

Plyometric training is intense and requires flexibility and agility. Exercises should be used only after stretching and a thorough warm-up (usually at the end of an exercise program). Three types of exercises are normally used: in-place, short-response, and long-response.[51] In-place activities include such activities as standing jumps, drop jumps, and hopping. Short-response actions are those such as the standing broad jump and box jumps. Long-response movements include bounding, hopping, and hurdle jumps. Machinery is becoming available that offers a combination of the safety inherent in an isokinetic system and the functional advantages of positive and negative acceleration.[67,77] Plyometrics has a role in late-stage rehabilitation and functional precompetitive testing following injury. Plyometric activity is used primarily for lower-limb training but can also be used for the upper limb and trunk.

☐ Conclusion

The lumbar spine, sacroiliac, and hip joint function as a mechanical unit and should not be assessed or treated in an isolated fashion. Many abnormalities presenting apparently simply as joint pain may be the expression of a comprehensive imbalance of the musculoskeletal system—articulations,[2,6,22,25] ligaments, muscles, fascial planes,[44] intermuscular septa, tendons, and aponeuroses, together with defective neuromuscular control.[30] The iliopsoas is usually the first contracture to develop and can affect the lumbar spine, pelvis, and hip. The inhibitory effect of a tight postural muscle is evidenced when weakness of the gluteus maximus accompanies tightness of the iliopsoas. Many patients with a lateral pelvic tilt of 1 to 2 cm present with early degenerative changes of the hip on the longer side as well as low back and sacroiliac problems.[21,22,55]

■ PASSIVE TREATMENT TECHNIQUES

☐ Joint Mobilization

Like the shoulder joint, techniques performed with the hip in a neutral position are used primarily to promote relaxation of the muscles controlling the joint, to relieve pain, and to prepare for more vigorous stretching techniques. The hip joint is, however, much more stable than the shoulder joint.

(For simplicity, the operator will be referred to as the male, the patient as the female. All the techniques described apply to the patient's *right* extremity, except where indicated. P—patient; O—operator; M—movement.)

  I. Hip Joint—Elevation and Relaxation
    A. *Inferior glide*—in neutral with a belt (Fig. 12-14*A*)
      P—Supine, with hip in resting position and knee extended. A stabilizing belt may be applied to the pelvis.
      O—Standing at the end of the treatment table. A belt describing a figure-of-eight is placed around the operator's waist and above the patient's ankle. The operator's hands are placed under the belt and around the distal end of the tibia and fibula.
      M—A distractive force is applied by leaning backward, thereby creating a pull through the belt to the operator's hands.
    B. *Inferior glide*—in abduction and external rotation (Fig. 12-14*B*)
      P—Supine. A belt may be used to keep the upper body from sliding inferiorly on the plinth. The leg is in slight abduction, external rotation, and flexion.
      O—Grasps the patient's ankle just proximal to the malleoli with the left hand, behind the back. He grasps the femur distally, just proximal to the condyles and from the medial aspect, with the right hand.
      M—The operator's arms remain fixed. An inferior glide is produced by leaning backward with the trunk. This may be done through various degrees of abduction. These techniques are used as general mobi-

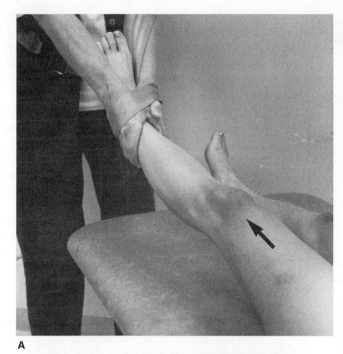

A

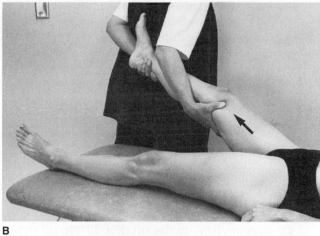

B

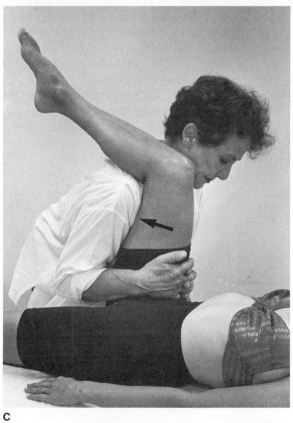

C

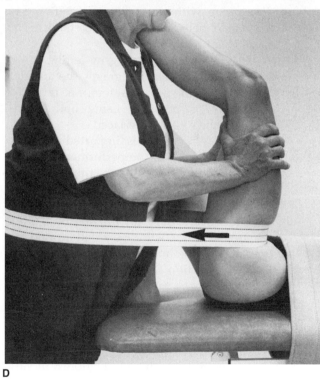

D

FIG. 12-14. Inferior glide of hip joint (**A**) in neutral with a belt, (**B**) in abduction and external rotation, (**C**) in flexion, and (**D**) in flexion with a belt.

lization to increase joint play. Inferior glide is a joint-play movement necessary for hip flexion and abduction. It is also used for relaxation of muscle spasm and pain relief and may be used before and after a treatment session and between other techniques. These procedures should be used on a continuing basis and in conjunction with the stretching techniques described in Techniques I,C and I,D.

Note: If there is a knee dysfunction, Techniques I,A and I,B should not be used; the evaluation position and hand-holds (see Fig. 12-10) may be used as an alternate technique.

C. *Inferior glide*—in flexion (Fig. 12-14C)

P—Supine, with hip and knee each flexed to 90°. A belt may be used to stabilize the upper body.

O—Supports the lower leg by letting it rest on his shoulder. He grasps the anterior aspect of the proximal femur as far proximally as possible, using both hands with the fingers interlaced.

M—An inferior glide is imparted with the hands. This may be performed while simultaneously rocking the thigh into flexion.

This technique is used to increase joint-play movement necessary for hip flexion. An alternate technique is to use a belt around the operator's trunk and the patient's thigh (Fig. 12-14D). Traction is applied via the operator's trunk.

D. *Inferior glide*—in extension

P—Supine. A belt may be used to keep the upper body from sliding inferiorly on the plinth. The leg is extended over the side of the plinth and positioned in various degrees of abduction and internal rotation.

O—Same as for Technique **I,B.**

M—The operator's arms remain fixed. An inferior glide is produced by leaning backward with the trunk. The leg may be progressively moved into various degrees of abduction and internal rotation combined with extension, working toward the close-packed position of the hip joint.

This technique is particularly useful for capsular stretching.

II. Hip Joint—Anterior Glide

A. *Anterior glide*—in supine (Fig. 12-15A)

P—Supine. A belt may be used to stabilize the pelvis.

O—Grasps around posteriorly with both hands to the posterior aspect of the proximal femur, level with the greater trochanter. The fingers are interlaced or overlapping. He stabilizes the distal thigh and knee against the plinth with his trunk.

M—The slack is taken up, and an anterior glide of the proximal femur is imparted with the hands.

This technique is used to increase the joint-play movement necessary for external rotation.

B. *Anterior glide*—in prone (Fig. 12-15B)

P—Prone, with the knee bent to 90°. A 1-inch thickness of toweling may be placed under the anterior aspect of the pelvis, just proximal to the acetabulum, for extra stabilization.

O—Supports the knee with the right hand by grasping around medially to the anterior aspect of the distal femur. He supports the lower leg by tucking it between his elbow and side. The left hand contacts the posterior aspect of the proximal femur with the heel of the hand. It is level with, and medial to, the greater trochanter.

M—The left hand imparts an anterior glide to the proximal femur. The right hand may simultaneously glide the leg into internal rotation or abduction.

Techniques II,B and II,C are considered more progressive than Technique II,A. They are used to increase joint play necessary for external rotation. They also provide a specific capsuloligamentous stretch by internally rotating the femoral head while simultaneously preventing its impingement on the acetabulum.

An alternate technique is to have the patient lie prone with the anterior pelvis at the edge of the table and the limb not being treated resting on the floor. In this position, a belt is placed around the operator's shoulder and the patient's thigh to help support the weight of the limb as force is applied in an anterior direction (Fig. 12-15C).

C. *Anterior glide*—in sidelying (Fig. 12-15D)

P—Lying on the left side, the bottom limb comfortably positioned and the right leg supported on the table near the limit of hip extension

O—Standing behind the patient. The pelvic girdle is supported with the cranial hand.

M—With the pelvis stabilized, posteroante-

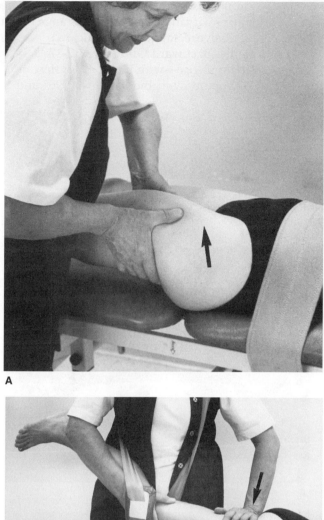

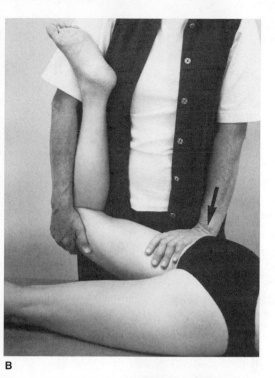

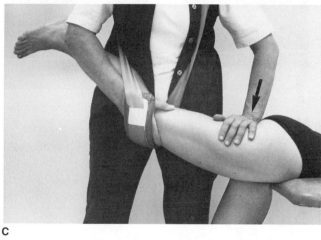

FIG. 12-15. Anterior glide of hip joint (**A**) in supine, (**B**) in prone, (**C**) in prone with a belt, and (**D**) in sidelying positions.

rior pressure of the femur is applied into the capsule with the caudal hand.

III. Hip Joint—Posterior Glide (Fig. 12-16A)

P—Supine. An inch of padding is placed beneath the pelvis just proximal and medial to the acetabulum.

O—Supports the knee and distal thigh with the right hand by grasping around medially to the posterior aspect. He con-

tacts the anterior aspect of the proximal femur with the heel of his left hand, with the forearm supinated.

M—A posterior glide is imparted with the operator's left hand by leaning forward with the trunk.

This technique is used to increase a joint-play movement necessary for internal rotation. An alternate technique is to have the patient

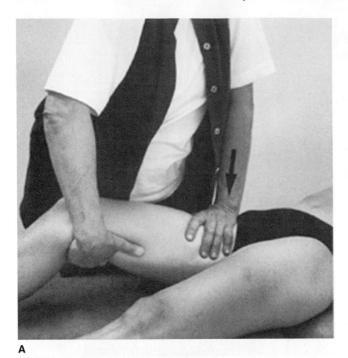

A

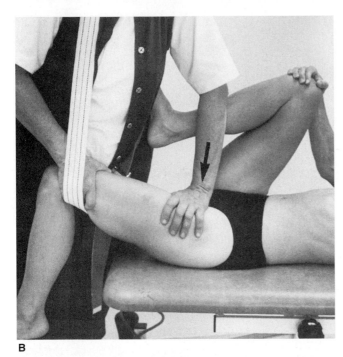

B

FIG. 12-16. Posterior glide of hip joint (**A**) in supine and (**B**) in supine with a belt.

supine, with the hips at the end of the table. The patient helps stabilize her pelvis by flexing the opposite hip and holding the thigh with the hands (Fig. 12-16B). A belt is placed around the operator's shoulder and under the patient's thigh to help support the weight of the limb. The cranial hand applies a posterior force to the patient's anterior proximal thigh. The hip joint is positioned in the resting posi-

tion if conservative techniques are indicated or approximating the restricted range if more aggressive techniques are indicated.

IV. Hip Joint—Backward Glide (Fig. 12-17A)
  A. *Backward glide*—with hip in 90º of flexion
    P—Supine, with the hip flexed 90° and the

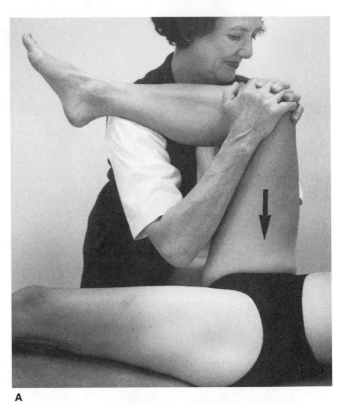

A

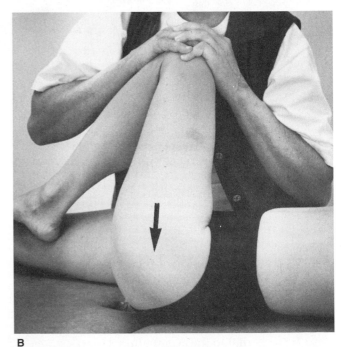

B

FIG. 12-17. Backward glide of the hip joint (**A**) with hip in 90° of flexion, (**B**) with the hip in flexion-adduction with compression.

lower leg supported comfortably on the crook of the operator's elbow

O—Both hands contact the distal end of the femur. He places one hand over the other to provide reinforcement.

M—A backward (dorsal) glide is effected by leaning forward with the trunk, and is assisted by the operator's body weight.

This technique is used to increase joint-play movement necessary for horizontal adduction of the thigh.

B. *Backward glide*—with the hip in flexion-adduction with compression (Fig. 12-17B)

P—Supine, with the hip flexed and adducted and the knee fully flexed

O—Standing on the opposite side of the table, hands clasped over the anterior knee

M—The operator begins by allowing body weight to compress through the long axis of the femur in a backward and lateral direction. The hip is taken into adduction until resistance is felt. The hip is moved further into flexion while adduction and compression are maintained.

Scouring (the quadrant test; see Fig. 12-12)

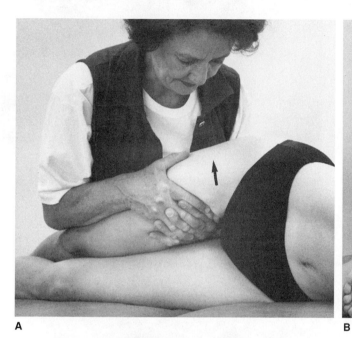

A

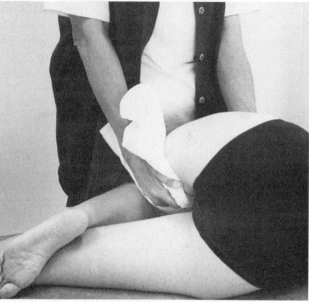

B

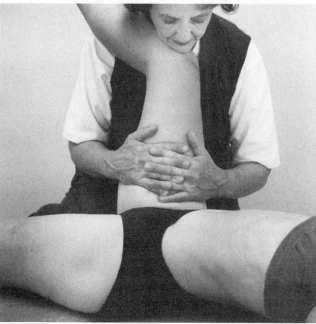

C

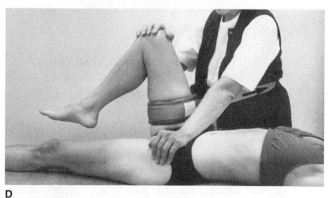

D

FIG. 12-18. Distraction of the femur (**A**) in neutral, (**B**) in neutral (alternative technique), (**C**) in flexion, and (**D**) in flexion with a belt.

may be used as a treatment technique. The operator attempts to identify the small arch of pain and stiffness. Once this arc is identified, the operator may rock back and forth over it, trying to smooth it out. This technique is useful in restoring osteokinematic function of the femur but should not be used when pain is the predominant factor.

V. **Distraction Techniques**

   A. *Distraction*—in neutral (Fig. 12-18A)

     P—Sidelying

     O—Standing behind the patient. The fingers are interlocked so that the anterior aspect of the forearm is in contact with the patient's thigh.

     M—The operator lifts (distracts) with his clasped hands while simultaneously depressing the patient's knee with his elbow. An alternate technique uses the patient's knee as a fulcrum against the operator's lower abdomen (Fig. 12-18B).[23] With the elbows extended, the operator contacts the medial aspect of the upper thigh (a towel is placed on the medial aspect). By backward leaning of the trunk, distraction is performed in the line of the head of the femur.

   B. *Distraction* (lateral glide)—in flexion (Fig. 12-18C)

     P—Supine, hip and knee flexed, leg positioned against the operator's trunk

     O—Both hands grasp the upper adductor mass with clasped hands.

     M—Mobilization force is applied by leaning at an angle lateral and distal (parallel with the neck of the femur). An alternate technique is to use a belt (Fig. 12-18D).

   Distraction techniques are used to increase range of motion into hip adduction and internal rotation, to increase joint play, and to decrease pain in the hip joint.

VI. **Medial Glide** (Fig. 12-19A)

     P—Sidelying with the lower leg bent, hip at end range abduction

     O—The caudal hand cradles the lower leg or knee and supports the weight of the limb. The cranial hand contacts the lateral aspect of the hip at the greater trochanter.

     M—Glide the femoral head inferiorly and medially.

   This is primarily a medial capsular stretch to help restore abduction. A more vigorous capsular stretch may be achieved by abducting and rotating the limb near its end range (Fig. 12-19B).

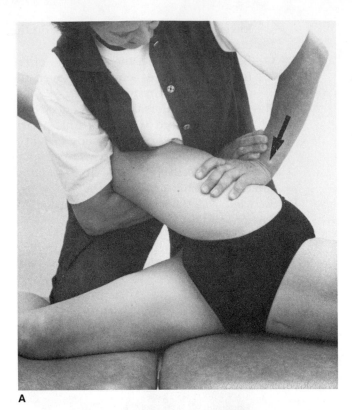

A

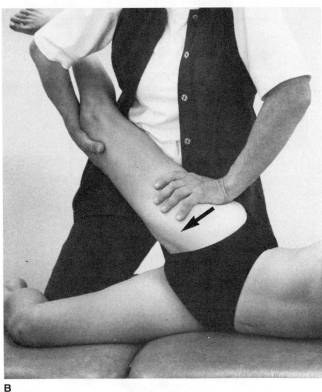

B

FIG. 12-19. *Medial glide of the femur.*

VII. Rotation Techniques

A. *Lateral rotation* (Fig. 12-20*A*)

P—Prone, knee flexed to 90°

O—Rotates the lower leg until the buttock rises slightly from the table

M—While maintaining the position of the lower leg, the cranial hand applies downward pressure over the ipsilateral buttocks to the table.

B. *Medial rotation* (Fig. 12-20*B*)

P—Prone, knee flexed to 90°

O—Rotates the lower leg until the contralateral buttock comes slightly off the table

M—While maintaining this position with the caudal hand, the cranial hand applies downward pressure toward the table over the contralateral buttock.

These techniques are used primarily to

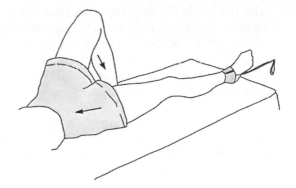

FIG. 12-21. Inferior glide or long-axis extension.

stretch the soft tissues of the hip joint, using a short lever system to help restore internal and external rotation.

☐ Self-Mobilization Techniques

I. Inferior Glide or Long-Axis Extension (Fig. 12-21)

P—A comfortable, snug-fitting ankle strap and a stationary wall or table hook for attachment to the ankle strap are needed. The patient lies supine with the right leg extended and the ankle strap attached to the end of the table or wall hook. The left lower extremity is flexed, with the foot on the table or floor.

M—The left leg pushes downward and upward to push the body away from the fixed point, thus transmitting a traction force on the right lower extremity.

II. Distraction in Sidelying (Fig. 12-22)

P—Lying on the right side, close to one side of the table. A firm pillow or blanket roll is placed between the legs in the groin area. The left hip is extended at the hip with the lower leg off the edge of the table. A sandbag or ankle cuff with a weight is applied to the left ankle.

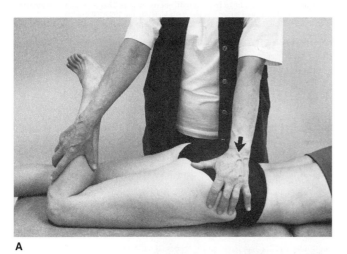

A

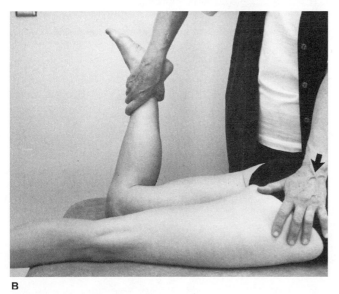

B

FIG. 12-20. Rotation techniques: (**A**) lateral, (**B**) medial rotations.

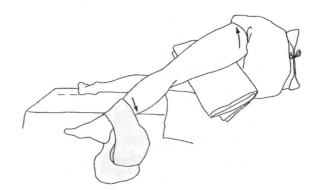

FIG. 12-22. Distraction in sidelying.

M—The left leg is actively raised against the pull of the weight and held for a few seconds; the patient then relaxes, allowing the leg to fall into adduction, with the hip in slight extension, over the edge of the table. Slight oscillatory motion will occur naturally at the end of range.

This technique is a combination of distraction and a muscle-strengthening exercise. In this case, the gluteus medius, which is commonly weak in most hip conditions, is exercised.

REFERENCES

1. Barnett CH: Effects of age on articular cartilage. Res Rev 4:183, 1963
2. Bartlett MD: Hip flexion contractors: A comparison of measurement methods. Arch Phys Med Rehabil 64:521, 1983
3. Beattie P, Isaacson K, Riddle DL, et al: Validity of derived measurement of leg-length differences obtained by use of a tape measure. Phys Ther 70:150–157, 1990
4. Burkett LN: Causative factors in hamstring strains. Med Sci Sports Exer 2:39–42, 1970
5. Burnie J, Brodie DA: Isokinetic measurement in preadolescent males. Int J Sports Med 7:205–209, 1986
5. Cameron HU, MacNab I: Observations on osteoarthritis of the hip joint. Clin Orthop 108:31–40, 1975
6. Chadwick P: The significance of spinal joint signs in the management of groin strain and patellofemoral pain by manual techniques. Physiotherapy 73:507–513, 1987
7. Clarke GR: Unequal leg length: An accurate method of detection and some clinical results. Rheumatol Phys Med 11:385–390, 1972
8. Corrigan B, Maitland GD: Practical Orthopedics. Boston, Butterworths, 1985
9. Cusick BD: Progressive Casting and Splinting for Lower-Extremity Deformities in Children with Neuromuscular Dysfunction. Tucson, AZ, Therapy Skill Builders, 1990
10. Cyriax JH, Cyriax PJ: Illustrated Manual of Orthopedic Medicine. Boston, Butterworths, 1983
11. Dee R: Mechanoreceptors of the hip joint capsule and their reflex contribution to posture. In Symposium on Osteoarthritis. St. Louis, CV Mosby, 1976:52–65
12. Ellison AE, Boland AL, DeHaven KE, et al (eds): Athletic Training and Sports Medicine. Chicago, American Academy of Orthopaedic Surgery, 1986
13. Fisk JW, Balgert ML: Clinical and radiological assessment of leg length. NZ Med J 81:477–480, 1975
14. Freeman MAR: The fatigue of cartilage in the pathogenesis of osteoarthritis. Acta Orthop Scand 46:323–328, 1975
15. Gamble JN: Strength and conditioning for the competitive athlete. In Kulund DN (ed): The Injured Athlete, 2nd ed. Philadelphia, JB Lippincott, 1988:11–150
16. Garrett WE, Mumma M, Lucareche CL: Ultrastructural differences in human skeletal muscle fiber types. Orthop Clin North Am 14:412–425, 1989
17. Gofton JP, Trueman GE: Studies in osteoarthritis of the hip: I. Classification. Can Med Assoc J 104:679–683, 1971
18. Gofton JP, Trueman GE: Studies in osteoarthritis of the hip: II. Osteoarthritis of the hip and leg-length disparity. Can Med Assoc J 104:791–799, 1971
19. Gofton JP, Trueman GE: Studies in osteoarthritis of the hip: III. Congenital subluxation and osteoarthritis of the hip disparity. Can Med Assoc J 104:911–915, 1971
20. Gofton JP, Trueman GE: Studies in osteoarthritis of the hip: IV. Biomechanics and clinical considerations. Can Med Assoc J 104:1007–1011, 1971
21. Grieve GP: The hip. Physiotherapy 69:196–204, 1983
22. Grieve GP: Common Vertebral Joint Problems. Edinburgh, Churchill Livingstone, 1981
23. Grieve GP: Mobilisation of the Spine: A Primary Handbook of Clinical Method, 5th ed. Edinburgh, Churchill Livingstone, 1991
24. Gruebel-Lee DM: Disorders of the Hip. Philadelphia, JB Lippincott, 1983
25. Gunn CC, Milbrandt WE: Bursitis around the hip. Am J Acupuncture 5:53–60, 1977
26. Hoagland FT: Osteoarthritis. Orthop Clin North Am 2:3–19, 1971
27. Hoppenfield S: Physical examination of the hip and pelvis. In Hoppenfield S (ed): Physical Examination of the Spine and Extremities. New York, Appleton-Century-Crofts, 1976
28. Inman VT: Functional aspects of abductor muscles of the hip. J Bone Joint Surg 29A:607–619, 1947
29. Janda V: Muscle Function Testing. Boston, Butterworths, 1983
30. Janda V: Muscles, central nervous motor regulation and back problems. In Knorr I (ed): The Neurobiologic Mechanisms in Manipulative Therapy. London, Plenum Press, 1978
31. Jensen K, DiFabio RP: Evaluation of eccentric exercise in treatment of patellar tendinitis. Phys Ther 69:211–216, 1989
32. Jonhagen S, Nemeth G, Eriksson E: Hamstring injuries in sprinters: The role of concentric and eccentric hamstring muscle strength and flexibility. Am J Sports Med 10:75–78, 1994
33. Jordon RP, Cusack J, Rosseque B: Foot function and its relationship to posture in the pediatric patient with cerebral palsy and other neuromuscular disorders. Lecture notes and instructional materials from Neurodevelopmental Treatment Association meeting, New York, 1983
34. Kannus P: Hamstring/quadriceps strength ratios in knees with medial collateral ligament insufficiency. J Sports Med Phys Fitness 29:194–198, 1989
35. Krejci V, Koch P: Muscle and tendon injuries in athletes. Chicago, Year Book Medical Publishers, 1979
36. Lambert SD: Athletic injuries to the hip. In Echternach JL (ed): Clinics in Physical Therapy: Physical Therapy of the Hip. New York, Churchill Livingstone, 1990:143–164
37. LeVeau B: Application of statics. In Lissner HR, Williams M (eds): Biomechanics of Human Motion, 2nd ed. Philadelphia, WB Saunders, 1977:100–102
38. Lissner HR, Williams M: Biomechanics of Human Motion. Philadelphia, WB Saunders, 1962:44–45
39. Lloyd-Roberts GC: The role of capsular changes in osteoarthritis of the hip joint. J Bone Joint Surg 35B:627–642, 1953
40. McCrea JD: Pediatric Orthopedics of the Lower Extremity: An Instructional Handbook. Mount Kisco, NY, Futura, 1985
41. Magee DJ: Orthopedic Physical Assessment. Philadelphia, WB Saunders, 1987
42. Mankin HJ: Biochemical and metabolic aspects of osteoarthritis. Orthop Clin North Am 2(1):19–31, 1971
43. Mankin HJ: Biochemical changes in articular cartilage in osteoarthritis. In Symposium on Osteoarthritis. St. Louis, CV Mosby, 1976:1–23
44. Mennell JB: Physical Treatment, Movement, Manipulation, and Massage. Philadelphia, Blakiston Co, 1947
45. Morris JM: Biomechanical aspects of the hip joint. Orthop Clin North Am 2:33–55, 1971
46. Morscher E, Figner B: Measurement of leg length. Prog Orthop Surg 1:21–27, 1977
47. Mundale MO, Hislop HJ, Rabideau RJ, Kottke FJ: Evaluation of extension of hip. Arch Phys Med Rehabil 37:75–80, 1956
48. Murray RO, Duncan C: Athletic activity in adolescence as an etiological factor in degenerative hip disease. J Bone Joint Surg 53B:406–419, 1971
49. Nichols PJ: The short leg syndrome. Br Med J 1:1963, 1960
50. Noble HB, Hajek MR, Porter M: Diagnosis and treatment of iliotibial band tightness in runners. Phys Sports Med 10:67–74, 1982
51. Norris CM: Physical training and injury. In Norris CM (ed): Sports Injuries: Diagnosis and Management for Physiotherapists. Oxford, Butterworth-Heinemann, 1993:89–116
52. Norris CM: The hip. In Norris CM (ed): Sports Injuries: Diagnosis and Management for Physiotherapists. Oxford, Butterworth-Heinemann, 1993:160–168
53. Ober FB: The role of the iliotibial and fascia lata as a factor in causation of low-back disabilities and sciatica. J Bone Joint Surg 18A: 105–110, 1936
54. O'Donoghue DH: Treatment of injuries to athletes, 4th ed. Philadelphia, WB Saunders, 1984
55. Patriquinn D: Differential diagnosis of lateral hip, inguinal and proximal anterior thigh pain. Proceedings of the 7th International Congress, Physical Medicine and Rehabilitation, Stockholm, 1980
56. Paul JP: Forces transmitted at the hip and knee of normal and disabled persons during a range of activities. Acta Orthop Belg [Suppl] 41(1):78–88, 1975
57. Puranen J, Orava S: The hamstring syndrome: A new diagnosis of gluteal sciatic pain. Am J Sports Med 16:517–521, 1988
58. Radin EL, Paul IL: Does cartilage compliance reduce skeletal impact loads? Arth Rheum 13(2):139–144, 1970
59. Radin El, Paul IL: The mechanics of joints as it relates to their degeneration. In Symposium on Osteoarthritis. St. Louis, CV Mosby, 1976:34–44
60. Radin El, Paul IL: Response of joints to impact loading. Arth Rheum 14:356–362, 1971
61. Reiman I, Mankin HJ: Quantitative histological analysis of articular cartilage and subchondral bone from osteoarthritic and normal human hips. Acta Orthop Scand 48:63–73, 1977
62. Renstram P, Petyerson L: Groin injuries in athletes. Br J Sports Med 14:30–36, 1980
63. Rydell N: Forces acting on the femoral head prosthesis: A study on strain-gauge supplied prostheses in living persons. Acta Orthop Scand [Suppl] 88:1–132, 1966
64. Sammarco G: The hip in dancers. Medical Problems of Performing Artists 2:5–14, 1987
65. Saudek CE: The hip. In Gould JA, Davies GJ (eds): Orthopedic and Sports Physical Therapy. St. Louis, CV Mosby, 1985
66. Schwane JA, Armstrong RB: Effect of training on skeletal muscle injury from downhill running in rats. J Appl Physiol 55:969–975, 1983
67. Seger JY, Westing SH, Hanson M, Karlson E, et al: A new dynamometer measuring concentric and eccentric muscle strength in accelerated, decelerated, or isokinetic movements. Eur J Appl Physiol 57:526–530, 1988
68. Sokoloff LS: The general pathology of osteoarthritis. In Symposium on Osteoarthritis. St. Louis, CV Mosby, 1976:23–24
69. Stanton P, Purdam C: Hamstring injuries in sprinting: The role of eccentric exercise. J Orthop Sports Phys Ther 10:343–349, 1989
70. Staheli LT: Prone hip extension test: Method of measuring hip flexion deformity. Clin Orthop 123:12–15, 1977
71. Thomas HO: Diseases of Hip, Knee, and Ankle Joints, with Their Deformities (Treated by New and Efficient Method), 2nd ed. Liverpool, Dobb, 1876
72. Van Roy P, Borms J, Haentjens A: Goniometric study of the maintenance of hip flexibility resulting from hamstring stretches. Physiotherapy Practice 3:52–59, 1987
73. Verhoshanski Y, Chornonson G: Jump exercises in sprint training. Track and Field Quarterly 9:1909, 1976
74. Vignon E, Arlot M, Meunier P, Vignon G: Quantitative histologic changes in osteoarthritic hip cartilage. Clin Orthop 103:269–278, 1974
75. Voight ML, Dravitch P: Plyometrics. In Albert MA (ed): Eccentric Muscle Training in Sports and Orthopaedics. London, Churchill Livingstone, 1991:45–73
76. Warren R, Kaye JJ, Saluiati EA: Arthrographic demonstration of an enlarged iliopsoas bursa complicating osteoarthritis of the hip: A case report. J Bone Joint Surg 57A:413–415, 1975
77. Westing SH, Thorstensson A: Iso-acceleration: A new concept in resistive exercise. Med Sci Sports Exer 23:631–635, 1991
78. Woerman AL, Binder-Macleod SA: Leg-length discrepancy assessment: Accuracy and precision in five clinical methods of evaluation. J Orthop Sports Phys Ther 5:230–236, 1983

The Knee

DARLENE HERTLING AND RANDOLPH M. KESSLER

REVIEW OF FUNCTIONAL ANATOMY

Osseous Structures

The distal end of the femur consists of two large condyles, separated posteriorly by the very deep intercondylar notch and anteriorly by the patellar groove, in which the patella glides. The anterior condylar surface is called the *trochlear surface* of the femur.

Looking anteriorly (Fig. 13-1), the medial condyle extends farther distally than does the lateral condyle, so that when standing with the distal surfaces of the condyles level, the femur and tibia form a valgus angle of about 10°. Both condyles have epicondyles extending from their sides. Medially, the adductor tu-

bercle lies just superior to the medial epicondyle. The articular cartilage extends farther superiorly on the anterior surface of the lateral condyle than it does on the same aspect of the medial condyle.

Looking inferiorly (Fig. 13-2), the articular surface of the distal femur forms a U about the deep intercondylar notch. The lateral condyle extends considerably farther anteriorly than does the medial condyle, helping to prevent lateral dislocation of the patella caused by the horizontal component of the direction of quadriceps pull. The medial condyle angles backward and medially. The lateral condyle lies in the sagittal plane.

Looking medially or laterally (Fig. 13-3), the condyles do not describe part of a circle; rather, their radius gradually decreases from anterior to posterior. The medial condyle is longer anteroposteriorly, with a

Darlene Hertling and Randolph M. Kessler: MANAGEMENT OF COMMON
MUSCULOSKELETAL DISORDERS: Physical Therapy Principles and Methods, 3rd ed.
© 1996 Lippincott-Raven Publishers.

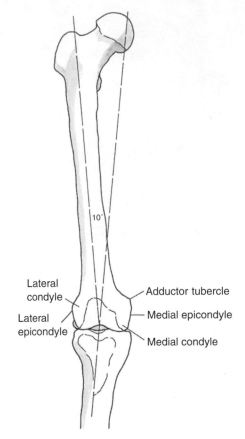

FIG. 13-1. Anterior view of the right femur.

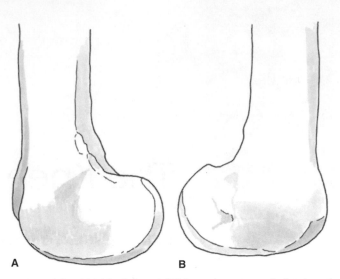

FIG. 13-3. (**A**) Medial and (**B**) lateral aspects of distal end of the right femur.

more gradual change in radius from back to front. The small lateral condyle tends to flatten sooner as one follows the curvature from back to front. The difference in the two condyles plays a part in the length rotation and locking mechanism of the knee, as discussed in the section on biomechanics.

The upper end of the tibia (Fig. 13-4) consists of two large condyles with joint surfaces superiorly for articulation with the femur. Both condyles are offset poste-

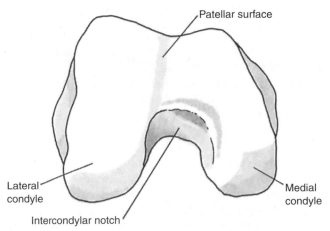

FIG. 13-2. Inferior aspect of the distal end of femur.

riorly to overhang the tibial shaft. They are also angulated 5° to 10° downward anteroposteriorly. The medial tibial condyle is larger; its superior surface is concave in all directions. The smaller lateral tibial condyle is actually convex anteroposteriorly. However, the lateral meniscus forms a concave articular surface for articulation with the convex lateral femoral condyle. Posterolaterally on the lateral tibial condyle is an articular facet for the head of the fibula, which faces somewhat downward. At the anteroinferior junction of the tibial condyles is the tibial tuberosity, an eminence onto which the patellar tendon inserts. Superiorly, between the condyles, is the roughened intercondylar area. The medial and lateral intercondylar tubercles, or eminences, lie centrally in the intercondylar area.

The patella (Fig. 13-5) is a triangular sesamoid bone, its apex lying inferiorly, embedded in the back of the quadriceps tendon. The posterior surface of the patella is cartilage-covered for articulation in the patellar groove of the femur, between the femoral condyles. The patellar articular surface consists of a lateral facet, a medial facet, and a small odd medial facet. The patella gives extra purchase to the quadriceps tendon in producing knee extension, especially toward the limits of extension.

☐ Menisci

The medial meniscus is semicircular, being larger posteriorly than anteriorly. Its anterior horn inserts onto the intercondylar area of the tibia, in front of the attachment of the anterior cruciate ligament (ACL), and its posterior horn inserts in front of the attachment of the posterior cruciate ligament (PCL). Peripherally, it

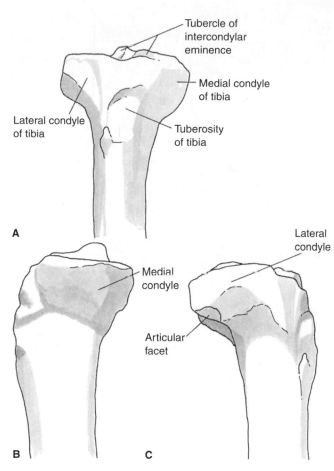

FIG. 13-4. Proximal end of the right tibia from (**A**) anterior aspect, (**B**) medial aspect, and (**C**) lateral aspect.

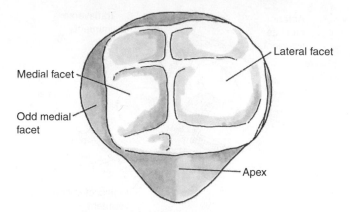

FIG. 13-5. Posterior aspect of the right patella.

In recent years the meniscus, formerly considered an unimportant appendage within the knee, has been recognized as one of the prime protectors of knee use and function.[157] The menisci serve several functions in the knee. They act as shock absorbers, spreading the stress over the joint surface and decreasing cartilage wear. They aid in the lubrication and nutrition of the joint, reduce friction during movement, and improve weight distribution by increasing the area of contact between the condyles. They are vascular in their cartilaginous inner two thirds and are partly vascular and fibrous in their outer third.[13] Because most recent literature indicates that removal of the total meniscus can lead to early degeneration of the joint,[66,167,230,241] most surgeons today remove only the torn portion of the meniscus, not the entire structure.

is attached to the joint capsule, to the short capsular fibers of the medial collateral ligament (MCL), and to the outer margin of the superior aspect of the medial tibial condyle by the coronary ligament. The coronary ligament constitutes the inferior aspect of the joint capsule (Fig. 13-6).

The medial meniscus forms part of a larger circle, but the lateral meniscus forms almost all of a smaller circle. Its two horns attach close to each other, just in front of and just behind the intercondylar eminence. The periphery of the lateral meniscus attaches to the tibia, the capsule, and a coronary ligament, but not to the lateral collateral ligament (LCL). The lateral meniscus is more mobile than the medial meniscus, due to its shape and less extensive peripheral attachments. A ligament usually runs from the posterior aspect of the lateral meniscus to the medial condyle of the femur. This meniscofemoral ligament runs behind the PCL, while another may run in front (Fig. 13-7). The popliteus tendon also attaches to the lateral meniscus; this attachment is said to assist in posterior movement of the meniscus during knee flexion.[160] Usually a transverse ligament connects the two menisci anteriorly.

☐ Ligaments

The MCL is a long, flat band attached above to the medial epicondyle and below to the medial aspect of the shaft of the tibia, about 4 cm below the joint line (Fig. 13-8). Its fibers run somewhat anteriorly, from top to bottom. Older descriptions often refer to *deep, shorter fibers* and *posterior oblique fibers* of the MCL, but these are both considered part of the joint capsule (see

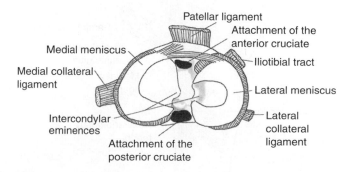

FIG. 13-6. Superior aspect of the right tibia, showing the menisci and tibial attachments of the cruciate ligaments.

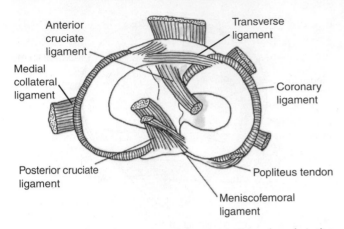

FIG. 13-7. Superior aspect of the right tibia, showing the ligaments.

below) in more recent literature.[119,284] The deep capsular fibers are attached to the medial meniscus.

The MCL becomes tight on extension of the knee, abduction of the tibia on the femur, and outward rotation of the tibia on the femur. Some of the anterior fibers become tight on knee flexion. The MCL also helps prevent anterior displacement of the tibia on the femur.

The LCL is a shorter, round bundle of fibers running from the lateral epicondyle to the fibular head (Fig. 13-9). It does not attach to the lateral meniscus. The popliteus tendon runs underneath the ligament between it and the meniscus. The LCL is largely covered by the tendon of the biceps femoris. The LCL runs slightly posteriorly from top to bottom and is tight on extension of the knee, adduction of the tibia

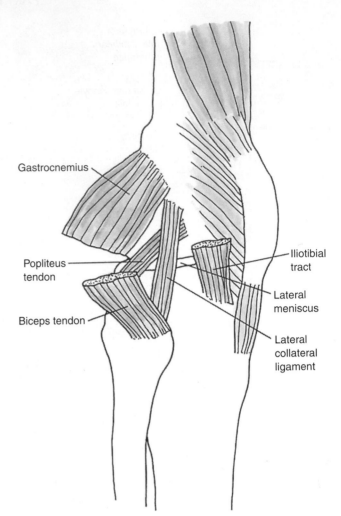

FIG. 13-9. Lateral aspect of the right knee.

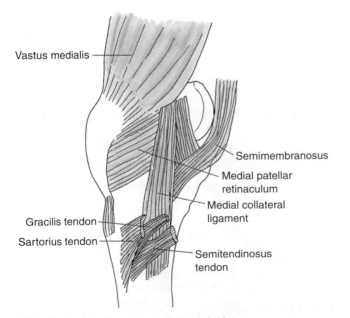

FIG. 13-8. Medial aspect of the right knee.

on the femur, and outward rotation of the tibia on the femur.

The ACL runs from the anterior intercondylar area of the tibia backward, upward, and laterally to the medial aspect of the lateral femoral condyle in the intercondylar notch (see Fig. 13-7).[89] It acts primarily to check extension of the knee, forward movement of the tibia on the femur, and internal rotation of the tibia on the femur. Because the ACL pulls tight on internal tibial rotation and as the knee extends, some have proposed that this ligament guides the tibia into outward rotation during knee extension.[242]

The PCL runs from the extreme posterior intercondylar area of the tibia forward, medially, and upward to the lateral aspect of the medial femoral condyle in the intercondylar notch (see Fig. 13-7). As it travels from the tibia to the femur, the ligament twists in a medial spiral. The posterolateral part of the ACL is taut in extension and the anteromedial portion is lax.[145,202,203] In flexion, all the fibers except the anteromedial portion are lax. It primarily checks backward movement of the tibia on the femur and helps check internal rotation of the tibia on the femur. It also tightens on full knee extension, although some fibers may be tight throughout the range of flexion–extension of the knee. It is aided by the popliteus muscle in checking forward sliding of the femur on the tibia when squatting.

The patellofemoral ligament is a thickening of the patellar retinaculum. It passes from the adductor tubercle of the femur to the medial aspect of the patella. Its femoral attachment often becomes irritated and tender in cases of patellofemoral tracking dysfunction.

A fibrous capsule surrounds the knee joint, attaching at the margins of articular cartilage. The superior aspect of the capsule runs from the articular margin of the femur to the periphery of the menisci. The inferior fibers run a short distance from the menisci to the tibia. The inferior capsule is often called the *coronary ligament*.

The fibrous capsule receives extensive passive and dynamic reinforcement (see Figs. 13-8 and 13-9). Passive reinforcement is provided by the above-mentioned ligaments and by what are referred to in older texts as the *deep layer* and *posterior oblique fibers* of the MCL. These are thickenings of the medial and posteromedial aspects of the joint capsule that provide added stabilization against valgus and external rotatory stresses. The posterior oblique fibers are now referred to simply as the *posteromedial capsule*. The short capsular fibers deep to the MCL are attached to the medial meniscus. There are also some thickenings of the capsule posteriorly, the *oblique* and *arcuate popliteal ligaments*.

Dynamic capsular reinforcement is provided to all aspects of the joint capsule. Anterior reinforcement is provided by the patellar tendon inferiorly and the quadriceps tendon superiorly. These constitute the anterior capsule because a fibrous capsule *per se* is absent anteriorly. Anteromedial and anterolateral reinforcements are provided by the medial and lateral patellar retinacula, which are superficial to and may blend with the fibrous capsule. These help stabilize the patellofemoral joint during loaded knee extension.

The distal aspect of the iliotibial band provides anterolateral reinforcement. This stabilizes against excessive internal rotation of the tibia on the femur and thus works in conjunction with the cruciates.

The pes anserinus tendons (semitendinosus, gracilis, and sartorius) and the semimembranosus tendon give medial and posteromedial reinforcement. These help prevent abnormal external rotation, abduction, and anterior displacement of the tibia on the femur. In doing so they dynamically reinforce the MCL, the posteromedial capsule, and to a certain extent the ACL.

Posterolateral support comes from the biceps femoris tendon. This helps check excessive internal rotation and anterior displacement of the tibia on the femur, providing reinforcement to the functions of the cruciates. It also may assist the LCL in preventing adduction of the tibia on the femur.

Finally, posterior reinforcement is provided by the insertions of the gastrocnemius muscles and from the popliteus muscle. The popliteus helps check external rotation of the tibia on the femur and backward displacement of the tibia on the femur.

☐ Bursae, Synovia, and Fat Pads

The synovium of the knee joint, in addition to lining the fibrous capsule, forms several large recesses (Fig. 13-10). Anteroinferiorly, it extends inward to line the back of the infrapatellar fat pad. The medial and lateral aspects of this lining unite centrally to form the ligamentum mucosa, which extends into the joint to attach to the intercondylar notch of the femur. Anterosuperiorly, the synovium runs from the superior aspect of the patella upward beneath the quadriceps

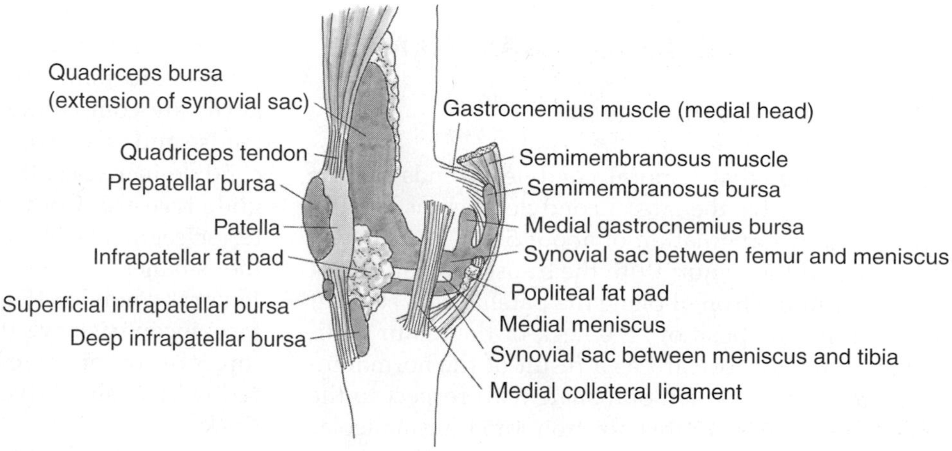

FIG. 13-10. *Medial aspect of the knee, showing the synovia and bursae.*

tendon, then folds back on itself to form a pouch, and inserts on the distal femur above the condyles. This suprapatellar pouch is part of the joint cavity and provides sufficient slack in the synovium to allow full knee flexion. Posteriorly, the synovium invaginates into the intercondylar notch to pass in front of the cruciates. In this way the cruciates are intracapsular but extrasynovial.

In addition to the suprapatellar pouch, which also serves as a bursa, there are three additional major bursae anteriorly. The prepatellar bursa lies over the patella, and may become inflamed with prolonged kneeling ("housemaid's knee"). A bursa also lies between the patellar tendon and the tibia (deep infrapatellar bursa) and between the patellar tendon and skin (superficial infrapatellar bursa).

Posteriorly, a main bursa lies between the semimembranosus tendon and the medial origin of the gastrocnemius muscle. This bursa often communicates with the joint and may become swollen with articular effusion ("Baker's cyst"). This bursa may also extend between the gastrocnemius and the capsule, or a separate bursa may be situated here.

Bursae may also exist beneath the tendons of the pes anserinus and the iliotibial band, just proximal to their insertions. These can become irritated with high levels of activity. There may also be other bursae about the knee joint, but these are of little clinical significance.

The large infrapatellar fat pad is situated deep to the patellar tendon and in front of the femoral condyles. When the knee is flexed, it fills the anterior aspect of the intercondylar notch. With the knee extended, it occupies the patellar groove and covers the trochlear surface of the femur. The back of the fat pad is lined with synovium. It is thought that as the fat pad sweeps across the condyles during knee flexion and extension, it helps to spread a lubricating layer of synovial fluid over the joint surface of the femur before contact with the tibia.

■ BIOMECHANICS OF THE FEMOROTIBIAL JOINT

☐ Structural Alignment

Because the medial femoral condyle extends farther distally than does the lateral condyle, there is usually a slight valgus angulation of about 5° to 10° between the tibia and the femur. With the transcondylar axis of the femur in the frontal plane the patella faces straight forward. In this position, the neck of the femur is directed about 20° forward as a result of the normal internal torsion of the femoral shaft with respect to the femoral neck. Also in this position, the transmalleolar axis at the ankle is rotated outward about 25° as a re-

sult of the normal external torsion of the tibial shaft, and the long axis of the foot is directed 5° to 10° outward.

☐ Movement

The knee is normally biaxial; it flexes and extends around an axis that is horizontally oriented in the frontal plane in the standing position, and it rotates about a vertical axis. Knee flexion–extension is polycentric, the axis of movement shifting backward along a curved centroid as the knee moves from extension into flexion.

FLEXION–EXTENSION

Osteokinematics. The total range of knee flexion–extension in the healthy knee is from about 5° to 10° of hyperextension to 140° to 150° of flexion. Flexion is limited by soft-tissue approximation of the calf and posterior thigh. Extension is terminated by locking of the joint in its close-packed position as the capsules and ligaments draw tight and become twisted. As the knee approaches full extension, it also assumes a valgus angulation because the medial femoral condyle extends farther distally than the lateral condyle.

Arthrokinematics. The femorotibial joint is markedly incongruent in positions of flexion, but becomes progressively more congruent as the knee extends. In the flexed position, the small convex radius of the posterior femoral condyles contacts a relatively large radius on the tibial condyles. In fact, the lateral tibial condyle is actually a convex surface. Because the radius of curvature of the femoral condyles progressively increases anteriorly, the joint becomes more congruent as the contacting area on the femur moves anteriorly during knee extension (Fig. 13-11).

The fibrocartilaginous menisci reduce joint surface incongruency. Their mobility and deformability allow them to conform to the shape of the contacting femoral joint surfaces. The anterior segments of the menisci are somewhat mobile, whereas the posterior horns are comparatively fixed. Thus, as the knee extends and the contacting radius of the femoral condyle increases, the anterior aspects of the menisci glide forward. Conversely, as the knee flexes, the anterior segments of the menisci recede to conform to the smaller radius of curvature of the contacting femoral condyles (Fig. 13-12). By reducing joint surface incongruency, the menisci help distribute the forces of compressive loading over a greater area, thus reducing compressive stresses to the joint surfaces of the knee.

As indicated by the instant centers of motion, flex-

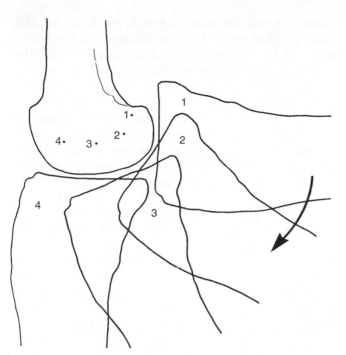

FIG. 13-11. Diagram showing loci of normal instant centers and congruency during flexion and extension of the knee.

ion and extension of the knee occur with a combination of rolling and sliding at the joint surfaces. The closer the instant center is to the contacting joint surfaces, the greater the amount of rolling that occurs at a particular point in the range of movement. An instant center that lies some distance from the contacting surfaces indicates considerable sliding between the surfaces. Because the normal axes of movement for flexion and extension of the knee lie within the condylar region of the femur—not on the joint surfaces or a long distance away—it follows that both sliding and rolling accompany the movement. It can be seen from the loci of normal instant centers that the axis of movement shifts farther away from the joint surface as the knee extends, indicating that relatively more sliding is occurring as extension takes place (see Fig. 13-11).[77,78] Considering that the tibia moves on the fixed femur, the direction of sliding and rolling of the tibial joint surface is anterior during extension and posterior during flexion.

TRANSVERSE ROTATION

Because the femorotibial joint surfaces are incongruent in all positions except full extension, and because the menisci are semimobile, the knee joint can undergo rotation in the transverse plane. This rotary movement can easily be produced actively or passively with the knee flexed, and is important for attenuation of rotary forces acting on the knee during normal function.

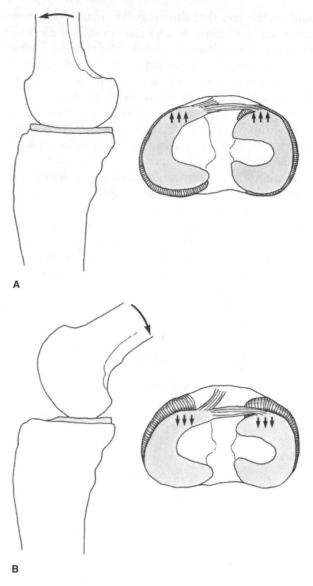

FIG. 13-12. (**A**) During extension, the menisci glide forward, while (**B**) during flexion, the menisci recede to conform to the radius of curvature of the connecting femoral condyles.

There is also an automatic, or conjunct, rotation at the knee that accompanies flexion and extension of the joint. This occurs as an external rotation of the tibia relative to the femur during the final 15° to 20° of extension, and an internal tibial rotation during the initial 15° or 20° of flexion from a fully extended position. Because the knee undergoes rotation and the menisci tend to move with the femur, much of the movement occurs between the menisci and the tibia.

Several factors contribute to the occurrence of knee rotation during flexion and extension.[16,242,263,277] First, and perhaps most important, is the shape and orientation of the medial femoral condyle. Looking at the femur end on, the medial condyle is curved and obliquely oriented, whereas the lateral condyle is situated in the sagittal plane (see Fig. 13-2). Also of significance is the fact that the articular surface of the medial condyle is longer, in an anteroposterior direction, than that of the lateral condyle. As the tibia moves into extension, the lateral side of the joint completes its movement before the medial side because of the difference in lengths of the respective femoral articular surfaces. When this occurs, the medial side of the tibia continues to move forward along the curved medial femoral condyle, while the lateral tibial joint surface undergoes a lateral spin. The net effect is an external rotary movement of the tibia on the femur. This movement reverses when the knee flexes from a fully extended position.

The cruciates are also thought to play a role in guiding rotary movement at the knee. The cruciates tighten as the knee extends and are twisted in a direction to rotate the tibia externally as they tighten.

☐ Pathomechanics

STRUCTURAL ALTERATIONS

Frontal Plane. Although the knee joint normally assumes a valgus angulation, the line of application representing the weight-bearing force acting on the knee

tends to bisect the joint. This is because the femoral head is offset medially from the shaft of the femur (Fig. 13-13). Excessive genu valgum causes the weight-bearing force to be shifted to the lateral side of the joint; genu varum results in a medial shift of the weight-bearing force line. Such alterations in force distribution may lead to accelerated wear on one side of the joint.[73] Common factors contributing to genu valgum are iliotibial band tightness, abnormal foot pronation, and femoral anteversion. Femoral retroversion tends to result in genu varum.

Transverse Plane. In increased femoral anteversion, the femoral condyles are rotated too far internally with respect to the femoral neck. Thus, with the hip joint in a neutral position, the condyles and patellae face inward, or, conversely, with the patellae and condyles facing forward, the hip joint assumes an externally rotated position. Since the tendency during gait is to maintain normal alignment of the hip joints, the person with increased femoral anteversion tends to walk with the knee rotated inward. This inward rotation may be transmitted to the foot as a toe-in stance or as abnormal foot pronation. At the knee, inward rotation results in a valgus angulation when the knee is semiflexed, as it is during most of the stance phase of

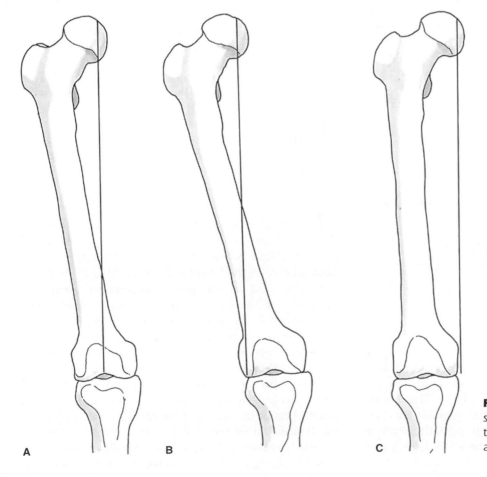

FIG. 13-13. Knee joint angulation showing (**A**) normal valgus angulation, (**B**) excessive valgus angulation, and (**C**) varus angulation.

A   B   C

gait. In a similar manner, abnormal retroversion of the hip causes a tendency for the patella to face outward during gait, for the knee to assume a varus position, and for the feet to either toe-out or supinate. In some persons with torsional deviations of the femur, compensatory structural rotation of the tibia develops. Thus, the child with femoral anteversion may also develop increased external tibial torsion to achieve normal foot placement. Similarly, internal tibial torsion may develop in association with femoral retroversion. Such torsional compensation at the tibia seems to enhance valgus–varus deviations.

INTRINSIC MOVEMENT ABNORMALITIES

Capsular Tightness. One of the most common causes of gross restriction of knee motion is capsular tightness. Fibrosis and subsequent loss of extensibility of the joint capsule frequently follow immobilization after trauma or surgery, and usually accompany the progression of chronic joint diseases such as degenerative joint disease (DJD) or rheumatoid arthritis. Capsular tightness at the knee results in a characteristic pattern of restriction in which knee extension is limited by 20° to 30°, and flexion is possible to only 80° or 100°. The functional disability resulting from capsular restriction varies with the patients's activity level, but ambulation is inevitably altered because nearly full knee extension is necessary for normal gait. According to Laubenthal and coworkers, the mean total flexion–extension necessary for the stance phase of gait is 21°; for the swing phase of gait, 67°; for stair climbing, 83°; and for sitting and rising, 83°.[161] Because capsular restriction at the knee typically allows only 50° to 80° of flexion–extension, some functional alteration is likely.

Of great significance during walking is the effect of reduced knee extension on the stresses imposed on the articular surfaces of the joint. Normally, during the stance phase of gait, peak weight-bearing forces are borne with the joint just short of full knee extension, a position in which the tibiofemoral contact area is greatest, and a position in which the joint capsule has not been drawn completely tight.[73,146] Since stress equals force divided by unit area, the compressive stress of weight-bearing is minimized by a relatively large tibiofemoral contact area. Furthermore, the joint is not "shock-loaded" by having the slack in the joint capsule suddenly taken up as the knee moves toward extension. If, however, knee extension is lacking due to capsular tightness, the joint cannot move to a position of maximal tibiofemoral contact, and as the knee extends, the joint capsule suddenly pulls tight. Stress to the joint surfaces is increased in magnitude and the joint is shock-loaded. The long-term effect is likely to be accelerated wear of joint surfaces.

Rotatory Dysfunction. A more subtle yet common movement disorder affecting the knee is loss of normal rotatory mechanics. The pathologic implications of rotatory dysfunction at the knee were proposed by Smillie[255] and confirmed by Frankel and Burstein.[78] The nature and the extent of rotation accompanying knee flexion and extension are governed by the shapes of the articular surfaces and are influenced by capsuloligamentous configurations. Alteration in normal rotatory mechanics may reflect articular surface abnormalities or capsuloligamentous disorders. Similarly, rotatory dysfunction produces abnormal stresses to the joint surfaces and the capsuloligamentous structures. Smillie proposed that since normal rotatory movement is small and occurs at the very limits of knee extension, full knee extension is possible in the absence of normal rotation, but at the expense of increased deformation to articular tissues.[255,256] Thus, knee extension occurring without normal external tibial rotation results in abnormal stresses to the medial joint surfaces, which are oriented to move into rotation, and increased tensile stresses to the cruciates, which pull tight on extension and internal tibial rotation. Furthermore, the tibia must rotate externally as the knee approaches full extension to prevent the lateral side of the medial femoral condyle from contacting the medial edge of the ACL.

Several types of disorders may cause altered rotatory mechanics at the knee. Smillie cites meniscal displacements, such as those associated with meniscus tears, as a frequent causative factor.[255,256] Because knee rotation, when combined with flexion or extension, requires meniscofemoral as well as meniscotibial movement, alterations in the structural configuration of the menisci probably interfere with normal rotatory mechanics.

Another common cause of restricted external tibial rotation is reduced extensibility of the medial or posteromedial capsuloligamentous structures. This typically occurs following injury or surgery, in which the posteromedial capsule or MCL may heal in an adhered or shortened state. Laxity of these same structures will also lead to abnormal rotatory mechanics, because external tibial rotation may be excessive or premature.[143,253] This would especially be true if a secondary external rotation contracture developed.

In recognition of the pathomechanics and pathologic implications of rotatory dysfunction at the knee, Helfet has described a simple means of detecting this problem clinically.[107] The method involves comparing femorotibial rotatory alignment in a semiflexed and fully extended position. Using this test, in addition to instant center analysis, Frankel and Burstein demonstrated a positive correlation between reduced femorotibial rotation and abnormal compression of the joint surfaces during terminal knee extension.[78] In most of the patients evaluated, meniscal derangement was the underlying cause. Arthrotomy revealed abnormal wearing in localized areas of the medial articular surfaces in 22 of 30 knees. These findings confirm the nature of the kinematic abnormality associated with altered rotatory mechanics and also suggest that such disorders, over a long period, may predispose to progressive DJD.

Smillie believes that kinematic disturbance resulting from rotatory dysfunction at the knee may also lead to fatigue disruption and fraying of the ACL.[255] He supports this contention with surgical case studies of isolated ACL lesions associated with chronic meniscal derangements.

The significance of rotatory dysfunction at the femorotibial articulation is becoming better appreciated as our knowledge of detailed knee biomechanics improves. Because the disturbance is subtle, it is not readily recognized unless femorotibial rotatory function is carefully examined. This type of assessment should become a routine component of knee examination in the rehabilitation period following capsuloligamentous injury or internal derangement.

☐ Pathomechanics of Common Loading Conditions

TRAUMA

Knee joint injuries are commonly of traumatic origin. This stems, in part, from the fact that the knee is freely movable in only the sagittal plane (flexion–extension). Thus, forces acting to move the knee in the frontal or transverse planes are largely attenuated by internal strain to the soft tissues about the joint. Furthermore, such forces may act over the relatively long lever arms provided by the femur and the tibia, thereby increasing the potential loading of the joint structures.

Valgus–External Rotation. Because of the exposure of the lateral side of the knee to external forces, compared with that of the protected medial aspect, traumatic valgus stresses are much more common than varus stresses. Usually such forces also involve components acting in the transverse and sagittal planes, thus causing rotatory and flexion–extension displacements. The knee is usually in some position of flexion when acted on by a force from the lateral aspect; thus, the direction of rotary movement is usually such that the tibia is rotated laterally with respect to the femur.

Valgus–external rotation injuries are most common in contact sports (especially football) and skiing. The degree of loading of the joint is accentuated by the fixation of the foot to the ground (*e.g.*, by a cleated shoe) and by forces acting over a long lever arm (*e.g.*, a ski). This does not allow rotary forces to be attenuated by movement of the foot with respect to the ground, and

more of the energy is absorbed as internal strain to joint structures. Because valgus and external rotation are primarily checked by the posteromedial capsule and the capsular and superficial fibers of the MCL, these structures are most commonly damaged. The menisci, especially the medial meniscus, may be injured because of the rotary stress component. With marked separation of the medial side of the joint, the ACL may be torn as well. With progressive force in a valgus–external rotation direction, first the deep capsular fibers of the MCL are torn, then the long superficial fibers of the MCL and the posteromedial capsule, and finally the ACL. A torn medial meniscus would complete the so-called terrible triad of O'Donoghue.

Hyperextension. Because the knee is used in a position close to its physiologic limits of extension for most functional activities, hyperextension injuries are quite common. Again, those involved in violent contact sports and skiers are particularly vulnerable to such injuries. Forced hyperextension of the knee results in tearing first of the posterior capsule, followed by the ACL, then the PCL.[145]

Anteroposterior Displacement. Forces producing a pure translatory movement between the tibia and femur in an anteroposterior direction are less common than the aforementioned injuries. Of these, perhaps the "dashboard injury" is most common: the victim, in a suddenly decelerating auto, is thrust forward, striking the tibial tubercle of the bent knee on the dashboard. The tibia is forced posteriorly on the femur, stressing the PCL, often to the point of rupture.

Isolated ACL tears, resulting from forces in the opposite direction, are rare; in fact, there is controversy over the frequency of isolated ACL lesions. The mechanism of injury is more likely to be a force stressing the tibia into internal rotation on the femur.[145,283]

Rotation. Forced external rotation of the tibia on the femur tends to stress the collateral ligaments and the posteromedial capsule. As mentioned above, these forces usually occur in conjunction with valgus stresses and therefore typically affect the medial stabilizing structures.

Internal rotation of the tibia on the femur is checked by the cruciate ligaments. It is believed that forced internal rotation is the primary mechanism in isolated ACL injuries.[145,283]

Forced rotation may also injure the menisci.[152] The medial meniscus, being less mobile by virtue of its attachment to the capsular fibers of the MCL, is much more frequently injured than the lateral meniscus. The menisci are particularly stressed when the knee is forced into rotation in an improper direction during flexion or extension. Thus, when the tibia, which is supposed to rotate internally during initial knee flexion, is forced externally as the knee goes into flexion,

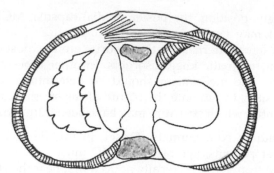

FIG. 13-14. *A longitudinal tear of the medial meniscus.*

the menisci are caught between trying to move into flexion with the tibia and into rotation (in the wrong direction) with the femur. The result is often excessive deformation and tearing of a meniscus. If, as typically occurs, there is a valgus component to the rotary force, the medial meniscus is additionally stressed through its attachment to the MCL.

Rotary stresses sufficient to produce meniscal damage do not necessarily require external forces: often the victim simply twists suddenly on the weight-bearing leg. This usually occurs during athletics, but may also occur with less vigorous activities. Occupations or activities involving rotation of the fully flexed knee (*e.g.,* wrestling, mining in cramped quarters) particularly predispose to meniscus tears because when the knee is fully flexed, the menisci reach their limit of posterior excursion. Rotation, which involves posterior movement of one condyle and simultaneous anterior movement of the other, may further stress one meniscus posteriorly or cause the condyle to grind over the relatively fixed meniscus.

Most traumatic medial meniscus tears affect the posterior segment of the meniscus, with the tear running in a longitudinal direction.[255] Successive injury to the same meniscus may cause the tear to extend sufficiently anteriorly to allow the lateral segment of the torn structure to flip centrally into the intercondylar region—a "bucket-handle" tear (Fig. 13-14). This produces a mechanical block to full knee extension, and the knee is locked; full extension can occur only at the expense of further damage to the meniscus or excessive stretching of the ACL.

■ EVALUATION

Many common lesions affect the knee joint. Traumatic injuries may be suffered by athletes as well as more sedentary persons. Symptomatic degenerative disorders involving the knee are not uncommon in middle-aged or older persons, and "overuse" fatigue syndromes may affect virtually any age group. The approach to the evaluation of knee disorders must be flexible enough to accommodate such a broad spectrum of disorders. Presented here is an assessment scheme that includes most of the evaluative procedures needed to perform a thorough clinical examination of virtually any patient presenting with a common knee disorder. Practically speaking, the therapist will rarely use all the tests and procedures outlined here in any one examination. However, he or she should become proficient in all the tests, and must know the rationale for each to perform the most efficient knee examination.

☐ History

The key to an efficient yet comprehensive examination of the knee is the patient interview. The information gained about the nature and extent of the physical problem is necessary so that the therapist can select the most appropriate objective evaluative procedures. Subjective data are also important in determining the degree of disability and in documenting a baseline.

Follow the format set out in Chapter 5, Assessment of Musculoskeletal Disorders, when conducting the subjective portion of the knee examination. Certain other questions depend on the nature of the disorder.

If the problem is of recent traumatic onset, ask:

1. What was the exact mechanism of injury? Did you feel a "pop"?
2. Did the knee swell? If so, how long after the injury did you notice the swelling? Where was it observed?
3. To what extent could you continue activities immediately after the injury? Could you walk? If the injury occurred during athletics, was a litter or some other form of passive or assisted transport required?

If the problem is of a chronic nature, ask:

1. Does the knee click, grind, grate, or pop? If so, was the onset of these symptoms associated with the onset of the present problem?
2. Has the knee ever locked, buckled, or given way? If so, under what specific circumstances? Is there some particular activity that tends to cause it?
3. Is going up or down stairs a problem?
4. Can you run? What is the effect of running backward, stopping quickly, or changing directions quickly?

☐ Interpretative Considerations

SITE OF PAIN

The knee joint receives innervation from the L3 through S2 segments of the spinal column, and depending on the site of the pathologic process, pain from knee disorders may be referred into any of these segments. Most common knee problems affect the anteromedial or medial aspect of the joint, which is largely innervated by L3. Because the L3 segment usually does not extend much below the knee, it is rare for a patient with a common knee disorder to experience pain radiating farther distally than midleg. It is more common for pain originating at the knee to be referred proximally into the anterior or anteromedial thigh. The anterior aspect of the hip joint is also innervated primarily by L3, so referred pain of hip joint origin may be similar in site to that arising from the knee. In fact, it is not unusual, especially in children, for a patient with a hip joint problem to complain of "knee pain."

In the patient with nontraumatic onset of pain about the knee, lesions situated elsewhere in the L3 through S2 segments must be ruled out. The two common sources of referred pain to the knee are the lumbosacral region and the hip region.

Pain felt over the posterior aspect of the knee is often secondary to effusion causing distention of the posterior capsule. Because the S1 and S2 segments, which innervate the posterior knee region, extend well down into the foot, posterior knee pain may be referred some distance distally.

Pain of nontraumatic onset felt over a generalized region at the anteromedial aspect of the knee is most commonly from patellofemoral joint dysfunction. This is especially likely when the pain is aggravated most by descending stairs and prolonged sitting with bent knees.

Localized anteromedial pain felt at the joint line, usually of sudden onset, is often related to meniscus injuries. The pain arises from the anteromedial coronary ligament. A sprain of the coronary ligament may be the sole lesion, or it may be associated with a tear of the body of the meniscus.

Medial knee pain of traumatic onset following a valgus or rotary strain is usually of capsuloligamentous origin. A tear of the meniscus must also be ruled out.

ONSET OF PAIN

Sudden, Traumatic Onset. Sudden injuries caused by trauma are common, especially from sports activities involving contact or sudden changes in direction. A sudden twisting injury, in which the tibia is rotated externally on the femur without an external source of force, may tear either the capsular fibers of the MCL (grade I tear), the coronary ligament (peripheral attachment of the meniscus), or the body of the medial meniscus. When some external force is involved, such as in contact sports, and the knee is also forced into valgus position, the posteromedial capsule, MCL, or ACL may also be damaged.

Valgus–external rotation injuries are the most common traumatic knee disorders. In other types of injuries the mechanism should be determined, when possible, to estimate the nature of the stresses and to identify which structure may have been traumatized.

Gradual, Nontraumatic Onset. In middle-aged and older patients, symptomatic DJD must be ruled out. Pain from DJD is typically noticed first near the end of the day or after long periods of walking. Later, pain and stiffness are felt on rising in the morning, easing somewhat after getting up and about.

Possible precipitating factors, such as recent immobilization, alteration in activities, past injuries, and previous surgeries, should be considered. Patellofemoral joint dysfunction, a common knee problem, is frequently related to quadriceps insufficiency. This may include true quadriceps weakness, as from disuse, or some increase in loaded knee-extension activities in the presence of inadequately trained quadriceps muscles. Typical activities would be hiking, bicycling, or skiing.

Effusion. Articular effusion commonly follows traumatic injury to the knee joint. This may be the result of blood filling the joint or of overproduction of synovial fluid. The time frame of the onset of the effusion often provides important insight into its nature. Hemarthrosis tends to develop over a relatively short period after injury, from several minutes to a few hours; synovial effusion occurs over a longer period of time, perhaps 6 to 12 hours, before it is noticed. Synovial effusion causes a dull, aching pain from the distention of the joint capsule. Hemarthrosis may be associated with more severe discomfort caused by chemical stimulation of capsular nociceptors.

Clinically it is important to differentiate the nature of the effusion, since in hemarthrosis an intra-articular fracture must be ruled out. Some relatively severe joint injuries, such as a complete rupture of the MCL, may not be followed by significant effusion because of leakage of fluid through the defect out from the confines of the joint capsule.

More subtle joint effusion may accompany chronic, nontraumatic knee disorders. The patient often describes posterior knee discomfort from posterior capsular distention.

NATURE OF PAIN AND OTHER SYMPTOMS

Pain of Traumatic Origin. Pain secondary to trauma is typically felt immediately at the time of injury. In ligamentous injuries the severity of the pain and resulting immediate disability do not necessarily reflect the severity of the injury. A minor or moderate sprain of the medial capsule or ligament is often more painful and more disabling at the time of injury than a complete MCL rupture.[212] This is because with a complete rupture, there are no longer intact fibers from which pain of mechanical origin can arise. Furthermore, later development of pain from joint effusion may not be significant because of leakage of fluid through the defect. Thus, after the initial pain from the ligament rupture, the patient may feel relatively little pain, especially if he or she is involved in a highly motivating activity such as an athletic competition.

Patellofemoral Joint Pain. Pain felt when sitting for long periods with the knee bent or when descending stairs is typical of patellofemoral joint problems.[21,95] These functions both involve high and prolonged patellofemoral compressive loading. Pain is felt more on descending than on ascending stairs because greater passive tension is developed in the quadriceps mechanism during eccentric contraction than during concentric contraction. Sitting is a problem because of prolonged patellofemoral compression. Bone, being viscoelastic, undergoes "creep" or continued deformation with prolonged loading.[79] Bone is also weaker, or more likely to yield, with slowly applied loads. Thus, the likelihood of trabecular breakdown is greater with loading over a long period of time than with a similar load applied quickly.

Morning Pain. Pain that is present on wakening, subsides with initial use of the joint, and then increases again after some period of use is typical of DJD.

Buckling or Giving Way. A joint that buckles or gives way suggests structural or functional instability. The common structural disorder that causes giving way is loss of ligamentous integrity. In such circumstances the patient may cite a particular activity that is a problem, usually one that stresses the joint in a direction the involved ligament is supposed to check. Thus, persons with chronic MCL ruptures find it difficult to turn abruptly away from the involved leg because of the valgus–external rotation stress imposed on the leg.[212,253] Similarly, persons with loss of cruciate integrity may have problems descending inclines or squatting.

Functional buckling occurs as a result of reflex muscle inhibition, presumably from abnormal joint receptor activity. A common cause is internal derangement from a meniscus tear or loose body. In such cases, an abnormality in arthrokinematics resulting from the mechanical derangement may reflexively incite a sudden inhibition of the quadriceps muscles, causing the joint to give way. The patient usually cannot attribute the incidence of buckling to any consistent situation or activity, but claims that the joint gives way for no apparent reason.

☐ Physical Examination

OBSERVATION

Record any functional deficits noted throughout the patient's visit. When possible, analyze and document the nature and extent of the deficit for future comparison. If the patient mentions a particular functional problem during the interview, ask him or her to attempt the particular activity or task to evaluate the problem more objectively. This is especially important for patients with relatively chronic problems who may not spontaneously demonstrate functional deficits during the evaluation.

Gait. Common gait abnormalities and their possible causes are discussed in Chapter 22, The Lumbosacral–Lower Extremity Scan Examination. The ability to hop, run, change directions quickly, stop abruptly, and climb stairs might be specifically evaluated.

Function. In a joint of low irritability, the patient may be asked to demonstrate the movements that produce the pain and the specific movement or action that produced the injury. With the patient squatting, note patellofemoral tracking—normally the patella should track freely and smoothly and describe a straight line over the second ray or midline of the foot. Also check to see if both knees flex symmetrically. Other useful maneuvers include having the patient squat and bounce, and stand from a sitting position; observing him or her climb and descend steps; having the patient change direction quickly or stop abruptly during movement; observing the patient run forward or backward, hop, and so forth; and having the patient jump into a full squat.

INSPECTION

Examine and record specific alterations in bony structure or alignment, soft-tissue configuration, and skin status.

   I. **Inspection of Bony Structure and Alignment.** The section on assessment of structural alignment in Chapter 22, The Lumbosacral–Lower Extremity Scan Examination, offers a complete discussion of this part of the examination. In many chronic knee problems, especially disorders of uncertain etiology, a complete structural assessment of the lower extremities and lumbosacral region should be done. In traumatic disorders of recent onset, the examination is often confined to the knee area. The following assessments are particularly relevant to examination of the knee:

A. *Standing examination*

1. *Frontal alignment.* The patient is viewed from behind. Use a plumb line that bisects the heels. Vertical or horizontal asymmetries in the frontal plane are detected by determining the positions of the navicular tubercles, medial malleoli, fibular heads, popliteal and gluteal folds, greater trochanters, posterosuperior iliac spines, and iliac crests. Document vertical disparities (leg-length differences) or lateral shifts from a plumb line that bisects the heels. Note abnormal or asymmetrical valgus–varus angulations. Differentiate tibial valgum or varum from genu valgum or varum; these are often confused. The knee is normally positioned in slight genu valgum because the medial condyle extends farther distally than the lateral condyle.

   a. Excessive genu valgum may be documented by measuring the distance between the malleoli, with the medial femoral condyles in contact.

   b. Excessive genu varum is noted by measuring the intercondylar distance at the knee, with the medial malleoli in contact.

   c. Vertical disparities are documented by measuring the distance from the lowest asymmetrical landmark to the floor.

   d. Horizontal deviations from the plumb line can be documented by measuring distances from the plumb line.

2. *Transverse rotary alignment.* The patient is viewed from the front with the feet at a normal stance width and pointed outward 5° to 10° from the sagittal plane.

   a. The intermalleolar line is normally rotated outward 25° to 30° from the frontal plane.

   b. The tibial tubercles should be in line with the midline or lateral half of the patellae.

   c. With the feet in normal stance position, the patellae should face straight forward. A "squinting" patella may indicate medial femoral or lateral tibial torsion. The normal patellar posture for exerting deceleration forces in the functional position of 45° knee flexion places the patellar articular surface squarely against the anterior femur; a lower posture represents patella baja, a higher posture patella alta. Normally, the length of the patella and patellar tendon should be roughly equal. In patella alta, the patellar tendon is excessively long (Fig. 13-15A). When viewed from the side, a "camel" or double hump may be apparent, resulting from the uncovered infrapatellar fat pad.[122] Patella alta makes the patella less efficient in exerting normal forces, and lateral displacement occurs easily.[122,127]

   d. The quadriceps angle (Q angle or patellofemoral angle) is formed by a line drawn from the center of the patella proximally toward the anterosuperior iliac spine, and a second line drawn from the center of the patella distally toward the tibial tubercle with the foot in the subtalar neutral position and the knee extended (weight-bearing). Normally the Q angle is 13° to 18° (13° for males, 18° for females). An angle above 14° indicates a tendency toward less patellar stability (Fig. 13-15B). An angle above 18° is often associated with patellar tracking dysfunction, subluxating patella, increased femoral anteversion, or increased lateral tibial torsion. Hughston[122] has advocated measuring the Q angle with the patient sitting and the quadriceps contracted; if the quadriceps is contracted and the knee fully extended, the normal Q angle is 8° to 10° (with 10° or more considered abnormal). If the patient is sitting and the quadriceps is relaxed (knee at 90°), the Q angle should be 0°.[122]

   e. A line drawn between the left and right anterosuperior iliac spines should be parallel to the frontal plane.

3. *Anteroposterior alignment.* The patient is viewed from the side. A plumb line facilitates assessment and measurement of deviations. In a relaxed standing position it is normal for the knee to assume a position of slight recurvatum. With the plumb line about 1 cm anterior to the lateral malleolus, the lateral femoral condyle should be slightly posterior to the plumb line. Abnormal angulation in

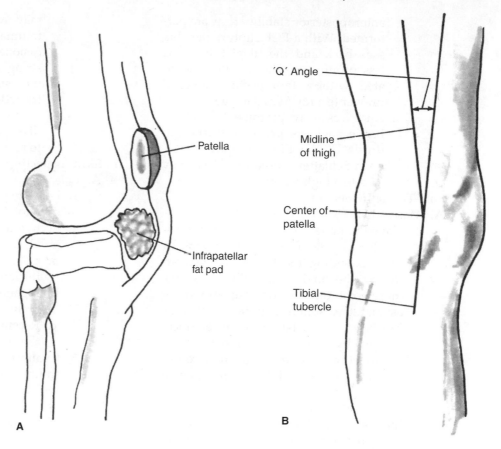

FIG. 13-15. Conditions predisposing the patient to recurrent subluxation of the patella. **(A)** The "camel" sign with a high-riding patella and uncovered fat pad. In a normal knee, the patella–patellar tendon ratio is approximately equal. **(B)** The quadriceps angle (Q angle) measures the divergence of the quadriceps from the sagittal plane. Normally, the Q angle should be 13° to 18° when the knee is straight and 0° in flexion.

the sagittal plane can be documented by measuring from some anatomic landmark to the plumb line.

  B. *Sitting examination.* The patient sits with the legs hanging freely over the edge of the plinth.
    1. *Femoropatellar alignment.* Assess the position and size of the patellae.
      a. A small, high-riding, outward-facing patella may predispose to a lateral patellar tracking disorder.
      b. A laterally facing patella suggests that the medial femoral condyle is considerably longer than the lateral condyle. This is likely to be associated with a valgus angulation when the knee is straightened.
      c. The inferior pole of the patella should be about level with the femorotibial joint line. A high-riding patella may be significant with respect to patellofemoral joint problems.[187]
    2. *Femorotibial alignment.* Assess the position of the tibial tubercles with respect to the patellae in the sitting, knee-bent position. The tubercle usually lines up with the midline or lateral half of the patella. Most important here is symmetry.

      a. A tubercle positioned too far medially may represent posteromedial capsular tightness, as may occur with healing of a sprain or rupture of one of the cruciate ligaments.
      b. A tubercle situated too far laterally may suggest laxity (*e.g.*, rupture) of the posteromedial capsule or MCL.
  C. *Supine examination*
    1. Legs straight
      a. Valgus–varus angulations may be measured with a goniometer.
      b. Leg-length disparities are documented by measuring from the anterosuperior iliac spines to the medial malleoli.
    2. Knees bent 60°, feet flat on the plinth
      a. Tibial lengths are compared by noting the heights of the tibial tubercles.
      b. Leg-length disparities of more proximate origin are detected by observing the lengths of the femurs. This is done by siting, from the side, a plane across the faces of the patellae.
      c. Anteroposterior femorotibial displacements are detected by comparing the prominences of the tibial tubercles. This must be done before

anteroposterior stability tests are performed. With a PCL rupture the tibia sags back and the tibial tubercle is less prominent. This is often associated with a false-positive anterior drawer test for ACL damage.

    d. An excessively prominent tibial tubercle suggests previous osteochondrosis of the tibial apophysis (Osgood-Schlatter disease). This may lead to a high-riding patella.

II. Soft-Tissue Inspection

A. *Muscle contours*

1. Have the patient maximally contract the quadriceps and calf muscle groups by fully extending the knees and plantarflexing the ankle. Carefully assess the muscle contours for obvious atrophy or asymmetry. Often significant atrophy can be observed before it can be documented by girth measurements. When asymmetries can be measured, record baseline values so changes can be noted later.

2. Assess other muscle groups in a similar manner, including the hamstrings and the anterior and lateral compartments of the leg.

B. *Swelling.* If significant swelling exists, record baseline girth measurements when possible.

1. Generalized edema of the lower leg may accompany various metabolic or vascular disorders. If it occurs soon after a surgical procedure, it may indicate venous thrombosis, in which case a physician should be notified. Edema persisting some time after trauma or surgery may be associated with a reflex sympathetic dystrophy.

2. Localized swelling may be articular or extra-articular.

    a. Articular effusion is manifest as swelling of the suprapatellar pouch and loss of definition of the peripatellar landmarks. Often the posterior capsule becomes distended, causing mild popliteal swelling. This swelling may be localized at the semimembranosus bursa, even in the case of articular effusion, since this bursa often communicates with the synovial cavity. If there is sufficient intracapsular swelling, the knee assumes a flexed or resting position (15° to 25°).

    b. Extra-articular effusion is most often noted in the prepatellar bursa. This may swell after sudden or repeated trauma (*e.g.*, housemaid's knee). Occasionally the distal belly of a hamstring muscle will herniate through the superficial fascia when contracted. This may appear as a pronounced popliteal "swelling," but disappears when the muscle is made to relax.

III. Skin Inspection

A. *Color*

1. Localized erythema may suggest an underlying inflammatory process.

2. Ecchymosis about the knee is most commonly associated with:

    a. Contusion. The injury is usually over the lateral aspect.

    b. Ligamentous damage, in which the ecchymosis is usually noted medially

    c. Recent patellar dislocation, in which the ecchymosis is seen medially

3. Cyanosis over the lower leg following trauma or surgery may be associated with a reflex sympathetic dystrophy.

B. *Scars.* The cause should be determined. If surgical, the reason for the surgery should be discovered.

C. *Texture.* In the presence of dystrophic changes, the skin of the lower leg becomes smooth and glossy.

IV. Selective Tissue Tension Tests

A. *Active movements*

1. Unilateral weight-bearing flexion–extension. If not contraindicated by recent trauma or significant disability, have the patient perform repeated one-legged half-squats. This yields some useful information concerning the functional capacity of the part. It is also a good way to compare the strength of the involved knee to the normal side, when possible; manual muscle testing is usually a poor test for quadriceps strength because the examiner may not be able to manually overcome even a significantly weak muscle. Note:

    a. The patient's ability to perform the movement. Can the knee be fully extended? How many repetitions can be performed before tiring? Compare this to the opposite leg.

    b. Any tendency toward giving way of the knee

    c. Patellofemoral or femorotibial crepitus. Palpate at the medial and lateral patellar margins for the former and at the femorotibial joint line for the latter. It is normal for a knee to "pop" or "snap" during this movement. A grinding similar to "sand in the joint" is more likely to indicate articular surface degenerative changes.

d. Provocation of pain. If pain is experienced, determine the point in the range of movement at which it is felt.

2. Non-weight-bearing flexion–extension. If the patient cannot perform weight-bearing flexion–extension or cannot do it through a full range of movement, assess flexion and extension in a supine position. For extension, have the patient straighten the knee, then tell him or her to hold it extended and attempt to raise the leg against gravity (straight-leg raise). Then have the patient flex the knee as far as possible. Note:

a. Range of motion. If the patient cannot fully flex or extend the knee, apply passive overpressure to determine whether the restriction is secondary to pain, weakness, or true tissue restriction. Compare the amount of passive extension to extension maintained against gravity. Document the degree of any "extensor lag."

b. Crepitus during movement. If joint crepitus is present determine whether it arises from the femorotibial or patellofemoral joint.

c. The presence of pain and the point in the range at which it is felt

d. If a capsular restriction exists, flexion is limited to 90° to 100° and extension is lacking by 20° to 30°.

e. Loss of knee extension in the presence of full flexion is most often caused by an internal derangement such as a bucket-handle meniscus tear.

f. Quadriceps lag. To complete the last 15° of knee extension, a 60% increase in force of the quadriceps muscles is required.[180] The loss of mechanical advantage, muscle atrophy, decreasing power of the muscle as it shortens, adhesion formation, effusion, or reflex inhibition may result in a quadriceps lag. This lag is usually associated with loss of accessory motion. Inability to extend the knee fully is assessed by having the patient lie supine, with the heel supported on a small firm pillow or block so that the knee can sag into full extension. Have the patient lift the heel off the support (it should be possible to do this before the knee starts to lift). If a quadriceps lag is present, the knee lifts first.[49]

g. Dynamic tibial rotatory function (Helfet test).[107] With the patient sitting, first assess the positions of the tibial tubercles, then passively extend each knee repetitively over the final 25° of extension. Assess rotation of the tibia during extension by observing the tibial tubercle during the movement; normally the tubercle should rotate laterally through an angle of 10° to 15° during the final phase of extension. Compare the involved side with the opposite knee. Loss of dynamic tibial rotation may be secondary to one of several factors:

   i. The tibia may already be rotated at the starting position.
   ii. Tightness or adhesion of the medial capsuloligamentous structures, as may occur with immobilization during healing of a sprain
   iii. An internal derangement such as a meniscus displacement or a cartilaginous loose body

h. Lateral and medial rotation of the tibia on the femur. With the patient seated and the knee flexed over the edge of the plinth, assess active axial rotation:

   i. Range of motion: Medial rotation should be about 30°, active lateral rotation about 40°.
   ii. Provocation of pain
   iii. End feel: The end normal feel of this movement is tissue stretch.

B. *Passive movements*

1. Osteokinematic movements

a. Flexion–extension. Passively flex and extend the knee and note:

   i. Range of motion. If movement is limited, determine whether the pattern of restriction is capsular or noncapsular.
   ii. Provocation of pain
   iii. End feel
   iv. Crepitus

b. Combined movement. Combined movements or quadrants can be tested. More information may be derived by testing passive range of motion in combination.

i. Flexion–adduction movements are the most helpful in eliciting pain.[181]

ii. Hyperextension.[49] With the patient lying supine, hold one hand over the patient's knee and use the other hand to lift the lower leg at the foot; repeat with the resting hand held over the tibial condyle. Normally up to 15° passive hyperextension is possible. Once the range of hyperextension has been determined, the test can be used in combination with abduction and adduction.

iii. Compare both lower extremities; determine the range and pain response of performing combinations of flexion and extension.

c. Passive lateral and medial rotation (axial rotation). To test axial rotation, the patient should be sitting. The knee is first flexed to 90°, then is nearly fully extended. The normal end feel of rotation of the tibia on the femur is tissue stretch. An increased range with the knee flexed may be associated with a rotatory instability of the knee. Loss of motion occurs in many intrinsic knee disorders.[49] With the patient supine, use a hand-hold at the foot, then rotate the tibia internally and externally on the femur, with the knee close to full extension.

i. Hypermobility of external rotation suggests an MCL or posteromedial capsule rupture.

ii. Pain on external rotation may be present with a sprain of the coronary ligament or MCL. A valgus stress can be used to differentiate the two: it will stress the MCL but not the coronary ligament.

d. Hip range of motion, including straight-leg raising and flexibility testing of adduction and abduction. The Ober test is used to assess iliotibial band tightness. The assessment for flexibility should include hip rotation, spine extension, and examination of the hamstrings, hip flexors, iliotibial band, and rectus femoris. To assess for tight hamstrings, have the supine patient flex the hip to 90°. While maintaining this flexion, see how far the patient can extend the knee. A measurement of 20° from full

knee extension is within normal limits.

According to Janda, the first priority of treatment of motor imbalance is to lengthen the tight antagonist.[133] Tight muscles not only increase the workload of the agonists, but also (according to Sherrington's law of reciprocal innervation) act in an inhibitory way on their antagonists.[245] This is an important factor in the quadriceps/hamstring relationship.[155,244,245]

2. Joint-play movements (stress tests). Assess the status of the capsuloligamentous structures by performing the following passive movements. Note the provocation of pain or muscle guarding and whether the movement is hypomobile or hypermobile. The latter can best be determined by comparing to a "normal" side, but experience is also helpful. Note and attempt to avoid eliciting protective muscle guarding when performing the joint-play tests; false-negative results may mask a serious injury that warrants immediate attention.

a. Anterior glide of the tibia on the femur (see Fig. 13-34A)

b. Posterior glide of the tibia on the femur (posterior drawer test) (see Fig. 13-33A)

c. Lateral-medial tilt (see Figs. 13-37 and 13-38)

d. Internal and external rotation of the tibia on the femur (see Figs. 13-35B and 13-36B)

e. Patellar mobility
  i. Medial-lateral (see Fig. 13-41A)
  ii. Superior-inferior (see Fig. 13-42A)

f. Distraction of the femorotibial joint (see Fig. 13-32A); compare with the unaffected side.

C. *Resisted isometric movements.* Lesions involving the muscles or tendons crossing the knee joint are not uncommon and are best detected by assessing the effect of maximal isometric contraction of the structure to be tested. Tendinitis most commonly affects the insertion of the iliotibial band, one of the pes anserinus tendons, or the insertion of the biceps femoris. The quadriceps are often contused in athletics, especially football.

Provide manual resistance to the isometric contraction and determine whether the contraction is strong or weak and whether it is painless or painful. The most important movements to resist are knee flexion (for the biceps femoris and pes anserinus tendons), knee extension (for the iliotibial tendon and quadriceps muscles), external rotation of the tibia on the femur (for the biceps femoris tendon), and internal rotation of the tibia on the femur (for the pes anserinus tendon).

If lesions involving other muscles or tendons are suspected, test the appropriate resisted movements. In relatively chronic tendinitis brought on by repetitive minor trauma (*e.g.*, long-distance running), pain may not be elicited on resisted movement testing unless the patient has recently engaged in the provoking activity. To avoid false-negative findings, it may help to have the patient perform the relevant activity just before testing. Also, testing repeated contractions of the suspected structure may increase the likelihood of eliciting discomfort in chronic cases.

V. **Ligamentous Instability Tests.** Because the knee, more than any other joint in the body, depends on ligaments to maintain its integrity, the status of the ligaments must be tested. In assessing joint laxity in the anterior, posterior, medial, or lateral direction, the four primary restraints by the MCL, LCL, ACL, and PCL are tested. The extent to which these four ligaments restrain their respective motions depends on the knee flexion angle. As the knee approaches extension, the participation of isolated ligaments lessens and the role of secondary restraints increases.[224]

When testing the ligaments of the knee, watch for one-plane instabilities as well as rotational instabilities. Evaluate anterior and posterior motions of the tibia in varying degrees of rotation. Always compare the measurements obtained with those from the normal knee.

It is important to grade the amount of laxity in a knee. In most clinical grading systems, grade I laxity represents up to 5 mm of motion; grade II, 6 to 10 mm; grade III, 11 to 15 mm; and grade IV, more than 15 mm.[224] However, instrumental measurements are challenging these concepts, and more accurate classification systems are being adopted.[43,185,186,200]

A. *Straight instabilities*

1. *Tests for anterior instability (one plane)*

   a. Straight anterior drawer test (see Fig. 13-34*B*). The classic anterior drawer tests are done in the supine position with the knee flexed 90° and the examiner sitting on the patient's foot to stabilize the tibia as described by

Slocum[253] and Furman,[85] or with the patient supported in a semireclining sitting position (lower leg over the edge of the table) with the patient's foot stabilized between the examiner's legs to prevent rotation.[112] In either test, the hamstring muscles must be relaxed. The examiner's hands are placed around the proximal tibia (over the gastrocnemius heads and hamstrings) with the thumbs over the tibial plateau and the joint line. The tibia is then drawn forward on the femur. The test is positive when the anterior displacement exceeds 6 mm. If the test is positive with both tibial condyles displaced anteriorly, the usual mechanism is a tear of the posterolateral and posteromedial medial capsule and the medial and lateral capsular ligaments. This produces a combined anteromedial/ anterolateral rotational instability. If the degree of subluxation is significant, the ACL is also ruptured.[203]

   b. Flexion–rotation drawer test. This test is performed exactly like the straight anterior drawer test except the foot and leg are first externally rotated beyond the neutral position and then internally rotated, allowing the examiner to assess rotatory instability as well. In each position, the examiner provides a gentle pull repeatedly in an anterior direction. The test is repeated with the foot in neutral. Each lower extremity is tested and the results are compared. A positive anterior drawer test with the foot in external rotation indicates anteromedial rotatory instability; with the foot in the neutral position, a positive test indicates anterolateral rotatory instability; and with the foot in internal rotation, a positive test indicates a cruciate tear. A reliability of 62% has been reported for the flexion–rotation drawer test, rising to 89% with the anesthetized patient.[134]

   c. Lachman test. The Lachman test, described by Tory and associates,[272] is considered the best indicator of ACL injury, especially the posterolateral band.[136,137,141,224] It is essentially an anterior drawer test with the knee near full extension (flexed 15° to 20°). The test can be performed with the patient in a semisitting position (with the back supported) and the ankle stabilized between the examiner's legs, or with the patient in supine. In the supine position one of the examiner's hands stabilizes the patient's femur while the proximal aspect of the tibia is moved forward with the other hand. Note the degree of anterior translation and the firmness of the end feel. The Lachman test is graded from 0 to 4+ (1+ = 5 mm; 2+ = 10 mm; 3+ = 15 mm; 4+ = 20 mm).[112] Fetto and Marshall[75] emphasize the importance of noting the type of end feel—for example, a 1+ Lachman test with a soft end feel is diagnostic of an ACL tear. Positive results from the Lachman test may also reflect possible injury of the posterior oblique ligament and the arcuate/popliteus complex.

According to Henning and associates,[112] the Lachman test is positive in 92% of acute ACL tears and in 99% of chronic tears. Positive results reflect anterior displacement, not reduction of a posteriorly displaced tibia.

The ACL has two functionally separate portions, so depending on the knee angle at the time of injury, only one portion may be damaged, thus resulting in a partial ligament tear.[202] If the posterolateral band is disrupted (more common), the anterior drawer test may be negative but the Lachman test positive, as the posterolateral band becomes tighter as the knee approaches extension. Similarly, if only the anteromedial band is damaged, the Lachman test may be negative but the anterior drawer test positive.

2. *Tests for posterior instability (one plane).* PCL instability is best measured by performing the posterior drawer test at 70° and 90° flexion.[224] When this ligament is torn, carefully observe the profile of the knee from the lateral view during the drop-back test and palpate the joint line during the posterior drawer test.

  a. Drop-back test (gravity drawer test) and Godfrey's chair test. Posterior tibial translation can be observed with the patient supine, the knee flexed 90° and the hip 45°, and the foot resting on a table, or with the heel supported on the seat of a chair with the hip and knee in 70° to 80° flexion (Fig. 13-16A,B).[70,92] Observe the positions of the patella and the tibial tubercle from the side. If the PCL is torn, the tibia will "drop back" or be displaced posteriorly on the femur.

  Next, with the patient's knees in full extension, elevate them by holding the great toes (Fig. 13-16C). Observe any external tibial rotation or recurvatum.[121] Compare one side with the other. Subtle degrees of hyperextension can be determined by holding the knee against the table and elevating the heel.[70] Measure the height of the heel above the table.

  b. Posterior drawer tests

  i. Passive posterior drawer test. The patient is placed in the same position as for the anterior drawer test with the hip flexed 45° and the knee 90° (see Fig. 13-33B). The unaffected leg is examined first to determine the normal degree of laxity. The patient's foot is fixed in neutral rotation, and the examiner sits on the dorsum of the foot to stabilize it. The hands are used to push the tibia to and fro to reveal any backward movements of the tibia on the femur. This test is positive after disruption of the PCL with a tear of the posterior capsular ligament.

  ii. Active posterior drawer test. For the 90° active drawer test, the patient is in the same position as for the passive drawer test, with the examiner holding the foot against the table.[224] Have the patient contract the quadriceps and try to extend the knee by pushing the foot down toward the end of the table. Normally the tibia will either remain in neutral or move slightly posteriorly. With a torn PCL, the tibia will move forward because of the unbalanced force vectors of the quadriceps and patellar tendon.[224]

3. *Valgus stress test for medial instability (one plane).* Medial instability is secondary to

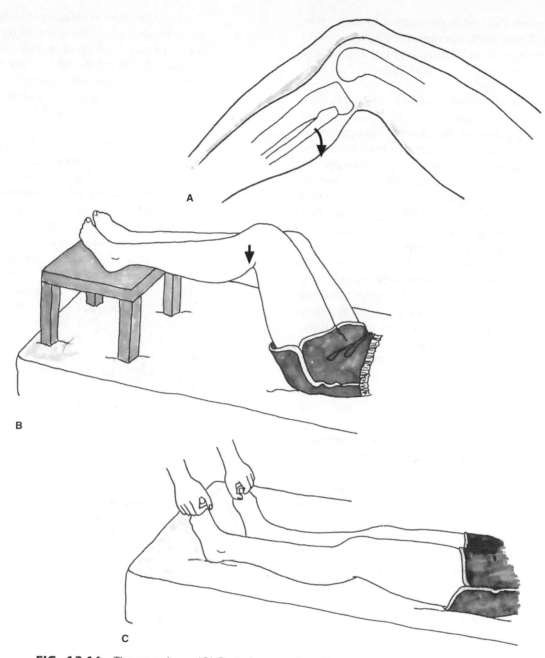

FIG. 13-16. The sag signs. (**A**) Posterior sag sign. Note profile of the two knees: the left (nearer) sags backward compared with the normal right knee. (**B**) The Godfrey chair test also is used to identify posterior sag of the tibia. (**C**) The external rotation recurvatum test; apparent recurvatum and external tibial rotation demonstrate posterolateral rotatory instability.

disruption of the ligaments of the medial tibiofemoral compartment and results in a valgus subluxation of the tibia on the femur. MCL laxity is best evaluated by the valgus stress test performed at 30° flexion and 0°.[224]

With the patient supine and the knee flexed 30°, apply a valgus stress at the knee (push the knee medially) while hugging the lower leg to steady it (see

Fig. 13-39B). Repeat the test with the knee at 0°.

If the test is positive with the knee flexed 30° but negative with the knee fully extended, the MCL has been damaged. If the test is positive with the knee at both 30° flexion and in full extension, both the medial capsular and cruciate ligaments are damaged.

If a stress roentgenogram is obtained

when the test is performed in full extension, a 5-mm opening indicates a grade I injury; up to 10 mm, grade II injury; and more than 10 mm, grade III injury.[112,142,197]

4. *Varus stress test for lateral instability (one plane).* Lateral instability is caused by disruption of the lateral compartment and results in a varus subluxation of the tibia on the femur. The varus stress test is similar to the valgus stress test, but the hands are changed to apply a varus stress (*i.e.,* lateral push) to the knee (see Fig. 13-39A). The test is done in 30° flexion and in full extension.

If the test is positive with the knee flexed to 30° but negative with the knee fully extended, the LCL probably has been injured to some degree. If it is also positive in extension, this implies damage to the cruciates and lateral capsule.

Laxity is graded the same as for the valgus stress test. When more than grade II laxity is present, there is a very high incidence of associated PCL and ACL laxity.[62]

B. *Rotatory instability.* Various rotational instabilities may be present in an injured knee. There may be an isolated rotatory instability, or one associated with other forms of straight instabilities. A rotatory instability secondary to a ligamentous injury results in an excessive degree of rotation of the tibia on the femur. Typically the patient presents with a history of the knee suddenly giving way without any warning. This may occur while descending stairs or when a runner suddenly changes direction.

1. *Anteromedial rotatory instability.* Anteromedial instability, initially described by Slocum and Larson,[253] is an anterior subluxation of the medial tibial condyle that also moves into external rotation on the femur. Anteromedial rotatory instability is increased with a tear of the capsular ligament of the medial joint compartment or with loss of the ACL or the medial meniscus.[166] This instability is diagnosed clinically in the presence of a positive anterior drawer test, performed while the tibia is held in external rotation.

2. *Anterolateral rotatory instability.* Anterolateral instability is caused by insufficiency of the ACL.[86,87,252] The degree of instability is increased if the LCL is also torn. Anterolateral rotatory instability results in anterior subluxation of the lateral tibial plateau, which also moves into internal rotation on the femur. Several tests are used to diagnose this condition. Tests demonstrating translation of the tibia include the presence of a 90° positive anterior drawer with the tibia held in neutral rotation[119,120] and the Lachman test with the knee in about 20° flexion.[203] Tests demonstrating anterolateral rotatory laxity include a 90° flexion–rotation drawer test with the tibia rotated medially by 15°[39,206] and various pivot-shift tests. The pivot-shift or jerk test, a confirmatory test of the ACL, results in the tibia being subluxed anteriorly when the knee is straighter than 125°.[75,86,87,129,170,173] One or more of these maneuvers can be used (pivot-shift test of MacIntosh and Galway,[86,87] the Losee test,[170,171] the Slocum test, the cross-over test, or Hughston's jerk test),[119,120,134] as well as the flexion–rotation drawer test designed to detect rotatory laxity.

a. Pivot-shift test[86] (Fig. 13-17). The patient is supine with the knee in full extension. The tibia of the affected knee is grasped at the proximal tibiofibular joint by the examiner's cranial hand. The caudal hand grasps the ankle and applies maximal internal rotation, subluxing the lateral tibial plateau (Fig. 13-17A). The knee is then slowly flexed as the proximal hand applies a valgus stress to the knee (Fig. 13-17B). If the test is positive, tension in the ITB will reduce the tibia, causing a sudden backward shift. The major disadvantage of this test is that the patient must be relaxed, which often is impossible because of pain. Donaldson and colleagues[67] tested more than 100 ACL-deficient knees and found that the pivot-shift test was positive in only 35% of cases. When the same test was done under anesthesia, the test gave 98% positive results. This test is reversed in the jerk test.

b. Slocum test. One advantage of the Slocum test over the previously described tests is that it allows hamstring and quadriceps relaxation.[197,252,253] The patient lies on the

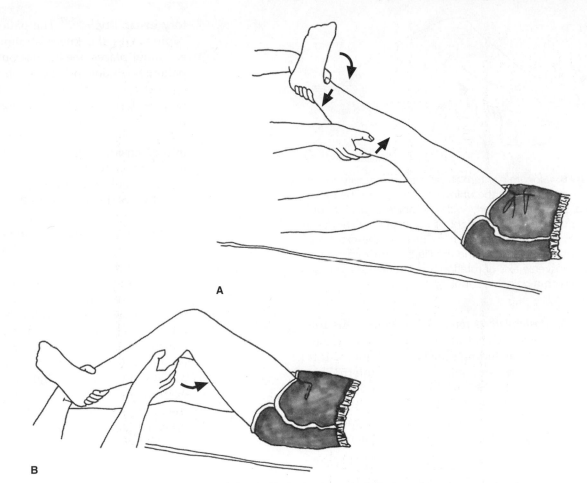

FIG. 13-17. The lateral pivot-shift. (**A**) With the knee in full extension, the examiner's cranial hand grasps the proximal tibia and applies a valgus force. The caudal hand grasps the ankle and maximally internally rotates the ankle. (**B**) The cranial hand then slowly flexes the knee. If the test is positive, a sudden posterior "shift" of the tibia on the femur will be noted.

unaffected side with the leg flexed 90° at the hip and knee (Fig. 13-18). The pelvis on the involved side is rotated slightly backward so that the weight of the leg, with the knee extended, is supported by the inner aspect of the foot and heel. The weight of the extremity creates a valgus stress at the knee, and the relative positions of the pelvis and foot cause a slight internal rotation of the leg. The examiner grasps the distal thigh with the cranial hand and the proximal part of the leg with the caudal hand while pressing behind the head of the fibula (with the caudal hand) and the femoral condyle (with the cranial hand). The examiner applies an additional valgus stress by pressing down on the tibia and femur while simultaneously flexing the knee from full ex-

tension to about 30° of flexion. When the test is positive, the lateral tibial plateau is reduced with a palpable "clunk" or thud as the iliotibial tract passes behind the transverse axis of rotation.

c. Cross-over test.[15] With the patient standing, the examiner fixes the foot of the affected leg by standing on it. The patient crosses the unaffected leg over the fixed foot and rotates the upper torso away from the fixed foot until it faces 90° in the opposite direction. When this position is achieved, the patient contracts the quadriceps muscle. The test is positive when the patient describes the same symptoms as in the jerk test. This functional cross-over test reproduces the pivot-shift and indicates anterolateral rotatory instability.[10,271]

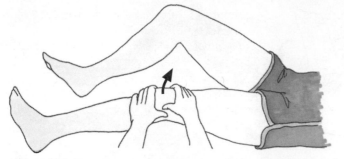

FIG. 13-18. Slocum's anterolateral rotary instability (ALRI) test. The patient lies on the uninvolved side, and the pelvis is rotated slightly posteriorly with the ankle and foot supported on the table. The weight of the extremity creates a valgus stress at the knee. When positive, as the extended knee is pushed into flexion and the iliotibial tract passes behind the transverse axis of rotation, the lateral tibial plateau is reduced with a palpable "clunk."

3. *Posterolateral rotatory instability.* This follows a tear of the arcuate ligament complex, including the PCL,[62,121] and results in posterior subluxation and internal rotation of the lateral tibial condyle. Several tests can be used to identify it.

   a. Reverse pivot-shift test, the primary test used to assess posterolateral rota-tory instability.[128,197] The patient lies supine with the knees straight. The examiner places one hand around the patient's ankle and places the foot against the examiner's pelvis. Beginning at 80° flexion, with the leg externally rotated and a slight valgus force applied, the leg is slowly brought into extension (Fig. 13-19). If the test is positive, the lateral tibial plateau will suddenly move forward and internally rotate at about 20° flexion. This is the opposite of what happens in the true pivot-shift test, where the tibia subluxates in extension and reduces in flexion.[30]

   b. Posterolateral drawer test. Hughston and Norwood described an alternate test for posterolateral rotatory instability.[121] The patient and examiner are in the same positions as for the previously described drawer tests, but the lower leg is slightly rotated externally. As the examiner pushes the tibia posteriorly, the lateral tibial condyle displaces posteriorly and the tibial tubercle displaces laterally.

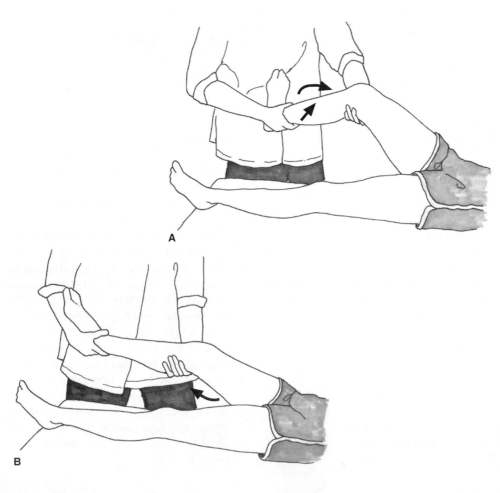

FIG. 13-19. Reverse pivot-shift test to detect posterolateral instability. Beginning at 80° flexion with the leg externally rotated and a slight valgus force applied (**A**), the leg is slowly brought into extension (**B**).

c. External recurvatum test. This is used to identify tears of the arcuate complex and the anteromedial and intermediate fibers of the ACL.[121] The patient lies supine with the knees straight, and the examiner lifts the legs by the toes to produce hyperextension at the knee. The test is positive when the tibia rotates externally with posterolateral displacement of the tibial tuberosity (see Fig. 13-16C).

VI. **Special Tests**

A. *Tests for meniscal injury.* Clinical diagnosis of meniscal tears has been discussed by several authors, notably McMurray,[190] Apley,[11] Noble,[201] Barry,[17] Anderson,[9] and Ricklin.[234] Most of these "meniscus signs" are known by the names of their initiators. The maneuvers can help differentiate meniscus lesions from other knee joint lesions. Although a positive test can help diagnose a meniscus lesion, a negative test does not necessarily exclude the diagnosis of a torn meniscus. Most of these tests are similar, so any one can be used, although McMurray's is considered the best manipulative test.[9] Only some of the better-known meniscus signs are described below.

1. *McMurray's test.*[190] Nearly full range of knee flexion must be present to perform McMurray's test. The knee is fully flexed and the tibia fully rotated either internally or externally. The examiner places the thumb and index finger over the medial and lateral femorotibial joint lines and, while maintaining rotation of the tibia, extends the knee to 90°. This test does not pertain to extension beyond 90°. Provocation of a painful area of movement and a palpable "click" elicited during the movement may indicate a positive test, although there is some question as to the reliability.[199]

2. *Apley's test.*[11] The patient is prone with the knee bent to 90°. Joint distraction or compression can be maintained to help differentiate between ligamentous injuries and injuries to the menisci or coronary ligaments. Pain elicited during external rotation with distraction suggests a collateral ligament injury. Pain on internal rotation with distraction may indicate a cruciate injury. Pain that is felt with rotation and compression, but not elicited when the joint is distracted, suggests a problem with a meniscus or a

meniscal attachment (coronary ligament).[116]

3. *Steinmann's sign.*[234] If localized tenderness is present along the anterior joint line, Steinmann's sign may be useful. In the presence of a possible meniscus tear, pain appears to move anteriorly when the knee is extended and posteriorly when the knee is flexed. Rotating the tibia one way and then the other with the knee flexed 90° may localize pain to the joint line.

B. *Plica Tests.* A pathologic process affecting the synovial plica can mimic a meniscal injury and cause symptoms similar to those of other common internal derangements of the knee; this makes the differential diagnosis more difficult.[19,26,105] A symptomatic mediopatellar plica can often be palpated as a tender, bandlike structure paralleling the medial border of the patella (see Fig. 13-31). A palpable and sometimes audible snap is present during flexion and extension.

With the patient supine, check for the presence of a pathologic synovial plica by passively flexing and extending the knee from 30° to 90° flexion. Produce pressure on the patella medially with the heel of the hand while palpating the medial femoral condyle with the fingers of the same hand. Then flex the knee and medially rotate the tibia slightly with the opposite hand on the foot. A tender fold may often be palpated that recreates the patient's familiar, painful popping sensation.

C. *Patellar Stability Tests*

1. *Apprehension test.* Patellar stability can be judged with the apprehension test performed at 15° to 20° flexion.[116] Try to push the patella laterally, noting the patient's reaction and the tendency toward subluxation (usually associated with medial patellar tenderness).

2. *Passive medial-lateral glide.* To determine the tightness of the medial and lateral restraints of the patellofemoral joint, perform passive glides (see Figs. 13-41A and 13-42). The tests can be performed in full extension and various degrees of flexion.

3. *Passive patellar tilt test.* To assess patellar laxity when the lateral patellar edge is elevated from the femoral condyle, passive patellar tilt is produced. A 0° or negative patellar tilt angle usually reflects excessive lateral retinacular tightness (Fig. 13-20A).[224]

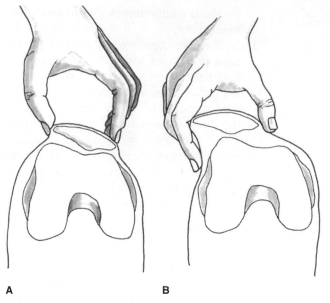

A **B**

FIG. 13-20. (**A**) Passive patellar tilt of +15°, and (**B**) passive lateral glide test, demonstrating a patella being subluxated laterally to half its width.

4. *Passive lateral glide test.* To estimate lateral patellar excursion, the width of the patella is divided into fourths. Longitudinally, lateral overhang in excess of half the width of the patella usually indicates lax or torn medial patellofemoral restraints (Fig. 13-20*B*).[224] A Q angle exceeding 14° indicates a tendency toward patellar instability.

VII. **Neuromuscular Testing.** Resisted isometric movements are used primarily to detect painful lesions of muscles or tendons; they give only general information as to muscle strength. To detect or quantify subtle losses in muscle strength—as may arise from disuse or segmental neurologic deficits—or strength increases resulting from training, repeated loading of the muscle to near-fatigue levels must be done. This is especially true for large-muscle groups such as the quadriceps and calf muscles. Various exercise equipment may be used for this purpose. A convenient but expensive method is the use of an isokinetic apparatus, which gives a torque-curve readout. A simpler but useful method for the quadriceps and calf groups is to have the patient perform repeated half-squats and toe-raises, respectively, in a standing position. Most current reports support a quadriceps:hamstring strength ratio of 3:2.[224] Manual tests for smaller groups, used especially to detect myotomic weaknesses associated with nerve-root lesions, are described in Chapter 22,

The Lumbosacral–Lower Limb Scan Examination.

Perform a scan examination of the key sensory areas and reflexes, and check the patellar (L3–L4) and medial hamstring (L5) reflexes. Note any differences in sensation. A stroking test and sensibility to pin prick may also be indicated (see Chapter 22, The Lumbosacral–Lower Limb Scan Examination).

VIII. **Palpation.** Clinically, palpation is best done in conjunction with inspection and is organized similarly.

A. *Bony structures and soft-tissue attachments.* Note any abnormalities in size, position, or integrity of bony structures. Determine the existence of tenderness, especially at tendon and ligament attachments, remembering that deep tenderness is often referred. With the patient sitting at the edge of the plinth, legs hanging freely, palpate the:

1. Patella
   a. Note size, shape, and position. A small, high-riding patella may be a predisposing factor in patellofemoral joint problems. The proximal lateral pole of the patella may be enlarged in the presence of bipartite patella.[98,214] The inferior pole of the patellar tendon is a common location for "jumper's knee." With the knee in extension, the fat pad is normally extruded to either side of the taut patellar tendon. Hoffa described tenderness on palpating the fat pad ("fat pad syndrome").[113]
   b. Palpate the superior and inferior poles, where the quadriceps and patellar tendons attach, for tenderness.
   c. Passively hold the knee extended, push the patella medially, and palpate the medial articular facets on the back side of the patella for tenderness.

2. Femoral condyles
   a. Note the prominence of the anterior aspect of the lateral condyle.
   b. Palpate the adductor tubercle, a major site of attachment for the medial retinaculum, as well as the site of insertion for the adductor magnus (see Fig. 13-1).
   c. Palpate the area over the medial femoral condyle for a snapping, tender medial patellar plica. Although a

medial patella plica is present to some degree in nearly every knee, it is rarely symptomatic.

d. Palpate the medial and lateral joint lines. Cysts of the lateral cartilage are felt as hard lumps and are prominent at 45° flexion but disappear at both full extension and 90° flexion.

3. Proximal tibia
   a. Palpate the area of insertion of the pes anserinus and MCL.
   b. Palpate the tibial tubercle, where the patellar tendon inserts.
   c. Palpate the lateral tibial tubercle, where the iliotibial band inserts.

4. Fibular head. The LCL inserts at its apex.

B. *Soft-tissue palpation*
   1. Muscles. Palpate the various muscle groups about the knee for:
      a. Mobility. This is especially important after surgery or prolonged immobilization, which may lead to the development of adhesions between muscle planes or between muscles and other tissues.
      b. Continuity. Severe trauma may cause palpable ruptures of muscles or tendons.
      c. Consistency. Prolonged disuse and reflex sympathetic dystrophy predispose to stringy, fibrotic muscles. Contusions of the quadriceps often resolve with heterotopic bone formation, which may be palpable.
   2. Ligaments
      a. Anteromedial coronary ligament (anteromedial border of the medial meniscus) (see Fig. 13-7). This is palpated at the anteromedial joint line. It becomes more prominent here when the tibia is passively rotated internally with respect to the femur. This is a site of point tenderness following medial meniscus tears or isolated coronary ligament sprains.
      b. MCL. The palpating finger follows the medial joint line from its anterior aspect a short distance posteriorly until it is felt to be obliterated by the anterior margin of the MCL (see Fig. 13-8). The posterior margin of the ligament can be similarly palpated where it crosses the joint line. Estimate the course of the ligament and palpate along its extent. It cannot be

distinguished as a discrete structure because of its flat configuration. Localized tenderness usually corresponds well with the site of MCL injuries.
      c. LCL. This is best palpated with the patient's ankle crossed over the opposite knee. It is felt as a well-defined, round structure, crossing the lateral joint line between the femur and the fibular head (see Fig. 13-9). This is one of the few sites at which a ligamentous rupture is palpable; however, at the LCL this is rare.

3. Tendons
   a. Patellar tendon. This is easily palpated from the inferior pole of the patella to its insertion on the tibial tubercle.
   b. Iliotibial band. From its insertion on the lateral tibial tubercle, the blunt, posterior edge of the iliotibial band can be felt well up into the lateral thigh region. Tenderness to palpation over the lateral femoral condyle in association with a tight iliotibial band suggests an iliotibial band friction syndrome (see Chapter 12, The Hip).[201,232]
   c. Popliteus tendon. Popliteus tendinitis is readily diagnosed by palpating the area of the fibular collateral ligament with the leg in the "figure four" position (see Fig. 13-9).[188]
   d. Biceps femoris. This prominent tendon is easily felt at the posterolateral corner of the knee, inserting into the fibular head (see Fig. 13-9).
   e. Patellar retinaculum. Palpate this structure for mobility and tenderness. Palpate the lateral patellar retinaculum while attempting to displace the patella medially. A tight lateral retinaculum has been described as an important factor causing patellar pain.[76] Tension in the medial retinaculum can be tested between the medial edge of the medial border of the patella and the edge of the medial condylar ridge. This area is often tender with patellofemoral joint dysfunction.
   f. Medial retinaculum. The retinaculum is flat and cannot be distinguished as a distinct structure. It is palpated in a

generalized area between the adductor tubercle and the medial border of the patella. It is often tender with patellofemoral joint dysfunction.

g. Pes anserinus tendons. The pes anserinus tendons join to give a flat tendinous insertion on the anteromedial aspect of the proximal tibia 5 to 7 cm below the joint line (see Fig. 13-8).

i. The semitendinosus tendon is easily felt as a prominent, cord-like structure at the posteromedial corner of the knee.

ii. The gracilis tendon is more difficult to distinguish, but can be felt as a "piano wire" between the semitendinosus tendon posteriorly and the sartorius tendon anteriorly.

iii. The sartorius tendon is a large, blunt structure crossing the posteromedial aspect of the knee, anterior to the semitendinosus and gracilis tendons.

h. Gastrocnemius heads. These are palpated deep in the popliteal fossa.

4. The popliteal space. The popliteal artery can usually be palpated at the midportion of the popliteal space. Comparing the popliteal artery pulse to the dorsal pedis and the posterior tibial pulses is helpful in assessing popliteal entrapment syndrome.[172] Swelling of the semimembranosus bursa (Baker's cyst) is best palpated with the knee fully extended.

5. Palpation for effusion. When a large volume of fluid accumulates within the confines of the synovial cavity, it is easily seen and palpated at the medial and lateral patellar margins, and distention of the posterior aspect of the joint is noted. Smaller quantities of fluid may be detected by:

a. Milking the fluid distally out of the suprapatellar pouch with one hand while palpating along the medial and lateral patellar margins with the other. Fluid will be felt to drain beneath the palpating fingers, and the patella may be felt to float up off the femoral condyles. Compare to the opposite knee.

b. After having milked the fluid distally, tap the patella posteriorly with the free hand. If fluid has caused the patella to float, a click will be felt as it is pushed down onto the femoral condyles. Palpate for distention of the semimembranosus bursa, which often communicates with the joint.

C. *Skin palpation.* Palpate the skin about the knee area and the distal aspect of the leg lightly with the back of the hand, noting:

1. Temperature. Localized areas of increased temperature may signify underlying inflammation. In reflex sympathetic dystrophy or other vascular problems, the leg may feel abnormally cool.

2. Tenderness. Burning dysesthesias may be associated with neural disorders, such as nerve-root impingements, or they may arise as referred tenderness from deep somatic pathologies.

3. Moisture. Hyperhidrosis is common with reflex sympathetic dystrophy. Abnormalities in skin moisture may also be associated with other vascular or metabolic disorders.

4. Mobility. Skin mobility is often impaired by adhesions following surgery or prolonged immobilization, and especially with development of a reflex sympathetic dystrophy.

☐ Summary of Evaluation Procedures

The knee evaluation presented here is lengthy when considered in the context of a busy clinical practice. The experienced examiner rarely uses all these tests, but chooses the appropriate examination procedures based on the patient interview and the general nature of the problem. To improve the efficiency of a knee examination, the clinician must organize the tests according to patient positioning. The standing tests are done first, then the sitting tests, the supine tests, and finally the prone tests. For each position, the relevant observations, inspection procedures, selective tissue tension tests, neuromuscular tests, and palpation procedures must be done before having the patient change position.

The following outline summarizes the knee evaluation according to patient positioning. It can be used as a checklist when performing the examination and as the basis for writing a knee evaluation form tailored to a particular clinical setting.

I. Standing
   A. *Observation*

1. Gait
2. Special functions—running, stair climbing, abrupt stops, abrupt turns, hopping, squatting, and so forth

B. *Inspection*
1. Standing structure and alignment
2. Soft-tissue contours
3. Swelling
4. Skin

C. *Selective tissue tension tests*—active weight-bearing flexion–extension

D. *Neuromuscular tests*
1. Repeated half-squats (L3) (same as weight-bearing flexion–extension)
2. Repeated toe-raises (S1–S2)

II. Sitting

A. *Inspection*
1. Patellar alignment and positioning
2. Femorotibial rotatory alignment
3. Muscle contours with maximal isometric contraction
4. Skin

B. *Resisted isometric movements*
1. Knee extension
2. Knee flexion
3. Internal tibial rotation
4. External tibial rotation

C. *Neuromuscular tests*—resisted hip flexion (L2, L3); patellar reflex (L3–L4)

D. *Palpation*
1. Bony structures and soft-tissue attachments
2. Tendons
3. Ligaments

III. Supine

A. *Inspection*
1. Tibial lengths (knees bent)
2. Anteroposterior tibial alignment (knees bent)
3. Femoral lengths (knees bent)
4. Leg-length measurement (anterosuperior iliac spine to medial malleolus)
5. Valgus–varus angulation
6. Swelling or atrophy (girth measurements)
7. Skin

B. *Selected tissue tension tests*
1. Non-weight-bearing (active–passive)
    a. Flexion–extension—measured with goniometer
    b. Lateral and medial rotation
2. Joint-play movements
    a. Anterior-posterior glide
    b. Valgus–varus tilt
    c. Internal–external rotation
    d. Patellar mobility

    e. Distraction
3. Ankle range of motion
4. Passive hip flexion–extension, abduction–adduction, and straight-leg raise
5. Special tests for:
    a. Ligamentous instability
    b. Meniscal tears
    c. Patellofemoral joint involvement

C. *Neuromuscular tests*—resisted dorsiflexion (L5)

D. *Palpation*
1. Muscles
2. Effusion
3. Skin

IV. Prone

A. *Inspection*
1. Soft tissues
2. Skin

B. *Selected tissue tension tests*
1. Passive hip internal–external rotation
2. Resisted knee flexion

C. *Neuromuscular tests*—medial hamstring reflex (L5)

D. *Palpation*
1. Muscles
2. Skin

A knee examination is never done in isolation. The knee is only a single component of the closed kinetic chain, and pathologic processes may exist proximal or distal to the knee. Pelvic obliquity or leg-length inequality must be recognized, because these problems affect the knee. Abnormal foot function is not uncommon and causes various knee ailments, including patellar tendinitis and lateral knee pain.[189] Increased pronation of the foot or a rigid, supinated configuration contributes to knee problems.[33,174–176,184] Failure to recognize that a foot abnormality is causing a knee problem may delay treatment and recovery.

A patient with knee problems should be evaluated frequently with a motion examination both on and off a treadmill (using various speeds). A foot that looks as though it is one configuration often will actually function as the opposite when in motion.[177] Videotapes or films also help in diagnosing difficult problems.[33]

■ BASIC REHABILITATION OF THE KNEE

The concept of knee injury and its treatment is constantly evolving, and staying current is a challenge to those who treat the knee. Many changes in treatment have resulted from arthroscopic techniques.[157] Because the knee is just one part of the closed kinetic chain of the spine and lower extremity, rehabilitation must always be directed toward the entire system as well as specific problems. Maintenance of optimal function as healing ensues is the cornerstone for rehabilitation. Unnecessary loss of strength and range of motion (ROM) must be minimized without imposing inappropriate stresses in the healing tissue. Throughout the entire program, appropriate warm-up and aerobic activities are performed to maintain cardiovascular fitness.

I. Management of Acute Joint Lesions

A. *Pain and swelling.* Ice is generally applied to minimize hemorrhage and swelling. Various forms of electrical stimulation, such as high-voltage pulsed galvanic stimulation and interferential current stimulators, are frequently used to decrease swelling.[198] A compressive bandage or splint is usually applied to provide rest and control swelling. A foam rubber or felt pad over the specific area of tissue damage may be helpful. Frequent elevation of the part should be encouraged to prevent fluid stasis, which may increase or prolong the swelling. Common methods to decrease pain include transcutaneous electrical stimulation and gentle joint-play oscillation techniques (grade I). After the acute phase, to further assist in the resolution of inflammation and to promote healing, heat (hot packs, whirlpool, ultrasound) or contrast treatments (hot pack, ice pack, or ice massage/ultrasound) might be considered.

B. *Prevention of deformity and protection of the joint*
   1. Often the patient is placed on crutches on a non-weight-bearing status initially (24 to 48 hours). Later canes or a walker may be necessary to distribute forces through the upper extremities while walking.
   2. Minimize stair climbing, sitting in deep chairs, or other activities of daily living that require forceful quadriceps contraction.

C. *Stiffness*
   1. If tolerated, perform grade I or II femorotibial distraction and joint-play motions with the joint in 15° flexion or near the resting position.
   2. Passive or active assistive ROM exercises are done several times a day. Wall slides are often helpful in increasing the range of knee flexion. The patient is positioned close enough to the wall that the involved foot remains in contact with the wall throughout knee ROM. The patient gains active range of flexion by sliding the injured leg down the wall and using the nor-

mal extremity to return it to the starting position with the knee extended.[246]

D. *Muscle atrophy and adhesions*
   1. Begin with quadriceps-setting exercises. To promote early quadriceps activity, an indirect approach that will facilitate overflow from uninvolved areas to the quadriceps may be appropriate; this helps avoid pain, which may result in reflexive inhibition.[59] The effect of isometric exercises can be further enhanced through the use of the "cross-over effect." By vigorously exercising the uninvolved contralateral leg, a cross-over strengthening effect can be obtained on the involved side.[108–110] Up to 50 repetitions of quadriceps exercises are encouraged each hour the patient is awake, but not to the point of increasing joint irritability. The patient may be sitting or supine. The foot and toes are dorsiflexed and the heel pushed away from the body. This helps to initiate the vastus medialis obliquus contraction. The length of the contraction (6 to 10 seconds) is important in developing a maximum isometric contraction.[23,196] A stronger contraction may be elicited by resisting dorsiflexion.
   2. Straight-leg raises (SLRs) represent a progression of isometric exercises to strengthen the quadriceps muscle when the patient can maintain the knee extended while lifting the extremity. Progress is limited, however, if the patient does not do the SLRs correctly. Optimal results are obtained if Gough and Ladley's[97] principles are applied with an isometric quadriceps set maintained throughout the exercise.[168,236,246] The patient tightens the quadriceps, holds for 2 seconds, then tightens the quadriceps harder and lifts the leg until the heel is 6 to 12 inches off the supporting surface. The extremity is held in that position for 2 seconds and then lowered slowly. The emphasis is on slow lowering of the leg to facilitate eccentric work, which is important in increasing strength.[1,31,45,46,151–153] The most effective resistance to the quadriceps is during the first few degrees of SLR.
   3. Hamstring-setting exercises are performed in long sitting with 50° to 60° knee flexion. The patient attempts to dig the heel down into the mat while pulling downward on the leg.

   Note: With progression of all isometric exercises the position of the knee must be altered in several ways to enhance isometric strengthening of the appropriate muscle groups at different angles and lengths in the pain-free range. Both submaximal and maximal isometric exercises must be performed at several angles, because isometrics are angle-specific and overflow is only about 15° in either direction.[169]

4. Hip exercises for proximal muscle strength include hip isotonic abduction strengthening (in sidelying), which contributes to lateral knee stability; hip isotonic extension (in prone, working from a flexed position to neutral); and hip adduction, performed isometrically by squeezing a towel roll between the legs. Clinically, patients can perform quadriceps-setting exercises better following isometric adduction exercises. This may be related to the fact that the vastus medialis obliquus has an attachment to the adductor muscle tendon.[110]

II. Management of Subacute and Chronic Joint Problems

A. *Stiffness.* To decrease the effect of stiffness from inactivity, have the patient perform active ROM.

B. *Pain from mechanical stress*
   1. Continue use of assistive devices for ambulation if necessary.
   2. Strengthen the quadriceps femoris.
      a. Begin with isometric exercises with the knee fully extended, because there is less patellar compression in extension.
      b. When tolerated, have the patient perform SLRs with resistance, using a short lever arm.
      c. Short-arc quadriceps exercises, with the patient sitting and a firm pad under the knee to limit flexion to less than 45°, are added once the patient can tolerate resistive SLR. If motion is not painful, light resistance is added at the ankle, as tolerated.

      Note: Resistance applied to knee extension at an angle greater than 45° flexion creates excessive patellofemoral compression forces.

C. *Function and strength.* To improve knee function and balance strength, there should be a gradual transition from isometric to isotonic work. Eccentric work is important in developing strength and is a good introduction to isotonic work.[63]
   1. Proprioceptive neuromuscular facilitation (PNF) patterns and techniques are effective in increasing isometric and eccentric control in the short range and in improving isometric and isotonic control of both

the quadriceps and hamstrings. If activity in the vastus medialis is a specific goal, one of two patterns should be emphasized:[268]
   a. Diagonal 1 flexion (D1F) pattern—pelvic protraction combining movements of flexion, adduction, and external rotation of the hip
   b. Diagonal 2 extension (D2E) pattern—pelvic depression combining movements of extension, adduction, and external rotation of the hip

   2. To selectively train and strengthen knee flexors, active isotonic knee flexion may be performed, with the patient standing, using ankle weights or a weighted boot and exercising through a range of 0° to 90°.[113] With the patient prone, resistance can be applied with a wall pulley, a boot, or manually; the inner and outer hamstrings can be selectively strengthened by working out of the cardinal plane in diagonal patterns. Balance of ratio between flexor and extensor strength should be obtained.[41,42] Normally knee flexion force is about 67% of knee extensor force.[263]

   3. Bilateral PNF patterns emphasizing knee control are most easily performed with the patient sitting. Techniques should first emphasize strengthening in the short range of knee extension and then be applied through gradual increments of range until resistance through full range of knee extension can be accomplished. To emphasize phasic control following slow controlled movement through the range, quick reversal motions with minimal resistance can be used.

   4. Isokinetic strength training. Because muscle strength varies with joint position and the speed at which the exercise is performed (subject to either considerable acceleration or deceleration), total muscle development is unpredictable. Thus, variable-resistance strength-training modalities have been developed. It is questionable how well these machines accomplish this goal, because muscle length/tension ratios vary from person to person.[219]

   When available, isokinetic strength training can be an important component of the strength-training program. Isokinetic exercise can be introduced before or after isotonic work. The patellofemoral forces should be considered in any rehabilitation program. If extensor mechanism problems exist, further restraints are put on activities requiring flexion–extension of the knee. Exercises with low forces and high repetitions will help prevent patellofemoral irritation.[182]

5. Endurance training. Strength and power are only part of the rehabilitation process; endurance and aerobic capacity training should also be included.[50] Two types of endurance must be developed in the rehabilitation process—cardiovascular and muscular endurance. To augment isokinetic effects, a stationary bicycle is useful. The seat can be lowered to decrease knee extension or raised to decrease knee flexion if motion limitations exist. Early on, endurance training can start with stationary cycling for the unaffected limb. To enhance endurance capabilities, cycling should be done at the initiation of the exercise program as well as at the end and should be performed to exhaustion. Swimming and other activities (*e.g.*, rowing machines) can also be used.

6. Functional and weight-bearing activities. The muscular support of the knee (as for any joint) depends on coordinated cocontraction of the muscles about the joint. With weight-bearing, unless the knee is in recurvatum, the quadriceps and hamstrings are the predominant muscles that must support the knee with dynamic cocontraction.[25] The tibia will shift neither posteriorly nor anteriorly but will be pressed to the femur, lessening the forces on the cruciate ligaments and secondary restraints. Cocontraction activities might include step-up exercises, bilateral sitting leg presses, or mini-squats (through 30° range of knee flexion). Active assistive (negative weights), free, or resistive activity (*e.g.*, wall pulleys, latissimus exercise bars) may be included. Isometric control of the quadriceps may be enhanced by manual resistance applied to the pelvis and by PNF techniques such as alternating isometrics and rhythmic stabilization, which increase the difficulty by challenging the quadriceps to maintain the knee in extension against the proximally applied force.

7. Proprioception and balance. Normal proprioception and balance are lost with a major knee injury, immobilization, or a lower extremity pathologic process.[80,281,290] Minimizing the atrophy of this system can begin with isometrics, which stimulate the mechanoreceptors.

These exercises are followed by limited weight-bearing activity using a balance board in sitting, then by assisted balance activities (using parallel bars) in standing. Eventually, one-foot balance with and without the eyes open is added, then standing balance on the toes with balance boards, and finally full weight-bearing balance activities outside the parallel bars or without arm support.

8. Timing and dynamic control. For patients who hope to return to strenuous athletic events, procedures to improve the timing of the muscular activity are necessary. This can be done when the injured knee has achieved 80% of quadriceps and hamstring strength of the normal extremity on Cybex testing.[246] Although fast bursts of activity can be promoted by some mechanical devices, to stimulate the control needed for most athletic endeavors and to emphasize a specificity of training, timing exercises in weight-bearing postures are important. Fast-alternating weight-bearing activities include running in place or on a treadmill or jogging on a trampoline. Quick changes in a variety of weight-bearing postures (*i.e.*, plantigrade, supine activities, bridging) and while running in place will further challenge the timing of the quadriceps activity with variation of the angle of knee flexion. In the plantigrade position, an excessive amount of knee flexion should be avoided because it may simulate the squat-thrusting exercises that can overstress the knee.[268] To further simulate control needed for specific athletic events, sideways, backward, and rotational movements may be added (see the discussion on plyometrics in Chapter 12, The Hip).

D. *Range of motion*
   1. Restore soft-tissue mobility by soft-tissue mobilization techniques (*i.e.*, connective tissue massage, pump massage, myofascial release, and friction massage). Restoring normal mobility of the connective tissue means that tissue will be allowed to move through a normal excursion without encroaching on the function of other adjacent tissues or producing painful stress.
   2. Restore ROM and joint play. As normal osteokinematic ROM and strength are regained, the therapist must also ensure that normal arthrokinematics are restored. Most importantly, normal femorotibial rotatory function must return and is gauged using the Helfet test. Occasionally a pa-

tient regains knee extension without concurrent return of external rotation, presumably because of residual tightness or adherence of part of the medial joint capsule. This may be a source of persistent chronic knee pain or eventual degenerative changes following an otherwise benign traumatic disorder. If such rotatory restrictions are detected, joint mobilization procedures should be instituted to correct them (see Chapter 6, Introduction to Manual Therapy).

Loss of knee extension is a common sequela to knee injury or surgery. Although loss of motion in either direction affects normal knee kinematics and can lead to a progressive arthrosis, loss of more than 10° of extension produces comparatively more complaints and alteration in normal gait patterns than a loss of flexion.[227] The infrapatellar contracture syndrome (with patellar entrapment resulting in patella infera or patella baja) is becoming more recognized in patients with a history of knee inflammation and swelling secondary to surgery or trauma associated with quadriceps weakness and knee immobility. A key finding is significant loss of superoinferior glide of the patellofemoral joint, particularly superior glide.[227]

Joint pain may be an expression of comprehensive imbalance of the musculoskeletal system, including defective neuromuscular control. The inhibitory effect of tight hamstrings (postural muscle) may vastly influence the strength of the vastus medialis and lateralis, which have mainly dynamic (phasic) functions.[132] Neglecting the close relationships between joints, soft tissue, muscles, and the nervous system lessens diagnostic as well as therapeutic possibilities.

The patient should be instructed in an isotonic home program to maintain strength levels over many months, and in proper warm-up and stretching techniques.

■ COMMON LESIONS

☐ Ligamentous Injuries

HISTORY

The patient will invariably recall the traumatic event. The therapist should attempt to determine the exact mechanism of injury.

Onset. One of the most common mechanisms occurs when a football player is tackled from the side with the foot planted and the knee slightly flexed. The victim is usually struck while trying to turn or "cut away." The forces on the knee include a valgus stress, external rotation of the tibia on the femur, and usually an anterior movement of the tibia on the femur. With sufficient force, the medial capsule is torn first, followed by the MCL, then the ACL.[143] The medial meniscus is invariably torn as well, completing the "terrible triad of O'Donoghue."

A minor medial ligament sprain is a common lesion that usually results from an external rotation strain of the tibia on the femur. An external force may or may not be involved.

A force against the anterior thigh, which can drive the femur backward on the tibia, while the knee is close to full extension, tends to stress the ACL. This is especially true if the tibia is in a position—or forced into a position—of internal rotation with respect to the femur. In fact, forced internal rotation of the tibia on the femur in itself may tear the ACL. Internal rotary strains are thought by some to be the primary cause of isolated ACL lesions.[145,283]

A force driving the tibia backward on the femur will stress the PCL. This seems to be true regardless of whether or not the knee is flexed, because the PCL remains relatively taut in most positions of the knee. An example of such an injury is the previously described "dashboard injury."

In the case of a force driving the knee into hyperextension, the posterior capsule tends to give way first, then the ACL, and finally the PCL.[145]

In cases of severe ligamentous injuries, sometimes the patient attempts to continue activities (*e.g.*, return to the field in a football game) immediately after the injury. This is especially true in the case of a complete MCL rupture, since no fibers remain intact from which pain can arise. The pain often subsides after a few minutes if the patient is in a highly motivating situation. No effusion ensues because the capsule is usually torn, allowing the fluid to leak out of the joint cavity. In partial ligamentous injuries, the patient is less likely to continue activity because of persisting pain after the injury.

In severe injuries the patient may describe painful effusion occurring within a few minutes after the injury; this is highly suggestive of hemarthrosis, and an intra-articular fracture must be ruled out by the physician. Slower development of effusion (*e.g.*, over several hours) suggests synovial effusion secondary to capsular irritation. This is common with mild and moderate ligamentous injuries.

Site of Pain. The patient usually will point to a localized area that corresponds well to the site of the tear as being the primary site of pain. The exception is an isolated ACL tear, which is relatively rare and may result in more generalized discomfort.

In the case of effusion, especially hemarthrosis, the entire knee area is likely to be painful; the patient is less able to localize the site of injury. Also, in severe injuries involving several structures, localization is less likely because of generalized pain.

The knee is largely innervated by the L3 segment, although it also receives contributions from L4 to S2. Referred pain into these segments is possible, although this does not seem to occur as frequently with acute ligamentous lesions as it does with chronic, degenerative problems.

Nature of Pain and Disability. In the absence of significant effusion, the pain is described as a continuous, deep, fairly localized pain, which is increased by any movement tending to further stress the ligament (partial tear). When considerable effusion exists, a more intense, aching, throbbing pain is described that is aggravated by weight-bearing and virtually any movement. Hemarthrosis is, as a rule, more painful than synovial effusion.

If a moderately severe tear or complete rupture is left to heal, the pain will largely subside. The patient may walk quite comfortably but cannot perform some particular activity such as running, jumping, cutting, walking down stairs, or squatting without having the knee give way. If carefully assessed, the particular disabilities will correspond to activities that tend to move the knee into directions that the stretched or ruptured ligament is meant to check. Some examples include:

1. Inability to turn quickly—MCL or LCL
2. Inability to run forward—ACL
3. Inability to descend stairs easily, squat, or run backward—PCL or posterior capsule.

An MCL rupture will usually result in considerable disability, whereas isolated cruciate tears may cause little or no disability if quadriceps muscle function is good.[187]

PHYSICAL EXAMINATION

In the acute stage, once joint effusion, considerable pain, and significant muscle guarding have developed, it may prove very difficult to perform some of the evaluation procedures. In any case, the knee must be examined, sparing the patient as much discomfort as possible and ensuring that no harm is imposed by the tests. The value of immediate, on-the-spot examination before the onset of effusion cannot be overemphasized.

I. **Acute Lesion With Effusion**
   A. *Observation.* The patient may hobble into the office, perhaps on crutches. The knee is held slightly flexed with only toe-touch weight-bearing, if any. The shoe, sock, and trousers are removed with difficulty.
   B. *Inspection.* Joint effusion is obvious, especially in the suprapatellar region. The patient stands with the leg held semiflexed, often unable to place the heel on the floor.
      1. The Helfet test cannot be done because the knee cannot be fully extended.
      2. Girth measurements at the suprapatellar region are increased from effusion.
      3. Some redness of the skin over the knee may be noticed. The skin may be somewhat shiny from being stretched.
   C. *Selective tissue tension tests*
      1. Active movement
         a. Weight-bearing flexion–extension is impossible.
         b. In the supine position, active movement is limited in a capsular pattern because of joint effusion, with pain especially at the extremes of both motions. Passive overpressure is met with a muscle-spasm end feel.
      2. Passive movements. Flexion–extension is limited in a capsular pattern (about 15° loss of extension and 60° to 90° loss of flexion) with no crepitus and a muscle-spasm end feel.
      3. Resisted movements
         a. Should be strong and painless, barring concurrent tendon injury
         b. Quantitative determination of muscle strength must be deferred because of the acute condition.
      4. Passive joint-play movements of the femorotibial joint may be hypermobile and painful. (Be aware of possible false-negative results from muscle guarding.)
         a. Anterior glide
         b. Posterior glide
         c. Medial-lateral glide
         d. Internal–external tibial rotation
         e. Patellar mobility cannot be validly assessed if significant effusion is present.
         f. Superior tibiofibular joint. Joint-play movement here may be painful in an LCL sprain.
   D. *Palpation*
      1. There is likely to be localized tenderness at the site of the tear. There may be referred tenderness in nearby areas as well.
      2. Effusion is easily confirmed by the tap test or by emptying the suprapatellar pouch while palpating the lateral patellar margins. Posterior capsular distention may

also be noted. Hemarthrosis may accompany (1) a cruciate tear, (2) a meniscus tear extending to the peripheral attachment, (3) a severe capsular tear, or (4) an intra-articular fracture.

    3. The joint is warm and slightly moist.

  E. *Ligamentous stability and special tests* (see Physical Examination, above)

II. Acute Lesion Without Effusion. Most ligament injuries at the knee are followed by some effusion, but the absence of significant effusion does not necessarily mean that the injury is mild. On the contrary, complete medial capsular ruptures, usually with tearing of all or part of the MCL, may not be followed by much joint effusion, since the fluid escapes the confines of the joint capsule through the defect.

There are two primary differences between a patient presenting with effusion and one presenting without. In the absence of effusion the patient presents with less of a gait disturbance—the knee is not maintained in as much flexion, and the patient may be able to walk without aids. Also, the available range of motion is greater. Generally, the patient who does not develop much joint swelling has less pain and disability. The clinician must carefully assess joint-play movements to determine whether the absence of effusion reflects a minor lesion or a very severe injury. Information acquired during the patient interview is also instructive.

If significant instability is present on one or more joint-play movements, a physician experienced in such injuries must be notified at once, because immediate surgery may be indicated.

III. Chronic Ligament Ruptures. Patients occasionally present with chronic ligament ruptures. The primary complaint is functional instability or giving way of the knee with particular activities. The patient may walk without a limp or obvious disability; the only significant findings may be (1) difficulty performing some specific function such as running, turning sharply, squatting, descending stairs, or running backward, (2) quadriceps muscle atrophy, especially if the joint was swollen or immobilized,[59] (3) hypermobility on one or more joint-play movements or ligamentous stability tests, and (4) a positive Helfet test.

Laxity of one of the medial stabilizing structures—the medial capsule or MCL—is most likely to result in some disability. Often this is combined with ACL rupture. The result is instability of anterior glide and external rotation of the tibia on the femur. Functionally, the patient cannot turn away from the involved side without the leg giving way, a real problem for a young, active

person. The medial meniscus may be torn at the time of injury or some time later from abnormal joint mechanics. The meniscus tear compounds the instability and the tendency for the knee to buckle.

MANAGEMENT

The approach to management of ligamentous injuries depends on several factors, including the patient's age and desired activity level and the nature of the pathologic process. It is important to determine the severity of the injury and whether the lesion is acute or chronic. Traditionally, ligamentous lesions have been graded as follows:

Grade I: Mild sprain, with no gross loss of integrity of the ligament fibers. On examination there is no joint-play hypermobility.

Grade II: Moderate tear, with partial loss of integrity of the ligament, manifested as mild joint-play instability

Grade III: Severe tear or complete rupture of the ligament, resulting in moderate to marked joint-play hypermobility.

This classification is useful for general communication purposes, but it cannot be used as an absolute guide to clinical management; it does not adequately represent the broad continuum of ligamentous injuries, nor does it take into account other individual factors such as the patient's age, activity level, motivational status, or the stage of the lesion.

The stage of the lesion—how acute or chronic it is—is also a somewhat arbitrary designation. For the sake of this discussion, we will base this classification on specific clinical criteria that may reflect the nature of the existing inflammatory process. In an *acute lesion*, the patient cannot bear weight without pain and a significant limp; there is significant loss of knee motion, with a painful, muscle-spasm end feel; and there is obvious swelling or effusion. In a *chronic lesion*, the patient can walk with minimal pain and without a significant limp; knee motion is relatively free, or, if restricted, is limited by stiffness (nonpainful end feel); and there is little or no swelling. A *subacute lesion* presents with some combination of acute or chronic criteria.

Grade I and II Sprains. Following a mild to moderate knee ligament injury, the patient should be able to return to a normal level of activity. In first-degree sprains, treatment is relatively unimportant and is designed mostly to prevent pain. In second-degree sprains, the critical factor in treatment is protection to allow healing. The rehabilitation program should be started early, with more progressive exercise techniques and functional activities added later (see Basic Knee Rehabilitation, above). The general strengthening exercises usually do not need to be modified, although for medial lesions care must be taken to avoid valgus stress at the knee, and for lateral lesions varus stress should be avoided.

Friction massage at the site of the lesion, applied transversely to the direction of the ligament fibers with the knee in different degrees of flexion–extension, may help prevent the healing ligament from adhering to adjacent tissues and may help align newly produced collagen along the normal lines of stress.[54] Take care not to apply friction at the proximal attachment of the MCL, because occasionally a periosteal disruption results here in the development of a bony outcropping (Pellegrini-Stieda syndrome).[278] (Although this is undoubtedly an inevitable result of the original injury, the use of massage may be held suspect should some medicolegal question develop.)

MCL Tear (Grade III Sprain). MCL tears do not usually require surgical repair.[24,72,106,114,237,261] The normal course for these injuries is re-examination under anesthesia followed by arthroscopy of the knee.[192] It is necessary, however, to prove that an isolated MCL injury is present, with no involvement of the meniscal or cruciate structures. The MCL has an excellent secondary support system. Weight-bearing forces tend to compress the medial side, thus aiding in stability, and the injury can be protected adequately with bracing.

Whether surgical repair is used or not, the knee is usually immobilized in a hinge cast or brace cast to minimize atrophy and prevent valgus stress.[101] Rehabilitation after most MCL injuries can progress fairly rapidly (2 to 8 weeks). The treatment program is similar to that for second-degree sprains. Weight-bearing with crutches is continued until knee extension to 10° is possible. Return to sports is not permitted until a normal gait pattern has been achieved.

ACL Tear (Grade III Sprain). Injuries of the ACL are problematic. In the nonsurgical patient, after control of swelling and pain, treatment begins with isometrics of the hamstrings and quadriceps to encourage cocontractions. Range of motion is limited and protected. Based on the studies of Daniels,[56,57] Henning,[111,112] and Paulos[227] and their associates, the range is limited from 90° of flexion to 45° of extension. This is because the ACL undergoes a deceleration strain at about 30° with maximum strain at 0° extension. A protected exercise program is allowed in this range. Isometric internal and external rotation exercises, added once the patient has 90° flexion, decrease any abnormal tibial rotation.[253,254] Special emphasis is placed on hamstring exercises. During all phases of the exercise program, electrical stimulation with maximum contraction is desirable to maintain muscle integrity.[198,264]

Functional knee braces have been suggested for permanent use in sports activities involving cutting or rotational stresses.[18,69,261,267,270] There are two types, featuring hinge posts with or without shells to encompass the thigh. Gait studies have shown that under low loading conditions, most functional knee braces limit excessive anterior tibial translation. However, under conditions of high loading that more closely simulate high activity levels, there is little or no control of anterior tibial translation.

ACL repair or reconstruction, like nonsurgical rehabilitation, typically demands a protocol that minimizes any quadriceps muscle activity involving anterior translation of the tibia. This means using midrange quadriceps work, avoiding terminal knee extension, and emphasizing hamstring strengthening to provide active stabilization. The advanced phase of treatment features eccentric quadriceps exercise and the removal of the extension stop of the rehabilitative brace.[8,48,69,270]

The operative methods of stabilization are intra-articular or extra-articular. In intra-articular procedures, the site must undergo revascularization followed by reorganization of collagen.[38,47,210] These procedures, therefore, necessitate a slower, longer rehabilitation process.[37,38,209,226,227,262]

With the use of securely fixed, high-strength, isometric grafts, the progressive rehabilitation protocol includes early protected motion, neuromuscular rehabilitation, and patellofemoral joint mobilization. Rehabilitation following ACL reconstruction is lengthy: an athlete with such an injury will usually require a year before returning to full activity.

The bone-patellar tendon-bone autograft is currently considered the gold standard.[64] Noyes and colleagues[207] reported that the patellar tendon graft had a strength of 168% of ACL, while the semitendinosus had 70%, the gracilis 49%, and the quadriceps/patellar retinaculum only 21%. Allogeneic tissue grafts from cadavers and amputation specimens pose an attractive option—they are readily available in various tissues (fasciae latae, hamstring tendons) and because of lack of rigid size constraints may be used in quantities that provide greater mechanical strength than the corresponding autogenous tissue.[64,94,126,164,195,205,225,247–250]

Synthetic tissues such as polytetrafluoroethylene (PTFE) are being used more frequently as research in this area has increased.[4,14,29,36,90] Artificial ligaments, prosthetic devices,[4,28,81,88,90,158,179,287,288] scaffold devices,[29,71] and ligament augmentation devices[102,238] are being used where intra-articular constructions have failed or when no biological alternative exists. Mobility may be attained more rapidly following surgery using theses materials. However, artificial materials used for prosthetic devices usually cannot adapt to stress-strains like biological grafts. A partially damaged graft will not heal and eventually will wear out.

Rehabilitation depends very much on the surgical procedure performed.[71,208,243,286] During the second rehabilitation phase (maximum protective phase, between 3 and 4 weeks after surgery), aquatic therapy programs[273,286] and closed-chain kinetic exercises are often emphasized.[217] The pool is often used to initiate a fast-paced walking or running program. A study by Tovin and associates[273] suggests that a rehabilitation program for patients with intra-articular ACL constructions performed in a pool is effective in reducing joint effusion and facilitating recovery of lower extremity function, as indicated by Lysholm scores.[178] The results also suggest that aquatic therapy is as effective as other exercise approaches for restoring knee ROM and quadriceps femoris muscle strength, but not as effective in restoring hamstring muscle strength.

Closed-chain exercises appear to be more effective than open-chain exercises at increasing the joint compressive forces and, thus, minimizing the anteroposterior translation of the tibia.[89,217,279,280] Closed-chain knee extension has been advocated as a safe exercise for patients after ACL reconstruction,[215] and research suggests that closed-chain exercises are safer than open-chain ones because there is less stress on the graft.[111,229,285] An open-chain action primarily emphasizes concentric work, but a closed-chain movement brings a more balanced action of concentric, eccentric, and isometric contraction.

Following the maximum protective phase, rehabilitation proceeds through a controlled ambulation phase, moderate protection phase, light activity phase, and return to activity phase. Closed-chain strengthening exercises are continued throughout. For the athlete, plyometrics are initiated during the final two phases.

PCL Tear (Grade III Sprain). Isolated PCL disruptions often have a good prognosis when treated nonoperatively.[51,55,60,219] Their prognosis after direct surgical repair is somewhat better than ACL repair because of a more generous blood supply. The knee with a torn ACL usually has symptoms of instability, but the knee with a torn PCL has symptoms of disability: medial compartment arthritis (60%), patellofemoral arthritis (70%), and swelling and pain related to activity.[219]

Acute PCL repair with augmentation appears to have a better success rate than does delayed reconstruction.[192,224] Unless synthetic ligaments are used, early postoperative motion after PCL repair usually is not recommended. A period of 4 to 6 weeks of immobilization is advocated to allow the bone grafts to heal

before initiating joint motion. The focus of rehabilitation for both surgical and nonsurgical patients is on quadriceps exercises. In conservative rehabilitation the hamstrings are omitted in the early exercise phase because they may accentuate posterior subluxation. Eccentric quadriceps exercises are started as soon as the patient can tolerate them.

A common surgical procedure for PCL repair is repositioning of the origin of the medial gastrocnemius muscle.[144] This transfer acts dynamically during weight-acceptance and the push-off phases of gait. In this case both quadriceps and gastrocnemius muscles are of primary importance with respect to exercise. Once the quadriceps have achieved 80% of the strength of the normal leg on Cybex or a similar testing device, hamstring exercises are added.[246] The length of time to return to sports is about the same as for injury of the ACL.

In addition to hamstring training to prevent anterior subluxation for ACL injuries and quadriceps training to increase structural stiffness and knee strength for PCL injuries,[91,135,280] it is important to include dynamic joint control training.[52,125,279] Even if the hamstrings and quadriceps are strengthened, it is important that they function quickly and adequately during unexpected trauma by improving neuromuscular coordination. Training should consist of balance and proprioception activities, functional development of the feet to grasp the ground, stabilization of the stance position, and improvement of reactions to sudden additional forces applied by the therapist.[125]

LCL Tears (Grade III Sprain). The LCL or fibular collateral ligament is not a very important stabilizing structure and can be treated nonsurgically.[192,224] However, when the secondary restraints, lateral capsule, and cruciates are torn, functional instability is common and surgical correction is usually required. Rehabilitation after repair follows the guidelines for PCL rehabilitation and for posterolateral rotatory instability. Athletes or other persons placing unusual demands on the functional capacity of the knee must undergo a more rigorous retraining program. For these patients especially, exercises should approximate the type of loading normally imposed on the joint. Most athletic activities, as well as routine activities of daily living, involve relatively high loading conditions. Isokinetic exercise equipment with variable speed adjustments is a convenient means of providing high-speed resistance to various muscle groups, while monitoring the percent of maximal torque output. Such exercises result in strengthening and also optimize the training effect of the exercise program.

Running, jumping, and athletic activities are not permitted until strength is nearly normal, ROM is full, and normal femorotibial rotation has returned. Such activities are gradually progressed from straight-ahead jogging to straight-ahead running, then running with gentle turns, and finally running with abrupt stops and turns. Clinical signs of healing, such as restoration of strength and ROM with no pain on stress testing, in no way signify return of normal strength to the injured ligament.[204] Restoration of ligamentous strength requires a maturation process of collagen aggregation and realignment that may take several months to a year.[3,211]

Any advantages of returning to activities involving intermittent high loading of the knee must be weighed against the risk that the still-weakened structure may give way prematurely, possibly resulting in a more serious injury than the original one. In making judgments about appropriate activity levels, the desires of the coach and the highly motivated young athlete must often take second priority to knowledge of the rate and mechanisms of tissue healing.

☐ Meniscus Lesions

Meniscus lesions affecting the knee are common, especially in athletes. Once it has been determined through examination that a meniscus lesion exists, it is important to classify the injury as a tear confined to the periphery or a tear involving the body of the meniscus. Often arthroscopy or arthrography will assist the physician in making this distinction. Most tears involving the body of the medial meniscus are accompanied by an anteromedial coronary ligament sprain.

HISTORY

Onset. The menisci move with the tibia in flexion–extension and with the femur in rotation. If, during flexion, external tibial rotation is forced instead of the internal rotation that should normally occur, abnormal stresses are applied to the menisci, and a tear is possible. The same, of course, applies to the case of forced internal tibial rotation during knee extension. Similarly, flexion or extension in the absence of the normal rotary movement that should accompany it may result in a meniscus tear. The medial meniscus, being less mobile, is more susceptible to injury. Because tibial rotation is impossible in the fully extended knee, the history is one of twisting on a semiflexed knee. Again, athletes, especially those wearing cleated shoes and involved in contact sports, are particularly prone to meniscus injuries, occasionally in conjunction with ligament tears.

Meniscus tears may also occur with hyperflexion of the knee, especially during weight-bearing. In this position, the femoral condyles have rolled back to articulate with the posterior aspects of the tibial articular surfaces. The menisci, then, must recede backward during flexion, but can recede only to a certain point before capsuloligamentous attachments restrict their further movement. If further flexion is forced once the menisci have reached their limit of backward movement, the menisci are susceptible to being ground between the femoral and tibial joint surfaces. This is especially true if rotation is forced in hyperflexion, because a rotary movement entails further backward movement of one condyle. Certain occupations, such as mining, in which one must move about in a squatting position, may predispose to development of meniscal tears from this mechanism. In athletics, the wrestler is classically prone to this type of injury.

Site of Pain. The person usually feels "something give" in the joint, often with an accompanying deep, sickening type of pain. If not masked by other injuries or extensive effusion, the patient often can point to the spot on the joint line corresponding to the site of the tear where the coronary ligament has been sprained.

Nature of Pain and Disability. The onset is usually sudden, with an immediate deep pain associated with giving way of the joint. If hemarthrosis occurs, pain is typically severe and generalized, arising within minutes of the injury. If a longitudinal tear of the medial meniscus extends anteriorly past the midpoint of the meniscus, the lateral portion may slip over the dome of the medial femoral condyle (see Fig. 13-14). This grossly interferes with normal knee mechanics, with a resultant immediate locking of the joint so that the last 20° to 30° of extension are lost. An injury involving such immediate locking is usually preceded by one or more previous minor incidences of giving way followed by effusion; the developing longitudinal tear finally extends anteriorly far enough to cause such locking.

The person suffering a meniscus tear hesitates to resume activity immediately after the injury, unlike the person suffering a ligamentous sprain. Synovial effusion, causing a generalized pressure sensation, may arise within hours after the injury. Effusion nearly always accompanies a medial meniscus tear, but not always a lateral tear.

In an untreated meniscus tear, the acute stage may completely subside with restoration of motion. The person may resume normal activities with little or no pain. The complaint, however, is one of intermittent buckling of the joint for no apparent reason, even during simple walking. Occasional or persistent clicking of the joint may be reported. Chronic or intermittent effusion may also occur, probably from altered joint mechanics resulting in undue stress to the joint capsule.

PHYSICAL EXAMINATION

I. Acute Stage

  A. *Observation*

  1. The patient may hobble in on crutches with the knee held slightly flexed and touching down only the toe.
  2. Obvious effusion may be present.
  3. The patient may have difficulty removing the shoe, sock, and trousers.

  B. *Inspection*

  1. Effusion may be noted, especially in the suprapatellar region.
  2. The patient stands with the knee held semiflexed.
  3. The Helfet test may not be performed because of incomplete extension.
  4. The suprapatellar girth measurement may be increased from effusion.
  5. The skin may appear slightly red and shiny.

  C. *Selective tissue tension tests*

  1. Active movements
    a. Weight-bearing flexion–extension is impossible.
    b. Flexion–extension in supine reveals:
      i. A capsular pattern if effusion is present
      ii. Considerable loss of extension if the knee is locked, causing a distorted capsular pattern if effusion is present, a noncapsular pattern if little or no effusion is present
    c. Passive overpressure reveals a muscle-guarding end feel at the extremes of flexion and extension.
    d. If the knee is locked, a springy-rebound end feel will be noted moving into extension.
  2. Passive movements
    a. Essentially the same as indicated above for active movement, with perhaps slightly greater range of movement
    b. McMurray's test may not be performed if considerable effusion restricts flexion, because it is applicable only from full flexion to 90°. If flexion is possible, a painful click may be elicited on combined external rotation and extension if a tear exists in the posterior portion of the medial meniscus, or on combined

internal rotation and extension if a posterior lateral meniscus lesion exists.
  3. Resisted isometric movements. These should be strong and painless unless a tendon or muscle has also been injured. Quantitative strength measurements cannot be made because of the acute condition.
  4. Passive joint-play movements
    a. Rotation opposite the side of the lesion may be painful, especially during Apley's test with compression applied. Distraction with rotation should relieve the pain.
    b. Otherwise, these movements should be relatively normal unless a ligamentous injury also exists.

  D. *Palpation*

  1. Tenderness is present at the joint line where a sprain of the peripheral attachment has occurred. This usually corresponds quite well with the side and site of the tear.
  2. Effusion, as mentioned, nearly always accompanies a medial meniscus tear, but not always a lateral tear. The tap test and emptying of the suprapatellar pouch will confirm the presence of minor effusion.
  3. The joint is warm, the skin somewhat moist.

II. Chronic Tear

  A. *History.* The patient describes intermittent giving way of the joint, often followed by some effusion, especially if the medial meniscus is at fault. There may be a history of locking with manipulative reduction by the patient, a friend, or physician, followed by immediate relief of pain and restoration of extension. The younger, active person is usually suffering from a longitudinal tear, beginning posteriorly and gradually extending anteriorly. The older person may have a "degenerative" horizontal tear, with sliding occurring between the upper and lower portions. Clicking is noted by the patient when the femoral condyle passes over a centrally protruding piece of a meniscus.

  B. *Objective signs*

  1. Quadriceps atrophy, especially involving the vastus medialis
  2. Full ROM, but perhaps some difficulty or apprehension when performing weight-bearing flexion–extension
  3. Possibly a positive Helfet test due to altered joint mechanics

4. Possibly a positive McMurray test if the posterior segment of the meniscus is torn
5. Pain on forced extension if the anterior segment of the meniscus is torn
6. Positive Apley test when the joint is compressed, but not when it is distracted
7. Tenderness to palpation at the joint line, usually corresponding to the site of the lesion
8. Perhaps some mild chronic effusion
9. Quantitative quadriceps weakness compared with the other leg
10. The clinical examination may be complemented by an arthrogram to give the examiner more information about the integrity of the menisci (Fig. 13-21).

III. Coronary Ligament Sprain

A. *History.* The patient usually describes a twisting injury followed by some minor swelling and pain over the anteromedial knee region. Rarely is the victim significantly disabled immediately after the injury; he or she usually does not seek medical attention in the acute stage. Acute symptoms usually subside within a few days. If the meniscus maintains good mobility during healing, the patient should have no further problems. However, often the coronary ligament becomes adhered to the anteromedial margin of the medial tibial condyle as it heals, resulting in reduced mobility of this part of the meniscus. In such cases, the person develops a more chronic problem characterized by intermittent twinging of the pain when the adhered tissue is stressed, usually with activities involving external rotation of the tibia on the femur. The persistent nature of the problem eventually prompts the person to seek medical assistance, even though the disorder is otherwise minor.

B. *Objective findings*
1. Consistent findings on physical examination:
   a. Point tenderness over the anteromedial joint line
   b. Pain on external rotation of the tibia on the femur, but no pain on valgus stress
2. Occasionally forced extension hurts as well. Rarely is effusion present by the time the person is seen clinically. There may be minimal quadriceps atrophy if the problem has been of long duration.

MANAGEMENT

Acute Tear of the Body of a Meniscus. If an acute meniscus tear is suspected on examination, the referring physician should be consulted and notified of the positive findings. Usually after arthroscopic evaluation of the knee joint, if an isolated tear is encountered (*i.e.*, one without concomitant ligament damage), a decision must be made as to whether repair or removal is the best treatment. Meniscal repair is a growing trend in orthopedics. Immobilization is necessary following meniscal repair. If the procedure is successful, recovery is expected in about 6 months. Most meniscal injuries still require removal of the torn portion of the meniscus; arthroscopy is the most effective way of doing this.[61,192]

If surgery is not planned, treatment in the acute stage is essentially the same as that discussed above for an acute, minor ligamentous sprain. Weight-bearing must not be allowed on a locked knee and should be restricted on a knee that cannot fully extend because of effusion. Extension must not be forced in the locked knee, because if the displaced piece of meniscus does not slip back, extension may occur only at the expense of the ACL or articular cartilage.

Chronic Tear of the Body of a Meniscus. Again, the physician should be notified if this is suspected. If arthroscopic surgery is not contemplated, the goal is restoration of optimal joint mechanics: mobilization, strengthening, and instruction in appropriate activity levels are necessary. A particular motion, especially extension, must not be encouraged if the restriction is secondary to an intra-articular block, as from a displaced piece of meniscus. Throughout meniscal rehabilitation, it is important to minimize compressive loading of the joint until adequate muscular protection and joint reorganization have been developed.

Coronary Ligament Tear. Persons with coronary ligament tears are generally seen in the chronic stage only because the acute pain and disability are usually

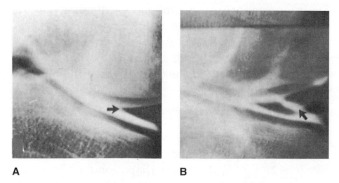

A   **B**

FIG. 13-21. (**A**) A normal meniscus appears as an uninterrupted dark wedge (*arrow*) on an arthrogram. An arthrogram of a torn meniscus (**B**) shows streaks of dye within the wedge. (Kulund DH: The Injured Athlete, 2nd ed. Philadelphia, JB Lippincott, 1988:176)

not severe. The persistent intermittent knee pain is the result of adherence of the anteromedial coronary ligament to the underlying tibia; the adhesion is broken with some sudden movement, then adherence recurs during healing. The objective of treatment is to restore mobility gradually to this part of the meniscus. This is accomplished with ultrasound and transverse friction massage applied directly to the site of the lesion. Five to 10 minutes of massage, over three or four treatment sessions, are usually sufficient. Attention should be paid to quadriceps weakness if present. The patient may be instructed in self-administered friction massage, to be applied before activity.

☐ Extensor Mechanism Disorders

Of all the knee problems presenting to the physical therapist, the most common are disorders of the extensor mechanism.[256] The term *extensor mechanism* encompasses several anatomic structures: the patella and its articular surface as well as the trochlear surface of the femur, the patellar tendon and its attachment to both patella and tibial tuberosity, all of the associated supporting soft tissues (such as the retinaculum, peripatellar synovium, and the structures known as synovial plica), the various parts of the quadriceps musculature, and the quadriceps tendon attachment into the patella.

PATELLAR TRACKING DYSFUNCTION (CHONDROMALACIA PATELLAE)

Disorders of the patellofemoral joint constitute a large percentage of chronic knee problems of nontraumatic origin. Nonacute patellofemoral joint dysfunctions tend to be referred to as "chondromalacia patellae," which literally means "softening of the articular cartilage of the patella." Because articular cartilage is not a pain-sensitive structure, the term "chondromalacia" does not adequately describe the clinically significant features of the pathologic process, nor does it take into account etiological considerations. In fact, surgical studies suggest that surface chondromalacia *per se* is a relatively normal characteristic of most adult patellae and probably has little relationship in cause or effect to symptomatic knee problems.[2,96,191,216,250,266]

BIOMECHANICAL CONSIDERATIONS

The patella is a triangular sesamoid bone receiving attachment from above by the quadriceps tendon, medially and laterally from the patellar retinacula, and inferiorly from the patellar tendon. The patella glides inferiorly with respect to the femoral condyles when the knee is flexed, and superiorly when the knee is extended.

Because the medial femoral condyle extends further distally than does the lateral condyle, most knee joints assume a slight valgus angulation in the standing position (see Figs. 13-1, 13-13, and 13-22). The direction of pull of the quadriceps musculature tends to be in line with the femur, whereas the pull of the patellar tendon is in line with the long axis of the tibia. The angle formed between the line of pull of the quadriceps muscle and the patellar tendon is the Q angle.

The vector that represents the pull on the patellar tendon during loaded knee extension can be resolved into a longitudinal component and a lateral component (Fig. 13-22). The longitudinal component is in line with the direction of pull of the quadriceps and with the long axis of the femur. The lateral vectorial component causes a tendency for the patella to be pulled laterally with respect to the long axis of the femur during loaded knee extension.

As the patella glides inferiorly and superiorly during knee flexion and extension, it should do so in line with the long axis of the femur. It is important then that excessive lateral patellar movement does not occur. Prevention of excessive lateral patellar move-

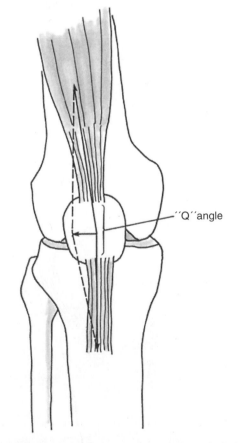

FIG. 13-22. Pull of the patellar tendon during loaded knee extension, showing the Q angle, and longitudinal and lateral vectorial components.

ment during loaded knee extension depends on structural and dynamic mechanisms of patellar stabilization. Structural factors include:

1. *Lateral femoral condyle*, which, because it is prominent anteriorly, provides some abutment against lateral patellar movement (see Fig. 13-2)
2. *Deep patellar groove of the femur*, in which the patella glides when the knee is in positions of flexion
3. *Angle between the pull of the quadriceps and the pull of the patellar tendon*. When the knee is in positions of flexion, there is an angle between the pull of the quadriceps and the pull of the patellar tendon, projected onto the sagittal plane (Fig. 13-23). The result of these pulls, represented vectorially, is a patellofemoral compressive force that holds the patella tightly against the patellar groove of the femur, disallowing extraneous movement.

The structural stabilizing mechanisms mentioned here are operational primarily in positions of some knee flexion. As the knee approaches full extension, the patella begins moving superiorly out of the deep part of the patellar groove of the femur. In this position the sagittally projected angulation between the quadriceps muscle and the patellar tendon decreases, thus reducing the patellofemoral compressive force that holds the patella firmly in the groove. As the knee moves into extension, especially when loaded, dynamic patellar stabilizing factors play an essential role.

The most important dynamic factor necessary to ensure normal patellofemoral joint function is contraction of the vastus medialis obliquus muscle. The distal fibers of the vastus medialis obliquus originate from the medial aspect of the distal femur and run almost horizontally to insert on the medial aspect of the patella. They attach to the patella by way of the medial retinaculum. The horizontal orientation of these fibers allows them to prevent excessive lateral movement of the patella during loaded knee extension (Fig. 13-24).

ETIOLOGY

Chronic patellar tracking dysfunction is a condition in which the patella tends to be pulled too far laterally each time the knee is extended under load. Causes, both structural and dynamic, might include:

1. An increase in the valgus angulation between the quadriceps muscle and the patellar tendon (in-

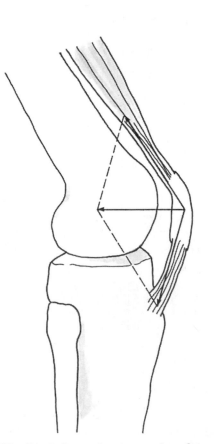

FIG. 13-23. Patellofemoral compression forces in the sagittal plane with the knee in a flexed position.

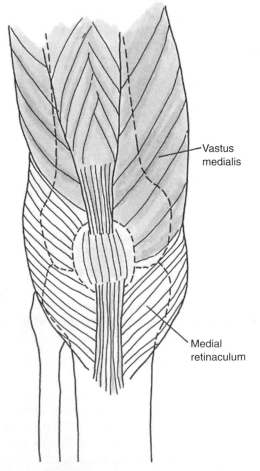

FIG. 13-24. Orientation of the fibers of the vastus medialis.

creased Q angle; see Fig. 13-22). Common causes are increased femoral anteversion, increased external tibial torsion, and increased foot pronation.

2. A lateral femoral condyle that is not sufficiently prominent anteriorly. This results in a loss of the abutment effect normally provided by the lateral condyle (Fig. 13-25).

3. A small, high-riding patella, often called *patella alta*. The more superiorly the patella moves on the femur during knee extension, the less time it spends in the deep portion of the patellar groove, where it is better stabilized.

Dynamically, the most important cause of reduced lateral patellar stabilization is vastus medialis obliquus insufficiency. This commonly occurs from disuse atrophy associated with immobilization or following knee injury. It may also occur when a person increases activities involving loaded knee extension, and the vastus medialis is not adequately conditioned to meet the added loads imposed on the extensor mechanism.

PATHOLOGIC PROCESS

To best understand the clinical manifestations of patellar tracking dysfunction, we must first discuss the pathologic implications of excessive lateral patellar movement. As the patella moves against the femoral condyles, the contact area on the back of the patella varies with the position of the knee. During normal knee function, both the medial and lateral facets of the patellar articular surface receive compressive stresses from contact with the femur. The small odd medial facet, however, makes contact only at extremes of knee flexion, a position that the knee seldom assumes during normal daily activities (Fig. 13-26).[96] Thus, during normal use of the knee, the odd medial facet is nonarticulating and does not receive much compressive stress. Because of this, the subchondral bone is less dense, softer, and weaker at the odd medial facet, compared with that of the rest of the patella (Fig. 13-27).[231,274–276]

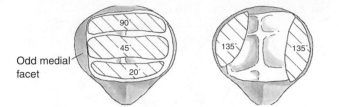

FIG. 13-26. Posterior aspect of the patella, showing contact areas of the facets during various degrees of flexion.

If the patella is pulled too far laterally during loaded knee extension, movement of the patella will follow the contour of the patellar groove of the femur. This causes the patella to undergo some rotation in the transverse plane, bringing the odd medial facet into a contacting position (Fig. 13-28). Under such conditions the relatively weak subchondral bone of the odd medial facet may be unable to withstand the loads imposed on it. This results in an increased rate of trabecular microfracturing, which may incite a low-grade, painful inflammatory response. Trabecular breakdown may be further enhanced by shear stresses between the soft odd medial facet and the stiffer medial facet during compressive deformation.[276] For a particular load, the odd medial facet would deform more than the medial facet, resulting in shearing when the two are compressed simultaneously. This would cause the pathologic process to progress into the medial facet of the patella.

Excessive lateral patellar movement during repeated knee extension may also cause abnormal tensile stresses to the medial retinaculum of the knee. This could also be a source of low-grade inflammation and pain associated with patellar tracking dysfunction.

CLINICAL MANIFESTATIONS

The patient presenting with patellar tracking dysfunction usually demonstrates characteristic symptoms and signs consistent with the etiological and pathologic factors mentioned. The consistent subjective complaints of a patient presenting with patellar tracking dysfunction include:

1. A gradual onset of pain. The patient often describes some recent increase in activities involving

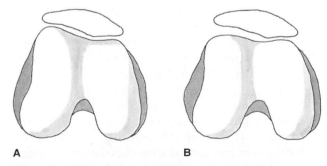

A   **B**

FIG. 13-25. Femoral condyles, showing (**A**) normal prominence of the lateral condyle and (**B**) insufficient prominence of the lateral condyle anteriorly.

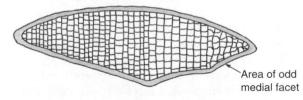

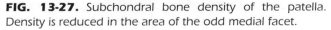

FIG. 13-27. Subchondral bone density of the patella. Density is reduced in the area of the odd medial facet.

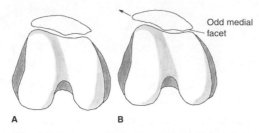

Odd medial facet

FIG. 13-28. (**A**) Position of patella during normal, loaded knee extension. (**B**) Abnormal lateral pull of the patella during loaded knee extension brings the odd medial facet into a contacting position.

loaded knee extension or may report some knee injury or disuse preceding the onset of the problem.

2. Pain is felt primarily in a generalized area over the medial aspect of the knee and in the peripatellar regions.

3. The pain is aggravated by activities involving increased patellofemoral compressive stresses. These typically include descending stairs and sitting with the knee bent for long periods of time. Slowly applied loads, such as those involved with sitting with the knees bent, are likely to cause more discomfort than running or walking. This is because bone is stronger under fast strain rates for loads of equal magnitude.

The objective findings on physical examination of patients with patellar tracking dysfunction might include:

1. Patellar malalignment. Quantifying the position of the patella is important because, as described above, excessive pressure on the odd facet may result if the patella's position is at fault. McConnell[189] described four abnormal patellar orientations: the glide component, tilt component, rotation component, and anteroposterior position (Fig. 13-29). By using the patellar poles as landmarks and comparing their positions with the planes of the femur, malalignment becomes apparent. These components can be assessed with the patient supine, knee extended, and quadriceps relaxed.

   Patellar glide occurs when the patella moves from a neutral position. The distance from the center of the patella to the medial and lateral femoral condyles is assessed (Fig. 13-29A).[12] Typically the patient shows lateralization of the patella due to tightness of the lateral retinaculum. Patellar tilt evaluates the position of the medial and lateral facets of the patella. Patients with patellar tracking dysfunction frequently exhibit a more prominent medial facet (Fig. 13-29B). Patellar rotation occurs when the inferior pole deviates

from the resting position. Rotations are described as internal (change to the medial side) or external (change to the lateral side) (Fig. 13-29C). Anteroposterior position is assessed during quadriceps contraction. Normally the inferior pole should remain inferior and not tilt above the plane of the superior pole (Fig. 13-29D).

Arno[12] attempted to quantify the patellar position with a description of the A angle (Fig. 13-30). He argued that an A angle above 35° constituted malalignment when the Q angle remained constant. DiVeta and Vogelbach[65] showed A angle measurement to be reliable, with an average value of 12.3° for normals and 23.2° for patients with patellar tracking dysfunction. This method relates patellar orientation to that of the tibial tubercle (see Fig. 13-30).

2. Some predisposing factors of patellar dysfunction include the rotatory limb malalignments—femoral anteversion, external tibial torsion and increased foot pronation. To ascertain the weight-bearing status of the foot and detect any excessive pronation, determine the neutral position of the subtalar joint (see Chapter 14, The Lower Leg, Ankle, and Foot). The normal weight-bearing foot should demonstrate a mild amount of pronation. If the patient is weight-bearing or running with the foot out of neutral position and near full pronation, an obligatory internal tibial rotation occurs and is actually prolonged, resulting in an increased force that is absorbed by the soft tissues of the knee.[130,131] Entities that produce compensatory subtalar pronation include genu varum, triceps surae contractures, hindfoot varus, and forefoot supination.[35,127,130,131]

3. Other structural factors include marked tibia vara, especially when the varus is sharply localized to the tibia. If the lateral angulation of the tibia to the floor angle exceeds 10°, the extremity requires an excessive amount of subtalar joint pronation to produce a plantigrade foot. This can occur in both genu varum and tibia vara and may be a cause of peripatellar pain.[44]

4. Congenital recurvatum, which may be associated with patella alta and with generalized joint laxity with relative patellar hypermobility.[228,282] Leg-length discrepancy may result in hyperextension on the shorter side during single-leg stance and at the push-off phase of gait, which may accelerate extensor mechanism difficulties.[27,279]

5. Abnormal patellar tracking and patellofemoral crepitus during weight-bearing (if the tissue breakdown has spread to surface layers of articular cartilage). Observation of lower extremity weight-bearing mechanics during gait, single-leg

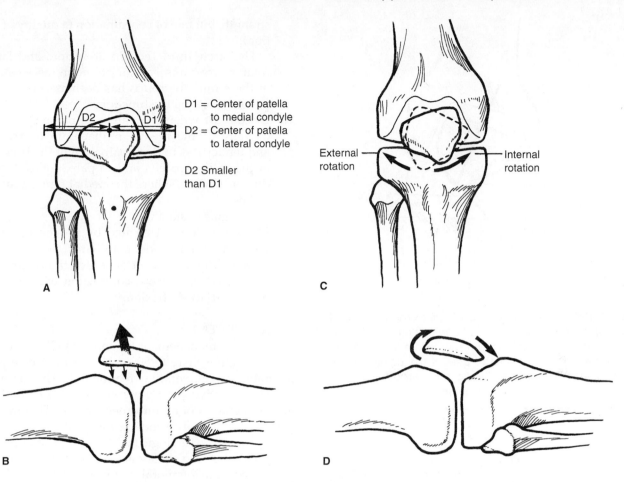

D1 = Center of patella
to medial condyle
D2 = Center of patella
to lateral condyle

D2 Smaller
than D1

External
rotation

Internal
rotation

FIG. 13-29. Assessment of patella position. (**A**) Patellar glide, (**B**) patellar tilt, (**C**) patellar rotation, and (**D**) antero-posterior position. (Arno A: A quantitative measurement of patella alignment. JOSPT 12:237–242, 1990)

squats, and step-downs may be the most helpful test of dynamic function. Careful analysis of gait allows the examiner to observe dynamic changes with respect to femoral and tibial torsions, knee position, and abnormal tracking and compensatory changes in the foot and ankle.

Abnormal patellar tracking may be observed in sitting as the patient flexes and extends the knee. The patella normally has 5 to 7 cm of longitudinal excursion with flexion and extension as it enters and exits the trochlear groove.[44] Normally there should be a smooth longitudinal trajectory, with a small amount of physiologic rotation.[159] Any abrupt or sudden movements at 10° to 30° flexion, as the patella enters or exits the femoral trochlea, are considered abnormal (*i.e.*, abrupt lateral translations just before or at the end of extension, or a semicircular route of the patella as if it were pivoting around the lateral trochlear facet).[76]

One other sign of abnormal position and track-

ing is the "grasshopper eye" patella. This is a combination of both high and lateral positions of the patella.[130]

6. Soft-tissue restrictions. One of the frequent findings in the patient with patellofemoral pain is lateral retinaculum tightness.[76,82,83,147,213] Overuse of the tensor fasciae latae may lead to increased tightness of the iliotibial band. This may in turn cause the lateral patellar retinaculum to tighten secondary to their anatomic connection.[20] According to Merchant,[194] the most common cause of lateral retinacular tightness is congenital. Other causes of lateral retinaculum tightness are posttraumatic scarring, postsurgical fibrosis, and reflex sympathetic dystrophy.[194] Tightness of the lateral retinaculum is noted when the patella is assessed for passive medial excursion or glide of the patella, and when the retinaculum is palpated.[84] Tightness of the hamstrings places increased demand on the quadriceps during knee

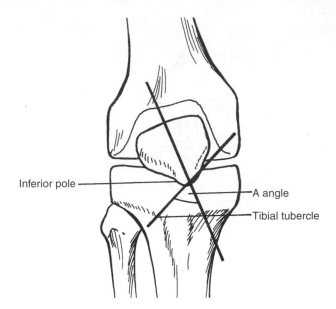

Inferior pole

A angle

Tibial tubercle

FIG. 13-30. *The A angle. To calculate the A angle, the poles of the patella are palpated and a line is drawn bisecting the patella. Another line is drawn from the tibial tubercle to the apex of the inferior pole of the patella, and the angle of intersection forms the A angle. (Arno A: A quantitative measurement of patella alignment. JOSPT 12:237–242, 1990)*

extension, which may increase patellofemoral joint reaction forces, while tight quadriceps increase compression of the patellofemoral joint.[20,118,202] A tight gastrocnemius may make the patient walk with a slightly flexed knee, thereby putting more stress on the extensor mechanism about the knee.[118]

7. Visible vastus medialis obliquus atrophy when the patient is asked to contract the quadriceps strongly against resistance at 30° or in the presence of terminal extension lag. A useful method proposed by Beck and Wildermuth[19] to assess a poorly functioning vastus medialis and to determine secondary substitutions is as follows. With the patient supine, the examiner places one rolled-up fist under the patient's knee to flex the leg 15° to 20°. Have the patient extend the knee but not lift the knee from the fist. If there is adequate vastus medialis function, the patient can maintain light contact with the fist without lifting the entire leg from the fist or pressing down on the fist. Substitutions that may occur include overuse of the proximal quadriceps, resulting in hip flexion with knee extension; or cocontraction by the hamstrings, exhibited by hip extension and the patient extending the knee with the upper quadriceps. In severe cases, the gluteals may be used; the patient lifts the entire pelvis off the table. The authors suggest that this is not a test of strength, but one of coordination (a quality of motion).

The strength of the hip abductors and lateral rotators warrants special attention, as weakness of these muscle groups has been associated with patellar tracking dysfunction.[20]

8. Discomfort when the patella is passively moved laterally (if the medial retinaculum is irritated) and tenderness to deep palpation of the back side of the medial patella and to palpation of the adductor tubercle, where the medial retinaculum attaches

9. Alterations in stability

10. Patellar discomfort elicited by provocation tests, which might include maintained inferior glide with an isometric contraction of the quadriceps, or resisted quadriceps contraction with the knee held at 30° to 45° flexion.

MANAGEMENT

The initial management for most patellar disorders is conservative. Sixty to 80% of knees treated respond favorably to nonoperative treatment.[147] The success of any conservative program relies on the compliance and cooperation of an informed patient. Treatment of patellar tracking dysfunction must take into account etiological and pathologic factors. The most important early measure is to reduce activities involving high or prolonged patellofemoral compressive loads. This is necessary to prevent continued tissue trauma. The patient must understand the deleterious affects of such activities as descending stairs or bent-knee sitting, because these activities do not necessarily cause immediate pain.

Particular attention should be paid to strengthening the vastus medialis. This may be necessary to correct insufficiency or as an attempt to compensate for structural causes of patellar tracking dysfunction. To strengthen the vastus medialis, it is often necessary to establish control of the muscle through techniques of neuromuscular facilitation (*i.e.*, quick-stretch, cross-limb reversal; repeated contractions) and electrical stimulation.[235,260,269] For training to be effective, the patient must not experience pain while exercising, because this will have a strong inhibitory effect on muscle function.[258,265]

Starting with quadriceps-setting exercises, the patient progresses to straight-leg raising. Straight-leg raising allows the least amount of patellofemoral contact force while maximally stressing the quadriceps muscle.[117,123] Vastus medialis activity is increased when performing straight-leg raising if the patient is instructed to "set" the quadriceps before lifting the leg.[162] Adding an adduction force while performing the exercise may facilitate the vastus medialis since muscle fibers have been found to originate from the tendon of the adductor magnus.[32,68,233] Doucette and Goble[68] describe this kind of vastus medialis exercise by performing straight-leg raising with the femur externally rotated. Selected hip adduction exercises have also been suggested as a means of increasing vastus medialis strength (squeezing a pillow between the knees positioned in about 20° of flexion).[32,34,104,233] Open-chain exercises usually progress to short-arc quadriceps exercises (starting eccentrically) and finally to concentric contractions (as tolerated, with range limitations of 0° to 30° terminal knee extension).

To enhance more normal tracking, the patella should be exercised during weight-bearing, and it should be firmly taped in the direction of normal tracking during these exercises.[189] The three components of the patella that must be assessed before taping are:

1. **Rotation.** The longitudinal axis of the femur and the patella should be in line with one another. To correct any alterations in alignment, firm taping from either the superior or inferior poles can be used. To correct external rotation of the inferior pole, tape from the middle inferior pole upward. For internal rotation of the inferior pole, tape from the middle superior pole downward.
2. **Tilt.** Most patients present with a positive tilt sign (0° or less) because of tightness of the deep lateral retinacular fibers (see Fig. 13-20A). Correction of this lateral tilt requires stretching and soft-tissue mobilization. The patella should be firmly taped from the midline of the patella medially to lift the lateral border and provide a passive stretch to the lateral structures.
3. **Glide.** Most patients require mobilization of the patella; usually medial glide of the patella is most restricted.

Weight-bearing training is very important because the knee primarily functions in a closed kinetic chain. Training in weight-bearing also places a major emphasis on eccentric control, thus facilitating muscle hypertrophy.[68,93,100] McConnell found the following exercises to be most useful:[189]

1. With the patient in a walk-stance position (symptomatic leg forward) and the knee flexed to 30°, have him or her contract the vastus medialis and hold for a period of 10 seconds or so while the foot is supinated past subtalar neutral and then allowed to slowly return to partial pronation (slightly out of the resting position of pronation). This is repeated several times, then the knee is straightened and the exercise repeated. The object is to train the invertors of the foot, thus decreasing pronation.
2. The same exercise is repeated but with the knee flexed to about 70°. If the patient has difficulty achieving vastus medialis control with either of

these exercises, a slightly turned-out position may facilitate control. Have the patient relax the vastus lateralis and hamstrings as much as possible with both these exercises. Pain-free progression may include half- and three-quarter squats as greater control of the quadriceps is achieved.
3. Descending stairs is performed as an exercise to further facilitate eccentric and concentric quadriceps control. The leg to be exercised remains on the top step while the patient steps down and then back up slowly, with the leg remaining on the step contracting eccentrically and concentrically. Emphasis is again placed on proper alignment and normal tracking. Progression can be made by altering the height of the step or providing resistance.
4. Hamstring exercises are generally included, starting with hamstring sets and progressing to hamstring curls (as tolerated) with flexion limitations of 90°. To facilitate cocontractions, weight-bearing mini-squats (up to 30° of knee flexion) and step-up exercises are most effective.

Assess the extensibility of the lateral retinaculum by noting the excursion of medial patellar movement with the knee close to full extension. If the lateral retinaculum appears tight, it should be stretched using the same technique as used to test its mobility. The effectiveness of stretching procedures may be enhanced by prior or simultaneous heating with ultrasound.

If the condition is associated with abnormal foot pronation and does not respond to the treatment measures mentioned, consider stabilizing the foot to control pronation. This may be done with various orthotic devices, such as a contoured arch support, or shoe modifications, such as a medial heel wedge or lateral sole wedge.

If a tight iliotibial band is found to contribute to functional valgus deviation at the knee, institute procedures to stretch the iliotibial band. A reverse Ober test may be used to manually stretch the entire band. This is best done passively with the patient lying on the involved side. Sit behind the patient's pelvis to stabilize it against rolling backward. Position the leg to be stretched with the hip in extension and neutral rotation and flex the knee to about 90°. While providing support under the patient's knee and preventing hip rotation or knee extension, stretch the iliotibial band by adducting the extended hip away from the plinth. Mennell's selective stretching of various parts of the band and muscle belly may be used as well as other soft-tissue mobilization techniques.[193] Strong medial glide techniques with the patient in sidelying have proved to be most effective at stretching the tight lateral structures around the knee.[189] According to McConnell, this maneuver facilitates vastus medialis training because patellar movements are no longer restricted.[189]

Tight hamstrings have long been recognized as a cause of various extensor mechanism disorders.[19,124] Efficient lengthening can be accomplished by gentle, nonballistic techniques (*i.e.,* reciprocal inhibition of antagonists: contract/relax, hold/relax), prolonged static stretch, and soft-tissue mobilization techniques.[58,74,240,259,268] In leg-length discrepancy and a hyperextended knee, abnormal gait can be corrected with a combination of a heel lift, gait training (using a program of resistive pelvic training/PNF techniques), and quadriceps control exercises.[149,150,209]

A final tool in the conservative management of patellar tracking dysfunction is some type of brace or external support. Taping or braces should be used with exercise and activity programs. Knee braces generally provide support for the knee, avoid direct pressure on the patella, prevent lateral subluxation, or create an uplift of the patella.[165,218]

Shoe orthoses may be helpful in patients who have patellofemoral pain associated with pronated feet.[257]

A few patients with patellar tracking dysfunction do not respond satisfactorily to a well-designed, appropriately instituted conservative treatment program. Common causes of failure include inadequate restriction of activities in the early stages of treatment and inadequate or inappropriate quadriceps strengthening.

The rare patient who does not respond satisfactorily to a well-instituted conservative program may be a surgical candidate.[22,96,127] Surgery may involve loosening a tight lateral retinaculum or reducing the Q angle by moving the attachment of the patellar tendon medially. Occasionally the medial structures of the extensor mechanism are tightened as well.

PLICA SYNDROME

The medial synovial plica is found in 20% to 60% of knees[7] but does not necessarily cause symptoms (Fig. 13-31).[156] Occasionally this plica may become thickened and fibrotic, causing anteromedial knee pain and snapping or clicking, mimicking a patellofemoral or meniscal problem. These tissue changes are often initiated by trauma that results in synovitis; this is more common in athletes.[202] Joggers and swimmers (breaststrokers) commonly have symptoms.[223] Pain is usually intermittent and increases with activity and descending stairs.

Amatuzzi and associates[7] found conservative treatment to be effective in 60% of cases. Conservative treatment using extensor mechanism rehabilitative techniques and ice massage may reverse tissue changes. Treatment is directed at reducing compres-

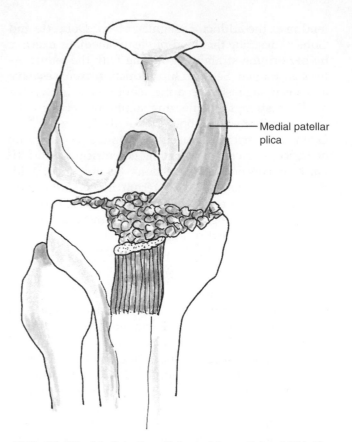

FIG. 13-31. *Medial plica. (Adapted from Kulund DN: The Injured Athlete, 2nd ed. Philadelphia, JP Lippincott, 1988:468)*

sion over the anterior compartment of the knee by using stretching exercises (*i.e.,* hamstrings, gastrocnemius, and quadriceps).

If conservative treatment fails, arthroscopic excision may be undertaken to relieve symptoms. It is often necessary to continue work on the extensor mechanism through exercise and perhaps external support. Several studies have found arthroscopic surgery to be efficacious in the treatment of pathologic plicae.[103,154,220–222]

PATELLAR TENDINITIS (JUMPER'S KNEE)

Repetitive jumping in sports such as volleyball and basketball can create chronic inflammatory changes of the patellar or quadriceps tendon. These changes are related primarily to overuse. Pain is the key complaint and is associated with swelling and joint tenderness.

Patellar tendinitis rarely, if ever, occurs in knees without predisposing physical findings found in tracking problems (*i.e.,* patella alta, vastus medialis dysplasia).[282] Many factors known to aggravate extensor mechanism disorders can accentuate the symptoms of patellar tendinitis (inflexibility of hamstrings or triceps surae).

Traditionally, extensor mechanism rehabilitation has been used with patellar tendinitis, but more recently work on the eccentric function of the quadriceps has been emphasized. The basis of this program is to use activities that place maximal stress on the tendon to increase its tensile stress by performing variations of quick mini-squats.[53] Biomechanical linkage with ankle mechanics has demonstrated that most patients present with weakness of the ankle dorsiflexors. Again, good results have been obtained with a program of eccentric work.[124,283]

Flexibility training is important: it increases the elasticity of the muscle–tendon unit and may increase the tensile strength of the tendon. Ice massage to the inflamed area and friction massage to the tendon are also helpful.

Popliteal and Semimembranosus Tendinitis

Tendinitis of the popliteal or semimembranosus tendons follows overuse injuries, usually from long-distance running. Hyperpronation of the foot may result in either popliteal or bicipital tendinitis at the knee secondary to overuse.

In popliteal tendinitis the patient complains of localized pain over the lateral aspect of the knee. With the knee in the "figure-four" position, the LCL and popliteal tendon are stretched and can be palpated. When the popliteal tendon is inflamed, joint tenderness is noticed at its insertion on the lateral surface of the femoral condyle.[124]

Tendinitis of the semimembranosus can mimic a meniscal injury because of its proximity to the joint line. The semimembranosus functions synergistically with the popliteus to prevent excessive external rotation of the tibia. Therefore, hyperpronating problems of the foot can stress the insertion of the semimembranosus.

Treatment consists of rest, ice for the first 72 hours, ultrasound, and flexibility and strengthening exercises. Proper training techniques and appropriate shoes should also be addressed.

Osgood-Schlatter Disease

Osgood-Schlatter disease used to be considered a form of osteochondritis associated with a partial avulsion of the patellar tendon at its insertion into the tibial tubercle before this apophysis unites. More re-

cently the process has been viewed as one part of the spectrum of mechanical problems related to the extensor mechanism.[282] Almost all patients with this condition have some mechanical inefficiency of the extensor mechanism. In fact, it is now thought that this is not really a "disease," but a form of tendinitis of the knee tendon. In young athletes, the tendon is attached to prebone, which is weaker than normal adult bone. With excessive stresses on the tendon from running and jumping, the structure becomes irritated and a tendinitis begins.

Objective findings include:

1. A tender swelling over the tibial tubercle
2. Pain is reproduced on resisting quadriceps extension; squatting may also reproduce the pain.
3. Decreased flexibility. Most patients have significant restriction in the hamstrings, triceps surae, and quadriceps muscles.

The mechanical inefficiencies of the extensor mechanism should be treated by appropriate rehabilitative exercises. Inflexibility should be addressed through stretching and ankle dorsiflexion strengthening if weakness is found. This condition usually resolves without any significant additional treatment. Complete immobilization is neither necessary nor practical. A simple patellar support, such as a Neoprene rubber knee sleeve, may help.

Osteoarthritis

Primary osteoarthritis has no known etiology; secondary osteoarthrosis can be traced to abnormal joint mechanics. Abnormal knee mechanics produce secondary changes in the articular cartilage, subchondral bone, and supportive structures of the knee. The knee is a common site of osteoarthritis of the femorotibial and patellofemoral joints, possibly because it is often subject to trauma.[140,183,251] Previous fractures of the joint surfaces, ligamentous instability, or tears of the meniscus may all be complicated by subsequent degenerative changes. Osteoarthritis may be a physiologic response to repetitive, longitudinal impulse-loading of the joint. Changes may involve either the medial or lateral tibiofemoral compartment, the patellofemoral joint, or any combination of these, or may be panarticular, involving all three areas.

Osteoarthritis usually begins in the medial or lateral tibiofemoral compartment, where it may be related to the articular cartilage damage that follows meniscal tears.[107] One of the compartments is usually involved if there is any knee deformity (*e.g.*, the medial compartment is associated with a varus deformity, the lateral compartment with valgus deformity). As the disease progresses, the degenerative changes in either compartment tend to increase the degree of the existing deformity. If there is a leg-length disparity, the knee on the longer side is usually involved.[66] A flexed knee gait often results on the longer side, if the shorter side is not compensated for with a built-up shoe. This results in increased patellofemoral forces, leading to excessive wear and degenerative changes in the joint.

The most common alteration in alignment of the osteoarthritic knee is a varus deformity. This results in increased forces in the medial compartment, which creates a degenerative lesion of the medial meniscus and subsequent degenerative changes of the medial compartment, and eventually becomes panarticular. Varus deformity is often associated with internal femoral torsion. Since these persons tend to walk with their feet pointed straight ahead by externally rotating the tibia, torsional malalignment also produces patellofemoral arthritis and subsequent abnormal mechanics of the extensor mechanism.

Any condition resulting in a loss of rotation at the hip will eliminate the screw-home mechanism of the knee. This results in vastus medialis atrophy, lateral tibial rotation, increased ligamentous laxity of the knee, and eventual genu valgum deformity and degenerative changes in the knee.

In the tibiofemoral compartment, the meniscus is also usually involved in the degenerative process. As the joint space narrows, increased pressure is carried by the weight-bearing surface of the meniscus, which develops increased degenerative changes and, occasionally, a horizontal cleavage type of tear. The meniscus is slowly ground away, and the anterior part of the meniscus may actually disappear.[255]

PHYSICAL EXAMINATION

The clinical features of primary and secondary osteoarthritis are the same. The major complaint is usually pain, which may be muscular, capsular, or perhaps venous in origin. Morning stiffness is also a common complaint. This is relieved after motion, but the knee becomes painful and stiff again once the weight-bearing tolerance of the joint is exceeded by prolonged standing or walking. The muscles of the thigh, particularly the quadriceps, become painful as a fixed flexion contracture of the knee develops with resulting instability. An insecure knee results in episodes of giving way, secondary to muscle fatigue, and transient severe pain, secondary to minor trauma (which may be the result of impingement of degenerated menisci, the presence loose bodies, or a misstep). Pain is aggravated by activity or weight-bearing, but may also be aggravated at rest, particularly if the knee is held in one position for a prolonged time.

Examination of the extensor mechanism may reveal quadriceps atrophy, parapatellar tenderness, retropatellar pain with compression, and retropatellar crepitation. If genu valgum is present, lateral subluxation of the patella is not unusual. In unicompartmental degenerative joint disease, joint compression with either a varus or valgus stress to the knee elicits pain. Marginal osteophytes along the femoral condyles may be palpable and are sites of capsular tenderness resulting from local irritation.

MANAGEMENT

The general management of patients with osteoarthritis of the knee is similar to that previously outlined for osteoarthritis of the hip and includes anti-inflammatory drugs, rest, weight loss, aids, and physical therapy (see Chapter 12, The Hip). Salicylates act as an enzyme inhibitor that prevents chondromalacia and, when given early and in adequate doses, prevents fibrillation. Ice for pain and spasm relief and heat applications are usually beneficial (hot moist packs or diathermy).[40] Patients also benefit from hydrotherapy. With bilateral involvement of the knees, weight loss allows muscle strengthening and re-education of gait in the presence of pain relief, with resultant functional improvement.

Mobilization techniques aid in easing knee pain and stiffness. Small-amplitude stretching movements used at the limit of range are of most value.[49] One of the most common changes in the osteoarthritic knee is knee flexion contracture, so patients should be taught early how to avoid contracture. Stretching of the tight hamstrings may be as important as strengthening of the vastus medialis. Tight gastrocnemius muscles (common in women who wear shoes with heels higher than 1 inch) can also be detrimental.[139] Although it can be difficult to accomplish, stretching of the gastrocnemius often helps prevent ankle plantar-flexion or knee flexion contractures.

Exercises to strengthen the quadriceps group should be a daily ritual, beginning with setting exercises and increasing to full progressive resistive exercises as tolerated. Biofeedback can be of great value in strengthening the vastus medialis.[148] A training regimen should incorporate several types of exercise and might include isotonic exercises (with eccentrics)[5] and isometric and isokinetic training.[6,163] Beneficial exercises include closed kinetic chain hamstring exercises (the patient stands and flexes one knee, then holds the contraction to the point of fatigue) and gastrocnemius/soleus exercises (the patient raises up on the toes bilaterally or unilaterally). Full-weight-bearing strengthening exercises should be used judiciously in subacute and chronic phases and avoided in the acute phase. Unloading[99,115] and weight-bearing in water[289] should be used as closed kinetic chain exercises in the more acute phases.

The patient's daily activities must be evaluated and if necessary changed. In the morning, active flexion and extension exercises should be done before weight-bearing activities. Walking should be encouraged for daily activities but not forced. Deep knee bends, sitting in low chairs, and remaining in the same position for prolonged periods should be avoided. Faulty posture that strains the stance should be corrected.

▪ PASSIVE TREATMENT TECHNIQUES

(For simplicity, the operator will be referred to as the male, the patient as the female. P—patient; O—operator; M—movement; MH—mobilizing hand.)

☐ Joint Mobilization Techniques

I. **Femorotibial Joint—Distraction**
  A. *Distraction in prone* (Fig. 13-32*A*)
    P—Prone with the thigh fixated with a belt
    O—Stands at the foot of the table and gently grasps the distal leg, proximal to the malleoli, with both hands. The present neutral (resting) position is found.
    M—Distraction is applied on the long axis of the tibia by the backward leaning of the operator's trunk.
    This technique is particularly well-suited for treating pain but should not be used with forces beyond grade 2 traction.[239]
  B. *Distraction in sitting* (Fig. 13-32*B*)
    P—Sitting on the edge of the plinth, with several layers of toweling supporting the underside of the distal thigh
    O—Stands at the patient's side facing the patient's feet so as to direct his forearms in the line of force. Both hands grasp the tibia proximal to the malleoli to gain a purchase on them.
    M—A long-axis distraction is produced by leaning forward with the trunk. This may be performed through varying degrees of flexion and extension.
    This technique is used as a general mobilization to increase femorotibial joint play for pain control. Distraction at this joint tends to occur when moving into flexion

(out of the close-packed position). As with any joint, if normal distraction does not occur, premature compression of joint surfaces will result when moving toward the close-packed position.

If conservative techniques are indicated, the resting position of the tibiofemoral joint is used; if more aggressive techniques are indicated, a position approximating the restricted range is used. An alternate technique is to use an ankle strap with a stirrup attachment for placement of the operator's foot to apply distraction (Fig. 13-32*C*).[137,138] This allows the operator's hands to be free to palpate the joint space as the distraction is applied or to use soft-tissue techniques (*i.e.*, to a restricted lateral retinaculum). The operator may be either standing or sitting. Starting positions include neutral and internal and external rotation of the tibia, with various degrees of flexion or approaching extension of the knee.

II. **Femorotibial Joint—Posterior Glide**
  A. *Posterior glide*—resting position (Fig. 13-33*A*)
    P—Supine, leg beyond the end of the table
    O—Stands facing the medial aspect of the leg and places his caudal hand around the distal end of the leg above the ankle. The cranial hand is placed on the proximal aspect of the tibia, with the ulnar aspect of the hand just distal to the joint line of the knee. The present neutral (rest) position is found.
    M—With the elbow extended, the cranial hand applies a posterior glide by the operator leaning his body weight onto the tibia or by flexing his knees. Grade 1 traction may be applied concurrently with the caudal hand.
    This technique is used for assessment and pain control and to increase joint-play movement necessary for flexion. The neutral position may change with the treatment, requiring repositioning.
  B. *Posterior glide*—of tibia on femur with knee flexed (Fig. 13-33*B*)
    P—Supine, with knee flexed 25° to 90°, foot flat on the plinth
    O—Stabilizes the anterior aspect of the distal femur by contacting it with his entire left hand. The forearm is directed horizontally. The operator contacts the proximal tibia with his caudal hand. The forearm is directed horizontally.
    M—The caudal hand produces a posterior

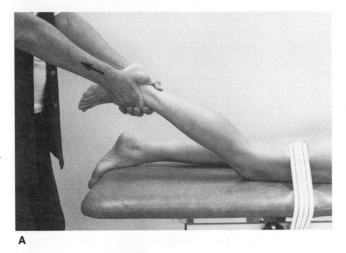

A

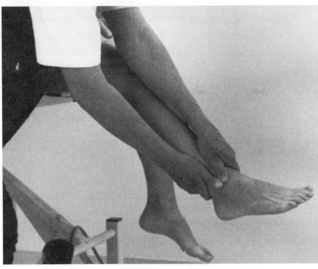

B

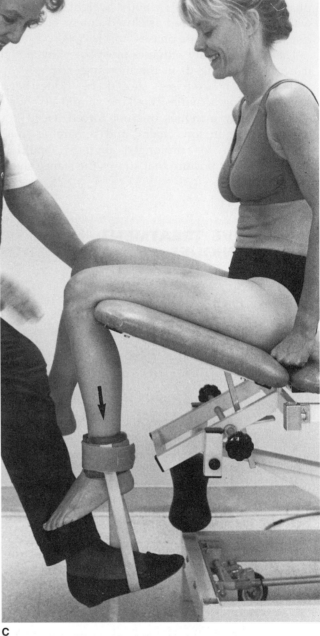

C

FIG. 13-32. Distraction of femorotibial joint: (**A**) in prone, (**B**) in sitting, (**C**) in sitting with use of an ankle strap.

glide of the tibia while the cranial hand stabilizes the femur.

This technique is used to increase joint-play movement necessary for knee flexion. This position is also used for the drawer test (knee in about 90º) to evaluate the PCL.

C. *Posterior glide*—of tibia on femur with knee approaching full extension (Fig. 13-33C)

    P—Supine, with knee slightly flexed from the limit of extension. A 1-inch thickness of toweling may be placed under the posterior aspect of the distal femur.

O—Supports the proximal tibia with the cranial hand placed over the distal femur. He uses the forearm to support and control the femur. The caudal hand is placed on the proximal aspect of the tibia just distal to the joint space.

M—A posterior glide is produced with the caudal hand by moving the lower leg dorsally.

This technique is used to increase joint-play movement necessary for knee flexion. Since the knee is approaching full extension

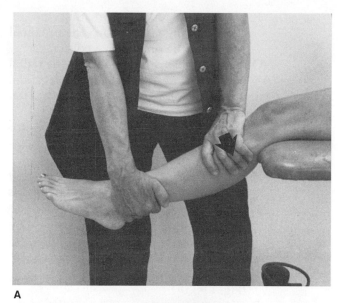

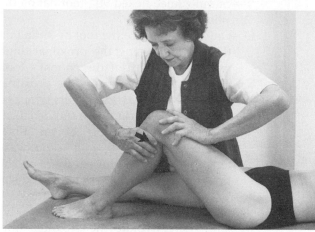

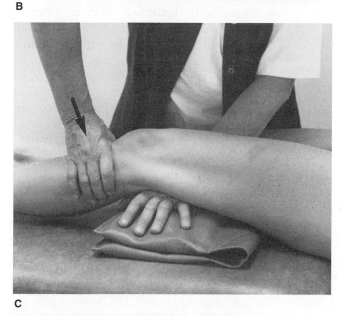

FIG. 13-33. Techniques for posterior glide of the femorotibial joint, tibia on femur: (**A**) near the resting position, (**B**) with the knee flexed (drawer test), and (**C**) with the knee approaching full extension.

(close-packed position), it is considered more vigorous than Technique II,B.

III. Femorotibial Joint—Anterior Glide

A. *Anterior glide*—of tibia on femur in prone, near the resting position (Fig. 13-34*A*)

P—Prone. A bolster may be placed under the distal femur for further stability and to prevent patellar compression

O—Kneels on the table and supports the patient's leg across his thigh. The caudal hand grasps the proximal tibia. The distal thigh is stabilized with the cranial hand. The present neutral position is found.

M—Keeping the arm straight, the operator leans forward, gliding the tibia anteriorly.

This technique is used to increase joint-play movement necessary for knee extension. The tibiofemoral joint is positioned in the resting position if conservative techniques are indicated or approximating the restricted range of extension if a more aggressive technique is indicated. If grade 1 traction is also desired, the operator removes his thigh, stands facing the lateral aspect of the patient's leg, and places his cranial (mobilizing) hand over the proximal tibia. The caudal hand grasps the distal aspect of the patient's leg. The cranial hand then glides the tibia in an anterior direction as the caudal hand applies traction.

B. *Anterior glide*—of tibia on femur with the knee flexed about 90° (Fig. 13-34*B*)

P—Supine, knee flexed about 90°, foot flat on the plinth

O—Stabilizes the foot and lower leg by partially sitting on the plinth, placing the proximal thigh over the dorsum of the patient's foot. He grasps the proximal tibia by wrapping the fingers of both hands around posteriorly and contacting the tibial tuberosity with both thumbs anteriorly.

M—Anterior glide is produced by keeping the arms fixed and leaning backward with the trunk.

This technique is used to increase joint-play movement necessary for knee extension. This position is also used for the drawer test (knee in about 90°) to evaluate the ACL and as a technique to restore joint-play movement for knee extension. The operator leans backward and glides the tibia anteriorly.

C. *Posterior glide of femur*—anterior tibia glide (Fig. 13-34*C*)

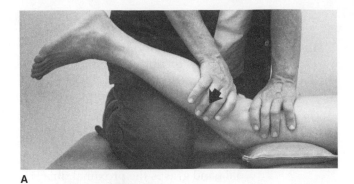

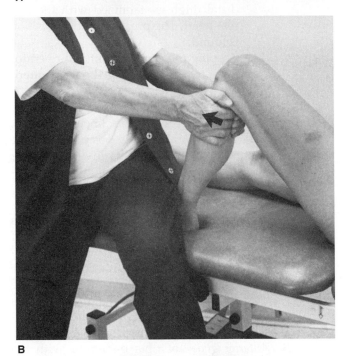

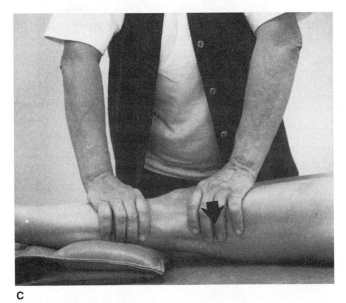

FIG. 13-34. Technique for anterior glide of the femorotibial joint, tibia on femur: (**A**) in prone near the resting position, (**B**) in supine with the knee flexed (drawer test), and (**C**) in extension (with posterior glide of the femur).

P—Supine, knee approximating the restricted range of motion. The proximal aspect of the tibia is on a bolster.

O—Grasps the distal femur with the radial aspect of the cranial hand. The caudal hand stabilizes the proximal tibia on the bolster.

M—Keeping the arm straight, the operator leans down on the cranial hand, gliding the femur posteriorly.

This technique is used to increase joint-play movement for extension. This technique is particularly useful when the patient lacks the last few degrees of terminal knee extension.

IV. **Femorotibial Joint—Internal Rotation**

A. *Internal rotation*—with the knee flexed about 90° (Fig. 13-35A)

P—Supine, knee flexed 90°, foot flat on the plinth

O—One may stabilize the foot by sitting on the plinth, placing the proximal thigh over the dorsum of the patient's foot. The cranial hand grasps the proximal tibia laterally, with the fingers wrapped around posteriorly, the thumb contacting the lateral aspect of the tibial tuberosity so as to gain a purchase against it. The caudal hand grasps the tibia anteriorly and medially, just distal to the cranial hand, gaining a purchase on the tibial crest.

M—Both hands rotate the proximal tibia medially (internal rotation), gaining purchase on the tibial tuberosity and lateral tibial condyle with the cranial hand, and the tibial crest and medial tibial condyle with the caudal hand.

This technique is used to increase a joint-play movement necessary for knee flexion.

B. *Internal rotation*—at varying degrees of flexion and extension (Fig. 13-35B)

P—Supine

O—Controls the distal thigh with the cranial hand grasping from the lateral aspect, the thumb wrapping around posteriorly and the fingers anteriorly. The caudal hand grasps the heel of the foot. He must place the ankle in the close-packed position by fully dorsiflexing it so that the rotary force is transmitted to the tibia, not the ankle joint. His forearm is kept in close alignment with the patient's tibia.

M—The caudal hand rotates the foot medially, transmitting the movement to the

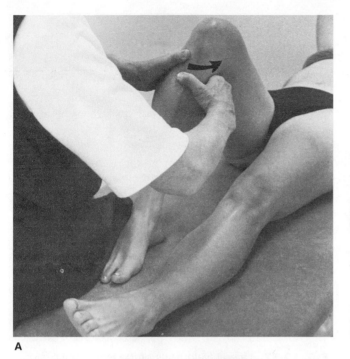

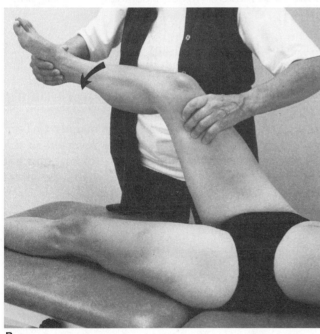

FIG. 13-35. Internal rotation of femorotibial joint: (**A**) with the knee flexed to about 90° and (**B**) at varying degrees of flexion–extension.

V. Femorotibial Joint—External Rotation

A. *External rotation*—with the knee flexed to about 90° (Fig. 13-36*A*)

This is performed in the same manner as Technique IV,A. The hand-holds are reversed, however, so that the cranial thumb

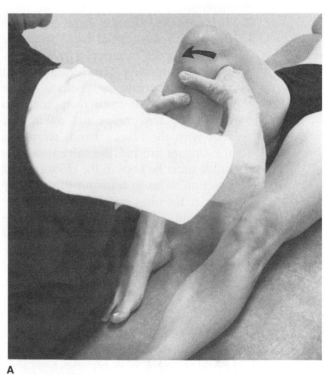

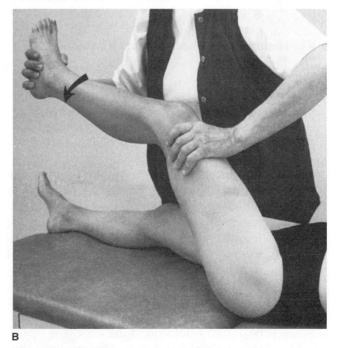

FIG. 13-36. External rotation of femorotibial joint: (**A**) with knee flexed to 90° and (**B**) at varying degrees of flexion–extension.

tibia through the close-packed ankle. Starting with the knee slightly flexed, the movement can be applied at various degrees of flexion and extension. Do not, however, rotate and simultaneously flex or extend.

This technique is considered more vigorous than Technique IV,A. It increases joint-play movement necessary for flexion.

contacts the tibial tuberosity medially, while the caudal hand grasps the tibial crest and lateral aspect of the proximal tibia. This technique is used to increase joint-play movement necessary for knee extension.

B. *External rotation*—applied in various positions approaching full extension (Fig. 13-36*B*)

P—Supine

O—Supports the knee and distal end of the thigh with the cranial hand from the medial aspect, wrapping the fingers around anteriorly. The cranial hand primarily controls the position of the knee, keeping it from dropping into extension. He grasps the ankle and foot with the caudal hand, wrapping the fingers around the calcaneus. The ankle must be kept in the close-packed position so as to transmit the rotatory force to the tibia, not the ankle joint.

M—The caudal hand and forearm rotate the foot and ankle externally (lateral rotation), keeping the ankle in the close-packed position. The cranial hand controls the position of the knee. This may be performed at various positions approaching full extension. Do not rotate and simultaneously flex or extend the knee.

This technique is used to increase joint-play movement necessary for knee extension. It is considered more vigorous than Technique V,A.

VI. Femorotibial Joint—Lateral (Varus) Tilt (Fig. 13-37)

P—Supine

O—Supports the lower leg by resting the leg on the proximal thigh. His knee is placed on the plinth. He supports the proximal tibia and knee with his caudal hand from the lateral side, wrapping the fingers around posteriorly and the thumb anteriorly. The cranial forearm is supinated and in line with the direction of force. The cranial hand contacts the medial aspect of the femoral and tibial condyles. The fingers wrap around posteriorly for additional support. The patient's knee is kept slightly flexed.

M—The cranial hand gently moves the knee into lateral tilt, taking care to avoid any flexion or extension of the knee. The operator's caudal hand supports the knee, but yields with the lateral movement.

This technique is used to increase joint play at

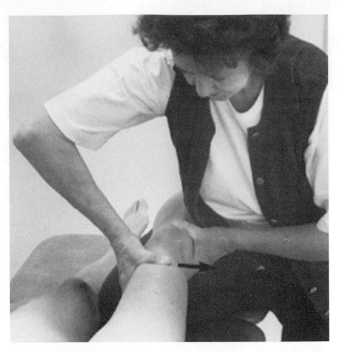

FIG. 13-37. *Lateral (valgus) tilt of the femorotibial joint.*

the knee. As with any joint-play movement, it must not be moved past normal anatomic limits.

VII. Femorotibial Joint—Medial (Valgus) Tilt (Fig. 13-38)

This is performed in a similar manner to Technique VI. The hand-holds are reversed so that the caudal hand supports the proximal tibia and the knee. The cranial hand contacts the lateral

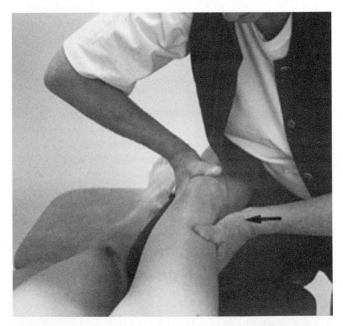

FIG. 13-38. *Medial (varus) tilt of the femorotibial joint.*

condyle. The cranial forearm comes around and is in line with the mobilizing hand, which moves the knee in a medial direction, thus creating a medial gapping at the joint line.

VIII. **Femorotibial Joint—Medial-Lateral Glide**
   A. *Medial (lateral) glide*—in supine (Fig. 13-39A)

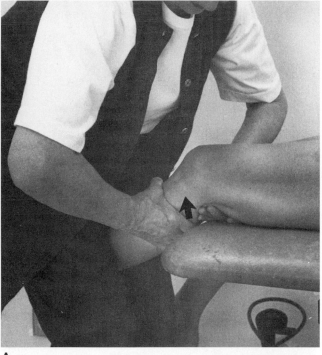

A

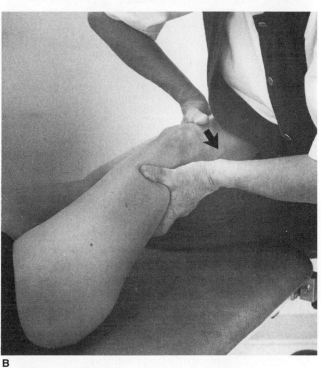

B

FIG. 13-39. Medial-lateral glide of the tibia: (**A**) medial glide, (**B**) lateral glide.

P—Supine, leg extending over the edge of the table. The tibiofemoral joint is positioned in the resting position if conservative treatment is indicated or approximating the restricted range if more aggressive techniques are indicated.

O—Stands at the foot of the table. The foot is held between his thighs or the lower leg is held between the arm and thorax. The cranial hand stabilizes the distal femur from the medial aspect. The caudal hand grips the proximal tibia and fibula from the lateral side.

M—The mobilizing hand glides the proximal tibia and fibula in a medial direction.

This technique is used to increase joint play at the knee. To perform lateral glide the hand-holds are reversed—the stabilizing hand grips the distal femur from the lateral aspect and the mobilizing hand grips the proximal tibia from the medial side (Fig. 13-39B). The mobilizing hand glides the tibia in a lateral direction while the trunk guides the motion.

   B. *Medial (lateral) glide*—in sidelying (Fig. 13-40A)[137,138]

P—Sidelying on the uninvolved side, involved leg extending over the edge of the table. A bolster is placed under the medial aspect of the distal thigh.

O—Stands facing the dorsal aspect of the leg. The caudal hand grasps the distal leg above the ankle. The cranial hand grips the proximal tibia and fibula from the lateral aspect. The knee is maintained in the resting position and the leg is held against the operator's trunk.

M—The tibia is glided in the medial direction indirectly through the fibula while the trunk guides the motion (by flexing the knees).

Lateral glide is performed in the same manner as above, but the hand-holds are reversed and the patient lies on the involved side (Fig. 13-40B). These techniques are used to restore joint play for restricted flexion or extension.

IX. **Patellofemoral Joint**
   A. *Medial-lateral glide (tilt)*—in supine (Fig. 13-41A)

P—Supine, knee slightly flexed over a firm support of toweling

O—Contacts the lateral patellar border

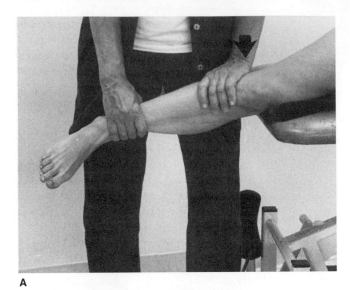

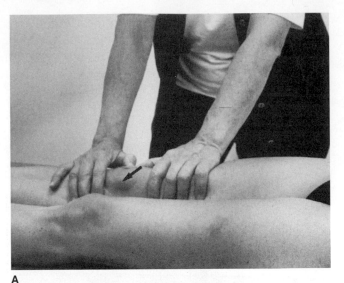

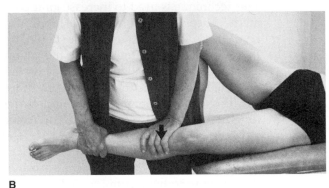

FIG. 13-40. Medial-lateral glide of femorotibial joint: (**A**) medial glide in sidelying, (**B**) lateral glide in sidelying.

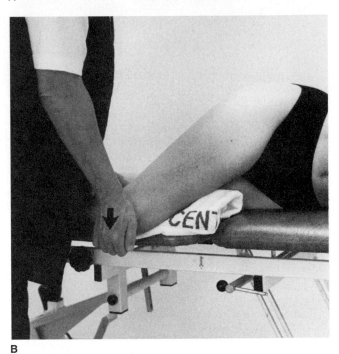

FIG. 13-41. (**A**) Medial-lateral tilt and (**B**) medial glide of the patellofemoral joint in sidelying.

with the thumb pads or the heel of the hand. The remaining fingers rest over the anterior aspect of the patient's leg to help support the operator's hands. He keeps the elbows close to full extension.

M—A medial glide of the patella is produced with both hands. A lateral glide is produced by using the pads of the index fingers. Both hands glide the patella in a lateral direction.

These techniques are used for general patellar mobilization in the presence of restricted patellar movement. Grades I and II should be applied to highly irritable joints where pain is predominant. In less irritable joints, where pain is a result of tight structures, grades III and IV should be considered.

B. *Medial glide*—in sidelying (Fig. 13-41*B*)

P—Lying on the unaffected side with the involved leg placed in hip and knee flexion. The affected patella is just over the edge of the table. A towel or bolster is placed under the knee.

O—Stands facing the leg. The stabilizing hand contacts the proximal tibia or distal femur. The mobilizing hand is positioned with the heel of the hand on the lateral border of the patella.

M—With the elbow extended, the mobilizing hand glides the patella in a medial direction. The force is produced by the operator's body weight.

In this position the lateral structures are under some degree of tension, allowing a more effective stretch to the lateral structures. Avoid compression.

X. Patellofemoral Joint—Superior-Inferior Glides

A. *Inferior glide*—in supine (Fig. 13-42A)

P—Supine, knee extended or in slight flexion with a towel under the knee

O—Stands next to the patient's thigh, facing her feet. The web space or heel of the near hand contacts the superior pole of the patella.

M—The mobilizing hand glides the patella in an inferior direction, parallel to the femur.

This technique is used to increase patellar mobility for knee flexion. Superior glide, to increase mobility for knee extension, is done in the reverse manner. The mobilizing hand is positioned with either the web space or the heel of the hand on the inferior pole of the patella. The patella is glided in the superior direction. Avoid compression of the patella into the femoral condyles. Grades I and II should be applied to highly irritable joints where pain is predominant. In less irritable joints, where pain is the result of tight structures, grades III and IV should be used.

B. *Inferior glide*—in knee flexion (Fig. 13-42B)

P—Supine, foot resting on the table, hip and knee in flexion

O—Stands next to the lower limb. The caudal hand stabilizes the leg by grasping the lower tibia. The heel of the mobilizing hand contacts the superior pole of the patella.

M—Glide the patella in a caudal direction, parallel to the femur.

This technique is considered more vigorous than Technique X,A. To selectively stretch the lateral or medial retinaculum, caudal glide may be directed in a more medial caudal or lateral caudal direction.

XI. Proximal Tibiofibular Joint (Fig. 13-43A)

A. *Anterior glide*

P—Assumes a half-kneeling position or stands at the side of the table, resting her leg on the table. The foot extends over the edge of the table.

O—Places the heel of the mobilizing hand over the posterior aspect of the fibular head. The other hand may be used to support or reinforce the mobilizing hand or stabilize the tibia. The thigh supports the patient's foot in plantarflexion (10°).

M—An anterior lateral glide of the fibula is produced by leaning forward with the trunk. The operator must prevent pain or fibular nerve compression.

This technique is used to increase joint play in the proximal tibiofibular joint and to reduce a dorsal positional fault of the fibula. Lateral knee pain is often present when the proximal tibiofibular joint is affected.[239]

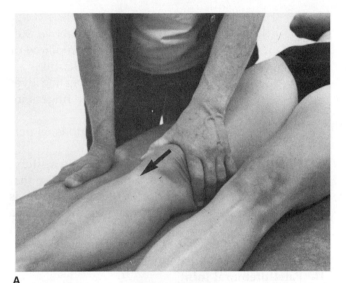

A

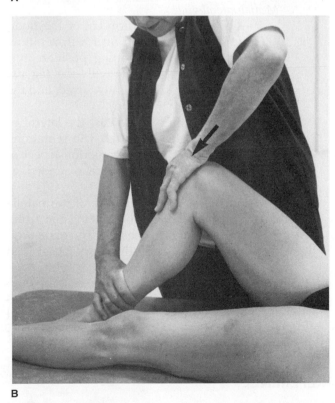

B

FIG. 13-42. *Superior-inferior glide of patellofemoral joint* (**A**) *with the knee in extension and* (**B**) *with the knee in flexion.*

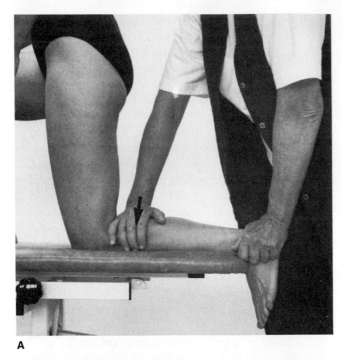

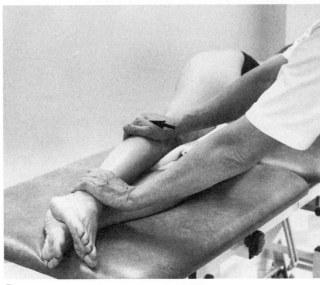

FIG. 13-43. Proximal tibiofibular joint: (**A**) anterior glide, (**B**) posterior glide.

Posterior mobilization may be performed in sidelying with the hip and knee slightly flexed (Fig. 13-43*B*). Both anterior and inferior glide may be performed in supine (see Fig. 14-40 in Chapter 14, The Lower Leg, Ankle, and Foot).

☐ *Self-Mobilization Techniques*

I. Femorotibial Joint
    A. *Forced (gentle) flexion* (Fig. 13-44)

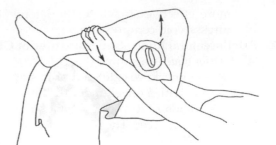

FIG. 13-44. Femorotibial joint—forced (gentle) flexion.

        P—Supine, hip flexed slightly above 90°. The knee is flexed over a firm pillow or towel roll, which acts as a fulcrum.
    MH—Both hands contact the lower leg over the anterior aspect, with the fingers interlaced.
      M—Gentle flexion, with oscillations, is performed.
Note: Forced flexion may also be done in a sitting position. The right hip is completely flexed so that the thigh is supported on the chest. The knee is flexed over the right forearm, which now acts as a fulcrum and gives additional support. The left MH contacts the lower leg over the anterior aspect and carries out gentle flexion of the knee.

II. Patellofemoral Joint
    A. *Medial-lateral glide*
        P—Long-sitting on a firm cot or the floor, knee slightly flexed over a firm pillow or towel roll. (A sitting position in a chair may be used, with the leg extended, the knee slightly flexed, and the foot fixed to the floor.)
    MH—Both thumb pads contact the lateral or medial patellar border. The remaining fingers rest over the anterior aspect of the leg. The elbows are extended as much as possible.
      M—A medial or lateral glide of the patella can be produced by leaning the trunk forward and to one side. The glide is effected by moving the trunk rather than any part of the hand.
Note: Superior-inferior glide may also be performed by contact of the thumb pads on the superior or inferior borders of the patella, with the rest of the hand resting over the medial and lateral aspects of the knee.

REFERENCES

1. Abbott B, Bigland B, Ritche JM: The physiological cost of negative work. J Physiol 117:380–390, 1952
2. Abernathy PJ, Townsend PR, Rose RM, Radin EL: Is chondromalacia patellae a separate clinical entity? J Bone Joint Surg 60B:205–210, 1978

3. Adams A: Effect of exercise upon ligament strength. Res Q 37:163–167, 1966
4. Ahlfeld SK, Larson RL, Collins HR: Anterior cruciate reconstruction in the chronically unstable knee using an expanded polytetrafluoroethylene (PTFE) prosthetic ligament. Am J Sports Med 15:326–330, 1987
5. Albert M: Eccentric Muscle Training in Sports and Orthopedics. London, Churchill Livingstone, 1991
6. Albert MS: Principles of exercise progression. In Greenfield BH: Rehabilitation of the Knee: A Problem-Solving Approach. Philadelphia, FA Davis, 1993:110–136
7. Amatuzzi MM, Fazzi A, Varella MH: Pathologic synovial plica of the knee. Am J Sports Med 18:466–469, 1990
8. American Academy of Orthopaedic Surgeons: Knee Braces—Seminar Report. Rosemont, IL, The Academy, 1985
9. Anderson AF, Lipscomb AB: Clinical diagnosis of meniscal tears—Description of a new manipulative test. Am J Sports Med 14:291–293, 1986
10. Andrews JR, Mc Leod WD, Ward T, Howard K: The cutting mechanism. Am J Sports Med 5:111–121, 1977
11. Apley G: The diagnosis of meniscus injuries. J Bone Joint Surg 29A:78–84, 1947
12. Arno S: The A angle: A quantitative measurement of patella alignment and realignment. J Orthop Sports Phys Ther 12:237–242, 1990
13. Arnoczky SP: The blood supply of the meniscus and its role in healing and repair. In American Association of Orthopedic Surgeons: Symposium on Sports Medicine: The Knee. St. Louis, CV Mosby, 1985
14. Arnoczky SP, Torzilli PA, Warren RF, et al: Biologic fixations of ligament prostheses and augmentations: An evaluation of bone ingrowth in the dog. Am J Sports Med 16:106–112, 1988
15. Arnold JA, Coker TP, Heaton LM, Park JP: Natural history of anterior cruciate tears. Am J Sports Med 7:305–313, 1979
16. Barnett CH: Locking at the knee joint. J Anat 87:91–95, 1953
17. Barry OCD, McManus F, McCauley P: Clinical assessment of suspected meniscal tears. Ir J Med Sci 152:149–151, 1983
18. Beck C, Drez D, Young J, Dilworth Cannon W, Stone ML: Instrumental testing of functional knee braces. Am J Sports Med 14:253–256, 1986
19. Beck JL, Wildermuth BP: The female athlete's knee. Clin Sports Med 4:345–366, 1985
20. Beckman M, Craig R, Lehman RC: Rehabilitation of patellofemoral dysfunction in the athlete. Clin Sports Med 8:841–860, 1989
21. Bentley GL: Chondromalacia patellae. J Bone Joint Surg 52A:221–232, 1970
22. Bentley GL: The surgical treatment of chondromalacia patellae. J Bone Joint Surg 60B:74–81, 1978
23. Berger RA, Mathus DL: Movement time with various resistance loads as a function of pretensed and prerelaxed muscular contraction. Res Q 40:456, 1969
24. Bergfeld J: Functional rehabilitation of isolated medial collateral ligament sprains. Am J Sports Med 7:207–209, 1979
25. Blackburn TA: Rehabilitation of ACL injuries. Orthop Clin North Am 16:141–269, 1985
26. Blackburn TA, Eiland WG, Brady WD: An introduction to the plica. J Orthop Sports Ther 3:171–177, 1982
27. Blustein M, D'Amico JC: Limb-length discrepancy: Identification, clinical significance and management. Phys Ther 75:200–206, 1985
28. Bolton CW, Bruchman WC: The Gore-Tex expanded polytetrafluoroethylene prosthetic ligament—An *in vitro* and *in vivo* evaluation. Clin Orthop 196: 202–213, 1985
29. Bonnarens FO, Drez D: Biomechanics of artificial ligaments and associated problems. In Jackson DW, Drez D (eds): The Anterior Cruciate Deficient Knee: New Concepts in Ligament Repair. St. Louis, CV Mosby, 1987
30. Bonnarens FO, Drez D: Clinical examination of the knee for ACL laxity. In Jackson DW, Drez D (eds): The Anterior Cruciate Deficient Knee: New Concepts in Ligament Repair. St. Louis, CV Mosby, 1987
31. Bosco C, Komi PV: Potentiation of the mechanical behavior of the human skeletal muscle through prestretching. Acta Physiol Scand 106:467–472, 1979
32. Bose K, Kanagasuntherum R, Osman M: Vastus medialis oblique: An anatomical and physiological study. Orthopaedics 3:880–883, 1980
33. Brody D: Techniques in the evaluation and treatment of the injured runner. Orthop Clin North Am 13:541–558, 1982
34. Brownstein BA, Lamb RL, Magine RE: Quadriceps torque and integrated electromyography. J Orthop Sports Ther 6:309–314, 1985
35. Brubaker CE, Jame SL: Injuries to runners. J Sports Med 2:189–198, 1974
36. Burri C, Hen Kemeyer H, Neugebauer R: Technique and results of allo-plastic carbon fibre ligament substitution. Aktuel Probl Chir Orthop 26:135–147, 1983
37. Cabaud HE, Feagin JA, Rodkey WG: Acute ACL injury and augmented repair. Am J Sports Med 8:395–401, 1980
38. Cabaud HE, Rodkey WG, Feagin JA: Experimental studies of acute ACL injury and repair. Am J Sports Med 7:18–22, 1979
39. Cabaud HE, Slocum DB: The diagnosis of chronic anterolateral rotary instability of the knee. Am J Sports Med 5:99–104, 1977
40. Cailliet R: Knee Pain and Disability, 2nd ed. Philadelphia, FA Davis, 1983
41. Campbell D, Glenn W: Foot-pound torque of the normal knee and the rehabilitated post-meniscectomy knee. Phys Ther 59:418–421, 1979
42. Campbell D, Glenn W: Rehabilitation of knee flexors and extensor muscle strength in patients with meniscectomies, ligamentous repairs, and chondromalacia. Phys Ther 62:10–15, 1982
43. Cannon WD: Follow-up of ACL reconstructions and studies with the knee laxity tester. Presented at the ACL Study Group Meeting, Steamboat Springs, Col., 1984
44. Carson WG: Diagnosis of extensor mechanical disorders. Clin Sports Med 4:231–246, 1985
45. Cavagna GA, Dusman B, Margaria R: Positive work done by a previously stretched muscle. J Appl Physiol 24:21–32, 1968
46. Cavagna GA, Saibene FP, Margaria R: Effects of negative work on the amount of positive work performed by an isolated muscle. J Appl Physiol 20: 157–158, 1965
47. Clancy WG, Nelson DA, Reider B, Narechania RJ: ACL reconstruction using one third of the patellar ligament augmented by extra-articular tendon transfers. J Bone Joint Surg 64A:352–359, 1982
48. Colville MR, Lee CL, Ciullo V: The Lenox Hill brace: An evaluation of effectiveness in treating knee instability. Am J Sports Med 14:257–261, 1986
49. Corrigan B, Maitland GD: Practical Orthopaedic Medicine. London, Butterworths, 1985
50. Costill DL: Muscle rehabilitation after knee surgery. Phys Sports Med 5:71–74, 1977
51. Cross MJ, Powell JF: Long-term follow-up of PCL rupture: A study of 116 cases. Am J Sports Med 12:282–297, 1984
52. Curt WW, Markey KL, Mitchell WA: Agility training following ACL reconstruction. Clin Orthop 172:133–136, 1983
53. Curwin S, Stanish WD: Tendinitis: Its etiology and treatment. Lexington, Mass., The Collamore Press, 1984
54. Cyriax J: Textbook of Orthopaedic Medicine, vol. II: Treatment by Manipulation, Massage and Injections, 10th ed. London, Bailliere Tindall, 1980
55. Dandy DJ, Pusey RJ: The long-term results of unrepaired tears of the PCL. J Bone Joint Surg 64B:92–94, 1984
56. Daniels DM: Instrumented measurement of anterior knee laxity. Presented at the ACL meeting, Steamboat Springs, Col., 1984
57. Daniels DM, Malcom LL, Losse G, et al: Instrumented measurement of anterior laxity of the knee. J Bone Joint Surg 67A:720–726, 1985
58. Davis VB: Flexibility conditioning for running. In D'Ambrosia R, Drez D (eds): Prevention and Treatment of Running Injuries. Thorofare, NJ, Slack, 1982
59. de Andrade JR, Grant C, Dixon A: Joint distension and reflex muscle inhibition in the knee. J Bone Joint Surg 47A:313–321, 1967
60. Degenhardt TC: Chronic PCL instability: Nonoperative management. Orthop Trans 5:486–487, 1981
61. DeHaven KE: Rationale for meniscus repair or excision. Clin Sports Med 4:267–273, 1985
62. DeLee JC, Riley MR, Rockwood CA: Acute straight lateral instability of the knee. Am J Sports Med 11:404–411, 1983
63. DeVries HA: Physiology of Exercise. Dubuque, Wm. C. Brown, 1974
64. DiStefano V: ACL reconstruction: Autograft or allograft? Clin Sports Med 12:1–11, 1993
65. DiVeta JA, Vobelbach WD: The clinical efficacy of the A-angle measuring patellar alignment. J Orthop Sports Phys Ther 16:136–139, 1992
66. Dixon ASJ: Factors in the development and presentation of osteoarthritis of the knee. In Progress in Clinical Rheumatoid Arthritis. London, J. & A. Churchill, 1965:313–329
67. Donaldson WF, Warren RF, Wickiewicz T: A comparison of acute ACL examinations. Am J Sports Med 13:57–10, 1985
68. Doucette SA, Goble EM: The effect of exercise on patellar tracking in lateral patellar compression syndrome. Am J Sports Med 20:434–440, 1992
69. Drez D: Knee braces. In Jackson DW (ed): The Anterior Cruciate Deficient Knee: New Concepts in Ligament Repair. St. Louis, CV Mosby, 1987
70. Drez D, Kinnard WH: Clinical examination. In Shahriaree H (ed): O'Connor's Textbook of Arthroscopic Surgery. Philadelphia, JB Lippincott, 1984
71. Einhorn AR, Sawyer M, Tovin B: Rehabilitation of intra-articular reconstruction. In Greenfield BH (ed): Rehabilitation of the Knee: A Problem-Solving Approach. Philadelphia, FA Davis, 1993:245–287
72. Ellsasser JC, Reynolds KC, Omohundro JR: The nonoperative treatment of collateral ligament injuries of the knee in professional football players. J Bone Joint Surg 56A:1185–1190, 1974
73. Engin AE, Korde MS: Mechanics of normal and abnormal knee joint. J Biomechanics 7:325–334, 1974
74. Evjenth E, Hamberg J: Muscle Stretching in Manual Therapy: A Clinical Manual, vol. 1: The Extremities. Alfta, Sweden, Alfta Rehab Forhaj, 1984
75. Fetto JF, Marshall JL: The natural history and diagnosis of ACL insufficiency. Clin Orthop 144:55, 1979
76. Ficat RP, Philippe T, Hangerford DS: Chondromalacia patellae. Clin Orthop 144:55–62, 1979
77. Frankel VH, Nordin M: Basic Biomechanics of the Skeletal System, 2nd ed. Philadelphia, Lea & Febiger, 1980
78. Frankel VH, Burstein AH: Orthopaedic Biomechanics. Philadelphia, Lea & Febiger, 1971
79. Frankel VH, Burstein AH, Brooks DB: Biomechanics of internal derangement of the knee. J Bone Joint Surg 53A:945–962, 1971
80. Freeman MAR, Dean MRE, Hanham IF: The etiology and prevention of functional instability of the foot. J Bone Joint Surg 47B:678–685, 1965
81. Friedmann MJ, Ferkel RD (eds): Prosthetic Ligament Reconstruction of the Knee. Philadelphia, WB Saunders, 1988
82. Fulkerson JP: Awareness of the retinaculum in evaluating patellofemoral pain. Am J Sports Med 10:147–149, 1982
83. Fulkerson JP: The etiology of patellofemoral pain in young active patients: A prospective study. Clin Orthop 179:129–133, 1983
84. Funk JF: Synthetic ligaments: Current status. Clin Orthop 219:107–111, 1987
85. Furman W, Marshall JL, Giris FG: The ACL: A functional analysis based on postmortem studies. J Bone Joint Surg 58B:179–185, 1976
86. Galway HR, Beaupre A, MacIntosh D: Pivot-shift: A clinical sign of symptomatic anterior cruciate insufficiency. J Bone Joint Surg 54B:763–764, 1972
87. Galway HR, MacIntosh DL: The lateral pivot-shift: A symptom and sign of ACL insufficiency. Clin Orthop 147:45–50, 1980
88. Gillquist J, Odensten M: Reconstruction of old ACL tears with a Dacron prosthesis: A prospective study. Am J Sports Med 21:358–366, 1993
89. Girgis FG, Marshall JL, Morajem ARS: The cruciate ligaments of the knee joint: Anatomical, functional, and experimental analysis. Clin Orthop 106:216–231, 1975
90. Glousman R, Shields C, Kerlan R, et al: Gore-Tex prosthetic ligament in anterior cruciate deficient knees. Am J Sports Med 16:321–331, 1988
91. Glove TP, Muller S, Barreck EK: Nonoperative treatment of the torn ACL. J Bone Joint Surg 65A:184–192, 1983
92. Godfrey JD: Ligament injuries of the knee. In Anstrom JP (ed): Current Practice in Orthopedic Surgery, vol. 5. St. Louis, CV Mosby, 1973
93. Goldberg A: Work-induced growth of skeletal muscle in normal and hypophysectomised rats. Am J Physiol 312:1193–1198, 1967
94. Good L, Odensten M, Gillquist J: Sagittal knee stability after ACL reconstruction with a patellar tendon strip: A 2-year follow-up study. Am J Sports Med 22:518–523, 1994
95. Goodfellow J, Hungerford DS, Woods C: Patellofemoral joint mechanics and pathology, Part 2: Chondromalacia patellae. J Bone Joint Surg 58B:291–299, 1976
96. Goodfellow J, Hungerford DS, Zindel M: Patellofemoral joint mechanics and pathology, Part 1: Functional anatomy of the patellofemoral joint. J Bone Joint Surg 58B:287–290, 1976

97. Gough JV, Ladley G: An investigation into effectiveness of various forms of quadriceps exercises. Physiotherapy 57:356–361, 1971
98. Green WR Jr: Painful bipartite patellae. Clin Orthop 110:197–200, 1975
99. Gustavsen R, Streeck R: Training Therapy: Prophylaxis and Rehabilitation, 2nd ed. Stuttgart, Georg Thieme Verlag, 1993
100. Gutman E, Schiaffino S, Hazlikova V: Mechanism of compensatory hypertrophy in skeletal muscles of the rat. Exp Neurol 31:451–464, 1971
101. Haggmark TN, Ericksson E: Cylinder or mobile cast brace after knee ligament surgery. Am J Sports Med 7:48–56, 1979
102. Hanley P, Lew WD, Lewis JL, et al: Load sharing and graft forces in ACL reconstructions with the Ligament Augmentation Device. Am J Sports Med 19:25–263, 1991
103. Hansen H, Boe S: The pathological plica in the knee—Results after arthroscopic resection. Arch Orthop Trauma Surg 108:282–284, 1989
104. Hanten WP, Schulthies SS: Exercise's effect on electromyographic activity of the vastus medialis oblique and vastus lateralis muscles. Phys Ther 70:561–565, 1990
105. Hardarkerwt WT, Whipple TL, Bassett FH: Diagnosis and treatment of the plica syndrome of the knee. J Bone Joint Surg 62A:222–225, 1980
106. Hastings DE: The nonoperative treatment of collateral ligament injuries of the knee joint. Clin Orthop 147:22–28, 1980
107. Helfet A: Disorders of the Knee. Philadelphia, JB Lippincott, 1974
108. Hellebrandt FA, Houtz SJ, Kirkorian AM: Influence of bimanual exercise on unilateral work capacity. J Appl Physiol 2:452–466, 1950
109. Hellebrandt FA, Houtz SJ, Partridge MJ, Walters EC: Tonic neck reflexes in exercises of stress in man. Am J Phys Med 35:144–157, 1956
110. Hellebrandt FA, Waterland JC: Indirect learning—the influence of unimanual exercise on related muscle groups of the same and the opposite side. Am J Phys Med 41:45–55, 1962
111. Henning CE, Lynch MA, Glick K: An *in vivo* strain gauge study of elongation of the ACL. Am J Sports Med 13:22–26, 1985
112. Henning CE, Lynch MA, Glick K: Physical examination of the knee. In Nicholas JA, Hershmann EB (eds): The Lower Extremity and Spine in Sports Medicine, vol. I. St. Louis, CV Mosby, 1986
113. Hoffa A: The influence of the adipose tissue with regards to the pathology of the knee joint. JAMA 43:795–796, 1904
114. Holden DL, Eggert AW, Butler JE: The nonoperative treatment of grade I and II medial collateral ligament injuries to the knee. Am J Sports Med 11:340–344, 1983
115. Holten O: Medisinsk Trenigsterapi Trykk Fugseth and Lorentzen. Medical Training Course, Salt Lake City, 1984
116. Hoppenfield S: Physical Examination of the Spine and Extremities. New York, Appleton-Century-Crofts, 1976
117. Huberti H, Hayes W: Patellofemoral contact pressures: The influence of the Q angle and tendofemoral contact. J Bone Joint Surg 66A:715–724, 1984
118. Hughston JC: Extensor mechanism examination. In Fox JM, Del Pizzo (eds): The Patellofemoral Joint. New York, McGraw-Hill, 1993:63–74
119. Hughston JC, Andrews JR, Cross MJ, Moschi A: Classification of knee ligament instability, Part I. J Bone Joint Surg 58A:159–172, 1976
120. Hughston JC, Andrews JR, Cross MJ, Moschi A: Classification of knee ligament instability, Part II. J Bone Joint Surg 58A:173–179, 1976
121. Hughston JC, Norwood LA: The posterolateral drawer test for posterolateral rotatory instability of the knee. Clin Orthop 147:82–87, 1980
122. Hughston JC, Walsh WM, Puddu G: Patellar Subluxation and Dislocation. Philadelphia, WB Saunders, 1984
123. Hungerford DS, Barry M: Biomechanics of the patellofemoral joint. Clin Orthop 144:9–15, 1979
124. Hunter SC, Poole RM: The chronically inflamed tendon. Clin Sports Med 6:371–388, 1987
125. Ihara H, Nakayama A: Dynamic joint control training for knee ligament injuries. Am J Sports Med 14:309–315, 1986
126. Indelicato PA, Linton RC, Huegel M: The results of fresh-frozen patellar tendon allografts for chronic ACL deficiency of the knee. Am J Sports Med 20:118–121, 1992
127. Insall J, Falvo KA, Wise DW: Chondromalacia patellae, a prospective study. J Bone Joint Surg 58A:1–8, 1976
128. Jakob RP: Observation on rotatory instability of the lateral compartment of the knee. Acta Orthop Scand (Suppl 191)52:1–32, 1981
129. Jakob RP, Staubli HU, Deland JT: Grading the pivot-shift. J Bone Joint Surg 69B:294–299, 1987
130. James SL: Chondromalacia patella. In Kennedy JC (ed): The Injured Adolescent Knee. Baltimore, Williams & Wilkins, 1979
131. James SL, Bates BT, Ostering LR: Injuries to runners. Am J Sports Med 6:40–50, 1978
132. Janda V: Muscles, central nervous motor regulation and back problems. In Korr I (ed): The Neurobiologic Mechanisms in Manipulative Therapy. London, Plenum Press, 1978
133. Janda V: Treatment of Patients. International Federation of Orthopedic Manipulative Therapists, 4th Conference, Christchurch, New Zealand, 1980
134. Jensen K: Manual laxity test for ACL injuries. J Orthop Sports Phys Ther 11:474–481, 1990
135. Jones AL: Rehabilitation for anterior instability of the knee—Preliminary report. J Orthop Sports Phys Therapy 3:121–128, 1982
136. Jonsson T, Alfhoff D, Peterson L, Renstrom P: Clinical diagnosis of ruptures of the ACL. Am J Sports Med 10:100–102, 1982
137. Kaltenborn FM: Manual Mobilization of the Extremity Joints, Vol. II: Advanced Treatment Techniques. Oslo, Olaf Norlis Bokhandel, 1986
138. Kaltenborn FM: Mobilization of the Extremity Joints, Vol. I: Examination and Basic Treatment Techniques. Oslo, Olaf Norlis Bokhandel, 1980
139. Kaplan PE, Tanner ED: Musculoskeletal Pain and Disability. Norwalk, CT, Appleton & Lange, 1989
140. Karzel RP, Del Pizzo W: Patellofemoral arthritis—General considerations. In Fox JM, Del Pizzo W (eds): The Patellofemoral Joint. New York, McGraw-Hill, 1993:243–248
141. Katz JW, Fingeroth RJ: The diagnostic accuracy of rupture of the ACL comparing the Lachman test, the anterior drawer sign, and the pivot-shift test in acute and chronic knee injuries. Am J Sports Med 14:88–91, 1986
142. Kennedy JC: The Injured Adolescent Knee. Baltimore, Williams & Wilkins, 1979
143. Kennedy JC, Fowler PJ: Medial and anterior instability of the knee. J Bone Joint Surg 53A:1257–1270, 1971
144. Kennedy JC, Galpin RD: The use of the medial head of the gastrocnemius muscle in the posterior cruciate-deficient knee: Indication, technique, results. Am J Sports Med 10:63–74, 1982
145. Kennedy JC, Weinberg HW, Wilson AS: The anatomy and function of the ACL, as determined by clinical and morphological studies. J Bone Joint Surg 56A:223–234, 1974
146. Kettelkamp DB: Clinical implications of knee biomechanics. Arch Surg 107:406–410, 1973
147. Kettelkamp DB: Current concepts review—Management of patellar malalignment. J Bone Joint Surg 63A:1344–1347, 1981
148. King AC, et al: EMG biofeedback-controlled exercise in chronic arthritic knee pain. Arch Phys Med Rehabil 65:341, 1984
149. Kisner C, Colby LA: Therapeutic Exercise—Foundations and Techniques. Philadelphia, FA Davis, 1985
150. Knott M, Voss D: Proprioceptive Neuromuscular Facilitation, 2nd ed. New York, Harper & Row, 1969
151. Komi PV: Measurement of the force-velocity relationship in human muscle under concentric and eccentric contractions. Med Sci Sport 8:224–229, 1973
152. Komi PV: Neuromuscular performance factors influencing force and speed production. Scand J Sports Sci 1:2–15, 1979
153. Komi PV, Bosco C: Utilization of stored elastic energy in leg extensor muscles by men and women. Med Sci Sports 10:261–265, 1978
154. Koshimo T, Okamoto R: Resection of painful shelf (plica synovialis mediopatellaris) under arthroscopy. Arthroscopy 1:136–141, 1985
155. Kottke FJ: Krusen's Handbook of Physical Medicine and Rehabilitation, 3rd ed. Philadelphia, WB Saunders, 1982
156. Kulund DK: The Knee. In Kulund DK: The Injured Athlete, 2nd ed. Philadelphia, JB Lippincott, 1988:435–512
157. Larson RL: Overview and philosophy of knee injuries. Clin Sports Med 4:209–215, 1985
158. Larson RL: Future of prosthetic ligament reconstruction. In Friedman MJ, Ferkel RD (eds): Prosthetic Ligament Reconstruction of the Knee. Philadelphia, WB Saunders, 1988
159. Larson RL, Cabaud HE, Slocum DB: The patella compression syndrome: Surgical treatment by lateral retinacular release. Clin Orthop 134:156–157, 1978
160. Last RJ: The popliteus muscle and lateral meniscus. J Bone Joint Surg 32B:93–99, 1950
161. Laubenthal KN, Smidt GL, Kettelkamp DB: A quantitative analysis of knee motion for activities of daily living. Phys Ther 52:34–42, 1972
162. LeBrier K, O'Neill DB: Patellofemoral stress syndrome. Sports Med 16:449–459, 1993
163. Lechner DE: Rehabilitation of the knee with arthritis. In Greenfield BH: Rehabilitation of the Knee: A Problem-Solving Approach. Philadelphia, FA Davis, 1993:206–241
164. Lephart SM, Kocher MS, Harner CD, et al: Quadriceps strength and functional capacity after ACL reconstruction: Patellar tendon autograft versus allograft. Am J Sports Med 21:738–743, 1993
165. Levine J, Splain S: Use of the infrapatellar strap in the treatment of patellofemoral pain. Clin Orthop 139:179–181, 1979
166. Levy IM, Torzilli PA, Warren RF: Effects of medial meniscectomy on anterior-posterior motion of the knee. J Bone Joint Surg 64A:883–888, 1982
167. Lewis RJ: Degenerative arthritis. In Nickel VL (ed): Orthopedic Rehabilitation. New York, Churchill Livingstone, 1982
168. Lieb F, Perry J: Quadriceps function, an electromyographic study under isometric contraction. J Bone Joint Surg 53A:749–758, 1971
169. Logan GA: Differential applications of resistance and resulting strength measured at varying degrees of knee flexion. Doctoral dissertation, USC, 1960
170. Losee RE: Concepts of the pivot-shift. Clin Orthop 172:45–51, 1983
171. Losee RE, Johnson TR, Southwick WO: Anterior subluxation of the lateral tibia plateau. J Bone Joint Surg 60A:1015–1030, 1978
172. Love JW, Whelan TJ: Popliteal artery entrapment syndrome. Am Med J Surg 109:620–624, 1965
173. Lucie RS, Wiedel JD, Messner DG: The acute pivot-shift: Clinical correlation. Am J Sports Med 12:189–191, 1984
174. Lutter L: Injuries in runners and joggers. Minn Med 63:45–51, 1980
175. Lutter L: Cavus foot in runners. Foot Ankle 1:225–228, 1981
176. Lutter L: The knee and running. Clin Sports Med 4:685–698, 1985
177. Lutter L: Running athlete in office practice. Foot Ankle 3:52–59, 1982
178. Lysholm J, Gillquist J: Evaluation of knee ligament surgery results with special emphasis on use of a scoring scale. Am J Sports Med 10:150–154, 1982
179. Macnicol MF, Penny ID, Sheppard L: Early results with the Leeds-Keio ACL replacement. J Bone Joint Surg 73B:377–380, 1991
180. Magee DJ: Orthopedic Physical Assessment. Philadelphia, WB Saunders, 1987
181. Maitland GD: Peripheral Manipulations. Sevenoaks, Butterworths, 1978
182. Malone T, Blackburn TA, Wallace LA: Knee rehabilitation. Phys Ther 66:1553–1639, 1980
183. Mankin HJ: Articular cartilage, cartilage injury and osteoarthritis. In Fox JM, Del Pizzo W (eds): The Patellofemoral Joint. New York, McGraw-Hill, 1993:49–62
184. Mann R, Baxter D, Lutter L: Running symposium. Foot Ankle 1:190–224, 1981
185. Markolf KL: Quantitative examination for anterior cruciate laxity. In Jackson DW, Drez D (eds): The Anterior Cruciate-Deficient Knee: New Concepts in Ligament Repair. St. Louis, CV Mosby, 1987
186. Markolf K, Graff-Radford A, Amstutz H: *In vivo* knee stability: A quantitative assessment using an instrumented clinical testing apparatus. J Bone Joint Surg 60A:664–674, 1978
187. Marks KE, Bentley G: Patella alta and chondromalacia. J Bone Joint Surg 60B:71–73, 1978
188. Mayfield G: Popliteus tendon tenosynovitis. Am Sports Med 5:31–36, 1977
189. McConnell J: The management of chondromalacia patellae: A long-term solution. Aus J Physiol 2:215–223, 1986
190. McMurray TP: The semilunar cartilage. Br J Surg 29:407–414, 1942
191. Meachim G, Emery IH: Quantitative aspects of patellofemoral cartilage fibrillation in Liverpool necropsies. Ann Rheum Dis 3:39–47, 1974

192. Mellion MB: Office Management of Sports Injuries and Athletic Problems. St. Louis, CV Mosby, 1988
193. Mennell JB: Physical Treatment by Movement, Manipulation and Massage, 5th ed. Philadelphia, Blakiston, 1947
194. Merchant AC: The lateral patellar compression syndrome. In Fox JM, Del Pizzo (eds): The Patellofemoral Joint. New York, McGraw-Hill, 1993:157–168
195. Meyer JF: Allograft reconstruction of the ACL. Clin Sports Med 10:487–498, 1991
196. Muller EA, Rohmert W: Die Geschwindigkeit der Muskelcraft Zunshme bei Isometricshe Training. Int Zeitschrift fur Angewandte Physiol 19:403–419, 1983
197. Muller W: The Knee: Form, Function and Ligament Reconstruction. New York, Springer-Verlag, 1983
198. Newton RA: Electrotherapeutic Treatment: Selecting Appropriate Waveform Characteristics. Clinton, NJ, JA Preston, 1984
199. Nicholas JA: Injuries to the menisci of the knee. Orthop Clin North Am 4:647–664, 1973
200. Nicholas JA, Hershmann EB (eds): The Lower Extremity and Spine in Sports Medicine, Vol. I. St. Louis, CV Mosby, 1986
201. Noble CA: Iliotibial band friction syndrome in runners. Am J Sports Med 8:232–234, 1980
202. Norris CM: The knee. In Norris CM: Sports Injuries: Diagnosis and Management of Physiotherapists. Oxford, Butterworth-Heinemann, 1993
203. Norwood LA, Cross MJ: The ACL: Functional anatomy of its bundles in rotatory instabilities. Am J Sports Med 7:23–26, 1979
204. Noyes FR: Functional properties of knee ligaments and alterations induced by immobilization—A correlative biomechanical and histological study in primates. Clin Orthop 123:210–242, 1977
205. Noyes FR, Barber SD, Mangine RE: Bone-patellar ligament-bone and fascia lata allografts for reconstruction of the ACL. J Bone Joint Surg 72A:1125–1136, 1990
206. Noyes FR, Bassett RW, Grood ES, Butler DL: Arthroscopy in acute traumatic hemarthrosis of the knee—Incidence of anterior cruciate tears and other injuries. J Bone Joint Surg 62A:687–695, 1980
207. Noyes FR, Butler DL, Grood ES: Biomechanical analysis of human ligament grafts used in knee ligament repairs and reconstructions. J Bone Joint Surg 66A 344–352, 1984
208. Noyes FR, Mangine RE, Barber S: Early knee motion after open and arthroscopic ACL reconstruction. Am J Sports Med 15:149–160, 1981
209. Noyes FR, Matthews DS, Mooar PA Grood ES: The symptomatic anterior cruciate-deficient knee, Part II: The result of rehabilitation activity modification and counseling on functional disability. J Bone Joint Surg 65A:163–174, 1983
210. Noyes FR, Mooar PA, Matthews DS, Butler DL: The symptomatic anterior cruciate-deficient knee, Part I: The long-term functional disability in athletically active individuals. J Bone Joint Surg 65A:154–162, 1983
211. Noyes FR, Torvik PJ, Hyde WB, Delucas JL: Biomechanics of ligament failure: II. An analysis of immobilization, exercise, and reconditioning effects in primates. J Bone Joint Surg 56A:1406–1418, 1974
212. O'Donoghue DH: Treatment of acute ligamentous injuries of the knee. Orthop Clin North Am 4:617–645, 1973
213. O'Neill DB, Micheli LJ, Warner JP: Patellofemoral stress: A prospective analysis of exercise treatment in adolescents and adults. Am J Sports Med 20:151–156, 1992
214. Ogden JA, McCarthy SM, Tokl P: The painful bipartite patella. J Pediatr Orthop 2:263–269, 1982
215. Ohkoshi Y, Yasada K: Biomechanical analysis of shear force exerted to ACL during half-squat exercise. Orthop Trans 13:310, 1989
216. Outerbridge REE: The etiology of chondromalacia patellae. J Bone Joint Surg 43B:752–757, 1961
217. Palmittier RA, An KN, Scott SG, et al: Kinetic chain exercise in knee rehabilitation. Sports Med 11:402–413, 1991
218. Palumba PM: Dynamic patellar brace: Patellofemoral disorders: A preliminary report. Am J Sports Med 9:45–49, 1979
219. Parolie JM, Bergfeld JA: Long-term results of nonoperative treatment of isolated PCL injuries in the athlete. Am J Sports Med 14:35–38, 1986
220. Patel D: Arthroscopy of the plicae-synovial fold and their significance. Am J Sports Med 6:217–225, 1978
221. Patel D: Plica as a cause of anterior knee pain. Orthop Clin North Am 17:273–277, 1986
222. Patel D: Synovial lesions: Plicae. In McGinty JB (ed): Operative Arthroscopy. New York, Raven Press, 1991:361–372
223. Patel D, Laurencin CT, Tsuchiya A, et al: Synovial folds—Plicae. In Fox JM, Del Pizzo W (eds): The Patellofemoral Joint. New York, McGraw-Hill, 1993:193–198
224. Paulos LE: Knee and leg: Soft-tissue trauma. In American Academy of Orthopedic Surgeons: Orthopedic Knowledge Update 2, 1987
225. Paulos LE, Cheri J, Rosenberg TD, et al: ACL reconstruction with autografts. Clin Sports Med 10:469–485, 1991
226. Paulos LE, Noyes FR, Grood E, Butler DL: Knee rehabilitation after ACL reconstruction and repair. Am J Sports Med 9:140–149, 1981
227. Paulos LE, Payne FC, Rosenbery TD: Rehabilitation after ACL surgery. In Jackson DW, Drez D (eds): The Anterior Cruciate-Deficient Knee: New Concepts in Ligament Repair. St. Louis, CV Mosby, 1987
228. Paulos L, Rusche K, Johnson C, Noyes FR: Patellar malalignment: A treatment rationale. Phys Ther 60:1627–1632, 1980
229. Pope MH, Stankewich CJ, Beynnon BD, et al: Effect of knee musculature on ACL strain *in vivo*. J Electromyog Kines 1:191–198, 1991
230. Radin EL, de Lamotte F, Maquet P: Role of the menisci in the distribution of stress in the knee. Clin Orthop Relat Res 185:290–294, 1984
231. Raux P, Townsend PR, Miegel R, Rose RM, Radin EL: Trabecular architecture of the human patella. J Biomech 8:1–7, 1975
232. Renne J: The iliotibial band friction syndrome. J Bone Joint Surg 57*A*:1110–1115, 1975
233. Reynolds LR, Levin TA, Mederios JM, et al: EMG activity of the vastus medialis oblique and the vastus lateralis in their role in patellar alignment. Am J Phys Med Rehabil 62:61–70, 1983
234. Ricklin P, Ruttmann A, Del Buno MS: Meniscus Lesions: Diagnosis, Differential Diagnosis, and Therapy, 2nd ed. Stuttgart, Thieme, 1983
235. Romero JA, Standford TL, Schroeder RV, Fahey TD: The effects of electrical stimulation of normal quadriceps on strength and girth. Med Sci Sports Exercise 14:194–197, 1982
236. Rosentswig J, Hinson MM: Comparison of isometric, isotonic and isokinetic exercises by electromyography. Arch Phys Med Rehabil 53:249–252, 1972
237. Sandberg R, Balkfors B, Nilsson B, Westlin N: Operative versus nonoperative treatment of recent injuries to the ligaments of the knee. J Bone Joint Surg 69A:1120–1126, 1987
238. Santi MD, Richardson AB: The ligament augmentation device in hamstring grafts for reconstruction of the ACL. Am J Sports Med 22:524–530, 1994
239. Schneider W, Dvorak J, Dvorak J, et al: Manual Medicine: Therapy. New York, Georg Thieme Verlag Stuttgart, 1988
240. Schultz P: Flexibility: The day of the static stretch. Phys Sports Med 7:109–117, 1979
241. Seedhom BB: Load-bearing function of the menisci. Physiotherapy 62:223–228, 1976
242. Shaw JA, Eng M, Murray DG: The longitudinal axis of the knee and the role of the cruciate ligaments in controlling transverse rotation. J Bone Joint Surg 56A:1603–1609, 1974
243. Shelbourne DK, Nitz PA: Accelerated rehabilitation after ACL reconstruction. Am J Sports Med 18:292–299, 1990
244. Shephard RJ: Physiology and Biochemistry of Exercise. New York, Praeger Press, 1982
245. Sherrington CS: The Integrative Actions of the Nervous System. New Haven, Yale University Press, 1906
246. Shields CL, Brewster CE, Morrissey MC: Rehabilitation of the knee in athletes. In Nichols JA, Hershmann EB (eds): The Lower Extremity and Spine in Sports Medicine, Vol. 1. St. Louis, CV Mosby, 1986
247. Shino K, Horibe S, Nagano J, et al: Quantitative assessment of anterior stability of the knee following ACL reconstruction using allogeneic tendon. Trans Orthop Res Soc 12:130, 1987
248. Shino K, Inoue M, Horibe S, et al: Reconstruction of the ACL using allogeneic tendon—Long-term follow-up. Am J Sports Med 18:457–465, 1990
249. Shino K, Nakata K, Horibe S, et al: Quantitative evaluation after arthroscopic ACL reconstruction: Allograft versus autograft. Am J Sports Med 21:609–616, 1993
250. Shino K, Oakes BW, Inoue M, et al: Human ACL allograft- collagen fibril population studied as a function of age of the graft. Trans Orthop Res Soc 15:520, 1990
251. Shoji H: Chondromalacia patellae: Histological and biochemical aspects. NY State J Med 74:507–510, 1974
252. Slocum DB, James SL, Larson RL, Singer KM: Clinical test for anterolateral rotary instability of the knee. Clin Orthop 118:63–69, 1976
253. Slocum DB, Larson RL: Rotary instability of the knee: Its pathogenesis and a clinical test to determine its presence. J Bone Joint Surg 50A:211-225, 1968
254. Slocum DB, Larson RL, James SL: Late reconstruction procedures used to stabilize the knee. Orthop Clin North Am 4:679–689, 1973
255. Smillie IS: Diseases of the Knee Joint, 2nd ed. Edinburgh, Churchill Livingstone, 1980
256. Smillie IS: Injuries of the Knee Joint. New York, Churchill Livingstone, 1978
257. Sonzogni JJ: Physical assessment of the injured knee. Emerg Med 20:74–92, 1988
258. Spencer J, Hayes K, Alexander I: Knee joint effusion and quadriceps reflex inhibition in man. Arch Phys Med Rehabil 65:171–177, 1984
259. Stanish WD: Neurophysiology of stretching. In D'Ambrosia R, Drez D (eds): Prevention and Treatment of Running Injuries. Thorofare, NJ, Slack, 1982
260. Steadman JR: Nonoperative methods for patellofemoral problems. Am J Sports Med 7:374–375, 1979
261. Steadman JR: Rehabilitation of first- and second-degree sprains of the medial collateral ligament. Am J Sports Med 7:300–302, 1979
262. Steadman JR: Rehabilitation of acute injuries of the ACL. Clin Orthop 172:129–132, 1983
263. Steindler A: Kinesiology of the Human Body. Springfield, Ill., Charles C. Thomas, 1955
264. Stillwell GK: Electrotherapy. In Kottke FS, Stillwell GK, Lehmann JF (eds): Krusen's Handbook of Physical Medicine and Rehabilitation, 3rd ed. Philadelphia, WB Saunders, 1982
265. Stokes M, Young A: Investigation of quadriceps inhibition: Implications for clinical practice. Physiotherapy 70:425–428, 1984
266. Storigord J: Chondromalacia of the patella: Physical signs in relation to operative findings. Acta Orthop Scand 46:685–694, 1975
267. Stuller J: Bracing the unstable knee. Phys Sports Med 13:142–156, 1985
268. Sullivan PE, Markos PD, Minor MAD: An Integrated Approach to Therapeutic Exercise—Therapy and Clinical Application. Reston, Va., Reston Publishing Co., 1982
269. Surburg RR: Proprioceptive neuromuscular facilitation. Phys Sports Med 9:115–127, 1981
270. Teitz C, Larson R: Health Maintenance. In American Academy of Orthopedic Surgeons: Orthopaedic Knowledge Update 2, 1987
271. Tibone J, Antich TJ, Fanton GS, Moynes DR, Perry J: Functional analysis of ACL instability. Am J Sports Med 14:276–283, 1986
272. Tory JS, Conrad W, Kalen V: Clinical diagnosis of ACL instability in the athlete. Am J Sports Med 4:84–93, 1976
273. Tovin BJ, Wolf SL, Greenfield BH, et al: Comparison of the effects of exercise in water and on land on the rehabilitation of patients with intra-articular ACL reconstruction. Phys Ther 74:710–719, 1994
274. Townsend PR, Miegel RE, Rose RM, Raux P, Radin EL: Structure and function of the human patella: The role of cancellous bone. J Biomed Mater Res 7:605–611, 1976
275. Townsend PR, Raux P, Rose RM, Miegel RE, Radin EL: The distribution and anisotrophy of the stiffness of cancellous bone in the human patella. J Biomech 8:363–367, 1975
276. Townsend PR, Rose RM, Radin EL, Raux P: The biomechanics of the human patella and its implications of chondromalacia. J Biomech 10:403–407, 1977
277. Turner W (ed): Anatomical Memoirs of John Goodsir. Edinburgh, Adam & Black, 1968
278. Vaey FB: The painful knee. In Germain BF: Osteoarthritis and Musculoskeletal Pain Syndromes. Hyde Park, NY, Medical Examination Pub. Co., 1983
279. Walker HL, Schreck RC: Relationship of hyperextended gait pattern to chondromalacia patellae. Physiotherapy 64:8–9, 1975
280. Walla DJ, Albright JP, McAuley E: Hamstring control and the unstable ACL-deficient knee. Am J Sports Med 13:34–49, 1985

281. Wallace L: Balance as a predictor of knee injury in football. Annual Meeting of APTA, Anaheim, 1982
282. Walsh WM: Office management of knee injuries. In Mellion MB (ed): Office Management of Sport Injuries and Athletic Problems. Philadelphia, CV Mosby, 1988
283. Wang YJB, Rubim RM, Marshall JL: A mechanism of isolated ACL rupture—Case report. J Bone Joint Surg 57A:411–413, 1975
284. Warren LF, Marshall JL: The supporting structures and layers on the medial side of the knee—An anatomic analysis. J Bone Joint Surg 61A:56–62, 1979
285. Whieldon T, Yack J, Collins C: Anterior tibial translation during weight-bearing and non-weight-bearing rehabilitation exercises in the anterior cruciate-deficient knee. Phys Ther 69:151, 1989

286. Wilk KE, Andrews JR: Current concepts in the treatment of ACL disruption. J Orthop Sports Phys Ther 15:279–292, 1992
287. Wilk RM, Richmond JC: Dacron ligament reconstruction for chronic ACL insufficiency. Am J Sports Med 21:374–379, 1993
288. Wood GA, Indelicato PA, Precot TJ: The Gore-Tex ACL prosthesis: 2- versus 3-year results. Am J Sports Med 19:48–55, 1991
289. Woolfenden JT: Aquatic physical therapy approaches for the extremities. Orthop Phys Ther Clin North Am 3:209–230, 1994
290. Wyke B: The neurology of joints. Ann R Coll Surg Engl 41:25–50, 1967

The Lower Leg, Ankle, and Foot

DARLENE HERTLING AND RANDOLPH M. KESSLER

■ **Functional Anatomy of the Joints**
Osteology
Ligaments and Capsules
Surface Anatomy

■ **Biomechanics**
Structural Alignment
Arthrokinematics of the Ankle–Foot Complex
Osteokinematics of the Ankle–Foot Complex

■ **Examination**
History
Physical Examination

■ **Common Lesions and Their Management**

Overuse Syndromes of the Leg
Ankle Sprain
Foot Injuries
Problems Related to Abnormal Foot Pronation
Problems Related to Abnormal Foot Supination
Orthoses

■ **Joint Mobilization Techniques**
Tibiofibular Joints
The Ankle
The Foot
The Toes

■ **FUNCTIONAL ANATOMY OF THE JOINTS**

□ **Osteology**

FIBULA AND TIBIA

The two bones of the lower leg, the tibia and fibula, along with their articulations (superior and inferior joints) form a functional unit that is involved in movements of the ankle (Fig. 14-1). The tibia transmits most of the body weight to the foot. Proximally, an oval facet indents the tibia posterolaterally and provides an articular surface where the fibula joins the tibia as the superior tibiofibular joint. The fibula, the lateral bone of the leg, is more slender than the tibia, for it is not called on to transmit body weight. With respect to the proximal end of the fibula, the medial part of the upper aspect of the head bears a circular articular sur-

face for the lateral condyle of the tibia (see Fig. 13-4). Although the facets are fairly flat and vary in configuration among individuals, a slight concavity to the fibular face and a slight convexity to the tibial facet seems to predominate.[45] The surface of the fibular facet faces forward, upward and medially. The shaft arches forward as it descends to the lateral malleolus.

The tibia or shin bone is, next to the femur, the longest and heaviest bone of the body.[55] The proximal end of the tibia (see Fig. 13-4) has been described earlier (see Chapter 13, The Knee).

The tibia flares at its distal end (see Fig. 14-1). As a result, the cross-section of the bone changes from triangular, in the region of the shaft, to quadrangular in the area of the distal metaphyseal portion of the bone. Medially there is a distal projection of the tibia, the medial malleolus; located laterally is the fibular notch, which is concave anteroposteriorly for articulation with the distal end of the fibula. Along the medial side

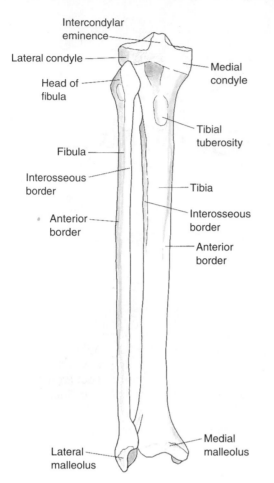

Intercondylar eminence

Lateral condyle

Head of fibula

Fibula

Interosseous border

Anterior border

Lateral malleolus

Medial condyle

Tibial tuberosity

Tibia

Interosseous border

Anterior border

Medial malleolus

FIG. 14-1. The two bones of the lower leg: anterior view.

of the posterior surface is a groove for the passage of the tibialis posterior tendon. The term *posterior malleolus* is often used to refer to the distal overhang of the posterior aspect of the tibia.

The lateral surface of the medial malleolus and the inferior surface of the tibia have a continuous cartilaginous covering for articulation with the talus. The articular surface of the inferior end of the tibia is concave anteroposteriorly. Mediolaterally, it is somewhat convex, having a crest centrally that corresponds to the central groove in the trochlear surface of the talus. This, then, is essentially a sellar joint surface. It is slightly wider anteriorly than posteriorly. The articular surface of the medial malleolus is comma shaped, with the "tail" of the comma extending posteriorly (see Fig. 14-1).

The fibula, which is quite narrow in the region of its shaft, becomes bulbous at its distal end (Fig. 14-2*A*). This distal portion of the bone, the lateral malleolus, is triangular in cross-section. When viewed from a lateral aspect, the fibula is somewhat pointed distally. The lateral malleolus extends farther distally and is situated more posteriorly than the medial malleolus.

The medial aspect of the lateral malleolus is covered by a triangular cartilaginous surface for articulation with the lateral side of the talus. Above this surface, the fibula contacts the tibia in the fibular notch of the tibia. The apex of this triangular surface points inferiorly. There is a fairly deep depression in the posteroinferior region of the lateral malleolus termed the *malleolar fossa* that can be easily palpated. The posterior talofibular ligament attaches in this fossa. There is a groove along the posterior aspect of the lateral malleolus through which the peroneus brevis tendon passes.

TALUS

The talus constitutes the link between the leg and the tarsus (Fig. 14-3). It consists of a body, anterior to which is the head. The body and head of the talus are connected by a short neck.

The superior surface of the body of the talus is covered with articular cartilage for articulation with the inferior surface of the tibia. This articular surface is continuous with the articular surfaces of the medial and lateral aspects of the talus. The superior surface is somewhat wider anteriorly than posteriorly. It is convex anteroposteriorly and slightly concave mediolaterally, corresponding to the sellar surface of the inferior end of the tibia mentioned previously. In this sense, the superior talar articular surface is trochlear, or pulley-like, and is often referred to as the trochlea.

The lateral aspect of the body of the talus is largely covered by articular cartilage for articulation with the distal end of the fibula (Fig. 14-4). This articular surface is triangular, with the apex situated inferiorly. Just below this apex is a lateral bony projection to which the lateral talocalcaneal ligament attaches.

The articular surface of the medial aspect of the talus is considerably smaller than that of the lateral side, and it faces slightly upward (Fig. 14-5). It contacts the articular surface of the medial malleolus on the tibia. It is comma shaped, with the tail of the comma extending posteriorly. The roughened area below the medial articular surface serves as an attachment for the deltoid ligament. The medial and lateral talar articular surfaces tend to converge posteriorly, leading to the wedge shape of the trochlea. It should be emphasized, however, that the lateral articular surface of the talus is perpendicular to the axis of movement at the ankle joint, whereas the medial surface is not. This has important biomechanical implications, which are discussed in the following section.

If one views the profiles of the lateral and medial sides of the trochlea, the lateral profile is seen as a section of a circle, whereas the medial profile may be viewed as sections of several circles of different radii;

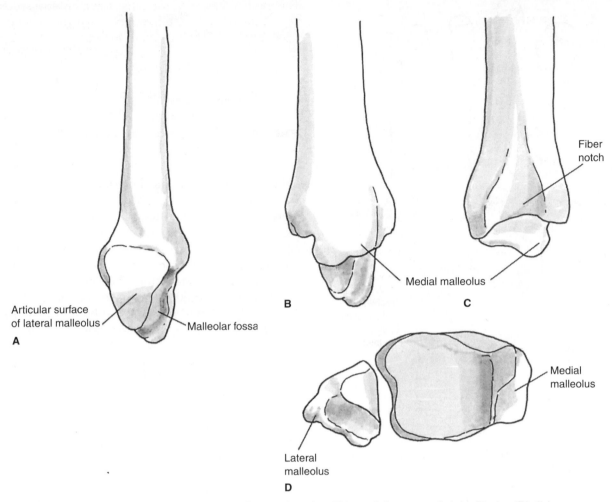

FIG. 14-2. Distal right tibia and fibula, showing (**A**) medial aspect of right fibula, (**B**) tibia from the medial aspect, (**C**) tibia from the lateral aspect, and (**D**) the inferior end of the fibula and tibia.

the medial profile is of smaller radius anteriorly than posteriorly.[76] More precisely stated, the contour medially is of gradually increasing radius anteroposteriorly, forming a cardioid profile. The importance of this is described in the section on biomechanics.

Posteriorly, the body of the talus is largely covered by a continuation of the trochlear articular surface as it slopes backward (Fig. 14-6). At the inferior extent of the posterior aspect is the nonarticular posterior process. The posterior process consists of a lateral and a smaller medial tubercle, with an intervening groove through which passes the tendon of the flexor hallucis longus. The posterior talofibular ligament attaches to the lateral tubercle. The medial talocalcaneal ligament and a posterior portion of the deltoid ligament attach to the medial tubercle.

The neck and head of the talus are positioned anteriorly to the body. They are directed slightly medially and downward with respect to the body. The head is covered with articular cartilage anteriorly for

articulation with the navicular and inferiorly for articulation with the spring ligament (plantar calcaneonavicular ligament).

The inferior surface of the talus has three cartilage-covered facets for articulation with the calcaneus (Fig. 14-7). The posterior facet, which is the largest of these, is concave inferiorly. The medial and anterior articular facets are continuous with each other and with the inferior articular surface of the head. Both the medial and the anterior facets are convex inferiorly and articulate with the superior aspect of the sustentaculum tali of the calcaneus. A deep groove, the sulcus tali, separates the posterior and medial facets on the inferior aspect of the talus. This groove runs obliquely from posteromedial to anterolateral. Where it is the deepest—posteromedially—it forms the *tarsal canal*; where it widens and opens out laterally it is referred to as the *sinus tarsi*. The interosseous talocalcaneal ligament and the cervical ligament occupy the sinus tarsi.

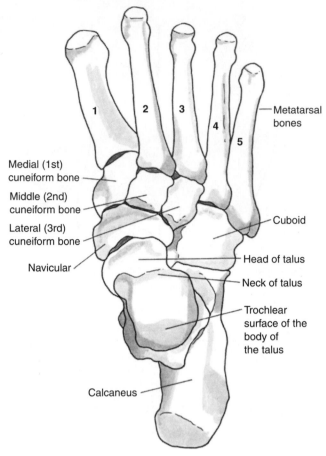

FIG. 14-3. *Dorsal aspect of the bones of the right foot.*

CALCANEUS

The calcaneus is situated beneath the talus in the standing position and provides a major contact point with the ground. It is the largest of the tarsal bones. The calcaneus articulates with the talus superiorly and with the cuboid anteriorly. Posteriorly it projects backward, providing considerable leverage for the plantar flexors of the ankle. The superior aspect of the calcaneus bears the posterior, medial, and anterior facets for articulation with the corresponding facets of the talus (Fig. 14-8). The posterior facet is convex,

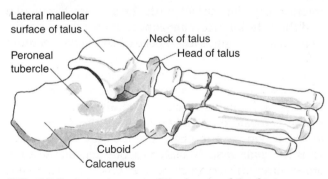

FIG. 14-4. *Lateral aspect of the bones of the foot.*

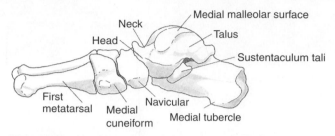

FIG. 14-5. *Medial aspect of the bones of the foot.*

whereas the medial and anterior facets are concave. The medial and anterior facets are situated on the superior aspect of the sustentaculum tali, which is a bony projection of the calcaneus that overhangs medially. As with the corresponding facets on the talus, the medial and anterior facets of the calcaneus are usually continuous with each other. The medial and anterior facets are separated from the posterior facet by the *sulcus calcanei*, which forms the bottom of the sinus tarsi and tarsal canal, thus corresponding to the sulcus tali of the talus.

The posterior aspect of the large posterior projection of the calcaneus contains a smooth superior surface, which slopes upward and forward, and a rough inferior surface, which slopes downward and forward. The upper surface is the site of attachment for the Achilles tendon (see Fig. 14-6). The lower surface blends inferiorly with the tuber calcanei, which is the point of contact of the calcaneus with the ground in the standing position.

The tuber calcanei on the inferior aspect of the calcaneus consists of a medial tubercle and a lateral tubercle, of which the medial is the larger. Anterior to the tuber calcanei is a roughened surface for the attachment of the long and short plantar ligaments (Fig.

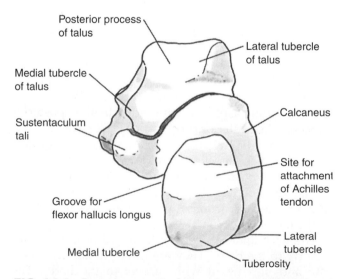

FIG. 14-6. *Posterior aspect of the calcaneus and talus.*

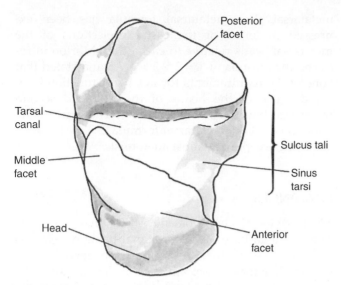

FIG. 14-7. *Inferior surface of the talus.*

14-9). At the anterior extent of the inferior surface of the calcaneus is the anterior tubercle, which also serves as a point of attachment for the long plantar ligament. On the inferior aspect of the medially projecting sustentaculum tali is a groove through which runs the flexor hallucis longus tendon.

The lateral aspect of the calcaneus is nearly flat. There is a small prominence, the peroneal trochlea, that is located just distal to the lateral malleolus (see Fig. 14-4). The peroneus brevis tendon travels downward and forward, just superior to this trochlea, while the peroneus longus tendon passes inferior to it. The calcaneofibular ligament attaches just posterior and slightly superior to the peroneal trochlea, at which point there may be a rounded prominence.

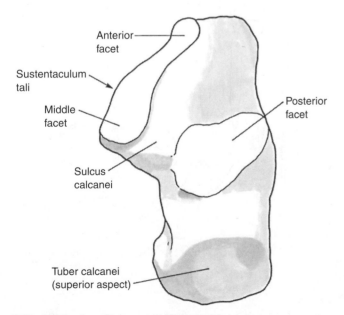

FIG. 14-8. *Superior aspect of the calcaneus.*

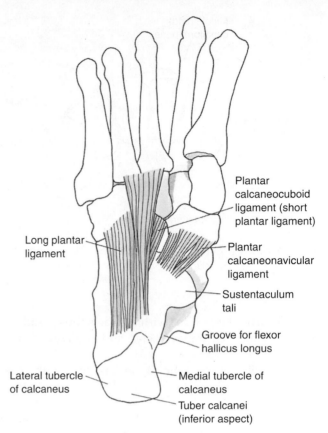

FIG. 14-9. *Plantar surface of the foot.*

From the anterosuperior extent of the medial aspect of the calcaneus, the sustentaculum tali projects in a medial direction (see Fig. 14-8). The sustentaculum tali may be palpated just below the medial malleolus.

On the narrowed anterior aspect of the calcaneus is the cartilage-covered articular surface that contacts the cuboid bone. This is a sellar joint surface, being concave superoinferiorly and convex mediolaterally (see Fig. 14-3).

LESSER TARSUS

Distally, the three cuneiform bones (medial [first], intermediate [second] and lateral [third]) are interposed between the navicular proximally, the first three metatarsals distally, and the cuboid laterally (see Fig. 14-3). The three cuneiforms and cuboid form an arcade or transverse arch that acts as a niche for the plantar musculotendinous and neurovascular structures (Fig. 14-10).[147] The middle cuneiform serves as the keystone. The cuneiforms, together with articulations of the metatarsal bones, form Lisfranc's joint.

The cuboid is intercalated between the calcaneus and the base of metatarsals 4 and 5 (Fig. 14-3). Medially, the cuboid has a fossa for the navicular and lateral cuneiform bones. On its plantar surface, there is a small groove for the peroneus longus tendon. Proxi-

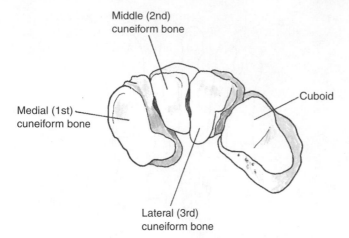

FIG. 14-10. *Transverse arch formed by the cuneiforms (C1, C2, C3) and the cuboid.*

mally, its articular surface with the calcaneus is saddle shaped, concave transversely and convex vertically.[147]

The navicular (scaphoid) articulates with the cuneiforms distally and with the talus proximally (see Fig. 14-3). It establishes minimal articular contact with the cuboid and is firmly bound with ligaments to the os calcis. It is an integral part of the talotarsal joint. The midtarsal joint is formed by the articulations between the navicular and talus and between the cuboid and calcaneus. The proximal articular surface is biconcave and in a few cases the surface is nearly flat.[105] It does not completely cover the navicular articular surface of the talus.[147] The distal articular surface to the three cuneiforms is faceted but is convex in its general contour.

METATARSALS

The metatarsals are the major stabilizers of the foot.[33] The five metatarsals articulate proximally with the three cuneiforms and the cuboid and form the tarsometatarsal or Lisfranc's joint (see Fig. 14-3). Proximally, the bases of the metatarsals are arranged in an arcuate fashion, forming a transverse arch. The apex of this arch corresponds to the base of the second metatarsal. The metatarsals are also flexed, thus contributing to the formation of longitudinal arches.[147] The first metatarsal diverges slightly from the second metatarsal. The intermetatarsal angle formed by the long axis of these two metatarsals is 3° to 9° in the adult.[159] Any measurement in excess of 10° is indicative of varus deformity of the first ray.[86] Of all hallux valgus cases, 80 percent are caused by metatarsal primus varus, in which the intermetatarsal angle is increased to more than 15°.[40,137]

The first metatarsal is shorter than the second

metatarsal. The metatarsal formula has been expressed in terms of the distal projections of the metatarsal heads relative to each other. Morton introduced the formula of 1 = 2 > 3 > 4 > 5 and stated that "one of the requirements for ideal foot function is an equidistance of the heads of the first and second metatarsal bones from the heel."[122] There are many variations, yet the metatarsal formula 2 > 3 > 1 > 4 > 5 is the one accepted by most anatomists.[83]

PHALANGES

The large toe has two phalanges: proximal and distal. The proximal base of the proximal phalanx bears an oval, concave articular surface with the glenoid cavity smaller than the corresponding articular surface of the metatarsal head (Fig. 14-11).[147] The articular surface of the head is trochlear and strongly convex in the dorsoplantar direction. The distal phalanx has an articular surface corresponding to the trochlear surface

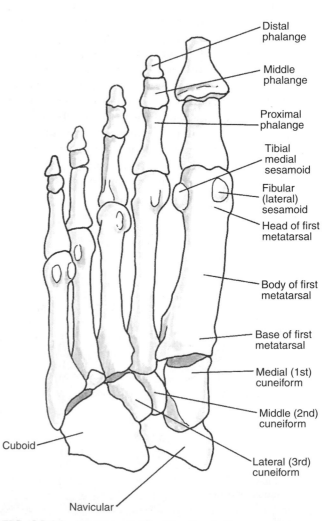

FIG. 14-11. *Plantar aspect of the forefoot.*

of the proximal phalangeal head. This surface is convex centrally and concave laterally.

The lesser toes have three phalanges: proximal, middle, and distal (see Fig. 14-11). The proximal phalanx is the longest of the three and the base has an oval (concave) articular surface for the metatarsal head. The head supports a trochlear type of articular surface. The base of the middle phalanx bears a transverse articular surface corresponding to the trochlear contour of the proximal phalangeal head.[147] The distal articular head presents a strong convexity in the dorsoplantar direction. The base of the distal phalanx corresponds to the head of the middle phalanx.

SESAMOIDS

The sesamoids are small, round bones so-named because they resemble sesame seeds (see Fig. 14-11). The sesamoids are embedded, partially or totally, in the substance of a corresponding tendon juxtaposed to articulations and are anatomically a part of a gliding or pressure-absorbing mechanism. Structurally, some sesamoids always ossify, whereas others remain cartilaginous or fibrocartilaginous for life. The tibial (medial) and fibular (lateral) sesamoids of the flexor hallucis brevis are always present plantar to the first metatarsal head. Other locations where sesamoids may be found are in the plantar plates of the metatarsophalangeal and interphalangeal joints, the intrinsic tendons of the lesser toes, or in the tendons of the tibialis anterior, tibialis posterior, or peroneus longus.

ACCESSORY BONES

The accessory bones are developmental anomalies and appear in the foot between the ages of 10 and 20.[130,163] The most commonly occurring accessory bones are the os trigonum at the posterior plantar surface of the talus, the os tibiale externum (an accessory of the navicular bone), and the os intermetatarseum 1–2.[147] These accessory bones as well as the sesamoids become sources of irritation and may require excision.[163] Comprehensive accounts of the accessory bones of the foot can be found in the studies of Dwight,[42] Kohler and Simmer,[89] Marti,[110] O'Rahilly,[130] and Trolle.[168]

☐ *Ligaments and Capsules*

SUPERIOR TIBIOFIBULAR JOINT

The superior tibiofibular joint is a plane synovial joint formed by the articulation of the head of the fibula with the posterolateral aspect of the tibia (Fig. 14-12A). In about 10 percent of the population, the synovial membrane is continuous with the knee joint through the subpopliteal bursa.[62] Motion has been described as superior and inferior sliding of the fibula, anteroposterior glide, and fibular rotation.[7,84,174]

An interosseous membrane binds the tibia and fibula throughout their length and separates the muscles on the front from those on the back of the leg (Fig. 14-12A). The interosseous membrane forms a "Y" proximally to surround the upper tibiofibular joint, the anterior division being called the anterosuperior tibiofibular ligament and the posterior division being called the posterosuperior tibiofibular ligament (Fig. 14-12A,B). A similar arrangement is formed below, where the interosseous membrane thickens and divides to surround the inferior tibiofibular syndesmosis (Fig. 14-12A,C). The two components are called the antero- and posteroinferior tibiofibular ligaments.

The interosseous membrane serves as the floor of the anterior compartment of the leg (Fig. 14-13). This is a closed space; the boundaries are the anterior fascia of the leg in front, the interosseous membrane behind, the fibula laterally, and the tibia medially. This space as well as the lateral compartment permits little, if any, expansion of the structures contained within, whereas the posterior compartment is a loosely contained space with a relaxed and redundant fascia. The tight fascial investment of the muscles contained in the anterior and lateral compartments helps to prevent undue swelling of the muscles during exercise and thereby facilitates venous return.[55]

The ligaments of the inferior tibiofibular articulation are oriented to prevent widening of the mortise. They are also important in preventing posterior displacement of the fibula at the syndesmosis, which tends to occur when the leg is forcibly internally rotated on the tarsus. It should be realized that complete sectioning of the inferior tibiofibular ligaments alone allows only a minimal increase in the intermalleolar space.[1] This is because the two bones are indirectly held together by their mutual connections to the talus by way of the medial and lateral ligaments of the ankle. Significant diastasis, then, is usually accompanied by rupture of one or more of the talocrural ligaments, usually the deltoid ligament.

INFERIOR TIBIOFIBULAR JOINT

The inferior tibiofibular joint is a syndesmosis and lacks articular cartilage and synovium. The distal fibula is situated in the fibular notch of the lateral aspect of the distal tibia and is bound to it by several ligaments (see Figs. 14-12A,C, 14-14 and 14-15). The anterior and posterior tibiofibular ligaments pass in front of and behind the syndesmosis. They are both directed downward and inward to check separation of the two bones. The inferior transverse ligament is a

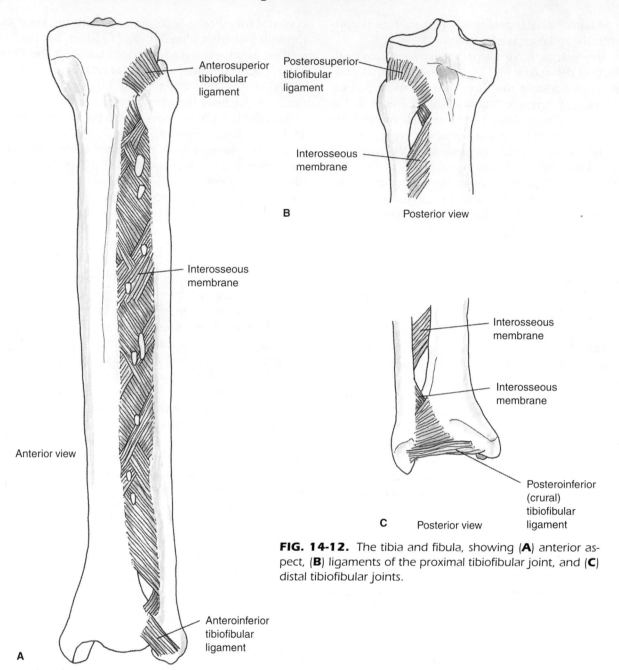

Anterosuperior tibiofibular ligament

Posterosuperior tibiofibular ligament

Interosseous membrane

B Posterior view

Interosseous membrane

Anterior view

Interosseous membrane

Interosseous membrane

Posteroinferior (crural) tibiofibular ligament

C Posterior view

Anteroinferior tibiofibular ligament

A

FIG. 14-12. The tibia and fibula, showing (**A**) anterior aspect, (**B**) ligaments of the proximal tibiofibular joint, and (**C**) distal tibiofibular joints.

thickened band of fibers that is closely related to the posterior tibiofibular ligament (see Fig. 14-12C). It passes from the posterior margin of the inferior tibial articular surface downward and laterally to the malleolar fossa of the fibula. This ligament is lined inferiorly with articular cartilage where it contacts the posterolateral talar articular surface during extreme plantar flexion. The interosseous ligament is a continuation of the interosseous membrane of the tibia and fibula (see Fig. 14-12C). It extends between the adjacent surfaces of the bones at the syndesmosis.

The tibiofibular interosseous ligaments are considered the strongest and most important of the ligaments at the distal tibiofibular joint (see Fig. 14-12C).[140]

The tibia and fibula are separated at the syndesmosis by a fat pad.

ANKLE JOINT
(Ankle Mortise or Talocrural Joint)

The ankle joint is formed by the superior portion of the body of the talus fitting within the mortise, or cavity, formed by the combined distal ends of the tibia and fibula. The medial, superior, and lateral articular surfaces of the talus are continuous, as are those of the medial malleolus, the distal end of the tibia, and the lateral malleolus.

The fibrous capsule attaches at the margins of the

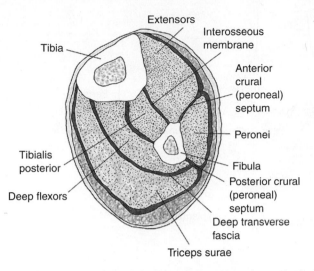

FIG. 14-13. Diagram of a horizontal section through the middle of the leg showing anterior compartment of the leg.

articular surfaces of the talus below and to the tibia and fibula above, except anteriorly, where a portion of the dorsal aspect of the neck of the talus is enclosed within the joint cavity. The capsule extends somewhat superiorly between the distal ends of the tibia and fibula, to just below the syndesmosis. The fibrous capsule is lined by a synovial membrane throughout its entirety. The capsule is well supported by ligaments, especially medially and laterally.

The medial ligaments are collectively referred to as the *deltoid ligament* (Fig. 14-16). The anterior portion of the deltoid ligament consists of the tibionavicular ligament, superficially, and the deeper anterior tibiotalar fibers. The tibionavicular ligament blends with the plantar calcaneonavicular (spring) ligament inferiorly. The middle fibers of the deltoid ligament constitute the tibiocalcaneal ligament, with some tibiotalar fibers

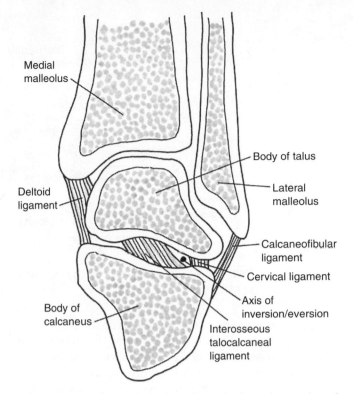

FIG. 14-15. Coronal section through the talocrural and subtalar joints.

deep to it. The posterior tibiotalar ligament forms the posterior portion of the deltoid ligament. The deltoid ligament as a whole attaches proximally to the medial aspect of the medial malleolus and fans out to achieve the distal attachments described above. In this way, it is somewhat triangular, with the apex at its proximal attachment.

The lateral ligaments, unlike those of the medial side, are separate bands of fibers diverging from their

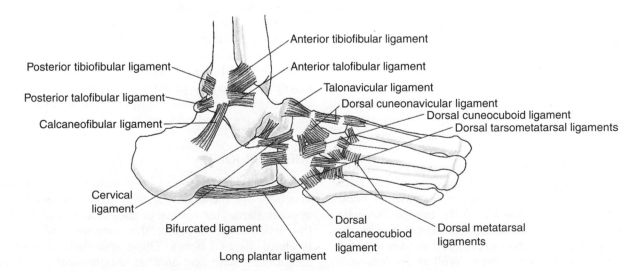

FIG. 14-14. Lateral view of the ligaments of the right talocrural, tarsal, and tarsometatarsal joints.

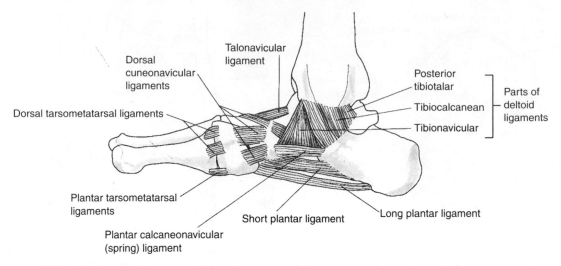

FIG. 14-16. *Medial view of the ligaments of the talocrural, tarsal, and first metatarsal joints.*

proximal attachment at the distal end of the fibula (see Fig. 14-14). The anterior talofibular ligament—the most frequently injured ligament about the ankle—passes medially, forward and downward, from the anterior aspect of the fibula to the lateral aspect of the neck of the talus. The calcaneofibular ligament runs from the tip of the lateral malleolus downward and backward to a small prominence on the upper lateral surface of the calcaneus. It is longer and narrower than the anterior and posterior talofibular ligaments. The posterior talofibular ligament passes from the malleolar fossa medially and slightly downward and backward to the lateral tubercle of the posterior aspect of the talus.

It should be noted that the proximal attachments of both the medial and lateral ligaments of the ankle are near the axis of movement for dorsiflexion and plantar flexion. For this reason, these ligaments are not pulled tight to any significant extent during normal movement at the talocrural joint.[70] Also, the calcaneofibular ligament, which crosses both the talocrural and the talocalcaneal joints, runs parallel to, and inserts close to, the axis of movement at the subtalar joint. It, then, plays little or no role in restricting inversion at the subtalar joint. This is true in all positions of dorsiflexion and plantar flexion, since it maintains a parallel orientation to the subtalar axis throughout the range of movement.

The ligaments about the talocrural joint primarily function to restrict tilting and rotation of the talus within the mortise and to restrict forward or backward displacement of the leg on the tarsus. The main exception to this is the tibiocalcaneal portion of the deltoid ligament, which is so oriented as to help check eversion at the subtalar joint as well as an "eversion tilt" of the talus in the mortise.

In the neutral position, the anterior talofibular ligament can check posterior movement of the leg on the tarsus and external rotation of the leg on the tarsus because it is directed forward and medially. With the foot in plantar flexion, the anterior talofibular ligament becomes more vertically oriented and is in a position to check inversion of the talus in the mortise. This ligament is the most commonly injured of the ligaments of the ankle, the mechanism of injury usually being a combined plantar flexion–inversion strain.

The calcaneofibular ligament is directed downward and backward when the foot is in the neutral position. When the foot is dorsiflexed, the ligament becomes more vertically oriented and is in a better position to check inversion of the tarsus with respect to the leg.

The posterior talofibular ligament is oriented so as to check internal rotation of the leg on the tarsus and forward displacement of the leg on the tarsus.

The deltoid ligament, considered as a whole, contributes to restriction of eversion, internal rotation, and external rotation, as well as forward and backward displacement of the tarsus. However, sectioning of the deltoid ligament alone apparently results primarily in instability of eversion of the tarsus on the tibia, the other motions being checked by other ligaments, as described previously.

SUBTALAR JOINT

Functionally, the subtalar joint includes the articulation between the posterior facet of the talus and the opposing articular surface of the calcaneus, as well as the articulation between the anterior and medial facets of the two bones. These articulations move in conjunction with one another. Anatomically, the anterior and medial articulations are actually part of the talocalcaneonavicular joint; they are enclosed within a joint capsule separate from that of the posterior talocalcaneal articulation.

The joint capsules of the posterior portion of the talocalcaneal joint and the talocalcaneonavicular portion of the subtalar joint are separated by the ligament of the tarsal canal. This ligament runs from the underside of the talus, at the sulcus tali, downward and laterally to the dorsum of the calcaneus, at the sulcus calcanei. Since it is situated medially to the axis of motion of inversion–eversion at the subtalar joint, it checks eversion.[155] This ligament is often referred to as the *interosseous talocalcaneal ligament* (see Fig. 14-15).

More laterally, in the sinus tarsi, is the cervical talocalcaneal ligament. It passes from the inferolateral aspect of the talar neck downward and laterally to the dorsum of the calcaneus. It occupies the anterior part of the sinus tarsi. Since the cervical ligament lies lateral to the subtalar joint axis, it restricts inversion of the calcaneus on the talus.[155]

Also, within the lateral aspect of the sinus tarsi, bands from the inferior aspect of the extensor retinaculum pass downward, as well as medially, to the calcaneus. These bands are considered part of the talocalcaneal ligament complex. They help check inversion at the subtalar joint.

MIDTARSAL JOINTS

TALOCALCANEONAVICULAR JOINT

The talocalcaneonavicular joint includes the articulation between the anterior and medial facets of the talus and calcaneus (described previously as part of the subtalar joint), the articulations between the inferior aspect of the head of the talus and the subjacent spring ligament, and the articulation between the anterior aspect of the head of the talus and the posterior articular surface of the navicular (Fig. 14-17). The combined talonavicular and talo-spring ligament portion of this joint is essentially a compound ball-and-socket joint; the head of the talus is the ball, while the superior surface of the spring ligament and the posterior surface of the navicular form the socket. It should be noted that the superior surface of the spring ligament is lined with articular cartilage. The talonavicular portion of this joint constitutes the medial half of the transverse tarsal joint.

The talocalcaneonavicular joint is enclosed by a joint capsule, the posterior aspect of which traverses the tarsal canal, forming the anterior wall of the canal. The capsule is reinforced by the spring ligament inferiorly, the calcaneonavicular portion of the bifurcate ligament laterally, and the tibionavicular portion of the deltoid ligament medially (see Figs. 14-14 and 14-16).

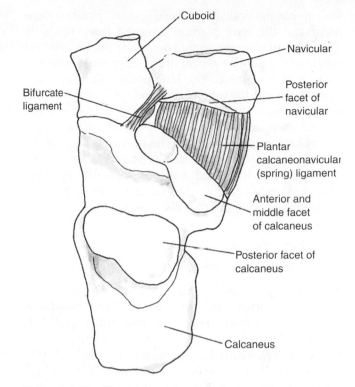

FIG. 14-17. The talocalcaneonavicular joint, superior view.

The spring ligament passes from the anterior and medial margins of the sustentaculum tali forward to the inferior and inferomedial aspect of the navicular. As mentioned, its superior surface articulates with the underside of the head of the talus. This ligament maintains apposition of the medial aspects of the forefoot and hindfoot and in so doing helps to maintain the normal arched configuration of the foot. Laxity of the ligament allows a medial separation between the calcaneus and forefoot, with the forefoot assuming an abducted position with respect to the hindfoot. At the same time, the foot is allowed to "untwist," which effectively lowers the normal arch of the foot, and the talar head is allowed to move medially and inferiorly. Further discussion of the twisted configuration and arching of the foot is included in the section on biomechanics.

CALCANEOCUBOID JOINT

The lateral portion of the transverse tarsal joint is the calcaneocuboid joint. The calcaneocuboid joint is a sellar joint in that the calcaneal joint surface is concave superoinferiorly and convex mediolaterally (see Figs. 14-3 and 14-4); the adjoining cuboid surface is reciprocally shaped. This joint is enclosed in a joint capsule distinct from that of the talocalcaneonavicular joint and constitutes the lateral half of the transverse tarsal joint. The joint capsule is reinforced inferiorly by the strong plantar calcaneocuboid (short plantar) ligament and the long plantar ligament (see Fig. 14-9). The short plantar ligament runs from the anterior tubercle of the plantar aspect of the calcaneus to the underside of the cuboid. The long plantar ligament runs from the posterior tubercles of the calcaneus forward to the bases of the fifth, fourth, third, and sometimes second metatarsals (see Fig. 14-9). Both of these ligaments support the normal arched configuration of the foot by helping to maintain a twisted relationship between the hindfoot and forefoot. Dorsally, the joint capsule is reinforced by the calcaneocuboid band of the bifurcate ligament (see Fig. 14-14).

ANTERIOR TARSAL AND TARSOMETATARSAL JOINTS

A common joint cavity connects the cuboid, navicular, three cuneiforms, and second and third metatarsal bones (Fig. 14-18). The first cuneiform and first metatarsal articulation has a separate cavity, as does the cuboid articulation with the fourth and fifth metatarsals.[174] Interosseous, dorsal, and plantar ligaments strengthen all of these small joints.

CUBONAVICULAR JOINT

The cubonavicular joint is usually a fibrous joint, but not infrequently the syndesmosis is replaced by a synovial joint of an almost plane variety, with the capsule and cavity continuous with the cuneonavicular joint.[62] Ligaments include the plantar cubonavicular ligament, interosseus ligament, and dorsal cubonavicular ligament, which strongly unite the cuboid and the navicular (Fig. 14-19).

CUNEONAVICULAR, CUNEOCUBOID, AND INTERCUNEIFORM JOINTS

The cuneonavicular, cuneocuboid, and intercuneiform joints have a common articular and synovial capsule (see Fig. 14-18). The navicular articulates with the three cuneiform bones and may be considered convex distally, being divided by low ridges into three facets which articulate with the first, second, and third cuneiforms to form the cuneonavicular joint.

TARSOMETATARSAL JOINTS

The tarsometatarsal (TMT) joints lie on a line, with the exception of the second cuneiform which is located 2 to 3 mm proximal to the first and third cuneiform. This creates the cuneiform mortise, which enhances the stability of Lisfranc's joint (see Fig. 14-18).[147]

The cuboid also shows three facets that articulate with the fifth metatarsal, the fourth metatarsal, and the lateral cuneiform (see Fig. 14-3). The cuboid is in a slight proximal recess of at least 2 mm relative to the third cuneiform; this creates a shallow metatarsal mortise.[147] The ligaments connecting the cuboid and the cuneiforms of the metatarsal bases are the dorsal, plantar, and interosseous ligaments.

The first TMT joint (the articulations between the first metatarsal and medial cuneiform) has its own articular capsule (see Fig. 14-18). The articular surface of the base of the first metatarsal presents a slight concavity transversely, the base of the second is concave with its articulation with the second cuneiform, the base of the third is flat, while the articular surface of the fourth is slightly convex with its articulation with the cuboid (see Fig. 14-3).[147] The base of the fifth

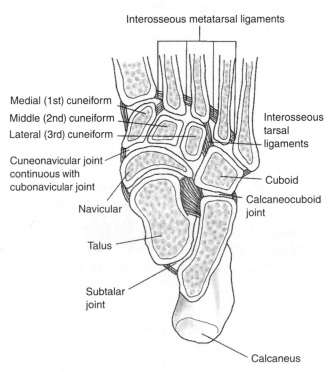

FIG. 14-18. Horizontal section through the foot joints from above.

Interosseous metatarsal ligaments

Medial (1st) cuneiform
Middle (2nd) cuneiform
Lateral (3rd) cuneiform

Interosseous tarsal ligaments

Cuneonavicular joint continuous with cubonavicular joint

Cuboid

Navicular

Calcaneocuboid joint

Talus

Subtalar joint

Calcaneus

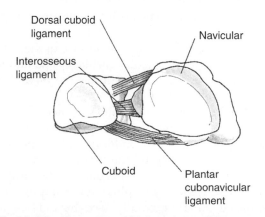

Dorsal cuboid ligament

Navicular

Interosseous ligament

Cuboid

Plantar cubonavicular ligament

FIG. 14-19. The cubonavicular joint and ligaments.

metatarsal is flat in a dorsoplantar direction and is projected laterally as the styloid apophysis or tubercle, which gives insertion to the peroneus brevis tendon.

The second TMT joint is the articulation of the base of the second metatarsal with a mortise formed by the middle cuneiform and the sides of the medial and lateral cuneiform (see Figs. 14-3 and 14-18). It is stronger and its motion more restricted than the other TMT joints. The third TMT joint shares its capsule with the second TMT joint, while the fourth and fifth TMT joints share a capsule with their articulation with the cuboid. There are small plane articulations between the bases of the metatarsals to permit motion of one metatarsal on the next. Slight gliding and rotation are possible at all of these joints. Although there is little movement between the individual tarsals and metatarsals, their collective movement can enhance either the foot's stability or flexibility. Dorsal and plantar ligaments join the bones (see Figs. 14-14, 14-16, and 14-20). The plantar ligaments of the cuneocuboid and

intercuneiform joints are strengthened by slips from the tendons of the tibialis posterior (Fig. 14-20).

METATARSOPHALANGEAL JOINTS

The first metatarsal head demonstrates a biconvex articular surface with its articular cap expanding inferiorly over the plantar condyles to the level of the anatomical neck and dorsally about one-third that distance.[173] The phalangeal base is correspondingly biconcave and the capsular ligament inserts in close proximity with its articular outer edge. The compartment formed is reinforced by collateral ligaments (medial and lateral) and metatarsophalangeal ligaments (Fig. 14-21).[134] The dorsal capsule is reinforced by the extensor hood expansion.[173] The plantar plate (equivalent to the hand's volar plates) is the fibrocartilaginous plantar metatarsophalangeal ligament and is continuous with the plantar aponeurosis, so that toe dorsiflexion tenses the plantar aponeurosis and stabilizes the foot's longitudinal arch.[173,174] The articular surface of the head of the first metatarsal presents with two fields in continuity: the superior phalangeal which is convex and the inferior sesamoidal whose two sloped surfaces are grooved, and each corresponds to a sesamoid.[147] The heads of the lesser metatarsals are convex or condylar (see Fig. 14-11).

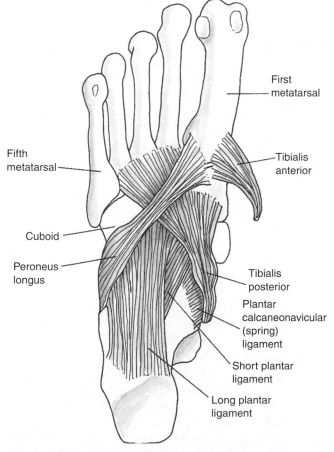

FIG. 14-20. *The tendons and ligaments of the foot, plantar aspect. Note the widespread insertion of the tibialis anterior.*

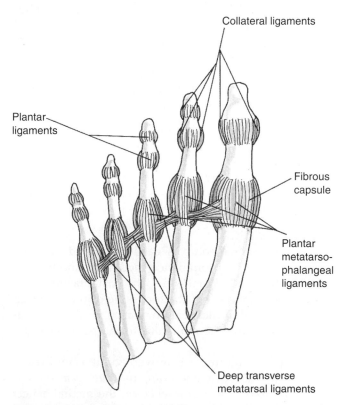

FIG. 14-21. *Ligaments of the metatarsophalangeal and interphalangeal joints.*

INTERPHALANGEAL JOINTS

The articulations of the phalanges of the toes are essentially similar to those of the fingers (see Fig. 14-11). On the plantar surface the capsule of each interphalangeal joint is thickened by a shallow concave plate, the plantar ligament; attached to its edges are the digital tendon sheaths as well as the lateral part of the fibrous capsule (see Fig. 14-21).[72] The collateral ligaments of the interphalangeal joints extend from the lateral aspect of the head of the corresponding phalanx to the base of the distally located phalanx (see Fig. 14-21). When sesamoid bones are present, they are an integral part of the plantar plate.[147]

PROXIMAL PHALANGEAL APPARATUS OF THE BIG TOE

The two sesamoids, embedded in the thick fibrous plantar plate and united to the proximal phalanx of the big toe, form an anatomical and functional unit called the *sesamophalangeal apparatus* (see Fig. 14-11).[61] The sesamoids are foci of insertion: the flexor hallucis brevis inserts on the proximal segment of each sesamoid; the lateral head of the flexor hallucis brevis and abductor hallucis inserts on the medial sesamoid; while the lateral sesamoid gives insertion to the oblique and transverse components of the adductor hallucis muscle.[147] The deep transverse metatarsal ligament attaches longitudinally along the lateral sesamoid (see Fig. 14-21). According to Sarrafian,[147] the sesamophalangeal apparatus moves backward or forward relative to the fixed metatarsal head; in hallux valgus the sesamoids follow the proximal phalanx and are displaced with the phalanx, not with the metatarsal head.

☐ **Surface Anatomy**

BONY PALPATION

MEDIAL ASPECT

The medial malleolus is easily palpated and observed as a large prominence medially. About 2 cm distal to the medial malleolus, the sustentaculum tali can be felt, especially if the foot is held in an everted position. The tibiocalcaneal portion of the deltoid ligament passes from the malleolus to the sustentaculum tali.

If the palpating finger is moved about 5 cm directly anterior to the sustentaculum, the *navicular tubercle* can be located as a prominence on the medial aspect of the arch of the foot. The tibionavicular portion of the deltoid ligament attaches just above the tubercle. Just superior and perhaps slightly posterior to the navicular tubercle, the medial aspect of the *talar head* can be palpated as a less prominent bony landmark. These two landmarks are important in assessing the structure of the foot with regard to the degree of twisting of the forefoot in relation to the hindfoot (the degree of "arching" of the foot).

The metatarsal can be felt to flare slightly at its base where it meets the first metatarsocuneiform joint. From the joint, one should probe distally along the medial shaft of the first metatarsal bone. The head of the first metatarsal bone and the metatarsophalangeal joint are palpable at the ball of the foot. The first metatarsophalangeal joint is the site of the common pathological condition, *hallux-abducto-valgus*, characterized by lateral deviation of the great toe. The first metatarsal shaft may be medially angulated (metatarsus primus varus) as well. The hallux abductus angle, intermetatarsal angle, and forefoot angles are increased and the first metatarsophalangeal joint is subluxed.[178]

DORSAL ASPECT

At the level of the malleoli, the anterior aspects of the distal ends of the tibia and fibula can be felt. The junction of the two bones, at the syndesmosis, can usually be distinguished, although it is considerably obscured by the distal tibiofibular ligament that overlies it. With the foot relaxed in some degree of plantar flexion, the dorsal aspect of the talar neck can be felt just distal to the end of the tibia. With the foot held inverted and plantarly flexed, the anterolateral aspect of the articular surface of the talus can be easily felt just distal and somewhat lateral to the syndesmosis. Between the dorsal aspect of the talar neck and the most prominent aspect of the dorsum of the foot farther distally, which is the first cuneiform, is the navicular bone, the dorsal aspect of which can be palpated.

The second and third cuneiform may be palpated distal to the navicular. One may palpate the cuboid by moving laterally from the third cuneiform or proximally from the styloid process at the base of the fifth metatarsal. By moving distally on the dorsum of the foot, the metatarsals and the phalangeal joints of each toe may be palpated.

LATERAL ASPECT

The lateral malleolus lies subcutaneously and so is easily palpated. The fairly flat lateral aspect of the calcaneus also has little soft-tissue covering it and can be felt throughout its extent. About 3 cm distal to the tip of the malleolus, a small prominence can be felt on the calcaneus. This is the peroneal tubercle (see Fig. 14-4). The peroneus brevis tendon passes superior to the tubercle, whereas the peroneus longus passes inferiorly. Occasionally a small prominence can be palpated just posterior to the peroneal tubercle; this is the point of insertion of the calcaneofibular ligament.

Just distal, and slightly anterior, to the malleolus, a rather marked depression can be felt if the foot is relaxed. This is the lateral opening of the sinus tarsi. Traversing the lateral aspect of the sinus tarsi are the inferior bands of the extensor retinaculum and the cervical talocalcaneal ligament. If the palpating finger is moved around dorsally and slightly superiorly from the sinus tarsi, the lateral aspect of the neck of the talus can be felt, where the often-injured anterior talofibular ligament attaches.

From the sinus tarsi, approximately one finger width distally, one may palpate the lateral aspect of the cuboid to the styloid process at the base of the fifth metatarsal bone. Proximal to the flare of the styloid one can appreciate the depression of the cuboid and the groove created by the peroneus longus muscle tendon as it runs to the medial plantar surface of the foot. As one probes distally along the lateral shaft of the fifth metatarsal to the head, the lateral aspect of the fifth head may demonstrate a bunionette deformity similar to that seen on the first toe called a *"tailor toe"* or tailor's bunion.[102] The deformity is characterized by a painful prominence of the lateral eminence of the fifth metatarsal head.

POSTERIOR ASPECT

At the posterior aspect of the heel is a prominent crest running horizontally between the upper and lower posterior calcaneal surfaces. The Achilles tendon gains attachment to the upper surface; the lower surface, covered by a fat pad, slopes forward to the medial and lateral tubercles on the inferior aspect of the calcaneus.

Palpation of the posterior aspect of the talus is obscured by the Achilles tendon, which overlies it prior to inserting on the calcaneus.

PLANTAR ASPECT

Palpation of the inferior aspect of the calcaneus is made difficult by the thick skin and fat pad that cover it. The weight-bearing medial tubercle can be vaguely distinguished posteriorly in most persons.

The calcaneus is palpated for point tenderness that may be due to calcaneus periostitis (bone bruise) and also for a possible calcaneal spur (traction osteophytes), which may develop just anterior to the medial tubercle of the calcaneus where the long plantar ligament attaches. This is also called *heel-spur syndrome* and is more proximal than mid-foot plantar fasciitis. Other bony structures that should be palpated include the sesamoid bones for possible sesamoiditis or displacement (which may occur in Morton's neuroma) and each metatarsal head. Metatarsalgia can develop if the transverse arch collapses, causing painful metatarsal heads and occa-

sionally pinched digital nerves. The cause may be vascular, avascular, neurogenic, or mechanical, such as when the transverse arch collapses.[63] Generalized metatarsalgia often occurs secondary to a tight Achilles tendon, which restricts dorsiflexion.[91]

Palpation of the plantar surface of the foot is difficult because of the overlying fascial bands and fat pads. One should palpate the shafts of the metatarsal bones and between the bones for evidence of pathology. Medially, on the plantar aspect of the first metatarsal, one may identify and palpate the two sesamoid bones just proximal to the head of the first metatarsal. This may be facilitated by dorsiflexing the big toe. In a similar fashion, the heads of the remaining four toes are palpated, and while doing so, it should be determined if any are disproportionately prominent. If one is more prominent, it may bear an unaccustomed amount of weight, characterized by excessive callosities (keratoses) due to increased pressure. The various etiologies of plantar keratoses are numerous and a significant differential diagnosis exists that needs to be taken into account when evaluating the patient.[102]

TENDONS AND VESSELS

MEDIAL ASPECT

The four ligaments that make up the deltoid (tibionavicular, tibiocalcaneal, and anterior and posterior tibiotalar) should be palpated for signs of pathology (see Fig. 14-16). Tenderness or pain elicited during palpation suggests an eversion ankle sprain.

The tendons of the tibialis posterior, flexor digitorum longus, and flexor hallucis longus muscles cross behind the medial malleolus (Fig. 14-22A). The tibialis posterior is the most anterior of these and is best visualized or palpated when plantar flexion and inversion are performed against some resistance. Posterior to the tibialis posterior tendon is the flexor digitorum longus tendon, which is less prominent. Palpation of the flexor digitorum is facilitated by providing some resistance to toe flexion. The flexor hallucis longus tendon is deeper and runs farther posteriorly; it is not usually palpable. Between the flexor digitorum and flexor hallucis longus tendons runs the posterior tibial artery. Its pulse is palpable behind the malleolus. The tibial nerve, which usually cannot be palpated, runs deep and posterior to the artery.

Just anterior to the medial malleolus is the long saphenous nerve; it can usually be visualized and palpated.

DORSAL ASPECT

Running along the medial side of the dorsum of the ankle is the tendon of the tibialis anterior, which is the most prominent tendon crossing the dorsal aspect of

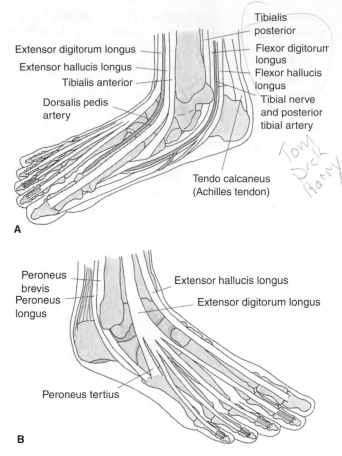

FIG. 14-22. (**A**) Medial and (**B**) lateral views of the tendons and vessels of the dorsum of foot.

the foot. It is made especially prominent by resisting inversion and dorsiflexion of the foot. It attaches to the medial aspect of the base of the first metatarsal.

Just lateral to the tibialis anterior tendon, the extensor hallucis longus tendon can easily be seen and palpated as the subject extends the big toe.

Running lateral to the extensor hallucis longus tendon, passing distally from where it emerges at the ankle, is the dorsalis pedis artery. Its pulse can best be palpated over the dorsum of the foot, at about the level of the navicular and first cuneiform bones.

Farther laterally, the common tendon of the extensor digitorum longus is seen and felt when the subject extends the toes (Fig. 14-22B). Its four branches can be distinguished where they develop, just distal to the ankle.

If the subject everts and dorsiflexes the foot, the tendon of the peroneus tertius is usually observable just proximal to its insertion at the dorsum of the base of the fifth metatarsal.

Returning to the area of the medial and lateral malleoli, one may palpate the area of the inferior tibiofibular joint and follow the crest of the tibia superiorly while palpating the muscles of the lateral com-

partment (peroneals and posterior tibialis) and anterior compartment (tibialis anterior and long extensors) for swelling, tenderness, and signs of pathology (*e.g.,* shin splints or stress fractures). About 75 percent of shin pain is due to overuse of the posterior tibial muscle.[56] Patients with flexor compartment chronic syndrome or medial shin syndrome complain of pain over the posterior tibial and flexor tendons anywhere from the medial malleolus up to the medial tibial plateau.[87] There are usually palpable areas of maximum tenderness and nodules that represent fibrosis and scar tissue formation.

LATERAL ASPECT

The peroneus longus and peroneus brevis tendons cross behind the lateral malleolus, with the brevis running more anteriorly. The brevis passes superior to the peroneal tubercle on the lateral aspect of the calcaneus; the longus passes inferior to the tubercle. Some resistance should be applied to the plantar flexion and eversion of the foot when palpating these tendons.

Also one should palpate the peroneal retinaculum, which holds the peroneal tendons in place, for tenderness. The lateral ligaments (anterior tibiofibular, anterior talofibular, calcaneofibular, posterior talofibular, and posterior tibiofibular) are palpated for tenderness and swelling (see Fig. 14-14). These ligaments will be point tender if they are sprained or partially torn. The most common sprain is of the anterior talofibular ligament. This injury occurs during plantar flexion and inversion. The bifurcate ligament (calcaneocuboid or calcaneonavicular portion) will be tender if sprained or partially torn from a plantar flexion injury (see Fig. 14-14).[67]

The surrounding area of the calcaneus should be palpated for exostosis (*e.g.,* pump bump) and swelling. Moving proximally, one may palpate the superficial (triceps surae) and posterior compartment muscles of the leg along their length. Ruptures or strains of the gastrocnemius usually occur to the medial muscle belly where the Achilles tendon joins the belly.[67] In addition to point tenderness, a gap can sometimes be felt in the muscle tissue.

POSTERIOR ASPECT AND POSTERIOR COMPARTMENT MUSCLES OF THE LEG

The Achilles tendon is quite prominent and is easily seen and felt proximal to its insertion on the calcaneus. Deep to the tendon, between the tendon and the upper surface of the posterior calcaneus, is the retrocalcaneal bursa. There is also a calcaneal bursa between the Achilles tendon and the skin. These bursae cannot be distinguished on palpation.

PLANTAR ASPECT

The intrinsic foot muscles and plantar aponeurosis (plantar fascia) should be palpated for tenderness, which may indicate mid-foot plantar fasciitis, and for nodules in the fascia, which may indicate Dupuytren's contracture.[73,163] The plantar aponeurosis should be palpated along its entire surface. Maintaining dorsiflexion of the toes will make the fascia more prominent and facilitate palpation. Nodules found on the skin, particularly on the ball of the foot (not usually on the weight-bearing area) are usually plantar warts.[102]

The plantar calcaneonavicular (spring) ligament is palpated for tenderness by applying pressure to the area immediately below the head of the talus, with the foot completely relaxed (see Figs. 14-9 and 14-16). This ligament, which helps to support the longitudinal arch, can become strained and painful from overuse. Also one should probe the region of the long and short plantar ligaments, which also support the longitudinal arch of the foot, for point tenderness (see Figs. 14-9 and 14-20). Foot pronation, sprain, or strain may result in acute pain.

■ BIOMECHANICS

The structural relationships and movements that occur at the ankle and hindfoot are complex. From a clinical standpoint, however, it is important that the clinician have at least a basic understanding of the biomechanics of this region. The joints of the foot and ankle constitute the first movable pivots in the weight-bearing extremity once the foot becomes fixed to the ground. Considered together, these joints must permit mobility in all planes to allow for minimal displacement of a person's center of gravity with respect to the base of support when walking over flat or uneven surfaces. In this sense, maintenance of balance and economy of energy consumption are, in part, dependent on proper functioning of the ankle–foot complex. Adequate mobility and proper structural alignment of these joints are also necessary for normal attenuation of forces transmitted from the ground to the weight-bearing extremity. Deviations in alignment and changes in mobility are likely to cause abnormal stresses to the joints of the foot and ankle as well as to the other weight-bearing joints. It follows that detection of biomechanical alterations in the ankle–foot region is often necessary for adequate interpretation of painful conditions affecting the foot and ankle, as well as conditions affecting the knee, hip, or lower spine, in some cases.

☐ Structural Alignment

In the normal standing position, the patella faces straight forward, the knee joint axis lies in the frontal plane, and the tibial tubercle is in line with the midline—or lateral half—of the patella. In this position, a line passing between the tips of the malleoli should make an angle of about 20° to 25° with the frontal plane.[7,69,76] This represents the normal amount of tibial torsion; the distal end of the tibia is rotated outward with respect to the proximal end. The lateral malleolus is positioned inferiorly with respect to the medial malleolus such that the intermalleolar line makes an angle of about 10° with the transverse plane.[76] The joint axis of the ankle mortise joint corresponds approximately to the intermalleolar line. With the patellae facing straight forward, the feet should be pointed outward about 5° to 10°.

If, when the feet are in normal standing alignment, the patellae face inward, increased femoral antetorsion, increased external tibial torsion, or both, may be present. Clinically, the fault can be differentiated by assessing rotational range of motion of the hips and estimating the degree of tibial torsion by noting the rotational alignment of the malleoli with respect to the patellae and tibial tubercles. In the presence of increased hip antetorsion, the total range of hip motion will be normal but skewed such that internal rotation is excessive and external rotation is restricted proportionally. Similar considerations hold for a situation in which the patellae face outward when the feet are normally aligned; femoral retrotorsion, internal tibial torsion, or both, are likely to exist.

With respect to the frontal plane, normal knee alignment may vary from slight genu valgum to some degree of genu varum. Since in most persons the medial femoral condyle extends farther distally than the lateral condyle, slight genu valgum tends to be more prevalent. At the hindfoot, the calcaneus should be positioned in vertical alignment with the tibia. A valgus or varus heel can usually be observed as a bowing of the Achilles tendon. A valgus positioning of the calcaneus on the talus is associated with pronation at the subtalar joint, whereas a varus hindfoot involves supination.

When considering the structure of the foot as a whole, it is helpful to compare it to a twisted plate (Fig. 14-23); the calcaneus, at one end, is positioned vertically when contacting the ground, whereas the metatarsal heads are positioned horizontally when making contact with a flat surface.[99] Thus, in the normal standing position on a flat, level surface, the metatarsal heads are twisted 90° with respect to the calcaneus.

To demonstrate this, a model can be constructed by taking a light rectangular piece of cardboard and twisting it so that one end lies flat on a table and the opposite end is perpendicular to the table top. Note the "arching" of the cardboard. This is analogous to the arching of the human foot. It should be realized

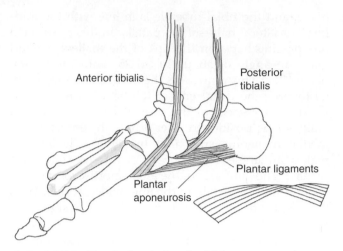

FIG. 14-23. The "twisted plate," which generates the medial arch.

that the term *arch* in this case applies to the configuration of the structure, which is dependent on the fact that it is twisted on itself. It does not refer to an arch in the true architectural sense, in which the arched configuration is dependent on the shapes of the component "building blocks." In the foot, both situations exist. On the medial side, there is little architectural arching and, therefore, little inherent stability of the

medial arch. The medial arch is dependent almost entirely on the twisted configuration of the foot, which is maintained statically by the short and long plantar ligaments and dynamically by the anterior and posterior tibialis muscles. In contrast, the lateral side of the foot represents a true architectural arch (Fig. 14-24).[99] Here the cuboid, being wedged between the calcaneus and metatarsals, serves as the structural keystone. Only a small component of the lateral arch is a result of the twisted configuration of the foot.

Referring back to the cardboard model, notice that when the cardboard is allowed to untwist—by inclining the vertical end in one direction and keeping the other end flat on the table—the arch flattens. Inclining the vertical end in the opposite direction increases the twist and increases the arch. In the foot, inclination of the vertical component of the structure, the calcaneus, will result in similar untwisting or twisting; this results in a respective decrease or increase in the arching of the foot, if the metatarsal heads remain in contact with the ground (Fig. 14-25). The person who stands with the heel in a valgus position will have a relatively "flat" or untwisted foot, whereas a person whose heel is in a varus position when standing will appear to have a "high" arch because of increased twisting between hindfoot and forefoot. The former

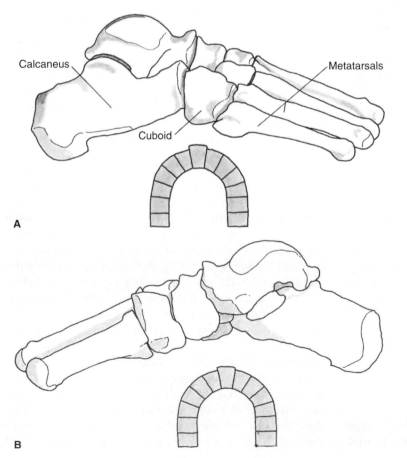

FIG. 14-24. (**A**) The lateral arch of the foot is a true arch. The calcaneus forms the ascending flank, the cuboid is the true keystone, and the fourth and fifth metatarsals are the descending flank. (**B**) The medial arch of the foot is not a true arch.

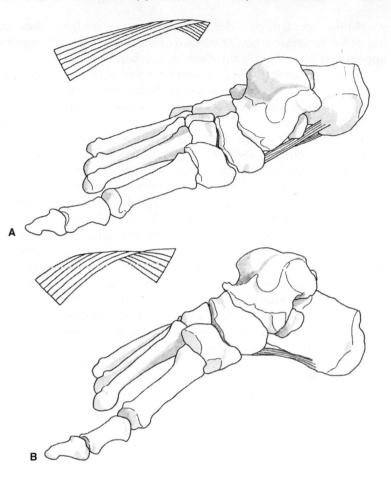

FIG. 14-25. The medial arch. (**A**) When it is allowed to "untwist," the arch flattens; (**B**) when the medial arch is "twisted" the arch increases.

situation is often termed a *pronated foot* or *flatfoot*, while the latter is termed a *supinated foot* or *pes cavus*. In the situation of the heel remaining in a vertical position but the metatarsal heads are inclined, as on an uneven surface, the effect will also be to twist or untwist the foot, thereby raising or lowering the arch. For example, if the inclination is such that the first metatarsal head is on a higher level than the fifth, the forefoot supinates on the hindfoot, untwisting the foot and lowering the arch. Note that supination of the forefoot with the hindfoot fixed is the same as pronation of the hindfoot with the forefoot fixed; they both involve untwisting of the tarsal skeleton from motion at the subtalar, transverse tarsal, and tarsal-metatarsal joints.

Reference is often made to a *transverse arch* of the foot, distinguishing it from the *longitudinal arch*. The cardboard model should help to make it clear that some transverse arching results from the twisted configuration of the foot. This is simply a transverse component of the arch discussed previously. This transverse component will increase and decrease along with twisting and untwisting of the foot. There is also a structural component to the transverse arching of the foot, resulting from the contours and relationships of the tarsals and metatarsals. It must be realized,

however, that at the level of the metatarsal heads in the standing subject, no transverse arch exists, since each of the heads makes contact with the floor.

☐ Arthrokinematics of the Ankle–Foot Complex

ANKLE MORTISE JOINT

The superior articular surface of the talus is wider anteriorly than posteriorly, the difference in widths being as much as 6 mm.[7,76] The articular surfaces of the tibial and fibular malleoli maintain a close fit against the medial and lateral articular surfaces of the talus in all positions of plantar flexion and dorsiflexion. As the foot moves from full plantar flexion into full dorsiflexion the talus rolls backward in the mortise. It would seem, then, that with ankle dorsiflexion the malleoli must separate in order to accommodate the greater anterior width of the talus. This separation could occur as a result of a lateral shift of the fibula, a lateral bending of the fibula, or both. However, it is found that the amount of separation that occurs between the malleoli during ankle dorsiflexion varies from none to only 2 mm, which is much less than would be expected, considering the amount of wedging of the superior articular surface of the talus. There appears to be a significant discrepancy between the difference in anterior and posterior widths of the trochlea of the talus and the amount of separation that occurs between the tibial and fibular malleoli with ankle dorsiflexion.

In understanding this apparent paradox, a closer look must be given to the structure of the trochlea and the type of movement the talus undergoes during ankle dorsiflexion. If both sides of the trochlea are examined it is evident that the lateral articular surface, which articulates with the fibular malleolus, is longer in its anteroposterior dimension than the medial articular surface. The reason for this is that the lateral malleolus moves over a greater excursion, with respect to the talus, during plantar flexion–dorsiflexion, than does the medial malleolus. This is partly because the axis of motion is farther from the superior trochlear articular surface laterally than medially. The corollary to this (and this is true of essentially all joints with sellar surfaces) is that the relatively trackbound movement that the talus undergoes on plantar flexion–dorsiflexion at the ankle is not a pure swing, but rather an impure swing; it involves an element of spin, or rotation, that results in a helical movement. Another way of conceptualizing this movement is to consider the talus as a section of a cone whose apex is situated medially rotating within the mortise about its own long axis, rather than a truly cylindrical body undergoing a simple rolling movement within the mortise (Fig. 14-26). As a result of this, the intermalleolar lines projected onto the superior trochlear articular surface at various positions of plantar flexion and dorsiflexion are not parallel lines. Therefore, the degree of wedging of the trochlea does not reflect the relative intermalleolar distances in dorsiflexion and plantar flexion of the ankle. The true intermalleolar distances are represented by the length of these nonparallel lines projected onto the superior trochlear surface. The projected line with the foot in plantar flexion is only slightly shorter, if at all, than that for dorsiflex-

ion, and the necessary separation of the malleoli during dorsiflexion is minimal.[76]

Up to this point, the ankle mortise joint axis has been considered as a fixed axis of motion. This has been done for the sake of simplicity and convenience using the approximate center of movement as the joint axis. But, as mentioned in Chapter 3, Arthrology, no joint moves about a stationary joint axis. As indicated by instant center analysis of knee joint motion, this is true of the ankle mortise joint as well.[145] The surface velocities determined from the instant centers of movement show that when moving from full plantar flexion to full dorsiflexion there is initially a momentary distraction of the tibiotalar joint surfaces, followed by a movement of combined rolling and sliding throughout most of the range, and terminating with an approximation of joint surfaces at the position of extreme dorsiflexion. These findings are consistent with the fact that the close-packed position of the ankle mortise joint is dorsiflexion; the tightening of the joint capsule that occurs with movement of any joint into its close-packed position produces an approximation of the joint surfaces.

SUBTALAR JOINT

As discussed previously, this is a compound joint with two distinct articulations. From the outset, movement at this joint is somewhat difficult to conceptualize because the posterior articulation between the talus and calcaneus is concave superiorly and convex inferiorly, while the anteromedial articulation is convex on concave. Understanding talocalcaneal movement is perhaps facilitated by considering it analogous to movement at the proximal and distal radioulnar joints. The radioulnar joints, like the talocalcaneal joints, move in conjunction with one another and have only one degree of freedom of motion. The posterior calcaneal facet moving against the opposing concave talar surface can be compared with the radial head moving within the radial notch of the ulna. As this movement occurs, the anteromedial facet of the talus must move in relation to the concave anteromedial surface of the calcaneus, just as the head of the ulna must move within the ulnar notch of the radius at the distal joint of the forearm. In at least some persons, this type of movement at the subtalar joint is accompanied by a slight forward displacement of the talus during pronation and a backward displacement on supination, thus making the total movement a helical, or screwlike, motion.[99]

NEUTRAL POSITION OF A JOINT

To facilitate arthrometric studies and to correlate function of the joints, it is necessary to assign to joints

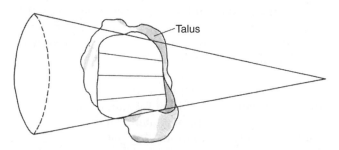

FIG. 14-26. Diagram to illustrate movement of the talus as a section of a cone, whose apex is situated medially, rotating within the mortise about its own long axis.

certain reference points called the neutral positions of those joints. By definition these neutral positions are purely reference points. They are, however, significant in that they make it possible to measure and define positional and structural variances.

The neutral position of the first ray is that position in which the first metatarsal head lies in the same transverse plane as the central three metatarsal heads when they are at their most dorsiflexed position.[141] From this neutral position, the first metatarsal can move an equal distance above and below the transverse plane of the lesser metatarsal heads when the first ray is moved through its full range.

Root and co-workers describe a neutral position of the subtalar joint as that position of the joint in which the foot is neither pronated nor supinated[141]; another way to state this is the position from which the subtalar joint could be maximally pronated and supinated. From this position, full supination of the normal subtalar inverts the calcaneus twice as many degrees as full pronation everts it. Subtalar neutral is two thirds from inversion and one third from eversion of the calcaneus.

Clinically this is important, since the subtalar neutral position provides a foundation for meaningful and valid measurements and observations with respect to the foot and entire leg. It is not only a basis for meaningful communication but is also the foundation for the application of precise therapy, such as the fabrication of an effective biomechanical orthotic device.[64] There is also a direct clinical correlation between the subtalar joint and the midtarsal joint. When the subtalar joint is held in its neutral position there is no longer the ability for the midtarsal joint to pronate. The midtarsal is unable to dorsiflex, evert, or abduct when the subtalar is in its neutral position. This position is termed the *normal locking position* of the midtarsal joint.

According to James, the talar head in a pronated foot can be palpated as a medial bulge; in a supinated foot the talar head bulges laterally. In the neutral position the talar head can be palpated equally on the medial and lateral aspects of the ankle.[79] The neutral position is usually present when the longitudinal axis of the lower limb and the vertical axis of the calcaneus are parallel. This method for establishing the subtalar neutral position is useful in both the open- and closed-chain positions.

A second method that is useful in the open-chain position involves visualizing and feeling the subtalar joint as it moves through its range of motion.[80] To begin, the examiner should place the ulnar surface of the thumb into the sulcus of the patient's fourth and fifth toes, moving the patient's foot from pronation to supination and back again. This movement is very similar in shape to that of a horse saddle, being very abrupt toward pronation and very flat and shallow to-

ward supination (Fig. 14-27A). The bottom of this saddle is the neutral position of the subtalar joint. This can be confirmed visually by observing the lateral curves above and below the malleolus (see Fig. 14-27B). If these curves are the same depth, this is the accurate neutral position. If the curve below the malleolus is deeper or shallower, then the foot is still in a pronated or supinated position and should be repositioned.

TALOCALCANEONAVICULAR JOINT

As the name implies, the talocalcaneonavicular (TCN) joint is a combination of the talonavicular joint and the subtalar (talocalcaneal) joint, which are both anatomically and functionally related (see Fig. 14-17).[129] The TCN synovial cavity is demarcated from the posterior subtalar cavity by the contents of the sinus and canalis tarsi. Ligamentous structures form an anatomical barrier between the posterior facet of the subtalar joint and its companion facets (the middle and anterior facets). This space houses the deep insertions of the inferior extensor retinaculum that cross anterior to the interosseous talocalcaneal ligament.

The plantar calcaneonavicular (spring) ligament spans the floor of this synovial cavity, enlarging the compartment and producing a functional anastomosis of sorts between the anterior portion of the sustenacu-

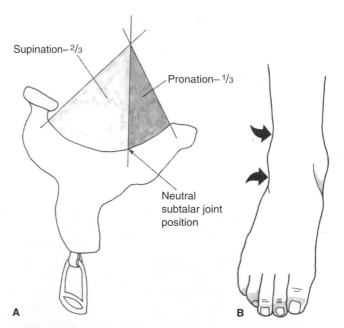

FIG. 14-27. *Subtalar movement is very similar in shape to that of a horse saddle, being very abrupt toward pronation and flat and shallow toward supination. The bottom position is the neutral position of the subtalar joint (**A**), which can be visually confirmed by observing the lateral curves above and below the malleolus (**B**). These curves should be of the same depth.*

lum tali and the navicular, known as the *acetabulum pedis.*[173] This unique space occupied by the talar head and neck is reinforced by the bifurcate ligaments laterally and the deltoid ligament medially.

The head of the talus and its large socket are enclosed by the same capsule that houses the anterior and middle facets of the subtalar joint. The capsule anatomically joins the subtalar joint and the talonavicular joints into the TCN joint.

The TCN joint, like its subtalar component, is a triplanar joint with 1° of freedom: supination and pronation.[129] Functionally, the subtalar joint and the talonavicular joint exist as components of the more complex TCN joint. The calcaneonavicular complex is a functional unit moving around the talus. The extracapsular ligaments of the sinus tarsi and tarsal canal are the major elements guiding the motion of the calcaneonavicular complex relative to the talus.

TRANSVERSE TARSAL JOINTS: TALONAVICULAR AND CALCANEOCUBOID

Although some movement may occur between the cuboid and navicular bones, movement of these two bones is considered here as a unit with respect to the calcaneus and the talus. The configuration of the talonavicular articulation is essentially that of a ball-and-socket joint. Because of this configuration, it potentially has 3° freedom of movement, allowing it to move in all planes. However, because the navicular is closely bound to the cuboid bone laterally, its freedom of movement is largely governed by the movement allowed at the calcaneocuboid joint.[46] The calcaneocuboid joint, having a sellar configuration, has 2° of freedom, each of which occurs about a distinct axis of motion. The axis of motion of most concern here is the axis of pronation and supination. This axis is similar in location and orientation to the subtalar joint axis, the major difference being that it is not inclined as much vertically. It passes through the talar head, backward, downward, and laterally. Such an orientation allows a movement of inversion–adduction–plantar flexion (supination) and eversion–abduction–dorsiflexion (pronation) of the forefoot. In the standing position, movement and positioning at the transverse tarsal joint occurs in conjunction with subtalar joint movement; when the subtalar joint pronates, the transverse tarsal joint supinates, and *vice versa.* Pronation of the forefoot causes close packing and locking of the transverse tarsal joint complex, whereas supination results in loose packing and a greater degree of freedom of movement.[99]

TARSOMETATARSAL JOINTS

The five metatarsals articulate with the three cuneiforms and the cuboid and form the tar-

sometatarsal (TMT) or Lisfranc's joint (see Fig. 14-10). They are plane synovial joints. Proximally, the bases of the metatarsals are disposed in an arcuate fashion forming a transverse arch that is high medially and low laterally. The apex of this arch corresponds to the base of the second metatarsal. The metatarsals are also flexed, thus contributing to the formation of the longitudinal arch.

The tarsometatarsal joints allow flexion and extension of the metatarsal bones and a certain degree of supination and pronation of the marginal rays.[35] Sarrafian[147] describes the supination and pronation of the first and fifth rays as longitudinal axial rotations. The combination of the sagittal motions and the axial rotations of the first and fifth rays results in a supination and pronation twist of the forefoot, as defined by Hicks.[69] A pronation twist of the forefoot is the result of first ray flexion (plantar flexed) and fifth ray extension (dorsiflexed), whereas a supination twist is a result of first ray extension and fifth ray flexion.[69,147]

METATARSOPHALANGEAL AND INTERPHALANGEAL JOINTS

The five metatarsophalangeal (MTP) joints have 2° of motion possible, either flexion/extension or abduction/adduction; the interphalangeal joints have 1° of motion, predominantly flexion and extension. In the weight-bearing foot, toe extension permits the body to pass over the foot while the toes dynamically balance the superimposed body weight as they press into the supporting surface through activity of the toe flexors.[129] The MTP joints serve primarily to allow the foot to "hinge" at the toes so that the heel may rise off the ground. This function is enhanced by the metatarsal break and the effect of MTP extension on the plantar aponeurosis (Fig. 14-28). The toes participate in weight-bearing in giving hold against the ground and in stabilizing the longitudinal arch by tensing the plantar aponeurosis during the push-off phase of the walking cycle. Approximately 40 percent of the body weight is borne by the toes in the final stages of foot contact.[103]

Weight-bearing forces to the toes are attenuated by the tension in the toe flexor tendons and the tendon sheaths. The interosseous and lumbrical muscles dynamically stabilize the toes on the floor in the tiptoe position.[172] Failure of these muscles to function accounts for toe deformities such as claw toe. The long flexors of the toes act as plantar flexors of the ankle and invertors of the talocalcaneonavicular joint, whereas the long extensors of the toes act as dorsiflexors of the ankle and evertors of the talocalcaneonavicular joint.[147] Dorsiflexion of the toes, especially the first MTP joint, is important to the windlass mechanism (see ankle and foot during gait). Sixty to seventy

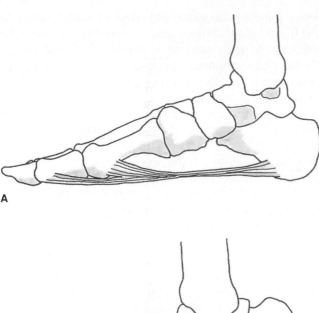

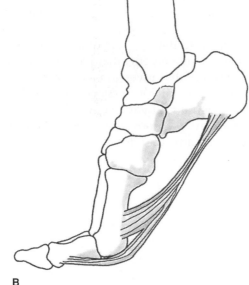

A

B

FIG. 14-28. (**A**) The foot is flat. (**B**) Toe standing causes the aponeurosis to tighten. Tightening the plantar aponeurosis raises the arch and adds to the rigidity of the tarsal skeleton.

degrees of dorsiflexion is necessary for tension to develop within the aponeurosis.[35]

☐ Osteokinematics of the Ankle–Foot Complex

TERMINOLOGY

At this point, some terms related to movement and positioning of various components of the ankle and foot must be clarified. Throughout this chapter the following definitions will hold:

Inversion–Eversion—Movement about a horizontal axis lying in the sagittal plane. Functionally, pure inversion and eversion rarely occur at any of the joints of ankle or foot. More often they occur as a component of supination or pronation.

Abduction–Adduction—Movement of the forefoot about a vertical axis or the movement of the forefoot that results from internal or external rotation of the hindfoot with respect to the leg.

Internal-External Rotation—Movement between the leg and hindfoot occurring about a vertical axis. Pure rotations do not occur functionally but rather occur as components of pronation and supination.

Plantarflexion–Dorsiflexion—Movement about a horizontal axis lying in the plane corresponding to the intermalleolar line. Functionally, these movements usually occurs in conjunction with other movements.

Pronation–Supination—Functional movements occurring around the obliquely situated subtalar or transverse tarsal joint axis. At both of these joints, pronation involves abduction, eversion, and some dorsiflexion; supination involves adduction, inversion, and plantar flexion of the distal segment on the proximal segment. This is because these joint axes are inclined backward, downward, and laterally. It must be appreciated that when the metatarsals are fixed to the ground, pronation of the hindfoot (subtalar joint) involves supination of the forefoot (transverse tarsal joint).

Pronated Foot–Supinated Foot—Traditionally, a pronated foot (in the standing position) is one in which the arched configuration of the foot is reduced; the hindfoot is pronated while the forefoot is supinated. In a supinated foot (standing) the arch is high, the hindfoot is supinated, and the forefoot is pronated.

Valgus–Varus—Terms used for alignment of parts. *Valgus* denotes inclination away from the midline of a segment with respect to its proximal neighbor, whereas *varus* is inclination toward the midline. At the hindfoot and forefoot, valgus refers to alignment in a pronated position and varus to alignment in a supinated position.

ORIENTATION OF JOINT AXES AND THE EFFECT ON MOVEMENT

In the normal standing position, the axis of movement for the knee joint is horizontal and in a frontal plane. With flexion and extension of the free-swinging tibia, movement will occur in a sagittal plane. The ankle mortise joint axis is directed backward mediolaterally about 25° from the frontal plane and downward from medial to lateral about 10° to 15° from horizontal. Movement of the free foot about this axis results in combined plantar flexion, adduction, and inversion or combined dorsiflexion, abduction, and eversion. Note that the above statements relate the movements at the respective joints to the orientations of the joint axes when the foot and leg are swinging freely. In this position, movements at one joint may occur independently of the other.

Therapists must be more concerned, however, with what happens when the foot becomes fixed to the ground and movement occurs simultaneously at the joints of the lower extremities. This is the situation during weight-bearing activities or normal functional activities involving the leg. The obvious question in this regard would be, how is it possible to move both the tibia and femur in the sagittal plane, such as when performing a knee bend with the knee pointed forward, when movement is occurring at the ankle and knee about two nonparallel axes? The heavy-weight lifter largely avoids the problem by pointing the knees outward, thus using external rotation and abduction at the hip. This brings the knee and ankle axes closer to parallel alignment. The fact remains, however, that it is possible to perform a deep knee bend with the knee directed forward, and through a considerable range. Since the knee joint axis lies horizontally in the frontal plane, no problem would be expected there, since it is ideally oriented to allow rotation of the bones in the sagittal plane. It would seem, then, that by performing such a knee bend an internal rotatory movement must be applied to the ankle, since the

ankle joint axis is externally rotated with respect to the frontal plane. Surely ankle mortise joints cannot be expected to withstand such stresses during daily activities. This apparent problem can be resolved by considering the orientation of the joint axis and associated movements at the subtalar joint.

The axis of motion for the subtalar joint is directed backward, downward, and laterally (Fig. 14-29).[21,76,106,108] The degree of inclination and mediolateral deviation of the axis varies greatly among persons. The average deviation from the midline of the foot is 16°, whereas the average deviation from the horizontal is 42°. Because the axis of motion for the subtalar joint deviates from the sagittal plane and from the horizontal plane, movement at this joint involves combined eversion, dorsiflexion, and abduction or combined inversion, plantar flexion, and adduction. Note that pure abduction and adduction of the foot are movements that would occur about a vertical axis and that inversion and eversion occur about a purely horizontal axis. Since the subtalar axis is positioned about midway between horizontal and vertical, it follows that movement about this axis would include elements of adduction–abduction as well as eversion–inversion.

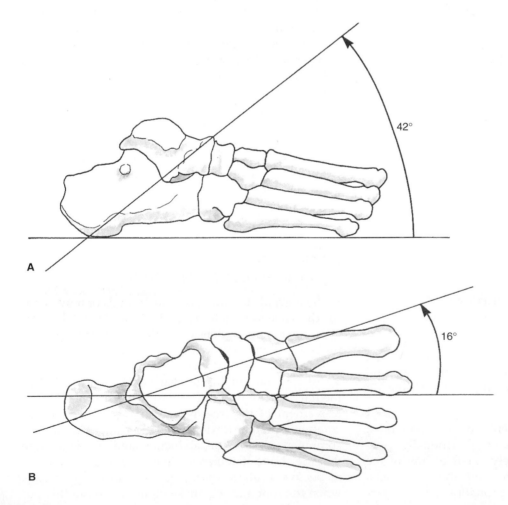

FIG. 14-29. Subtalar joint axis of movement. The subtalar joint axis is 42° from the transverse and 16° from the foot's midline, so the axis, as well as movement, is triplanar.

Consider again a situation of simultaneous knee and ankle flexion in the sagittal plane with the foot fixed (*e.g.*, a deep knee bend). It was indicated that with such a movement an internal rotatory moment of the tibia on the talus would be applied to the ankle. Because the subtalar axis allows an element of movement about a vertical axis (rotation in the horizontal plane), this internal rotatory moment can be transmitted to the subtalar joint. Internal rotation of the tibia on the foot is, of course, equivalent to external rotation of the foot on the leg, which is referred to as abduction of the foot. Subtalar movement is essentially uniaxial, so that any movement occurring at the joint may occur only in conjunction with its component movements; that is, abduction can only occur in conjunction with eversion and dorsiflexion, the three together constituting pronation at the subtalar joint. Thus, with the foot fixed, simultaneous dorsiflexion of the ankle and flexion of the knee, keeping the leg in the sagittal plane, requires pronation at the subtalar joint. As a corollary to this, with such a movement, if pronation at the subtalar joint is restricted, an abnormal internal tibial rotatory stress will occur at the ankle mortise joint or an internal femoral rotatory stress will be placed on the knee, or both. The need for subtalar movement can be reduced by moving the leg out of the sagittal plane (by pointing the knee outward) and bringing the knee and ankle axes into closer alignment.

Similar considerations apply to the situation of a person rotating the leg over a fixed foot. Any rotation imparted to the tibia is transmitted to the subtalar joint (Fig. 14-30). For example, if one rotates the leg externally over a foot that is fixed to the ground, the subtalar joint undergoes a movement of supination. This is analogous to movement about a mitered hinge; movement of one component about a vertical axis is transmitted to the second component as movement about a horizontal axis. Supination causes the calcaneus to assume a varus position, which, since the metatarsals remain flat on the ground, increases the twist in the foot and raises the arch.[21] The opposite occurs with internal tibial rotation; pronation of the hindfoot causes a relative supination of the forefoot; the foot untwists and the arch flattens. This can easily be observed if one attempts to rotate the leg with the foot fixed to the ground. With respect to the structural alignment, then, a person with excessive internal tibial torsion will tend to have a pronated hindfoot (calcaneus in valgus position) and a forefoot that is supinated with respect to the hindfoot. The resultant untwisting of the foot causes a flatfoot on standing. The person with excessive external tibial torsion will tend to have a varus heel and a high arch.

The degree of twisting and untwisting of the foot also varies with stance width.[99] When standing with the feet far apart, the heel tends to deviate into a valgus position with respect to the floor and the metatarsal heads remain flat; the metatarsals assume a position of supination with respect to the heel, thus untwisting the foot. The opposite occurs when standing with the legs crossed.

It should be noted that when standing with the hindfoot in pronation and the forefoot in supination, the medial metatarsals assume a position closer to dorsiflexion.[69] Since the joint axis of the first metatarsal is obliquely oriented (from anterolateral to posteromedial), dorsiflexion of the first metatarsal involves a component of abduction away from the midline of the foot. Therefore, in a pronated foot, the first metatarsal is usually positioned in varus. On the other hand, a person with metatarsus primus varus, a condition in which the first metatarsal deviates into varus position, the foot will tend to assume a pronated position. This is because in order for the first metatarsal to be in a varus angle, it must also be in some dorsiflexion. This causes supination of the forefoot, which necessitates pronation of the hindfoot in order for the person to stand with the metatarsal head and calcaneus in contact with the ground.

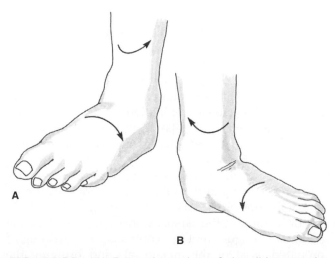

FIG. 14-30. (A) External rotation of the tibia over the fixed foot imparts a movement of supination to the foot, increasing the arch. **(B)** Internal tibial rotation flattens, or pronates, the fixed foot.

ANKLE AND FOOT DURING GAIT

Clinicians must be concerned with the function of the joints of the ankle and foot during normal daily activities. The prime consideration here, of course, is walking. Again, because these are weight-bearing joints and because the foot becomes fixed to the ground during the stance phase, an understanding of the biomechanical interrelationships between these joints and the other joints of the lower extremity is necessary.

During the gait cycle, the leg progresses through space in a sagittal plane. In order to minimize energy expenditure, the center of gravity must undergo minimal vertical displacement. This is largely accomplished by angular movement of the lower extremity components in the sagittal plane, that is, flexion–extension at the hip, knee, and ankle complex. The hip has no trouble accommodating such movement since it is multiaxial, allowing some movement in all vertical planes. The knee, although essentially uniaxial, allows flexion and extension in the sagittal plane because its axis of movement is perpendicular to this plane and horizontally oriented. The ankle mortise joint, however, cannot allow a pure sagittal movement between the leg and foot because its axis of motion is not perpendicular to the sagittal plane; it is rotated outward about 25°. During the normal gait cycle, however, movement between the foot and leg in the sagittal plane does occur. This is only possible through participation of another joint, the subtalar joint. Movement of the tibia in a parasagittal plane over a fixed foot requires simultaneous movement at the subtalar and ankle mortise joints. This is consistent with the fact that no muscles attach to the talus. Those muscles that affect movement at the ankle mortise joint also cross the subtalar joint, moving it as well.

In considering the various movements occurring at each of the segments of the lower extremity during gait, it is convenient to speak of three intervals of stance phase; these are (1) the interval from heel-strike to foot-flat, (2) midstance (foot-flat), and (3) the interval from the beginning of heel-rise to toe-off.

During the first interval, each of the segments of the lower extremity rotates internally with respect to its more proximal neighboring segment; the pelvis rotates internally in space, the femur rotates internally on the pelvis, and the tibia rotates internally on the femur (Fig. 14-31*A*).[93,95,148] It follows that the entire lower limb rotates during this phase and that distal segments rotate more, in space, than the more proximally situated segments. At the point of heel-strike, the foot becomes partially fixed to the ground, so that only minimal internal torsion between the heel and the ground takes place. Much of this internal rotation is absorbed at the subtalar joint as pronation (Fig. 14-31*B*).[161,180] Internal rotation of the leg with respect to the foot, occurring at the subtalar joint, makes the axis of the ankle mortise joint more perpendicular to the plane of progression. This allows the ankle mortise joint to provide for movement in the sagittal plane, which, of course, is the plantar flexion occurring at the ankle during this interval (Fig. 14-31*C*).

Note that the foot tends to deviate slightly medially in this stage of stance phase. This is because the obliquity of the ankle axis, in the coronal plane, imposes a component of adduction of the foot during plantar flexion.

At heel-strike, a moment-arm equal to the distance between the point of heel contact and the ankle joint develops. The reactive force of the ground acting on the foot at heel-strike across this moment-arm will tend to swing the tibia forward in the sagittal plane. This results in some flexion at the knee, which is consistent with the fact that the tibia is rotating internally with respect to the femur. Knee flexion, from an extended position, involves a component of internal tibial rotation.

Note that at heel-strike, the hindfoot moves into pronation while the tibialis anterior muscle contracts to bring the forefoot into supination. This causes the foot to untwist, the transverse tarsal joint to unlock, and the joints to assume a loose-packed position. The foot at this point is in a position favorable for free mobility and is, therefore, at its greatest potential to adapt to variations in the contour of the ground.[46,180]

Once the foot becomes flat on the ground, movement at the ankle mortise joint changes abruptly from plantar flexion to dorsiflexion.[124,135] Through the early period of foot-flat, during which most of dorsiflexion occurs, the segments of the lower extremity continue to rotate internally. This rotation is transmitted to the joints of the ankle, since the foot is now fixed to the ground. Some internal rotation of the tibia automatically occurs at the ankle mortise joint during dorsiflexion with the foot fixed, since the joint axis is inclined about 15° from horizontal, downward and laterally. However, most of the internal rotation takes place at the subtalar joint as a component of pronation.[21,180]

Throughout most of the period during which the foot is flat on the ground, the segments of the lower extremity rotate externally; the more distal segments rotate externally to a greater degree than their proximal neighbors.[96] Again, because the foot is fixed to the ground, the tibia rotates externally with respect to the foot. This occurs as supination at the subtalar joint. The change during foot-flat, from internal rotation to external rotation, takes place after most of ankle dorsiflexion is complete.

Because the forefoot is fixed to the ground, the inversion occurring at the subtalar joint imposes pronation at the transverse tarsal joint, causing a close-packing or locking of the tarsus. Consistent with this, the peroneus longus muscle contracts, maintaining a pronated twist of the metatarsals and bringing the foot as a whole toward its twisted configuration. The foot at this point is being converted into an intrinsi-

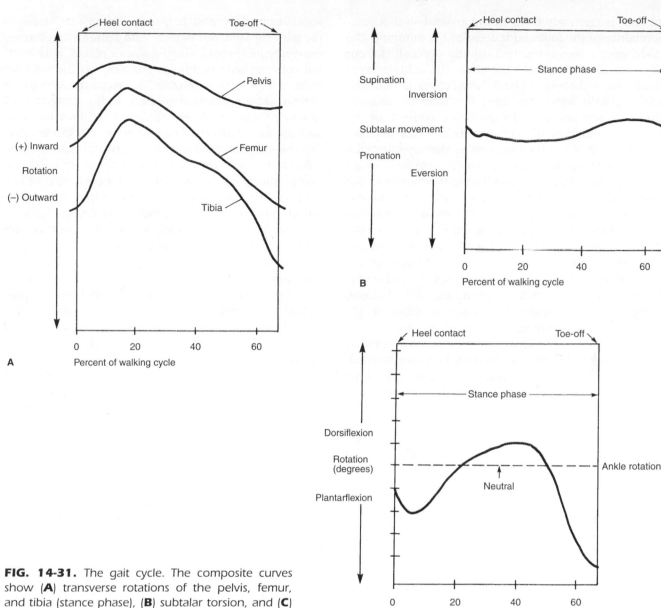

FIG. 14-31. The gait cycle. The composite curves show (**A**) transverse rotations of the pelvis, femur, and tibia (stance phase), (**B**) subtalar torsion, and (**C**) ankle mortise rotation (sagittal plane).

cally stable lever capable of providing for the thrust of pushing off.

During the final interval of stance phase, from heel-rise to toe-off, the segments of the lower limb continue to rotate externally. This external rotation of the tibia is again transmitted to the subtalar joint as supination of the hindfoot. With contraction of the calf muscle, the ankle begins plantar flexion, creating a thrust for push-off. This again creates a moment-arm acting on the knee, this time moving the tibia into extension with respect to the femur. Note that this is consistent with the external rotation of the tibia occurring during this phase, since knee extension involves a component of external tibial rotation.

The extension of the metatarsophalangeal joints, oc-

curring with heel-rise, causes a tightening of the plantar aponeurosis through a windlass effect, since the distal attachment of the aponeurosis crosses the plantar aspect of the joints (see Fig. 14-28).[70] This tightening of the aponeurosis further raises the arch and adds to the rigidity of the tarsal skeleton.

It should be emphasized that during this final phase of stance, the joint movements that occur automatically convert the foot into a stable lever system and require little, if any, muscle contraction in order to accomplish this.

In summary, then, the transverse rotations of the segments of the lower extremity that occur during stance phase of the gait cycle are transmitted to the ankle joints. This is because during the stance phase the foot is relatively fixed to the ground so that rotation between the foot and the ground is minimal. The ankle mortise axis is inclined slightly vertically (about 15° from the horizontal axis) while the subtalar joint axis is situated about midway between horizontal and vertical. Both joints are able to "absorb" rotatory movements transmitted to the ankle because of the vertical inclination of the joint axes. With the foot fixed to the ground, the tibia rotates slightly internally at the ankle mortise during dorsiflexion and externally during plantar flexion. Internal rotation of the talus with respect to the calcaneus occurs as pronation, while external rotation results in supination at the subtalar joint. Also, once the foot becomes flat on the ground, the metatarsal heads become fixed and the twisting and untwisting of the foot becomes dependent on the position of the hindfoot. At heel-strike, the tibia rotates internally, pronating the hindfoot, while the tibialis anterior contracts to supinate the forefoot; this results in an untwisted foot. During midstance, as the tibia rotates externally and the subtalar joint gradually supinates, the foot becomes twisted. This twisting is further increased by tightening of the plantar aponeurosis. The twisted configuration results in maximal joint stability with minimal participation of the intrinsic foot muscles. It is the twisted foot, then, that is best suited for weight-bearing and propulsion. During midstance there is little activity of the intrinsic muscles in the normal foot because the twisted configuration confers a passive, or intrinsic, stability on the foot. However, in the flat-footed person, considerably more muscle action is required since the foot is relatively untwisted.[99] The flat-footed person must rely more on extrinsic stabilization by the muscles. An untwisted configuration is desirable in situations in which the foot must be mobile, such as in adapting to surface contours of the ground. Consistent with this is the fact that at heel-strike, the foot assumes an untwisted state in preparation for conformation to the contacting surface.

A relatively common condition that illustrates the biomechanical interdependency of the weight-bearing joints is femoral antetorsion. A person with femoral antetorsion must stand with the leg internally rotated in order to position the hip joint in normal (neutral) alignment. Conversely, if the leg is positioned in normal alignment with the patella facing straight forward, the hip joint assumes a position of relative external rotation. External rotation at the hip decreases the congruity of the joint surfaces. During stance phase, as the femur externally rotates on the pelvis, the hip of the person with femoral antetorsion will tend to go into too much external rotation. As the slack is taken up in the part of the joint capsule that pulls tight on external rotation, the joint receptors sense the excessive movement. To avoid excessive joint incongruity and to prevent abnormal stress to the joint capsule, the person with femoral antetorsion must *internally* rotate during stance phase. This internal rotation is transmitted primarily to the subtalar joint, which is best oriented to accommodate transverse rotations. Internal rotation at the subtalar joint causes pronation of the hindfoot; the foot untwists and the arch flattens. Thus, femoral antetorsion predisposes to pronation of the foot. Also, because of the internal rotatory movement transmitted through the knee, femoral antetorsion may also be a causative factor in certain knee disorders. For example, internal rotation imposed on a semiflexed knee causes the knee to assume an increased valgus position. This may predispose to patellar tracking dysfunction (see Chapter 13, The Knee). Since there is a tendency for the person with femoral antetorsion to walk with increased hip joint incongruity, the force of weight-bearing is transmitted to a smaller area of contact at the articular surface of the hip. The result may be accelerated wear of the hip joint surfaces, perhaps leading to degenerative hip disease.

Femoral antetorsion provides a good example of how a structural abnormality in one region may lead to localized biomechanical disturbances as well as altered mechanics at joints some distance away. This, again, is especially true of the lower extremity and should emphasize that when evaluating many patients with foot disorders it may be appropriate, if not necessary, to examine the structure and function of the knee, hip, and lower back. Conversely, foot or ankle dysfunction may precipitate disturbances in more proximal joints.

■ EXAMINATION

The L4, L5, S1, and S2 segments contribute to the ankle and foot. Symptoms arising in the more proximal regions of these segments may refer to the ankle and foot, the most common of which might be paresthesias arising from lumbar nerve root irritation. Actual pain of more proximal origin is rarely felt in the foot. Rather, foot and ankle pain usually arise from local pathological processes. Pain arising from tissues of the foot or ankle may be referred a short distance proximally but almost never to the knee or above.

The common lesions affecting the ankle are of acute, traumatic onset, whereas those affecting the foot are more likely to be chronic disorders resulting from stress overload. Because of the biomechanical interdependency of the weight-bearing joints, attention must often be directed to the structure and function of more proximally situated joints during examination of patients with chronic or subtle foot disorders. Similarly, examination of the foot may well be in order in patients with disorders affecting more proximal regions.

☐ History

A patient interview designed to elicit specific information related to the patient's pain, functional status, and other associated symptoms, as set out in Chapter 5, Assessment of Musculoskeletal Disorders and Concepts of Management, should be carried out. The following are general concepts that apply to information that may be elicited when a therapist interviews patients with common foot or ankle disorders.

If the disorder was of an acute, traumatic onset, an attempt can be made to determine the exact mechanism of injury. Plantar flexion–inversion strains are more likely to result in capsuloligamentous injury, whereas forces moving the foot into dorsiflexion and external rotation (abduction) are more likely to produce a fracture.

If the disorder is of a more chronic nature and of insidious onset, the therapist can attempt to determine whether a change in activity level or footwear may be associated with the onset of the problem. The effect of changing footwear should be ascertained. For example, a therapist might determine the effect of variations in heel height, including whether the problem is affected, for better or for worse, by going barefoot.

Chronic stress overload (fatigue) disorders may be classified as (1) those due to high levels of activity in which the frequency or high rate of tissue stress is such that the body is unable to keep up with the increased rate of tissue microtrauma (the rate of tissue breakdown exceeds the rate of repair and the tissue gradually fatigues) and (2) those that occur with normal activity levels and are due to some structural or biomechanical abnormality that subjects the affected tissue to mildly increased stresses over a long period of time. Such stresses may produce pain on an intermittent basis and, over a long period of time, may induce tissue hypertrophy. Since these are mild stresses acting over a long period, the body is able to respond by laying down an excessive amount of tissue in an attempt to strengthen itself against these abnormal stresses. Tissue hypertrophy such as corns and calluses may, in itself, lead to pain by allowing localized areas of stress concentration.

Patients incurring tissue damage from high stresses acting over a relatively short time period are typically persons who have increased their activity level significantly. Often, but not always, the patient will blame a particular activity for contributing to the onset of the problem. Keep in mind that in such instances the patient may or may not be correct; the particular disorder may have been developing over some period of time, perhaps as a result of a biomechanical abnormality, and may simply be aggravated by a particular activity. By evaluating the mechanical effects of activities that reproduce the pain, the examiner can often find important clues as to the nature of a particular disorder.

Shoes tend to provide support for the twisted or arched configuration of the foot to varying degrees. A high heel causes the toes to dorsiflex when standing with the feet in contact with the ground. This raises the arch by tightening the plantar aponeurosis that crosses the plantar surface of the metatarsophalangeal joints (see Fig. 14-28). Heels also reduce the passive tension on the Achilles tendon and gastrocnemius-soleus group and, by effectively reducing the toe lever-arm of the foot, reduce the active tension developed in the gastrocnemius-soleus muscle-tendon complex. Most shoes also provide some contoured base of support for the "arch" of the foot. This maximizes the contacting surface area of the foot and, therefore, distributes the stresses of weight-bearing over most of the sole of the foot. Proper contouring of a shoe also minimizes the amount of tension that needs to be developed in the plantar aponeurosis, long and short plantar ligaments, tarsal joint capsules, and intrinsic muscles to maintain a normal twisted configuration to the foot. When a person walks barefoot, the effects of the heel and contoured support are lost. This usually creates no problem in a person with good bony alignment and ligamentous support. However, in a person with a tendency toward pronation (untwisting of the foot), the added tension to the plantar ligaments may lead to pain. Or, if the ligaments are already lax, increased intrinsic muscle activity will be necessary. If such muscular activity is prolonged, pain may also arise from muscular fatigue. These persons are often more comfortable wearing shoes than going barefoot. Even persons with normal foot structure may experience some foot pain with lower heel heights if they are accustomed to wearing a shoe with a heel. Lowering the heel reduces the support provided by the plantar aponeurosis, putting more tension on the plantar ligaments and joint capsules and calling for increased activity of the intrinsic muscles of the foot. This is why flat-soled shoes, especially, must have well-contoured "arch supports."

Shoes also provide an interface for shear and compressive stresses. Foot pain arising from localized pressure concentration, from shear stresses between the skin and an exterior surface, or from shearing between skin and subcutaneous tissue may be alleviated by going barefoot. This is primarily true in cases in which such stresses occur over all but the soles of the feet. Pain from pressure concentration over the sole of the foot, as frequently occurs over the head of the second metatarsal, may be reduced by wearing shoes, since the contouring of the shoe may serve to distribute the pressures of weight-bearing over a broader area.

Complaints of cramping of the foot may accompany muscular fatigue usually associated with some biomechanical disturbance. Cramping may also accompany intermittent claudication from arterial insufficiency. Claudication should always be suspect when the patient relates a history of pain or cramping of the feet, and usually of the lower leg, after walking some distance, but the pain is relieved with rest. Cramping may accompany disk protrusions, presumably from altered conduction of fibers subserving motor control or muscle reflexes. This cramping is noticed more often at night.

☐ Physical Examination

I. Observation

A. *General appearance and body build.* Weight-bearing stresses will be increased in the presence of obesity.

B. *Activities of daily living.* Dressing, grooming, gait, and transfer activities (see gait analysis discussion under Lumbosacral–lower limb scan examination). With localized foot or ankle disorders, usually only the gait is affected. Observe the patient walking with and without shoes. An antalgic gait associated with foot or ankle lesions is typically one in which heel-strike or push-off, or both, are lacking. This results in a shortened stride on the affected side, which is accentuated at faster paces. Chronic disorders may produce no obvious gait disturbances. However, one should look carefully for more subtle gait deviations, indicating a possible biomechanical abnormality of one or more of the weight-bearing joints that may be related to a foot problem. It is of primary importance to observe for abnormal rotatory movements of the weight-bearing segments. To assess rotations of the hindfoot into pronation and supination, look at the following:

1. The patellae to judge rotary movements of the femur
2. The position of the malleoli with respect to each other or the tibia
3. The position of the calcanei
4. The degree of toeing-in or toeing-out
5. The degree of motion in ankle dorsiflexion and plantar flexion

6. The angle and base of gait. Normally, this angle does not exceed 15° from the midline of the body.[141]
7. Point of heel contact. The position of the calcaneus in either eversion or inversion during heel-strike[114]
8. The approximate time of pronation. Normally, pronation will occur 15% to 20% into the contact phase of gait.[142,152]
9. The approximate time of supination. Normally this will occur in the last half of stance.[141,152]
10. For the foot, the critical periods to identify during gait include[74]
    a. Contact (heel- or rear foot-strike to foot-flat)
    b. Midstance
    c. Lift-off (heel-rise to toe-off)
    The patient's gait should be reviewed during both walking and running. Very frequently a foot that looks as though it is one configuration will actually function as the opposite in motion.[9] Videotape or film analysis with slow motion and the use of a treadmill, if available, are invaluable in diagnosing difficult problems.[98] The practical advantage of a treadmill is control of speed.

II. Inspection

A. *Skin and nails*

1. If areas of abnormal callosities, redness, or actual skin breakdown are noted, suggesting excessive shear or compression forces, document the size of the involved area to serve as a baseline measurement. This can easily be done by tracing the perimeter of the involved area on a piece of acetate (such as old roentgenographic film).
2. Excessive dryness or moisture may suggest abnormal vascularity or abnormal sympathetic activity to the part, or both.
3. Note the site and size of hypertrophic skin changes, such as corns and calluses. These suggest mildly increased shear or compression forces acting over a longer period of time than those that might produce localized inflammation or actual breakdown. Keep in mind that a painful callus is one in which the underlying tissue is in the process of breaking down.
4. Diffuse ecchymosis may be associated with common ankle sprains as well as more serious trauma.
5. Inspect the toe nails for splitting, over-

growth, inappropriate trimming, and inflammation of the nail beds.

B. *Soft tissue*
  1. Swelling (see under palpation)
  2. Wasting of isolated or generalized muscle groups
  3. General contours

C. *Bony structure and alignment*
  1. Note toe and metatarsal deformities such as claw toes, hammer toes, and varus–valgus deviations.[116]

    a. Claw toes are usually associated with a pes cavus deformity and may accompany certain neurological disorders. The metatarsophalangeal joints are positioned in extension and the interphalangeal joints in flexion (Fig. 14-32A). Contracture of the long toe-extensors causes extension of the toes, which increases the passive tension on the long toe-flexors. The intrinsic muscles are overbalanced, both actively and passively, by these muscle groups.

    b. Hammer toes are a result of capsular contracture of the proximal interphalangeal joints (Fig. 14-32B). The involved joint or joints are fixed in some degree of flexion.

    Typically there is hyperextension of the metatarsophalangeal joint and distal interphalangeal joints and flexion of the proximal interphalangeal joint. It is usually only seen in one toe—the second toe, occasionally the third.

    c. Mallet toe is associated with a flexion deformity of the distal interphalangeal joint (Fig. 14-32C). The metatarsophalangeal joint and proximal interphalangeal joints usually are normal. There is usually a callus formation under the tip of the toe or a deformity of the nail.

    d. Tailor's bunions ("bunionette") are caused by irritation and pressure of the fifth metatarsal head. There may be an overlapping fifth toe or quinti varus deformity (often congenital) of the fifth toe (Fig. 14-32D).

    e. A hallux valgus is the most common deformity of the first metatarsophalangeal (M-P) joint. Pathologically it is a lateral deviation of the proximal phalanx and medial deviation of the first metatarsal bone in relation to the center of the body (Fig. 14-32E). It may be associated with a pronated foot and is found most frequently in older women. The joint surfaces are no longer congruent and some may even go on to subluxation. Note the presence of any bursa over the M-P joint (bunion) and whether active inflammatory changes are present. The toe may be rotated with the toe nail pointed inward.

    f. Assess the length of the metatarsals (Fig. 14-33). A line across the metatarsals should form a smooth parabola. The so-called Morton's, Grecian, or atavistic foot is a hereditary type, in which the second toe is longer than the first. With this condition, normal balance is disturbed and weight stress falls toward the inside arch (pronation).[71] This tends to produce hypermobility of the first ray, displacement of the sesamoid bones, and increased stress on the second metatarsal head.

  2. If indicated, assess pronation of the foot, manifested by a flattening of the medial longitudinal arch. The relative position of the navicular tuberosity in the weight-bearing and non-weight-bearing position is examined. A line (Feiss' line) is drawn from the tip of the medial malleolus to the plantar aspect of the first metatarsophalangeal joint.[133] The navicular tubercle should be within one third of the perpendicular distance between this line and the ground. If the navicular falls one third of the distance to the floor, the condition is referred to as first-degree flatfoot; if it rests on the floor, a third-degree flatfoot.

  3. The calcanei should be positioned vertically with little or no inward or outward bowing of the Achilles tendon.

  4. The general configuration of the foot should be assessed in standing and sitting positions.

    a. When standing, an untwisted foot is one in which the hindfoot is in pronation and the forefoot is in supination. The calcaneus will be in valgus position and the navicular tubercle will be sunken and often prominent. The talar head also becomes prominent medially, and the forefoot often assumes an abducted position with respect to the hindfoot. There is often an associated valgus deformity of the first metatarsal-phalangeal joint.

    With excessive twisting of the foot

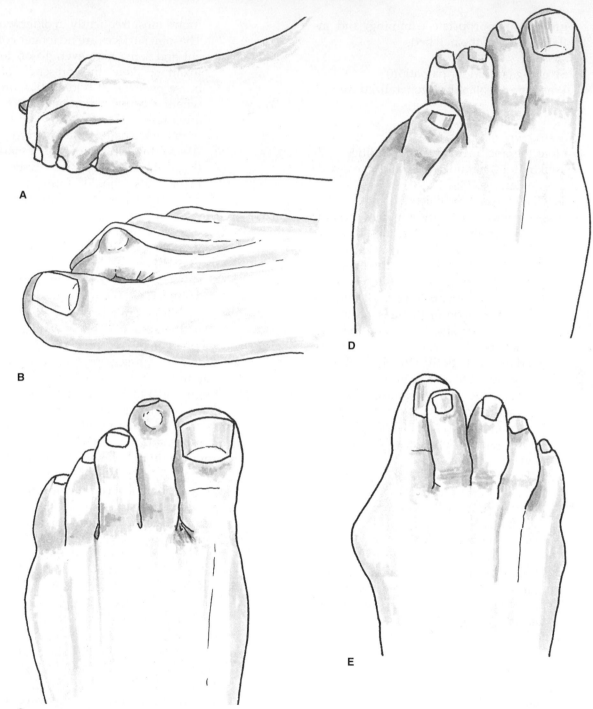

FIG. 14-32. Toe deformities: (**A**) claw toes, (**B**) hammer toe, (**C**) mallet toe (second toe), (**D**) an overlapping fifth toe or *quinti varus* deformity, and (**E**) *hallux valgus* with a bunion and overlapped second toe.

(pes cavus) the calcaneus assumes a varus position and the medial arch is well formed, with the navicular tubercle positioned well superiorly. There is often a tendency toward clawing of the toes in a cavus foot.

b. When sitting, the foot should relax into a position of plantar flexion, inversion, and adduction. A "supple" or "mobile" flat-foot will take on a more normal configuration in sitting with the force of weight-bearing relieved. A "fixed"

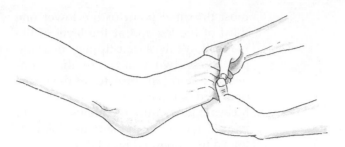

FIG. 14-33. Inspection of toes: Flex the toes and note the relative length of the metatarsals. Abnormally short first or fifth metatarsals are a potential cause of forefoot imbalance. When both are short, there is often a painful callus under the second metatarsal.

or "structural" flat-foot will maintain its planus (untwisted) state.

5. Perform a complete structural examination of the remainder of the lower extremities, the pelvis, and the lower back, as discussed in Chapter 22, Lumbosacral–Lower Limb Scan Examination. Any structural deviations or asymmetries should be noted, and the possible effects on the biomechanics of the foot considered.

6. Inspect the shoes, inside and out, for wear patterns that may offer clues as to the presence of persistent biomechanical disturbances and localized areas of pressure. Also inspect for other possible sources of pain arising from the shoe, such as nails protruding through the insole and prominent seams.

    a. On the outer sole, the wear pattern should be displaced somewhat laterally at the heel. Over the front sole, the wear pattern should be spread fairly evenly across the area corresponding to the level of the first, second, and third metatarsophalangeal joints, with less wear laterally. There should be an even wear pattern across the rest of the medial side of the sole. Areas of localized excessive wear should be noted as well as abnormal wear patterns.

    b. The upper portion of the shoe should show a gently curved transverse crease line at the level of the metatarsophalangeal joints. Excessive curling of the vamp of the shoe and the front part of the sole may occur in a shoe that is too long, too narrow, or both. A crease line that runs obliquely, from forward and

medial to backward and lateral, may arise from a stiff first metatarsophalangeal joint.

Localized prominences of the vamp commonly occur medially in the presence of hallux valgus or dorsally with hammer toes or claw toes. Such prominences should be noted.

Inspect for excessive overhanging of the upper shoe with respect to the sole. This is likely to be observed medially in shoes of patients with pronation of the hindfoot.

When viewed from behind, the cup formed by the counter of the shoe should rise vertically and symmetrically from the sole. Inclination of the counter medially, with bulging of the lateral lip of the counter, will be seen in shoes of patients with pronated feet.

Areas of excessive scuffing of the upper shoe should be noted. Scuffing of the toe of the shoe may occur with weak dorsiflexors or restriction of motion toward dorsiflexion.

    c. When inspecting the inside of the shoe, feel along the inner surface of the seams for prominent areas that may give rise to pressure concentration. Also feel along the entire surface of the inner sole for prominent areas that might be caused by protruding nails.

The wear pattern on the inside of the shoe should also be examined. There should be evidence of an even distribution of pressure over the medial and lateral sides of the heel counter, over the inner sole at the heel, and over the inner sole at the metatarsal heads.

III. **Selective Tissue Tension Tests**

A. *Active movements (functional movements)*

    1. Barefoot walking

        a. Normal gait

        b. On toes. If unable to do so, determine whether it is because of pain, weakness, or restriction of motion. The heel should invert and the arch should rise.

        c. On heels. If unable to do so, determine whether it is because of pain, weakness, or restriction of motion.

    2. Standing with feet fixed

        a. Externally rotate the leg with respect to the foot. This should cause some varus deviation of the heels and raising of the arches. Compare one foot to the other.

b. Internally rotate the legs on the feet. This should result in some valgus deviation of the heels and flattening of the arches. Compare one foot to the other.
3. Standing, keeping knees extended
   a. Evert the feet by standing on medial borders of feet.
   b. Invert the feet by standing on lateral borders of feet.
4. Sitting, with legs hanging freely. Compare range of motion of one foot to the other. Assess pain, range of motion, and crepitus.
   a. Dorsiflexion
   b. Plantar flexion
   c. Inversion
   d. Eversion
   e. Toe movements

B. *Passive physiological movements*
1. Standing, before measurements are taken, determine the dynamic angle and base of walking using the patient's own line of progression as a reference.[115] A paper walkway (approximately 20 to 24 feet long) on which the patient's footprints can be recorded (after walking in a normal fashion) is most convenient.[11,115,153] Using the line of progression as a reference, select one left and one right footprint from the middle of the progression to use to construct a paper template of the footprints adjacent to each other. The dynamic foot angle and the distance between the middle of each heel are maintained (Fig. 14-34).

   Note: The paper walkway recording can be used for additional data collection such as stride length, velocity, and cadence in the gait analysis.
2. Measurement of subtalar joint in relaxed standing
   a. With a felt-tipped marking pen, bisect the middle one third of the posterior calcaneus.[141] Extend the bisection line plantarly to the base of the supporting surface and from the middle one third of the calcaneus superiorly approximately 1 inch; the point of bifurcation is located at the junction of the proximal and middle one third of the bisected calcaneus.
   b. Next, bisect the distal one third of the lower extremity just proximal to the malleoli. Extension of this line superiorly should bisect the knee joint within the popliteal space. Calipers may be used to determine the center of the most proximal point of the lower one third of the leg and at the level of the malleoli. With a felt-tipped marking pen, these two points are then connected to form the bisector of the lower one third of the leg.
   c. Measure the neutral calcaneus stance (a relaxed foot with the subtalar joint allowed to pronate) (Fig. 14-35).
      i. Have the patient stand in a normal angle and base of gait (see **B.1.** above) and facing away from the examiner.[141] Using a goniometer or protractor, place the straight arm along the supporting surface (transverse plane). The center point of the goniometer or protractor is placed at the apex point of the angle created by the calcaneal bisection and the supporting surface (frontal plane). Rearfoot valgus is then measured to the nearest degree.
      ii. The normal weight-bearing foot should demonstrate a mild amount of pronation but should still allow for additional pronation.[12] If the patient is bearing weight or walking with the foot out of neutral position and near full pronation, an obligatory internal tibial rotation occurs and is prolonged, resulting in an increased force that is absorbed by the soft tissues of the knee.[79,80]
3. Measurement of tibia varum
   a. Measure tibia varum (tibiofibular varum), if indicated. If a lateral angulation of the tibia-to-floor angle is 10° or greater, the extremity requires an excessive amount of subtalar joint pronation to produce a plantigrade foot (Fig. 14-36).
      i. Have the client stand in a normal angle and base of gait. With the feet in a resting calcaneal stance position, recheck the bisections of the calcaneus and lower leg. When the bisections are acceptable, measure the frontal plane relationship of the tibia to the transverse plane (or level ground). If a gravity goniometer is used, the angle between the bisection of the leg and vertical is read on the face of the

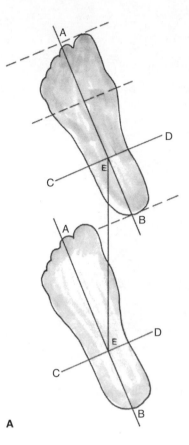

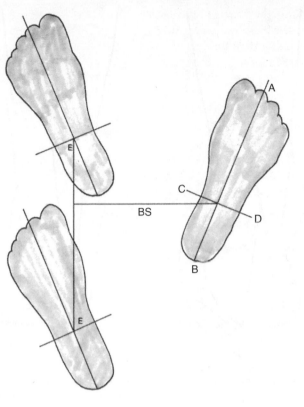

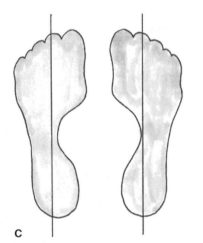

FIG. 14-34. (**A**) Computation of foot angle (AB—longitudinal line bisecting each foot; CD—horizontal line through posterior third of foot perpendicular to line AB; EE—connecting line of intersections of CD and AB of two ipsilateral feet [line of progression]; resulting angle is foot angle). (**B**) Computation of the base of support [BS—line drawn from intersection of CD and AB of contralateral foot perpendicular to line EE). (**C**) Computation of dynamic angle and base of walking template.

goniometer. Tibia varum is present when the distal end of the bisecting line of the leg is closer to the midsagittal plane than the proximal end. Tibia valgum is present if the leg is angulated in the opposite direction.

Note: Tibia varum (tibiofibular varum) measurements can also be performed with the foot positioned in subtalar neutral by palpating for talar congruency as the patient rotates the trunk to the left and right,

allowing the tibia to externally and internally rotate, thus supinating and pronating the subtalar joint. Once subtalar neutral is reached, the subject is then asked to maintain this position while measurements are recorded. According to McPoil and co-workers the best patient position for clinical measurement of tibiofibular varum is the neutral calcaneal stance position. It would appear that the measurement of true tibia varum cannot be

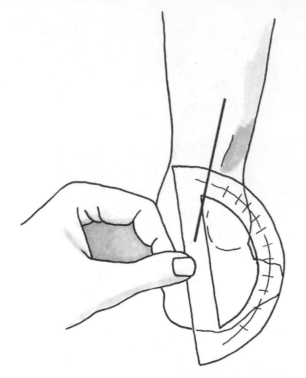

FIG. 14-35. Measurement of neutral calcaneal stance (a relaxed foot with subtalar joint allowed to pronate).

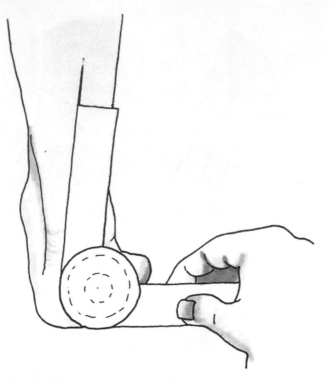

FIG. 14-36. Measurement of tibia varum in the resting calcaneal stance position.

done without obtaining roentgenograms of the lower extremities taken during weight-bearing.[115]

4. Measurement of great toe extension
   a. Measurement of great toe extension can be made while the person is standing. The great toe is extended actively and assisted passively without dorsiflexing the first ray. Forty-five degrees has been found to be adequate for general ambulation.[104]
   b. Great toe extension test. Passive extension of the great toe at the metatarsophalangeal joint in the normal weight-bearing foot has two effects: elevation of the medial longitudinal arch (windlass effect) and lateral rotation of the tibia. The test is normal when both effects are seen (Fig. 14-37).[143]
5. Passive range of motion. The patient sits with legs hanging freely. Compare range of motion of one foot to the other. Note the presence of pain or crepitus. Note abnormalities or asymmetries in range of motion. Note the presence of pathological end feels.
   a. Hindfoot
      i. Plantar flexion
      ii. Inversion

iii. Eversion
   b. Transverse tarsal
      i. Plantar flexion
      ii. Pronation (eversion)
      iii. Supination (inversion)
      iv. Abduction
      v. Adduction
6. Supine
   a. Hip flexion–extension
   b. Knee flexion–extension
   c. First ray: position and mobility
      i. Place the foot in a neutral subtalar position (see Fig. 14-27). Load the forefoot (see **7.c.i** below). While maintaining the foot in neutral position, grasp the metatarsal heads (between the thumb and forefinger) with the loading hand. Grasp the first metatarsal head with the other hand.
      ii. Assess the position of the first metatarsal head in relationship to its neutral position and assess the end-range position of the first metatarsal head in relationship to the second metatarsal head.[142]
      iii. While maintaining the foot in neutral subtalar position, manually plantar flex and dorsiflex the first

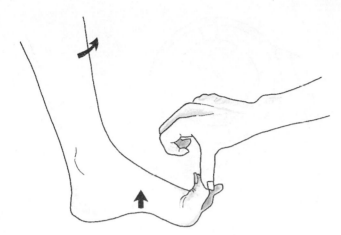

FIG. 14-37. Great toe extension test.

ray. Assess the motion of the first ray in relationship to its neutral position.

    iv. Limited range may result from a combination of biomechanical factors such as excessive pronation or a short tendon or from restriction of the joint proper.[51]

7. Prone, with the feet over the edge of the table.

    a. Hip internal and external rotation with the knees flexed to 90°.

    b. Supination and pronation of the calcaneus. The amount of supination and pronation that is available can be measured by lining up the longitudinal axis of the lower limb and vertical axis of the calcaneus (Fig. 14-38).[79,142] Passive movement of the calcaneus into inversion (amount of supination) is normally 20°.[142] Conversely, the amount of eversion (pronation) is normally 10°.[142]

    c. Forefoot valgus–forefoot varus. The subtalar should be positioned in subtalar neutral and the forefoot locked (Fig. 14-39).

        i. In order to accomplish locking of the forefoot in the open-chain position the forefoot must be loaded against the neutral subtalar rearfoot. This is accomplished by applying a dorsiflectory force against the fourth and fifth metatarsal heads so that the forefoot is fully pronated on a neutral rearfoot. In order to fully lock the forefoot, also called loading the forefoot, at the midtarsal joint the dorsiflectory

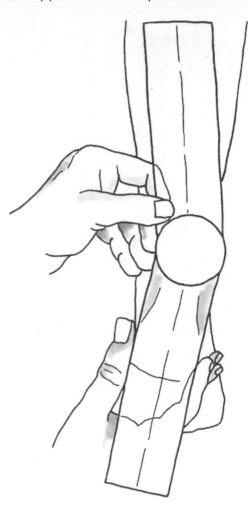

FIG. 14-38. Measurement of supination and pronation of the calcaneus (hindfoot inversion and eversion [non–weight bearing]).

force should be applied only until resistance is appreciated. The relationship of the neutral subtalar position and a fully pronated forefoot against the rearfoot results in the neutral position of the foot in the open-chain position. It is not necessary to dorsiflex the foot to 90° or lift the leg from the supporting surface. Slightly adduct the forefoot to ensure complete midtarsal joint pronation.

    ii. Place one arm of the goniometer along the posterior calcaneal bisection and the other arm along the plantar aspect of the heel (see Fig. 14-39A). Align the latter arm with the plane of the forefoot (an imaginary line from the head of the fifth metatarsal to the head of the first) and read the degrees of forefoot

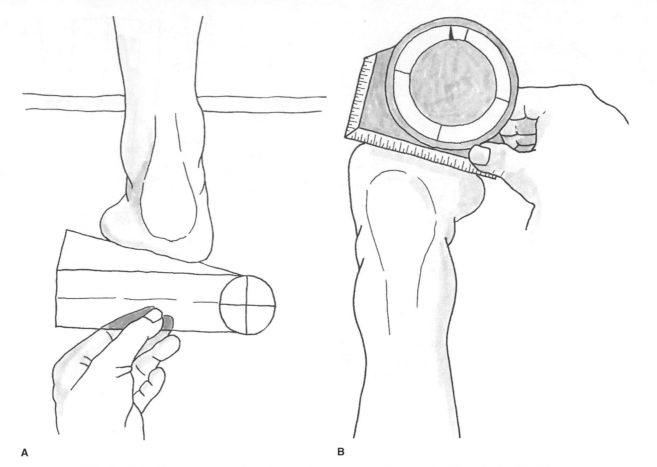

A   **B**

FIG. 14-39. Measurement of forefoot valgus or varus (non–weight bearing) with (**A**) goniometer or (**B**) inclinometer.

deviation. An inclinometer may also be used with the knee in 90° of flexion (see Fig. 14-39*B*). Deviation from a normal perpendicular relationship with a line bisecting the calcaneus represents a difference between alignment of forefoot to hindfoot.

iii. Forefoot valgus is commonly found in the varus foot. Forefoot varus may require increased pronation to adequately contact the surface while running or walking.[80,166]

iv. The calcaneal position, varus or valgus, can also be determined at this time.

d. Dorsiflexion

  i. Position the patient prone with his foot over the edge of the table. Place a 4-inch roll underneath the distal anterior thigh to ensure full knee extension. Place the foot into subtalar neutral. While maintaining subtalar neutral, manually assist dorsiflexion of the foot on the leg while the patient actively dorsiflexes the foot to its end range.

  ii. Repeat with the knee flexed to 90°.

  iii. Dorsiflexion is measured to the nearest degree.

  Note: The subtalar joint must be maintained in a neutral position during these motions. Pressure applied to the first ray will help prevent pronation.[117]

C. _Resisted isometric movements._ Resisted isometrics are done in the supine or sitting position. Resisted isometric knee flexion should be included because of the triceps surae action on the knee. With the patient's foot placed in the anatomical position, the movements tested are as follows.

1. _Dorsiflexion._ Pain may be due to a tendinitis. Painless weakness associated with a

footdrop may be due to a lesion of the lateral popliteal or the L5 nerve root. Painful resisted dorsiflexion and inversion occurs in tendinitis of the anterior tibialis.

2. *Plantar flexion.* Test in weight-bearing. Pain may be due to a lesion of the Achilles tendon or a tear in the gastrocnemius. A painless weakness may be due to S1 nerve-root pressure.

3. *Inversion.* A painful weakness of inversion is usually due to tenosynovitis or tendinitis of the posterior tibialis muscle. Painless weakness may be due to a tendon rupture or L4 nerve root compression.

4. *Extension of the great toe.* A painful weakness occurs with tenosynovitis of the extensor hallucis longus muscle. Painless weakness may indicate an L5 nerve root compression.

5. *Toe extension.* A painful weakness may indicate a tenosynovitis of the extensor digitorum longus; painless weakness occurs in an L5 nerve root lesion.

D. *Joint-play movements.* Assess for hypermobility or hypomobility and presence or absence of pain.

1. Distal tibiofibular joint–anteroposterior glide (see Fig. 14-41)

2. Ankle mortise (talocrural) joint
   a. Distraction of talus (see Fig. 14-42)
   b. Anterior and posterior glide of talus. Anterior glide is an important test for integrity of the anterior talofibular ligament. The patient is supine. Place one hand over the dorsum of the distal tibia and cup the other hand around the back of the calcaneus. The talus by way of the calcaneus is pulled forward in the mortise, and the movement is compared with the movement on the opposite side.
      i. Hypermobility will be present in the case of a chronic anterior talofibular ligament rupture.
      ii. Pain will be reproduced from a talofibular ligament sprain or adhesion.

3. Subtalar joint
   a. Distraction of calcaneus
   b. Dorsal rock of calcaneus, plantar rock of calcaneus (see Figs. 14-47 and 14-48)
   c. Varus-valgus tilts of calcaneus (see Figs. 14-45 and 14-46). The range of calcaneal inversion and eversion is assessed and the two feet are compared.

Capsular restriction will result in a greater loss of inversion than eversion.

4. Transverse tarsal joint—dorsal-plantar glides (see Fig. 14-49)

5. Naviculocuneiform joint—dorsal-plantar glides (see Fig. 14-50)

6. Cuneiform-metatarsal joints
   a. Dorsal-plantar glides
   b. Pronation–supination (see Fig. 14-51)

7. Cuboid–fifth metatarsal joint—dorsal-plantar glides

8. Intermetatarsal and tarsometatarsal joints—dorsal-plantar glides (see Fig. 14-53)

9. Metatarsophalangeal and interphalangeal joints
   a. Dorsal-plantar glides (see Fig. 14-55)
   b. Internal-external rotations
   c. Medial-lateral tilts
   d. Distraction (see Fig. 14-54)

IV. **Neuromuscular Tests**

There are few localized neurological problems that affect the foot. If a disorder affecting a relevant nerve root (L4, L5, S1, or S2) is suspected, or if a problem affecting a peripheral nerve supplying the foot is suspected, the necessary sensory, motor, and reflex testing should be performed. The segmental and peripheral nerve innervations, as well as the related reflexes, are listed in Chapter 4, Assessment of Musculoskeletal Disorders and Concepts of Management.

V. **Palpation**

A. *Skin*

1. Moisture or dryness. Abnormal moisture, usually associated with pain and joint restriction, may accompany a reflex sympathetic dystrophy. Vascular disorders may also cause changes in the moisture or texture of the skin.

2. Texture

3. Mobility. Skin mobility may be restricted after prolonged immobilization, especially following a surgical procedure.

4. Temperature. Inflammatory lesions will often result in increased skin temperature over the site of the lesion. Fairly precise documentation of the degree of inflammation may be made by using a thermistor probe. This often offers a convenient guide as to the effect of treatment procedures on the state of the lesion as well as a guide to the state of the inflammatory process in general. For example, a baseline reading can be documented and measurements taken before and after each treatment ses-

sion (these must be taken over precisely the same point and at the same time of day). A slight elevation of, say, 1°C can be expected after any treatment that imposes some mechanical stress, such as mobilization, massage, or exercise. However, it is important that the elevation does not persist over more than a few hours. If so, the treatment program may be too vigorous. If some decline in temperature is noted, it may be a sign that resolution is taking place. Thermistor readings, as with most tests, are significant when compared with a normal side.

B. *Soft tissue*
1. Swelling
   a. Localized extra-articular swelling may accompany ankle sprains, usually involving the lateral aspect of the ankle below the lateral malleolus.
   b. Localized articular effusion of the ankle mortise joint manifests as a loss of definition over the malleolar regions. Subtle joint effusion can be detected by applying firm pressure with the thumb and index fingers over the regions below the medial and lateral malleoli simultaneously. This will force the fluid into the anterior capsular region and cause a fullness over the dorsum of the ankle.
   c. Generalized edema of the foot may follow major trauma, or it may accompany systemic, more generalized vascular or metabolic disorders.
2. Mobility
3. Consistency
4. Pulses
   a. The pulse of the dorsalis pedis artery may be palpated just lateral to the tendon of the extensor hallucis longus over the dorsum of the foot.
   b. The pulse of the posterior tibial artery is palpated behind the tendons of the flexor digitorum longus and flexor hallucis longus posterosuperior to the medial malleolus.
5. Other specific tendons, ligaments, and muscles should be palpated, as indicated by findings up to this point in the examination. A guide to palpation of these structures is included in the section on surface anatomy in this chapter.

C. *Bony structures and tendon and ligament attachments*
1. Palpate joint margins to assess structural

alignment and to note any hypertrophic changes.
2. Palpate tendon and ligament attachments as indicated in the section on surface anatomy.

■ COMMON LESIONS AND THEIR MANAGEMENT

Probably the most common lower limb problem in amateur and professional athletics is that of overuse syndromes. The frequency of overuse injuries ensures that they will be a significant portion of the practice of the sports medicine clinic and the general orthopedic clinic. Overuse injuries affect different anatomical sites and tissues and are usually secondary to training errors and accumulated microtrauma. In the lower leg group, specific syndromes include tibial stress syndrome, Achilles tendinitis, shin splints, tibial stress fractures, and compartment syndromes.

The common disorders affecting the foot are in the majority of cases the result of some biomechanical disturbance. As indicated in the preceding section, such biomechanical disorders may be of local origin, or the primary problem may involve one of the other weight-bearing segments. For this reason, evaluation of chronic, subtle foot disorders requires that structural and functional assessments of the other weight-bearing joints be made. Similarly, evaluation of patients with problems in these other regions may necessitate examination of the foot. In understanding the rationale of the evaluative and treatment procedures related to foot disorders, it is essential that the practitioner have a basic knowledge of the biomechanics of the foot and how they relate to the biomechanics of the other weight-bearing joints.

Because the numerous joints of the foot contribute to make it a very mobile structure as a whole, it has the ability to attenuate the energy of forces applied to it. For this reason, traumatic lesions affecting the foot are relatively rare. On the other hand, the common lesions affecting the ankle are usually of traumatic origin.[17] While the individual joints making up the ankle are relatively trackbound or uniaxial, the ankle complex allows some movement in the sagittal, frontal, and transverse planes. However, transverse rotations are of limited range because they do not occur about a true vertical axis. Also, eversion is normally quite restricted because the fibular malleolus extends distally to create an abutment that limits this movement. Forces that move the ankle past its physiological limits of motion will tend to cause damage, usually to the osseus or ligamentous components of the ankle complex, or to both. Excessive forces to the ankle producing such damage are often the result of forces from the ground acting over the lever-arm provided by the foot or forces of the center of gravity of the body acting over the lever-arm of the lower extremity with the foot fixed. Because of these lever-arms over which forces acting on the ankle may be applied and because certain ankle motions are normally limited, the ankle is often the site of acute traumatic injuries such as sprains and fractures.

Except in situations in which there is malalignment of bony constituents, such as after healing of a fracture, or in situations in which there is marked restriction of movement of one of the ankle joints, such as after arthrodesis of the subtalar joints, degenerative joint disease affecting the ankle is rare. Rheumatoid arthritis often affects the foot but less often the ankle.

Both the foot and ankle may be the site of fatigue disorders. Such disorders result from abnormally high stresses occurring over relatively short periods of time or from mildly abnormal stresses occurring over a long period of time. The former situation usually occurs in athletes or others who have undergone an abrupt increase in activity level. In such cases, the degree of microtrauma affecting certain tissues exceeds the rate at which the body is able to repair itself; the result is a fatigue-induced yielding of the involved tissue. Examples are stress fractures, blisters, and many of the tendinitis conditions affecting this region. Milder stresses occurring over longer periods of time tend to result in tissue hypertrophy that may contribute to certain painful disorders. Typical examples are heel spurs and various callus formations.

☐ Overuse Syndromes of the Leg

The pathophysiology of overuse injuries is a local inflammatory response to stress. The causes of overuse injuries are either intrinsic (malalignment syndromes, muscle imbalances) or extrinsic (training error).[65] A systematic musculoskeletal assessment is necessary in order to differentiate overuse injuries and to clarify the etiological factors. Effective treatment is predicated on recognizing and correcting the underlying predisposing, precipitating or perpetuating etiological factors.

SHIN SPLINTS

The term *shin splints* is considered by many to be a catch-all phrase applied to a number of different conditions limited to the legs and has generated much confusion.[144,154,156] Shin splints (idiopathic compartment syndrome) is used here to mean an etiological subset of exercise-induced pain: mechanical inflammation due to repetitive stress of the broad proximal portion of any of the musculotendinous units origi-

nating from the lower part of the leg or tibia during weight-bearing.[87,154,175] This narrower definition is consistent with American Medical Association terminology.[2]

Depending on the affected muscles, shin splints can be anterolateral or posteromedial.[5,87,175] Anterolateral shin splints cause pain and tenderness lateral to the tibia over the anterior compartment and involve the pretibial muscles, including the anterior tibialis, extensor hallucis longus, and extensor digitorum longus. Anterolateral shin splints may occur secondary to heel contact on hard surfaces, or to wearing a shoe with a hard heel, or to biomechanical abnormalities such as forefoot varus.[65,87] A muscle imbalance between a weak pre-tibial muscle group and tight gastrocnemius-soleus muscles may result in overactivation of these muscles during heel-strike and swing phase.

Posteromedial shin splints cause symptoms along the posteromedial border of the middle to lower tibia over the posterior compartment, which is appreciated more during toe-off.[128] Research has shown a strong positive correlation between excessive pronation and posteromedial shin splints.[171]

In anterolateral and posteromedial shin splints, there is typically weakness of the affected muscles and pain reproduced by resisted active motion.[128]

MEDIAL TIBIAL STRESS SYNDROME

Medial tibial stress syndrome (MTSS) or tibial periostitis presents as exercise-induced pain localized to the distal posteromedial border of the tibia. According to Walker,[175] the clinical distinction between posteromedial shin splints and MTSS is hazy, but the latter is usually more focal and more painful. The precise pathophysiology of MTSS is controversial, but it is most likely periosteal inflammation (periostitis) near the origin of the posterior tibialis or the medial soleus.[123] The soleus muscle syndrome has been identified as a cause of posteriomedial shin splints through cadaver electromyography (EMG) and open biopsy analysis by Michael and Holder.[120]

Examination reveals a well-localized 3- to 6-cm area of tenderness over the posteromedial edge of the distal one third of the tibia.[82] Active resisted plantar flexion and inversion of the foot reproduce the pain.

STRESS FRACTURE OF THE TIBIA

Stress fractures of the lower limbs account for 95 percent of all stress fractures in athletes.[131] About one half occur in the tibia or fibula. Stress fractures result from fatigue failure within the bone, although the surrounding muscle may actually fatigue first.[175] Increased or different activity results in an altered relationship of bone growth and repair (Wolff's law). The resulting stress fracture may run the spectrum from a microfracture with simple cortical hypertrophy to rupture of bony cortices with a fracture line.[107]

The factors that seem to be most clearly associated with the development of stress fractures are repetitiveness of activity and muscle forces acting across the bone. The muscle forces, or torque, across the bone may stress that bone if an imbalance between antagonistic muscles exists.[32]

Symptoms of stress fracture are usually gradual in onset over a 2- to 3-week period.[107] The patient complains of pain which initially occurs during activity and is relieved by rest. In the next stage the pain continues for hours, perhaps through the night, or it might become worse during the night, which is highly suggestive of bone pain.[147] Swelling may occur particularly after activity.

On clinical examination, localized tenderness with or without swelling is almost always present over the fracture. Common sites are the medial aspect of the tibia and 2 to 3 inches above the tip of the fibular malleolus above the joint line.[87] A positive percussion sign (transmission of pain to the fracture site area on percussion of the bone at a distance) and the tuning fork test may help to add weight to the presumptive diagnosis of stress fracture. The use of ultrasound over a stress fracture often causes rather acute pain 1 to 2 hours after the patient leaves a therapy session. This is felt to be secondary to increased hyperemia of the bone containing the stress fracture.[87]

A stress fracture may not be visible on ordinary x-ray films for 2 to 8 weeks after symptoms commence. Therefore, a technetium-99 diphosphonate bone scan is the gold standard in diagnosing stress fracture.[175] An increased uptake or "hot spot" on a positive bone scan can be seen within the first few days of the symptoms presenting and false-positive scans are infrequent.[26,60,107,136]

TENDINITIS

Another common lower leg overuse injury about the ankle is tendinitis. Achilles tendinitis is the most common form of tendinitis seen in athletes.[44,79,91] Because the Achilles tendon does not have a synovial sheath, this condition cannot be considered to be tenosynovitis. Inflammation, resulting from stress, often occurs in the loose connective tissue about the tendon known as the *paratenon*. Classification is based on whether this tissue, or the tendon itself, is involved.[146] Seen more often in men than women, Achilles tendinitis, with or without peritendinitis (involving the paratenon; see below) is often associated with repetitive or high-impact sports such as running, basketball, or volleyball.[20]

When overuse is a contributing factor, there will a characteristic history of gradual onset of pain that may be accentuated by excessive pronation or supination.[163] Clement and colleagues[20] found that 56 percent of 109 runners with Achilles tendinitis displayed excessive pronation. Training errors, poor flexibility, and weakness of the Achilles tendon have also been implicated as predisposing factors in Achilles tendinitis.[65] The pain may also be associated with underlying hyperostosis of the posterior surface of the calcaneus (Haglund's deformity or "pump bump") or inflammation of the infratendinous or supratendinous bursa.[91,163] Bursitis alone may be present and should be included in the differential diagnosis for posterior heel and ankle pain. One should also consider in the differential diagnosis os trigonum problems.[163]

As with other overuse injuries, pain is aggravated by activity and relieved by rest. The patient presents with pain several centimeters proximal to the insertion of the tendon into the calcaneus, the area of poorest blood supply.[91] A presentation of considerable swelling and lumpiness of the Achilles tendon usually points to intratendinous damage. When there are superficial, isolated areas of pain and crepitation that are palpable, one may be sure of the diagnosis of paratenonitis. Dorsiflexion causes pain, and crepitus may be felt along the tendon at the most tender area.[91] If there is pain on excessive plantar flexion, especially with palpation at the lateral posterior aspect of the ankle, an os trigonum injury should be suspected.[163]

Treatment follows similar lines as that of other overuse injuries. Chronic paratenon lesions that do not respond to appropriate physical therapy, rest, and other adjunct measures will require a surgical tenolysis. Tendinosis or intratendinous lesions may require surgical exploration. Necrotic tissue is cureted and the tendon is repaired.[163] A rupture of the Achilles tendon requires immediate referral for consideration of a surgical repair.

TREATMENT OF OVERUSE INJURIES

The principles of treatment and rehabilitation of overuse injuries are the same as those related to the management of abnormal foot pronation and supination (see pages 427 and 433). Rest of the affected muscle-tendon-bone unit is the mainstay of treatment in phase I. Both shin splints and medial tibial stress syndrome can progress to stress fracture, and stress fractures may progress to complete cortical break.[107] The duration of rest varies from 1 to 2 days for mild shin splints to several months for severe stress fractures.

In phase I, analogous to treatment of traumatic injuries (see management of ankle sprains, page 421), ice, compression, and elevation are used to reduce swelling and inflammation. Nonsteroidal anti-inflammatory drugs (NSAIDs) are believed to be beneficial in most types of overuse injury.[175] However, in stress fractures, they may have no advantage over simple analgesics.[111]

To prevent recurrence of overuse injury, it is imperative to review and correct faulty training methods and to evaluate for biomechanical factors. Of all running injuries, 60 percent result from training errors such as running on hard, uneven, or inclined surfaces, improper footwear, and overzealous training.[23]

☐ Ankle Sprain

The most common lesion affecting the ankle is a sprain or tear of one of the ligaments.[17,52] The anterior talofibular ligament is the most commonly sprained ligament at the ankle and is probably the most commonly sprained ligament in the body. The next most frequently sprained ligaments at the ankle are the calcaneocuboid and the calcaneofibular ligaments. Portions of the deltoid ligament may also be sprained, but more often a forceful eversion stress will result in an avulsion of the tibial malleolus rather than damage to the ligament.[18,31]

I. History

A. *Onset of pain.* The patient will invariably recall the traumatic incident. The common mechanism of injury for an anterior talofibular ligament sprain is a plantar flexion-inversion stress.[57,66,88,127] Typical examples include an athlete who lands from a jump on the lateral border of the plantarly flexed foot, a person wearing high-heeled shoes or walking on uneven ground who catches a toe on the lateral side of the foot, or a person stepping off a curb or step who rolls over the lateral side of the plantarly flexed foot. If the forefoot is forced into supination or adduction, the calcaneocuboid ligament may be injured instead or as well. The calcaneofibular ligament restricts inversion with the foot in a more neutral or dorsiflexed position. It may be injured along with the talofibular ligament if, at the time of injury, the person retains good contact of the foot with the ground but continues to force the foot into inversion.

When torn, the deltoid ligament is usually injured because the foot is forced into external rotation and eversion with respect to the leg. As mentioned, it is more common for a portion of the tibial malleolus to avulse with the deltoid ligament attachment. The anterior tibiofibular ligament may be torn with a similar mechanism, since as the talus rotates within the mortise, it tends to wedge the tibia and fibula apart, producing a diastasis.[1,18,31] In order for the talus to rotate enough to produce a diastasis and to tear the anterior tibiofibular ligament, the deltoid ligament is torn or the tibial malleolus is avulsed as well.[1]

B. *Site of pain.* This usually corresponds well with the approximate location of the injury. Some pain may be referred distally into the foot or proximally into the lower leg.

C. *Nature of pain or disability.* Similar to ligamentous lesions at the knee, the degree of pain and disability immediately following an injury to an ankle ligament does not necessarily correlate well with the severity of the lesion.[78] A person sustaining a mild or moderate sprain may describe more pain and be more reluctant to continue a particular activity than one who completely ruptures a ligament. This is because in the event of a rupture there is complete loss of continuity of the structure and there are no longer intact fibers to be stressed and from which pain can be elicited.

Repeated episodes of anterior talofibular ligament sprains are not uncommon. Usually the initial injury results in somewhat more pain and disability than with subsequent occurrences. These patients typically describe intermittent giving way of the ankle, often during athletic activities, followed by pain and effusion lasting for a few days.[49,158]

II. Physical Examination

A. *Observation.* A patient seen soon after injury may hobble into the office walking with a characteristic "foot flat," short-stance gait; both heel-strike and push-off are lacking. If the pain is more severe, the patient may walk in with the aid of crutches or hop on one leg.

B. *Inspection.* Localized swelling over the region of the involved ligament is usually present within several hours after the injury. Since the anterior talofibular ligament and the deep fibers of the deltoid ligament blend with the ankle mortise joint capsule, there may be some associated articular effusion. Within a day or so following most ankle sprains, there is diffuse ecchymosis in the region of the injury, which may extravasate distally into the foot.

C. *Selective tissue tension tests*

1. Active movements. In the acute stage there is likely to be considerable difficulty in heel and toe walking and other weight-bearing activities involving ankle movements. The examiner must exercise judgment in requesting the patient to perform

these movements to avoid undue discomfort or stress to the part.

2. Passive movements and joint-play movements (key objective tests)

   a. If the ankle mortise joint capsule has been stressed with subsequent articular effusion, the ankle movements will be limited in a capsular pattern; plantar flexion will be slightly more restricted than dorsiflexion.

   b. In the case of a mild or moderate ligamentous sprain, pain will be reproduced with movements that stress the involved ligament. There will usually be an associated muscle-spasm end feel. Painless hypermobility will be noted in the presence of chronic ruptures. Acute ruptures will also demonstrate hypermobility; however, a false-negative finding may be elicited because of protective muscle spasm. Take care to ensure maximal relaxation of the part when performing passive movements. The common ligaments injured and the passive movements used to test their integrity are as follows:

      i. Anterior talofibular ligament. Combined plantar flexion-inversion-adduction of the hindfoot and anterior glide of the talus on the tibia[17,97]

      ii. Calcaneocuboid ligament. Combined supination–adduction of the forefoot

      iii. Calcaneofibular ligament. Inversion of the hindfoot in a neutral position of plantar flexion–dorsiflexion

      iv. Deltoid ligament. Anterior fibers: combined plantar flexion-eversion-abduction of the hindfoot; middle fibers: eversion of the hindfoot

3. Resisted movements. These should be strong and painless. Occasionally the peroneal tendons are strained in conjunction with an inversion ligamentous strain. In this case, isometric resistance to eversion will be strong and painful.

D. *Neuromuscular tests.* Results are noncontributory.

E. *Palpation*

   1. Tenderness will usually correspond to the site of the lesion in acute injuries. There is also likely to be diffuse tenderness in the presence of marked swelling from extravasation of blood into the tissues.

   2. Joint effusion from synovitis or extra-articular swelling will be palpable in the acute stages.

   3. Skin temperature will be elevated over the region of the involved structure in the acute stages.

III. **Management**

   A. *Acute sprains—immediate measures.* At this early stage, there is little that needs to be done to, or for, the patient that he cannot do on his own. Ice, elevation, compression, mobility exercises, and strengthening can be carried out easily at home by most patients. This does, however, require very clear and precise instruction by the therapist. Do not spare words or time in making sure that the patient understands exactly what he should or should not be doing with the ankle. A follow-up visit after 2 or 3 days should be scheduled so that a reassessment can be made and the program appropriately progressed. At this point, there should be evidence of reduction of the acute inflammatory process; pain, temperature, and swelling should be decreased. It is important, in the subacute stage, to carefully reassess joint-play movements, since at this stage the therapist can determine more easily whether there has been some loss of integrity of the involved structure. Often in the acute stage, muscle spasm precludes accurate determination of the extent of the damage.

      1. Reduction of stress to the ligament to allow healing without undue lengthening.

         a. Ankle strapping will help reduce movement in response to mild (non-weight-bearing) stresses. Swelling should have stabilized by the time of application. A felt or foam rubber horseshoe pad should be used to fill in the submalleolar depressions to obtain even compressions of the area with tape or an elastic bandage.

         b. Crutches should be used to relieve stress and pain during ambulation. A three-point, partial-weight-bearing crutch gait should be instituted; non-weight-bearing is usually not necessary and should be avoided because of its nonfunctional nature.

      2. Reduction of the acute inflammatory process to reduce pain and to prevent undue tissue damage from localized pressure and proteolytic cellular responses

         a. Ice—To decrease blood flow and reduce capillary hydrostatic pressure, thus reducing extravasation of blood fluids

         b. Compression—Increased external pressure to the area will minimize capillary leakage by effectively reducing the volume of the tissue spaces. This can be maintained by appropriate application of an elastic bandage with a horseshoe pad below the malleolus.

c. Elevation—Reduces capillary hydrostatic pressure to minimize fluid loss and assists the venous and lymphatic return.

3. Prevention of residual disability

a. Motion of the part is instituted in planes that do not stress the healing ligament to minimize residual loss of movement and optimize circulation in the area.

b. *Isometric exercises* to the muscles in the area should be started as early as pain allows, to maintain strength of the muscles of the lower leg and foot.

B. *Acute sprains—subsequent measures*

1. Mild sprains. In the case of a simple sprain, in which there is no hypermobility on the associated passive movement tests, gradual return to normal activities should be allowed as the inflammatory process resolves. Weight-bearing should be increased and the crutches discarded, usually by the fifth day. Range of motion, strength, and joint play should be restored to normal. Most patients may regain normal motion and strength with careful instruction in home exercises. Before discharging the patient from care, the therapist must ascertain that normal joint play has returned. If it has not, the restricted movements must be restored with passive joint mobilization techniques. Friction massage, initiated in the subacute stage, may promote healing of the ligament in a mobile state and prevent adherence to adjacent tissue.

As the swelling subsides in the subacute stage, strapping should be substituted for the elastic bandage to provide support and to increase proprioceptive feedback as the patient resumes functional use of the part. Use of strapping should continue until good strength, range of motion, and joint play are restored. The athlete should continue to strap the ankle when participating in vigorous activities. Studies suggest that ankle strapping does play a role in preventing ankle sprains.[37] This is probably not due to actual mechanical support provided by the tape, since movement of the bones within the skin (to which the tape is

adhered) is probably still sufficient to allow a ligament to be stretched. However, the added proprioceptive input provided by the tape may enhance protective reflexes (such as contraction of the peroneal muscles) in response to forces tending to stress the ankle ligaments.

Return to vigorous activity must be gradual. Clinical evidence of healing does not indicate that a ligament has regained normal strength. In fact, maturation of the new collagen laid down during healing may take weeks or months. The necessary stimulus for maturation and restoration of normal ligamentous strength is stress to the ligament produced by functional use of the part. This induces formation of the appropriate collagen cross-links and realignment of the new collagen fibers along the normal lines of stress. However, the ligament must not be overstressed before normal strength is regained, since it is susceptible at this point to reinjury. The athlete should begin by jogging, then running, in straight lines. When normal muscle strength and joint motion have been regained, figure-of-eight patterns that impose some lateral stress to the part may be initiated. Gradually, the patient should progress to sharp cutting drills. When these can be performed well and without pain, competitive activity may be resumed.

Also during the later stages of rehabilitation, balance drills should be instituted to facilitate the restoration of normal protective reflexes.[48,50] Progression may proceed from challenging one-legged standing to one-legged standing on a rocking board to one-legged standing on a board supported on half a sphere (free to tilt in all planes).

2. Moderate sprains and complete ruptures. The related literature reflects some controversy regarding the management of ruptured ligaments at the ankle. Most authorities would agree that injuries involving extensive damage, with rupture of both the anterior talofibular and calcaneofibular ligaments, should be repaired surgically to restore passive stability to the ankle.[4,158] Good results are favored by early surgery, since the torn ends will tend to atrophy and retract with time, making apposition and suturing technically difficult or impossible. Similar considerations apply to rupture of the deltoid ligament.

There is more divergence of opinion, however, with respect to management of isolated ruptures, in which some hypermobility of anterior glide of the talus in the mortise is demonstrable. While some clinicians favor early surgical intervention to suture the torn ends and minimize residual and structural instability, others favor early return to function following some period of restricted activity and immobilization. There is evidence from studies by Freeman that suturing of the ligament does result in a more stable joint, but in the end, the functional status of those undergoing surgery is really no better than those treated "conservatively."[48–50] In fact, those patients treated conservatively returned to normal function significantly sooner than those undergoing surgery, if they were not immobilized in plaster for a prolonged period of time. Of those treated conservatively, there was very little difference in residual mechanical stability between those who were immobilized in plaster for 6 weeks and those treated with strapping and early mobilization. The incidence of residual pain and swelling several months following injury was highest in the surgical group. The only way to guarantee increased mechanical stability following rupture of the anterior talofibular ligament is to reappose the torn ends with sutures. However, it seems that the residual disability resulting from prolonged immobilization in those treated with surgery outweighs whatever advantage this form of management may have in producing a more stable ankle. Further studies by Freeman suggest that there is no correlation between mechanical instability, as determined by stress roentgenograms, and the incidence of residual disability resulting from chronic swelling and pain.[48–50]

Conservative (nonsurgical) management of patients in whom there is evidence of actual loss of integrity of the ligament should follow the same approach as management for less serious injuries; the primary difference should be that those ankles with more extensive damage will need to be protected, by crutches and strapping, somewhat longer, perhaps as long as 2 weeks. However, early motion and strengthening at pain-free intensities should be initiated as resolution of the acute inflammatory process ensues. Also, in cases of more extensive damage, return to normal and, especially, to vigorous activity levels should be more gradual. Again, it must be emphasized that although new collagen is laid down within the first 1 or 2 weeks following injury, it takes months for this new tissue to mature to normal strength. During the period of maturation, the ligament is weaker than normal and, therefore, more susceptible to reinjury.

C. *Chronic recurrent ankle sprains.* Following initial injury, especially to the anterior talofibular ligament, a certain number of patients will suffer recurrent giving way of the ankle, with subsequent pain and swelling. There are three possible causes of this to be considered and to which assessment should be directed.

1. Healing of the ligament with adherence to adjacent tissues. In this situation, the healed ligament does not allow the joint play necessary for normal functioning of the part.[31] With repetitive stress to the tightened structure, pain and swelling will result from a fatigue phenomenon. With forceful stress to the structure, the adhesion will rupture, producing another sprain. This type of problem will present as a painful, minor restriction on passive plantar flexion–inversion of the hindfoot and on anterior glide of the talus. Treatment consists of deep, transverse friction massage to the ligament and specific joint mobilization in the directions of restriction. Normal mobility to the ligament is thus gradually restored.

2. Loss of protective reflex muscle stabilization. Normally, stress to some aspect of a joint capsule or to a joint ligament results in firing of specific receptors in the structure, through a reflex arc, to produce contraction of the muscles overlying the stressed structure. This "booster" mechanism of dynamic joint stabilization protects joint ligaments from injury under conditions of heavy loading. Thus, when the anterior talofibular ligament is stressed, the peroneus tertius is called to reduce the load to the ligament. Damage to a ligament with subsequent immobilization may result in interference of this protective mechanism. Freeman has shown good results in management of such cases by instituting a program of balance training, as described.[48] The therapist must also make sure that good muscle strength has been restored.

3. Gross mechanical instability of the joint. If both the anterior talofibular ligament and the calcaneofibular ligament are ruptured, or if there has been extensive capsular disruption with an anterior talofibular ligament rupture, the resultant mechanical instability of the joint may not allow certain functional weight-bearing activities to be performed without giving way. Such patients will present with obvious hypermobility on joint-play movement tests. If an aggressive muscle strengthening and balance training program is not sufficient to compensate for the instability, surgical reconstruction may be contemplated.

Thus, the therapist should direct assessment of the chronically unstable ankle toward determining if there is some residual increase or decrease in joint play, if good muscle strength has been regained, and whether the person is able to balance well during one-legged standing under various unstable conditions (*e.g.,* on a tilt board). It is important to realize that giving way of the joint is not necessarily the result of structural instability and that some degree of structural instability can be compensated for by muscle strengthening or balance training.

☐ Foot Injuries

CUBOID DYSFUNCTION

Cuboid dysfunction also may be referred to as subluxation or the cuboid syndrome. The etiology is uncertain but may be related to dysfunction of the calcaneocuboid joint or abnormal pull of the peroneus longus tendon through a groove on the inferior aspect of the cuboid dorsally, causing the medial aspect of the cuboid to sublux plantarward.[126] Newell and Woodie[126] found that 80 percent of cuboid subluxations occur in pronated feet. The patient presents with fairly acute, severe pain and sometimes swelling localized to the calcaneocuboid joint. He or she is unable to run, cut (do a lateral shift), jump, or dance without a marked increase in pain. There is localized tenderness to palpation in the plantar aspect of the foot and laterally over the joint.[144] Roentgenograms are negative.

Treatment by manipulation of the cuboid using one of a number of methods, usually brings immediate relief (see Fig. 14-52).[29,54,91,100,108,109,118] Release of the long dorsiflexors and peroneals with deep massage should be performed prior to manipulation.[108] This should be followed by placement of a felt pad beneath the cuboid on the plantar surface of the foot, along with a low-dye strapping procedure (see Appendix B) to give the arch added support for 1 or 2 weeks.[91] In longstanding cases resistant to other forms of therapy, surgical exploration of the cuboid and peroneus longus tendon has been undertaken.[144]

METATARSALGIA

Metatarsalgia is a syndrome describing pain over the metatarsal heads or in the metatarsophalangeal (MTP) joints. The cause may be vascular, avascular, neurogenic, or mechanical.[63] Scranton[149] classifies metatarsalgia according to whether a weight-bearing imbalance exists between the metatarsals (primary) or whether the forefoot pain is due to other factors, such as stress fractures or rheumatoid arthritis (secondary). Both primary and secondary metatarsalgia have characteristic associated keratosis. A third classification of forefoot pain is that without reactive keratosis such as neuromas, gout, and plantar fasciitis.[77]

Many theories have been developed to attempt to explain the etiology of primary or generalized metatarsalgia. One theory suggests that a short first metatarsal will cause the second to have to bear a disproportionate amount of weight as the body propels over the foot and thereby result in ultimate dysfunction and the development of a painful callus.[77] A subluxing second or third MTP joint, or failure of the transverse metatarsal arch to be maintained by the transverse metatarsal ligaments and the transverse head of the adductor hallucis muscle, may also be the cause of metatarsalgia.

According to Kraeger,[91] generalized metatarsalgia often occurs secondary to a tight Achilles tendon, which restricts dorsiflexion. The loss of full dorsiflexion loads the weight onto the forefoot, thus applying pressure to the MTP joints. Any tendency toward excessive pronation will lead to hypermobile functioning of the first and fifth ray and thereby cause a relative depression of the transverse metatarsal arch. Metatarsalgia is common in middle-aged persons with a pronation tendency.[14] Other extrinsic factors such as excessive weight gain and wearing high-heeled shoes have been suggested as causes for, or aggravating circumstances of the condition.

The patient presents with an antalgic gait including diminished push-off. In some cases the patient may prevent any weight shift across the metatarsal heads by weight-bearing exclusively on the lateral border of the foot.[77] Pain may occur at night, but the patient typically reports pain only on weight-bearing. Pressure to the involved metatarsal head will elicit pain.

Treatment of the different causes of metatarsalgia are similar, although it must be individualized to the exact problem. Treatment should include heel cord stretching and exercises to strengthen the intrinsic toe flexors. Mobilization is suggested in order to reduce secondary fibrositis from spasm and joint dysfunction.[29] Metatarsophalangeal decompression (traction) and manipulation of the metatarsals (metatarsal whip) are recommended treatments. Metatarsal pads just proximal to the second or third metatarsal head or an external metatarsal pad should be considered. Another option is to place a pad beneath the first metatarsal to allow it to bear more weight.[91] Orthotics, shoe modification, or a reduction in heel height should be considered.

PLANTAR FASCIITIS

Plantar fasciitis is an inflammation of the plantar fascia and the perifascial structures. Chronic stress to the origin of this fascia on the calcaneus may cause calcium to deposit, forming a spur (plantar calcaneal spurs). Since plantar calcaneal spurs and plantar fasciitis involve basically the same symptoms, develop via similar mechanisms, and are treated in the same manner, these common pathologies are often considered together. Frequently, heel spurs are not symptomatic. This has been shown to be the case with the discovery of calcaneal spurs on x-ray studies of nonsymptomatic heels. Roentgenograms may show big spurs without plantar fasciitis or no spurs in the patient with severe plantar fasciitis.

As is typical of any overuse injury, plantar fasciitis can be caused by an acute injury (strain) from excessive loading of the foot. More often the mechanical cause is due to chronic irritation from an excessive amount of pronation or prolonged duration of pronation, resulting in microtears at the plantar fascial origin. A cavus or high-arched foot with its limited subtalar excursion is also at risk, because a tight plantar fascia is usually present in this type of foot. A cavus foot may develop plantar fasciitis owing to its intrinsic inability to dissipate force (lack of pronation) from heel-strike to mid stance, resulting in increased load in the plantar fascia.[92]

Plantar fasciitis is a common cause of heel pain. It occurs in patients of either sex, usually over the age of 40 except in active sportsmen when the patient, usually male, may be in his twenties.[25] It is commonly found in people whose occupation involves prolonged standing or walking. Pain is made worse by activity, such as climbing stairs, walking, or running, may be present at night, and is often present when first getting out of the bed in the morning. It tends to be relieved by rest.

Clinical examination usually localizes tenderness at the plantar fascial attachment of the calcaneus, just distal to this attachment, in the medial arch area and in the abductor hallucis muscle. Pain to palpation of the posterior inferior origin of the abductor hallucis muscle has been theorized to be the result of overuse of the abductor hallucis muscle in its role to aid in producing forefoot supination to decrease loading on the plantar fascia.[19] Chronic partial ruptures have abundant scar tissue, which is palpable near the attachment of the plantar fascia to the plantar tubercle of the calcaneus or more distally, toward the mid aspect of the foot.[163] Pain may be reproduced by stretching the fascia on full dorsiflexion of the ankle or big toe. Range of motion of the great toe is usually limited in dorsiflexion, and ankle dorsiflexion is often less then 90°.[91] Swelling is rare, but occasionally a small granuloma is palpated on the medial fascial origin. With increased pain, the patient changes his gait pattern, keeping the foot in a rather supinated or inverted posture from foot-strike through to toe-off to minimize pain.[19]

This injury must be differentiated from tarsal tunnel syndrome, and entrapment of the first lateral branch of the posterior tibialis nerve. Those with tarsal tunnel syndrome may also complain of burning pain with paresthesias of the heel. They usually have a positive Tinel sign and do not have pain to direct palpation of the plantar fascia. The etiology in younger patients, particularly when the symptoms are bilateral and are unresponsive to the usual conservative treatments, may be seropositive and seronegative collagen vascular disorders (*e.g.*, rheumatoid arthritis, spondylitis, and Reiter's syndrome).[13,58,59,151,170] The older patient with heel pain may have gout or osteomalacia.[132]

When dealing with a mechanical etiology, the treatment plan is directed at both a short-term goal (to control inflammation at the insertion of the fascia into the calcaneus in conjunction with relieving undue stress in the plantar fascia itself) and a long-term goal (correction of mechanical factors). Ice-massage, rest, and anti-inflammatory medications should be used initially. Ultrasound and phonophoresis with 10 percent hydrocortisone has been used with limited success to control acute inflammation and pain.[77] A period of non-weight-bearing is recommended until symptoms subside. Excessive pronation should be limited by use of low-dye strapping and, if this is beneficial, an in-shoe orthotic device or over-the-counter arch support is recommended. The use of tension night splints has shown promising results. There are also an assortment of heel pads made specifically for heel pain.[169] In the case of a high-arched foot, a carefully selected in-shoe orthotic device with good shock absorbency can be used. Soft tissue techniques that stretch the plantar fascia, friction massage at the origin of the fascia to break down the scar tissue, and joint mobilizations which mobilize the hind foot, subtalar joint, and inferior navicular are usually the most effective treatment methods.[25,29] Local corticosteroid injections should be used judiciously. Surgery is rarely indicated.

☐ Problems Related to Abnormal Foot Pronation

Pronation of the hindfoot with respect to the forefoot is a relatively common disorder that may or may not give rise to foot pain. Also, because of the biomechanical interplay between the foot and other weight-bearing segments, the pronated foot may result in dysfunction in other regions of the lower extremity, especially the knee. Similarly, a pronated foot may be caused by some local structural abnormality of the tarsal skeleton, or it may be caused by some structural deviation in segments either distal or proximal to the hindfoot.

Pain resulting from a pronated foot is usually of the fatigue type from prolonged increased stress on the affected tissues. In some patients, pain may arise with normal activity levels, while others may get along well until they engage in some activity, such as jogging, that involves increased stress levels or frequency. Pain of local origin usually has its source in one of the plantar structures responsible for maintaining the twisted configuration of the foot—the plantar aponeurosis, the short plantar ligament, or the long plantar ligament. Pain may also arise from fatigue of the intrinsic muscles of the foot, in which activity may be increased in an attempt to prevent undue stress to the plantar aponeurosis and ligaments. In association with increased tensile stress to the plantar aponeurosis, a calcaneal periostitis may develop from the added pull to the proximal attachment of the aponeurosis on the plantar surface of the calcaneus. Excessive pulling on the periosteum in this region occasionally results in a bony outcropping (heel spur) that in itself may give rise to localized pressure to the overlying soft tissue. Periostitis and eventually osteophyte formation should be considered as resulting from increased stress to the plantar aponeurosis. It must be emphasized that spurring can develop in the absence of pain and that a cartilaginous spur may be present that is not visible in roentgenograms. Another source of local pain occurring in association with a pronated foot is pressure from the shoes against the talar head or the navicular, which becomes prominent medially when the foot untwists.

A pronated foot may be the cause of, or be associated with, pain in the forefoot, leg, or the knee. Pain from pressure over the first one or two metatarsal heads may result from increased weight-bearing over the medial side of the forefoot. This occurs if the talar head and navicular drop downward and inward, shifting the center of gravity line medially. Since hal-lux valgus often accompanies pronation of the hindfoot, either as a cause or as a result, pressure over a prominent first metatarsophalangeal joint may also occur with increased pronation of the foot. Leg pain may result from increased tension on the anterior or posterior tibialis muscles, which are dynamic supporters of the arch of the foot. Chronic periostitis at the proximal attachment of these muscles may result and is often referred to as shin splints. The knee tends to assume a valgus position when the foot pronates. Such an angulation tends to increase the lateral pull on the patella during loaded quadriceps contraction. This may predispose to pain from patellar tracking dysfunction at the knee (see Chapter 13, The Knee).

As mentioned, pronation of the hindfoot may occur from some local structural disorder or from structural deviations elsewhere. The common local causes are capsuloligamentous laxity and bony abnormalities. Capsuloligamentous laxity may be a hereditary condition, or it may accompany some specific disease state, such as rheumatoid arthritis. The common *bony* anomaly resulting in flatfoot is tarsal coalition, in which the talus and calcaneus are fixed to one another in a pronated orientation through fibrous or osseous union.[43] The common malalignment problems affecting other regions that predispose to abnormal pronation of the hindfoot are femoral antetorsion, internal tibial torsion, a shortened Achilles tendon, and adduction of the first metatarsal. The excessive internal rotation imposed by antetorsion of the femur or internal tibial torsion during stance phase is at least partially absorbed by the subtalar joint, bringing the hindfoot into pronation. In the presence of a short Achilles tendon, the midtarsal joint attempts to compensate for lack of dorsiflexion at the ankle; in order to do so, the foot must untwist to unlock the midtarsal joints. Because of the oblique orientation of the first cuneiform–first metatarsal joint, adduction of the first metatarsal also involves a component of dorsiflexion. This effectively supinates the forefoot, which necessitates a compensatory pronation of the hindfoot in order to get the foot flat on the ground. Each of these possible causes must be considered when examining the patient with a pronated foot.

Finally, it must be remembered that abnormal foot pronation during gait is not always associated with a "pronated foot" seen on structural examination with the patient standing. The typical example is a person with increased tibial varum. The foot usually appears normal or even supinated during relaxed standing. However, when running or walking there is a tendency to heel-strike on the lateral border of the heel, causing the foot to undergo increased hindfoot pronation in order to press the heel flat on the ground. Even though the foot appears not to be pronated, it will be subject to increased pronatory stresses. Similar considerations apply to the patient with either femoral retrotorsion or external tibial torsion, in which the cause of pronation is not localized to the foot itself.

I. History

A. *Onset of pain* is usually insidious, since the pathological tissue conditions associated with biomechanical abnormalities such as a pronated foot are typically fatigue phenomena. Often the onset can be related to some increased activity level, such as long-distance running. Another common predisposing factor is a period of disuse, such as immobilization of the foot in a cast. In such cases, the muscles of the foot weaken, and when activity is resumed, they no longer contribute their share to stabilizing the arch of the foot. This results in increased stress to the capsuloligamentous structures. Occasionally, a change in footwear, for example, to a lower heel height, can be related to the onset. Lowering the heel height increases the tension on the Achilles tendon, which may in turn result in increased pronation of the hindfoot in the same way as described for a shortened Achilles tendon. A lowered heel also results in reduced dorsiflexion of the toes during the stance, decreasing the windlass effect on the plantar aponeurosis and reducing the twisted configuration of the foot.

B. *Site of pain.* Foot pain associated with abnormal pronation usually is felt over the plantar aspect of the foot. Pain from calcaneal periostitis and heel spurs is fairly well localized over the bottom of the heel, often more medially; it may be referred anteriorly into the sole of the foot. Pain from fatigue stress to the plantar ligament or aponeurosis is felt over the sole of the foot, usually more medially. Keep in mind that the bony and soft-tissue pathological processes referred to previously may occur concurrently.

Forefoot pain arising secondary to a pronated foot condition may be felt in the region of the medial metatarsal heads, if due to abnormal weight distribution, or it may be felt over the medial aspect of the first metatarsophalangeal joint, if caused by pressure over the joint resulting from a hallux valgus deformity.

Knee pain related to a pronated foot is typically from patellofemoral joint problems (see section on patellar tracking dysfunction in Chapter 13, The Knee).

C. *Nature of pain.* Pain is from increased stress to the plantar ligaments, fascia, capsules, or calcaneal periosteum under conditions in which increased untwisting of the foot takes place. This typically occurs in a person whose foot undergoes an abnormal degree of pronation during stance phase or whose foot remains in a pronated position during prolonged standing. The muscles controlling the twist, or arch, of the foot will protect these structures for a certain period of time. However, once the muscles fatigue, more stress is transmitted to the ligaments and fascia, which are responsible for the passive stabilization of the arched configuration of the foot. In some cases, this may occur with normal activity levels, such as after walking some distance or after standing for a long period of time. In others, increased activity, such as long-distance running, provides the added stress to bring on the pain. Once a low-grade inflammation develops, the pain is brought on with less stress and may be relatively continuous during weight-bearing. In these more severe cases, pain is typically pronounced on initial weight-bearing, subsiding somewhat as the muscles contract more to protect the painful structures, then increasing again as the muscles fatigue.

II. Physical Examination

A. *Observation and inspection of structural alignment.* Evidence of excessive pronation of the foot and associated biomechanical abnormalities may be noted when the patient walks or stands.

1. Flattening of the medial arch. The region of the navicular and the talar head may appear to be prominent medially and depressed inferiorly.
2. Abduction of the forefoot on the rearfoot.
3. Adduction of the first metatarsal, perhaps with a valgus deformity of the first metatarsophalangeal joint.
4. Valgus position of the heel maintained throughout stance phase.
5. Internal tibial torsion. The feet may be pointed inward while the patellae face straight forward.
6. Femoral antetorsion. The patellae face inward when the feet are in normal alignment. This must be differentiated from external tibial torsion, which may present similarly. External tibial torsion is evidenced by an increased external rotation of the intermalleolar line with respect to the frontal plane (in excess of about 25°).

Femoral antetorsion is suggested when the total range of motion at the hip is about normal, but the range of internal rotation is increased and the range of external rotation is proportionally decreased.

7. Genu valgum. This often exists in conjunction with femoral anteversion.

B. *Inspection (supine)*
1. Structural alignment
   a. Forefoot varus. This is the most common intrinsic deformity resulting from abnormal pronation.[33,142,167] Root and co-workers describe it as a frontal plane deformity that is compensated at the subtalar joint by eversion or a valgus position of the calcaneus in weight-bearing.[141]
   b. Dorsiflexed and hypermobile first ray producing hallux valgus, which is subluxation of the metatarsophalangeal joint of the big toe in the sagittal and transverse plane.[141]
2. Skin. Inspected for signs of pressure over the navicular tubercle, first metatarsophalangeal joint, and medial metatarsal head. As a result of first ray insufficiency, callus or keratosis may develop under the head of the second metatarsal.[75]
3. Soft tissue. Inspected for muscle atrophy that may relate to loss of dynamic support of the arch of the foot.
4. Inspection of shoes (see page 411).

C. *Selective tissue tension tests*
1. Active movements. If inspection of structural alignment reveals a pronated position of the hindfoot, the patient is observed while raising up on the toes and externally rotating the leg over the fixed foot. Both of these movements should decrease the pronation and cause an increased twisting and arching of the foot. If not, a rigid flatfoot, caused by some fixed structural abnormality such as tarsal coalition, probably exists.
2. Passive movements. Unless a rigid flatfoot exists (a relatively rare condition), a pronated foot is usually a hypermobile foot. Hypermobility, especially of the midtarsal joints, may be noted.
   a. If a tight heel cord or restricted ankle mortise joint capsule is a contributing cause, dorsiflexion of the hindfoot will be restricted. One must lock the foot by supinating the calcaneus and pronating the forefoot when testing ankle dorsiflexion to avoid misinterpreting move-

ment of the forefoot as being movement at the ankle. There should be about 10° to 20° of dorsiflexion. If dorsiflexion and plantar flexion are both restricted, the joint capsule is probably at fault. If dorsiflexion is restricted with the knee straight, but not with the knee bent, the gastrocnemius is tight. If dorsiflexion is restricted regardless of the position of the knee, the soleus is probably at fault.
   b. If antetorsion of the hip is a contributing factor, hip range of motion will be relatively normal but skewed toward internal rotation with restriction of external rotation.
   c. Joint play. Movements of the tarsal joints are likely to be hypermobile. Excessive arthrokinematic movements typically occur between four bones: calcaneus, talus, navicular, and cuboid.[33]
   d. Pain from low-grade inflammation of the plantar fascia or ligaments, or from calcaneal periostitis, may be reproduced by passively everting the heel, supinating the foot, and dorsiflexing the toes.
3. Resisted movements. Results are usually noncontributory.

D. *Neuromuscular tests.* Determine whether weakness, either neurogenic or atrophic, of any of the muscles controlling movement and stability of the foot exists.

E. *Palpation.* Localized tender areas may exist that relate to areas of low-grade inflammation occurring in response to abnormal tissue stresses. As usual, the finding of localized tenderness to palpation, in itself, must not be taken to be diagnostic of any specific disorder because of the common phenomenon of referred tenderness associated with lesions of deep somatic tissue.

Typical areas of tenderness associated with abnormal foot pronation might include the calcaneal attachment of the plantar fascia and long plantar ligament, especially at the medial tubercle; the plantar fascia, usually over the medial aspect of the sole of the foot; the navicular tubercle; the spring ligament, between the sustentaculum tali and the navicular tubercle; the medial one or two metatarsal heads; and the medial aspect of the first metatarsophalangeal joint.

Areas of skin or subcutaneous tissue hypertrophy may be distinguished on palpation as localized indurated regions. Such calluses, associated with pronation, might be found over the medial one or two metatarsal heads or over the medial aspect of the first metatarsalphalangeal joint.

III. Management

Symptoms arising in association with abnormal foot pronation are the result of increased stress to some pain-sensitive tissue. Proper management, then, must involve selective reduction of abnormal stresses. The approach used must be in accordance with findings on evaluation, including information relating to the patient's activity level. In developing a program of management, it must be kept in mind that the tissue pathology resulting in the painful condition may be due to normal stresses occurring at too great a frequency, to abnormally high stresses occurring at normal frequencies, or to some combination thereof. Either situation may result in tissue fatigue in which the rate of tissue breakdown exceeds the rate at which the tissue is able to repair itself. However, the approach to management will differ, depending on which condition prevails. In general, management of conditions associated with pronation of the foot involves measures to reduce either the frequency or the magnitude of stresses, or both.

In the case of the pronated foot, forces are typically increased by structural malalignments that cause changes in the direction in which forces occur and changes in the degree of movement of skeletal parts during functional activities. The most common postural malalignment causing abnormal foot pronation is probably increased femoral antetorsion, which is usually accompanied by increased genu valgum (knock knees). As mentioned earlier, the other common structural deviations predisposing to increased pronation of the foot are adduction of the first metatarsal and increased internal tibial torsion. Each of these conditions results in untwisting of the tarsal skeleton during ambulation, such that a greater tensile stress is imposed on the plantar ligaments, fascia, and joint capsules. Under such conditions, the foot loses the typical passive stability normally produced by becoming twisted during stance phase. To compensate, the intrinsic muscles of the foot must contract more to prepare the foot for push-off. Pain may arise from increased stress to the plantar capsuloligamentous structures, from fatigue of the abnormally contracting muscles, or both.

Persons with long-standing pronation from a congenital structural malalignment or from a malalignment acquired early in life are likely to have a permanent hypermobility of the joints of the foot. The ligaments and joint capsules will have been elongated from the chronic increased stresses applied to them throughout development. By the time they are adults, these persons are not likely to have pain arising from the already lengthened ligaments and fascia during normal activity levels. They are, however, likely to have feet that tire easily from increased activity of the intrinsics and other muscles supporting the arch during gait. They are also more predisposed to developing problems elsewhere, such as metatarsalgia, hallux valgus, and patellofemoral joint dysfunction.

Persons with more subtle structural deviations resulting in an increased tendency toward pronation are likely to have problems only with increased activity levels, such as long-distance running, that increase the magnitude and frequency of pronatory stresses. The mobility of the joints of the foot in these persons allowed by the capsules and ligaments is likely to be fairly normal. It is especially important in patients experiencing pain suggestive of increased pronation, but who have relatively normal structural alignment, to consider nonstructural causes. The most common of these would include a tight heel cord and inappropriate footwear. It is these patients, having subtle structural deviations or nonstructural causes of increased pronation, who are likely to experience pain and develop pathological lesions associated with increased strain to specific tissues. The most common tissues involved are the supporting plantar structures of the foot, including the periosteum of the plantar aspect of the calcaneus, and the Achilles tendon.

A. *Techniques*

1. Instruction in appropriate activity levels. As in any common musculoskeletal disorder, appropriate instruction in exactly what the patient should and should not do, and to what degree, is an essential component of the treatment program too often overlooked. With respect to problems related to increased foot pronation, this is especially important in the person experiencing problems primarily with increased activity levels. Treatment of the long-distance runner experiencing pain from plantar fasciitis, Achilles tendinitis, or other pronation-related disorders simply involves advising the patient to not run so much. But this is not adequate management of the problem since, as with any disorder, the therapist must be concerned

primarily with restoring optimal function. From the patient's standpoint, optimal function may be running long distances!

The role of the therapist should be first to decide whether the patient's functional expectations are realistic. The patient with considerably increased femoral antetorsion, knock knees, and hypermobile flat feet probably should not be engaging in activities, such as long-distance running, that involve high-frequency, weight-bearing stresses. However, this condition should not prevent the person from engaging in other vigorous conditioning exercise, such as swimming and bicycling.

If there are no gross structural malalignments predisposing to pronation-type problems, the therapist must then determine what can be done to reduce the stresses to the involved tissues, to allow them to heal, and to prevent further pathological processes and pain. As far as healing is concerned, the most important step to be taken is to reduce the stresses that caused the problem. The most reliable method of doing this is to reduce the activity level. The long-distance runner experiencing chronic, persistent pain must be advised to markedly reduce or stop running for a period of 1 to 2 weeks to allow the tissue to heal. Complete immobilization, however, is seldom, if ever, indicated for fatigue disorders such as these. During this period of relative rest the therapist should determine what can be done to reduce stresses when the activity is resumed. Other procedures to help restore the involved tissue to its normal state may also be instituted.

2. Muscle strengthening and conditioning. Strengthening and endurance exercises for the intrinsic muscles of the foot as well as for the extrinsic muscles, such as the anterior and posterior tibialis that help maintain a twisted configuration of the foot, are important in the management of virtually all foot problems resulting from abnormal pronation. Improving the function of these muscles will allow the person with the hypermobile flat foot to stand or walk for longer periods of time before muscle fatigue sets in. It will also help relieve strain on the plantar fascia and ligaments in patients suffering from strain of these structures by increasing the dynamic support of the arch, thus allowing the muscles to take a greater portion of the load.

3. Proprioceptive balance training
   a. Because the pedal intrinsic muscles appear to function similarly to the plantar fascia in stabilization of the foot, pedal intrinsic strengthening exercises should be prescribed.[108] Foot doming is a particularly beneficial exercise.[36,108]
   b. Dorsiflexors are often found to be weak. Before strengthening, according to Janda, it is better to stretch the tight structures (gastrocnemius–soleus). Both eccentric and concentric exercises should be included.[81]
   c. The tibialis posterior, flexor digitorum longus, and flexor hallucis longus exert a supinatory force at the subtalar joint. These muscles help control pronation by working eccentrically. Marshall prefers to strengthen the supinators eccentrically by using the BAPS balance board (Camp International, Inc., Jackson, Michigan).[108]

4. Strapping. Strong muscles are of little use unless they contract with sufficient force and at the appropriate time to perform the desired function. Abnormal foot pronation can be controlled to varying degrees by contraction of the muscles that cause an increased twisted configuration of the foot. Most important among these are the anterior and posterior tibialis muscles and the peroneus longus. Theoretically, muscle function can be enhanced by providing additional input along the afferent limb of the reflex arcs that normally invoke muscle contraction during functional activities. One method of doing so is to strap the part in a manner that will cause increased tension to the straps, and therefore the skin, when movement occurs in the undesired direction. The added afferent input from the tension and pressure produced by the straps serves to enhance activity of muscles that normally check the undesired movement. This is apparently the means by which ankle strapping helps to "stabilize" the ankle against inversion sprains.[52] Although empirically there seems to be evidence for the efficacy of such procedures, electromyographical studies have yet to be performed to substantiate the proposed mechanism.

For an excellent review of the literature,

the reader is referred to the work of Metcalf and Denegar.[119] The low-dye strapping technique that was designed by Ralph Dye in an attempt to provide functional mechanical support of the joints of the feet is recommended by Newell and Nutler[125] and by others[3,6,39,71,90,150,177,179] to restrict abnormal foot pronation. The ability of low-dye strapping to modify forces on the medial arch during weight-bearing has been clearly demonstrated by Scranton and colleagues.[150] It is meant to bring the ground up to the foot to eliminate the need for the foot to pronate to reach it.[177] It may be used to protect the passive stabilizing structures of the foot, such as the plantar fascia and associated structures, during the rehabilitation phase following injuries and to assess the effect of more permanent stabilizing measures, such as a biomechanical functional foot orthosis or shoe modification.

A number of variations have been developed (modified low-dye, cross-X technique, Herzog taping) and used in rehabilitating posterior tibial syndrome, posterior tibial tendinitis, peripatellar compression pain, Achilles tendon problems, and jumper's knee.[80,125,176,177] James and associates demonstrated effectiveness of this type of treatment for overuse injuries when combined with rehabilitation exercises.[80] These procedures pull the medial aspect of the foot toward the supportive surface and secure it in this position with tape (see Appendix B for one variation of this technique).

5. Ultrasound and friction massage. These may be important treatment measures in cases of plantar fasciitis, Achilles tendinitis, and tibialis periostitis. The resultant increased blood flow may assist in the healing process. Transverse frictions will promote the development of a mobile structure and help prevent adhesions as healing ensues.

6. Achilles tendon stretching. This is especially important when evaluation reveals a tight heel cord as a possible contributing cause of the patient's problem, and in cases of Achilles tendinitis.

McCluskey and co-workers were one of the first groups to report the beneficial effects of calf muscle stretching to reduce ankle injuries.[112] Ten degrees of dorsiflexion with the knee extended and the subtalar in neutral is the amount considered necessary for normal walking.[142] James suggests at least 15° talocrural joint dorsiflexion is required for running.[79] One must take care to ensure that the stretching force is applied to the hindfoot, since using the forefoot as a lever to stretch the heel cord will result in dorsiflexion of the transverse tarsal joint in addition to dorsiflexion at the ankle mortise (talocrural) joint. This may result in hypermobility of the transverse tarsal joint, which may add further to a tendency toward pronation of the foot.

When stretching of the calf muscle is attempted, it is important that the subtalar joint is maintained in a neutral position. To ensure that this position is maintained, the patient should either stretch out in a biomechanical orthotic device or place a lift under the medial aspect of the bare foot during stretch.

In the more acute stages of Achilles tendinitis, the therapist must not be overly vigorous in restoring mobility to the heel cord, since the condition could be aggravated. However, since most cases of Achilles tendinitis are fatigue disorders, an acute stage never exists. Some gentle stretching may be initiated carefully from the outset; the slow, short-termed stress produced by such stretching procedures in no way approximates the high-frequency, high strain-rate stresses that produce this type of disorder. In fact, early stretching, performed judiciously, will help prevent the fibers from healing in a shortened state.

Increasing the load and speed of contraction with an emphasis on eccentric training has been found to be particularly helpful.[157] This can be carried out with the rear foot over the edge of a step to allow for greater range of dorsiflexion–plantar flexion and eccentric control. To ensure normal weight-bearing alignment, a tennis ball can be placed between the patient's medial malleoli; the patient is instructed not to lose contact with the ball throughout the exercise, since this may invoke excessive supination or pronation.[121]

7. Shoe inserts and modifications. When abnormal foot pronation is due to some structural malalignment, whether marked or subtle, only surgery can remedy the true cause of the disorder. However, non-surgical management is effective in the

majority of cases. In order to optimize function, while at the same time preventing stresses sufficient to cause painful pathologic processes, the excessive untwisting of the foot must be reduced. This can be accomplished by altering the orientation of the segments of the foot as they contact the ground during stance phase or by producing direct support to the arched configuration of the foot, or by both.

If the joint capsules and ligaments of the foot are not elongated, as in the hypermobile flat foot accompanying gross malalignment, the twist in the foot during stance phase can be increased by increasing the pronatory orientation of the forefoot or by increasing the supinatory orientation of the hindfoot. This can be done by providing a lateral wedge for the forefoot or a medial wedge for the heel. A trial, temporary insert can be made by cutting such a wedge from a piece of felt, $1/8$- to $3/16$-inch thick, to fit inside the shoe. However, if it is to be used on a permanent basis, the wedge should be incorporated into the sole or heel of the shoe by one experienced in shoe modifications or should be incorporated into an orthosis.

If the tarsal joints of the foot are lax, then the twisted configuration cannot be restored by indirect means such as wedging, since these rely on taking up the slack in the joint capsules to effect a twisting of the tarsal skeleton. In the case of a hypermobile, pronated foot, some direct support must be provided to prevent the head of the talus and navicular from dropping downward and medially in a pronatory fashion. For the severely pronated foot, an arch support may be used in conjunction with wedging of the sole or heel. Such wedging may be built into the orthosis or into the shoe. Regardless of the type of shoe modification or insert used, in order for the support to be effective the calcaneus must be stabilized by a firm shoe counter or a calcaneal cup built into an orthosis. If the calcaneus is not held firmly, it will tend to compensate for attempts to increase the twist of the foot by rolling farther over into a valgus position (pronation). Thus, many orthoses now in use have a heel cup incorporated into the orthosis itself, obviating the need for an extra-firm shoe counter. Such an orthosis can be used, for example, in athletic shoes, which often do not have very stiff counters.

When chondromalacia of the knee occurs as a result of abnormal pronation of the foot, the use of arch supports or shoe modification may be a necessary component of the treatment program.

The progression of a hallux valgus deformity may also be retarded by use of orthoses or shoe modifications, if the adduction of the first metatarsal is a result of abnormal foot pronation.

In cases of metatarsalgia, if reducing the degree of pronation with appropriate orthotic devices or shoe modification does not adequately relieve the pressure over the metatarsal heads, a metatarsal insert may be used. This simply reduces the stress to the metatarsal heads by increasing the weight-bearing surface area behind the heads. Metatarsal pads are available with an adhesive backing, or a metatarsal support may be incorporated into an arch-supporting orthosis. To place the pad properly in the shoe, tape it to the patient's foot in place just behind the metatarsal heads with the widest dimension of the pad forward. Outline the bottom of the pad with lipstick or some substance that will leave a mark on the insole of the shoe when the patient steps down. The patient then puts on the shoes and walks about to make sure they are reasonably comfortable, realizing, of course, that they will at first feel somewhat peculiar. The shoes are then removed and the pad adhered to the insole of the shoe in the appropriate place as indicated by the marks left on the insole by the lipstick.

Several devices designed to modify forces in the foot have been reported to be helpful for the patient with plantar heel pain. Heel pads have been used to reduce the shock of weight-bearing and to shift vertical forces forward and away from the heel.[6,8,53] Some authors have suggested the use of a heel cup to prevent calcaneal eversion and thus reduce tension on the plantar fascia.[15,41,85,150]

☐ Problems Related to Abnormal Foot Supination

Abnormal supination of the entire foot occurs when the subtalar joint functions in a supinated position.[142]

There are three basic classifications for abnormal supination: pes equinovarus, pes cavus, and pes cavovarus.[101,166] A pes equinovarus foot demonstrates a fixed plantar flexed forefoot and an inverted forefoot; the rear foot in weight-bearing is in neutral.[33] A pes cavovarus foot demonstrates a fixed medial column or first ray. In the weight-bearing position the calcaneus is in varus or inverted.[33]

Root and co-workers define forefoot valgus as eversion of the forefoot on the rear foot with the subtalar joint in neutral.[142] The compensation for a forefoot valgus is inversion of the calcaneus in the weight-bearing position.[138,166] Forefoot valgus and a fixed plantar-flexed first ray are the most common intrinsic deformities resulting in abnormal supination of the subtalar joint.

Functionally abnormal supination is a failure of the foot to pronate, resulting in a foot unable to compensate normally. There is prolonged supination during the stance phase and a delayed pronation during the gait cycle. Stress fractures, metatarsalgia, plantar fasciitis, and Achilles tendinitis are common in this type of foot.

In general, treatment consists of stretching, mobilization, exercises, and orthoses.[167] The flexible cavus foot responds well to conventional biomechanical orthotic foot control. The rigid cavus foot requires a special orthosis or a shoe with shock-absorbing materials such as Spenco Insoles (SpencoMedical Corp., Waco, Texas) and Sorbothane Inserts (Spectrum Sports, Twinsburg, Ohio) to lessen the strain on the lower extremities.

☐ Orthoses

Ultimately, the patient exhibiting a true intrinsic biomechanical fault should be fitted with a custom-made functional biomechanical orthosis to correctly balance the foot during weight-bearing activities. Orthotic devices are most often used to correct excessive pronation and thus may be effective in the management of related shin splints, chondromalacia, and, occasionally, trochanteric bursitis.

The orthosis made from a positive mold of the foot in its neutral position is designed for restoration of normal alignment of the subtalar and midtarsal joint by controlling excessive pronation and supination and reducing the abnormal forces through the kinetic chain. In basic terms, it is directed toward preventing the foot from compensating and allowing normal motion to take place in its proper sequence.

When the orthosis is in place, the foot should function near its neutral position. It is important to evaluate muscle imbalances extrinsic and intrinsic to the foot, in addition to evaluating forefoot and rear foot deformities. Softer flexible types of orthoses can be fabricated in the clinic as a temporary measure or may be made of flexible materials molded to a positive cast of the patient's foot. Most clinics are not equipped for fabrication of the rigid orthosis, which must be custom-made (from a positive model). There are a number of podiatry laboratories specializing in these types of orthotic appliances. Many excellent texts and articles have described orthotic fabrication and shoe modifications.*

Shoe styles and features are constantly being changed by the manufacturers so that it is almost impossible for the clinician to keep abreast of current shoe models, particularly the athletic shoe. The basic functions of any quality shoes are to enhance shock absorption and foot control and to provide good traction and protection. Lasting or curve of the sole of the shoe should generally conform to the patient's own foot shape. In general, most patients will do well with a relatively straight last. Many manufacturers now provide information on shoes that have been selectively designed to limit common foot abnormalities such as overpronation or oversupination of the subtalar joint.

Since foot problems and related disorders are common and because alteration of footwear is often an important component of management of these problems, it is important that the therapist develop a close working relationship with an orthotist, podiatrist, or other professional possessing these skills.

■ JOINT MOBILIZATION TECHNIQUES

Note: For the sake of simplicity, the operator will be referred to as the male, and the patient as the female. All of the techniques described apply to the patient's left extremity except where indicated. (P = patient; O = operator; M = movement)

☐ Tibiofibular Joint

1. *The Proximal Tibiofibular Joint*—Anteroposterior glide (Fig. 14-40)
    P—Supine, with knee flexed about 90°, the foot flat on the plinth
    O—Stabilizes the knee with the right hand contacting the medial aspect of the knee area. He grasps the head and neck of the proximal fibula with the left hand, the thumb contacting anteriorly, the index and long finger pads con-

---

*See references 10, 12, 15, 22, 24, 27, 28, 37, 38, 47, 68, 80, 92, 94, 108, 114, 139, 160, and 176.

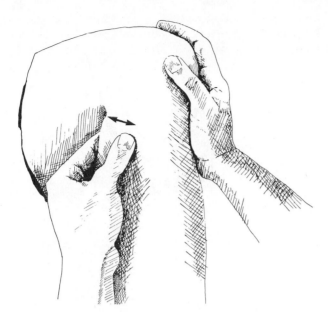

FIG. 14-40. *The proximal tibiofibular joint: anteroposterior glide.*

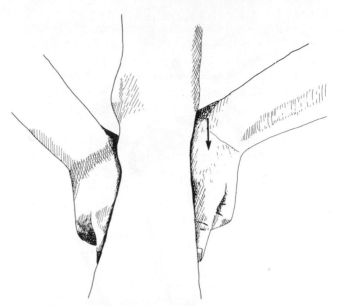

FIG. 14-41. *The distal tibiofibular joint: anteroposterior glide.*

tacting posteriorly. He takes care to avoid direct pressure to the common peroneal nerve.

M—The left hand may move the proximal fibula posteriorly or anteriorly. This should be performed through a movement of flexion and extension at the shoulder, rather than through finger or wrist movements.

This technique is used to increase joint play at the tibiofemoral joint. The fibular head must move forward on knee flexion and backward on knee extension. Dysfunction at the proximal tibiofibular joint commonly causes symptoms distally in the leg or ankle rather then proximally.

2. *The Distal Tibiofibular Joint*—Anteroposterior glide (Fig. 14-41)

P—Supine

O—Cradles the ankle in his right hand, fixing it to the plinth, so that the fingers wrap around the heel posteriorly. The medial malleolus rests over the palmar aspect of his dorsiflexed wrist. The left hand contacts the lateral malleolus anteriorly with the heel of the hand.

M—While the operator's right hand prevents downward movement of the medial malleolus, the left hand glides the lateral malleolus posteriorly in relation to the medial malleolus. The handholds may be reversed to move the medial malleolus posteriorly on the lateral malleolus.

These techniques are used to increase joint play at the distal tibiofibular joint. This joint must spread slightly during ankle dorsiflexion, since the talus is wider anteriorly than posteriorly. Although spreading cannot be performed passively by the operator, increasing anteroposterior movement is likely to increase other joint-play movements such as spreading.

☐ The Ankle

1. *The Talocrural Joint*—Distraction (Fig. 14-42)

P—Supine, with the knee flexed about 90°, the hip flexed and somewhat abducted

O—Half-sits on the edge of the plinth, with his back to the patient. He wraps the patient's leg around his right side to support the knee on his iliac crest, tucking the lower leg between his elbow and side (Fig. 14-42*A*). The operator grasps the ankle with both hands so that the thumbs wrap around medially and the fingers laterally. The web of his right hand contacts the neck of the talus dorsally; the web of his left hand contacts the calcaneus posteriorly. The forearms are kept in line with the direction of force (Fig. 14-42*B*).

M—A distraction is imparted with both hands. The ankle may be slightly everted to help lock the subtalar joint.

This technique is used to increase joint play at the ankle mortise joint. Distraction must occur here during plantar flexion, and is necessary for full movement toward the close-packed position, which is dorsiflexion.

2. *The Talocrural Joint*—Posterior glide of tibia on talus (or anterior glide of talus on tibia) (Fig. 14-43)

P—Supine

O—Stabilizes the talus and foot by grasping

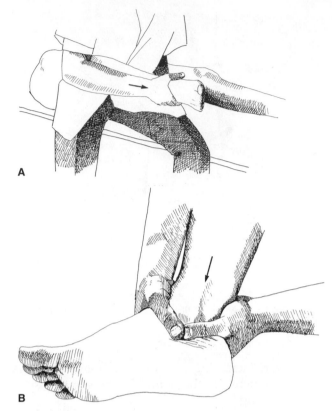

FIG. 14-42. The talocrural joint. Distraction: (**A**) position of the operator; (**B**) view of the operator's grip at the ankle.

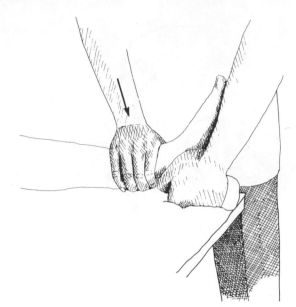

FIG. 14-43. The talocrural joint (left foot): posterior glide of tibia on talus.

around medially to the posterior aspect of the calcaneus with the left hand. He contacts the distal tibia by placing his right hand over the anterior distal aspect of the tibia, just proximal to the malleoli.

M—The tibia is glided posteriorly on the talus with the right hand.

Note: An anterior glide of the talus on the tibia may be performed by stabilizing the tibia with the right hand and moving the talus anteriorly. When this technique is used, it is important to keep the subtalar joint slightly everted to lock the calcaneus on the talus. The talus is glided anteriorly on the tibia via the calcaneus at the ankle mortise. This is a slightly more difficult technique, because the operator must work against gravity.

Both of these techniques are used to increase joint-play movements necessary for plantar flexion at the ankle mortise joint.

3. *The Talocrural Joint*—Posterior glide of the talus on the tibia (Fig. 14-44)
   P—Supine, with the calcaneus hanging over the end of the plinth
   O—Stabilizes the distal tibia against the plinth by grasping it with the left hand, wrapping the fingers around posteriorly. The left forearm rests over the dorsum of the patient's lower leg to prevent it from rising up from the plinth

during the movement. He contacts the neck of the talus dorsally with the web of the right hand, bringing the thumb around laterally and the index finger medially. The remaining three fingers of the right hand wrap around the sole of the foot for support and control of the degree of plantar flexion.

M—The right hand moves the talus posteriorly on the tibia.

This technique is used to increase a joint-play movement necessary for ankle dorsiflexion.

4. *The Subtalar Joint*—Distraction (not illustrated)
   This is performed in the same manner as distraction at the talocrural (refer to technique 1), except that the dorsal handhold moves distally to contact

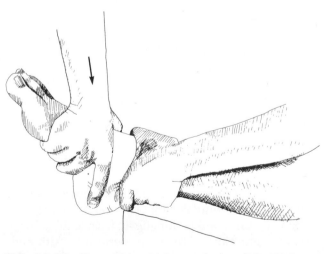

FIG. 14-44. The talocrural joint: posterior glide of talus on tibia.

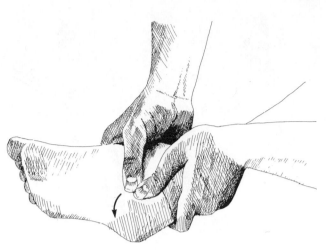

FIG. 14-45. The subtalar joint: valgus tilt (eversion).

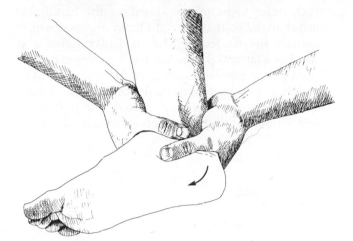

FIG. 14-47. Dorsal rock of the calcaneus on the talus.

the navicular. In this way the calcaneus is distracted from the talus by the navicular and cuboid.

5. *The Subtalar Joint*—Valgus tilt (eversion) (Fig. 14-45)

   P—Supine, with the knee flexed about 90°, the hip flexed and somewhat abducted

   O—Assumes the same position as for distraction (see Fig. 14-42*A*) and grasps the ankle so that the thumb pads contact the medial aspect of the calcaneus and the remaining finger pads contact laterally, just proximal to the calcaneus and level with the sinus tarsi.

   M—A valgus tilt of the calcaneus is produced by ulnar deviation of the wrists, transmitting the force through the thumb pads. The finger pads act as a fulcrum about which the movement occurs. This technique is used to increase eversion at the subtalar joint.

6. *The Subtalar Joint*—Varus tilt (inversion) (Fig. 14-46)

   This is carried out in the same manner as valgus tilt (refer to technique 5). The operator's thumb pads move just proximal to the calcaneus; the finger pads move distally to contact the calcaneus laterally. The finger pads move the calcaneus into inversion about a fulcrum created by the thumb pads.

This technique is used to increase inversion at the subtalar joint.

7. *The Subtalar Joint*—Dorsal rock of the calcaneus on the talus (Fig. 14-47)

   P—Supine, with the knee flexed about 90°, the hip flexed and somewhat abducted

   O—Assumes the same position as for distraction (see Fig. 14-42*A*) and stabilizes the talus dorsally with the web of the right hand, wrapping the thumb around medially and the fingers laterally. He contacts the upper border of the calcaneus posteriorly with the web of his left hand in a similar fashion.

   M—While the right hand stabilizes the talus, the left hand rocks the calcaneus forward and dorsally.

Note: According to Mennell, a small amount of movement must occur at the subtalar joint at the extremes of plantar flexion and dorsiflexion. This technique, and the one that follows, have been developed to restore that movement.[118]

8. *The Subtalar Joint*—Plantar rock of the calcaneus on the talus (Fig. 14-48)

   This is carried out in the same manner as dorsal

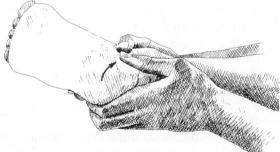

FIG. 14-46. The subtalar joint: varus tilt (inversion).

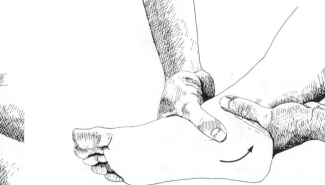

FIG. 14-48. Plantar rock of the calcaneus on the talus.

rock (refer to technique 7), except the handholds are changed so that the right hand moves down to contact the navicular. The navicular tubercle is used as a landmark. The left hand moves just proximal to the posterior aspect of the calcaneus. The right hand rocks the calcaneus backward and plantarly via the navicular and cuboid. The web of the left hand acts as a fulcrum about which movement occurs.

☐ The Foot

1. *The Transverse Tarsal Joints (talonavicular and calcaneocuboid joints)*—Dorsal-plantar glide (Fig. 14-49)

   P—Supine, with the knee bent about 60°, the heel resting on the plinth

   O—The left hand fixes the calcaneus and talus to the plinth by grasping dorsally at the level of the talar neck, the thumb wrapping around laterally and the rest of the fingers medially. The right hand grasps the navicular, using the navicular tubercle as a landmark. The web and the thumb contact dorsally, and the hand and fingers wrap around the foot medially and plantarly.

   M—As the left hand stabilizes and prevents movement at the ankle, the right hand may move the navicular dorsally or plantarly on the talus. The cuboid is moved in a similar manner, with one hand fixating the calcaneus and talus while the other hand moves the cuboid dorsally or plantarly on the calcaneus. These techniques are used to increase joint play at the forefoot.

2. **The Naviculocuneiform Joint**—Dorsal-plantar glide (Fig. 14-50)

   This is performed in the same manner as dorsal-plantar glide at the talonavicular joint (refer to technique 1), with the handholds moved distally.

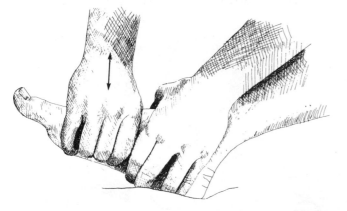

FIG. 14-49. The transverse tarsal joints: dorsal-plantar glide.

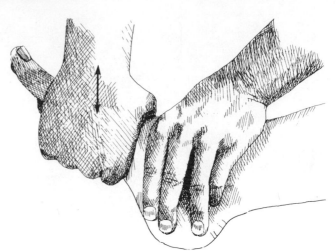

FIG. 14-50. The naviculocuneiform joint: dorsal-plantar glide.

The left hand stabilizes the navicular while the right hand moves the cuneiforms.

This technique is used to increase joint play at the forefoot.

3. **The Cuneiform–Metatarsal Joints**—Dorsal-plantar glide (not illustrated)

   This technique is also performed in the same manner as for the talonavicular joint, with the handholds shifted distally. The right hand grasps the cuneiforms and provides stabilization while the left hand moves the metatarsal joints.

   This technique, like techniques 1 and 2 for the talonavicular and naviculocuneiform joints, is used to increase joint play of the forefoot.

4. **The Cuneiform–Metatarsal and Cuboid–Metatarsal Joints**—Rotation (pronation and supination) (Fig. 14-51)

   P—Supine, with the knee bent about 70°, the heel resting on the plinth

   O—Stabilizes the cuneiforms and cuboid with the left hand, the thumb wrapping around the foot dorsally, the fingers plantarly. For *pronation*, the operator's right hand grasps the proximal metatarsal shafts from the lateral aspect, with the thumb contacting dorsally and the fingers plantarly. His forearm is supinated (see Fig. 14-51*A*). For *supination*, the operator's right hand grasps the proximal metatarsal shafts from the medial aspect, with the thumb contacting dorsally and the fingers plantarly. His forearm is pronated (see Fig. 14-51*B*).

   M—The right hand rotates the metatarsals, as a unit, into pronation or supination.

   These techniques are used to restore pronation and supination to the forefoot.

5. **The Cuboid–Metatarsal Joint:** Dorsal-plantar glide

   This technique is performed as dorsal-plantar

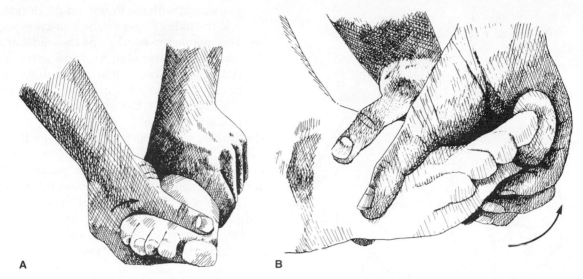

FIG. 14-51. Rotation of cuneiform-metatarsal and cubometatarsal joints: (**A**) pronation and (**B**) supination.

glide at the calcaneocuboid joint (refer to technique 1), with the handholds moved distally. The proximal hand stabilizes the cuboid while the distal hand moves the fourth and fifth metatarsal joints. This technique, like technique 3 for the cuneiform–metatarsal joints, is used to increase joint play of the forefoot.

6. **Manipulation of the Cuboid and Navicular Joints:** Whip and squeeze techniques (Fig. 14-52)

   P—Prone with the thigh and leg beyond the table and flexed at 30° or, even better, standing and leaning forward on the table (see Fig. 14-52*A*).

   O—Standing at the foot end of the table, the operator holds the foot, pressing on the cuboid with both thumbs superimposed (see Fig. 14-52*B*).

   M—The arms of the operator are extended so that the pressure on the cuboid causes knee flexion and dorsiflexion. Finally when the foot is relaxed, a thrusting movement similar to cracking a whip, is performed (tractional plantar-flexion thrust) laterally at a 45° angle.

This action usually allows the subluxed cuboid (inferolateral) to move dorsally back into place. Treatment is identical to that of the cuboid for manipulation of an inferior navicular when present in the pronated foot. Dorsal glide of the cuboid or navicular joints can be effectively applied in the prone position. Marshall and Hamilton[109] believe that a technique called the "cuboid squeeze" is far more effective than the cuboid whip. To perform the squeeze technique, the clinician gradually stretches the foot and ankle into maximum plantar flexion. When the operator feels the soft tissues relax, the cuboid is reduced with a final squeeze of the thumbs.

These techniques should be followed with a low-

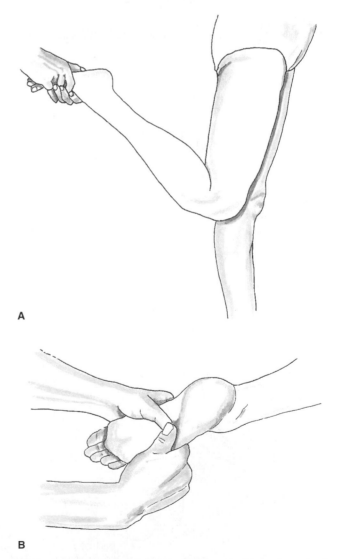

FIG. 14-52. Manipulation of the cuboid and navicular joints: (**A**) whip and (**B**) squeeze techniques.

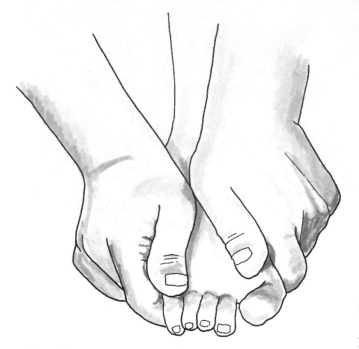

FIG. 14-53. Intermetatarsal and tarsometatarsal joints: dorsal-plantar glide.

dye strapping procedure to give added arch support for 1 to 2 weeks.[175] The management of chronic subluxations should include instruction in self-mobilization techniques.

7. **Intermetatarsal and Tarsometatarsal Joints:** Dorsal-medial glide (Fig. 14-53)

P—Supine, with the foot in a neutral position

O—Facing the dorsal surface of the foot, the stabilizing hand grips the midshaft of one metatarsal with the thumb on the dorsal aspect and the index finger on the plantar aspect.

M—The mobilizing hand grips the midshaft of the adjacent metatarsal in the same manner as the stabilizing hand. While the stabilizing hand holds one metatarsal in position, the mobilizing hand glides the metatarsal in a dorsal or plantar direction.

Movements can be performed between the second and first, the third and the fourth, and the fourth and fifth metatarsal bones. The purpose is to restore or increase joint play in the intermetatarsal articulations in the presence of hypomobility and to decrease pain in the forefoot. Movements will simultaneously take place in the tarsometatarsal joints and between the MTP joints.

□ The Toes

Note: The use of a surgical glove, athletic underwrap used in adhesive taping, or a tongue blade taped to the toe may assist the operator in obtaining a stronger grip by reducing slippage and in directing a more precise mobilization of the toes.

1. *Metatarsophalangeal (MTP) Joints*—Distraction (Fig. 14-54)

P—Supine

O—Facing the dorsal aspect of the foot, the stabilizing hand holds the midfoot securely, while the thumb and forefinger of the mobilizing hand grasp the first phalanx at the MTP joint. The MTP joint is positioned in the resting posi-

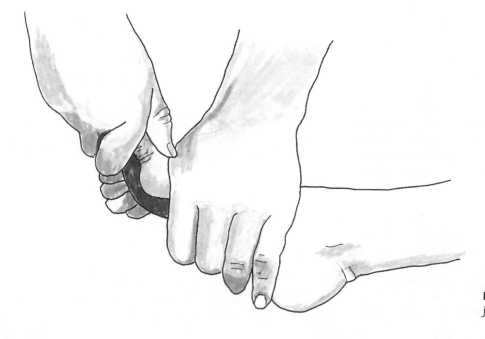

FIG. 14-54. Metatarsophalangeal joints: distraction.

tion if conservative techniques are indicated or near the restricted end range if more aggressive techniques are indicated.

M—The mobilizing hand moves the base of the proximal phalanx distally.

This is a useful technique in increasing joint play in the MTP joint and overall range of motion. A hallux valgus deformity is usually caused by improperly fitting shoes or has a genetic origin. Because of this, the treatment of choice is mechanical, such as orthotics or surgery. However, along with this, mobilization should be used in order to help increase the abduction of the first MTP joint.[29] Mobilization of the MTP joint—with oscillatory movements in dorsal-plantar glide, medial-lateral glide, abduction, adduction, rotation and compression—may provide pain relief.

1. **Metatarsophalangeal Joints:** Dorsal-plantar glide (Fig 14-55)

   P—Prone or supine with the forefoot supported on the table or with a sandbag or wedge, toes extended over the edge of the table

   O—Standing beside the patient and facing the foot, the stabilizing hand grips the head of the metatarsal between the thumb and index finger.

   M—The mobilizing hand grips the proximal phalanx (dorsal and plantar aspect) between the thumb and index fingers. The MTP joint is po-

sitioned in the resting position or approximating the restricted range if more aggressive techniques are indicated. The mobilizing hand glides the proximal phalanx in a dorsal direction (Fig. 14-55A, patient prone) or plantar direction (Fig. 14-55B, patient supine) while employing grade 1 traction.

The purpose of these techniques is to increase joint play in the MTP joints; plantar glide for restricted flexion and dorsal glide for restricted extension.

As to the remaining joints of the foot, the interphalangeal joints may be mobilized in the same manner as that described for the corresponding joints of the hand. Self-mobilization should be considered in chronic conditions.

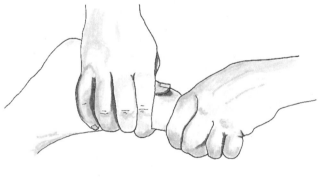

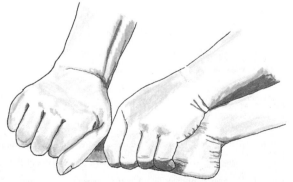

FIG. 14-55. Metatarsophalangeal joints: (**A**) dorsal and (**B**) plantar glide.

REFERENCES

1. Alldredge RH: Diastases of the distal tibiofibular joint and associated lesions. JAMA 115:2136–2140, 1940
2. American Medical Association, Subcommittee on Classification of Sports Injuries. Standard Nomenclature of Athletic Injuries, pp 122–126. Chicago, American Medical Association, 1966
3. Anderson JL, George F, Krakauer LJ, et al: Year Book of Sports Medicine. Chicago, Year Book Medical Publishers Inc, 1982
4. Anderson KJ, LeCocq JF: Operative treatment of injuries to the fibular collateral ligament of the ankle. J Bone Joint Surg 36(A):825–832, 1954
5. Andrews JR: Overuse syndromes of the lower extremity. Clin Sports Med 2:139–148, 1983
6. Appenzeller O, Atkinson R: Sports Medicine: Fitness Training, Injuries, 2nd ed, pp 413–414. Baltimore, Urban & Schwarzenberg, 1983
7. Barnett CH, Napier JR: The axis of rotation at the ankle joint in man: Its influence upon the form of the mobility of the fibula. J Anat 86:1–9, 1952
8. Bateman JE: The adult heel. In Jahss MH (ed): Disorders of the Foot, vol 1, ch 27. Philadelphia, WB Saunders, 1982
9. Bates B: Running biomechanics. Presented at American Orthopedic Foot Society Meeting, New Orleans, 1982
10. Bates BT, Osternig LR, James MS, et al: Foot orthotic devices to modify selected aspects of lower extremity mechanics. Am J Sports Med 7:338–342, 1979
11. Boeing DD: Evaluation of a clinical method of gait analysis. Phys Ther 57:795–798, 1977
12. Brody DM: Running injuries. Clinical Symp 32:2–36, 1980
13. Bywater EG: Heel lesions of rheumatoid arthritis. Ann Rheum Dis 13:42–51, 1953
14. Cailliet R: Foot and Ankle Pain, 2nd ed. Philadelphia, FA Davis, 1983
15. Campbell JW, Inman VT: Treatment of plantar fasciitis and calcaneal spurs with the UC-BL shoe insert. Clin Orthop 103:57–62, 1974
16. Carson WG: Diagnosis of extensor mechanism disorders. Clin Sports Med 4:231–246, 1985
17. Cedell CA: Supination-outward rotation injuries of the ankle. Acta Orthop Scand (Suppl) 110:1–148, 1967
18. Cedell CA: Ankle lesions. Acta Orthop Scand 46:425–445, 1976
19. Clancy WG: Tendinitis and plantar fasciitis in runners. In D'Ambrosia R, Drez D (eds): Prevention and Treatment of Running Injuries, pp 77–87. Thorofare, NJ, Slack, 1982
20. Clement DB, Taunton JE, Smart GW: Achilles tendinitis and peritendinitis: Etiology and treatment. Am J Sports Med 12:179–184, 1984
21. Close JR, Inman VT, Poor PM, et al: The function of the subtalar joint. Clin Orthop 50:159–179, 1967
22. Colson JW, Berglund G: An effective orthotic design for controlling the unstable subtalar joint. Orthotics and Prosthetics 33:39–49, 1979
23. Cook SD, Brinker MR, Poche M: Running shoes: Their relationship to running injuries. Sports Med 10:1–8, 1990
24. Cook SD, Kester MA, et al: Biomechanics of running shoe performance. Clin Sports Med 4:619–626, 1985
25. Corrigan B, Maitland GD: Practical Orthopaedic Medicine, pp 212–213. London, Butterworth, 1985
26. Daffner RH: Stress fractures: Current concepts. Skeletal Radiol 2:221–229, 1978
27. D'Ambrosia RD: Orthotic devices in running injuries. Clin Sports Med 4:611–618, 1985
28. D'Ambrosia RD, Drez D: Orthotics. In D'Ambrosia RD, Drez D (eds): Prevention and Treatment of Running Injuries. Thorofare, NJ, Slack, 1982
29. Davis DG: Manipulation of the lower extremity. In Subotnick SI (ed): Sports Medicine of the Lower Extremity, pp 397–417. New York, Churchill Livingstone, 1989
30. Day RW, Wildermuth BP: Proprioceptive training in the rehabilitation of lower extremity injuries. Adv Sports Med Fitness 1:241, 1988
31. De Souza Dias DL, Foerster TP: Traumatic lesions of the ankle joint: The supination external rotation mechanism. Clin Orthop 100:219–224, 1974
32. Devas M: Stress Fractures, pp 224–227. London, Churchill Livingstone, 1975
33. Donatelli R: Normal biomechanics of the foot and ankle. J Orthop Sports Phys Ther 7:91–95, 1985

34. Donatelli R: Abnormal biomechanics of the foot and ankle. J Orthop Phys Sports Ther 9:11–16, 1987
35. Donatelli R: Normal anatomy and biomechanics. In Donatelli R, Wolf SL (eds): The Biomechanics of the Foot and Ankle. Philadelphia, FA Davis, 1990
36. Dowd I: In honor of the foot. Contact Q (Fall):33–39, 1986
37. Doxey GE: The semi-flexible foot orthotic, fabrication and guidelines for use. J Orthop Sports Phys Ther 5:26–29, 1983
38. Drez D: Running footwear. Am J Sports Med 8:140–141, 1980
39. Duggar GE: Plantar fasciitis and heel spurs. In McGlawry ED (ed): Reconstructive Surgery of the Foot and Leg, pp 67–73. New York, Intercontinental Medical Book Co, 1974
40. Durman DC: Metatarsus primus varus and hallux valgus. Arch Surg 74:128–135, 1957
41. DuVries HL: Surgery of the Foot, 4th ed, pp 287–291. St Louis, CV Mosby Co, 1959
42. Dwight T: Variations of the Bones of the Hands and Feet: A Clinical Atlas, pp 14–23. Philadelphia, JB Lippincott, 1907
43. Dwyer FC: Causes, significance and treatment of stiffness in the subtaloid joint. Proc R Soc Med 69:97–102, 1976
44. Eggnold JF: Orthotics in the prevention of runner's overuse injuries. Phys Sports Med 9:125–128, 1981
45. Eichenblat M, Nathan H: The proximal tibiofibular joint. Int Orthop 7:31–39, 1983
46. Eltman H: The transverse tarsal joint and its control. Clin Orthop 16:41–46, 1960
47. Festa S, Schuster R: Ask the expert what the doctor says. Runner 9:61, 1986
48. Freeman M: Treatment of ruptures of the lateral ligament of the ankle. J Bone Joint Surg 47(B):661–668, 1965
49. Freeman M: Instability of the foot after injuries to the lateral ligament of the ankle. J Bone Joint Surg 47(B):669–677, 1965
50. Freeman M: The etiology and prevention of instability of the foot. J Bone Joint Surg 47(B):678–685, 1965
51. Fromherz WA: Examination. In Hunt GC (ed): Physical Therapy of the Foot and Ankle, pp 59–90. New York, Churchill Livingstone, 1988
52. Fulp MJ: Ankle joint injuries. J Am Podiatry Assoc 65:889–911, 1975
53. Furey JG: Plantar fasciitis: The painful heel syndrome. J Bone Joint Surg 57(A):672–673, 1975
54. Garbalosa JC: Physical therapy. In Donatelli R, Wolf SL (eds): The Biomechanics of the Foot and Ankle, pp 217–247. Philadelphia, FA Davis, 1990
55. Gardner E, Gray DJ, O'Rahilly R: Anatomy: A Regional Study of Human Structure, 4th ed. Philadelphia, WB Saunders, 1978
56. Garrick JG, Requa RK: Role of external support in the prevention of ankle sprains. Med Sci Sports 5:200–203, 1973
57. Gerbert J: Ligament injuries of the ankle joint. J Am Podiatr Assoc 65(9):802–815, 1975
58. Gerster JC: Plantar fasciitis and Achilles tendinitis among 150 cases of seronegative spondarthritis. Rheum Rehabil 9:218–222, 1980
59. Gerster JC, Vischer TL, Bennani A: The painful heel. Ann Rheum Dis 36:343–348, 1977
60. Geslien GE, Thrall JH, Espinosa JL: Early detection of stress fractures using 99m Tc-polyphosphate. Radiology 121:683–687, 1976
61. Gillette: Des os sesamoides chez l'homme. J Anat Physiol 8:506–538, 1872
62. Gorman D: The Body Moveable. Guelp, Ontario, Ampersand Press, 1981
63. Gould JS: Metatarsalgia. Orthop Clin North Am 20:553–562, 1989
64. Gray GW: When the Foot Hits the Ground Everything Changes. Toledo, OH, The American Physical Rehabilitation Network, 1984
65. Greenfield B: Evaluation of overuse syndromes. In Donatelli R, Wolf SL (eds): The Biomechanics of the Foot and Ankle, pp 153–177. Philadelphia, FA Davis, 1990
66. Gross AE, MacIntosh DL: Injuries to the lateral ligaments of the ankle: A clinical study. Can J Surg 16:115–117, 1973
67. Hartley A: Knee assessment. In Hartley A (ed): Practical Joint Assessment. St Louis, Mosby Year Book, 1990
68. Henderson WH, Campbell JW: UC-BL shoe inserts: Casting and fabrication. Bull Prosthet Res 10:11:215–235, 1969
69. Hicks JH: The mechanics of the foot: I. The joints. J Anat 87:345–357, 1953
70. Hicks JH: The mechanics of the foot: II. The plantar aponeurosis and the arch. J Anat 88:25–30, 1954
71. Hlavac HF: The Foot Book. Mountain View, CA, World Publications, 1977
72. Hollinshead WH: Leg and foot. In Hollinshead WH (ed): Textbook of Anatomy, 3rd ed, p 483. Hagerstown, MD, Harper & Row, 1974
73. Hoppenfeld S: Physical examination of the foot and ankle. In Hoppenfeld S (ed): Physical Examination of the Spine and Extremities. New York, Appleton-Century-Crofts, 1976
74. Hunt GC: Examination of lower extremity dysfunction. In Gould JA, Davies GJ (eds): Orthopaedic and Sports Physical Therapy. St Louis, CV Mosby, 1985
75. Hutton WC, Dhanedran M: The mechanics of normal and hallux valgus feet: A quantitative study. Clin Orthop 157:7–13, 1981
76. Inman VT: The Joints of the Ankle. Baltimore, Williams & Wilkins, 1976
77. Jablonowski GJ: Foot and ankle dysfunction. In Kaplan PE, Tanner ED (eds): Musculoskeletal Pain and Disability, pp 203–242. Norwal, CT, Appleton & Lange, 1989
78. Jackson DW: Ankle sprains in young athletes: Relation of severity and disability. Clin Orthop 101:201–219, 1974
79. James SI: Chondromalacia of the patella in the adolescent. In Kennedy JC (ed): The Injured Adolescent Knee, pp 214–228. Baltimore, Williams & Wilkins, 1979
80. James SI, Bates BT, Ostery LR: Injuries to runners. Am J Sports Med 6:40–50, 1978
81. Janda V: Muscle Function Testing. Boston, Butterworth, 1983
82. Jones DC, James SL: Overuse injuries of the lower extremity. Clin Sports Med 6:273–290, 1987
83. Jones FW: Structure and Function as Seen in the Foot, 2nd ed. London, Bailiere, Tindall & Cox, 1949
84. Kapandji IA: The Physiology of Joints: Vol 2. The Lower Limb. Edinburgh, Churchill Livingstone, 1970
85. Katoh Y, Chao EY, Morrey BF, et al: Objective technique for evaluating painful heel syndrome and its treatment. Foot Ankle 3:227–237, 1983
86. Kelikian H: Hallux valgus: Allied Deformities of the Forefoot and Metatarsalgia, pp 102–112. Philadelphia, WB Saunders, 1965
87. Key J, Jarvis G, Johnson D, et al: Leg injuries. In Subotnick SI (ed): Sports Medicine of the Lower Extremity, pp 187–296. New York, Churchill Livingstone, 1989

88. Kleiger B: Mechanisms of ankle injury. Orthop Clin North Am 5:153–176, 1974
89. Kohler A, Simmer EA: Borderlands of the Normal and Early Pathologic in Skeletal Roentgenology, 3rd ed. New York, Grune & Stratton, 1968
90. Kosmahl EM, Kosmahl HE: Painful plantar heel, plantar fasciitis, and calcaneal spur: Etiology and treatment. J Orthop Sports Phys Ther 9:17–24, 1987
91. Kraeger DR: Foot injuries. In Lillegard WA, Rucker KS (eds): Handbook of Sports Medicine: A Symptom-Oriented Approach, pp 159–171. Boston, Andover Medical Publishers, 1993
92. Kwong PK, Kay D, Voner RT, et al: Plantar fasciitis: Mechanics and pathomechanics of treatment. Clin Sports Med 7:119–126, 1988
93. Lamoreux L: Kinematic measurements in the study of human walking. Bull Pros Res 10–15:3–84, 1971
94. Langer S: Posting: Theory and practice. Langer Lab Bio Mech New Lett 1:3, 1973
95. Leonard MH: Injuries of the lateral ligaments of the ankle: A clinical and experimental study. J Bone Joint Surg 31(A):373–377, 1949
96. Level AS, Inman VT, Blosser JA: Transverse rotation of the segments of the lower extremity in locomotion. J Bone Joint Surg 30(A):859–872, 1948
97. Lindstrand A: New aspects in the diagnosis of lateral ankle sprains. Orthop Clin North Am 7:247–249, 1976
98. Lutter LD: The knee and running. Clin Sports Med 4:685–698, 1985
99. MacConnaill MA, Basmajian JV: Muscles and Movements: A Basis for Human Kinesiology, pp 74–84. Baltimore, Williams & Wilkins, 1969
100. Maigne R: Manipulations and mobilization of the limbs. In Rogoff JB (ed): Manipulation, Traction and Massage, 2nd ed, pp 121–139. Baltimore, Williams & Wilkins, 1980
101. Mann RA: Biomechanics of running. In Mack (ed): Symposium on the Foot and Leg in Running Sports, pp 1–29. St Louis, CV Mosby, 1982
102. Mann RA, Coughlin MJ: Keratotic disorders of the plantar skin. In Mann RA, Coughlin MJ: Surgery of the Foot and Ankle, 6th ed, vol 1. St Louis, CV Mosby, 1993
103. Mann RA, Hagy JL: The function of the toes in walking, jogging and running. Clin Orthop 142:24–29, 1979
104. Mann RA, Hagy JL: Running, jogging and walking: A comparative electromyographic and biomechanical study. In Bateman JE, Trott AW (eds): The Foot and Ankle. New York, Brian C Decker, 1980
105. Manner-Smith T: A study of the cuboid and os peroneum in the primate foot. J Anat Physiol 42:399–414, 1908
106. Manter JT: Movements of the subtalar and transverse tarsal joints. Anat Rec 80:397–410, 1941
107. Markey KL: Stress fractures. Clin Sports Med 6:405–425, 1987
108. Marshall P: The rehabilitation of overuse foot injuries in athletes and dancers. Clin Sports Med 7:175–191, 1988
109. Marshall P, Hamilton WG: Cuboid subluxation in ballet dancers. Am J Sports Med 20:169–175, 1992
110. Marti T: Die Skeletvarietaten des Fusses ihre Klinische und Unfallmedizinische Bedentug, pp 27–111. Berne, Hans Uber, 1947
111. McBryde A: Stress fractures in runners. In D'Ambrosia RD, Drez D (eds): Prevention and Treatment of Running Injuries. Thorofare, NJ, Slack, 1982
112. McCluskey GM, Blackburn TA, Lewis T: Treatment of ankle sprains. Am J Sports Med 4:158–161, 1976
113. McKenzie DC, Clements DB, Taunton JE: Running shoes, orthotics and injuries. Sports Med 2:334–347, 1985
114. McPoil TG, Brocato RS: The foot and ankle: Biomechanical evaluation and treatment. In Gould JA, Davies GL (eds): Orthopaedic and Sports Physical Therapy. St Louis, CV Mosby, 1985
115. McPoil TG, Schuit D, Knecht HG: A comparison of three positions used to evaluate tibial varum. J Am Podiatr Med Assoc 78:22–28, 1988
116. McRae R: Clinical Orthopedics. New York, Churchill Livingstone, 1983
117. Melillo TV: Gastrocnemius equinus: Its diagnosis and treatment. Arch Podiatr Med Foot Surg 2:159–205, 1975
118. Mennell JM: Joint Pain. Boston, Little, Brown and Co, 1964
119. Metcalf GR, Denegar CR: A critical review of ankle taping. Athletic Training 187:121, 1983
120. Michael RH, Holder LE: The soleus syndrome: A cause of medial tibial stress (shin splints). Am J Sports Med 13:87–98, 1985
121. Molnar ME: Rehabilitation of the injured ankle. Clin Sports Med 7:193–204, 1988
122. Morton DJ: The Human Foot: Its Evolution, Physiology & Functional Disorders, p 179. New York, Columbia University Press, 1935
123. Mubarak SJ, Gould RN, Lee YF, et al: The medial tibial stress syndrome. Am J Sports Med 10:201–205, 1982
124. Murray MP, Draught AP, Kory RC: Walking patterns in normal men. J Bone Joint Surg 46(A):335–360, 1964
125. Newell SG, Nutler S: Conservative treatment of plantar fascial strain. Phys Sports Med 5:68–73, 1977
126. Newell SG, Woodie A: Cuboid syndrome. Phys Sports Med 9(4):71–76, 1981
127. Nicholas JA: Ankle injuries in athletes. Orthop Clin North Am 5:153–176, 1974
128. Nicholas JA, Hershmann EB (eds): The Lower Extremity and Spine in Sports Medicine, pp 601–655. St Louis, CV Mosby, 1986
129. Norkin CC, Levangie PK: The ankle–foot complex. In Norkin CC, Levangie PK (eds): Joint Structure and Function, 2nd ed, pp 379–418. Philadelphia, FA Davis, 1992
130. O'Rahilly R: Developmental deviations in the carpus and tarsus. Clin Orthop 10:9–18, 1957
131. Orava PJ, Puranene J, Ala-Ketola L: Stress fractures caused by physical exercise. Acta Orthop Scand 49:19–27, 1970
132. Paice EW, Hoffbrand BI: Nutritional osteomalacia presenting with plantar fasciitis. J Bone Joint Surg 69(B):38–40, 1987
133. Palmer ML, Epler M: Ankle and foot region. In Palmer ML, Epler M (eds): Clinical Assessment in Physical Therapy, p 326. Philadelphia, JB Lippincott, 1990
134. Patton GW, Tursi FJ, Zelichowski JE: The dorsal fold of the first metatarsal phalangeal joint. J Am Podiatr Med Assoc 26:210, 1987
135. Peiyer E, Wright DW, Mason L: Human locomotion. Bull Pros Res 10–12:48–105, 1969
136. Prather JL, Nusynowitz ML, Snowdy HA, et al: Scintigraphic findings in stress fractures. J Bone Joint Surg 59A:869–974, 1977
137. Price GFW: Metatarsus primus varus—including various clinicoradiologic features of the female foot. Clin Orthop Relat Res 145:217–223, 1979

138. Ramig D, Shadle J, Watkins A, et al: The foot and sports medicine: Biomechanical foot faults as related to chondromalacia patellae. J Orthop Sports Phys Ther 2:48–50, 1980

139. Reed JK: Orthotic devices, shoes and modifications. In Hunt GC (ed): Physical Therapy of the Foot and Ankle. New York, Churchill Livingstone, 1988

140. Rocce D: The leg, ankle and foot. In Rocce D (ed): The Musculoskeletal System in Health and Disease. Hagerstown, MD, Harper & Row, 1980

141. Root ML, Orien WP, Weed JH: Biomechanical Examination of the Foot, vol 1. Los Angles, Clinical Biomechanics Corp, 1971

142. Root ML, Orien WP, Weed JN: Clinical Biomechanics, vol II. Normal and Abnormal Function of the Foot. Los Angeles, Clinical Biomechanic Corp, 1977

143. Rose GK, Welton EA, Marshall T: The diagnosis of flat foot in the child. J Bone Joint Surg 67(B):71–78, 1985

144. Roy SM, Irvin R: Injuries to the running athlete—Particularly the long-distance runner. In Roy SM, Irvin R (eds): Sports Medicine: Prevention, Evaluation, Management, and Rehabilitation, pp 433–435. Englewood Cliffs, NJ, Prentice-Hall, 1983

145. Sammarco GJ, Burstein AH, Frankel VH: Biomechanics of the ankle: A kinematic study. Orthop Clin North Am 4:75–95, 1973

146. Santilli G: Achilles tendinopathies and paratendinopathies. J Sports Med 19:245–259, 1979

147. Sarrafian SK: Anatomy of the Foot and Ankle, 2nd ed. Philadelphia, JB Lippincott, 1993

148. Saunders JB, Dec M, Inman VT, Eberhart HD: The major determinants in normal and pathological gait. J Bone Joint Surg 35(A):543–558, 1953

149. Scranton PE: Metatarsalgia diagnosis and treatment. J Bone Joint Surg 62(A):723–732, 1980

150. Scranton PE, Pedegana LR, Whitsel JP: Gait analysis: Alterations in support phase using supportive devices. Am J Sports Med 10.6–11, 1982

151. Sewell JR, Black CM, Statham J: Quantitative scintigraphy in diagnosis and management of plantar fasciitis (calcaneal periostitis): Concise communication. J Nucl Med 21:633–636, 1980

152. Sgarlato TE: A Compendium of Podiatric Biomechanics. San Francisco, CA, College of Podiatric Medicine Press, 1971

153. Shore M: Footprint analysis in gait documentation: An instructional sheet format. Phys Ther 60:1163–1167, 1980

154. Slocum DB: The shin splint syndrome: Medical aspects and differential diagnosis. Am J Surg 114:875–881, 1967

155. Smith JW: The ligamentous structures in the canalis and sinus tarsi. J Anat 92:616–620, 1958

156. Southmayd W, Marshall H: The lower leg. In Southmayd W, Marshall H (eds): Sports Health: The Complete Book of Athletic Injuries. New York, Quick Fox, 1981

157. Standish WD, Curwin S, Rubinovich M: Tendinitis: The analysis and treatment for running. Clin Sports Med 4:593–609, 1985

158. Staples OS: Ruptures of the fibular collateral ligaments of the ankle: Result study of immediate surgical treatment. J Bone Joint Surg 57(A):101–107, 1975

159. Straus WL Jr: Growth of the human foot and its evolutionary significance. Contrib Embryol 19:101–116, 1927

160. Subotnick SI: Orthotic foot control and the overuse syndrome. Phys Sports Med 3(1):75–79, 1975

161. Subotnick SI: Biomechanics of the subtalar and midtarsal joints. J Am Podiatr Med Assoc 65:756–764, 1975

162. Subotnick SI: The cavus foot. Phys Sports Med 8:53–55, 1980

163. Subotinick SI: Foot injuries. In Subotnick SI (ed): Sports Medicine of the Lower Extremities, pp 237–239. New York, Churchill Livingstone, 1989

164. Subotnick SI: Ankle injuries. In Subotnick SI (ed): Sports Medicine of the Lower Extremities, pp 277–278. New York, Churchill Livingstone, 1989

165. Subotnick SI, Jones RE: Normal anatomy. In Subotnick SI (ed): Sports Medicine of the Lower Extremities, pp 74–112. New York, Churchill Livingstone, 1989

166. Subotnick SI, Newell SG: Podiatric sports medicine. In Fielding MD (ed): Podiatric Medicine and Surgery. Mount Kisko, NY, Futura, 1975

167. Tax H: Flexible flatfoot in children. J Am Podiatry Assoc 67:616–619, 1977

168. Trolle D: Accessory Bones of the Human Foot: A Radiological, Histo-embryological, Comparative Anatomical and Genetic Study. Copenhagen, Munksgaard, 1948

169. Van Pelt WL: Accommodating, strapping, and bracing. In Subotnick SI (ed): Sports Medicine of the Lower Extremity. New York, Churchill Livingstone, 1989

170. Vidigal E, Jacoby RK, Dixon AJ: The foot in chronic rheumatoid arthritis. Ann Rheum Dis 34:292–297, 1975

171. Viitasale JT, Kust M: Some biomechanical aspects of the foot and ankle in athletes with and without shin splints. Am J Sports Med 11:125–130, 1983

172. Viladot A: The metatarsals. In Jahss MH (ed): Disorders of the Foot, vol 1, pp 659–710. Philadelphia, WB Saunders, 1982

173. Vogler HW, Bauer GR: Contrast studies of the foot and ankle. In Weissman SD: Radiology of the Foot, 2nd ed, pp 439–495. Baltimore, Williams & Wilkins, 1989

174. Wadsworth CT: Manual Examination and Treatment of the Spine and Extremities. Baltimore, Williams & Wilkins, 1988

175. Walker WC: Lower leg pain. In Lillegard WA, Rucker KS (eds): Handbook of Sports Medicine: A Symptom-Oriented Approach, pp 150–158. Boston, Andover Medical Pub, 1993

176. Wallace L: Lower quarter pain: Mechanical evaluation and treatment (Continuing education course). Bellingham, WA, 1984

177. Wallace L: Foot pronation and knee pain. In Hunt GC (ed): Physical Therapy of the Foot and Ankle, pp 101–122. New York, Churchill Livingstone, 1988

178. Weissman SD: Podiatric pathology. In Weissman SD (ed): Radiology of the Foot, pp 106–109. Baltimore, Williams & Wilkins, 1988

179. Whitesel J, Newell SG: Modified low-dye strapping. Phys Sports Med 8:129–131, 1980

180. Wright DG, Desai SM, Henderson WH: Action of the subtalar and ankle complex during stance phase of walking. J Bone Joint Surg 469(A):361–382, 1964

15
CHAPTER

The Temporomandibular Joint

DARLENE HERTLING

TEMPOROMANDIBULAR JOINT AND THE STOMATOGNATHIC SYSTEM

Disease and dysfunction of the temporomandibular joints and the adjacent structures affect a large number of persons. Over 20 percent of the average population at one time or another has symptoms relating to the temporomandibular joint.[127] Practitioners of dentistry and medicine have long been aware that the temporomandibular joints are among the few joints in the body that, like the vertebral joints, function as a unit in a sliding–gliding action because of the mandible, which links the two condyles together.

However, the many intricacies of the temporomandibular joint are just beginning to be appreciated.

In referring to the temporomandibular joints, the masticatory systems, its component structures, and all the tissues related to it, the term *stomatognathic system* is used. The designation includes a number of systematically related organs and tissues that function as a whole. The components of this system include the following:

- Bones of the skull, mandible, maxilla, hyoid, clavicle, and sternum
- Temporomandibular and dentoalveolar joints
- Muscles and soft tissues of the head and neck and the muscles of the cheeks, lips, and tongue

- Vascular, lymphatic, and nerve supply systems
- Teeth

The stomatognathic system functions almost continuously, not only in mastication and swallowing but also in respiration and speech. It also directs the intricate postural relationships of the head, neck, tongue, and hyoid bone, as well as movements of the mandible. One must remember that the entire system governs the movements of the mandible. Impaired physiological function results in breakdown not only of an individual tissue but also of the interdependent structures and eventual function of the other parts, thus setting up a chain reaction.

The relationship of the head and neck must be considered. Postural maintenance must consider the shoulder girdle, clavicle, sternum, and scapulae as the fixed base of operation. The head may be said virtually to teeter on the atlanto-occipital joint. Since the center of gravity of the head lies in front of the occipital condyles, it follows that a balanced force must be applied to hold the head erect. That force is provided by the large posterior muscles of the neck. Normal balance of the head and neck unit requires normal balance of the anterior and posterior muscles, mandible and cranial relationship, and occlusion of the teeth. If one element is off balance, the normal relationship is broken, leading to eventual dysfunction. To restore balance, the entire system must be evaluated and treated.

A faulty relationship of the mandible and maxilla may result in faulty posture of the cranium on the first and second cervical vertebrae, or an imbalance between these vertebrae may result in symptoms referable to the mouth, ear, face, or even the thoracic cavity. Furthermore, faulty curvature of the cervical spine, along with the strains it produces, often is responsible for pain and dysfunction of the head, temporomandibular joints, shoulders, upper extremities, and chest.[14]

Management of the stomatognathic system is not limited to the discipline of any one particular field but encompasses in part nearly every specialty within dentistry and medicine. Treatment involves a team approach that may include physical, myofunctional, and speech therapists; the general dentist; oral-maxillofacial surgeon; orthodontist; otolaryngologist; psychologist; neurologist; allergist; and others.

■ FUNCTIONAL ANATOMY

☐ Osteology

The mandible, the largest and strongest bone of the face, articulates with the two temporal bones and accommodates the lower teeth. It is composed of a hori-

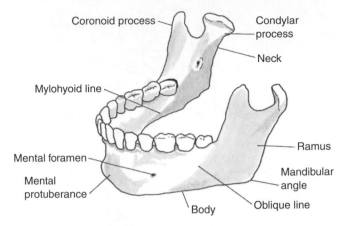

FIG. 15-1. *Lateral and frontal aspects of the mandible.*

zontal portion, the body, and two perpendicular portions, the rami, which unite with ends of the body nearly at right angles (Fig. 15-1).

The external surface of the body is marked by a midline, the mental protuberance, bilateral mental foramina (for passage of the mental artery and nerve), and the oblique line. Muscle attachments include the platysma, depressor anguli oris, depressor labii inferioris, mentalis, and buccinator. The internal surface is concave from side to side. The superior or alveolar border, wider posteriorly than anteriorly, consists of the dentoalveolar cavities for reception of the teeth. Extending upward and backward on either side of the internal surface is the mylohyoid line, to which the mylohyoid muscle attaches (see Fig. 15-1). Other muscle attachments include the digastric and medial pterygoid muscles.

The ramus, which is quadrilateral in shape, has two processes, the coronoid process and the condylar process. The coronoid process serves as an insertion for the temporalis and masseter muscles. The triangular eminence varies in shape and size; its anterior border is convex, and its posterior border is concave. The condylar process consists of two portions, the neck and the condyle. The condyle, which is convex in shape, articulates with the meniscus of the temporomandibular joint. The mandibular condyle is 15 to 20 mm long and 8 to 10 mm thick and resembles a little cylinder laid on its side. Its long axis is directed medially and slightly backward. An imaginary line drawn through the axis to the middle line would meet a line from the opposite condyle near the anterior margin of the foramen magnum (Fig. 15-2).* The lateral pterygoid inserts into a depression on the anterior portion of the neck of the condyle.

---

*This relationship is an important consideration in the application of mobilization techniques.

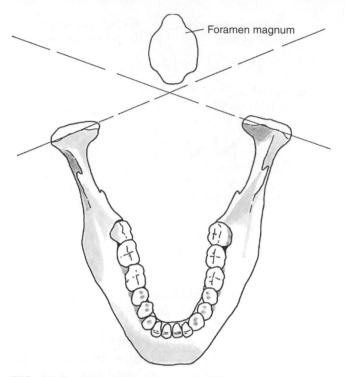

FIG. 15-2. Schematic representation illustrates how extensions of the long axis of the condyles meet near the anterior margin of the foramen magnum.

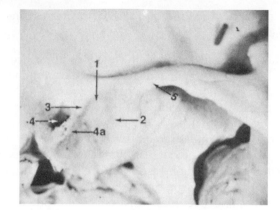

FIG. 15-3. Temporal bone, articular area: Temporal fossa (1), articular eminence (2), post-glenoid process (3), external auditory meatus (4), tympanic bone (4a), and zygomatic arch (5). (Alderman MM: Disorders of the temporomandibular joint and related structures. In Lynch MA [ed]: Burket's Oral Medicine: Diagnosis and Treatment, 7th ed. Philadelphia, JB Lippincott, 1977)

☐ The Joint Proper

The temporomandibular joint is located between the temporal fossa (glenoid fossa) on the inferior surface of the temporal bone and the condylar process of the mandibular bone (Figs. 15-3 and 15-4). Just posterior to the joint is the external auditory meatus. The temporal portion consists of the temporal fossa, which is concave, and an anteriorly placed articular eminence, which is convex.

The temporal fossa is bounded in front by the articular eminence (tubercle) and posteriorly by the post-glenoid process (spine) (see Figs. 15-3 and 15-4). The post-glenoid process separates the articular surface of the temporal fossa from the anterior margin of the tympanic part of the temporal bone (see Fig. 15-3). The temporal fossa (squamous part of the temporal bone) is made up of thin compact bone. The articular surface, which is smooth, oval, and deeply concave, articulates with the articular disk or meniscus of the temporomandibular joint. The average person after his mid-twenties has no more fibrocartilage in the posterior portion of the mandibular fossa.*

From a functional point of view, the concave fossa

serves as a receptacle for the condyles when the jaws are approximated and as a functional component in lateral movements of the jaw. During opening, closing, protrusion, and retrusion, the convex surface of the condylar head must move across the convex surface of the articular eminence. The existence of the interarticular disk (meniscus) compensates functionally for the incongruity of the two opposing convex bony surfaces. In addition, the disk divides the joint into two portions, sometimes referred to as the upper and lower joints. The disk is concavoconvex on its superior surface to accommodate the form of the mandibular fossa and the articular tubercle. The inferior sur-

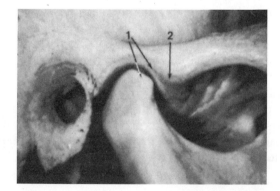

FIG. 15-4. Temporomandibular joint, right view of bony relations. Note the mandibular condyle and the incongruity of the articular surfaces (1) and the lateral view of articular eminence of temporal bone (2). (Alderman MM: Disorders of the temporomandibular joint and related structures. In Lynch MA [ed]: Burket's Oral Medicine: Diagnosis and Treatment, 7th ed. Philadelphia, JB Lippincott, 1977)

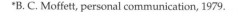

*B. C. Moffett, personal communication, 1979.

face is concave over the condyle. In function both the condylar head and articular eminence of the temporal bone are not in contact with each other but with the opposing surfaces of the disk. The upper cavity is the larger of the two. The outer edges of the disk are connected to the capsule. Synovial membranes line the two cavities above and below the disk (Fig. 15-5). The superior portion of the joint acts as a gliding joint that allows forward, backward, and lateral movements of the joint. During horizontal lateral jaw movements, the ipsilateral condyle rotates with a slight lateral shift (Bennett movement), with a corresponding forward translation and rotation of the other condylar head. On opening of the mouth, the disk rotates and translates forward under the articular eminence. The lower joint, consisting of the mandible caudally and the disk cranially, is primarily responsible for rotation while the upper joint is primarily responsible for translation.

The disk follows the condyle closely in normal function, being pulled forward as the lateral pterygoid contracts to open the mouth and back by the elasticity of its posterior attachment. Arthrography has shown that the disk also changes shape during function while it moves bodily.[82]

Rees has described the disk or meniscus as having three parts: (1) a thick anterior band (pes meniscus), (2) a thicker posterior band (pars posterior), and (3) a thin intermediate zone (pars gracilis) between the two bands (Fig. 15-6).[143] It is the intermediate band that is

both avascular and aneural, with its fibrous tissue being most dense. The intermediate band is positioned between the pressure-bearing articulating surfaces of the temporal bone and the mandibular condyle. The anterior and posterior bands have both vascular and neural elements present.

The disk envelops the condyle much as a cap envelops the head of a jockey, with the anterior and posterior bands converging medially and laterally to be inserted rigidly onto the medial and lateral poles.[108] The two terms *meniscus* and *disk* usually given to this structure do not describe it adequately. It is not the shape of a meniscus (a crescent-shaped body) or a disk (suggesting a flat structure interposed between the bony surfaces).[92] The articular disk or meniscus has the following attachments:[92,108,142]

- **Anterior attachment** (see Fig. 15-6). Anteriorly, the disk is attached to the capsule. Fibers from the upper head of the lateral pterygoid muscle attach through the capsule into the medial part of the anterior edge of the disk.
- **Medial and lateral attachments** (Fig. 15-7). Medially and laterally, the disk inserts into the corresponding poles of the mandibular condyle, via the medial and lateral collateral ligaments.
- **Posterior attachments** (see Figs. 15-6 and 15-7).[108,142] The posterior-superior disk attaches to the superior stratum, which then attaches to the

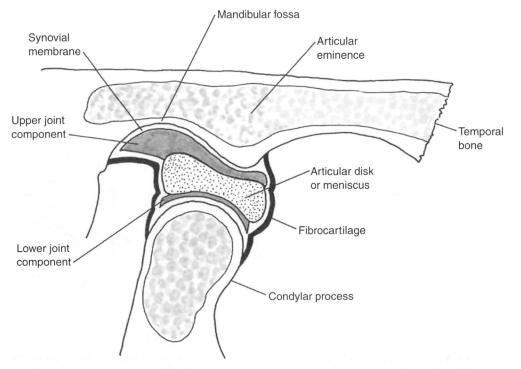

FIG. 15-5. Articular structures of the temporomandibular joint in the closed position.

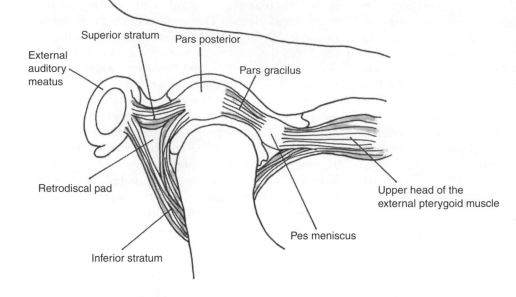

FIG. 15-6. Parasagittal section of the temporomandibular joint. The lower lamina of the bilaminar zone is inserted into the condylar neck, and the upper lamina is inserted into the squamotympanic fissure.

post-glenoid spine. The posterior-inferior disk attaches to the inferior stratum, which then attaches to the neck of the mandibular condyle. The disk also attaches to the posterior capsule. The superior and inferior (lower) strata or laminae enclose an area termed the *bilaminar zone*.[143] This bilaminar zone consists of loose neurovascular connective tissue referred to as the retrodiskal pad.[76] Since the retrodiskal pad consists of both vascularized and innervated tissue within the capsule it may be a source of nonarthritic intracapsular inflammation and arthralgia.

An excellent comprehensive study by Rees provides a more detailed analysis of the function and structure of the temporomandibular joint.[143]

☐ Ligamentous Structures

The ligamentous structures around the temporomandibular joint include the following:

- Articular capsule (capsular ligament)
- Lateral ligament (temporomandibular ligament)
- Sphenomandibular ligament (internal lateral ligament)
- Stylomandibular ligament

The capsular ligament is attached to the circumference of the mandibular fossa and the articular tubercle superiorly and to the neck of the mandibular condyle inferiorly (Fig. 15-8). It is a sleeve of thin, loose, fibrous connective tissue. The capsule is especially lax

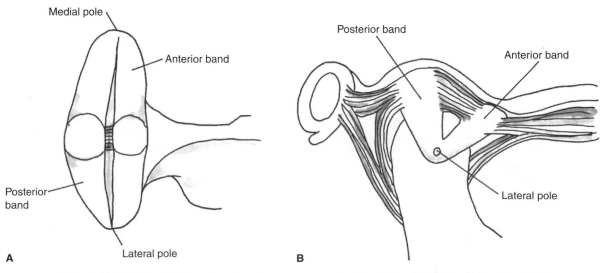

FIG. 15-7. Schematic drawing showing the normal disk (right side) seen from above (**A**) and from the side (**B**). The posterior and anterior bands are seen converging, to be inserted at the medial and lateral poles.

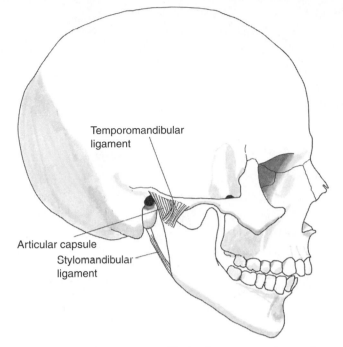

FIG. 15-8. Temporomandibular ligament and capsule.

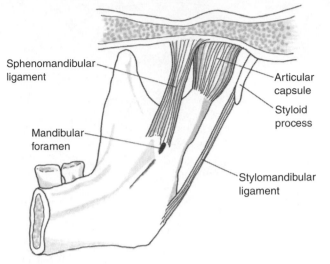

FIG. 15-9. Sphenomandibular and stylomandibular ligaments as viewed from the medial aspect of the mandible.

anteriorly in the superior cavity but very taut in the inferior cavity between the head and disk. Therefore, when the condyle moves forward, the disk follows.

The temporomandibular ligament, a thickening of the joint capsule, is attached superiorly to the lateral surface of the zygomatic arch and articular eminence; inferiorly it attaches to the lateral surface and the posterior border of the neck of the mandible (see Fig. 15-8). The ligament prevents extensive forward, backward, and lateral movements and is the main suspensory ligament of the mandible during moderate opening movements.

The sphenomandibular ligament, an accessory ligament, originates from the spine of the sphenoid and attaches to the lingula of the mandible at the mandibular foramen (Fig. 15-9). This ligament serves as a suspensory ligament of the mandible during wide opening. After moderate opening, the temporomandibular ligament relaxes and the sphenomandibular ligament becomes taut. The medial pterygoid is associated with the medial surface of the sphenomandibular ligament.

The stylomandibular ligament is also considered an accessory ligament (see Fig. 15-9). It runs from the styloid process of the temporal bone to the posterior portion of the ramus of the mandible and separates the masseter and medial pterygoid muscles. It acts as a stop for the mandible during extreme opening, preventing excessive anterior movement.

The mandibular-malleolar ligament has been demonstrated by Pinto and others.[136] This ligamentous structure connects the neck and anterior process of the malleus to the medioposterior part of the joint capsule, the disk, and the sphenomandibular ligament. According to Ermshar this anatomical association of the joint and middle ear may well explain many of the middle ear complaints associated with temporomandibular dysfunction.[52]

☐ **Mandibular Musculature**

Function of all of the muscles of the upper quadrant need to be understood because of their impact on temporomandibular joint function and dysfunction. Movements of the mandible are a result of the action of the cervical and jaw muscles. The cervical muscles stabilize the head to increase the efficiency of the mandibular movements.

The three major closing muscles of the mandible are the temporalis, the masseter, and the medial pterygoid. The superior head of the lateral pterygoid is also actively involved in mandibular closure.[107,119]

The *temporalis* muscle, which is fan shaped, arises from the temporal fossa and deep surface of the temporal fascia. The anterior fibers of the muscle are vertical, the middle are oblique, and the posterior are nearly horizontal. The fibers converge as they descend, becoming tendinous, and insert into the medial and anterior aspects of the coronoid process of the ramus (Fig. 15-10). The temporalis muscle functions primarily as an elevator of the mandible, moving the jaw vertically and diagonally upward. The posterior fibers also retract the mandible and maintain the condyles posteriorly.

The *masseter* is a thick quadrilateral muscle com-

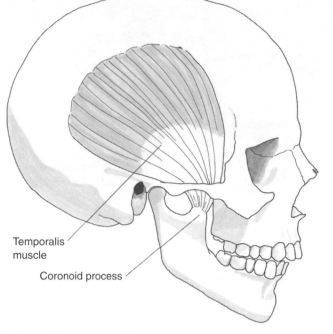

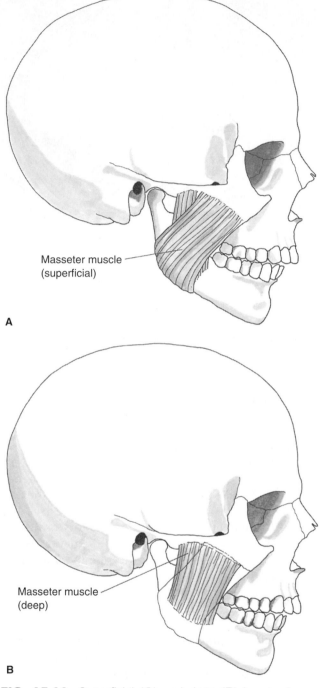

FIG. 15-10. Temporalis muscle.

FIG. 15-11. Superficial (**A**) and deep (**B**) layers of masseter muscle.

posed of two bellies, the deep and superficial. The superficial portion arises from the lower border of the zygomatic arch and maxillary process; it extends down and back and inserts into the angle and the inferior half of the lateral surface of the ramus. The muscle itself is formed by an intricate arrangement of tendinous and fleshy bundles that make it extremely powerful (Fig. 15-11*A*). The smaller, deeper portion is fused anteriorly to the superficial portion but is separated from it posteriorly. It arises from the entire length of the zygomatic arch and passes anteriorly and inferiorly, inserting in the lateral surface of the coronoid process and superior half of the ramus (Fig. 15-11*B*). The masseter functions primarily as an elevator of the mandible. The superficial fibers also protrude the jaw a little, with the deep portion acting as a retractor as well.

The *medial pterygoid* is located on the medial aspect of the ramus. Although less powerful than the masseter, its construction is similar to the masseter in that it is characterized by an alternation of fleshy and tendinous parts. The medial pterygoid, which is quadrilateral in shape, arises from the medial surface of the lateral pterygoid plate and pyramidal process of the palatine bone. The fibers pass laterally, posteriorly, and inferiorly and insert onto the medial surface of the ramus and angle of the mandible (Fig. 15-12). Its primary function is closing and elevating the mandible. It also protrudes and laterally deviates the jaw.

The major muscles that depress the mandible are the lateral pterygoids and the anterior strap muscles,

the suprahyoid and infrahyoid groups. The suprahyoid muscles are the digastric, stylohyoid, mylohyoid, and geniohyoid. They are all either opposed or assisted synergically by the infrahyoid muscles.

The *lateral pterygoid* is a thick conical muscle and consists of two bellies (see Fig. 15-12). The superior head arises from the infratemporal crest of the greater wing of the sphenoid bone. The inferior head arises from the lateral surface of the pterygoid plate. The

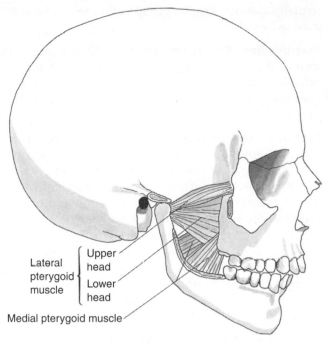

Lateral pterygoid muscle { Upper head / Lower head

Medial pterygoid muscle

FIG. 15-12. Medial and lateral pterygoid muscles.

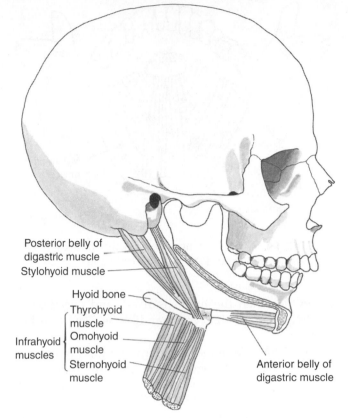

Posterior belly of digastric muscle

Stylohyoid muscle

Hyoid bone

Infrahyoid muscles { Thyrohyoid muscle / Omohyoid muscle / Sternohyoid muscle

Anterior belly of digastric muscle

FIG. 15-13. Digastric, stylohyoid, and infrahyoid muscles.

two heads form a tendinous insertion in front of the temporomandibular joint. The lower fibers run horizontally and insert on the neck of the condyle, with some fibers attaching to the medial portion of the condyle as well. Fibers from the superior head are attached to the articular disk and capsule as well as to the condylar head.[119,138] The attachment of the lateral pterygoid to the condyle and disk is significant in stabilizing the temporomandibular joint during bilateral protrusion, retrusion, and closing of the mandible. Lateral movement of the mandible is achieved by the action of the lateral and medial pterygoid on one side and the contralateral temporalis muscle. The lateral pterygoid, especially its inferior head, is also the primary muscle used in opening the mouth, and in protruding the mandible. The superior head is believed to play an important role in stabilizing the condylar head and disk against the articular eminence during closing movement of the mandible.[119] This muscle is particularly important in cases of temporomandibular joint dysfunction and is the muscle most frequently involved.

The *digastric* muscle consists of an anterior and posterior belly connected by a strong round tendon. The anterior belly arises from the lower border of the mandible close to the symphysis. The posterior belly, which is considerably longer than the anterior one, arises from the mastoid process of the temporal bone. Both bellies descend toward the hyoid bone and are united by the intermediate tendon, which is connected to the hyoid bone by a loop of fibrous tissue (Fig. 15-13). The function of the digastric is to pull the

mandible back and down. The digastric, assisted by the suprahyoids, plays a dominant role in forced opening of the mandible when the hyoid bone is fixed by the infrahyoid muscle group. It also aids in retraction of the jaw and elevation of the hyoid bone.

The *stylohyoid* muscle arises from the styloid process of the temporal bone and inserts on the hyoid bone. Along with the geniohyoid it determines the length of the floor of the mouth. It also acts in initiating and assisting jaw opening and draws the hyoid bone upward and backward when the mandible is fixed (see Fig. 15-13).

The *geniohyoid* is a narrow muscle, wider posteriorly than anteriorly, that lies adjacent to the midline of the floor of the mouth and above the mylohyoid muscle. It arises from the symphysis of the mandible and inserts onto the anterior surface of the hyoid bone (Fig. 15-14). Like the digastric, it acts to pull the mandible down and back when the hyoid bone is fixed and assists in elevation of the hyoid bone.

The *mylohyoid* muscle arises from the whole length of the medial surface of the mandible, from the symphysis to the last molar teeth, and makes up the floor of the mouth. The fibers pass downward, with some meeting in the median raphe and some attaching directly to the hyoid bone. The mylohyoid elevates the floor of the mouth. It also assists in depression of the

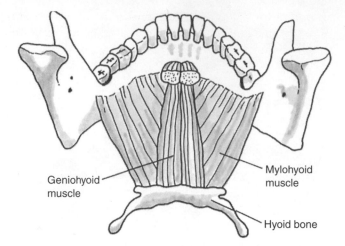

FIG. 15-14. Mylohyoid and geniohyoid muscles viewed from above and behind the floor of the mouth.

mandible when the hyoid is fixed, and elevation of the hyoid bone when the mandible is fixed (see Fig. 15-14).

The *infrahyoid* muscles (sternohyoid, thyrohyoid, and omohyoid) act together to steady the hyoid bone or depress it, thus allowing the suprahyoids to act on the mandible (see Fig. 15-13). Of the extrinsic muscles of mastication, only the digastric and geniohyoid muscles exert a direct pull on the mandible, pulling it in a posterior and inferior direction, thereby retruding and depressing the mandible.[24]

Other muscles that have a close neurophysiological relationship to the temporomandibular joint and that are innervated by the fifth cranial nerve include

Tensor tympani—Controls movement of the tympanic membrane. It is contained in the bony canal superior to the bony part of the auditory tube, from which it is separated by a thin bony septum.

Tensor veli palatini—Controls diameter of the eustachian tube. This thin triangular muscle lies lateral to the medial pterygoid plate, the auditory tube, and the levator veli palatini. Its lateral surface is in contact with the upper and anterior part of the medial pterygoid.

Abnormal muscle contraction or spasms of any of the temporomandibular muscles, including clenching of the jaw, may affect the tensor veli palatini and tensor tympani muscles and, indirectly, the stapedius muscle of the ear.[32,89]

☐ Muscle Group Action

Mandibular movements are complicated because of the wide range of positions that the mandible can po-

tentially assume. Briefly, group action might be summarized as follows:

Mandibular Elevators. The mandibular elevators include the coordinated action of the masseter, temporalis (for retrusion), superior head of the lateral pterygoid (for stabilization), and the medial pterygoid (for protrusion).

Mandibular Opening. The inferior head of the lateral pterygoid and the anterior head of the digastric are considered the primary muscles used in opening the mandible. The inferior head of the lateral pterygoid acts synergistically with the suprahyoid muscle group in the translation of the condylar head downward, inferiorly, and contralaterally during opening movements. Opening is assisted by the other suprahyoid muscles, which also act in initiating motion when the hyoid bone is fixed by the infrahyoid muscles. The masseter and the medial pterygoid muscles also help draw the jaw slightly forward.

Retrusion of the Mandible. The posterior fibers of the temporalis draw the condyles backward during retrusion and are assisted by the digastric and suprahyoids.

Protrusion of the Mandible. Protrusion is performed by the masseter and medial and lateral pterygoids.

Lateral Movements. Action is achieved primarily by the lateral and medial pterygoids on one side and the temporalis muscle on the contralateral side (see Fig. 15-16). When the mandible moves to the right side, the left lateral pterygoid and medial pterygoid move the chin across the midline toward the right side. The digastric, geniohyoid, and mylohyoid also are actively involved.

☐ Dynamics of the Mandible and Temporomandibular Joints

POSITIONS OF THE MANDIBLE

Before evaluating the dynamics of the various mandibular movements, certain physiological positions of the jaw should be defined. These are the rest position, occlusal positions, hinge position, and centric position. The terminology of some of these positions is confusing and controversial. No basic terminology has been universally adopted, and each investigator has had to establish his or her own.

The *rest position* of the mandible is considered the position the jaw assumes when there is minimal muscle-action potential. It usually implies that the head is also in its normal rest position when the person is in an upright posture. The mandibular rest position is considered to be an equilibrium between the tonus of the gravity, or jaw-opening muscles, and that of the antigravity, or jaw-closing muscles. The residual tension of the muscles at rest is termed *resting tonus*. In this position there is no occlusal contact between the maxillary and mandibular teeth. The space between the upper and lower teeth is called the *free-way space* or *interocclusal clearance*. It normally measures from 2 to 5 mm between incisors.

The rest position of the tongue, often referred to as the *postural position*, is up against the palate of the mouth.[58] The most anterosuperior tip of the tongue lies in the area against the palate just posterior to the back side of the upper central incisors. The rest position of the tongue by way of neuroreflexors (jaw–tongue reflex) provides a foundation for the resting muscle tone of the elevator muscles of the mandible and for the resting activity of the tongue.[5]

The importance of the rest position lies in the fact that it permits the tissues of the stomatognathic system to rest and thus repair themselves. If the vertical dimension is abnormally decreased (eliminating the interocclusal space), the teeth will be in constant contact. This eliminates the rest position and creates constant muscular tension and stress on the supporting structures and teeth. Factors that influence muscle tonus and the rest position are function, sleep, pathological conditions, and the normal aging process.

Occlusal positions are functional positions in which contact between some or all of the teeth occur. One occlusal position, termed *median occlusal position* by Sicher and DuBrul, is highly significant.[160] This is the position in which the jaws are closed so that all upper and lower teeth meet, resulting in full occlusion with a balanced intercuspation of the upper and lower dental arches. From the median occlusal position, the mandible can move forward into protrusive occlusal positions, laterally, and backward to a limited extent in all normal jaws. Absent or abnormally positioned teeth can displace the mandible from the normal median occlusal position, disturbing the complete balance between the teeth, temporomandibular joints, and the musculature.

The *hinge position* is the position of the mandible from which a pure hinge opening and closing of the jaw can be made.[160] In the hinge position, the condyles are in the most retruded position that the muscles of the jaw can accomplish; it is determined by the length of the temporomandibular ligaments. The position is considered a retruded position or "strained relationship," which the mandible can assume actively or passively. Determination of this position is useful for some clinical procedures.

Centric position, or centric-relation occlusion, denotes a concept of normal mandibular posture. Centric position implies the most retruded, unstrained position of the mandible from which lateral movements are possible and the components of the oral apparatus are in balance. Normal centric position is slightly forward of the most posterior position that the mandibular musculature can actually achieve. Ideally, median occlusal position should coincide with centric position.

MOVEMENT PATTERNS

Mandibular movements are complicated because of the wide range of positions that the mandible can assume. Involved and integrated in mandibular movements are the shape of the fossae, the degree of tension of the associated ligaments, the menisci, the neuromuscular system, and the guiding incline of the teeth.

Kinematically, the mandible may be considered a free body that can rotate in any angular direction. It has, therefore, three degrees of freedom; each of these degrees of freedom of motion is associated with a separate axis of rotation.[181] The two basic movements required for functional motion are rotation and translation. The mandible is capable of affecting these movements in three planes: sagittal, horizontal, and frontal. The joint has three functional motions: opening and closing, protrusion and retrusion, and lateral motions. A considerable degree of rotation is also possible.

When the mouth is opened, the condyles first rotate around a horizontal axis. This motion is then combined with gliding of the condyles forward and downward with the lower surface of the disk at the same time as the disk slides forward and downward on the temporal bone. This movement results from the attachment of the disk to the medial and lateral poles of the head of the mandible and from the contraction of the lateral pterygoid, which carries the condyle with the disk onto the articular eminence. The forward sliding of the disk ceases when the fibroelastic tissue attached to the temporal bone posteriorly has been stretched to the limits. Thereafter, there is some further hinging and gliding forward of the condyle until it articulates with the most anterior part of the disk and the mouth is fully opened. The condyles essentially rotate on an axis in the horizontal plane and translate against the posterior slope of the articular eminence in the sagittal plane.

Opening movements of the mandible are caused by the synergistic action of the lateral pterygoid muscles and the depressors of the mandible. Although the lateral pterygoid pulls the condylar head and disk forward, the digastric and geniohyoid muscles pull the mandible downward and backward, affecting rotation. This blending of muscle action makes possible the rotatory and translatory movements of jaw opening. This motion affects all the other muscles anchored to the mandible. The elevators of the mandible must lengthen to ensure smoothness of performance, and the muscles of the cranium and hyoid bone must act as holders to establish a fixed position (Fig. 15-15).

In mandibular closure, the movements are reversed. In the first phase of the movement, the condyles glide backward and then hinge on the disks, which are held forward by the lateral pterygoids. The backward glide of the mandible results from interaction between the retracting portions of the masseter and temporalis muscles and the retracting portions of the depressors. During the second phase, the inferior head of the lateral pterygoids relaxes while the upper head allows the disks to glide backward and upward on the temporal bone along with the condyles.[107] The second phase begins with the contraction of the masseter, the medial pterygoid, and temporalis muscles; it ends with intercuspation of the teeth. The onset of superior head or lateral pterygoid function is usually concurrent with that of the elevator musculature.[119]

In protrusion, the teeth are retained throughout in the occlusal position, so far as possible, and the lower teeth are drawn forward over the upper teeth by both lateral pterygoids. In contrast to opening movements, the condyles and disks move downward and forward along the articular eminences without rotation of the condyles around a transverse axis. To prevent the mandible from falling, the elevating muscles exhibit some degree of contraction. They must make the necessary adjustment with the balancing depressor–retractors as they lengthen to allow the mandible to slide forward just free of the interlocking dentition.

In retraction, the mandible is drawn backward by the deep portion of the masseter muscles and by the posterior fibers of the temporalis muscles to the rest position. At the same time, the geniohyoid, the digastric muscles, and the elevators synergistically balance each other to maintain the mandible in the horizontal position.

In lateral movements of the mandible, asymmetrical muscular patterns develop on both sides. In this movement, one condyle and disk slide downward and forward in the sagittal plane and medially in the horizontal plane along the articular eminence. At the same time, the other condyle rotates laterally on a sagittal plane around a shifting vertical axis and translates medially in the horizontal plane while remaining in the fossa. The condylar translation in the horizontal plane is known as the Bennett movement.[160,183,186] If one views the mandible from above, it will be seen that the medial pole of the condyle juts far medially from the plane of the jaw, while the coronoid process leans laterally. The lateral pterygoid muscle, inserted on the medial pole of the condyle, pulls inward and forward in the horizontal plane, while the horizontal fibers of the temporalis muscle, inserted on the coronoid process, pull outward and backward (Fig. 15-16). These muscles, operating as a *force couple,* contribute to the torque of rotating the condyle that is necessary to effect chewing on this side. This condyle is known as the working-side condyle. Therefore, in lateral deviation to the left, the lateral pterygoid on the right, together with the right and left anterior bellies of the digastric and geniohyoid, contract. This causes the right condyle to move downward, forward, and medially, while the actions of the left temporalis and the lateral pterygoid rotate the left condyle in the fossa and displace the mandible to the left. This is described as *left lateral excursion with a Bennett shift to the left.* The

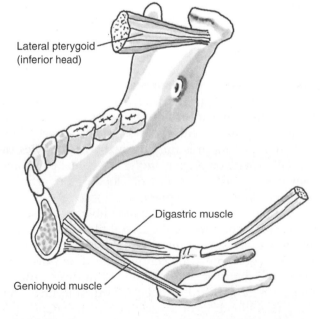

Lateral pterygoid
(inferior head)

Digastric muscle

Geniohyoid muscle

FIG. 15-15. *Mandibular muscles involved in opening.*

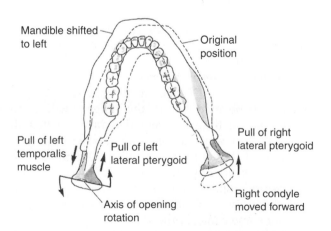

Mandible shifted to left

Original position

Pull of left temporalis muscle

Pull of left lateral pterygoid

Pull of right lateral pterygoid

Right condyle moved forward

Axis of opening rotation

FIG. 15-16. *Mandibular muscles involved in lateral movement of the mandible to the left. The suprahyoid muscles are not shown.*

left condyle is called the *working-side condyle* and the right condyle is the *nonworking condyle* or balancing condyle. Basic types of working condylar motions include the following:[184]

- Rotation with no lateral shift (Fig. 15-17A)
- Rotation with movement backward, upward, and/or laterally (Fig. 15-17B)
- Rotation with movement downward, forward, and laterally (Fig. 15-17C)
- Rotation with a lateral shift (Fig. 15-17D)
- Rotation with movement downward, backward, and laterally (Fig. 15-17E)

It is apparent that the right lateral pterygoid has also entered into the force-couple system. In the closing stroke, the force couple changes in direction and components. Thus, in the rotatory movements of grinding or chewing, these alternating movements swing the mandible from side to side.

Although masticatory movements are highly complex, they become automatic in each person as a result of the integration of the proprioceptive mechanism and muscular action. All of the muscles of mastication are involved in the act of chewing because it involves all four movements of the mandible—elevation, depression, protrusion, and retrusion.

☐ Nerve Supply

The innervation of the temporomandibular joint is supplied by three nerves that are part of the mandibular division of the fifth cranial nerve. The posterior deep temporal and masseteric nerves supply the medial and anterior regions of the joint. The auriculotemporal nerve supplies the posterior and lateral regions of the joint (see Fig. 17-11). The auriculotemporal nerve is the major nerve innervating the posterior lateral capsule, the retrodiskal pad, the temporomandibular ligaments, and the capsular blood vessels. The auriculotemporal nerve also sends a few branches to the tympanic membrane, the external auditory

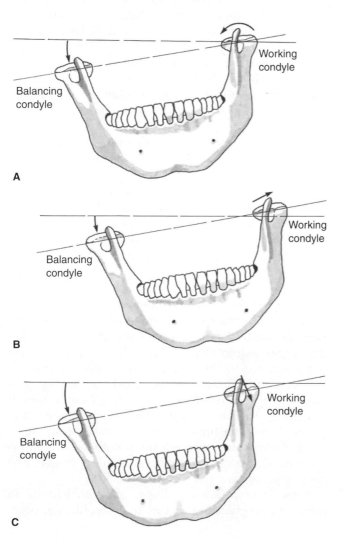

A

B

C

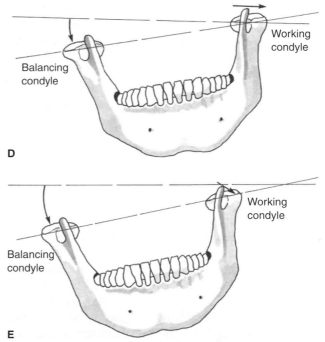

D

E

FIG. 15-17. The basic types of working condylar motions are (**A**) rotation with no lateral shift; (**B**) rotation with movement backward, upward, and/or laterally; (**C**) rotation with movement downward, forward, and laterally; (**D**) rotation with a lateral shift; and (**E**) rotation with movement downward, backward and laterally. (After Weinberg LA: An evaluation of basic articulators and their concepts: I. Basic concepts. J Prosthet Dent 13:622–644, 1963.)

meatus, the superior one half of the auricle on its lateral aspect, and the skin of the temples and scalp.[44,74] The central part of the disk is not innervated.[142]

All four types of joint mechanoreceptors have been identified with respect to the joint structures of the temporomandibular joint. For a detailed understanding of their morphological and functional characteristics see Chapter 3, Arthrology, and articles by Clark,[36] Klineberg,[97] and Wyke.[191] The general characteristics of mechanoreceptors types I, II, and III are postural and kinesthetic perception, reflexive influence on motor neuron pool activity, and inhibition of nociceptor-mechanoreceptor activity. The major contribution to position sense of the mandible is believed to come from these joint receptors, although the presence of spindles in the muscles of mastication and pain impulses from the periodontal membrane also contribute to afferent information. This mechanoreceptor system is polysynaptic and heavily influences the reflex coordination of masticatory activity (both inhibitory and facilitory).

There is also an abundant supply of type IV, nonadapting, high-threshold pain receptors, which are nonactive under normal conditions. Abnormal activity of these receptors results when related tissue is subject to marked deformation or other noxious mechanical or chemical stimulation (*e.g.*, intracapsular pressure changes, capsular tightness, and strained positions of the mandibular condyles).[94] As a result there will be altered perception of mandibular movement and positioning as well as altered muscle activity of those muscles innervated by the fifth cranial nerve.

■ APPLIED ANATOMY

☐ Relation of Head Posture to Rest Position of the Mandible

Functionally the temporomandibular joint, the cervical spine, and the articulations between the teeth are intimately related. The neuromuscular influence of the cervical and masticatory region actively participate in the function of mandibular movement and cervical positioning.[81,135,173,191] Many factors influence the masticatory muscles and affect the rest position and path of mandibular closure.[99,122,125,139,141] A change in head position caused by cervical muscles changes the mandibular position.[37,42,71,125,144] This change affects occlusion and the masticatory muscles, and the masticatory muscles then affect the temporomandibular joint.[63,149] The balance between the flexors and extensors of the head and neck is affected by the muscles of mastication and the suprahyoid and in-

frahyoid muscles.[146] Dysfunction in either the muscles of mastication or the cervical muscles can easily disturb this normal balance.

Cervical posture change affects the mandibular path of closure,[139] the mandibular rest position,[37] masticatory muscle activity,[81,117,139] and, subsequently, the occlusal contact pattern. Neurologically the cervical apophyseal joints and increased gravitational forces on the head can directly alter muscular activity about the jaw. Electromyographical studies have indicated increased masticatory levels with cervical backward bending and cervical flexion: backward bending increases activity of the temporalis muscles and cervical flexion increases activity of the masseter and digastric.[25,27]

A common postural defect that increases the gravitational forces on the head and may lead to hyperextension of the head on the neck is *forward head posture* (FHP). When the head is held anteriorly, the line of vision will extend downward if the normal angle at which the head and neck meet is maintained. To correct for visual needs there is a tilting of the head backwards (posterior cranial rotation [PCR]), flexion of the neck over the thorax, and posterior migration of the mandible.[149] The posterior cervical muscles are shortened isometrically and are forced to contract excessively to maintain the head in this position while the anterior submandibular muscles are stretched to cause retrusive forces on the mandible and an altered occlusal contact pattern. The mandible is forced posteriorly by the rebound effect of the stretched platysma and other anterior cervical muscles.[64] The contracted posterior cervical muscles may entrap the greater occipital nerve and refer pain to the head.[31] Excessive mandibular shuttling between opening and closing, necessary for functional activities such as eating, leads to joint hypermobility because the temporomandibular joint capsule is stretched.[63] Increased muscular activity in the anterior cervical (longus colli) and hyoid muscles will in turn cause tightness in the throat and difficulty swallowing.[149]

Among important environmental factors contributing to the forward head posture are the many occupations and activities of daily living that require that the upper extremities and the head be positioned more anterior to the trunk than is either normal or comfortable (improper home, work, or driving postures).[43,49,112,113] Another contributing factor is mouth breathing. Various investigations have shown that postural relationships change to meet respiratory needs.[43] Breathing through the mouth facilitates forward head posture, lowered mandibular position, and a low and forward tongue position.[84,140]

Acute trauma (such as hyperextension injuries, in which reflex guarding of the longus colli, sternocleidomastoid, and scalenes occurs) is usually associated with a decrease in the cervical spine curvature approaching total flattening out of the cervical lordosis; a straight form of FHP without PCR (Fig. 15-18B).[111,116] Any forward deviation of the head out of the long axis of the body should be considered pathological, as this reduces the potential mobility of the cervical spine. Total flattening out of the physiological cervical lordosis and any kyphosis of the lower cervical spine (cervical or neck kyphosis) must also be considered pathological.[96] Kyphosis of the neck affects, roughly, the C5–T3 segments. It is seen in connection with a pronounced thoracic flat back, particularly in the mid-thoracic spine. Motions of all segments affected by the kyphosis of the neck are considerably restricted.

In the presence of an FHP with no significant PCR the suprahyoids shorten and the infrahyoids lengthen, consequently decreasing or eliminating the free-way space.[100,155] The hyoid bone is repositioned superiorly and the degree of elevation is proportional to the decrease in the cervical lordosis or increase in FHP.[100,145,148] An opposite action occurs at the mandibular condyles as they are forced to elevate and translate forward at the same time the mentum is depressed and retruded.[59,165] These repositioning effects are maximized when the FHP is associated with a significant degree of PCR.[113]

As the mandibular condyles assumes a retro position in the joint, the superior head of the lateral pterygoid becomes stretched.[43] By reflex action, this stretch may lead to premature contraction, causing the disk to become anteriorly displaced.[29,72] With changes in the mandibular position and the length–tension relationship of the hyoid, the occlusal contact pattern and the arthrokinematics of the temporomandibular joint also change.[28,65,125,140] Mouth breathing may compound the situation with the tongue assuming a lowered position and causing abnormal swallowing patterns (Fig. 15-19).[9] The position of the scapula, to which the omohyoid muscle is attached, will also influence the length–tension relationship of the hyoid muscles.[145,146] Shoulder girdle posture relates to the position of the head and neck in the same way that the sacral base rules the position of the lumbar spine.[146]

The effects of abnormal FHP may lead to an excessive amount of tension in the masticatory musculature, teeth, and supporting structures.[5] Abnormal position may lead to eventual osteoarthrosis and remodeling of the temporomandibular joint.[67,125]

One of the common neuroanatomical sequelae involving FHP is suboccipital impingement or entrapment. The neuroanatomical studies by Bogduk[21–23] have clarified the numerous possibilities for muscular, osseous, and facial entrapments of C1, C2, and C3.

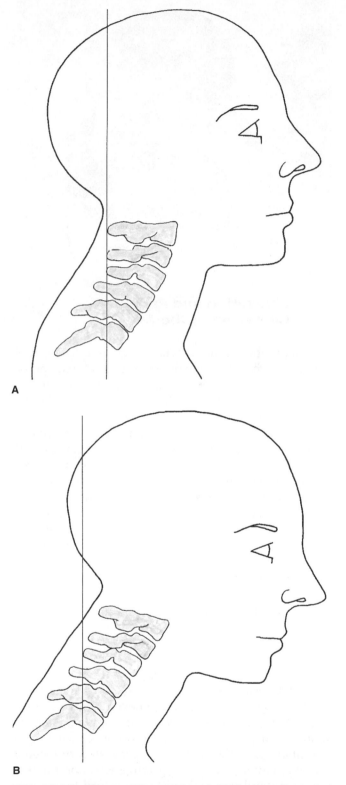

FIG. 15-18. Types of forward head: (**A**) increased cervical lordosis with posterior cranial rotation, and (**B**) total flattening out of the cervical lordosis without posterior cranial rotation.

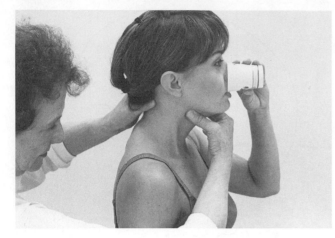

FIG. 15-19. *Examination of altered swallowing sequence.*

Subluxation and Premature Translation of the Jaw

The temporomandibular joint can subluxate itself through its own muscular dynamics. Subluxation occurs when the condyle translates onto the articular tubercle and then back to the articular eminence. Predisposing factors that allow the subluxation to occur more easily in some persons than others is a decrease in the slope of the articular eminence or a flattened articular eminence (see Figs. 15-4 and 15-5) and stretching of the ligamentous attachments of the meniscus into the condylar pole.[91,92,192] Signs of subluxation include excessive mandibular opening (greater than 40 mm), movement of the lateral poles too far anteriorly (too much translation), and joint noise at the beginning of closing. If unilateral subluxation occurs, there will be a quick deviation from midline to the contralateral side at the end of opening.

In premature translation during jaw opening, translation occurs within the first 11 mm of opening. Such a movement is contrary to normal arthrokinematic movements of the jaw, in which translation begins only after the first 11 mm of opening.

Both translation occurring too soon and subluxations are conditions that are believed to involve muscle imbalances. There may be no actual temporomandibular joint dysfunction present with these two conditions, and they may occur separately or together in some patients. Their long-range effect on the temporomandibular joint, however, can lead to temporomandibular joint dysfunction. If either or both of these conditions are observed, it is important to control them to minimize the stress placed on the intracapsular tissues and prevent the perpetuation of temporomandibular joint dysfunction that is present and may be a hindering factor to treatment.

Dislocation of the Jaw

Dislocation may result from actual trauma to the chin during opening of the mouth, or it may occur without actual trauma, such as with a sudden muscular spasm during a yawn. This dislocation is always anterior and may be unilateral or bilateral, resulting in displacement of one or both condyles forward into the infratemporal fossa anterior to the articular eminences.[158] In bilateral dislocations, the chin is displaced forward so that the patient shows some degree of prognathism with an open bite. In unilateral dislocation the mandible is displaced toward the non-injured side.

Reduction is accomplished unilaterally by depressing the mandible with the thumb placed on the last molar teeth and at the same time elevating the chin. The downward pressure overcomes the spasm of the elevating muscles, and elevating the chin repositions the condyles backward behind the articular eminences. Reduction is usually followed by several days of rest.[156]

Habitual dislocation, subluxations, or self-reducing dislocations are not especially rare. According to Dufourmentel and Axhausen, there are two kinds of habitual subluxation that patients themselves may learn to adjust either by a special jaw movement or with the hand. These are luxation in the upper cavity (meniscotemporal) and luxation in the lower cavity (meniscocondylar).[7,48]

Derangement of the Disk

Trauma, overclosure of the mouth with backward displacement of the condyle, or malocclusion may cause derangement of the disk. Trauma to the disk can vary from an inflammatory condition to a complete or partial tearing of the disk from its capsular attachment. If the disk remains attached to the anterior capsule and the external pterygoid, an anterior dislocation of the disk occurs. It may be manifested by displacement of the mandible toward the affected side and possible blockage of mandibular opening and closing.[158] If the disk remains attached to the posterior capsule, a painful blockage in closing the mandible results.[158]

The most widely accepted view is that clicking is the result of derangement of the disk. However, many investigators have reported various other theories of its etiology in addition to derangement of the disk. Among these are incoordinate contraction of the two bodies of the lateral pterygoid, so that the disk snaps over the condyle rather than following the movement smoothly and coordinately when the mouth is open;

deterioration of the disk and cartilaginous surfaces; and stretching of the joint ligaments by frequent subluxation.[159]

Clicking may occur as one or more clicks in one joint, or clicking may occur in both joints; it may or may not be associated with pain. Various types of clicking noises have been observed during sagittal opening, including an opening click, an intermediate click during the opening phase, and a full opening click. Each of these clicks appears to be associated with various pathological occlusions.

An opening click is believed to be due to an anterior displacement of the disk, with the condyle displaced posteriorly and superiorly. As the mandible opens, the condyle must pass over the posterior surface of the disk.[159]

Clicking during various parts of the opening of the mandible is believed to result from incoordinate movements of the upper and lower heads of the external pterygoid, so that the condyle cannot remain in its normal relationship with the disk.[159] More likely causes are possible anteroposterior displacement of the disk and ruptures or rents of the disk.[188]

A final click occurring in the full opening phase may be caused by the condyle passing over the anterior portion of the disk, by the disk being pulled forward of the condyle, or by both the disk or condyle passing over the articular eminence.[159]

In addition to clicks produced during mandibular opening, clicks may be produced by eccentric movements. Again, these may be largely due to structural changes in disks or incoordinate functioning of the parts of the joint.[159]

Crepitus has been associated with perforation of the disk. Moffett and co-workers demonstrated that perforation of the disk is usually followed by osteoarthritic change on the condylar surface, which is, in turn, followed by similar bony alterations on the opposing surface of the fossa.[124] The most common disk–condyle derangements that present clinically are anterior disk derangements in which there are anterior disk dislocations that reduce and those that do not reduce.[55]

The classic signs of the type of anterior disk dislocation that reduces are (1) a distinguished, sometimes loud click or pop during mandibular opening, signifying that the disk has relocated itself with respect to the condyle, and (2) a more subtle click usually occurring during mandibular closing and signifying that the disk has displaced itself anterior to the mandibular condyle. The sign of an anterior disk dislocation that does not reduce is the absence of joint noises with a series of reproducible restrictions during mandibular movements. These restrictions are due to the disk blocking translatory glide.

TEMPOROMANDIBULAR EVALUATION

I. History

The general format of the initial evaluation should follow the same lines of questioning as set out in Chapter 5. Information on when the problem started and how it occurred as well as previous management and the results obtained is helpful. If the problem was caused by injury or surgical procedure, the therapist will need to know what was done by the attending personnel and physicians. A most important aspect of taking the history is the attempt to clarify any emotional factors in the patient's background that may provoke habitual protrusion or muscular tension.

The history may be handwritten from answers to verbal questions. A more complete history may be obtained, however, by using a personal history form, which is completed by the patient. After reviewing the form, all pertinent facts may be reviewed in detail with the patient. The work of Day,[45] Shore,[159] and Morgan and Rosen[128] provides excellent detailed outlines and the rationale for obtaining such information as a means of compiling a complete history relating specifically to temporomandibular joint disorders. Such forms have been designed to include most of the information that will be found useful in treating temporomandibular joint disorders and related orofacial problems. Certainly no specific set of questions is adequate, and more detailed questioning will usually be necessary. It is also unlikely that the therapist will obtain all relevant information at the initial evaluation. A few pertinent questions that apply particularly to temporomandibular joint disorders include the following:

1. Does the joint grate, click, pop, snap, or lock?
2. Do you have difficulty opening and closing your mouth?
3. Do you have frequent headaches? What area of the head? How long do they last?
4. Have you ever had a severe blow to the head or a whiplash injury?
5. Are your jaws clenched or your teeth sore when you awaken from sleep?

Perhaps one of the most common complaints of head pain is what is generally termed *tension headache*. Berry had studied 100 patients with mandibular dysfunction pain and reports that over 50 percent of his patients had headaches and pain in the neck, back, and shoulders.[15] This condition may be the result of structural cervical disease, may be associated with vascular pain syndrome, or may occur as a separate entity.[14,45]

II. Physical Examination

A. *Observation.* Record significant findings. The physical examination, in a sense, occurs simultaneously when the clinician takes the history. The appearance, general posture, and characteristics of bodily movements are often revealing. Physically the typical patient with temporomandibular joint pain–dysfunction, with an emotional overlay, has a posture of elevated shoulders, forward head, stiff neck and back, and shallow, restricted breathing.[86] The patient is observed for facial expression and habits of the jaw (*e.g.,* clenching or grinding the teeth, biting the fingers, or twitching the masseter).

The most common abnormality in the cervical spine with direct impact on the temporomandibular joint, cranial facial area, and temporomandibular area is the FHP. Any increase in the sternocleidomastoid (SCM) angulation or distance from the thoracic apex to mid-cervical region manifested by forward inclination of the head and neck constitutes a FHP (see Fig. 17-16). Angulation of the sternocleidomastoid is considered to be minimal at 60°, moderate at 60° to 75°, and maximal at 75° to 90°.[112] Internal rotation of the glenohumeral joint and protraction of the shoulder girdle may also be observed. The scapulae may be protracted, retracted, elevated, or winged.

B. *Inspection of the head, face, and neck.* Record significant findings.

1. *Skin.* Examine the face for blemishes, moles, pigmentations, scars, and texture.

2. *Soft tissue.* Note any swelling. Swelling of the joint must be moderate or marked before it is apparent on inspection. If swelling is detectable, it appears as a rounded bulge just anterior to the external meatus. The face should be further examined for atrophies and hypertrophies. Asking the patient to clench his jaws together may help to disclose asymmetry.

3. *Bony structure and alignment.* Record significant findings. The profile of the face in both the frontal and sagittal planes will reveal the relative development of the skull, face, and mandible. The size of the mandible should be compared with that of the skull and abnormal positions or asymmetry of the jaw noted. Asymmetry may be indicative of a growth or developmental problem or unusual muscular activity. Take particular note of the occlusal and rest positions of the jaw. An abnormal protrusive position may be associated with tongue thrust (deviant swallowing) or habitual protrusion. The evaluation described by Kraus to determine the presence of an acquired adult tongue thrust is helpful.[99] The patient is asked to swallow water several times, pausing between each swallow while the therapist palpates the hyoid bone and the suboccipital muscles (see Fig. 15-19). Normally a quick up and down movement of the hyoid should be felt with minimal contraction of the suboccipital muscles. With an acquired anterior adult tongue thrust, a slow up and down movement of the hyoid bone is felt along with significant suboccipital muscle contraction. Excessive forward movement of the entire head and neck and lip may be noted.

The examiner should briefly inspect the upper spine, shoulder girdles, and arms for obvious muscle atrophy or deformities.

C. *Selective tissue tension tests.* Record significant findings. Before examining the temporomandibular joint movements, the resting position of the mandible and tongue is noted by the clinician by parting the patient's lips (or using a lip separator) to reveal the alignment of the incisors as well as any evidence of abnormal resting position of the tongue or a deviant swallow (see section on dynamics of the mandible and temporomandibular joint).

1. *Active movements* (with passive overpressure). Observe the general patterns of active movements (depression, elevation, lateral deviation, protraction, retraction) for freedom of movement, range, and symmetry. Ascertain if any pain accompanies active movements and in what part of the range it occurs and where. Pain may be felt in the area of the joint and about the ear, but often it is felt diffusely through the face, teeth, jaws, and mouth. Masticatory pain is typically not well localized. (During the palpation portion of the examination, actual sites of tenderness can be established.)

Abnormal movements such as "jumps" or "facet slips" should be noted. In particular the patient is asked to open his mouth to a limited extent (about 1 cm) while the examiner observes whether the mandible is making an initial rotation or translatory movement. Forward movement will be revealed by a reduction in incisal overjet and by excessive prominence of the condylar heads.

The restriction of movement, deviations to one side, and asynchronous patterns of movement are recorded; the maximum opening the patient can achieve without pain is measured. Lateral movements to the left and right, using the bite position as the control as well as protrusion–retrusion, again using normal bite as control, should be recorded when restricted. Lateral motions may be lost earlier and to a greater degree than vertical motions.

A T bar is often used for recording active motion and abnormal tracking of the mandible during opening.

a. *Mandibular opening and closing:* The client should be able to put at least two of his or her knuckles between the upper and lower incisors for normal jaw opening. Measurement of maximal voluntary mandibular opening can be obtained by measuring between the maxillary and mandibular incisal edges with a ruler scaled in millimeters (Fig. 15-20). Measurements may be recorded on the vertical plane of the T bar. Normal mandibular opening has been reported to be between 35 to 50 mm[1,2,79] when using this method, or from 48 to 52 mm when measured from acquired occlusion (including vertical overlap).[54,55,88] To complete 40 mm of functional range, 25 mm is rotational and 15 mm occurs with anterior and inferior translational glide.[84,129,147]

The vertical path of the mandible during opening and closing should be recorded for deviations or deflections. A deviation is defined as a lateral movement of the mandible that returns to midline prior to maximal opening, whereas a deflection is a lateral movement without return to midline.[189] If deflection occurs to the right on opening with limited motion, the right temporomandibular joint is said to be hypomobile (see Fig. 15-20). If the mandible abnormally tracks (deviates) out of midline (*i.e.*, in an S-type curve) the problem is probably due to muscle imbalance (see Fig. 15-20).

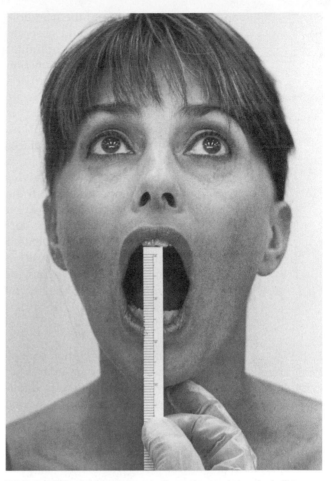

FIG. 15-20. Measurement of maximum intercisal distance.

b. *Lateral characteristics* (ROM and deviations or deflections): Lateral movements are normally 8 to 10 mm when the midline of the maxillary and mandibular incisors are viewed in the normal adult.[189] Movement of 50 percent or less is indicative of an intracapsular restriction in the temporomandibular joint contralateral to the side of lateral movement.[189] Measurements may be recorded on the horizontal plane of the T bar.

c. *Protrusion characteristics* (ROM and deviations or deflections): Protrusion is defined as the distance through which the lower teeth can move horizontally past the maxillary teeth. It may be measured by the distance between the upper and lower central incisor teeth. The normal adult should have 5 mm of movement from the position of centric occlusion in which the front teeth are opposed.[176] Loss of movement in one temporomandibular joint will result in an ipsilateral deviation of the mandible ascertained by palpation and observation. Pain at the end of range or limitation can be due to joint dysfunction (*e.g.*, synovitis or a capsular sprain) or a displaced disk.[14,84]

d. *Retrusion characteristics:* Retrusion is measured the same way as protrusion. Full retrusion, or centric relation, places the temporomandibular joints in a close-packed position with the condyles resting on the center of the disk in the uppermost and most posterior position in the fossa. Graber[72] states that normally there is 3 to 4 mm of movement from the position of rest to the position of centric relation. Pain, weakness, or limitation of range can be caused by the muscles or their nerve supply. Intracapsular injury causes pain at the end of active retrusion.[14]

It should be noted whether pain is provoked when the jaws are in firm occlusion and when the patient is asked to bite against a tongue blade on one side. Such tests help distinguish muscle spasms from diskitis and retrodiskitis.[14]

2. *Passive movements* (anatomical ranges). With passive movements, in addition to seeing how easily the jaw can be moved and making a comparison with active range of motion, note the type of end feel as well as the presence of pain and spasms. To determine the nature of the end feel, have the patient open his mouth and then apply additional pressure with the thumbs and index fingers on the edge of the upper and lower teeth, noting the type of end feel present. Passive movements should routinely include depression, elevation, protraction, retraction, and lateral movements.

One of the most common intracapsular dysfunctions of the temporomandibular joint is internal derangement of the articular disk. This is characterized by a posterior-superior displacement of the condyle and anterior displacement of the disk. The most common signs of internal derangements are (1) reciprocal clicking, (2) disk displacement without reduction (locking), or (3) subluxation indicating condyle/disk incoordination.[168]

Two specific pathological conditions of the temporomandibular joint should be

recognized: (1) hypermobility with excessive translational glide, clicking, and subluxation; and (2) locking of the joint that is characterized by hypomobility. Locking can be of two major types and present with different types of end feel.[24]

a. The first type of locking is due to shortening of the periarticular connective tissues as a defensive mechanism. With passive stretch there is gummy end feel and a considerable increase in range of motion after stretching.

b. Closed-lock caused by anterior displacement of the disk is characterized by a hard end-feel with limited motion. Passive stretch will produce little or no increase in range of motion.

3. *Resisted movement* (static tests). Determine the strength and presence of pain by applying resistance to mandibular opening, protrusion, and lateral deviations. Pain arising in the pterygoid muscles may be provoked by resisted deviation to the painful side as well as clenching the teeth. Weakness of the muscles that close the mouth is rather uncommon, since strength is usually maintained by mastication.

It is not necessary to employ all such tests in the examination of every patient, although they are often helpful in localizing pain and should be done when indicated. Tests which are particularly important include:

a. *Resisted mandible depression:* Resistance is applied to the underside of the mandible while the client attempts to keep the mouth open (1–2 cm). The lateral pterygoids and hyoids can present with pain or weakness caused by injury to the muscle or nerve supply. Imbalance problems may cause temporomandibular joint problems or result from temporomandibular joint dysfunction.

b. *Resisted mandible lateral excursion:* With good stabilization of the head, the examiner should ask the patient to open her jaw slightly and then resist lateral excursion to each side. A weak lateral pterygoid may not be obvious on resisted depression but becomes evident with resisted excursion when compared bilaterally.

c. *Resisted protrusion:* This motion tests the lateral and medial pterygoids, not the suprahyoids. It can confirm a suspected weakness from resisted mandible depression.

4. *Passive joint-play movements:* Since movements are small and difficult to feel, one can obtain more information by applying repeated gentle oscillations. The movements are classified as normal, hypomobile, or hypermobile. Many of the joint mobilizations for the temporomandibular joint are extensions of the mobility testing. For more details of carrying out the tests, see the joint mobilization section (see Figs. 15-29 to 15-33). The most common accessory movements tested are:

   a. Caudal traction, produced by distraction of the joint by pressure over the lower mandible.

   b. Ventral glide (protrusion), produced by placing the index and third finger over the angle of the ramus.

   c. Medial-lateral glide, produced by the fingers and hypothenar eminence around the patient's mandible.

   d. Medial-lateral glide, produced by placing the thumb in the patient's mouth and over the medial surface of the mandible head.

   e. Medial glide applied directly to the condyle by thumb pressure.[110,177]

      Note stability, mobility, presence of pain, guarding, spasm, and behavior.

D. *Palpation*

   1. *Skin.* Palpate for warmth, tenderness, temperature, moisture, and mobility.

   2. *Muscles.* Palpate for consistency, mobility, continuity, tenderness, pain, and signs of spasm. Palpation of the muscles of mastication should routinely include the origin and insertion of the masseter, temporalis, internal pterygoid, and the insertion of the external pterygoid (see Fig. 17-28).[156]

      When indicated, all the muscles of the maxillary facial region should be palpated including the facial muscles, sublingual, suprahyoids and the cervical muscles, especially the sternocleidomastoid and longus colli (See Figs. 17-27 to 17-29). Various structural or functional cervical diseases may result in spasms of the masticatory muscles. A comprehensive thesis on the musculature and differential diagnosis of orofacial pain is described by Bell.[14] Always compare bilaterally. With respect to the temporomandibular joint itself, musculature and insertions that should be included are the following:

a. *Insertion of the temporalis:* Palpation of the insertion on the coronoid process is best achieved intraorally by placing the finger lateral to the first mandibular molar and following the ramus of the mandible in a posterior direction until the tip of the coronoid can be felt (Fig. 15-21). Tenderness is often due to overuse of the muscles of mastication or bruxism.

b. *Medial pterygoid:* Palpate externally on the anterior edge of the ramus and intraorally to the lower medial surfaces of the ramus (Fig. 15-22).

c. *Lateral pterygoid:* Intraorally, use the index finger to palpate this muscle behind the last molar toward the neck of the mandible. Slide a finger along the buccal aspect of the maxillary dentition until the tuberosity region is reached and then palpate superiorly and medially in the region of the hamular process of the pterygoid process (Fig. 15-23). Wide opening will elicit point tenderness of the muscle.[30]

d. *Digastric:* Palpation of the anterior digastric is accomplished by having the patient open the jaw against resistance and finding the body of the muscle medial and also most parallel to the inferior border of the mandible (Fig. 15-24A). For the posterior aspect of the digastric, palpate near the angle of the ramus while instructing the patient to swallow (Fig. 15-24B). The muscle felt to be contracting is the digastric. The hyoid bone can also be checked for mo-

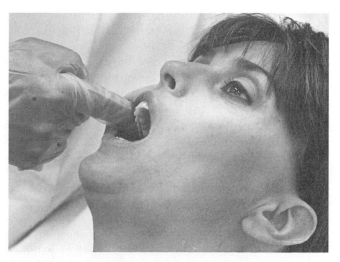

FIG. 15-21. Palpation of the insertion of the temporalis.

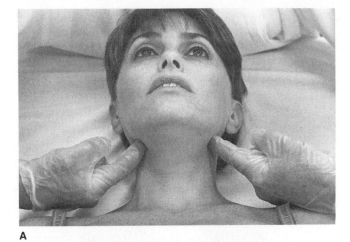

A

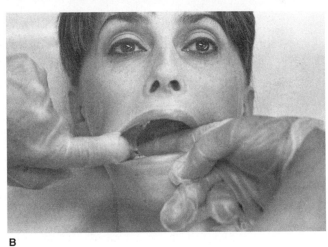

B

FIG. 15-22. Palpation of the medial pterygoid: (**A**) external palpation and (**B**) interorally.

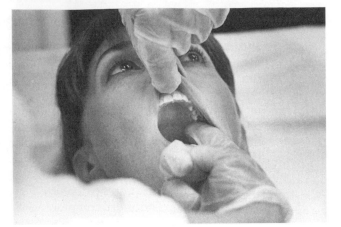

FIG. 15-23. Palpation of the lateral pterygoid.

bility by manipulating it while asking the patient to swallow (see Fig. 15-19). If there is greater tension of the digastric on one side, there may be lateral deviation of the hyoid and thyroid cartilage, and increased resistance to shifting of midline structures away from the deviating side.

　e. *Mylohyoid:* This muscle, which forms the floor of the mouth, can be easily palpated intraorally as well as extraorally.

3. *Temporomandibular joint.* First, palpate the condylar heads laterally with the mouth closed; then palpate the distal aspect with the jaw apart for tenderness. Determine if any such tenderness is definitely accentuated when the mandible is moved contralaterally. This maneuver brings the condyle more firmly under the palpating finger. The posterior aspect can be palpated through the external auditory meatus with

the palpating finger. Pain and tenderness on palpation suggests a capsulitis, particularly if tenderness is found posteriorly. Abnormal capsular thickening, warmth, and swelling should also be noted. Moderate degrees of swelling in the joint prevent the fingertip from entering the depressed area overlying the joint. Swelling of a marked degree may be palpable as a rounded, often fluctuant mass overlying the joint.

The range and dynamics of condylar motion can also be ascertained by means of palpation. From a position behind the patient, the examiner's forefingers are placed on the lateral aspects of the condylar heads as the patient actively opens his mouth. Inability to feel protrusion of the condylar head suggests a lack of forward movement.

The examiner can determine the presence and the amount of rotation by placing the fingertips in the ear. Palpation should be done bilaterally so that a comparison of both joints can be made and any asymmetrical movements ascertained. Palpable snapping, clicking, or jumps should also be noted.

During jaw opening, translation and rotation should occur simultaneously and at a similar ratio to one another throughout range of motion.[120] The relative contribution of these two motions should be analyzed. Distraction techniques are somewhat more effective in restoring rotation while ventral glide is more helpful in restoring translation when it appears to be deficient.

4. *Bony palpation:* Palpate the posterior structures of the neck (spinous processes, facet

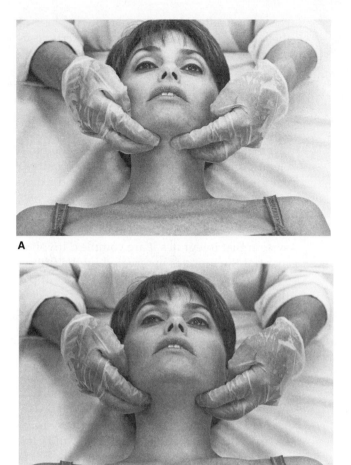

A

B

FIG. 15-24. Palpation of the (**A**) anterior digastric and (**B**) posterior digastric.

joints) and the bones of the skull and temporal bone (including the mastoid process) for tenderness, deformity, and symmetry. Palpate along the entire length of the mandible, maxilla, and zygomatic bone for bony asymmetry, growth irregularities, and suspected fracture sites.

Anteriorly, palpate the hyoid bone and note its relations to C2–C3. In FHP with shortening of the suprahyoids it is often elevated and may be displaced somewhat posteriorly. Ask the patient to swallow. Normally, the hyoid bone should move and cause no pain. With the neck in a neutral position, the thyroid cartilage can be easily moved back and forth with the index finger and thumb (see Fig. 17-28H). Motion may be limited with loss of normal crepitations following traumatic injury to the cervical spine and under circumstances of overuse (*e.g.*, musicians who play wind instruments).[110] Bony palpation should in-

clude palpation of the zygomatic arch, the hyoid bone, and the upper cervical spine.

5.   *Auscultation.* Palpation of the temporomandibular movements often reveals the presence of clicking or crepitus. However, such sounds can be more accurately evaluated with the bell of a stethoscope placed over the condylar head as the patient actively opens his mouth. Note the type of sound associated with the movements and particular phase of movement in which it occurs. All movements—opening, closing, lateral deviation, protrusion, and retrusion—should be assessed.

The placement of a tongue depressor between the molar teeth, onto which the patient bites, occasionally eliminates the click, possibly because its presence frees the disk from the condyle prior to opening fully.[30]

E.   *Selective loading of the temporomandibular joint can aid in determining intracapsular pathological conditions.*

Tests may include the following:

1.   *Dynamic loading of one joint.* Have the patient bite forcefully on a cotton roll or tongue blade on one side. This procedure loads the contralateral temporomandibular joint and may elicit pain.

2.   *Posterior loading (compression) of both temporomandibular joints.* Grasp the mandible with both hands. The thumbs are placed on the most distal molars or alveolar ridge with the fingers beneath the mandible. The mandible is then tipped down and back to compress the joints. The mandible may also be moved forward or backward to localize tenderness in the posterior or inferior parts of the joint.

3.   *Distraction (unloading) or caudal traction.* Using the same handhold as above, distraction of both joints is performed at the same time or caudal traction of each joint is performed separately (see Fig. 15-29).

Frequently the incisors are not aligned, with the mandible being deviated to one side. To assess the relevance of this deformity to the patient's symptoms, the examiner passively attempts to correct the deformity.[177] If the deviation is a protective deformity, then this test will increase the pain.

F.   *Dental and oral examination.* Make a general survey of the oral cavity, since both facial pain as well as temporomandibular joint disorders may have their origin in dental or oral lesions.[118] The examination of the teeth and their supporting structures, other oral structures, and mucosa is important.

By having the patient open his mouth maximally, the examiner is able to observe the oropharynx, tonsillar areas, and surfaces of the palate and tongue. Any alteration in the color and texture of the lingual tissues is noted. Palpations are included.

Cavities and restored and missing teeth should be noted. Wear of biting edges and chewing surfaces that appears excessive for the patient's age often points to tensional oral habits such as bruxism. Also, the occlusion of the teeth, premature contact, overclosure of the vertical dimension, and the degree of overjet are noted.[38] Detailed occlusal analysis should always be deferred until muscle relaxation has been achieved.

Faulty occlusion may be the most common cause of temporomandibular joint dysfunction and pain. Malocclusion patterns are categorized according to the relationship of the first molars (upper and lower) to each other.

Class I: Mesiodistal first molar relationship is normal but there are tooth irregularities elsewhere.

Class II, division 1: The lower first molar is posterior to the upper first molar, causing mandibular retrusion which is usually reflected in the client's profile.

Class II, division 2: The lower first molar is posterior to the upper first molar but greater than in division 1, causing a large overbite.

Class III: The lower first molar is anterior to upper first molar, causing an underbite with mandibular protrusion.

A bimaxillary protrusion exists when the occlusion is normal but the entire dentition is forward with respect to the facial profile. When a vertical space exists between the upper and lower anterior teeth in centric occlusion, the condition is called an open bite.

Malocclusion can lead to temporomandibular disk problems, joint deterioration, and muscle imbalances. Individuals with class II malocclusion are more prone to muscle and joint dysfunction than clients with class I or class III.[84] Both the bimaxillary protrusion and anterior open bite encourage soft tissue disorders of the tongue and lips.

Other types of malocclusion causing temporomandibular symptoms include the loss of posterior teeth without replacement, loss of the vertical dimension of the jaw (*vertical dimension* is the distance from the bottom of the nose to the tip of the chin), and an off-center bite. Decreased vertical dimension will lead to excessive temporomandibular joint compression and shortening of the muscles of mastication, whereas an off-center bite (which can originate from or cause overwork to the muscles on one side of the jaw) typically results in compression on the shortened side and extension on the opposite side.

G. *Sensory and motor response.* Masticatory and orofacial functioning and the neurological system that integrates it are complex. Involvement of the muscles innervated by the fifth to 12th cranial nerves and at least the upper three cervical spinal nerves may be reflected in masticatory malfunctioning or pain. Not only the chief masticatory and secondary muscles but also the muscles of the lips, cheeks, tongue, floor of the mouth, neck, palate, and pharynx may be involved. Sensory as well as motor function testing may be indicated.

The characteristic muscular imbalance is increased activity in the masticatory muscles, which are tight, whereas the muscles that govern the opening of the mouth (mainly the digastric and the deep neck flexors) are relatively weak.[105]

Sensory testing of the cutaneous nerve supply of the face, scalp, and neck should be included if a neural deficit or neural problem is suspected (Fig. 15-25). The examiner must be aware of the dermatomal pattern for the head and neck as well. Upper limb reflexes (see Fig. 17-22) and the jaw reflex should be tested for

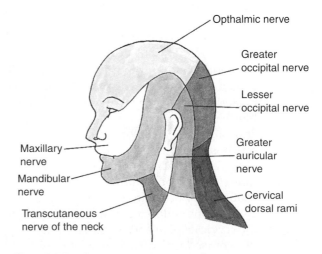

FIG. 15-25. Cutaneous nerve supply.

possible damage to the fifth cranial nerve. To test the jaw reflex, the examiner's thumb is placed on the patient's chin with his or her mouth slightly open. Tapping is done with the finger or reflex hammer (Fig. 15-26).

H. *Other tests.* A cervical–upper extremity scan examination is frequently indicated in the evaluation of temporomandibular joint disorders (see Chapter 18, The Cervical–Upper Limb Scan Examination). It should be noted that the upper cervical spinal nerves are more likely sources of pain that refers or spreads to the masticatory region than are the lower cervical nerves. The upper cervical joints (occipito-atlantal, atlanto-axial) and suboccipital muscles that are supplied by C1 to C3 nerves have been shown to refer pain into the frontal, retro-orbital, temporal, and occipital areas of the head.[39,56,63,104] Passive movements (physiological) and passive joint-play movements of the upper cervical spine should be included (see Chapter 17, The Cervical Spine).[110,177]

Adjuncts, such as roentgenography and electromyography, may be indicated. Only electromyography can reveal how a muscle acts at any point during mandibular movements and postures; some researchers believe that electromyography is more reliable diagnostically than roentgenograms of the temporomandibular joints.[18,110,127]

Analgesic blocking of tender muscles of the joint proper may be needed to confirm the source of pain as well as to help identify secondary pain effects.[14]

Examination of the ear, nose, and throat may be necessary to exclude a variety of diagnosable and treatable conditions that may be confused with temporomandibular joint pathology. In addition to the history and clinical examination, further procedures are often necessary to evaluate tinnitus, hearing loss, and vertigo to establish or rule out an otological or neurological cause for these symptoms.

III. Interpretation of Findings

Bourbon[24] and others have found the use of the three types of syndromes of the spine, described by McKenzie, helpful in identifying the source of pain and a plan of care to reduce or eliminate pain and the effects of the pathological mechanism in mechanical dysfunction of the temporomandibular joint. They are described below as they relate to temporomandibular joint pathology.

A. *Derangement syndrome:* The temporomandibular joint in which normal articular alignments are disrupted is prone to internal derangements. These are defined as some type of mechanical restriction that alters the temporomandibular joint function. Disk displacement with reduction (clicking) may manifest itself by the disk displacing in any of several directions. The most common direction of displacement is anteromedial.[168] Locking occurs when the disk becomes lodged anterior to the condyle.

B. *The postural syndrome:* A postural syndrome presenting as prolonged FHP is a classic example of a condition causing increasing stress to the joint and causing pain. Restoration of normal posture may help to normalize the joint. However, adaptive changes often lead to a dysfunction syndrome.

C. *Dysfunction syndromes* typically present with abnormal ranges of motion as the result of changes in the surrounding tissue. There are two major categories: hypermobility and hypomobility. Osteoarthritis, skeletal limitations, and reduced vertical dimensions secondary to poor posture are often followed by capsular restriction and muscle tightness leading to limited range of motion.

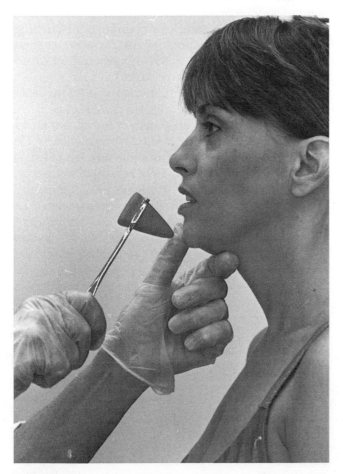

FIG. 15-26. Testing of the jaw reflex.

■ COMMON LESIONS

□ Temporomandibular Joint Dysfunction Syndrome

A common temporomandibular joint disorder found clinically is temporomandibular joint dysfunction syndrome, also referred to as mandibular pain–dysfunction syndrome, arthrosis temporomandibularis,[159] temporomandibular joint arthrosis, and myofascial pain syndrome.

Temporomandibular joint dysfunction syndrome cannot be considered a disease of aging or senility, since it commonly occurs in patients between the ages of 20 and 40 years.[156] It is most frequently found among women. The early incoordination phase associated with clicking, subluxation, and recurrent dislocation is most commonly found among women in the third to fourth decade of life and in men during the third decade. The later limitation phase occurs most frequently in women in the fourth to fifth decade of life.[157]

Signs and symptoms of the early incoordination phase are usually unilateral but may be bilateral. They may include muscular tenderness, limited motion, and a dull aching pain in the periarticular area often radiating to the ear, face, head, neck, and shoulders and aggravated by function. Usually, the syndrome first manifests itself in the form of functional incoordination of the mandibular muscles with symptoms of clicking in the temporomandibular joint, which is otherwise asymptomatic, and subluxation or recurrent dislocation. Additionally, clinical examination often reveals hypermobility of the joints or a tendency to protrude the mandible or both during the initial opening movement.[166] These symptoms are followed in many cases by spasms of the masticatory muscles characterized by pain on movement of the joint, especially during mastication. Gradually, the pain becomes worse and is accompanied by decreased mobility. Pain and mobility tend to be worse in the morning. In unilateral conditions, the mandible deviates to the symptomatic side, resulting in compensation of the contralateral joint by hypermobility, subluxation, and irregular mandibular opening and closing movements. Mandibular "catching" or "locking" in certain positions may also occur on opening. Often pain may accompany movement of the hypermobile joint and may require treatment as well.

The temporomandibular joint dysfunction syndrome is usually reversible, but its perpetuation may and often does result in organic changes. When spontaneous recovery does not occur and when spasm is not relieved by treatment, such spasm may set up a sustaining cycle. If dysfunction is of a long duration, contracture of the masticatory muscles with limited painless mandibular movement may occur. This is referred to as the *limitation phase*. At this stage, pathological changes are noted and are mainly degenerative. They are located in the fibrous covering of the articular eminence, in the condylar head, and in the fibrous articular disk. There is, however, little evidence to support the view that there is a relationship between degenerative changes within the joint and symptoms of temporomandibular joint dysfunction.[156] Marked changes are often seen without symptoms, and frequently marked symptoms are seen without radiographic evidence of changes in structure. When arthrosis of the temporomandibular joint shows extreme changes in the structure of the joint or joints, the disease is sometimes referred to as *arthrosis temporomandibularis deformans*.[159]

It is generally accepted that temporomandibular joint dysfunction–pain syndrome is a neuromuscular or joint dysfunction and that the etiology of pain is multicausal. The five major causes of pain may be neurological, vascular, the joint itself, muscular, or hysterical conversion.[187] Pain that originates from the joints themselves can be caused by infection, disk derangement, condylar displacement, microtrauma, and traumatic injury.[185] Many patients, particularly those with painful limited mandibular movements, complain of sudden onset of symptoms on awaking, after rapid or extensive mandibular opening (*e.g.*, yawning, or after a long dental appointment), or when changes are made in occlusion (*e.g.*, through restoration, grinding, or the use of a dental appliance).

Many authors point out that many conditions called temporomandibular joint disorders are not, in the strict sense of the word, disorders of the joint at all but simply dysfunction of the masticatory muscles.[131] The presence of painful areas within the muscles and signs of mandibular dysfunction were Schwartz's most constant finding.[156] Such painful areas and accompanying dysfunction have been given various names such as *myalgia, myositis, fibrositis*, and *myofascial pain syndromes*. The precipitating factor is believed to be motion that stretches the muscle, setting off a self-sustaining cycle of pain, spasm, and pain. The muscles that are commonly involved are the masseters, medial and lateral pterygoids, temporalis, suprahyoids, infrahyoids, sternocleidomastoids, scaleni, and rhomboids. The muscles most frequently involved are the lateral pterygoids.

Myofascial pain syndrome (MPS) has been defined as a regional pain syndrome accompanied by trigger point(s).[33,61,62,161,175] Diagrams have been published depicting the areas of trigger points and the zones of referred pain on palpation of these points.[61,62,161,174,175] Friction and co-workers[60,61] quantified the areas of pain with their trigger points among patients seen in a temporomandibular joint and craniofacial clinic. A large majority of the patients understandably had pain in the jaw (63 percent) and the temporomandibular joint area (56 percent).

Rheumatologists and clinicians have attempted to categorize myofascial pain into distinct syndromes, with specific criteria applying to each one. For categorization purposes, the syndromes are generally classified into two distinct categories, each with specific criteria: MPS and primary fibromyalgia (fibromyalgia syndrome) (Table 15-1).[33,190,193–195] The fibromyalgia syndrome (FMS) is considered a form of nonarticular rheumatism characterized by widespread musculoskeletal aching and stiffness, as well as tenderness on palpation at characteristic sites, called *tender points*.[163,190,194] It occurs predominantly among females; only 5 to 20 percent of the patients are males.[70,190,193–195]

The most common and characteristic symptoms of fibromyalgia are generalized pain, stiffness, fatigue, poor sleep, edema, and paresthesia. Associated symptoms include chronic headache, primary dysmenorrhea, and irritable bowel syndrome.[193,194] Common sites of pain or stiffness are the neck, scapular girdle and shoulder region, arm, hand, low back, pelvic girdle, hips, and knees[194]; however, many other sites including the anterior chest[134,194] and temporomandibular joint may be involved.[19,20,51,114,130,179,182] The most significant finding related to FMS is the presence of multiple tender points.[162,163,190,195]

Myofascial manipulations, flexibility, and low-grade strength training, cardiovascular training, transcutaneous nerve stimulation, biofeedback, cryotherapy, acupressure, stress management, and patient education all apply to the management of FMS and MPS. Myofascial manipulations become more regional than global in the management of MPS with specific emphasis on trigger point areas. It is possible to stimulate trigger points in a number of ways. These include deep pressure (acupressure), ultrasound, massage with an ice cube, dry needling with a hypodermic or acupuncture needle, laser therapy, and strain–counterstrain.[26,90,102] Another method, developed by Travel, is to spray the area from the trigger point to the reference zone with a vapocoolant spray while at the same time stretching the muscle to its fullest length. This is best followed by the application of moist heat and a home stretching exercise program. Since postural and muscle imbalances are more common in MPS, strengthening and elongation are emphasized.[33]

Emotional tension may also play a predominant role. With stress, the tension of the skeletal muscles increases, often with clenching of the teeth or bruxism resulting in local disharmony of the masticatory apparatus. When hypertonicity occurs in the masticatory muscles for a long period of time, pain-dysfunction syndrome, occlusal wear, and tooth mobility may be evident. Once the pattern is established, it appears to be self-perpetuating. Other habit manifestations seen in these patients that cause pathological occlusal contact are numerous and include unilateral mastication, abnormal swallowing, and "tooth doodling" during the waking hours.[68,166] What the patient does to his occlusion in reaction to stress seems to be more important than any existing malocclusion. Certainly malocclusion, by mechanically increasing the amount of force or altering its direction, can make the chance of injury more likely. More important than the type of malocclusion, however, may be the amount and kind of muscular activity and the reaction of the person to such activity. In some persons, change in proprioception, no matter how slight, seems to be more important than a long-standing malocclusion, no matter how irregular.

Diagnostic procedures to establish the presence of temporomandibular joint dysfunction and a definitive diagnosis include

- An accurate history
- Determination of the patient's emotional state and daily habits
- Examination of mandibular movements
- Measurement of mandibular opening, lateral deviation, and protrusion
- Palpation of the temporomandibular joint and muscles of mastication
- Dental and oral examination
- Occlusal analysis
- Roentgenograms
- Electromyography

TABLE 15-1 SOME DIFFERENCES BETWEEN MYOFASCIAL PAIN SYNDROME (MPS) AND FIBROMYALGIA SYNDROME (FMS)

FEATURES	MPS	FMS
Pain quality	Regional pain	Diffuse, global pain
Physical signs		
Tender-point palpation	Referred	Local
Tender-point anatomy	Muscle belly	Muscle–tendon junction
Stiffness	Regional	Widespread
Sleep patterns	Alpha; disruption of delta sleep in some cases	Alpha; disruption of delta sleep in most cases
Fatigue	Usually absent	Debilitating
Prognosis	Moderately poor; better than FMS	Poor, seldom cured

- Physical examination of related structures (cervical spine)
- Neurological testing

The primary methods of therapy revolve around the correction of occlusal disharmonies and tension habits, as well as physical therapy to eliminate spasm and increase range of motion through therapeutic exercise and mobilization techniques.

☐ Hypermobility

Hypermobility of the temporomandibular joint is defined as a laxity of the articular ligaments. It may be localized or be part of a generalized hypermobility syndrome.[168] Localized hypermobility of the temporomandibular joint is believed to be the most common mechanical disorder.[129] It is characterized by early or excessive anterior translation, or both. Unfortunately, this permits hypertranslation of the condyle, which can lead to dysfunction. This excessive anterior glide results in the laxity of the surrounding capsule and ligaments. It is interesting to note that the temporomandibular joint has no capsule on the medial half of the anterior aspect.[84] The breakdown of these structures enables disk derangement in one or both temporomandibular joints. Ultimately, pain, functional loss, and possibly arthritic changes set in.

Generalized hypermobility, a disorder of increased mobility of multiple joints, has been suggested to be a predisposing factor in the development of degenerative temporomandibular joint disorders.[4,10,11,47,75,83,103,121,137,164,167,170] The results of a study by Dijkstra and colleagues,[46] however, did not support the hypothesis that generalized hypermobility predisposes to temporomandibular joint osteoarthrosis and internal derangement. Future research is necessary in order to determine whether local hypermobility of the temporomandibular joint may be a predisposing factor.

Parafunctional habits that appear to contribute to localized hypermobility of the temporomandibular joint include gum chewing, nail biting, mouth breathing, nocturnal bruxism, prolonged bottle feeding, and pacifier use.[88,151] Hypermobility can also occur when the joint is stretched by trauma subluxations and dislocations.

Presenting signs and symptoms clinically demonstrated by patients with temporomandibular joint hypermobility include the following[84,129]:

1. The ability to insert three or four knuckles between the incisors
2. Excessive joint mobility often characterized by large anterior translation at the beginning of opening when rotation should be occurring

3. Lateral deviation of the mandible during depression or elevation
4. Clicking, popping, or cracking with mandibular depression or elevation
5. Closed or open locking
6. Pain in one or both temporomandibular joints and the surrounding masticatory muscles
7. Tinnitus

Structures that are overstretched in hypermobile joints should be identified and stabilized. A program of muscle retraining in the control of joint rotation and translation and mandibular stabilization should be implemented. Avoiding excessive anterior translation and reestablishing normal head, neck, and shoulder girdle posture have been found to be particularly beneficial, as have splint therapy and stress management.[129]

Existing programs stress exercises that help normalize the position of the jaw, regain normal tracking, and restore the proper sequence of movement. According to Rocabado and Iglarsh,[151] hypermobile joints are best treated by avoiding excessive anterior translational glides of the condyle, controlling rotation, stabilizing the joint, and reestablishing normal head, neck, and shoulder girdle posture.

☐ Degenerative Joint Disease—Osteoarthritis

Although osteoarthritis may occur at any age, it is considered primarily a disease of middle or old age. It affects an estimated 80 to 90 percent of the population over 60 years of age.[78,127]

The etiology is generally believed to be the result of normal wear and tear associated with aging and function, as well as the result of repeated minor trauma. The damage is speculated to consist primarily of degeneration of the chondroitin–collagen-protein complex.[77] Roentgenographic examination may reveal narrowing of the temporomandibular joint space with condensation of bone in the region of the articular cortex, spur formation, and marginal lipping at the articular margins of the condylar head.[77] In some cases there is considerable thickening of the synovial membrane due to chronic synovitis. There may be perforation of the disk without bony changes. Erosion of the condylar head, articular eminence, and fossa may be noted.

Symptoms do not seem to be related to the extent of articular damage. Osteoarthritis may be asymptomatic even in the presence of extensive articular damage, while on the other hand, articular findings may be completely absent in patients with acute symptoms. The onset is generally insidious with mild symptoms. Pain, which is usually a dull aching in or around the joint, is usually not constant. Typically, painful stiffness of the jaw muscles is noted in the morning or following periods of rest. With use, the symptoms may disappear and then reappear with fatigue at the end of the day. Pain may be precipitated on opening or during mastication. Crepitation, crackling, or clicking may occur in one or both joints. Subluxation and locking of one or both joints during certain movements are common complaints. The patient may also complain of symptoms of the ear, impaired hearing, frequent headaches, and dizziness. At the onset, symptoms are usually short-lived, but as degeneration progresses they occur more frequently and last longer. Crepitation and limited motion are the most constant findings.

Diagnostic procedures to establish the presence of osteoarthritis can be difficult but again depend on an accurate history, the determination of the patient's emotional state, physical examination, and roentgenograms. Physical examination may or may not reveal discrete painful areas in the musculature; minimal emotional tension may be noted. Loss of movement is greatest in the upper joint compartment. There is limitation in a capsular pattern of restriction. In unilateral conditions, contralateral excursions and opening are most restricted; protrusion and retrusion are both restricted. There is an ipsilateral deviation of the mandible at the extreme range of opening. Accessory movements are limited and reproduce temporomandibular pain.

The primary method of therapy is directed at symptoms and may involve correcting the occlusion of the teeth or prosthesis, drug therapy, and physical therapy. During the painful phase, the application of hot packs may help to reduce muscle spasm and pain. Active range-of-motion exercises (often in conjunction with ultrasound), passive range-of-motion exercises, mobilization techniques (preceded by deep friction massage to the capsule[40]), and stretching may be used during the chronic phase. Graded exercises involving a few simple movements performed frequently during the day are often prescribed as a home treatment. Advanced bony changes within the joint may necessitate arthroplasty with joint debridement.

Rheumatoid Arthritis

There is little agreement regarding the incidence of patients with rheumatoid arthritis who also develop the disease in the temporomandibular joints; estimates vary from 20 to 51 percent.[77] Women are affected more often than men.

There are three groups of symptoms: transitory, acute, and chronic. Transitory symptoms include limitation of motion and referred pain. Acute symptoms consist of transitory symptoms plus joint pain, swelling, and warmth lasting 6 to 10 weeks. Chronic symptoms are characterized by severe pain and limitation of motion. The joint and muscle symptoms are most severe in the morning and diminish with the day's activity. Inflammatory changes are noted in the synovial membrane and periarticular structures by atrophy and rarefaction of bone. A serious sequela of ankylosis may restrict or even eliminate movement. If symptoms are not relieved by conservative management, surgical intervention may be indicated.

The primary method of therapy is directed at symptoms and may involve drug therapy, if indicated by specific signs and symptoms, and physical therapy. In the acute phase, immobilization is contraindicated but rest in the form of a soft or liquid diet is advocated. After inflammation has subsided, treatment is directed at reducing muscle spasm and restoring mandibular movements by corrective exercises.

Surgical procedures such as condylectomies and condylotomies frequently used in the past are now believed to be obsolete for the most part but are occasionally performed.[153] After surgery, corrective exercises and exercises of mandibular excursions, using mouth props to ensure that range of motion is not compromised, should be performed several times a day.[109]

Trauma and Disorders of Limitation

One of the most frequent causes of temporomandibular joint dysfunction is a direct or indirect blow to the area, including resultant fracture in the region of the condyle. When there is no fracture, injuries may result in edema and possible soft-tissue damage, such as tearing of the capsular ligaments or disk and simple dislocations and subluxations. Other causes of limitation include postoperative trismus following tooth extraction and whiplash injuries.

There is adequate proof that whiplash injuries are responsible for many temporomandibular joint dysfunctions. Whiplash can be explained as a deceleration effect on the mandible and thus on the temporomandibular joint either through direct injury or through neurological involvement. When the head is snapped back abruptly, the mouth flies open, evoking a stretch reflex of the masseter. The capsule, ligaments, and inter-articular disk act as a restraining ligament; tearing or stretching of these tissues may result. Immediately following, the jaw snaps shut; this may strain the attachment of the disk if malocclusion is present. Cervical traction, commonly used in the management of the cervical spine, may also produce temporomandibular joint dysfunction, or the primary temporomandibular joint dysfunction may be aggravated.

Treatment and management of such injuries will depend on the structures involved, the extent of displacement, the effect on function, and the degree of pain. During the acute phase, soft and liquid diets, head bandages or intermaxillary immobilization, and splints may be used to rest the joint. Surgical procedures, open and closed reduction, and manipulations may be necessary.

Physical therapy may consist of heat and other methods to reduce pain and muscle spasm, early mobility exercises after surgery or after immobilization to ensure range of motion is not compromised, and muscle re-education and corrective exercises. Stretching and mobilization techniques may be necessary to treat contracture of the musculature or capsules. When mechanical cervical traction is considered necessary in the treatment of neck and whiplash injuries, the temporomandibular joint should be protected with bite plates or soft splints and the proper use of traction.

☐ Other Conditions

Other conditions that may cause temporomandibular joint dysfunction include a variety of neurological and muscular disorders, bone disease, tumors, infections, psychogenic disorders, growth and developmental disorders, diseases causing disturbance of the occlusion of the teeth or supporting structures, faulty habits of the jaw, and orofacial imbalance.

■ TREATMENT TECHNIQUES

Temporomandibular joint dysfunction, arthritic conditions, ankylosing diseases, traumatic injuries, and postsurgical entities may be a few of the causes that bring a patient to the physical therapist.

When degenerative disease, bony or fibrous ankylosis, fractures, occlusal disharmony, and other conditions necessitate surgery, follow-up physical therapy may become necessary to maintain or regain motion, as well as regain normal mandibular osteokinematics. In the majority of postsurgical cases, muscle tonus remains good, except after long-term ankylosis or degenerative joint disease. In these cases there is greater possibility that the muscles have atrophied, making rehabilitation more difficult and necessitating a more extensive program of therapeutic exercises to increase the physiological elasticity and strength of the muscles.

After condylectomy the attachment of the lateral pterygoid to the condyle has been severed, so that the jaw will increasingly deviate ipsilaterally. Postoperative rehabilitation for the lost function should encourage the similarly functioning muscles of the masseter, temporalis, and suprahyoid muscles on the healthy side to perform with increased strength. At least partial use of the lateral pterygoid muscle should be stressed so that it is able to contribute to contralateral mandibular excursion and to prevent posterior drifting of the ramus in its tonic state.

Signs and symptoms of the temporomandibular joint syndrome vary but generally include a cluster of symptoms:

- Pain and tenderness of the masticatory muscles
- Limited or altered mandibular function (*i.e.,* hypermobility or a tendency to protrude the mandible in the initial opening phase)
- Crepitation or clicking
- Deviation of the mandible on opening
- Disturbed chewing patterns
- Locking of the jaw
- Vague, remote subjective complaints

The means of treatment of temporomandibular joint syndrome is basically like that for other myofascial pain syndromes—anesthetics, exercise, and physical and pharmacological agents. There are, however, additional considerations. There are two traditional concepts of the etiology of temporomandibular joint dysfunction. Some clinicians stress malocclusion as the causal factor. They advocate treatment involving mainly mechanical methods, such as equilibration of the occlusion.[40,80] Others emphasize that psychological factors, especially response to stress, and harmful habits of the jaw may influence both the onset and course of symptoms. They advocate patient education, the elimination of habitual protrusion or other harmful habits, and muscular relaxation.

The effective management of temporomandibular joint disorders requires first of all a diagnosis based on a complete history, thorough physical examination, and when indicated, adjuncts such as a detailed study of the patient's occlusion, roentgenography, and electromyography.

SOFT TISSUE TECHNIQUES

Soft tissue mobilization techniques may include deep friction massage to the capsule of the joint,[40] gentle kneading or stroking techniques interorally to inhibit pain (to the insertion of the temporalis and medial and lateral pterygoid musculature) (see Figs. 15-21 to 15-23), deep pressure joint massage,[35,115,154,171] connective tissue massage,[172] strain–counterstrain,[90] craniosacral therapy,[180] myofascial release, muscle energy or post-isometric relation techniques,[105,106,123] and stretching techniques.

Myofascial release techniques have been found to be particularly helpful to release a tight masseter, the temporalis masseter complex, and supra- and infrahyoid musculature.[49] Suprahyoid and infrahyoid release techniques are indicated for patients with lack of craniocervical extensibility and restriction of the infrahyoid muscles. These techniques assist in proper placement of the tongue in patients with abnormal tongue position or swallowing habits and are useful in patients with FHP either after traumatic injury or overuse through maladaptation.[49,180] Gentle tractions are held for a number of seconds to a minute or longer until a giving way is sensed (Fig. 15-27). Infrahyoid release may be used to decrease spasms in the overstretched infrahyoid muscles, often seen in the postcervical whiplash patient.

A useful muscle energy technique for increased tension of the digastric on one side (the main antagonist of the masticatory muscles) is to have the patient assume a supine position.[105] In this position, with one hand the therapist resists the opening of the mouth while the thumb of the other exerts minimal pressure on the hyoid on the side of increased tension (Fig. 15-28A). The patient is instructed to open the mouth gently and breathe in, to hold the breath, and then to breathe out and relax. During relaxation, resistance in the digastric will automatically give way under the therapist's thumb. There is also a useful self-treatment (Fig. 15-28B).

☐ Treatment of Limitation Disorders

STRETCHING TECHNIQUES

To increase limited mandibular movements, a variety of exercises involving the muscles of mastication may be employed. They are used, on one hand, to help break up the muscle spasm, and on the other, to main-

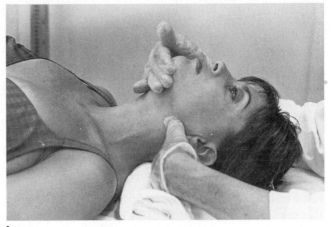

A

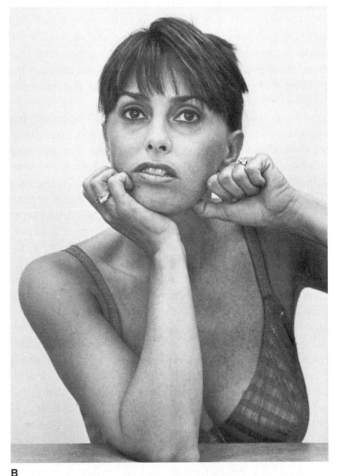

B

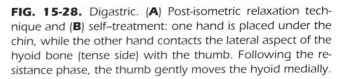

FIG. 15-28. Digastric. (**A**) Post-isometric relaxation technique and (**B**) self–treatment: one hand is placed under the chin, while the other hand contacts the lateral aspect of the hyoid bone (tense side) with the thumb. Following the resistance phase, the thumb gently moves the hyoid medially.

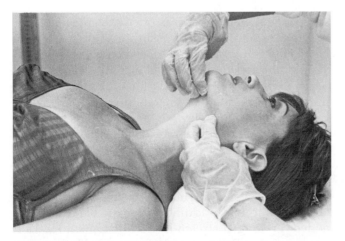

FIG. 15-27. Suprahyoid release technique.

tain and increase limited jaw movement to full physiological function.

ACTIVE STRETCH

The patient actively opens his mouth as wide as possible several times following a series of warm-up exercises.[157] By having the patient repeat a gentle, rhythmic, hingelike movement a number of times before active stretch, muscle spasm can be physiologically diminished or eliminated. With the patient in a comfortable, relaxed, reclining position or in a recliner chair, have her place her tongue in contact with the hard palate as posteriorly as possible, while keeping the mandible in a retruded position. In this position with the tongue on the hard palate, the patient's articular movements are mainly rotatory and early protrusion is avoided. It is helpful to have the patient palpate the condyles so that she can feel the movement. If glide occurs too early, with little or no rotatory motion, there is an early protrusion problem. Instruct the patient to open her mouth slowly and rhythmically within this limited range 10 times or so in succession. She then performs active stretch by opening her mouth as wide as possible within the pain-free limit, as slowly as she can two or three times. The opening position should be held for 5 seconds, followed by relaxation in the rest position for 5 seconds. In the case of a unilateral limitation, the tip of the tongue is positioned on the palatal surface behind the canine teeth on the contralateral side. The application of a vapocoolant spray or ultrasound may be an effective adjunct during active stretch.

During normal mandibular opening, translation begins beyond 11 mm.[99] Improving translation is therefore accomplished by having the patient place a finger (six or so tongue blades, or a wooden pencil) horizontally between the teeth, which will open the mandible approximately 11 mm. The patient can then actively practice protrusive, retrusive, and lateral excursions of the mandible but avoid any jamming effects that might occur if translation is done within the first 11 mm of opening.

Lateral excursion exercises are frequently used during postoperative physical therapy. During the repair phase, lateral deviations should be limited to 5 mm on the side opposite the surgery to prevent overstretching of the repair site.[17,87,150,151]

Yawning is recommended as a home program exercise. It is an active stretching movement that is accomplished by strong reflex inhibition of the mandibular elevators.

These active exercises should be repeated often during the day for brief periods. These procedures must be applied cautiously in the presence of roentgenographic evidence of temporomandibular joint arthropathy and if done soon after disk plication or graft.

A variety of neuromuscular facilitation exercises may be used when range of motion is limited by shortening, contracture, or spasm.[97,156,188] One of the most frequently used methods is hold–relax to make stretching of the masticatory muscles more effective. This technique implies a contraction of the antagonist against maximal resistance, followed by relaxation, and then active or assistive stretch of the agonist. For example, to increase mandibular opening, the patient is asked to close his mouth tightly as resistance is applied gently and slowly to the mandible. This is followed by a relaxation and then by active or passive motion. Isometric contraction of the mouth elevator muscles facilitates their relaxation. The resultant stimulation of the jaw-opening muscles permits increased active or passive stretch. The therapist might use the following commands:

1. "Just hold your jaw closed and don't let me move it." (Apply resistance gently and slowly to the mandible.)
2. "Let go." (Maintain gentle support of the mandible and wait for relaxation to occur.)
3. "Open your mouth." (Have the patient move the mandible actively with or without resistance.)

Unresisted reversing movements may also be used as a follow-up procedure by either active or assistive stretch.

A variety of similar techniques such as maximal resistance superimposed on an isotonic or isometric contraction, slow-reversal–hold, and contract–relax may be used.[97,156,188] Such exercises may also be used for increasing range of protrusion, retrusion, and lateral deviation. The therapist provides resistance, or the patient may be asked to do so with his own hand.[156] By using resistance, the patient effects an increased relaxation of the antagonist muscles. This sets up a reflex mechanism called *reciprocal inhibition*.

PASSIVE STRETCH

Prolonged static stretch is often advantageous and may be accomplished by using a series of tongue blades built up, one on top of the other, between the anterior incisors for bilateral limitation or between the upper and lower teeth (far back on the involved side) in the case of unilateral limitation.[110] This places the capsule and tight elevator muscles on moderate stretch. The tongue blades are not meant to be used as a forced stretch but rather to take up the slack and maintain the mandible in a relaxed open position. The use of cold (ice or vapocoolant spray) or ultrasound may be administered while on passive stretch. As the jaw begins to relax, additional tongue blades may be added. Prolonged stretch is usually applied for 15 to 20 minutes. Following temporomandibular joint surgery, no more than 1 or 2 minutes of stretching is recommended.

Tongue blades can also be used for home treatment, both as a static stretch and for briefer periods of active and passive stretch. Tongue blades, however, must be used with caution since too vigorous application may cause injury. Shore recommended the use of a tapered cork.[159] The cork, which is approximately 15 mm at its narrow end and 30 mm at its widest end, is gradually inserted (small end first) into the patient's mouth until the jaws are separated. Once the jaw begins to relax, the cork can be placed farther into the mouth, thus progressively opening the jaw wider and wider. Shore recommends using this technique as a home treatment for 30-second periods every 2 hours.

ASSISTIVE STRETCH (DIRECT METHOD)

With the patient sitting, the therapist stands behind and places both thumbs over the patient's lower teeth and his index fingers over the upper teeth. A sterile gauze or a cloth may be placed over the lower teeth. The patient is instructed to support the mandible with one hand under the chin. The mandible is then opened with gentle but maximal effort. If a less vigorous stretch is indicated, the therapist uses one hand, with the index finger and thumb in the same position, and supports the patient's mandible with the opposite hand.[156]

The patient may be taught to use this method as a form of self-treatment, using the thumb and index finger in a reverse position and supporting the mandible with one or both hands.[156]

All of these exercises should emphasize movement without pain or undue force. Stretching should be done slowly and can be done actively (with or without resistance to the mandible) or passively.

Reflex relaxation of the elevator muscles followed by active stretch, as used for the opening movement, as well as passive and assistive stretch may also be applied to lateral, protrusive, and retrusive movements. With instruction, the patient can carry out many of these exercises alone.

MOBILIZATION TECHNIQUES

Mobilization techniques in the treatment of temporomandibular joint disorders are aimed at restoring normal joint mechanics in order to allow full, pain-free osteokinematics of the mandible to occur. The techniques described are based on courses presented by Rocabado and the works of Kaltenborn.[93,145] They are restricted to a description of manual techniques, which are best learned and practiced under supervision in a postgraduate course or in physical therapy schools.

1. **Caudal Traction (Fig. 15-29)**
   Note: P—patient; O—operator; M—movement.

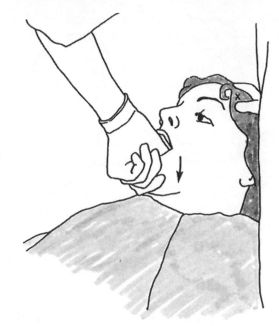

FIG. 15-29. Caudal traction.

P—Lies supine on a semi-reclining table or in dental chair that supports the head and trunk.

O—Stands at patient's side and faces left side of patient's head. Right hand and forearm are placed around patient's head, fixating head against the table. (A stabilizing belt across the forehead may be used instead.) Left hand holds, with thumb in the mouth over the left inferior molars and with the fingers outside around the patient's jaw.

M—Ask patient to swallow. While maintaining the forearm in a straight line (hand and forearm act as a unit), apply traction caudally. Reverse for the opposite side.

Note: Caudal traction may be combined with ventral and dorsal glide (protraction and retraction). The mandible is first distracted caudally, and while traction is maintained the mandible is glided ventrally, then dorsally, followed by a gradual release of caudal traction.

2. **Protrusion**—Ventral glide (Fig. 15-30)

P—Lies supine on a semi-reclining table or in dental chair that supports the head and trunk.

O—Stands at patient's side and faces left side of patient's head. Right hand and forearm are placed around the patient's head, fixating against the operator's body. Left hand holds onto the angle of the ramus with index and third finger. The rest of the hand contacts the patient's jaw.

M—Ask patient to swallow. While maintaining the forearm in a straight line, glide the mandible ventrally into protrusion. Reverse for the opposite side.

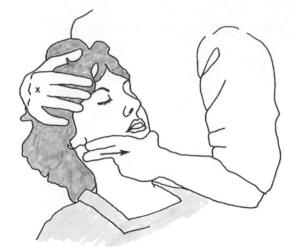

FIG. 15-30. Protrusion.

Note: An alternative handhold would be to place the thumb in the mouth on the right inferior molars and the fingers outside around the right side of patient's jaw. This same handhold can be used for retrusion (dorsal glide).

Gliding movements ventrally may be combined with a little rotation. The right mandible is first glided forward, as described, and then rotated to the left by rotation of operator's body.

3. **Medial-Lateral Glide (Fig. 15-31)**
   a. Rotation of the left joint and forward glide of the right joint
      P—Lies supine on a semi-reclining table or dental chair that supports the head and trunk.
      O—Stands behind patient. Right hand holds around the patient's head, fixating head against table. Left hand is positioned so that the hypothenar eminence is placed just caudal to the left temporomandibular joint with the fingers wrapped around the patient's jaw.
      M—Ask patient to swallow. The hypothenar eminence acts as a pivot point as the mandible is glided forward and medially to the left. Reverse for opposite side.
   b. Alternative technique (Fig. 15-32)
      P—Lies supine on a semi-reclining table or in dental chair that supports the head and neck.
      O—Stands at patient's side and faces left side of patient's head. Right hand is placed around patient's head, fixating head against table. Left hand holds with thumb in mouth on medial aspect of body of mandible near the right inferior molars, with the fingers (outside) wrapped around the jaw.
      M—Ask patient to swallow. With the thumb acting as a pivot point, move the wrist ulnarly so that the right condyle moves outward, forward, and laterally as the mandible is moved medially to the left. Reverse for opposite side.

Many of the semi-reclining techniques described above may be carried out in a sitting position. The patient's head may be stabilized against the operator's body and supported with the free hand. However, the semi-reclining or supine position is preferred, since the head and mandible are in a better position for fixation. Furthermore, if a stabilizing belt is used, the operator's other hand is free to assist the mobilizing

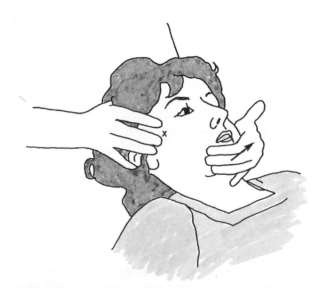

FIG. 15-31. Medial-lateral glide.

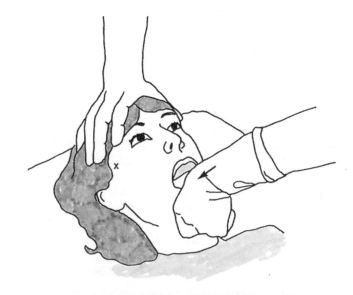

FIG. 15-32. Medial-lateral glide (alternative technique).

hand or to palpate the joint to determine if correct motion is obtained. Mobilization techniques using pressures against the head of the mandible, which have been developed by Maitland, are particularly useful (Fig. 15-33).[110,176] One of the greatest difficulties encountered when mobilizing the jaw is the patient's inability to relax the jaw completely. By mobilizing the condyle directly rather than through the mandible (which involves large movements), the patient is often able to relax more readily and treatment is often more successful. Also, overstretching of the upper joint compartment is avoided. Medial glide is particularly useful in restoring rotation (lower joint compartment).

☐ Treatment of Temporomandibular Joint Dysfunction Syndromes, Disk Derangement, or Condylar Displacement

Signs and symptoms of early temporomandibular joint dysfunction include primarily muscular hyperactivity and pain, disturbed chewing habits, clicking, "catching" or "locking" of the jaw (recurrent subluxations), and limited motion or hypermobility of the joints. Palliative therapy is directed at reducing muscle spasm (the pain–spasm–pain cycle) and relieving intrajoint symptoms caused by trauma, inflammation,

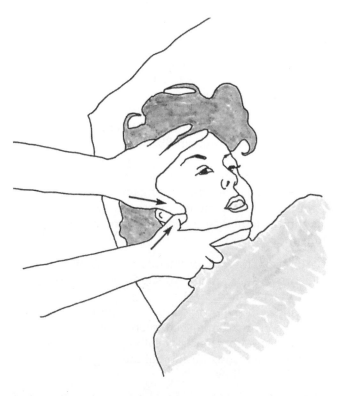

FIG. 15-33. Mobilization techniques (here a medial glide) may be applied directly to the condyle.

condylar displacement, or disk derangement.[187] Treatment may include drug therapy, injections, application of various forms of heat or cold, disengagement of the occlusion by prostheses or voluntarily, and alterations in dietary and oral habits.

Causative therapy procedures may include manipulations and joint mobilization techniques to restore normal joint mechanics; correction of condylar displacements with the use of occlusal repositioning splints or occlusal equilibration; and correction of disk derangement by mandibular manipulations or repositioning appliances.[101,110,132,159,187] Occasionally, surgical correction may be necessary.

Adjunctive therapy may include the use of ultrasound, electrical stimulation, patient education, relaxation techniques, psychotherapy, biofeedback, and exercises. According to Somers, treatment directed toward patient education, the elimination of poor oral habits, and the acquisition of muscle relaxation is often all that is required to relieve the patient's symptoms.[166]

PATIENT EDUCATION

A most important step is to educate patients regarding the functioning of their joints, the reason for their symptoms, and the means of removing those symptoms. Advice should include reassurance, which is often simply gained by understanding the anatomy of the joint and the physiological mechanisms at work.

Use of a skull, the patient's roentgenograms, or simple diagrams will help the therapist to explain the structure and function of the temporomandibular joints and the rationale for the various procedures that must be undertaken. Instructions should emphasize diet and careful use of the jaw.[159] The harmful effects of wide opening, yawning, biting off large mouthfuls of hard food, habitual protrusion, diurnal clenching, or nocturnal bruxism should be explained. Because an emotional overlay is often present, counseling on how emotional conflicts are translated into muscle tension and pain is usually an important consideration. Point out that methods to achieve muscle relaxation and abolish well-established patterns of inappropriate muscular activity and methods to acquire new ones are important means of eliminating symptoms.

RELAXATION TRAINING

In addition to patient education, relaxation training for jaw and facial muscles is often considered, although it may be difficult to achieve. Muscle tension is one of the most important contributing causes of muscular derangements of the temporomandibular joint, whether or not the derangement occurred through trauma. A report by Heiberg and colleagues indicates that of a group of patients with a diagnosis of temporomandibular joint syndrome, almost all exhibited tense muscles in the neck and back as well, indicating that muscular tension is not confined to the masticatory muscles alone. Increased muscular tension, especially in the erector trunci, was present in 95 percent of these patients.[86] Typically they presented with a tightly closed jaw, stiffened neck and back, elevated shoulders, and a forward head. Faulty respiration patterns were also a common finding.

Relaxation of the whole body or body regions is frequently indicated in the treatment of these overly tense patients. More often than not, general relaxation techniques will have to precede training for local relaxation. (See Chapter 8, Relaxation and Related Techniques.) Relaxation exercises such as those modified from Jacobson, autogenic training, and reflex relaxation exercises may all be used.

The therapist can show the patient the presence of unnecessary muscular contraction at the end of the initial physical examination or during the first treatment session. Most patients are unable to relax the jaw muscles so that the mandible can be moved freely by the therapist. They are unable to let the head loll back when the shoulders are supported, since the neck muscles remain rigid. They cannot permit their elevated arm to fall limply to the treatment table when requested by the examiner.

Perhaps one of the hardest of all relaxation procedures to achieve is elimination of overcontraction of the jaw muscles. An example of a local technique using a modification of Jacobson's approach follows:

- Clench the jaw firmly and concentrate on feeling the sense of tightness in the temples as well as the jaw itself.
- Switch off and let the jaw fall open.
- Push the jaw open against the pressure of an assistant's hand.
- Relax completely.
- Move the jaw sideways to the left as far as possible with or without resistance and experience the sensation this gives to the jaw and temples before relaxing.
- Repeat the same exercise to the right.
- Complete the sequence by clenching the jaw firmly again, and let the jaw drop open loosely.

Somers suggests that total relaxation cannot be assumed until the assistant can take the patient's chin between the thumb and forefinger and tap the teeth together rapidly without any opposition from the jaw muscles.[166] It is often most helpful for the patient to adapt this method for use from time to time to assess the degree of tension and his progress in attempting to achieve relaxation. Autosuggestion techniques to guard against clenching and tooth contact are also helpful. He may be told to repeat the following after each meal: "Lips together, teeth apart." He should also be instructed to make frequent checks during the day for jaw clenching and to attempt to maintain the rest position of the mandible in which only the lips touch while the teeth are held apart. These methods of treatment are often considered the first line of defense against clenching and nocturnal bruxism.[159]

The use of biofeedback methods to guide the patient in controlling muscle activity and promoting relaxation has increased in recent years.[80,133,177,178] Feedback from electromyography of the frontal, temporal, and masseter muscles has been popular.

POSTURE AWARENESS AND BALANCING THE UPPER QUADRANT

In addition to relaxation training and patient education, the therapist must spend time instructing the patient in good body mechanics, postural control, and correct body positioning for maximum relaxation of the cervical spine and masticatory muscles. Cervical traction, exercises, and mobilization may also be indicated when associated cervical symptoms or pathological processes coexist. Occlusal splints may be indicated to create relaxation of the elevator muscles and to disorient an acquired noxious occlusal sensory input. Splints may also be used to disorient the sensory input in patients who clench, by changing the quality of afferent touch information.[101,159] Occlusal analysis and equilibration, if indicated, are usually best deferred until relaxation has been achieved.

Many clinical manifestations of pain in the upper quarter have their source not in an isolated joint disorder but in chronic upper quarter dysfunction spanning several body segments. It is estimated that 70 percent of patients presenting with craniomandibular dysfunction (temporomandibular disorders) will also present with craniocervical dysfunction.[146] Based on clinical studies and experience of numerous practitioners, there are several findings that are common to a population of patients presenting with temporomandibular joint dysfunction. Some of the findings include the following:

- Abnormal forward or lateral head postures
- Compensatory abnormal shoulder girdle postures (protracted shoulders)
- Changes in the position of the mandible (condylar retrusion and diminished interocclusal distance)[50]
- Mouth and upper chest breathing
- Abnormal resting position of the tongue
- Deviant swallow

Postural or orthostatic evaluation and treatment of these patients is extremely important, because an altered biomechanical relationship will always produce accommodations and even subsequent adaptations if the accommodations are maintained.[126,149]

A system of upper quarter re-education methods has been developed by Rocabado[149] and Kraus[99] that addresses these common imbalances. Methods of treatment encompass correcting abnormal head posture and craniocervical dysfunction, instructions in the normal sequence of swallowing and the proper resting position of the tongue and mandible, and techniques to enhance proper use of the diaphragm (naso-diaphragmatic breathing) and thoracic spine mobility.[50,99,145,149]

SWALLOW SEQUENCE

The presence of a residual pediatric tongue thrust or an acquired adult anterior tongue thrust secondary to FHP can affect the response to all treatment of the temporomandibular joint.[49,151] Treatment should include instruction in the normal resting position of the tongue and proper swallowing. Maintenance of the correct head-on-neck posture is essential. The evaluation method (see Fig. 15-19) of "water-sipping" can be used as an exercise in retraining aberrant swallowing patterns. As water is sipped during the initial phase of swallowing, the tip of the tongue should return to its resting position without putting pressure on the teeth. The main force of swallowing should be against the palate and is maintained by the middle third of the tongue.[49] The patient should sense a wavelike motion that starts at the tip of the tongue and ends with the middle third of the tongue against, and putting pressure on, the posterior part of the palate.[42,99,145]

A useful exercise to learn to alleviate symptoms of FHP and cervical syndromes in the region of the anterior neck (larynx and pharynx) and to facilitate normal swallowing is talking with a cork in the mouth (Fig. 15-34).[96] The musculature of the temporomandibular joint is designed not only to provide power (for chewing) but intricate control, as in speech.[13]

DIAPHRAGMATIC BREATHING

Proper diaphragmatic breathing is also important. Patients with allergies, asthma, or nasal obstructions often breathe through their mouths with increased activity of the accessory muscles of respiration (scalenes and sternocleidomastoids), which leads to FHP with posterior cranial rotation.[169] The patient should be instructed in nasodiaphragmatic breathing, which is best learned supine, followed by sitting, and finally standing.[8,34,95]

Attempts to alter breathing patterns are often difficult. However, a more normal breathing pattern can be facilitated by altering the head and neck posture. An exercise proposed by Fielding[57] may help: A soft ball or equivalent is placed behind the patient's back

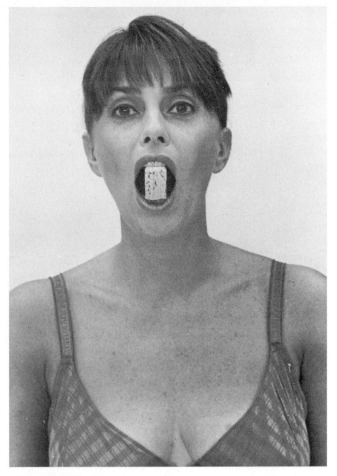

FIG. 15-34. Articulating with a cork exercise. The height of the cork depends on how far the patient can open her mouth (she should only open it halfway). The patient reads aloud or simply improvises for about 2 minutes; then, with the cork out of the mouth, she repeats what she just said and feels how easy it is now to articulate.

at the level of the scapula as she sits in a straight chair (Fig. 15-35). The mechanism for this is not clear, but the patient is observed to reduce cervical lordosis, close the mouth, lower the elevation of the shoulders, and breathe at a slower deeper rate. A more normal breathing pattern can also be accomplished by suggesting that while sitting relaxed, the patient make a conscientious effort to keep the tongue on the roof of the mouth. Some patients do this well, thereby resulting in a return to breathing with a closed mouth.[57]

EXERCISE THERAPY

The use of retraining exercises to overcome spasm and incoordination of the mandibular musculature, to promote harmonious coordinated mechanisms, to reduce momentary luxation of the disk, and to increase muscle strength have long been advocated; however, they are now considered controversial.[16,41,132,156,157]

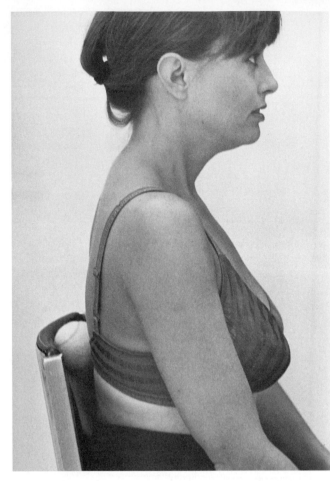

FIG. 15-35. Posterior contraction using a ball to facilitate a more normal breathing pattern.

Cyriax believed that clicking of the jaw due to momentary luxation of the intra-articular disk can usually be relieved by strengthening the muscles of mastication. Opening, protrusion, and lateral resistive movements are performed. It is usually not necessary, he believes, to develop the jaw-closing muscles, since most patients usually maintain normal strength of these muscles by chewing.[40]

Schwartz and Bertoft recommend a training program of exercises against resistance to promote reflex relaxation of the antagonistic muscles. This stimulates the maximum number of motor units within the lateral pterygoids during opening and lateral mandibular movements.[16,156,157]

Paris advises that major derangements should be treated in the same manner as subluxations by mobilization techniques. Minor derangements, however, are best treated by isometrics to the lateral pterygoids (*i.e.*, protrusion and lateral movements).[132] Regardless of the type of exercises used, they should always be carried out without clicking and pain.

Such strengthening-resistive exercises, according to

Weinberg, are not indicated in the temporomandibular joint pain–dysfunction syndrome because the neuromuscular mechanism involved is associated with overfunction rather than underfunction.[185,186] Such exercises do not seem to have a rational basis as an effective therapy. Strengthening and re-education exercises may be indicated when true muscle weakness is found (as in the limitation phase) or when habits such as deviant swallowing or habitual protrusion reverses normal muscle function and contributes to the temporomandibular joint pain–dysfunction syndrome.[166,187]

☐ Treatment of Orofacial Imbalances

Muscles of the entire stomatognathic system and the orofacial complex play a major role in proper balance and function of the temporomandibular joint. It should be kept in mind that the orofacial muscles are under stress 24 hours a day. Swallowing takes place 2000 times a day as a reflexive act. Forces during eating, drinking, speech, and the rest position of the tongue must be taken into consideration. If there is an imbalance of forces, there will be a tremendous amount of pressure against the temporomandibular joint that can cause malfunction of the joint apparatus.

Protrusion of the mandible resulting in an abnormal palatal swallow may be caused by ankylotic tongue, shortened frenulum, or abnormal use of facial muscles, particularly the mentalis.[66,73] Abnormal use or position of the tongue at rest, muscle imbalance of the masseter, decreased strength of the orbicularis oris, neuromuscular problems, post-traumatic and surgical conditions (*e.g.,* unilateral condylectomies), pain conditions of the head, face, or cervical spine, and other pathological processes can result in malfunction of the temporomandibular joint.

In many of these conditions, real or apparent reduction in muscle strength of one or more muscles may be disclosed during examination. This may point to lack of use (*e.g.,* in unilateral function), atrophy of muscle fibers, muscular fibrositis, and other pathological conditions localized in or near the muscle and its tendon, causing pain on contraction. Although strengthening–resistive exercises are usually not indicated in muscles that are already refusing to relax, they do need to be considered in the proper balance and function of the temporomandibular joint complex when weakness exists, from whatever cause.

FACILITORY EXERCISES

There is a wide variety of well-known facilitory and strengthening-resistive exercises that are at the therapist's disposal.[53,66,98,152,156,157] Exercises employing postural reflexes, brushing, vibration, synergistic muscle action of the facial and cervical muscles, and activities of daily living may be used as facilitory techniques. Stimuli—consisting of stretch, maximal resistance, pressures, stroking, or tapping—may be given manually. Popping or clucking of the tongue on the hard palate may be used to strengthen the muscle of the tongue and encourage greater range of motion of the jaw. Gargling after each brushing helps facilitate mandibular depressors. Resistive tongue exercises may be used to facilitate the three major jaw muscles. Resisted neck motion may facilitate tongue motions as well as mandibular motions. In general, facial and mandibular motions that require depression or downward motions are facilitated by neck flexion; conversely, facial and mandibular motions that require elevation and upward motions are facilitated by neck extension. Neck rotation reinforces motion on the side of the face or the mandible toward which the head is turned.

NEUROMUSCULAR COORDINATION OF THE TEMPOROMANDIBULAR JOINT

Early protrusion of the mandible during opening that is due to an imbalance of the synergistic action of the suprahyoids and lateral pterygoids is often revealed during examination. A translatory rather than a rotatory movement is occurring; its abolition should be a major step in management. An excellent, initial exercise requires the patient to place his tongue as posteriorly as possible in contact with the hard palate, to effect retrusion (Fig. 15-36). By assuming this position, protrusion of the lower jaw is eliminated, since the patient's articular movements are mainly rotatory and limited by the constraints of the internal pterygoids. By limiting the movement to the interocclusal clearance, any subsequent translatory movement is eliminated. Instruct the patient to open his mouth slowly and rhythmically within the pain limits several times in succession. He should practice this simple exercise frequently during the day.

The next step is to instruct the patient to repeat this exercise with the addition of one critical modification, voluntary resistance. The patient should grasp the chin firmly or position a closed fist under the mandible to resist the motion of pressing the jaw down and back.

Both of these exercises rely on synergistic action of the suprahyoids and lower bodies of the lateral pterygoids. In normal opening, all of these muscle pairs contract strongly. However, when the lateral pterygoids contract more strongly than the suprahyoids,

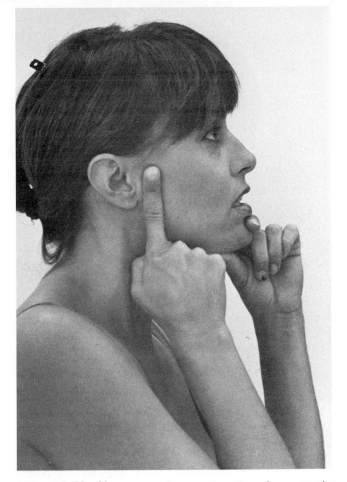

FIG. 15-36. Neuromuscular re-education for excessive translation. The index finger of one hand palpates the lateral aspect of the condyle of the temporomandibular joint, while the other hand contacts the chin. With the tongue on the hard palate, the patient practices mandibular opening with only condylar motions occurring.

the mandible will protrude. These exercises are believed to help train the suprahyoids to contract more forcefully than the lateral pterygoids.

Another useful exercise for the development of the suprahyoids, described by Shore, consists of teaching the patient to perform isometric contraction of these muscles in front of a mirror (Fig. 15-37).[159] The patient is taught to contract these muscles with the mouth closed and the teeth in light contact. She then makes a conscious effort to retrude the jaw and depress the floor of the mouth without actually moving it. Once acute spasms have subsided, the patient repeats the exercise with the mouth slightly open. Each day she can gradually increase the extent of mouth opening until coordinated mandibular muscular action is achieved.

Once the patient has mastered rotation during limited opening without forward condylar movement,

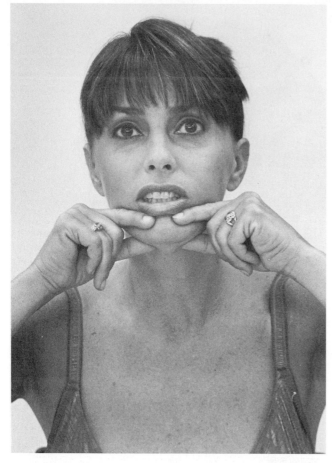

FIG. 15-37. Isometric coordinating exercise. The patient places the tip of the tongue against the hard palate and attempts to retrude and depress the floor of the mouth without moving it (additional isometrics can be performed moving the mandibule in all directions).

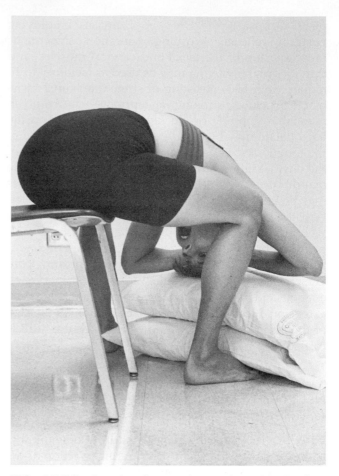

FIG. 15-38. Opening-the-mouth exercise with the long axis of the body inverted.

the range of opening is gradually increased. While the patient is looking in a mirror, she is asked to place her index finger over each condylar head, or her palms over the sides of the face, to monitor and correct any abnormal protrusion of the condylar head during opening and closing. She should also note any irregular movements such as one condylar head preceding movement of the other. Keeping the hands in place, the patient is instructed to carry out slow rhythmic full opening and closing within the pain-free range, avoiding any clicking, abnormal protrusion, or lateral deviation of the jaw. If abnormal deviation or protrusion does occur, she is taught to guide the motion with her thumb or forefinger positioned on her chin so that the mandible moves smoothly in a coordinated hingelike fashion without protrusion. Initially, this exercise should be performed with the therapist, who assists by guiding the motion of the mandible as the patient actively opens and closes her mouth.

An interesting variation of this exercise (for patients

who can assume the position) is learning to move the temporomandibular joints freely and with precision with the head in the inverted position (Fig. 15-38).[96] Opening of the mouth in this position must be performed against gravity, providing eccentric isotonic work of the masseter muscle in opening and making its concentric work in closing superfluous.

In the absence of obvious malocclusion and organic disease, simple exercises have been found to alleviate the annoying problem of temporomandibular joint clicking. Gerschmann[69] found that simple exercises such as lower jaw thrust exercises, in a forward, backward or anteroposterior direction with teeth disengaged, and the "chewing the pencil" exercise could alleviate this problem in about 2 weeks. The latter exercise consists of using a soft cylindrical rod (1.5 to 2 cm) placed horizontally at the back of the mouth so that the molars grasp the object with the mandible thrust forward. The patient then rhythmically bites on the object with a grinding like movement (Fig. 15-39). Au and Klineberg[6] in a study in young adults found that clicking was a reversible condition that could be

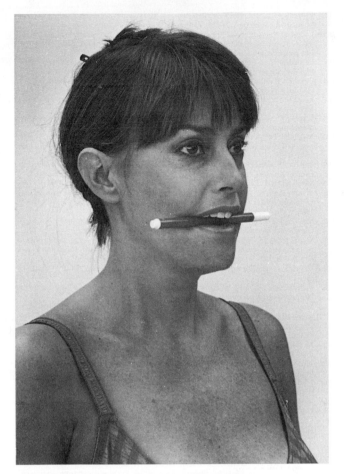

FIG. 15-39. "Chewing the pencil" exercise.

treated successfully with noninvasive isometric exercises (jaw opening as a hinge movement and lateral deviations), which helps to confirm that there is a neuromuscular cause for many temporomandibular joint clicking problems.

REFERENCES

1. Agerberg G: Maximal mandibular movements in young men and women. Sven Tandlak Tidskr 67:81–100, 1974
2. Agerberg G, Osterberg T: Maximal mandibular movements and symptoms of mandibular dysfunction in 70 year old men and women. Sven Tandlak Tidskr 67:147–163, 1974
3. Alderman MM: Disorders of the temporomandibular joint and related structures. In Lynch MA (ed): Burket's Oral Medicine. Diagnosis and Treatment, 7th ed. Philadelphia, JB Lippincott, 1977
4. Annandale T: Displacement of the inter-articular cartilage of the lower jaw, and its treatment by operation. Lancet 1:411, 1987
5. Atwood DA: A critique of research of the rest position of the mandible. J Prosthet Dent 16:848–854, 1966
6. Au AR, Klineberg IJ: Isokinetic exercise management of temporomandibular joint clicking in young adults. J Prosthet Dent 70:33–38, 1993
7. Axhausen G: Pathology and therapy of the temporomandibular joint. Fortschrite der Zahnaerz 6:101–215, 1932
8. Barlow W: Learning the principle. In Barlow W: The Alexander Technique, pp 185–199. New York, Warner Communications Company, 1973
9. Barrett R, Hanson M: Oral Myofascial Disorders. St. Louis, CV Mosby Co, 1978
10. Bates R, Stewart CM, Atkinson WB: The relationship between internal derangements of the temporomandibular joint and systemic joint laxity. J Am Dent Assoc 109:446–447, 1984
11. Beighton P, Graham R, Bird HA: Hypermobility of Joints. Berlin, Springer Verlag, 1989
12. Bell WE: Orofacial Pains—Differential Diagnosis. Dallas, Denedco of Dallas, 1973
13. Bell WE: Temporomandibular Disorders: Classification, Diagnosis, Management, 3rd ed. Chicago, Yearbook Medical Publishers, 1990
14. Bell WE: Orofacial Pains: Classification, Diagnosis, Management, 4th ed. Chicago, Yearbook Medical Publishers, 1989
15. Berry DC: Mandibular dysfunction pain and chronic minor illness. Br Dent J 127:170–175, 1969
16. Bertoft G: The effect of physical training on temporomandibular joint clicking. Odontologisk Revy 23:297–304, 1972
17. Bertolucci LE: Postoperative physical therapy in temporomandibular joint arthroplasty. J Craniomand Pract 10:211–220, 1992
18. Bessette RW, Mohl ND, DiCosimo CJ: Comparison of results of electromyographic and radiographic examination in patients with myofascial pain-dysfunction syndrome. J Am Dent Assoc 89:1358–1364, 1974
19. Blasberg B, Chalmers A: Temporomandibular pain and dysfunction syndrome associated with generalized musculoskeletal pain. A retrospective study. J Rheumatol Suppl 19:87–90, 1989
20. Block SR: Fibromyalgia and rheumatisms. Common sense and sensibility. Rheum Dis Clin North Am 19:61–78, 1993
21. Bogduk N: The clinical anatomy of the cervical dorsal rami. Spine 7:319–330, 1982
22. Bogduk N: The cervical zygapophyseal joints as a source of neck pain. Spine 13:610–617, 1988
23. Bogduk N, Corrigan B, Kelly P, et al: Cervical headache. Med J Aust 143:2–207, 1985
24. Bourbon B: Musculoskeletal analysis: The temporomandibular joint and cervical spine. In Scully RM, Barnes MR (eds): Physical Therapy, pp 415–420. Philadelphia, JB Lippincott, 1989
25. Boyd CH: The effect of head position on electromyographic evaluations of representative mandibular positioning of muscle groups. J Craniomandib Pract 5.51–53, 1987
26. Bradley JA: Acupuncture, acupressure, and trigger point therapy. In Peat M (ed): Current Physical Therapy, pp 228–234. Toronto, BC Decker, 1988
27. Bratzlavsky M, HanderEecken H: Postural reflexes in cranial muscles in man. Acta Neurol Belg 77:5–11, 1977
28. Brenman HS, Amsterdam M: Postural effects on occlusion. Dent Progress 4:43–47, 1963
29. Bronstein SL, Tomasetti BL, Ryan DE: Etiology of internal derangement of the temporomandibular joint: Correlation of arthrography with surgical findings. J Oral Surg 39:572–584, 1981
30. Brooke RI, Lapointe HJ: Temporomandibular joint disorders following whiplash. Spine: State of Art Review 7:443–454, 1993
31. Cailliet R: Neck and Arm Pain, 3rd ed. FA Davis, 1991
32. Campbell CD, Loft GH, Davis H, Hart DL: TMJ symptoms and referred pain patterns. J Prosthet Dent 47(4):430–433, 1982
33. Cantu RI, Grodin AJ: Myofascial Manipulation: Theory and Clinical Application. Gaithersburg, MD, Aspen Pub, 1992
34. Caplin D: Breathing correctly to ease back pain. Gainesville, FL, Triad Publishing Co, 1987
35. Chin LC, Jiang YH, Shen WW, et al: Kinesic press–finger compress method for TMJ treatment. J Craniomandib Pract 5:261–267, 1987
36. Clark R, Wyke B: Contributions of temporomandibular articular mechanoreceptors to the control of mandibular posture: An experimental study. J Dent 2:121–129, 1974
37. Cohen S: A cephalometric study of rest position in edentulous persons: Influence of variations in head position. J Prosthet Dent 7(4):467–472, 1957
38. Curnutte DC: The role of occlusion in diagnosis and treatment. In Morgan DH, Hall WP, Vamvas SV (eds): Disease of the Temporomandibular Apparatus: A Multidisciplinary Approach, 2nd ed. St Louis, CV Mosby, 1982
39. Cyriax J: Rheumatic headache. Br Med J 2:1367–1368, 1938
40. Cyriax J: Textbook of Orthopedic Medicine: Diagnosis of Soft Tissue Lesions, vol 1, 8th ed. London, Bailliere Tindall, 1982
41. Dachi SF: Diagnosis and management of temporomandibular dysfunction syndrome. J Prosthet Dent 2:53–61, 1968
42. Darling DW, Kraus S, Glasheen-Wray MB: Relationship of head posture and the rest position of the mandible. J Prosthet Dent 52:111–115, 1984
43. Darnell M: A proposed chronology for events for forward head posture. J Craniomandib Pract 1:50–54, 1983
44. Davis D: Gray's Anatomy Descriptive and Applied, 34th ed. London, Longmans Green, 1967
45. Day LD: History taking. In Morgan DH, Hall WP, Vamvas SV (eds): Disease of the Temporomandibular Apparatus: A Multidisciplinary Approach. St Louis, CV Mosby, 1977
46. Dijkstra PU, Lambert GM, de Bont LGM, et al: Temporomandibular joint osteoarthrosis and generalized joint hypermobility. J Craniomandib Pract 10:221–227, 1992
47. Dolwick F, Katzberg RW, Helms CA: Internal derangement of the temporomandibular joint: Facts or fiction. J Prosthet Dent 49:315–418, 1983
48. Dufourmentel L: Chirugie de l'articulation temporo-maxillaire. Paris, Masson, 1920
49. Dunn J: Physical therapy. In Kaplan AS, Assael LA (eds): Temporomandibular Disorders: Diagnosis and Treatment, pp 455–500, 1991
50. Ellis JJ, Makofsky HW: Balancing the upper quarter through awareness of RTTPB. Clin Management 7:20–23, 1987
51. Eriksson PO, Lindman R, Stal P, et al: Symptoms and signs of mandibular dysfunction in primary fibromyalgia syndrome (PSF) patients. Swed Dent J 12:141–149, 1988
52. Ermshar CB: Anatomy and neuroanatomy. In Morgan DH, Hall WP, Vamvas SV (eds): Disease of the Temporomandibular Apparatus: A Multidisciplinary Approach. St Louis, CV Mosby, 1977
53. Farber SD: Sensorimotor Evaluation and Treatment Procedures, 2nd ed. Bloomington, Indiana University Press, 1974
54. Farrar WB: Characteristics of the condylar path in internal derangements of the TMJ. J Prosthet Dent 39:219–323, 1978
55. Farrar W, McCarty W Jr.: Outline of Temporomandibular Joint Diagnosis and Treatment, 6th ed. Montgomery, AL, Normandy Study Group, 1980
56. Feinstein B, Lanton NJK, Jameson RM, Schiller F: Experiments on pain referred from deep somatic tissues. J Bone Joint Surg 36(A):981–997, 1954
57. Fielding M: Physical therapy in chronic airway limitation. In Peat M (ed): Current Physical Therapy, pp 12–14. Toronto, BC Decker, 1988
58. Fish F: The functional anatomy of the rest position of the mandible. Dent Prac 11:178, 1961

59. Forsberg CM, Hellsing E, Linder-Aronson S, et al: EMG activity in the neck and masticatory muscles in relation to extension and flexion of the head. Eur J Orthod 7:177, 1985
60. Friction J, Hathaway K, Bromaghim C: Interdisciplinary management of patients with TMJ and craniofacial pain: Characteristics and outcome. J Craniomandib Dis 1:115–122, 1987
61. Friction J, Kroening R, Haley D: Myofascial pain syndrome of the head and neck: A review of clinical characteristics of 164 patients. Oral Surg 60:615–623, 1985
62. Friction J, Kroening RJ, Hathaway KM: TMJ and Craniofacial Pain: Diagnosis and Management. St Louis, Ishiyaku EuroAmerica, 1988
63. Friedman MH, Weisberg J: Temporomandibular Joint Disorders: Diagnosis and Treatment. Chicago, Quintessence, 1985
64. Friedman MH, Weisberg J, Agus B: Diagnosis and treatment of inflammation of the temporomandibular joint. Semin Arthritis Rheum 12:44–51, 1982
65. Funakoshi M, Fujita N, Takehana S: Relations between occlusal interference and jaw muscle activities in response to changes in head posture. J Dent Res 55:684–690, 1976
66. Garliner D: Myofunctional Therapy. Philadelphia, WB Saunders, 1976
67. Gattozzi JG, Nicol BR, Somes GW, et al: Variations in mandibular rest position with and without dentures in place. J Prosthet Dent 36:159–163, 1978
68. Gelb H: The craniomandibular syndrome. In Garliner D (ed): Myofunctional Therapy. Philadelphia, WB Saunders, 1976
69. Gerschmann JA: Temporomandibular dysfunction. Aust Fam Phys 17:274, 1988
70. Goldenberg DL, Felson DT, Dinerman H: A randomized, control trail of amitriptyline and naproxen in the treatment of patients with fibromyalgia. Arthritis Rheum 31:1535–1542, 1986
71. Goldstein DF, Kraus SL, Williams WB, Glasheen-Wray M: Influence of cervical posture on mandibular movement. J Prosthet Dent 52:421–426, 1984
72. Graber TM: Over-bite: The dentists' challenge. J Am Dent Assoc 79:1135–1139, 1969
73. Greene BJ: Myofunctional Therapy. In Morgan DH, Hall WB, Vamvas SJ (eds): Disease of the Temporomandibular Apparatus: A Multidisciplinary Approach, 2nd ed. St Louis, CV Mosby, 1982
74. Greenfield B, Wyke B: Reflex innervation of the temporomandibular joint. Nature 211:940–941, 1966
75. Greenwood LF: Is temporomandibular joint dysfunction associated with generalized hypermobility? J Prosthet Dent 58:701–703, 1987
76. Griffen C: A neuro-myo-arterial glomus in the temporomandibular meniscus. Med J Austr 48:113–116, 1961
77. Grokoest A: Osteoarthritis. In Schwartz L (ed): Disorders of the Temporomandibular Joint. Philadelphia, WB Saunders, 1959
78. Grokoest A, Chayes CM: Rheumatic disease. In Schwartz L, Chayes CM (eds): Facial Pain and Mandibular Dysfunction. Philadelphia, WB Saunders, 1968
79. Gross A, Gale EN: A prevalence study of the clinical signs associated with mandibular dysfunction. J Am Dent Assoc 107:932–936, 1983
80. Grossan M: Biofeedback. In Morgan DH, Hall WP, Vamvas SJ (eds): Disease of the Temporomandibular Apparatus: A Multidisciplinary Approach, 2nd ed. St Louis, CV Mosby, 1982
81. Halbert R: Electromyographic study of head position. J Can Dent Assoc 23:11–23, 1958
82. Hargreaves A: Dysfunction of the temporomandibular joints. Physiotherapy 72:209–212, 1986
83. Harinstein D, Buckingham RB, Braun T, et al: Systemic joint laxity (the hypermobile joint syndrome) is associated with temporomandibular joint dysfunction. Arthritis Rheum 31:1259–1264, 1988
84. Hartley A: Temporomandibular assessment. In Hartley A (ed): Practical Joint Assessment: A Sports Medicine Manual, pp 33–43. St Louis, Mosby Year Book, 1990
85. Harvold EP: Primate experiments on oral respiration. Am J Orthod 79:359–372, 1981
86. Heiberg AN, Heloe B, Krogstad BS: The myofascial pain dysfunction: Dental symptoms and psychological and muscular function: An overview. Psychother Psychosom 30:81–97, 1978
87. Iglarsh Z, Snyder-Mackler L: Temporomandibular joint and cervical spine. In Richardson JK, Iglarsh ZA (eds): Clinical Orthopaedic Physical Therapy, pp 1–72. Philadelphia, WB Saunders, 1994
88. Isberg-Holm A, Ivarsson R: The movement pattern of the mandibular condyle in individuals with and without clicking: A clinical cineradiologic study. Dentomaxillofac Radiol 9:55–65, 1980
89. Jonck LM: Ear symptoms in temporomandibular joint disturbance. South Afr Med J 54:782–786, 1978
90. Jones LH: Strain and counterstrain. Colorado Springs, CO, American Academy of Osteopathy, 1981
91. Juniper RD: Temporomandibular joint dysfunction: A theory based upon electromyographic studies of the lateral pterygoid. Br J Oral Maxillofac Surg 22:1–8, 1984
92. Juniper RD: The pathogenesis and investigation of TMJ dysfunction. Br J Oral Maxillofac Surg 25:105–112, 1987
93. Kaltenborn F: Manual Therapy for the Extremity Joints. Oslo, Olaf Norlis Bokhandel, 1974
94. Kawamura Y, Majina T, Kato I: Physiologic role of deep mechanoreceptors in temporomandibular joint capsule. J Osaka Univ Dent School 7:63–76, 1967
95. Kisner C, Colby LA: Chest therapy. In Kisner C, Colby LA (eds): Therapeutic Exercise: Foundation and Techniques, pp 577–616. Philadelphia, FA Davis, 1990
96. Klein-Volgelbach S: Functional Kinetics: Observing, Analyzing, and Teaching Human Movement. Berlin, Springer-Verlag, 1990
97. Klineberg I: Structure and function of temporomandibular joint innervation. Ann R Coll Surg 49:268–288, 1971
98. Knott M, Voss DE: Proprioceptive Neuromuscular Facilitation. New York, Harper & Row, 1962
99. Kraus SL: Physical therapy management of TMJ dysfunction. In Kraus SL (ed): TMJ Disorders: Management of Craniomandibular Complex, pp 139–173. New York, Churchill Livingstone, 1988
100. Kraus SL: Cervical spine influences on the craniomandibular region. In Kraus SL (ed): TMJ Disorders: Management of the Craniomandibular Complex, pp 367–404. New York, Churchill Livingstone, 1988
101. Krogh-Poulsen WG: Management of the occlusion of the teeth. In Schwartz L, Chayes CM (eds): Facial Pain and Mandibular Dysfunction. Philadelphia, WB Saunders, 1968
102. Kusunose RS: Strain and counterstrain. In Basmajian JV, Nyberg R (eds): Rational Manual Therapies, pp 329–333. Baltimore, Williams & Wilkins, 1993
103. Laskin DM : Surgery of the temporomandibular joint. In Solberg WK, Clark GT (eds): Temporomandibular Joint Problems. Biologic Diagnosis and Treatment. Chicago, Quintessence, 1980
104. Lazorthes G, Gaubert J: L'innervation des articulations interapophysaires vertebrales. Comptes Rendus de l'Association des Anatomistes, 1956, pp 488–494
105. Lewit K: Manipulative Therapy in Rehabilitation of the Locomotor System, 2nd ed. Oxford, Butterworth-Heinemann Ltd, 1991
106. Lewit K, Simons DG: Myofascial pain: Relief by post isometric relaxation. Arch Phys Med Rehabil 64:452–456, 1984
107. Luschei ES, Goodwin GM: Patterns of mandibular movement and muscle activity during mastication in the monkey. J Neurophysiol 35(5):954–966, 1974
108. Mahan P: Temporomandibular problems. Biologic diagnosis and treatment. In Solberg WK, Clark GT (eds): Temporomandibular Joint Problems. Chicago, Quintessence, 1980
109. Mahan PE, Kreutziger KL: Diagnosis and management of temporomandibular joint pain. In Alling C, Mahan P (eds): Facial Pain. Philadelphia, Lea & Febiger, 1977
110. Maitland GDP: Peripheral Manipulations, 3rd ed. Boston, Butterworth, 1991
111. Mannheimer JS, Attanasio R, Cinotti WR, et al: Cervical strain and mandibular whiplash: Effects upon the craniomandibular apparatus. Clin Prev Dent 11:29–32, 1989
112. Mannheimer JS, Dunn J: Cervical spine. In Kaplan AS, Assael LA (eds): Temporomandibular Disorders, pp 50–94. Philadelphia, WB Saunders, 1991
113. Mannheimer JS, Rosenthal RM: Acute and chronic postural abnormalities as related to craniofacial pain and temporomandibular disorders. Dent Clin North Am 35:185–208, 1991
114. Marylon F: Fibrositis (fibromyalgia syndrome) and the dental clinician. Cranial 9:63–70, 1991
115. Masunaga S, Ohashi W: Zen Shiatsu: How to Harmonize Yin and Yang for Better Health. New York, Japan Pub Inc, 1977
116. McCall J: Electromyography of muscles of posture: Posterior vertebral muscles in man. J Physiol (London) 157:33, 1961
117. McLean LF, Brenman HS, Friedman MGF: Effects of changing body position on dental occlusion. J Dent Res 52:1041–1050, 1973
118. McNamara DC: Examination, diagnosis and treatment of occlusion pain-dysfunction. Aust Dent J 23:50–55, 1978
119. McNamara JA: The independent function of the two heads of the lateral pterygoid muscle. Am J Anat 138:197–205, 1973
120. Merlini L, Palla S: The relationship between condylar rotation and anterior translation in healthy and clicking temporomandibular joints. Schweiz Monatsschr Zahnmed 98:119, 1988
121. Merrill RG: Arthroscopic lysis, lavage, manipulation and chemical sclerotherapy of the TMJ for hypermobility and recurrent dislocation. In Clark GT, Sanders B, Bertolami CN: Advances in Diagnostic and Surgical Arthroscopy of the Temporomandibular Joint. Philadelphia, WB Saunders, 1992
122. Mintz VW: The orthopedic influence. In Morgan DH, Hall WP, Vamvas SJ (eds): Disease of the Temporomandibular Apparatus: A Multidisciplinary Approach. St Louis, CV Mosby Co, 1977
123. Mitchell FL Jr, Moran PS, Pruzzo NA: An Evaluation and Treatment Manual of Osteopathic and Muscle Energy Procedures. Valley Park, MO, Mitchell, Moran and Pruzzo, 1979
124. Moffett BC, Johnson LC, McCabe JB, Askew HC: Articular remodeling in the adult human temporomandibular joint. Am J Anat 115:10–130, 1964
125. Mohl ND: Head posture and its role in occlusion. NY State Dent J 42:17–23, 1976
126. Mohl ND: The role of head posture in mandibular function. In Solberg W, Clark G (eds): Abnormal Jaw Mechanics: Diagnosis and Treatment. Chicago, Quintessence, 1984
127. Morgan DH, Hall WP, Vamvas SJ (eds): Disease of the Temporomandibular Apparatus: A Multidisciplinary Approach, 2nd ed. St Louis, CV Mosby, 1982
128. Morgan DH, Rosen LM: Interpretation of radiograph. In Morgan DH, Hall WP, Vamvas SJ (eds): Disease of the Temporomandibular Apparatus: A Multidisciplinary Approach, 2nd ed. St Louis, CV Mosby, 1982
129. Morrone L, Makofsky H: TMJ home exercise program. Clin Management 11:20–26, 1991
130. Muller W: The fibrositis syndrome: Diagnosis, differential diagnosis and pathogenesis. Scand J Rheumatol Suppl 65:40–53, 1987
131. Munro RR: Electromyography of the masseter and anterior temporalis muscle in the open-close-clench cycle in the temporomandibular joint dysfunction. Monogr Oral Sci 4:117–125, 1975
132. Paris SV: The Spinal Lesion. Christchurch, New Zealand, Pegasus Press, 1965
133. Peck C, Kraft G: Electromyographic biofeedback for pain related to muscle tension: A study of tension headache, back, and jaw pain. Arch Surg 112:889–895, 1977
134. Pellegrino MJ: Atypical chest pain as an initial presentation of primary fibromyalgia. Arch Phys Med Rehabil 71:526–528, 1990
135. Perry C: Neuromuscular control of mandibular movements. J Prosthet Dent 30:714–720, 1973
136. Pinto OF: A new structure related to the temporomandibular joint and the middle ear. J Prosthet Dent 12(1):95–103, 1962
137. Plunkett GAJ, West, VC: Systemic joint laxity and mandibular range of movement. J Craniomandib Pract 6:320–326, 1988
138. Porter MR: The attachment of the lateral pterygoid muscle of the meniscus. J Prosthet Dent 24:555–562, 1970
139. Prieskel HW: Some observations on the postural position of the mandible. J Prosthet Dent 15:625–633, 1965
140. Profitt WR: Equalization theory revisited: Factors influencing position of the teeth. Am J Orthod 48:175–186, 1978
141. Ramfjord SP: Dysfunctional temporomandibular joint and muscle pain. J Prosthet Dent 11:353–374, 1961
142. Rayne J: Functional anatomy of the temporomandibular joint. Br J Oral Maxillofac Surg 25:92–99, 1987
143. Rees LA: The structure and function of the temporomandibular joint. Br Dent J 96:125–133, 1954
144. Robinson MJ: The influence of head position on TMJ dysfunction. J Prosthet Dent 16:169–172, 1966

145. Rocabado M: Management of the temporomandibular joint. Presented at a course on physical therapy in dentistry. Vail, CO, January, 1978

146. Rocabado M: Advanced Upper Quarter Manual. Rocabado Institute, Tacoma, WA, 1981

147. Rocabado M: Arthrokinematics of the temporomandibular joint. Dent Clin North Am 27(3):573–594, 1983

148. Rocabado M: Biomechanical relationship of the cranial, cervical and hyoid region. J Craniomandib Pract 1:61–66, 1983

149. Rocabado M: Diagnosis and treatment of abnormal craniomandibular mechanics. In Solberg W, Clark G (eds): Abnormal Jaw Mechanics: Diagnosis and Treatment. Chicago, Quintessence, 1984

150. Rocabado M: Physical therapy for the post surgical TMJ patient. J Craniomandib Pract 3:75–82, 1989

151. Rocabado M, Iglarsh ZA: Musculoskeletal Approach to Maxillo-facial Pain. Philadelphia, JB Lippincott, 1991

152. Rood M: Neurophysiological reactions as a basis for physical therapy. Phys Ther 34:444–449, 1954

153. Scherman P: Surgery of the temporomandibular articulation. In Gelb H (ed): Clinical Management of Head, Neck and TMJ Pain and Dysfunction: A Multidisciplinary Approach to Diagnosis and Treatment. Philadelphia, WB Saunders, 1977

154. Schultz W: Shiatsu: Japanese Finger Pressure Therapy. New York, Bell, 1976

155. Schwartz AM: Positions of the head and malrelationships of the jaws. Int J Ortho Oral Surg Radiol 14:56–88, 1928

156. Schwartz L (ed): Disorders of the Temporomandibular Joint. Philadelphia, WB Saunders, 1959

157. Schwartz L, Chayes CM (eds): Facial Pain and Mandibular Dysfunction. Philadelphia, WB Saunders, 1968

158. Shira RB, Alling CC: Traumatic injuries involving the temporomandibular joint articulation. In Schwartz L, Chayes CM (eds): Facial Pain and Muscular Dysfunction. Philadelphia, WB Saunders, 1968

159. Shore MA: Temporomandibular Joint Dysfunction and Occlusal Equilibration. Philadelphia, JB Lippincott, 1976

160. Sicher H, DuBrul EL: Oral Anatomy, 8th ed. St Louis, CV Mosby, 1988

161. Simons DG: Muscular pain syndromes. In Friction JR, Awad EA (eds): Advances in Pain Research and Therapy, vol 1, pp 1–41. New York, Raven Press, 1990

162. Smythe HA: Non-articular rheumatism and fibrositis. In McCarty DJ (ed): Arthritis and Allied Conditions: A Textbook of Rheumatology, pp 874–884. Philadelphia, Lea & Febiger, 1972

163. Smythe HA: Non-articular rheumatism and psychogenic musculoskeletal syndromes. In McCarty DJ (ed): Arthritis and Allied Conditions: A Textbook of Rheumatology, pp 881–891, 2nd ed. Philadelphia, Lea & Febiger, 1979

164. Solberg WK: Temporomandibular disorders: Clinical significance of TMJ changes. Br Dent J 160:231–236, 1986

165. Solow B, Kreiberg S: Soft tissue stretching: A possible control factor in craniofacial morphogenesis. Scand J Dent Res 85:505–507, 1977

166. Somers N: An approach to the management of temporomandibular joint dysfunction. Aust Dent J 23(1):37–41, 1978

167. Speck JE, Zarb GA: Temporomandibular dysfunction: A suggested classification and treatment. J Can Dent Assoc 6:305–310, 1976

168. Talley RL, Murphy GJ, Smith SD, et al: Standards for the history, examination, diagnosis and treatment of temporomandibular disorders (TMJ): A position paper. J Craniomandib Pract 8:60–77, 1990

169. Tallgren A, Solow B: Hyoid bone position, facial morphology and head posture in adults. Eur J Orthod 9:1–8, 1987

170. Tanaka TT: A rational approach to the differential diagnosis of arthritic disorders. J Prosthet Dent 56:727–731, 1986

171. Tappan FM: Finger pressure to acupuncture points. In Tappan FM (ed): Healing Massage Techniques: Holistic, Classic and Emerging Methods, 2nd ed, pp 133–166. Norwalk, CO, Appleton & Lange, 1988

172. Tappan FM: The bindegewebmassage system. In Tappan FM (ed): Healing Massage Techniques: Holistic, Classic, and Emerging Methods, 2nd ed, pp 219–260. Norwalk, CO, Appleton & Lange, 1988

173. Thompson JR, Brodie AG: Factors in the position of the mandible. J Am Dent Assoc 29:925–941, 1942

174. Travel JG, Rinzler SH: The myofascial genesis of pain. Postgrad Med 11:425–434, 1952

175. Travel JG, Simons DG: Myofascial Pain and Dysfunction: The Trigger Point Manual. Baltimore, Williams & Wilkins, 1983

176. Trott PH: Examination of the temporomandibular joint. In Grieves GP (ed): Modern Manual Therapy of the Vertebral Column, pp 521–529. New York, Churchill Livingstone, 1986

177. Trott PH: Passive movements and allied techniques in the management of dental patients. In Grieves GP (ed): Modern Manual Therapy of the Vertebral Column, pp 691–699. New York, Churchill Livingstone, 1986

178. Trott PH, Goss AN: Physiotherapy in diagnosis and treatment of the myofascial dysfunction syndrome. Int J Oral Surg 7(4):360–365, 1978

179. Truta MP, Santucci ET: Head and neck fibromyalgia and temporomandibular arthralgia. Otolaryngol Clin North Am 22:1159–1171, 1989

180. Upledger JE, Vredevoogd JD: Craniosacral Therapy. Chicago, Eastland Press, 1983

181. Viener AE: Oral surgery. In Garliner D (ed): Myofunctional Therapy. Philadelphia, WB Saunders, 1976

182. Waylonnis GW, Heck W: Fibromyalgia syndrome. New associations. Am J Phys Med Rehabil 71:343–348, 1992

183. Weinberg LA: An evaluation of basic articulators and their concepts: I. Basic concepts. J Prosthet Dent 13:622–644, 1963

184. Weinberg LA: The etiology, diagnosis, and treatment of TMJ dysfunction-pain syndrome: I. Etiology. J Prosthet Dent 42(6):654–664, 1979

185. Weinberg LA: The etiology, diagnosis and treatment of TMJ dysfunction-pain syndrome: II. Differential diagnosis. J Prosthet Dent 43(2):50–70, 1980

186. Weinberg LA: The etiology and treatment of TMJ dysfunction-pain syndrome: III. Treatment. J Prosthet Dent 43(2):186–196, 1980

187. Wetzler G: Physical therapy. In Morgan DH, Hall WP Vamvas SV (eds): Disease of the Temporomandibular Apparatus: A Multidisciplinary Approach, 2nd ed. St Louis, CV Mosby, 1982

188. Whinery JG: Examination of patients with facial pain. In Alling C, Mahan P (eds): Facial Pain. Philadelphia, Lea & Febiger, 1977

189. Widmer CG: Evaluation of temporomandibular disorders. In Kraus SL (ed): TMJ Disorders: Management of the Craniomandibular Complex, pp 79–111. Edinburgh, Churchill Livingstone, 1988

190. Wolfe F, Smythe HA, Yunus MB, et al: The American College of Rheumatology 1990 criteria for classification of fibromyalgia: Report of the Multicenter Criteria Committee. Arthritis Rheum 33:160–172, 1990

191. Wyke BD: Neuromuscular mechanisms influencing mandibular posture: A Neurologist's review of current concepts. J Dent 2:111–120, 1972

192. Yale S, Allison B, Hauptfuehrer J: An epidemiological assessment of mandibular condyle morphology. Oral Surg 21:169–177, 1966

193. Yunus MB: Fibromyalgia syndrome and myofascial pain syndrome: Clinical features, laboratory tests, diagnosis, and pathophysiologic mechanisms. In Rachlin ES: Myofascial Pain and Fibromyalgia, pp 3–29. St Louis, CV Mosby, 1994

194. Yunus MB, Masi AT: Fibromyalgia, restless legs syndrome, periodic limb movement disorder and psychogenic pain. In McCarty DJ JR, Koopman WJ (eds): Arthritis and Allied Conditions. A Textbook of Rheumatology, pp 1383–1405. Philadelphia, Lea & Febiger 1992

195. Yunus MB, Masi AT, Calbro JJ, et al: Primary fibromyalgia (fibrositis): Clinical study of 50 patients with matched normal controls. Semin Arthritis Rheum 11:151–171, 1981

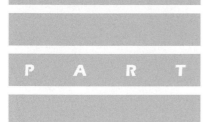

PART THREE

Clinical Applications— The Spine

16
CHAPTER

The Spine—General Structure and Biomechanical Considerations

DARLENE HERTLING

GENERAL STRUCTURE

The spine is divided into five regions: cervical, thoracic (or dorsal), lumbar, sacral, and coccygeal (the "tail" or coccyx). The spine usually has 33 segments—seven cervical, 12 thoracic, five lumbar, five sacral, and four coccygeal (Fig. 16-1). The sacral vertebrae are fused together and serve as an attachment to the pelvic girdle. The "presacral" vertebrae, with which we are most concerned clinically, most often total 24.

Occasionally there are supernumerary thoracic or lumbar vertebrae, or perhaps an unfused sacral vertebra, rather than an actual additional segment. It is questionable whether these variations hold much clinical significance, although a spine in which a lumbar vertebra is sacralized is felt to gain stability at the expense of mobility, and a spine in which a sacral vertebra is not fused tends to be mobile but less stable.[6,33,60] Unilateral sacralization or lumbarization, in which only one side of the vertebra is involved, is often thought to be of more significance, presumably leading to asymmetry in mobility and stability. However, this may not always be the case, because osseous fusion on one side is often accompanied by fibrous fusion (not evident on roentgenograms) on the opposite side. Another not uncommon finding is fusion of two upper cervical vertebrae, which again may have little clinical significance.[29,56,63]

The spine is a flexible, multi-curved column. When viewed in the sagittal plane, the cervical and lumbar regions are in lordosis (lordotic curve); the thoracic, sacral, and coccygeal regions are in kyphosis (kyphotic curve) (Fig. 16-1C). These normal anatomical curves give the spinal column increased flexibility and augmented shock-absorbing capacity while at the same time maintaining adequate stiffness and stability at the intervertebral joints.[3,179] In humans, the thoracic spine is partially splinted by the rib cage. The thoracic curve is structural and is secondary to less vertical height at the anterior thoracic vertebral border, as opposed to the posterior border. This is also true of the sacral curve. Although the sacrum is rigid, slight motions occur *in vivo* in the sacroiliac joint, which decrease with age (see Fig. 16-1).[39,55,139,142,215] The coccyx, which is not well developed in humans, has no functional role (Fig. 16-1A,C).

Darlene Hertling and Randolph M. Kessler: MANAGEMENT OF COMMON MUSCULOSKELETAL DISORDERS: Physical Therapy Principles and Methods, 3rd ed.
© 1996 Lippincott-Raven Publishers.

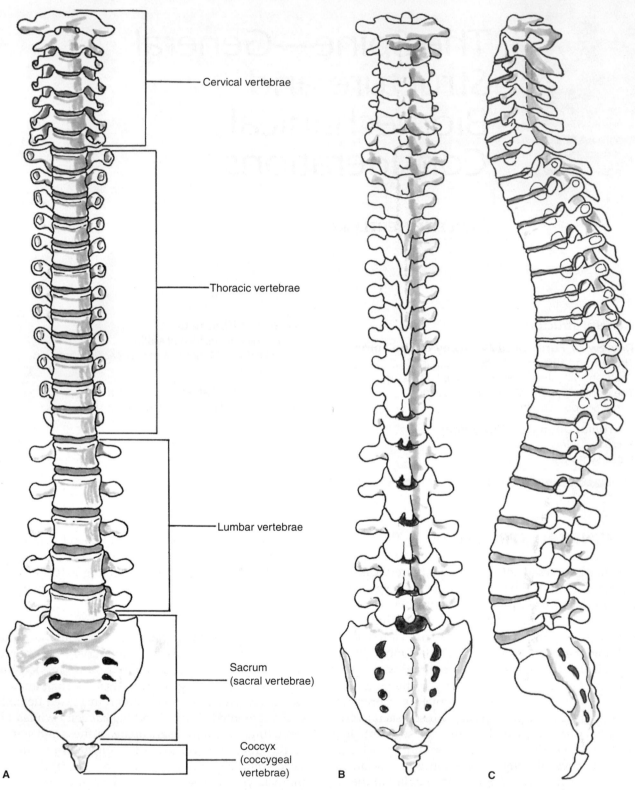

FIG. 16-1. The vertebral column, including the sacrum and coccyx, as seen on (**A**) anterior, (**B**) posterior, and (**C**) left sagittal views.

In contrast, the cervical spine and lumbar spine are quite flexible, yet still are able to support heavy loads. The demanding functional role they play is felt to be a major reason why these regions of the spine are the most likely to become symptomatic. Curvature of the cervical and lumbar regions is largely due to the wedge-shaped intervertebral disks.[220] These disks are entirely responsible for the existence of a normal cervical lordosis, because the cervical vertebral bodies are actually shorter in height anteriorly than posteriorly (Fig. 16-1C). They are largely responsible for the lumbar lordosis in the upper lumbar spine, but less so in the lower lumbar spine, where the vertebral bodies are wedge-shaped so as to form the lordosis. Thus, in both the cervical and lumbar regions the disks are of greater height anteriorly than posteriorly. In the thoracic spine the kyphosis is almost entirely caused by the shape of the vertebral bodies—the disks being of equal height anteriorly and posteriorly.

The spine has at least four biomechanical functions: 1) housing and protection, 2) support, 3) mobility, and 4) control.[179,220] Its most important function is to protect the delicate spinal cord from potentially damaging forces or motions. From a support standpoint, it transfers the weight and bending movements of the head and trunk to the pelvis. Facilitated by the ribs, it functions as a framework for attachment of the internal organs.

The human neck has been described as a cylindrical conduit that supports the head and renders it mobile.[125] It provides avenues of passage for essential connections in the respiratory, gastrointestinal, nervous, and vascular systems and serves as a locus for vital ductless glands and for the organs of phonation, vocalization, and ventilation. As such, it is a compact aggregate of numerous critical structures related to the cervical spine, which serves as the major architectural member. The cervical spine is a highly mobile structure that functions principally to position the head in space, permitting effective adaptation of the organism to the environment. Motions of the neck are therefore inseparably linked with motions of the head, and this linkage is a critical concept in both normal and pathological states.[125]

Mobility allows for physiological motion to occur between the parts of the spine. Thus, instead of a single rigid column, the spine is a flexible stack of rigid blocks with flexible soft tissue in between. The basic functional unit of the spine is the *spinal motion segment,* which may be defined as comprising the adjacent halves of two vertebrae, the interposed disk and articular facet joints, as well as the supporting structures (*i.e.,* ligaments, blood vessels, nerves, and muscles).[56,173,179,195] It should be noted that in the cervical spine there are no disks between the atlas and the occiput and the atlas and the axis. The disks permit intervertebral movement, while the posterior articulations control the amplitude and direction of the movement. This concept leads to a more functional than anatomical approach to pathology.

REVIEW OF FUNCTIONAL ANATOMY OF THE SPINE

Although a detailed description of the anatomy of the spine is beyond the scope of this chapter, the reader is referred to several other, comprehensive sources.[60,67,109,151,191,192,220] Briefly, the following constituents of the spinal segment and how they respond to motion and load are reviewed:

1. Support system—Vertebral bodies, posterior elements, articular facet (apophyseal) joints, intervertebral disks, and vertebral foramen
2. Control system—Both contractile (muscles) and noncontractile (ligaments, fascia, capsules, and vertebral innervations)
3. Other support systems—Intra-abdominal and thoracic pressures

The Support System: Individual Structures

VERTEBRAE

The special anatomical features of the vertebrae are probably best described in relation to their biomechanical functions. Probably the earliest biomechanical study of the human spine with respect to strength measurements of the vertebrae was conducted by Messerer more than 100 years ago.[141]

Each vertebra consists of two major parts—the anterior vertebral body, which is the major weight-bearing structure of the vertebra, and the posterior vertebral arch (Fig. 16-2). The vertebral arch is composed of the pedicle, which joins the arch to the body and to which the superior articular process is attached. This superior process articulates with the inferior articular process by means of the articular facet (apophyseal) joint and the transverse and spinous processes.

The basic design of the vertebrae in the various regions of the spine is the same. The size and mass of the vertebral bodies increase all the way from the first cervical to the last lumbar vertebra (see Fig. 16-1A); this is a mechanical adaptation to the progressively increasing loads to which the vertebrae are subjected.[220] There are individual differences in the various regions of the spine. Unique to the typical cervical vertebrae (C2–C7) are lateral prominences called *uncinate processes;* the transverse processes contain *foramina* (foramina transversarii) through which the vertebral

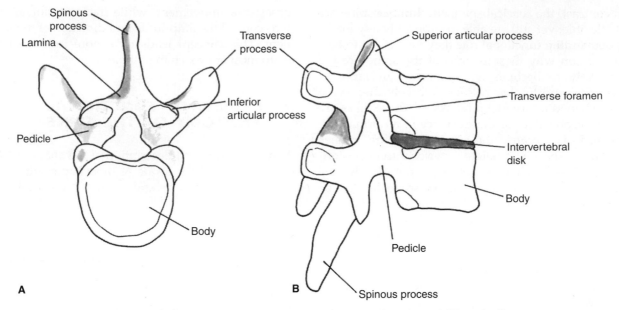

FIG. 16-2. Parts of a vertebra, viewed from (**A**) inferiorly and (**B**) sagittally.

artery passes (Fig. 16-3B,C). The thoracic vertebrae have articular facets for the ribs (Fig. 16-4A,C) and the lumbar spine has *mammary processes* (roughened raised areas on each articular pillar that serve for muscle attachment for the multifidi) (Fig. 16-5A,C). Of course the sacral spine, being fused, is unique.

ANTERIOR PORTION OF THE MOTION SEGMENT

Although the articular facets carry some compressive load, it is the vertebral bodies that are primarily de-

signed to sustain these loads. A compressive load is transmitted from the superior end-plate of a vertebra to the inferior end-plate by way of two paths, the *cortical shell* and the *cancellous core*. The body consists of spongy bone covered with a thin, dense bony cortex, whereas the neural arch and its processes are thinner and have proportionally more cortical bone. The cortical bone of the upper and lower surfaces of the bodies (vertebral plateaus) reflects the structure of the overlying cartilaginous end-plate, with a somewhat concave center and a more dense, ringed epiphyseal plate peripherally. As the superimposed weight of the

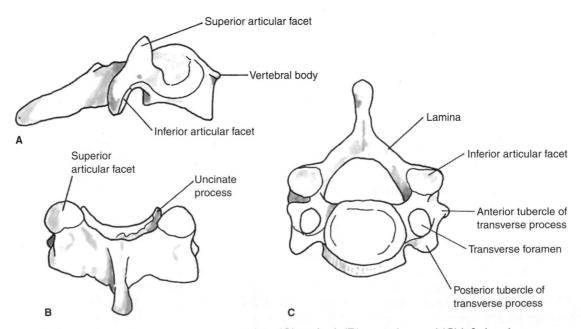

FIG. 16-3. Typical lower cervical vertebra: (**A**) sagittal, (**B**) posterior, and (**C**) inferior views.

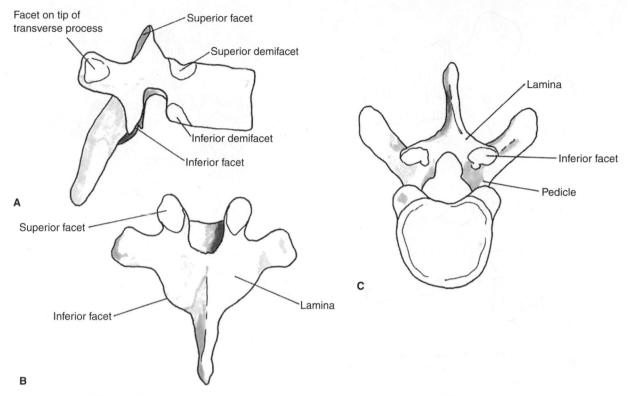

FIG. 16-4. Typical thoracic vertebra: (**A**) lateral, (**B**) posterior, and (**C**) inferior views.

upper body increases, the vertebral bodies become larger. The bodies in the lumbar spine have a greater height and cross-sectional area than those in the thoracic and cervical spine; their increased size allows them to sustain the greater loads to which this part of the spine is subjected.[129]

The vertebral bodies are about six times stiffer and three times thicker than the disks. Thus the vertebral bodies deform about half as much as the disks under compression. Because the vertebrae are filled with blood, it is possible that they behave like hydraulically strengthened shock absorbers.[111,112]

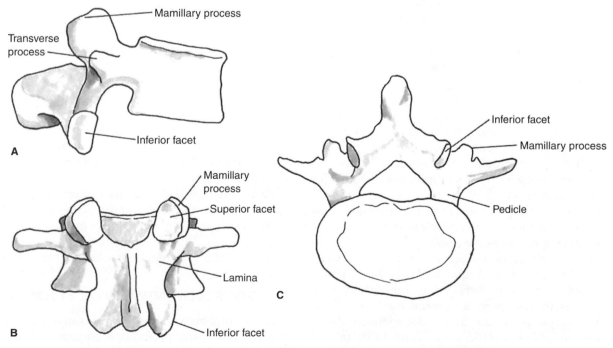

FIG. 16-5. Typical lumbar vertebra: (**A**) lateral, (**B**) posterior, and (**C**) inferior views.

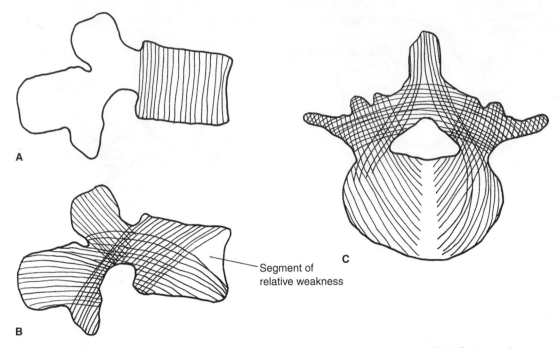

FIG. 16-6. Trabecular arrangement of vertebrae: (**A**) vertical trabeculae, (**B**) inferior and superior oblique patterns (note segment of relative weakness), and (**C**) oblique patterns viewed from above.

Vertical and oblique trabecular systems that correspond to the stresses placed on the bodies are found within the spongy bone (Fig. 16-6).[71,109] Vertically directed trabeculae mainly support the body and the compressive forces and help to sustain the body weight (Fig. 16-6A). The other trabecular systems help to resist shearing forces. At both the lower and upper surfaces of the body there are oblique trabeculae, which aid in compressive load-bearing function and also serve to resist the bending and tensile forces that occur at the pedicles and spinous processes (Fig. 16-6B,C). In osteoporosis there is a greater loss of horizontal trabeculae in comparison to the vertical trabeculae of cancellous bone; the effect on the strength of the vertebrae is considerable. In pathological processes of the spine, the type of failure may be related to whether the spine was loaded in flexion or extension, with flexion tending to cause anterior collapse where the trabeculae are weakest.[179] This also explains the wedge-shaped compression fracture of the vertebrae that occurs.[109]

Krenz and Troup found that the pressure was higher in the center of the end-plate than in the periphery during compressive loading.[123] This is a common site for failure in which the nucleus apparently ruptures the end-plate. Again, this may be a significant problem for those who have diminished bone strength, as in osteoporosis. Central fractures of the end-plate typically occur in nondegenerated disks, whereas peripheral fractures are found to be related to degenerated disks.[175,176,190]

Regionally, the lumbar vertebral bodies alter in shape from the first lumbar vertebra (more squared) to the fifth lumbar vertebra (more rectangular), giving the articular end-plate a broader surface area (see Fig. 16-5C). The bodies of the middle thoracic vertebrae are almost heart-shaped because of the pressure of the descending aorta (see Fig. 16-4C). The thoracic vertebral bodies are proportionally higher than the lumbar vertebrae and more squared in the transverse plane. Unique to the cervical spine (C2–C7) are lateral uncinate processes on the superior surface of each vertebral body, which articulate with the beveled edge of the inferior surface of the proximal vertebral body (see Fig. 16-3B). At this junction there is usually a synovial joint called the *joint of Luschka*.[87,212]

The atypical cervical vertebrae (C1 and C2) are characterized by the absence of a vertebral body at C1 (the *atlas*) and by the embryological fusion of the C1 body with C2 (the *axis*), forming a prominent pillar on the surface of C2 known as the *odontoid process* or *dens* (Fig. 16-7B–D).[212]

Each vertebral body has its primary nutrient foramen located in the center of the posterior aspect, and *in situ* it is covered by the *posterior longitudinal ligament* (Fig. 16-8A,B).[191,192] In general the upper and lower surfaces of the vertebral bodies are slightly concave.

POSTERIOR ELEMENTS AND FACET JOINTS

The vertebral arch is more complex than the body, because it has many projections, including four articulating facet (apophyseal) joints and three processes (see Fig. 16-2). The processes, two transverse and one

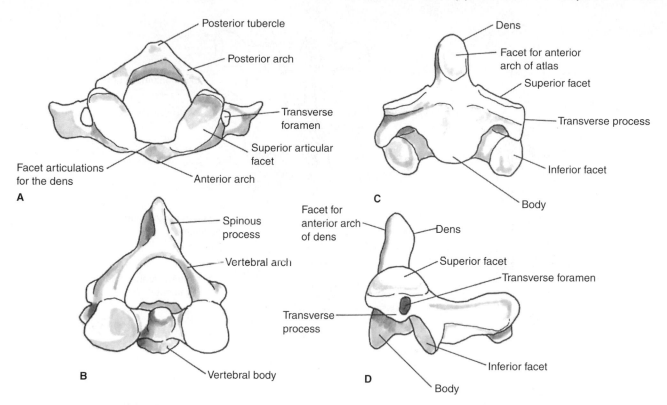

FIG. 16-7. *First and second cervical vertebrae: (**A**) the atlas (C1), as viewed from above; (**B**) the axis (C2), as viewed from above; (**C**) anterior view of axis; and (**D**) sagittal view of axis.*

spinous, provide for the attachment of ligaments and muscles. The arch is divided into a short anterior portion and a long posterior portion by the articulating projections and transverse processes. The anterior half of the arch consists of the pedicles, which attach the arch anteriorly to the upper posterior wall of the vertebral body (see Fig. 16-2). The laminae join to form the peak of the arch and continue to form the spinous process. At the site where the lamina takes origin from the pedicle, the lamina is narrowed, an area referred to as the *pars interarticularis* or *isthmus* (see Fig. 16-5*B*). Whereas pedicles rarely fracture, the pars is a frequent site of a distinctive fracture, apparently secondary to fatigue of bone rather than a sudden or acute fracture; this defect is commonly found in athletes.[3] Because the pars interarticularis is actually part of the neural arch forming a part of the posterolateral boundary of the arch, these lesions are often referred to as *neural arch defects.*[80] These defects are known as either *spondylolysis,* which consists of a single fracture of the pars, or as *spondylolisthesis,* which consists of a bilateral fracture often accompanied by some degree of forward slippage of the vertebral body (see Chapter 20, The Lumbar Spine).

The trabecular systems of the vertebral arch extend into the vertebral body (see Fig. 16-6). The area where the transverse process and articular facets arise is reinforced by many crossing trabeculae. The alignment of the trabeculae in the vertebral body and posterior

element indicates that the facet articulations must function to some extent as a fulcrum between the anterior vertebral body and the laminae and spinous processes, although the compression forces applied to the posterior elements in direct axial compression are markedly relieved by the compression strength of the body and disk system and by the potential for tensile elongation of the ligaments and muscles posteriorly.[109]

The articular facet joints are extensions of the laminae and are covered with hyaline cartilage on their articulating surfaces (Fig. 16-9*A,B*). The articular facets are particularly important in resisting torsion and shear, but they also play a role in compression. They may carry large compressive loads (25 to 33 percent), depending on the body posture, and they also provide (in equal proportion to the disk) 45 percent of the torsional strength of a motion segment.[60,99,115,131]

The amount of load-bearing by the articular facet joints is related to whether the motion segment is loaded in flexion or extension. Differences in interdiskal loading between erect sitting and standing can be explained in part by load-bearing of the articular facet joints while in extension or lordosis. Theoretically, the disk would be protected from both torsional and compressive loads when the motion segment is in extension. However, excessive loading of the spine in extension may cause failure of this secondary load-bearing mechanism; that is, loads transmitted through

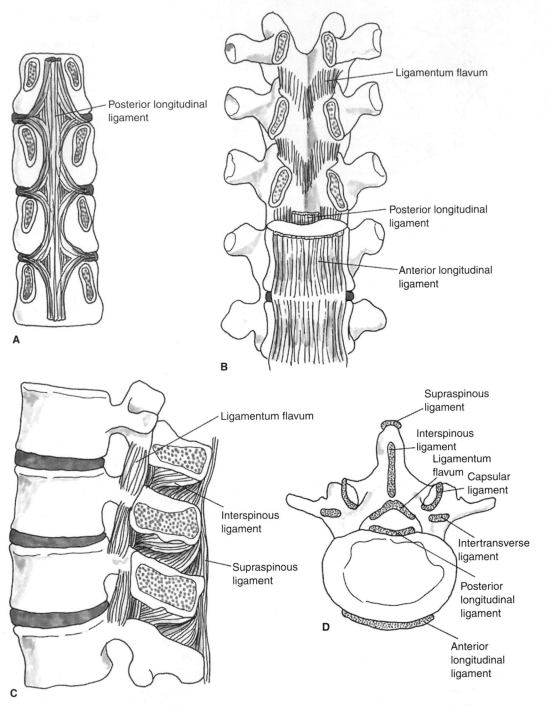

FIG. 16-8. The ligaments of the vertebral column include (**A**) the posterior longitudinal ligament (posterior view); (**B**) the ligamentum flavum and anterior longitudinal ligament (anterior view); (**C**) the supraspinous ligaments (sagittal view); and (**D**) the intertransverse ligaments (superior view).

the articular facet joints may produce high strains in the pars interarticularis, leading to spondylolysis.

The apophyseal or articular facet joints are usually described as *plane diarthrodial synovial joints* (except for the joints between the first two cervical vertebrae), although there is a "meniscus" (fatty synovial mass) in most of the joints (see Fig. 16-9A,B).[116] The superior

processes (prezygapophyseal) always bear an articulating facet whose surface is directed dorsally to some degree (see Figs. 16-3A,B; 16-4A,B; and 16-5A,B); the inferior articulating processes (postzygapophyseal) direct their articulating surfaces ventrally (see Figs. 16-3A, 16-4A, and 16-5A).[191,192] The joint consists of a cartilaginous articular surface, a fluid-filled capsule,

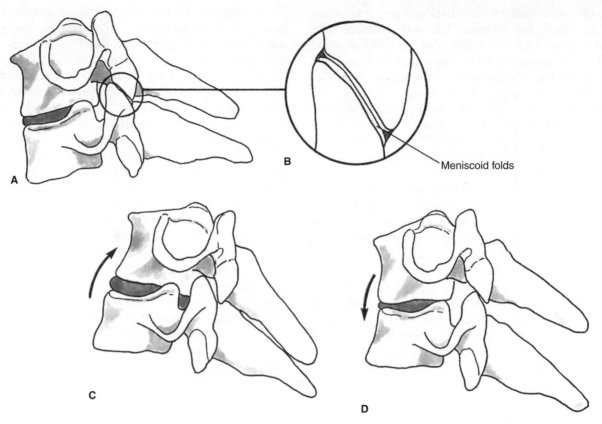

FIG. 16-9. *Sagittal section of an articular facet joint (**A**), with an enlarged view (**B**) showing the mensicoid folds. The articular surfaces tend to approximate during extension (**C**) and separate during flexion (**D**).*

and numerous ligaments surrounding and reinforcing the capsule. In degeneration the synovium is redundant, and the capsule frequently is redundant or torn and may contribute to malfunction as trapped menisci do in other joints.[117,173]

Generally motion between two vertebrae is extremely limited and consists of a small amount of gliding or sliding. The net effect of small amounts of gliding in a series of vertebrae produces a considerably large range of motion for the spinal column as a whole. The motions available to the column may be likened to that of a joint with three planes of motion: flexion–extension, lateral flexion (sidebending), and rotation.[166] In addition, a small amount of vertical compression and distraction is possible. The type and amount of motion that are available differ from region to region and depend on the orientation of the facets and the fluidity, elasticity, and thickness of the intervertebral joint. Although the degree of movement at the spinal segment is largely determined by the disks, the patterns of movement of the spine depend on the shape and orientation of the articular facet joint surfaces. If the superior and inferior articular facets of the three adjacent vertebrae lie in the sagittal plane, the motions of flexion and extension are facilitated. Conversely, if the articular facets are placed in the frontal plane, the predominant motion is that of lateral flexion or sidebending.

Regionally (except for C1 and C2, whose articular facets are oriented in the transverse plane), the articular facets of the intervertebral joints of the cervical spine are oriented at 45° to the transverse plane and parallel to the frontal plane (see Fig. 16-3A). This alignment of the intervertebral joints allows flexion, extension, sidebending, and rotation. The angle increases at descending levels, approaching vertical at C7 in the frontal plane. The superior articular facet surface is convex, and the inferior facet surface is concave. The articular facet joint surfaces tend to separate during forward bending and approximate during backward bending (see Fig. 16-9C,D). Sidebending and rotation occur together to the same side. This is because the articular facet joint surfaces are positioned approximately halfway between the frontal and transverse planes. As one articular facet joint slides forward and upward, its mate slides backward and downward, translating to a sidebending component in the frontal plane and a rotatory component in the frontal plane and in the transverse plane. In this way, sidebending and rotation from C2–C3 to about

T1 involve essentially an identical movement between articular facet joint surfaces. The only difference between sidebending and rotation of the cervical spine results from differences in movement at the upper cervical spine. The unique joint configuration found in the alanto-axial complex is discussed in Chapter 17, The Cervical Spine. According to Kapandji, combined movement of flexion and extension for these segments is approximately 100° to 110°.[109] When combined with movement of the atlanto-axial complex, the total range of motion is 130°.

In the erect spine, sidebending and rotation in the thoracic and lumbar regions tend to occur to opposite sides. The reasons may be more complex than at the cervical spine, but again seem to be largely the result of the orientation of the articular facet planes (see Figs. 16-4A and 16-5A). In the thoracic spine, all 12 thoracic vertebrae support ribs and show facets for the articulation of these structures. Unlike the spinous processes in the lumbar and cervical areas, where the tip of the spinous process is found directly posterior to the body of the vertebra, the tip of the spinous process lies posteriorly and inferiorly to the body (see Fig. 16-4A,B). The spinous processes are long and triangular in section. Those of the upper and lower four thoracic vertebrae are more bladelike and are directed downward at an angle of 60° so that their spines completely overlap the next lower segment (see Fig. 16-1C).[191,192] This elongation limits the amount of extension possible at each segment. The thoracic pedicles are longer than in the cervical and lumbar areas, giving the vertebral canal an oval appearance and diminishing the possibility of stenosis of the canal (see Fig. 16-4C). The transverse processes are characterized by having a concave facet that receives the tuberculum of the rib and being angled backward; this encourages rotatory movements by the attached muscles.

The articular facets of the thoracic vertebrae are oriented 60° to the transverse plane and 20° to the frontal plane (see Fig. 16-4A,B),[119,129,135] which allows sidebending, rotation, and some flexion and extension. Because of the articular facet alignment and stabilization of the vertebral bodies laterally, rotation is the most accessible movement. Gregersen and Lucas concluded from a study on rotation of the trunk that approximately 74° of rotation occurred between the first and twelfth thoracic vertebrae (the average cumulative rotation from the sacrum to the first thoracic vertebrae was 102°).[81] The superior articular facets form a stout, shelflike projection. The ovoid surfaces of the superior articular facets are slightly convex, whereas the inferior articular facets are slightly concave (similar to the articular facet joint surfaces in the cervical spine), which is opposite to the articular facets in the lumbar spine.[76]

The majority of thoracic vertebrae adhere to the basic structural design of all vertebrae, except for some minor variations. The C7–T3 segments are a transitional zone between the cervical lordosis and thoracic kyphosis, with all ranges being diminished, although flexion and extension are freer than in the lower thoracic spine. The first thoracic vertebra is considered the transitional vertebra, whereas the second thoracic vertebra, which can be distinguished by an enlarged pedicle, is thought to be developed to carry that portion of the weight borne by the articular facets into a more forward position, so that at levels below the second thoracic vertebra the weight is carried principally by the vertebral bodies and disks.[173] The physiological movement combinations are the same as for the typical cervical regions (i.e., sidebending accompanied by rotation).[84] At the T3–T10 segments, both sidebending and rotation are limited by the bony thorax. Amplitudes of movement, especially in the sagittal range, increase progressively as the restriction offered by the ribs begins to decrease. The T11–L1 segments are a transitional zone between the thoracic kyphosis and lumbar lordosis. While the articular facet joints remain vertically oriented, they begin to change from the frontal to the sagittal plane. The last thoracic vertebra (T12), acting as a bridge between the thoracic and lumbar regions, has its inferior articular facets in the sagittal plane to match those of L1.[109]

RIB CAGE ARTICULATIONS

According to Maigne, involvement of the rib cage in pathological processes is often neglected. Yet costal sprain is very frequent and is expressed by thoracic or upper lumbar pain.[135] It follows either a contusion, an unusual effort, or a faulty movement (generally in rotation). The ribs are thus mechanically significant articulations of the thoracic spine. The 12 pairs of thin arc-shaped bones form a protective cavity for the heart, lungs, and great vessels.[42] They also provide attachment for muscles necessary for respiration, posture, and arm function. The rib cage has several important biomechanical functions related to the spine. It acts as a protective barrier for any traumatic impact directed from the sides or anterior aspect, and it stiffens and strengthens the thoracic spine. The moment of inertia provided by the rib cage is its most important biomechanical aspect, according to White and Panjabi.[220] The increased moment of inertia stiffens the spine when it is subjected to any kind of rotatory forces, such as bending movements and torques.

The transverse dimensions of the thoracic spine are increased manifold by the inclusion of the sternum and ribs. Cartilaginous junctions fix the ribs to the sternum. Characterized as *true ribs*, the first seven are attached to the sternum by individual cartilages (Fig. 16-10*A*). The eighth, ninth, and tenth ribs have a common junction with the sternum and are called *false ribs*.

The ends of the true ribs join this costal cartilage by means of the costochondral joint. The first rib is joined firmly to the manubrium by a cartilaginous joint, while the second rib articulates with demifacets on both the manubrium and the body of the sternum by way of synovial joints (see Fig. 16-10*A*). The cartilages of the third to seventh ribs have small synovial joints

which attach to the body of the sternum.[220] Later in life these joints become ankylosed or obliterated.[84]

The ribs and vertebrae are united at two locations. The radiate ligament anchors each rib head to two adjacent vertebral bodies and the disk between them (see Fig. 16-10*B,C*).[177] This occurs at the superior and inferior costal demifacets located at the junction of the vertebral body and posterior arch, and forms the costovertebral joint (a synovial joint) (see Fig. 16-10*B*). Costotransverse ligaments join the rib tubercle and corresponding vertebral transverse process (see Fig.

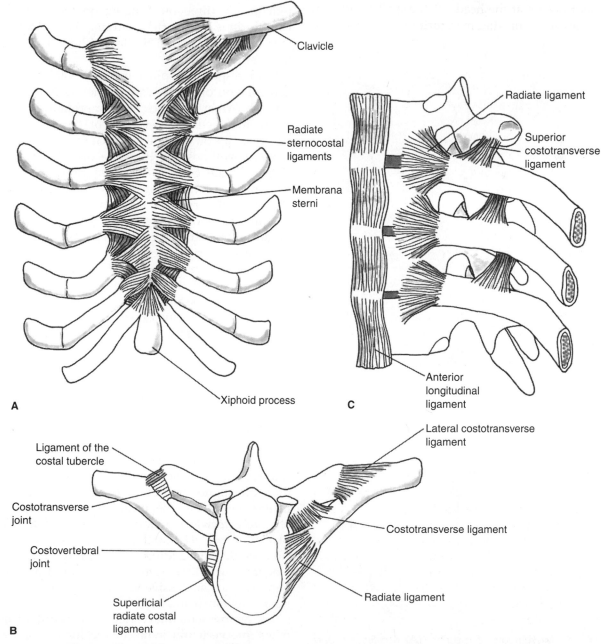

FIG. 16-10. Joints of the ribs: (**A**) costosternal joints and connections; (**B,C**) costovertebral joints, on superior and sagittal views.

16-10*B,C*). To accommodate this articulation, each long transverse process is capped by a costal facet. The costotransverse joint is also a synovial joint surrounded by a capsule, but it is primarily strengthened by three costotransverse ligaments.[109]

Each rib is a curved lever which has its fulcrum immediately lateral to the costotransverse joint, and each has its own range and direction of movement differing slightly from the others. Although it is fair to surmise that each rib has its own pattern of movement, certain generalizations can be made. The first ribs form a firm horseshoe-shaped arch, which moves upward and forward as a unit (Fig. 16-11*A,B*). This movement occurs at the heads of these ribs and is a simple elevation of the manubrium upward and

forward.[134] The false ribs combine the elevation of their anterior ends with a caliper-like opening (Fig. 16-11*C*).[134] Following direct trauma or secondary to some attempts at trunk rotation, the false ribs induce pain somewhat analogous to that of lumbago. The pain is typically located in the lumbar fossa, radiating toward the groin, and is acutely intensified by certain movements.[135]

The final two (eleventh and twelfth) ribs are free floating (termed *floating ribs*) and simply end in the trunk musculature of the abdominal wall. Their loose attachment at their heads and lack of union with the transverse processes leaves them subject to push and pull in any direction, hinging on the head.[134] The twelfth rib is the shortest and may be so short that it fails to project beyond the lateral border of the back muscles that cover it.[97]

With respect to spinal motion, both sidebending and rotation of the thoracic spine are limited by the rib cage. When a thoracic vertebra rotates, the motion is accompanied by distortion of the associated rib pair. The ribs on the side to which the body rotates become convex posteriorly, while the ribs on the contralateral side become flattened posteriorly.[166] The amount of rotation that is possible depends on the ability of the ribs to undergo distortion and the amount of motion available in the costovertebral, costotransverse, and costochondral joints.

Because the rib cage actually encloses the thoracic spine, any external stabilizing force must be indirectly applied through the ribs. Because of their size and configuration, the ribs are more plastic than the vertebral bodies.[188] As such they readily yield to applied forces, and their shape will be altered before any corrective effect is noted on a rigid spine.[42]

LUMBAR ARTICULATIONS

The average plane of inclination of the lumbar articular facets is almost 90° to the transverse plane and 45° to the frontal plane (see Fig. 16-5*A,B*). The articular facets face in almost a lateromedial direction and are therefore aligned in the sagittal plane, whereas the articular facets of the fifth lumbar vertebra face obliquely forward and laterally toward the frontal plane.[191,192,220] This alignment allows flexion, extension, and sidebending, but almost no rotation. Sidebending is limited to a range of approximately 5° between each successive vertebra, whereas rotation is limited to approximately 3°.[3]

The lumbosacral intervertebral joints differ from the other intervertebral joints in the lumbar spine. The orientation and shape of the facets at this level allow more rotation.[132] Most L4–L5 articular facet joints are angled about 43° from the coronal or frontal plane,

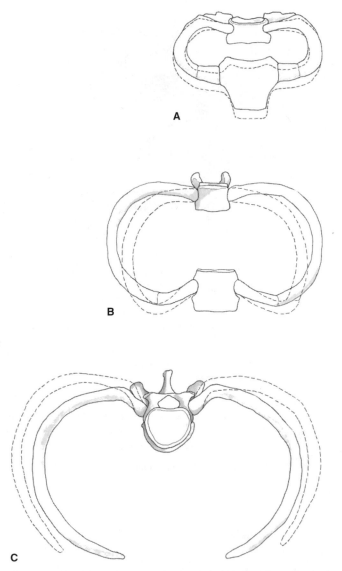

FIG. 16-11. Movements of the ribs: (**A**) the first rib and manubrium with upward and forward movement; (**B**) the typical vertebrosternal ribs with bucket-handle movement; and (**C**) the caliper-like movements of the lower ribs

while most L5–S1 articular facets are angled about 52°. Unlike the more superior lumbar joints, the articular facets of the inferior articulating process of the L5 vertebra face forward and slightly downward to engage the reciprocally corresponding articular processes of the sacrum. The most essential function of the lumbosacral articulations involves their role as buttresses against the forward and downward displacement of the L5 vertebra relative to the sacrum.[191,192] Because the sacrovertebral angle produces the most abrupt change of direction in the column, and the center of gravity which passes through the L5 segment falls anterior to the sacrum, there is a marked tendency for the thick, "wedge-shaped" fifth lumbar disk to give way to the shearing vector that the lumbosacral angularity produces. The resulting condition, spondylolisthesis, most frequently reveals a deficiency in the laminae that fails to anchor L5 to the sacrum and allows it to displace forward.

All of the articular pillars of the lumbar vertebrae have convex surfaces on the inferior articular process, forming in most cases one third or one half of a sphere with a greater curvature in the transverse than in the longitudinal section. The superior articular process carries a corresponding concave surface so that the joints have two principal movements—translation (slide) and distraction (gapping). Unlike the intervertebral disks, which allow motion in all planes, the articular facet joints restrict the motion segment, assisted by the ligaments. The capsules of the lumabr articular facets are quite fibrous and extend upward and medially onto the laminae above, which enables them to restrict forward bending.[48,173]

According to White and Panjabi, "mechanical load-sharing" between the facets and disks is rather complex.[220] Other authors have made quantitative estimates of the biomechanics, including Nachemson who found that 18% of the compressive load is borne by the articular facet,[155] King who reported that 0 to 33 percent of the axial load was borne by the facet, depending on the position or posture of the joint[115]; and Farfan who attributed 45 percent of torsional stiffness to the articular facets and capsules.[60] The articular facet joints make a major contribution to the rotational stiffness of the lumbar spine; this is important because *in vitro* testing of loaded motion segments in rotation alone and rotation with either flexion or sidebending can produce the types of disk lesions seen clinically. The importance of asymmetrical articular facet orientation for pathological processes of the intervertebral disk has been well documented by Farfan and Sullivan, who established a highly significant correlation between asymmetry of the articular facet joints and the level of disk involvement, and between the side of the more oblique articular facet orientation and side of sciatica.[62] Most articular facet planes have a difference

in angle of less than 10°, but "gross" asymmetry is seen in about 25 percent of an essentially random population by conventional roentgenography.[60] This may be associated with asymmetrical vertebral bodies or with unilateral laminar hypertrophy and is clearly associated with early disk degeneration at the level of the asymmetry. When such asymmetry is present, it is the side with the most oblique articular facet that acquires early posterolateral annular damage.

INTERVERTEBRAL DISKS

The spine, which is composed of alternating rigid and elastic elements, possesses a considerable degree of flexibility that is primarily attributable to the intervertebral disks. The amount of flexibility depends on the material characteristics, the size and shape of the disk, and the amount of restraint offered by the invertebral ligaments. Normally the disks may be considered to act as universal joints, permitting motion in four directions between vertebral bodies: (1) translational motion in the long axis of the spine, occurring because of compressibility of the disk; (2) rotary motion about a vertical axis; (3) anteroposterior bending; and (4) lateral bending.[151]

VERTEBRAL BODY RELATIONSHIP

Each successive vertebral body is linked by an intervertebral disk, which acts as a symphysis between the vertebrae. There are no disks between the occiput and atlas nor between the atlas and axis. The disk "spaces" in the young adult contribute to as much as 20 to 33 percent of total vertebral column height. The ratio between the height of the disk and the corresponding vertebral bodies, in part, determines the amount of motion that may occur in a particular region. Flexibility has been shown to vary directly with the square of the vertical height of the disk and indirectly with the square of the horizontal diameter of the body.[153] Because of the proportionally greater height in the lumbar region, the range of intervertebral motion is greater in the lumbar region, but because of the greater horizontal diameter, the flexibility is less than in the thoracic region.[151] Motion is greatest in the cervical spine. The unique composition of the intervertebral disks allows for a more even distribution of weight transmitted to the adjacent vertebral bodies during movement.

It is often mentioned that the disks act as shock absorbers during vertical compressive loading. While this may be true to some extent, shock absorption on vertical loading is largely related to the fact that the spine is a curved, "spring-loaded," flexible column, rather than a rigid, rodlike structure.

The cervical disks are largely responsible for the existence of a normal cervical lordosis in the upper spine; the lumbar disks are somewhat less responsible for the normal lumbar lordosis, which is mostly caused by the wedged-shaped vertebral bodies. In the thoracic spine the normal kyphosis is almost entirely caused by the shape of the vertebral bodies.

DISK STRUCTURE

The disk is composed of several structures, including the nucleus pulposus, which is the central fluid-filled portion of the disk, and the annulus fibrosus, the series of elastic fibers that surround the nucleus (Fig. 16-12). The disk is bounded above and below by cartilaginous end-plates, to which the annular fibers are firmly anchored. These end-plates are then attached to the body surface of the vertebral bodies. The inner fluid nucleus (a remnant of the embryonic notochordal tissue) is surrounded by a zone of irregular connective tissue bands that are also rich in fluid and are, in turn, surrounded by the lamellae of the annulus fibrosus.[173] The overall shape of the nucleus mimics that of the body, and takes up about 25 percent of the disk area.[60] The fluid mass of the nucleus pulposus is composed of a colloidal gel rich in water-binding glucosaminoglycans with a few collagen fibers randomly embedded within. It is centrally located in the disk, except in the lower lumbar segments where it is located more posteriorly.

NUCLEUS PULPOSUS AND FLUID EXCHANGE

Both the relative size of the nucleus pulposus and its capacity to take on water and swell are greatest in the cervical and lumbar spine. It is well suited for its essential function to resist and redistribute compressive forces within the spine. Because of its high water content and plastic nature, its functions follow closely the laws of hydrodynamics. Typically, the nucleus pulposus occupies an eccentric position within the confines of the annulus, usually close to the posterior margin of the disk (Fig. 16-12B). Being avascular, the nucleus depends on nutrition from its exchange of fluid across the cartilaginous end-plate with the vascularized vertebral body. The tendency of imbibition of fluid by the nucleus is greatest when weight-bearing is reduced through the disk (as in sleeping). As a result, a young person tends to be taller ($1/4$ to $3/4$ inch) in the morning than at the end of the day. During the day the disk fluid is expressed from the disk to complete the nutrient cycle. In addition to being expressed, the disk fluid can be relocated by the assumption of specific postures.[120] Examples of this include the loss of normal lordosis after assuming a flexed position when gardening, or a lateral shift associated with low back injury.[173] The mucopolysaccharide gel changes in its biochemical characteristics with damage and age. These biochemical changes decrease the water-binding capability of the nucleus. Hendry demonstrated that a disk will give up water more readily if it is degenerated because of damage or age.[93] Normally, the nucleus contains between 70 and 88 percent water, which makes it nearly incompressible, and thus it acts as a distributor of force at the vertebral level. As the disk becomes drier and its elasticity decreases, it loses its ability to store energy and to distribute stresses and is therefore less capable of resisting loads.

ANNULUS FIBROSUS

The annulus fibrosus consists of fibroid cartilage with bundles of collagen fibers arranged in a crisscross pattern, which allows them to withstand high bending and torsional loads (see Fig. 16-12A). These fibers run obliquely between vertebral bodies such that the fibers in one layer run in the opposite direction to the fibers in adjacent layers. The outer layer of fibers blends with the posterior longitudinal ligament

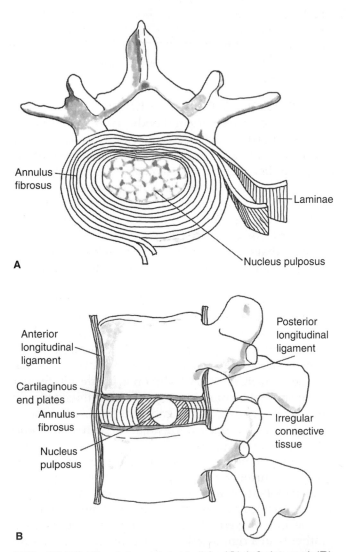

Annulus fibrosus

Laminae

Nucleus pulposus

A

Anterior longitudinal ligament

Posterior longitudinal ligament

Cartilaginous end plates

Annulus fibrosus

Irregular connective tissue

Nucleus pulposus

B

FIG. 16-12. The intervertebral disk: (**A**) inferior and (**B**) sagittal views.

posteriorly and with the anterior longitudinal ligament anteriorly. These outer fibers attach superiorly and inferiorly to the margins of the vertebral bodies by Sharpey's fibers. The fibers of the outermost ring of the annulus extend beyond the confines of the disk and blend with the vertebral periosteum and longitudinal ligaments. The inner fibers attach superiorly and inferiorly to the cartilaginous end-plates. The cartilaginous end-plate is composed of hyaline cartilage that separates the outer two components of the disk from the vertebral body (see Fig. 16-12B). In addition to absorbing forces, the annulus contains the nucleus pulposus, which acts as the fulcrum of movement for the three planes of motion available at each vertebral level.[109] One of the major functions of the annulus is to withstand tension, whether the tensile forces are from the horizontal extension of the compressed nucleus, from torsional stress of the column, or from the separation of the vertebral bodies on the convex side of spinal flexion.[191,192] The entire unit is then ensheathed by the periosteum, which extends over the vertebrae (and, in effect, the intervertebral disks), displaying a thickening both anteriorly (anterior longitudinal ligament) and posteriorly (posterior longitudinal ligament).[199] According to Paris, the area of the disk covered by this sheath has been found to be both innervated and vascularized and possesses, in effect, a neurovascular capsule.[173] Innervation from the sinuvertebral nerve has been substantiated by findings of Cloward and others. It is proposed that the diseased disk, in which parts of the annulus have been torn and repaired, contains a richer innervation from the ingrowth of nerve tissue with granulation.[38] This may be of some importance clinically in patients with spinal pain. Surgically removed disk tissue has been reported to contain some complex as well as free nerve endings.

DISK PRESSURES

The young healthy disk maintains a positive pressure within the nucleus pulposus at rest, which increases as loads are applied to the spine. This pressure approximates 1.5 times the mean applied pressure over the entire area of the end-plate.[163] These pressures have importance therapeutically when activity and exercise programs for patients with disk problems are being designed. Disk pressures have been extensively studied in various postures and seating configurations. A more detailed description can be found in other sources and will not be covered here.* The "preloaded" spinal column in the healthy nucleus maintains a continuous pressure to separate the adjacent vertebrae. This preloaded condition and the in-

*See references 5, 7—15, 82, 84, 85, 88, 89, 147, 150, 152, 155, 157–161, and 163.

compressibility of the nucleus serve to form a self-righting system: with a compressive force or angular movement in any direction, the resultant intradiskal pressure changes are such that the disk favors movement back to the "neutral" position. Note, however, that this self-righting system also depends on the tensile strength and the elasticity of the annulus. Tensile strength or stiffness must be provided in the horizontal direction in order to withstand the intermittent stresses applied to it from the nucleus. Elasticity of the annulus or movement between adjacent planes of annular fibers is necessary in a vertical direction to allow angular movement between adjacent vertebral bodies. Loss of a balance between this extensibility and stability of the annular fibers is probably a contributing factor in disk disorders.

In axial compression, the increased intradiskal pressure is counteracted by annular fiber tension and disk bulge, rather analogous to inflating a tire (Fig. 16-13A).[179] Some disk-space narrowing also occurs. Because of the incompressibility of the fluid-like nucleus, forces acting on the nucleus will act to move it, change its shape, or both. In flexion, extension, and lateral bending, the same process occurs. Because the annular fibers are somewhat elastic and because the annulus allows vertical and tangential movements between vertebral bodies, the nucleus in the healthy disk may either change in shape or move within the limits allowed by the annulus.[197] Its volume, however, must remain the same. Displacement of the nucleus within the disk has been disputed more recently.[84,118] Because the nucleus is roughly spherical, some have considered it as a ball that allows one vertebra to rotate over its neighbor. The nucleus is said to move backward during flexion and forward during extension. However, others have not confirmed this observation, and Krag and associates found little motion of the nucleus.[118]

In the consideration of an angular movement forward (flexion) of one vertebral body on another in a weight-bearing situation, the forward shift of weight will result in an increased compressive force on the anterior aspect of the disk. This causes the anterior annular fibers to bulge backward and causes the nucleus to shift backward, transferring the vertical compressive force to a horizontally directed force backward against the posterior annulus (Fig. 16-13B). Because the healthy nucleus is fluid-like, an even distribution of pressure results across the inner annular layers. The posterior annular fibers, which are normally bulged somewhat backward in the neutral position, tend to straighten because of the increase in distance between the posterior vertebral bodies. However, because of the pressure against the posterior annulus by the nucleus, there is also a tendency to maintain this posterior bulge and thus bring the vertebrae back to a neu-

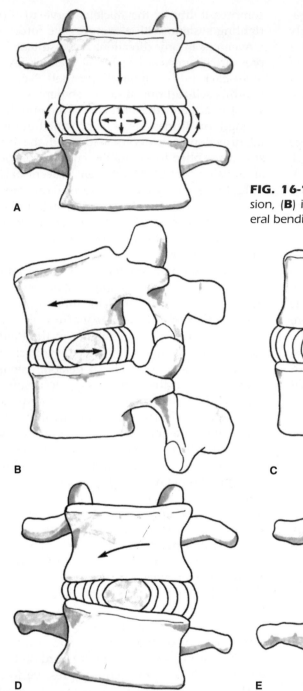

A

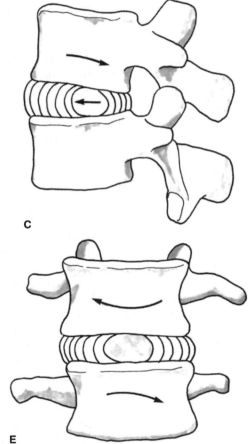

FIG. 16-13. Nucleus pulposus: (**A**) during axial compression, (**B**) in spine flexion, (**C**) in spine extension, (**D**) in lateral bending, and (**E**) during axial rotation.

B

C

D

E

tral relationship (the self-righting mechanism discussed earlier). Looking at it from another perspective, the straightening of the annular fibers tends to increase the counterpressure against the posteriorly bulging nucleus, which effects a counterforce against the original vertical compressive force. In this way an equilibrium must be reached between the transformation of the vertical loading to a horizontal pressure against the annulus and the tendency for the annulus to reconvert this pressure, in a self-righting manner, to counter the compressive loading. In extension

and lateral bending, the same process occurs (Fig. 16-13C,D). Of clinical significance is the fact that changes in this equilibrium favor pathological changes in the related tissues, while, conversely, pathological tissue changes result in a change in the equilibrium; the resultant cycle of events should be obvious. For example, a weakening of the annular fibers results in less tendency to resist the horizontal forces exerted by the nucleus, which will result in further weakening of the annulus. Osteoporosis of the vertebral bodies results in a decreased ability to withstand reactive vertical forces with erosion of disk material into the vertebral bodies; the so-called vacuum phenomenon.

In axial rotation, a compressive force causes an increase in intradiskal pressure and tends to narrow the joint space (Fig. 16-13E). When rotation occurs, the annular fibers—which are oriented in the direction of rotary movement—become taut, while the fibers oriented in the opposite direction tend to slacken. Mathematical models based on the geometry of the disk demonstrate that torsion produces stress concentrated on the region of the posterior lateral annulus, which is a common site of disk herniation.[121,204] Torsional loading of spinal segments *in vitro* produces fissures in the annulus in the same posterolateral location and is thought to be one of the common early causes of acute low back pain.[180] During daily activities the disk is loaded in a complex manner, usually by a combination of compression, bending, and torsion. Flexion, extension, and lateral flexion of the spine produce mainly tensile and compressive stresses in the disk, whereas rotation produces shear stress. The tensile stress in the posterior part of the annulus fibrosus in the lumbar spine has been estimated to be four to five times the applied axial load.[70,155] The thoracic annuli fibrosi are subjected to less tensile stress than the lumbar annuli fibrosi because of their geometric difference. The ratio of disk diameter to height is higher in the thoracic disk than the lumbar disk.[124]

The entire intervertebral disk in the adult is avascular. Up to the time of skeletal maturity, blood vessels do enter the disk from the vertebral bodies through the cartilaginous end-plates. These vessels are gradually obliterated, leaving scars in the end-plate where they penetrated.

INTERVERTEBRAL FORAMINA

The *intervertebral foramen* is the aperture that gives exit to the segmental spinal nerves and entrance to the vessel and nerve branches that supply the bone and soft tissues of the vertebral canal. This aperture or canal is superiorly and inferiorly bounded by the respective pedicles of the adjacent vertebrae (see Fig. 16-2). Its ventral and dorsal relations involve the two major intervertebral articulations. Ventrally it is bounded by the dorsum of the intervertebral disk, covered by the posterior longitudinal ligament, and dorsally by the capsule of the articular facet and ligamentum flavum (see Fig. 16-8). Spur formation within the foramen can decrease the available space and create compression forces on the spinal nerves exiting through the foramen or on the structures that reenter the foramen, such as the sinu-vertebral nerve, which

innervates the posterior longitudinal ligament (see later, Vertebral Innervation, page 509).

Nerve-root entrapment may also result from closure or narrowing of the vertebral foramen, through any of the following mechanisms: (1) approximation of the pedicles resulting from narrowing of the intervertebral disk; (2) hypertrophic degenerative arthritic changes of the articular facet joints; and (3) thickening of the ligamentum flavum. The existence of additional ligamentous elements in relation to the intervertebral foramen (*e.g.*, the transforaminal ligaments, found frequently in the lumbar region) could be critical.[33,191,192] The transforaminal ligaments are strong, unyielding cords of collagenous tissue that pass anteriorly from various parts of the neural arch to the body of the same or adjacent vertebra.

☐ The Control System: Noncontractile Soft Tissues

LIGAMENTS

The ligaments are vital for the structural stability of the spinal system. Their principle role is to prevent excessive motion. The ligaments are also the principal tensile load-bearing elements and, along with the apophyseal capsules, provide the central nervous system with information in regard to posture and movement.[225] Unlike muscles, ligaments are passive structures so that their tension depends on their length. Ligaments are viscoelastic in nature, with their deformation and type of failure being dependent on the rate of loading. Like all materials, ligaments fatigue and can fail with repetitive loading.[179,216] They readily resist tensile forces but buckle when subject to compression.

The ligaments that connect the anterior elements of the spine are the broad *anterior longitudinal ligament*, which extends from the basiocciput to the sacrum, and the *posterior longitudinal ligament*, which also extends from the basiocciput to the sacrum on the anterior aspect of the neural canal, behind the vertebral bodies. These ligaments are interlinked at each level by the disk, which adds support to the disk and vertebral body network (see Fig. 16-8). The annulus fibrosus of the intervertebral disk may be considered a part of the ligamentous structure. These ligaments deform with separation of the vertebrae and bulging of the disk.[220] Richly supported by nerve fibers, they respond to painful stimuli. The remaining ligaments of the spine support and link the posterior elements.

ANTERIOR LONGITUDINAL LIGAMENT

The anterior longitudinal ligament is one ligamentous structure placed anterior to the center of rotation of the intervertebral joint. It thus acts to prevent hyperextension, along with the capsular ligament of the articular facet joint (see Fig. 16-8). It begins as a rather narrow band from the basiocciput and broadens as it descends from C3 to the sacrum. It consists of long fibers along its length and short, arched fibers coursing between individual vertebrae and inserting into the anterior aspect of the intervertebral disk (see Fig. 16-10C).[109] Considered perhaps the strongest ligament in the body (with a tensile strength of nearly 3000 pounds per square inch), the anterior longitudinal ligament, along with the muscles about the spine, keeps a preload beam condition in the spine that helps to strengthen the spine during lifting.[59] In the lumbar spine it also resists the weight of the spine in its tendency to slip into the pelvic cavity.[173] Because of its breadth and tensile strength, this ligament provides strong support and reinforcement to the anterior disk during lifting, and Harrington and others have used the strength of the anterior ligament combined with Harrington rods to apply traction to fracture dislocations of the low back.[220]

POSTERIOR LONGITUDINAL LIGAMENT

The posterior longitudinal ligament extends from the basiocciput to the sacrum on the anterior aspect of the neural canal behind the vertebral bodies (see Fig. 16-8A,B,D). It is densely attached to the posterior annulus fibrosus at each level, with both vertical and transverse fibers that spread across the posterior annulus; however, as the posterior longitudinal ligament passes the vertebral bodies, it narrows and is not attached to them except at their margins.[191,192] This allows entrant arteries, veins, and lymphatics to pass in and out of the posterior portion of the vertebral bodies. In flexion the posterior longitudinal ligament becomes taut and serves as a valve on these vessels, which do not have a valve mechanism of their own. It, like the anterior longitudinal ligament, is thickest in the thoracic (dorsal) spine. It is often reduced to a cord-shaped filament in the lumbar spine. The lateral expansions over the disks are thin, whereas the central portions are much thicker. This is presumably why most posterior protrusions of the disk soon move laterally to become posterolateral protrusions. Although the posterior longitudinal ligament is not as massive as the anterior longitudinal ligament in terms of cross-sectional area, the tensile strength per unit area seems to be the same for both structures.[209] Functionally, the ligament limits forward bending and gives support to the disks except in the lumbar region. Of interest is that in the midline the ligament does have a small amount of elastic tissue.[173] In the cervical spine the ligament is a broad band on the entire posterior aspect of the bodies, but because it is attached only in the region of the disk, with disk degeneration it produces folds that can press into the spinal canal

on backward bending; this movement is therefore to be avoided in such conditions.

SEGMENTAL LIGAMENTS

The segmental ligaments of the spine include the *ligamentum flavum*, the *interspinous* and *intertransverse ligaments*, and the *anterior and posterior capsular ligaments of the articular facet joints*. The biomechanical significance of these structures depends on their strength, stiffness, and distance from the axis of rotation of the joints they span.[220]

LIGAMENTUM FLAVUM

The ligamentum flavum extends from the anteroinferior border of the laminae above to the posterior border of the laminae below (see Fig. 16-8B,C,D). It connects the laminae from C2 to S1. The medial edges fuse with the contralateral ligament in midline and completely close the vertebral canal (a slight septum is provided for the passage of arteries and veins). At its lateral border, the ligamentum flavum blends with the capsules of the articular facets, particularly in the lumbar region (see Fig. 16-8B,C).[96] Histologically, the ligamentum flavum has the highest percentage of elastic fibers of any tissue in the body.[31,162] It checks the movement of the articular facet joints by exerting a constant pull on the capsule and thus assists in preventing the synovial lining and intra-articular menisci from being painfully nipped between the articular joint surfaces.[173] It owes much of this function to its yellow elastic fibers (hence, *flavum*, meaning yellow).

During forward bending the ligamentum flavum permits considerable range and assists in return to neutral or the resting position of the spinal segments without the development of folds. It thus serves to protect the spinal canal from encroachment by soft tissues on flexion and extension. Nachemson and Evans found that in neutral the ligamentum flavum is prestrained by about 15 percent and that full physiological flexion can stretch it an additional 30 to 35 percent, while it retains a 5 percent stretch in full physiological extension.[162] This elasticity is lost to some extent in normal aging, but if the instant axis of rotation for flexion is in the region of the posterior annulus, the flexion–extension torque resistance in the ligamentum flavum is significant. There is appreciable strain of the ligamentum flavum on sidebending or lateral flexion.[171] The ligamentum flavum also provides some preloading of the disk (leading to disk nucleus pressures greater than atmospheric), even when there is no external load on the spine, which may reduce slack in the motion segment. In patients with severe spine degeneration, the ligamentum flavum may be thickened and less elastic and may produce narrowing of the spinal canal in extension. This narrowing occurs because of the buckling of the ligament. Thus, at the time of surgery for spinal stenosis, its excision may be necessary.

INTERTRANSVERSE AND INTERSPINOUS LIGAMENTS

The intertransverse ligaments are well developed in the thoracic spine and are intimately connected with the deep muscles of the back.[220] They pass between the transverse processes and are characterized as rounded cords. These ligaments are barely mentioned in many texts on functional anatomy, particularly with respect to the lumbar spine, as being significant. Functionally, they tend to limit sidebending and rotation.

The interspinous ligaments, which connect the spinous processes, are important for the stability of the spinal column. They are reinforced, especially at the level of the thoracic and lumbar spine, by the supraspinous ligaments (see Fig. 16-8C,D). Their attachments extend from the root to the apex of each spinous process, proceeding in an upward and backward direction, *not* an upward and foreword direction, as often illustrated.[173] This upward and backward orientation permits increased range of motion during flexion while still resisting excessive range. Panjabi and associates found high strain in both the interspinous and supraspinous ligaments with flexion while these were relatively unstrained in rotation.[171] The interspinous ligaments are narrow and elongated in the thoracic region, only slightly developed in the cervical spine, and thicker in the lumbar spine.[220] In 90 percent of cadavers over 40 years of age, Rissanen noted that the interspinous ligament between L4 and L5 had degenerated or was completely ruptured.[187]

The supraspinous ligament is a strong fibrous cord that connects the apices of the spines from the C7 to L4, and occasionally to L5 (see Fig. 16-8C,D).[173] At this level it is replaced by the interlocking fibers of the somewhat stronger erector spinae tendons of insertion. The supraspinous ligament is thicker and broader in the lumbar region than the thoracic, and it is intimately blended in both areas with the neighboring fascia. Between the spine of C7 and the external occipital protuberance, it is much expanded and called the *ligamentum nuchae* (see Fig. 17-4).[212] In the cervical region the spinous processes are buried deeply between the heavy muscles on the back of the neck so that the supraspinous ligament is represented by a thin septum between the musculature of the two sides. In quadrupeds with heavy heads, the ligamentum nuchae is a strong, thick band of elastic tissue which aids the muscles in holding up the head.[97] In humans, however, the supraspinous and interspinous ligaments and the ligamentum nuchae are largely collagenous tissue, relatively inelastic and of little strength; in the cervical and lumbar regions, where they should be most important in limiting segmental flexion, the interspinous ligaments are frequently defective or lacking in one or several interspaces.[97] Because the supraspinous ligament is the most superficial of the spinal ligaments and farthest from the axis of flexion, it has a greater potential for sprains.[109]

FASCIAL ANATOMY

THORACOLUMBAR REGION

Although not technically a ligament, the thoracolumbar (lumbodorsal) fascia has a tensile strength of nearly 2000 pounds per square inch and serves as one of the most important noncontractile structures in the lumbar spine (Fig. 16-14A).[60]

The thoracolumbar fascia consists of three layers (anterior, middle and posterior) that arise from the transverse and spinous processes and blend with other tissues. The anterior layer is derived from the fascia of the quadratus lumborum muscle. The middle layer lies posterior to it. The posterior layer consists of two laminae, one with fibers oriented caudomedially and the other oriented caudolaterally.[25] The two laminae of the posterior layers fuse with the transversus abdominus muscle to the lumbar spinous processes. Gracovetsky, Farfan, and Helleur[78] have designated the anterior part of the thoracolumbar fascia as the "passive" part and the posterior layer as the "active" part. The passive part serves to transmit tension from contraction of the hip flexors to the spinous processes. The active part is activated by the transversus abdominus muscle, which tightens the fascia. The tension in the fascia transmits longitudinal tension to the tips of the spinous processes of L1–L4 and may help the spinal extensor muscles to resist an applied load.

In the lower thoracic and lumbar regions this fascia is much thicker than the rest of the spinal area, for it represents not only fascial tissue but the fused aponeuroses of several muscles.[97] It functions in many respects as a ligament, because it invests epaxial muscles that course along the spinous processes and is reinforced by the aponeurotic origin of the latissimus dorsi cranially and by the attachment of the erector spinae (epaxial paravertebral) muscle mass caudally into the sacrum and sacral ligaments. It spans the area from the iliac crest and sacrum up to the thoracic cage. The posterior layer is reinforced by the latissimus dorsi superficially and by the attachment of the sacrospinalis to its deep surface. The fascial aponeurotic sheet encloses the erector spinae muscle mass between the thoracic spines and the interspinous ligaments medially, and the laminae and ligamentum flavum anteriorly.

Because the thorocolumbar fascia encloses a space on each side of the spine, contraction of the erector

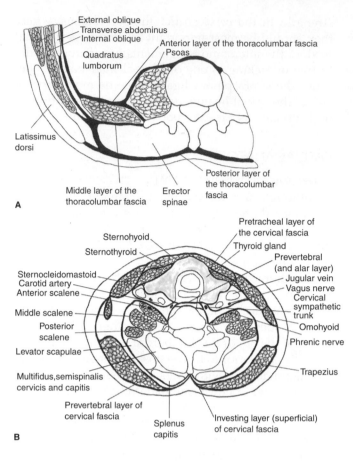

A

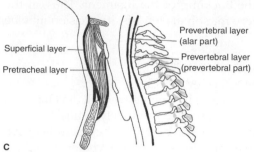

C

FIG. 16-14. (**A**) The thoracolumbar fascia, (**B**) a cross-section of the neck, and (**C**) a longitudinal section of the fascial layers of the neck.

B

spinae muscle mass (with a consequent increase in the transverse muscle area) tends to greatly tighten the thoracolumbar fascia, so that it functions as part of an active mechanism for pulling the vertebrae posteriorly and controlling shear and flexion during lifting. On full flexion, as the muscles become electrically silent, the thoracolumbar fascia becomes the major force against further flexion.[134] On extension from a fully flexed position the gluteus maximus and hamstrings act in concert with the thoracolumbar fascia to initiate extension.[76] With increased activity of these muscles the fascia serves to increase their efficiency.[79] It also serves as a protective ligament against excessive flexion, and as the muscle mass contracts, the increased diameter of the muscle exerts a wedging effect on the aponeurosis, which may relieve some of the shear load on the articular facet joints and disks in flexion–extension movements of the spine.[61]

It has been further demonstrated on the basis of dissections and histological observations that the muscles of the abdomen have the potential to stabilize the vertebral column through the action of the thoracolumbar fascia. This can be brought about, according to Tesh and associates, by (1) the intrinsic nature of the fascia without direct involvement of the vertebral

ligaments; (2) muscle contraction modifying longitudinal ligament tension by the thoracolumbar fascia; or (3) a combination of both mechanisms.[208]

CERVICAL REGION

The cervical spine, with its investing musculature, is housed within the vertebral compartment, situated centrally and posteriorly. The contents of this compartment provide points of anchorage and suspension for fascial layers defining all remaining compartments (see Fig. 16-14B).[125]

The superficial (investing) layer embeds all the muscles of the neck except the platysma. The primary layers of the deep cervical fascia are the pretrachial layer and prevertebral fascia. The pretrachial layer is connected with the connective tissue sheath around the neurovascular bundle (common carotid artery, internal jugular vein, and vagus nerve as the carotid sheath) and embeds the infra- and suprahyoid muscles. It is firmly adherent to the clavicle and deeper still to the layer or lamina of the prevertebral fascia. Although these fascial layers provide stabilization to their contents, they are normally sufficiently lax to permit motion of the neck as a unit, as well as motion of one compartment relative to another.

PREVERTEBRAL FASCIA

The prevertebral fascia (see Fig. 16-14*B,C*) is a firm membrane lying anteriorly to the prevertebral muscles (longus colli; longus capitis; anterior, middle, and posterior scalenes; and rectus capitis). It is attached to the base of the skull just anterior to the capitis muscles and descends downward and laterally to ultimately blend with the fascia of the trapezius muscles. In its course it covers the scalene muscles and also binds down the subclavian artery and the three trunks of the brachial plexus. The prevertebral fascia crosses medially to the transverse processes of the cervical vertebrae and covers all the cervical nerve roots. The fascia does not ensheath the subclavian or axillary veins, and therefore does not cause venous congestion. The fascia is firmly adherent to the anterior aspects of the cervical vertebrae.

In the posture causing scapulocostal syndrome symptoms, the depressed scapula places strain on the fascia as well as the scapular musculature.[33] Obliteration of the radial pulse, as observed in Adson's maneuver, can be attributed to the tension of the cervical fascia on rotation of the head and neck. Traction on the lower trunk of the brachial plexus may well cause pain and numbness in the ulnar distribution of the hand, which is common in this syndrome.[211]

CAPSULES

The joint capsule of the spinal articular facet joint is composed of two layers, an outer layer known as the *stratum fibrosum* and an inner layer called the *stratum synovium*. The outer layer is attached to the periosteum of the component bone by Sharpey's fibers and is reinforced by musculotendinous and ligamentous structures that cross the joint. The outer layer is poorly vascularized but richly innervated. The nerve endings that are located in and around the joint capsule are sensitive to the rate and direction of motion, tension and to compression and vibration.[86]

In contrast to the outer layer, the inner layer of the capsule is highly vascularized but poorly innervated.[94] The stratum synovium is insensitive to pain but undergoes vasodilatation and vasoconstriction in response to heat and cold. It produces the hyaluronic acid component of the synovial fluid and serves as an entry point for nutrients and an exit point for waste material.[94] The capsules of the articular facet joints possess two noteworthy recesses, one superior and one inferior, through which the synovium may distend during effusion or backward bending.[52,136] The superior recess is the weaker, and effusion here may protrude sufficiently to press on the mixed spinal nerve as it enters the intervertebral foramen.[52]

Capsules encompass all the articular facet joints in the spine including the articulation of the head with the atlas.[150] The capsules include separate thickenings which have different functional roles. The capsules and their ligaments guide and restrict the motion segments. Because they are far from the disks and therefore act on long moment arms, these ligaments have an important functional role in resisting spinal flexion.[179] In full flexion of the lumbar spine, the capsules support 40 percent of the body weight.[76] These fibers are generally oriented in a direction perpendicular to the plane of the articular facet joints. They are broader and more taut in the cervical region than the rest of the spine.[171] The capsules of the lumbar spine, which are often illustrated as being short and bunchy, in fact have a considerable medial extent and are quite fibrous, possessing an upward and medial direction that ideally suits them to restricting forward bending.[173] The capsular ligaments, along with the anterior longitudinal ligament, also act to prevent hyperextension of the spine.[60]

Capsules are an important consideration with respect to the loose- and close-packed positions of the articular facet joints of the spine.[46,76] The concept of loose- and close-packed positions is useful in understanding when a joint may be less stable and more vulnerable. Loose-packed positions are those positions in a joint's range of motion in which the ligaments and capsules are slack; the area of contact with the articular surfaces is generally low and the joints are more vulnerable and less able to resist an external force. Close-packed positions, on the other hand, are those in which there is maximum contact between articular surfaces and maximum tautness of the ligaments.[2] The close-packed position of the articular facet joints from C3 to L5 is extension, whereas the close-packed position for the atlas and axis is full flexion.[76] The close-packed position is often lost following a pathological process, trauma, or prolonged periods of poor posture. Inability to assume a full close-packed position results in the potential for increased dysfunction, and as a result a more unstable, loose-packed position is maintained.

VERTEBRAL INNERVATION

Because of the high frequency of patients presenting clinically with complaints of spinal pain or pain appearing to be of spinal origin, it is necessary for the clinician to have a thorough knowledge of spinal innervation. More specifically, the clinician must be aware of what structures appear to lack innervation totally. This information must be combined with an understanding of common pathological processes and their clinical manifestations. In this way a more reliable understanding may be acquired as to the nature and extent of various disorders and perhaps a better understanding of the often bizarre symptoms and signs that result.

Information relating to spinal innervation and pain-sensitive spinal tissues has come from two types of investigations: (1) actual experiments with human subjects in which attempts are made to isolate noxious stimuli to a particular tissue; and (2) laboratory tissue studies in which sensory endings are identified and attempts are made to trace the afferent pathways from these endings to central connections. For obvious reasons, those studies belonging to the first category of investigation are relatively few and results have at times been inconsistent or highly criticized. There have been numerous studies of the second type, however, and the results, for the most part, seem to be consistent. One must realize, however, that there is a limit as to how much can be inferred from tissue studies with respect to clinical significance. This is especially true when considering pain-sensitive tissue, because there is no direct correlation between the type of ending found within a particular tissue and the capacity for the tissue, when stimulated, to send signals to higher centers, which result in the perception of pain (see Chapter 4, Pain).

Presented here will be a summary of what seem to be reasonably well-accepted findings relating to spinal neurology. Spinal structures receive innervation largely from two sources, the sinu-vertebral (recurrent meningeal) nerves and the medial branches of the posterior primary divisions of the segmental spinal nerves (Fig. 16-15A,B). Endings found in the dura mater and blood vessels are primarily of the free nerve plexus type (see Chapter 3, Arthrology). Endings found in the posterior longitudinal ligament and periosteum include free nerve endings and plexuses as well as encapsulated and nonencapsulated nerve endings. It is assumed that the larger encapsulated nerve endings act primarily as mechanoreceptors. It is important to realize that each sinu-vertebral nerve tends to innervate the tissues at its own level as well as send ascending and descending branches to levels above and below (Fig. 16-15A). It follows that stimulation of endings supplied by a particular sinu-vertebral nerve may result in the perception of pain or in reflex changes in muscle tone at levels of the spine other than the level at which the lesion lies. Also, because it is well documented that stimulation of deep somatic tissues often results in segmentally referred pain, one may assume that pain may be referred into a segment not corresponding to the vertebral segment (level) at which the lesion lies.

The posterior division of the spinal nerve divides into lateral, intermediate, and medial branches (Fig. 16-16). The lateral branch innervates the skin and deep muscles of the back segmentally, while the medial branch innervates the articular facet joint cap-

sules, the posterior aspect of the ligamentum flavum, the interspinous ligaments, the supraspinous ligaments, and the blood vessels supplying the vertebrae. The medial branches of the posterior division also send ascending and descending branches to (usually) one level above and one level below, with the same clinical implications as discussed for the overlapping sinu-vertebral nerves. Receptors found in the facet joint capsules, sending signals along the medial branch of the posterior division, include all four of the receptors discussed in the section on joint neurology (see Chapter 3, Arthrology).

Afferent fibers from both the sinu-vertebral nerve and the medial branch of the posterior primary division approach the spinal cord through the dorsal roots. In the dorsal roots the small unmyelinated fibers, thought to be largely responsible for transmission of noxious stimuli, aggregate toward the anterior aspect of the dorsal root. These enter the spinal cord and send branches to Lissauer's tract, where they may ascend or descend for a few segments before sending fibers to the substantia gelatinosa at the tip of the dorsal horn (see Chapter 4, Pain). Other fibers may pass directly to the base of the dorsal horn of the gray matter. From here they may ascend along the spinoreticulothalamic tract or through internuncial neurons and synapse with alpha motor neurons of segmentally related muscles (see Fig. 16-15A). In this way, noxious stimulation of sensitive spinal tissues may result in reflex muscle spasm (or perhaps inhibition) of segmentally related muscles. Thus, muscle spasms—which are often a part of this clinical syndrome—may result from this proposed pathway or by yet an undetermined sensory or motor-reflex pathway.[69] Note again that because of the overlapping distribution of sensory fibers, muscles of more than one segment are likely to be affected. The previously mentioned ascending tract tends to cross within a few segments before ascending, with only a few ascending ipsilaterally. Signals traveling along this tract are thought to contribute to the conscious awareness of pain.

The larger-diameter afferent fibers reach the spinal cord through the posterior rami of the dorsal roots. These contribute to the dorsal columns of the spinal cord, which supply information to higher centers, including proprioceptive and "fast-pain" input. Other large fibers synapse at the tip of the dorsal horn of the gray matter, the substantia gelatinosa, to contribute to modulation of afferent input to higher centers, as discussed in Chapter 4, Pain. Recall, however, that ultimate perception of pain is, in part, determined by the relative balance of large-fiber and small-fiber input to the substantia gelatinosa, and that an imbalance in favor of small-fiber input tends to facilitate pain perception.

Selective stimulation of spinal structures has been

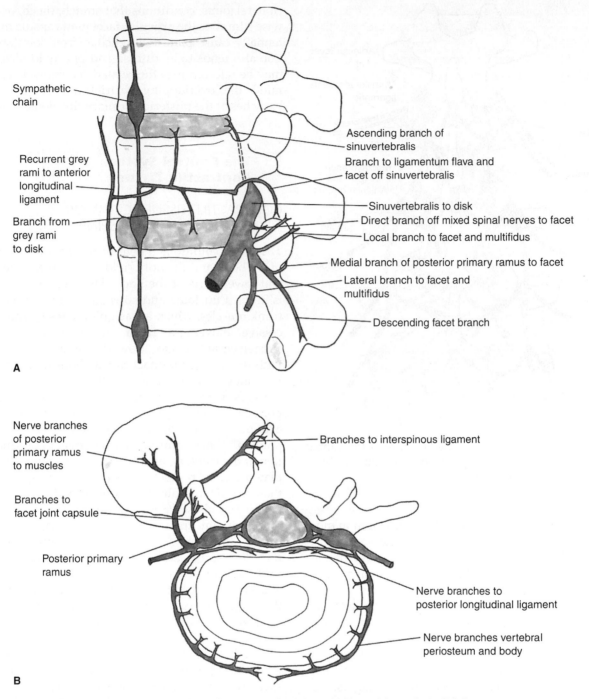

Sympathetic chain

Recurrent grey rami to anterior longitudinal ligament

Branch from grey rami to disk

Ascending branch of sinuvertebralis

Branch to ligamentum flava and facet off sinuvertebralis

Sinuvertebralis to disk

Direct branch off mixed spinal nerves to facet

Local branch to facet and multifidus

Medial branch of posterior primary ramus to facet

Lateral branch to facet and multifidus

Descending facet branch

A

Nerve branches of posterior primary ramus to muscles

Branches to facet joint capsule

Posterior primary ramus

Branches to interspinous ligament

Nerve branches to posterior longitudinal ligament

Nerve branches vertebral periosteum and body

B

FIG. 16-15. (**A**) Innervation of the posterior joints. (Adapted from Paris SV: Anatomy as related to function and pain. Orthop Clin North Am 14:476, 486, 1983.) (**B**) Innervation of the spinal structures.

carried out in a number of investigations. These studies include distention of normal and pathological disks, needling of various aspects of intervertebral disks, injection of hypertonic saline into interspinous ligaments, injections of facet joints, and mechanical stimulation of nerve roots and other structures during surgery carried out under local anesthesia. Back pain can be reproduced by injecting hypertonic saline into

the supraspinatus, interspinous, and longitudinal ligaments; the ligamentum flavum; and facet capsules.[95,128,138] These structures and the peripheral third of the annulus fibrosus are innervated by nociceptive nerve fibers, which are afferent branches of the posterior primary rami.[23,226] The studies in which the intervertebral disks were distended by injection of dye during diskography suggests that, indeed, pain can re-

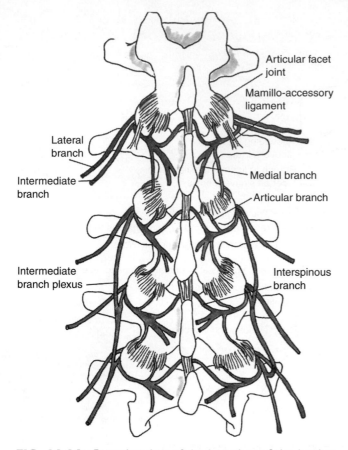

FIG. 16-16. Posterior view of the branches of the lumbar posterior rami. The mamillo-accessory ligament has been left *in situ* covering the L2 branch.

sult from distention of the disk. It is noted that in most cases distention of a pathologically degenerated or protruded disk resulted in much more severe pain than injection of a normal disk. In most cases pain was referred into the shoulder or hip girdles with cervical and lumbar injections, respectively, and often into the limbs. It was usually described as a deep, aching, poorly localized pain, whereas direct stimulation of a nerve root tends to result in a sharp, lancinating pain well localized to the related dermatome. On the basis of such findings, Rothman and Simeone distinguish between scleratogenous pain of spinal origin and neurogenic pain.[191,192] The former usually results from stimulation of the sinu-vertebral nerve from a nuclear protrusion, putting abnormal mechanical pressure on the outer annular layers or the posterior longitudinal ligament. This results in a deep, aching, somewhat diffuse pain which may be referred to any part, or all, of the relevant sclerotomes. The latter, neurogenic pain, is that of sharp, well-localized pain felt in a dermatomal distribution, resulting from actual nerve-root pressure.

Studies also show the spinal joints to be sensitive to pain.[225] Because the fibrous capsule is a primary pain-sensitive structure of the spinal joints, as it is in the pe-

ripheral joints, conditions that stretch, pinch, or otherwise stimulate the articular facet joint capsule may potentially cause pain. Pain elicited from joint stimulation also tends to be diffuse and poorly localized and may be referred into the related segments, keeping in mind the overlapping distribution of the medial branches of the posterior primary divisions.

☐ The Control System: Contractile Tissues

CONTRACTILE TISSUES COMMON TO MOST AREAS OF THE SPINE

The spinal column is the vertical supporting structure of the body and the only rigid link between the upper and lower parts of the body. However, this structure is in itself unstable and so is supported by the major trunk muscles, which act as guidewires to prevent excessive movement in a direction of imbalance. Gregersen and Lucas showed how an excised spine, with the ligaments intact but without muscles, buckles under even very small compressive forces, whereas a muscled spine can, with abdominal support, carry the weight of the trunk, head, and upper extremities in addition to hundreds of added pounds.[81] These muscles also contract to produce motion of the trunk against the forces of gravity and may play a role in protecting the spine during trauma, if there is time for voluntary control, and possibly in the post-injury phase.[220] From a preventive and therapeutic standpoint, the muscles are very important structures of the spine. Under voluntary control they position the spine and stabilize it during awkward postures and provide the power necessary for lifting and carrying. Chaffin and Park have demonstrated that workers with inadequate lifting strength who work in relatively stressful lifting tasks have higher low-back injury rates than workers with equally stressful lifting tasks but better strength.[36] Apparently when lifting near the strength limit of these muscles, excessive strain may be transmitted to the other soft tissues, such as ligaments and disks.

The proper functioning of the mobile segment demands perfect synergy of the different muscles. A movement that is not anticipated or is poorly estimated can bring about a harmful distribution of forces on the intervertebral joints. Certain elements of the joints may be submitted to traction or compression forces beyond their capacity for resistance. Spasms of these muscles undoubtedly constitute a major factor in the genesis of the painful spine, which is amenable to treatment by manual therapy.

The motor elements of the mobile segment comprise short and long paraspinal muscles. The former exert their action directly, whereas the latter act indirectly by affecting distal segments. These muscles are innervated by the posterior branches of the spinal nerves, which thus play a very important part in invertebral mechanical pathological processes. Only a brief description of the musculature is appropriate here.

The posterior (epaxial) muscles in humans are organized in three planes with the shortest (myomeric) muscles being the deepest (see Chapter 1, Embryology of the Musculoskeletal System). The semispinalis, multifidi, and rotatores, although they have different sources, are often called the *tranversospinalis muscles* (Fig. 16-17). Clearly there are fibers that course from spinous process to adjacent transverse process (inter-spinous), from transverse process to adjacent transverse process (intertransversalis), from transverse process to spinous process (multifidus), from transverse processes below to laminae above (musculi rotatores), and, in the thoracic region, from transverse processes to ribs (musculi levatores costrum).

The intermediate layer of the posterior musculature is massive and courses from transverse process to spinous processes two to four segments above (multifidi) or multisegmentally (see Fig. 16-17). According to their regions, they are the multifidus (lumbosacral), thoracis, semispinalis cervicis, and semispinalis capitis (cervical). The deep and intermediate layers are of most interest to the motion segment; in particular, the com-

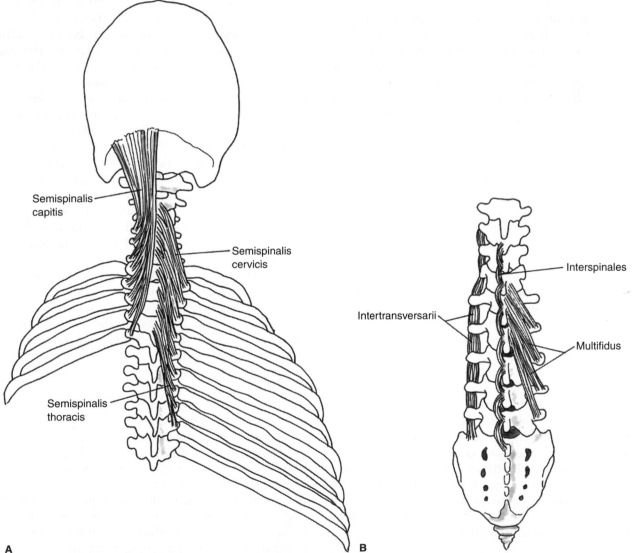

FIG. 16-17. Deep muscles of the back. The medial group (the tranversospinalis, interspinalis, and intertransversarii) includes (**A**) the semispinalis (head, neck, and thoracic sections) and (**B**) the intertransversarii, interspinales, and multifidus. (Note: These muscles are only partially illustrated in each section so that their relation to the bony structures of the spine can be seen.)

plex multifidus in the lumbosacral region. The multifidus is bipennate in both origin and insertion and is functionally significant with respect to its posterior insertion to the capsule of the articular facet joint.[173]

Overlying the multifidi are the longer and more lateral muscles that arise from the sacrum and adjacent connections to insert on the lower six or seven ribs (iliocostalis) and the longest and most medial muscles that share the same origin but insert into the medial portions of the nine or ten lowest ribs and the transverse processes of the lower thoracic vertebrae (longissimus) (Fig. 16-18B). These superficial and posterior muscles are collectively called the *erector spinae*. The active function of these muscles working together is to extend and stabilize the spine, while in groups they can rotate or sidebend it, often working with muscles in other groups.

The rotator muscles, although present at other levels, are most prominent in the thoracic region.[88] These muscles bring about rotation of the vertebrae in the direction opposite the side of the muscle and have a sensory role in monitoring rotation. Morris and colleagues found the longissimus thoracis and rotatores spinae to be continuously active during standing.[152] The trapezius and latissimus dorsi are common to most areas of the spine (Fig. 16-19 and Fig. 17-6). Combined, the origin of the trapezius and latissimus dorsi spans the entire spine from occiput to sacrum. The trapezius spans from the occiput to T12, and the latissimus overlaps the six segments from T6 to the sacrum. The trapezius then inserts on the stable portion of the shoulder complex (the scapula), whereas the latissimus dorsi inserts onto the mobile humerus. Together they act to position the shoulder and retract it during lifting, spreading the load of the upper extremity across the entire span rather than concentrating the force in the upper thoracic region.[76] The latissimus dorsi also produces extension of the lumbar spine, along with the serratus posterior. In addition, it acts in concert with the transverse abdominus, internal oblique, and gluteus maximus muscles as a dynamic stabilizer of the low back, by way of their attachments to the lumbodorsal fasciae or aponeuroses (see Figs. 16-14 and 16-19). The trapezius also serves as one of the suspensor motors of the shoulder girdle, along with the rhomboids and the levator scapulae (see Fig. 17-6). These muscles, taking origin from the cervical and thoracic spine, suspend and mobilize the scapula and thereby link cervical and thoracic spine motions with upper limb motions.[125]

MUSCLES OF THE THORACOLUMBAR SPINE

The lateral muscles of the trunk originate from the hypaxial portion of the lateral mesoderm, the quadratus lumborum, and psoas. The quadratus is the more posterior and is complex, filling the space between the iliac crest and the twelfth rib, while also attaching to the transverse processes of the lumbar vertebrae. It is a primary lateral bender of the lumbar vertebrae, assisted by the psoas muscle. It is also described as a "hip hiker" that is active in gait, during the swing phase, to hold the pelvis in a neutral position.[100] If painfully restricted, it can limit chest or rib cage expansion and can contribute to a leg-length discrepancy.

The psoas is more ventral and is considered, by some, primarily a limb muscle,[97] but as Michele has stated, it is also a potential extensor of the spine and a flexor of the lumbar spine on the pelvis depending on the relative positions of the spine, pelvis, and femur.[143] The *psoas major* arises from the anterolateral aspect of the lumbar vertebral bodies and transverse processes, and then crosses the hip before inserting with the iliacus on the lesser trochanter. The *psoas minor* (not always present) lies ventral to the psoas major and courses from the vertebrae of the thoracolumbar junction to insert on the superior pubis ramus, which allows it to work with the abdominal muscles in upward tilting of the pelvis.

The extensive fascial attachment of the gluteus maximus muscle, both at its origin and insertion, is well known (Fig. 16-19). The crescent-shaped origin has widespread bony aponeurotic and ligamentous attachments. Approximately two thirds of the gluteus maximus muscle ends in a thick tendinous lamina, which inserts into the iliotibial band of the fascia lata. This offers strong control of the lower extremity during stressful activity. A comparison of the magnitude of action potentials elicited in the gluteus maximus muscle during a variety of exercises and activities demonstrates that the greatest electrical activity occurs during muscle-setting contractions; these include exercises of hyperextension of the thigh accompanied by resistance, external rotation or abduction, and vigorous hyperextension of the trunk from the erect position.[64] The muscle seems to lack a major postural function in symmetrical upright positions at rest. Rotation of the trunk in a standing position activates the gluteus maximus contralateral to the direction of rotation, which is the corresponding function as an outward rotator of the leg when the trunk is flexed. Anteflexion of the trunk in the hip joint is attended by gluteus maximus activity, whose function probably is to fix the pelvis in its anteverted attitude.[110] Extension of the flexed thigh is performed primarily by action of the hamstrings, while extension beyond the relaxed standing position is associated with strong contraction of the gluteus maximus. Electromyographic studies recorded during lifting activities indicate that hamstrings are activated earlier and to a greater ex-

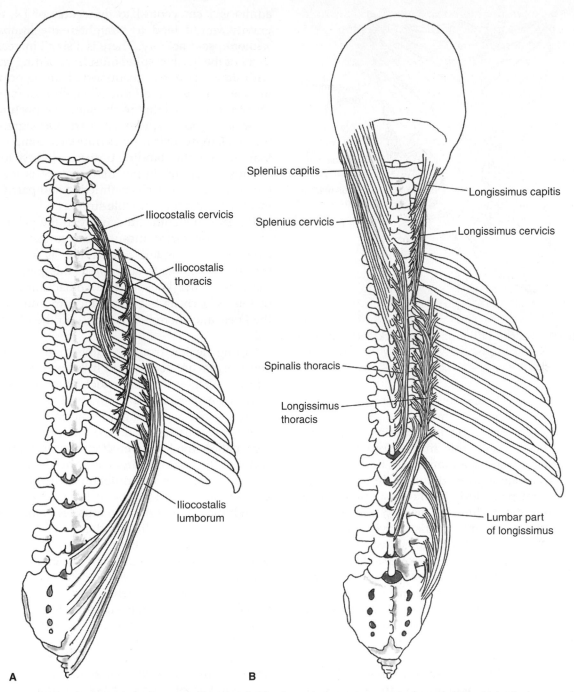

Splenius capitis

Longissimus capitis

Splenius cervicis

Longissimus cervicis

Iliocostalis cervicis

Iliocostalis thoracis

Spinalis thoracis

Longissimus thoracis

Iliocostalis lumborum

Lumbar part of longissimus

A   **B**

FIG. 16-18. Deep muscles of the back. The lateral group (erector spinae and the splenius) includes (**A**) the iliocostalis (cervical, thoracic, and lumbar sections) and (**B**) the longissimus (head and neck sections), splenius (head and neck sections), and spinalis thoracis. (Note: These muscles are only partially illustrated in each section so that their relation to the bony structures of the spine and ribs can be seen.)

tent during straight-knee lifts than during flexed-knee lifts. In contrast, the gluteus maximus and adductor magnus are more activated initially in the flexed-knee lift than the straight-leg lift.[64,164,165,174]

The human abdominal wall is developed from the body wall portion of the hyaxial mass of the lateral embryonic mesoderm. The two paired rectus muscles run alongside the midline from the sternum and costal cartilages to the pubis and, although they flex the spine powerfully, they do not increase interabdominal pressure. The transverse abdominus is the deepest of the lateral abdominal muscles, and runs from the lumbar vertebrae forward around the abdominal wall to merge with the contralateral trans-

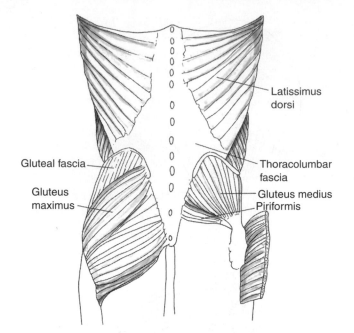

FIG. 16-19. Muscles of the posterior back and gluteal region.

verse abdominus. In the lower abdomen the lower fibers of the transverse abdominus and those of the internal oblique muscle form the conjoint tendon. The transverse has a major role in developing intra-abdominal pressure and is an important tie between the muscle–fascia column formed anteriorly by the rectus abdominus and posteriorly by the sacrospinalis muscles and the thoracolumbar fascia.[88] The internal oblique muscle is the intermediate layer and has its fibers from the iliac crest to the lower ribs and the lateral margin of the rectus sheath oriented to flex the trunk and turn the upper body to the contracting side. The external oblique muscle is the most superficial abdominal muscle layer, and its fibers also run from the lower ribs to the rectus, the pubis, and the iliac crest. However, these fibers flex and rotate the trunk away from the side that is contracting. When the oblique muscles contract bilaterally and symmetrically, they also raise the intra-abdominal pressure[179] (see Other Support Structures, page 517).

There is a fair concurrence of opinion about muscular activity in human posture based on electromyographic studies by many investigators.[60,97,156,220] Briefly, the activity of the lumbar spine muscles is low in relaxed standing and alternates with low levels of activity during body sway. There seems to be somewhat more constant activity in the paralumbar portion of the psoas major, both in standing and sitting, which provides additional preload to the spine and helps to maintain normal lumbar lordosis. Roentgenographic studies have shown that the line of gravity in most adults is 1 cm ventral to the center of L4, and that gravity would tend to straighten the lumbar spine without psoas activity. There is a small increase in activity of the lumbar spine muscles in sitting compared with standing. In the unsupported sitting posture, the muscle activity in the lumbar region was found to be about the same as that in the standing posture. In the thoracic region, Anderson and Örtengren found higher activity of the back muscles compared with that found in the standing posture.[7,9] These low levels of muscle activity imply that posture is maintained partly by active muscle contraction and partly by ligamentous and noncontractile support.

The lack of significant activity in the pelvic portion of the psoas major means that truncal equilibrium over the pelvis is fairly stable and is maintained by the strong ligaments anterior to this joint, as is also the case at the knee and sacroiliac joints. The line of force clearly falls behind the hip and in front of the knee, and there is no activity in the glutei at rest, either.

During flexion from standing to sitting the glutei and erectors are active until full flexion is reached, at which time they are again quiet. They are active while initiating extension and again at full extension. As the erector spinae muscles grade the rate of flexion, the abdominal muscles grade the rate of extension. During rotation, the longer erector muscles on the ipsilateral side, the short rotators and multifidi on the contralateral side, and the glutei on both sides are active, as is the tensor fascia lata on the ipsilateral side. Although the internal oblique muscles could assist with this motion, there is little abdominal activity in active rotation without resistance. Return to neutral is accomplished without significant muscular activity, evidently recovering some of the deforming force stored in the soft tissue. Sidebending is accomplished with ipsilateral activity of the back muscles, unless the person is very tall and limber or is supporting external weight, in which case the contralateral muscles become active as soon as the equilibrium position is overcome by ipsilateral contraction.

A number of studies have scrutinized muscular function in control of the spine.* Several of the more recent studies have also reported results in patients with back disorders.† Most would concede the importance of muscular function during both posture and functional activities. Whether or not injury to these muscles is a common cause of spinal pain is still controversial.

*See references 5, 7–15, 30, 65, 75, 101–107, 152, 153, 167–169, 171, 174, 183, 202, 213, 223, and 224.
†See references 20, 40, 43, 65, 75, 77, 98, 122, 140, 179, 184, 198, 202, 203, and 224.

MUSCLES OF THE CERVICAL SPINE

In the cervical area special attention must be paid to a balance of the length and strength of posterior, anterior, and lateral musculature that control head-on-neck and neck-on-thorax movements.[109] The muscles of the cervical spine may be categorized into four groups:

1. Cervicocapital motors
2. Visceral motors
3. Suspensor motors of the first ribs
4. Suspensor motors of the shoulder girdle[125]

The cervicocapital motor muscles consist of three groups, all of which move the cervical spine and skull. The first of these groups lies extrinsically to the spine, passing from the shoulder girdle to the skull in peripheral regions of the neck and producing primary motion of the head on the neck. The major members of this group are the sternocleidomastoid muscles (see Fig. 17-8). The sternocleidomastoid group is especially important with respect to the position of the head and, when restricted, facilitates a forward head position and limits rotation toward the side of the tight muscle. The remaining two groups of cervicocapital muscles have origins directly from the spine and insertions onto either the spine or skull, and thus are intrinsic to the spine. They occur in right and left pairs and act to rotate and tilt the head and neck. One of these groups is located entirely anteriorly (the prevertebral muscles) and includes the longus muscles (cervicis, capitis) and the rectus capitis anterior and lateralis. When its members contract in concert, flexion occurs. The longus capitis and the longus colli (see Fig. 17-10) lie deep to the esophagus and are positioned in such a way that head and neck flexion and extension, rotation, and sidebending are resisted or assisted by the oblique or vertical fibers that make up these muscles.[109] The remaining cervicocapital muscles are located entirely posteriorly, comprising the erector spinae and splenius muscles, which produce head and neck extension and often act in concert (see Figs. 16-18 and 17-6).

The long cervicocapital motor muscles are supplemented by smaller muscles in the atlanto-axial region, which produce discrete motion (or fine tuning) of the structures in this special region (see Fig. 17-7). The four muscles that compose the suboccipitals are the rectus major and minor and the obliquus superior and inferior. The rectus minor and the obliquus superior originate on the atlas and insert on the occiput. This places them in a good position to monitor and move the head into extension. The rectus major and the obliquus inferior act to move the head and C1 in rota-

tion and are important in small neck movements (see Chapter 17, The Cervical Spine).

The visceral motors of the neck include those muscles associated with the pharynx, larynx, trachea, hyoid bone, thyroid bone, and thyroid gland. The suspensor motors of the first ribs are the scalene muscles, which pass from the spine to cover the domes of the thoracic cavities; thus, they have an intimate relationship with vessels emerging to supply the head and upper limbs (see Fig. 17-8). The brachial plexus gains access to the thoracic outlet region by separating the muscle bundles of the scalene muscles. The scalene muscles, if unable to maintain their proper length, have a constrictive effect on the subclavian artery and veins as well as on the brachial plexus, all of which exit from the thoracic cavity and neck and go to the upper extremity.[88]

The suspensor motor group of the shoulder girdle includes the trapezius, rhomboids, and levator scapulae (see Fig. 17-6). These muscles, originating from the cervical and thoracic spine, suspend and mobilize the scapulae and thereby link neck motions with upper limb motions. The levator scapulae is clinically important in two ways. First, its origin (which arises from the dorsal tubercles of the transverse process of the first to fourth cervical vertebrae) allows the muscle to move the C1–C2 area, especially when the shoulder is fixed. Second, it has a propensity for transferring symptoms from the upper cervical area to its insertion on the superior angle of the scapula.[83] Pain in the upper cervical area creates an increased tension in the levator, which acts to elevate, migrate forward, and rotate downward the scapulae, resulting in rounded shoulders.

The muscles that serve the function of ventilation, mastication, vocalization, and phonation are collectively known as the *suprahyoids* and *infrahyoids* (see Figs. 15-13–15-15, 17-8, and 17-9).

☐ **Other Support Structures**

Intra-abdominal pressure has been regarded as important for stabilization and relief of the spine when it is exposed to heavy loads, as when lifting. Both the abdominal and thoracic cavities have been shown to become pressurized during strenuous activity. The abdominal cavity can be pressurized by mechanical contraction of the muscles of the abdominal wall together with the diaphragm. Associated closing of the glottis (Valsalva maneuver) results in further pressurization.[49,50] This increased pressure tends to force the pelvic wall (floor of the abdominal cavity) and the lung's diaphragm (roof of the abdominal cavity) apart. This intra-abdominal pressure has been regarded as important for the stabilization and relief of the lumbar spine when carrying out heavy tasks (*e.g.,* lifting) by extending the spine and thus reducing the contraction force required in the extensor muscles. Bartelink showed that the rectus was not active, but that the transverse and oblique muscles were.[19] He maintained that strengthening of the rectus may have a positive effect on posture, but does little or nothing to brace the spine during lifting. Farfan has suggested that the thoracolumbar fascia can change the length of the dorsal ligament by means of a laterally directed force from the oblique musculature. This is said to shorten these ligaments.[60] He postulated that this is the mechanism by which intra-abdominal pressure creates an extension moment about the spine, and that this assists in compressive load-bearing. Other investigators have also shown that strengthening of the abdominal muscles does not generally affect intra-abdominal pressure during lifting.[90,127]

Recently, Hemborg and co-workers have conducted a number of studies with respect to intra-abdominal pressure and trunk muscle activity during lifting in both healthy subjects and low-back patients.[90–92] Various breathing techniques were assessed in order to elucidate the causal factors of increased intra-abdominal pressure during lifting and the effects of respiration. The intra-abdominal and intrathoracic pressures and the electromyographic activity of the oblique abdominals, the erector spinae, and at times, the puborectalis muscles were recorded. The transdiaphragmatic pressure was calculated both during lifting and during the Müller maneuver.[73,193] The increase in intra-abdominal pressure during lifting seems to be correlated to coordination between the muscles surrounding the abdominal cavity. Of these the diaphragm seems to be the most important for the level of pressure. Closure of the glottis seems to be less important during lifting. Stillwell feels that the hydropneumatic effect of the abdominal support is facilitated by the bifolate shape of the diaphragm and by the change in shape of the abdominal wall that accompanies a deep breath taken before lifting.[205]

The general concept of spinal support from the abdomen has lead to a rationale for flexion exercises and protection of the spine by wearing a corset.[179] Davis has used this concept in determining safe loads to be used in industry.[51] In lifting there is a linear relationship between the amount of weight lifted and the intra-abdominal pressure that can be measured in the stomach or rectum.[12,82] However, in a position of spinal flexion or axial rotation with altered mechanics, Gilbertson and associates have shown that an increase in intra-abdominal pressure may not decrease the activity of the dorsal musculature and therefore may not reduce the net axial loading of the disk.[74]

It is accurate to say that lifting is associated with high abdominal and thoracic pressures and that these pressures may reduce spinal compressive loads. However, it should be pointed out that lifting is only one type of loading that leads to spinal injury. Manning and co-workers have shown that slipping on wet or slippery floors is one of the most common events leading to a significant back injury; it is hard to see how strong abdominals and a deep breath can be used to prevent such an unexpected turn of events.[137] Other factors that protect the back in lifting include

- Stabilization of the vertebral column through the action of the thoracolumbar fascia (see Fascial Anatomy, p. 507)
- The lever action of the thoracolumbar fascia, erector spinae muscles, and supraspinous ligaments. These structures pass some distance posteriorly to the spinous processes (and far posterior to the anterior column of the spine); however, they are firmly attached to them, and thus passive stretch of these structures can reduce the tendency toward flexion and forward shear of the lumbar vertebrae that would otherwise occur during lifting because of the orientation of the spinal elements. A shear resistance is created by the curve of the back, which imparts a posteriorly directed vector to the pull of the erector spinae muscles and the posterior ligaments of the lumbar vertebrae. Although this mechanical feature is lost in the upper lumbar spine with flexion, it is preserved in the lower lumbar spine.[1,60]
- According to Adams and Hutton, the flexion position may strengthen the spine and obviate the need for a great amount of relief from increased abdominal pressure.[1] It is thought that the posture adopted by experienced weight-lifters (*i.e.,* flexed lower lumbar spine, extended thoracic spine, and weight as close to the body as possible to reduce the bending moment) is the most efficient one biomechanically. The authors do not feel their studies negate the importance of abdominal pressure in increasing the margin of safety; rather, they state that the role of abdominal pressure is better defined as increasing the margin of safety, not making the lift possible in the first place, as others have implied.[1]
- The lumbosacral rhythm, in which the spine does not perform its segmental motions in the most disadvantageous position of full trunk flexion, but waits until after the hip extensors have brought the trunk to approximately 45° and reduced the lever arm
- Action of the external and internal oblique muscles when asymmetrical loads are encountered. Although the line of action of these muscles is anterior to the axis of rotation for flexion, these mus-

cles are critical in preventing buckling and overrotation with asymmetrical loading.

SACROILIAC JOINT AND BONY PELVIS

The base of support for spinal movement is the pelvis, to which many of the back muscles attach and through which the muscles of the thigh exert their influence on posture. The pelvis supports the abdomen and links the vertebral column to the lower limbs. It is a closed osteoarticular ring made up of three bony parts and three joints. The three bony parts are the two iliac bones and the sacrum, a solid piece of bone resulting from fusion of the five sacral vertebrae. The three joints consist of the two sacroiliac joints and the pubic symphysis, which links the iliac bones anteriorly (Fig. 16-20).[109,212]

Sacroiliac Joints

The major forces through the sacroiliac joints are borne by ligaments that tend to bind the sacrum into the ilia and lock together the unusually shaped articular surfaces (narrow, curving in an earlike shape in their plane, and deeply modified by depressions and elevations). The pelvis is usually described as a ring or arch with the innominate bones as lateral pillars and the sacrum as the keystone. This analogy only holds if it is appreciated that the sacroiliac ligaments hold the arch together; in usual engineering practice it is the superimposed and lateral masses that hold an arch together and there is usually no tension member. The pelvis is an extremely stable system of joints maintained by some of the strongest ligaments in the body.

Movement of the sacroiliac joints has been described by many authors, with considerable effort being expended to try to precisely measure these movements by roentgenographic and physical means (*e.g.,* pins placed in bones).[37,39,55,132] It is quite clear from this latter type of study that some motion does occur, but it is of small amplitude, while at least one roentgenographic study indicated the potential for "significant" deflection of bones of the pelvis during various static manipulations.[68,222] Even if the motions of the joint are of small amplitude, the joint is located and constructed to serve as a shock absorber and thus there is little reason that it should fuse. In fact, careful anatomical studies indicate that although the joint undergoes severe degenerative changes, fusion is relatively unusual, except in ankylosing spondylitis.[28] With respect to degenerative changes it is interesting that the iliac articular surface is fibrocartilaginous throughout life, whereas the sacral surface is hyaline cartilage. In general, the sacral cartilage is also about three times thicker in early adult life than the iliac cartilage. Resnick and associates found that early degenerative changes occurred on the iliac surface rather than on both surfaces of the joint simultaneously.[186]

Mitchell, in describing normal motion in the sacroiliac joints and in gait, suggests that the ilium rotates in a posterior direction at heel-strike and gradually moves from a posterior to an anterior direction as the person proceeds through the stance phase.[145] Elaborate descriptions of the possible axes and degree of motion have been postulated. These include a transverse axis through the pubic symphysis with rotation of the pubis to allow ilial motion in walking; a superior transverse axis, in the appropriate line of the second sacral segment, where some gross flexion occurs; a middle transverse axis, where additional gross flexion occurs; an inferior transverse axis, held to be the site of reciprocal motions of the joint during ambulation; and a set of oblique axes from the upper portion of one side of the sacrum to the lower portion of the contralateral joint.[145,217] Work by Weisl and others are not in total agreement about the amount and planes of motion.[39,214,222]

Kapandji describes the movements of nutation and counternutation (flexion and extension) of the sacrum

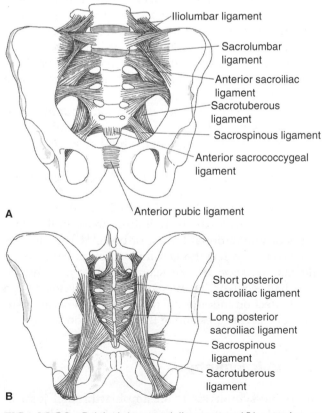

FIG. 16-20. Pelvic joints and ligaments: (**A**) anterior aspect; (**B**) posterior aspect.

Labels for **A**:
Iliolumbar ligament
Sacrolumbar ligament
Anterior sacroiliac ligament
Sacrotuberous ligament
Sacrospinous ligament
Anterior sacrococcygeal ligament
Anterior pubic ligament

Labels for **B**:
Short posterior sacroiliac ligament
Long posterior sacroiliac ligament
Sacrospinous ligament
Sacrotuberous ligament

within the ilia as being about a transverse axis posterior to the joint at the sacral tuberosity where the sacroiliac ligaments insert.[109] During nutation (flexion), movement of the sacral promontory is anterior and inferior, while the apex of the sacrum moves posteriorly. The iliac bones approximate and the ischial tuberosities move apart. Conversely, during counternutation (extension), the sacral promontory moves superiorly and posteriorly and the apex of the sacrum moves anteriorly. The iliac bones move apart while the ischial tuberosities approximate each other. These movements occur normally during the gait cycle and during activities such as forward and backward bending.

Understanding the position of the sacrum and ilia during gait and various body positions will help give the clinician an appreciation of the sacroiliac joint pain that may occur with locomotion. Despite differences of opinion regarding the movement center, most researchers agree that nutation and counternutation of the sacrum correspond to movements of the spine.[68,215] Therefore, in forward bending there is initially a backward bending (counternutation) of the sacrum, and as the spine completely flexes there is a resultant forward bending (nutation) of the sacrum. Whereas the position of the sacrum is determined by a force that reaches it from above, the ilium is controlled by movement of the femur. In standing, the base of the sacrum moves anteriorly. At heel-strike, the ipsilateral ilium is in a posteriorly rotated position. During the initial stance phase, sacral torsion occurs to that side. At midstance, increased tension of the iliopsoas encourages the ilium to move toward anterior rotation.[146]

Movement of the stable pelvic structure is made possible by the pelvic joints, consisting of the paired L5–S1 articular facet joints, the two sacroiliac joints, and the pubic symphysis. The two synovial sacroiliac joints are L-shaped when viewed from the side. The shorter and disposed cephalic limb of the sacral articulation is borne by the first sacral segment, while the longer and horizontally directed caudal limb is borne by the second and third sacral segments. Weisl has extensively studied these joints and has shown that a central depression can often be found at the junction of the two segments.[214,215] It has been noted that the cephalic limb of the sacral articular surface is more angled or wedged and is essentially vertical until it flares again inferiorly, as if to prevent it from sliding upward against the ilia.[203] The horizontal section of the sacrum has been described by Solonen as wedged dorsally in the upper portion of the joint and ventrally in the lower portion, whereas the ilial surface is convex superiorly and concave inferiorly.[203] The articular capsule is attached close to the margin of the articular surfaces of the sacrum and ilium.

The ligaments of the sacrum are a network of fibrous bands that fuse and intermingle to give added strength to the wedge of the pelvis. There are three main intrinsic and three main extrinsic ligaments. The three main *intrinsic ligaments* are the anterior sacroiliac, short posterior sacroiliac, and long posterior sacroiliac ligaments (see Fig. 16-20A,B).

The *anterior sacroilac ligaments* represent a thickening of the anterior and inferior parts of the fibrous capsule. They are particularly well developed at the level of the articular line but are thin elsewhere.[212] They stretch and tear easily upon slight pubic separation and allow the sacroiliac joints to gap during pregnancy.[194]

The *short posterior sacroiliac ligaments* pass from the first and second transverse tubercle on the dorsum of the sacrum to the posterior ilium. They prevent anterior (flexion) motion of the sacrum (see Fig. 16-20B).

The *long posterior sacroiliac ligaments* attach from the third transverse tubercle of the dorsum of the sacrum and the posterosuperior iliac spine, where they merge with the superior part of the sacrotuberous ligament and counteract the motion of downward slipping of the sacrum into the pelvis (see Fig. 16-20B).

The three main *extrinsic ligaments* are the sacrospinous, sacrotuberous, and iliolumbar ligaments (see Fig. 16-20A,B). The *sacrospinous ligaments,* which attach to the ischial spine and cross over to the anterior sacrum, and the *sacrotuberous ligaments,* which attach at the ischial tuberosity and traverse to the inferior sacrum, strongly stabilize the pelvis and anterior motion of the sacrum.

The *iliolumbar ligament* attaches from the iliac crest to the transverse processes of L4 and L5. It resists posterior rotation of the ilium and forward gliding of L5 on the sacrum (see Fig. 16-20A). According to Kapandji, the function of the superior band of the iliolumbar ligament is to check forward flexion of the vertebrae while the inferior or second band checks extension of the vertebral bodies.[109] Both bands of the iliolumbar ligament are also thought to be involved in lateral flexion (sidebending) and rotation of the lumbar spine.[182]

While the strongest muscles of the body surround the sacroiliac joint, none are intrinsic to it and so do not play a major part in directly moving the sacrum between the ilia. According to Mitchell, sacral movement is a result of forces carried to it through the pull of ligaments or gravitational forces, or both.[145] The muscles will indirectly affect the sacrum by their pull on the ilia and maintenance of poor sacral position after movement has occurred. Conversely, these muscles have a direct effect on innominate movement. They can instigate or cause progression of iliosacral lesions.

☐ Pubic Symphysis

The pubic symphysis is an amphiarthrodial joint in the anterior aspect of the pelvis that forms a fibrocartilaginous union between the two pubic bones. The osseous surfaces are covered by a thin layer of hyaline cartilage and the joint is formed by a fibrocartilaginous disk that joins the bones. The four ligaments associated with the joint are the *anterior pubic ligament* (Fig. 16-20*A*), *superior pubic ligament,* the *inferior arcuate ligament* (see Fig. 21-1), and the *posterior ligament.*[126] The thick inferior pubic ligament or arcuate ligament forms an arch that spans both inferior rami and stabilizes the joint from rotatory, tensile, and shear forces.[78] Kapandji[109] describes the muscle expansions as forming an anterior ligament consisting of the internal obliquus abduminus, rectus abdominus, transversus abdominus, and the adductor longus.[109]

The pubic symphysis permits tissue deformation and small translatory movements as a result of muscle, ground reaction, and trunk forces.[181] Many forces act on this joint, especially those exerted by the muscles of the lower extremity when the foot is fixed to the ground. The pubic symphysis can be affected by excess motion in the sacroiliac joints and can be a source of symptoms.

Not unlike the shoulder girdle, the pelvic girdle serves as the fixed base of support of operation of the lumbar and thoracic spine. Static and dynamic disorders which alter this fixed base of support, such as differences in leg length (real or apparent) or malpositions of the pelvic bones, may often elicit symptoms over time and result in degenerative changes of the lumbar spine, hip, and sacroiliac joints. One should bear in mind that the sacroiliac joint is a common site for referred pain and tenderness derived from segmental diskogenic backache.

■ KINEMATICS

Motion in the spine is produced by the coordinated action of nerves and muscles. *Agonistic* muscles initiate and carry out motion, whereas *antagonistic* muscles often control and modify it. While the degree of movement at spinal segments is largely determined by the disk–vertebral height ratio, the types of movement that may occur depend on the orientation of the articular facets of the intervertebral joints at each level. The motion between two vertebrae is small and does not occur independently. Obviously, the degree and combination of the individual types of motion vary considerably in the different vertebral regions.

Skeletal structures that influence motion of the spine are the rib cage, which limits thoracic motion, and the pelvis, whose tilting increases trunk motion.

□ *Ranges of Segmental Motion*

In three-dimensional space, the spine has six planes of freedom. A vertebra may rotate about or translate along a transverse, a sagittal, or a longitudinal axis or move in various combinations of these motions.[84,221]

Although the range of motion in an individual segment of the spine has been found to vary in different studies using autopsy material or roentgenographic *in vivo* measurements, there is agreement on the relative amount of motion at different levels of the spine. The phenomenon of *coupling,* in which two or more individual motions occur at the same time, has been well documented experimentally.[17,61,81,130,189,196,206,210] Frequently three motions will simultaneously take place during normal physiological spinal movement or function. The coupling effect occurs in the thoracic spine,[170,218,219] but is more common in the cervical[133] and lumbar spine.[119,172]

Pure movement in any of the three principle planes very seldom occurs, because orientation of facet joint surfaces does not exactly coincide with the plane of motion and therefore modifies it to a greater or lesser extent.[84] For example, when the lumbar motion segment is rotated axially, it simultaneously bends in the sagittal plane and rotates axially.[220] Spinal movement is complex, and the intricacies of changing relationships observed on cineradiographical and other studies are sometimes difficult to explain.[84]

The occipito-atlanto-axial joints are the most complex joints of the axial skeleton, both anatomically and kinematically. Although there have been some thorough investigations of this region, there is considerable controversy about some of the basic biomechanical characteristics. (In Chapter 17, The Cervical Spine, the best available information is analyzed with some discussion of representative values of range of segmental motion.)

Representative values of other parts of the spine are presented here to allow a comparison of motion at various levels of the lower cervical (C2–C7), thoracic, and lumbar spine.[220] A representative value for flexion–extension is 8° at C2–C3, 13° at C3–C4, and 17° at C5–C6. A representative value for flexion–extension is 4° at T1–T4, 6° at T5–T10, and 12° at T11–T12. The range of flexion–extension progressively increases in the lumbar motion segments, reaching a maximum of 20° at the lumbosacral level (Fig. 16-21).

Lateral flexion shows the greatest range in the C3–C4 and C4–C5 segments, which reach 11°. The greatest range in the thoracic spine is in the lower segments, where 8° to 9° is possible. In the lumbar spine, 6° of lateral flexion is common, except for the lumbosacral segments, where only 3° of lateral flexion occurs (Fig. 16-21).[220]

Axial rotation is greatest in the midcervical spine, where 10° to 12° of motion is found. In the thoracic spine, axial rotation is greatest in the upper segments, where 9° is possible. The range of motion progressively decreases caudally, reaching 2° in the lower segments of the lumbar spine, but it again increases in the lumbosacral segment to 5° (Fig. 16-21).[220]

Segmental motion cannot be measured clinically and

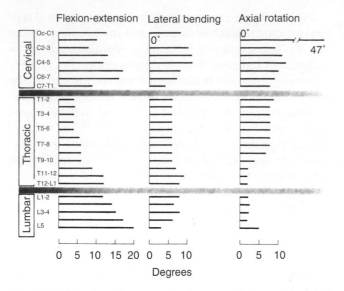

FIG. 16-21. *Average ranges of segmental movement of the spinal joints. (From White AA III, Panjabi MM: The basic kinematics of the human spine: A review of past and current knowledge. Spine 3:16, 1978.)*

motion of the spine is a combined action of several segments. The degree of movement in the spinal segment has clinical meaning in relation to its immediate neighbor and in general terms of the patient's body type.

Regional movement characteristics should also be appreciated. In general it can be said that in all sagittal starting positions of the cervical spine and in the flexed thoracic (below T3) and lumbar spines, sidebending is unavoidably accompanied by rotation to the same side; in the neutral or extended thoracic (below T3) and lumbar spines, sidebending is accompanied by rotation to the opposite side.[84]

In the upper thoracic spine there appears to be less consistency. According to White, the direction of coupled axial rotation is probably dominated by the middle sections of the thoracic spine, but sometimes the reverse is true.[218]

☐ Functional Motions of the Thoracolumbar Spine

Normal values of functional range of motion of the spine do not exist because there are great variations among individuals. In fact, the range of motion in each of the three planes shows a gaussian distribution, according to Lindl.[129] The range of motion also differs between the sexes and is strongly age dependent, decreasing by about 50 percent in old age.[147]

FLEXION–EXTENSION

Flexion is the most pronounced movement of the vertebral column as a whole. It requires an anterior com-

pression of the intervertebral disks and a gliding separation of the articular facets, in which the inferior set of an individual vertebra tends to move upward and forward over the opposing superior set of the adjacent inferior vertebra. The movement is checked mainly by the posterior ligaments and epaxial muscles. With respect to the thoracolumbar spine, the first 50° to 60° of spinal flexion occurs in the lumbar spine, mainly in the lower motion segments.[61] Forward tilting of the pelvis allows further flexion. There is an interconnection of movement between the spine and pelvis, particularly in total forward bending. Normally there is a synchronous movement in a rhythmical ratio of the lumbar spine to that of pelvic rotation about the hips. As forward bending progresses, the lumbar curve reverses itself from concave to flat to convex. The sacrum is also moving within the ilia during forward bending. Initially, the sacrum flexes. As the pelvis rotates anteriorly over the hips, the sacrum begins to counter-extend within the ilia. The thoracic spine contributes little to flexion of the total spine because of the orientation of the facets, the almost-vertical orientation of the spinous processes, and the restriction of the rib cage. Flexion is initiated by the abdominal muscles and the vertebral portion of the psoas. The weight of the upper body then produces further flexion, which is controlled by the gradually increasing activity of the erector muscles as the movement force increases.

Extension tends to be a more limited motion, producing posterior compression of the disk with the inferior articular process gliding posteriorly and downward over the superior set below. It is checked by the anterior longitudinal ligament and all the ventral muscles that directly or indirectly flex the spine. The laminae and spinous processes may also limit extension.[191,192] A reverse sequence of flexion is observed as the trunk returns from full flexion to the upright position. The lumbar spine becomes concave and the pelvis derotates and shifts forward as the spine extends. In some studies the concentric work performed by the muscles involved in raising the trunk has been shown to be greater than the eccentric work performed by the muscles during flexion.[68,108] When the trunk is extended from the upright position, the back muscles are active during the initial phase of motion. Activity decreases during further extension, and the abdominal muscles become active to control and modify motion.[129]

This arc of movement in forward and backward bending should normally be smooth and rhythmical, with a balance between lumbar reversal and pelvic rotation.[33]

LATERAL FLEXION

Lateral flexion is accompanied by some degree of rotation. It involves a rocking of the vertebral bodies upon their disks, with a sliding separation of the articular facets on the convex side and overriding of the articular facets related to the concavity.[191,192] Lateral flexion is limited by the intertransverse ligaments and the extension of the ribs. During lateral flexion, rotation may predominate in the thoracic or lumbar spine. In the lumbar spine the wedge-shaped spaces of the intervertebral joints show variation during motion.[185] The spinotransversal and transversospinal systems of the erector spinae are active in lateral flexion of the spine. The motion is initiated by ipsilateral contraction of these muscles and modified by the contralateral side.[129]

☐ Rotation

Rotation is consistently combined with lateral flexion. The entire vertebral column rotates approximately 90° to either side of the sagittal plane, but most of this transversion is accomplished in the cervical and thoracic spines. With respect to the thoracic spine, the combined motion is most marked in the upper segments. The vertebral body rotates toward the concavity of the lateral curve of the spine.[218] A combined pattern of rotation and lateral flexion also exists in the lumbar spine.[144] In this region the vertebral body rotates toward the convexity of the curve. Lumbar rotation is extremely limited at the lumbosacral level because of the orientation of the facets. Pelvic motion is essential to increase the range of trunk rotation. During rotation, back and abdominal muscles are active on both sides of the spine as both ipsilateral and contralateral muscles cooperate.[129]

Measurements obtained during walking indicate that the pelvis and lumbar spine rotate as a functional unit.[81] In the lower thoracic spine, rotation diminishes gradually up to T7. This vertebra represents the area of transition from vertebral rotation in the direction of the pelvis to rotation in the opposite direction—that of the shoulder girdle.

■ COMMON PATTERNS OF SPINAL PAIN

☐ Anatomical and Pathological Considerations

THE FACET (APOPHYSEAL) JOINTS

The facets have been clearly shown to be a source of referred pain. Like the synovial joints elsewhere in the body, the apophyseal joints can be a source of pain caused by trauma and various forms of arthritis, including degenerative arthritis. Inflammation of these joints produces dull to severe pain, depending on the extent of the inflammation. Inflammation can also lead to associated muscle spasm, which in itself is capable of causing pain.[35]

The cervical facet joint syndrome can cause both local and referred pain and is often indistinguishable from cervical disk disease.[16] Upper cervical facet joint irritation may be responsible for symptoms of upper neck pain, with referral to the occipital region and ipsilateral frontal area. Associated symptoms are occipital and vascular headaches.[200] Lower cervical facet joint irritation is characterized by referred pain to the shoulder and scapular girdle.[26] Often, cervical facet and disk disorders occur together. Facet joint irritation most commonly arises from facet joint thickening and hypertrophy initiated by trauma, spondylosis, excessive load-bearing stress, or disk degeneration.[24]

Each lumbar apophyseal joint is innervated by two or three adjacent nerves originating from the dorsal nerves, which originate from the dorsal primary rami.[23,24,27,113,149,150] The joint capsules are also innervated by free nerve endings. Immunohistochemical studies of degenerated facets in low-back-pain patients have revealed erosion channels extending through the subchondral bone and calcified cartilage into the articular cartilage containing substance P nerve fibers.[21] This confirms that a component of low back pain resides in the facets.[35] Pain from these joints can be referred to any part of the lower limb as far distal as the calf and ankle, but most commonly to the gluteal region, groin, and proximal thigh.[114]

THE INTERVERTEBRAL DISK

Until recently, the intervertebral disk was generally believed to be a non-pain-sensitive structure. Recently it has been found that the superficial layer (outer third) of the annulus fibrosis has significant innervation from the sinu-vertebral nerves and stimulation of these nerves may result in pain.[27] Their function has not been clarified, but they appear to have a proprioceptive and nociceptive function. Thus, internal disk disruption may cause intrinsic disk pain.

However, the disk more commonly causes pain by its effect on pain-sensitive structures such as the anterior dura mater and posterior longitudinal ligament or by a posterior lateral prolapse against a nerve root. When a prolapsed disk exerts pressure on the posterior longitudinal ligament and the dura, the consequence is spondylogenic referred pain, which is usually experienced locally but can be referred over a wider area. The pain is usually dull, deep, and poorly localized. In the lumbar spinal region, the pain is typically experienced in the low back, buttocks, and sacroiliac. Less commonly it may be referred to both legs and to the calf but is not referred to the ankle or foot.

The concept of dural pain was introduced by Cyriax[45] and further expanded on in his many-editioned *Textbook of Orthopaedic Medicine*[46,47] (see Fig. 19-2). On the basis of its innervation by the sinu-vertebral nerve, dura mater has also been suggested as a source of primary pain by Edgar and Nundy,[54] Murphy,[154] Bogduk,[23] and Cuatico and co-workers.[44] Some elements of this concept may be usefully criticized, but there are many aspects of the interpretation of dural pain that are relevant and useful in assessment and treatment.[34]

According to Cyriax[47] and Cailliet,[33] if the disk exerts pressure on the dural sleeve of the nerve root only, the radicular pain is experienced along the course of the nerve root. Pain can be experienced in any part of the dermatome of the affected nerve root (see Fig. 4-4). It should be pointed out that it is unusual to see actual pain in the hand or foot due to nerve root compression.[53] Rather, the radicular pain is proximal while only numbness is felt distally. With further mechanical pressure on the nerve dura there may be no pain and the following may occur:[114]

1. Motor weakness
2. Diminished or absent reflexes
3. Anesthesia or paresthesia in the distal end of the dermatome

■ TYPES OF SPINAL PAIN

The two basic types of mechanical spinal pain may be classified simply as radicular pain and non-radicular (or spondylogenic) pain.

Radicular pain is that caused by disorders of the spinal nerves and their root. Radicular pain is common in the cervical and lumbar spine but very rare in the thoracic spine.[114] Although the roots as they exit from the spinal canal can be compressed by numerous factors, by far the most common source of such irritation is either an acute disk herniation or a degenerative disk that in turn has caused focal osteoarthritic changes with foraminal stenosis.[18] The terms *soft* and *hard disk* disorders are commonly used. The soft disk (herniation) disorders tend to occur in patients under the age of 50 while the hard disk/osteoarthritis tends to occur in the older population. The onset is often acute. Pain may be sharp, stabbing, or lancinating, and accompanied by anesthesia and numbness. It is often superimposed on the dull ache of referred pain.

Non-radicular (spondylogenic) pain is produced by stimuli within deep skeletal structures such as muscle attachments, ligaments, fascia, periosteum, joints, dura mater, and the intervertebral disk. Non-radicular pain tends to be a deep, dull, aching type of pain, vaguely localized, referring over a great distance and relatively prolonged in duration. It is relieved by rest.

There are no neurological signs, dermatome reference, or localizing features. Such pain is usually insidious in onset.

Spinal pain is a complex phenomenon and it is not always possible to determine its source reliably. The possible causes are numerous and frequently originate from sources outside the spine. Nevertheless, diagnosis is possible in the majority of cases but depends on an orderly evaluation, including a careful history, a thorough physical examination, and routine laboratory and x-ray studies. At times, diagnostic tests such as nerve and joint blockade and computed tomographic scanning may be necessary to help establish the origin of the problem.

REFERENCES

1. Adams M, Hutton WC: Prolapsed intervertebral disc: A hyperflexion injury. Spine 7:184–191, 1982
2. Akeson WH, Amiel D, Woo SL: Immobility effect on synovial joints: The pathomechanics of joint contracture. Biorheology 17:95–110, 1980
3. Alexander MJL: Biomechanical aspects of the lumbar spine injuries in athletes: A review. Can J Appl Sci 10:1–20, 1985
4. Allen CEL: Muscle action potentials used in the study of dynamic anatomy. Br J Phy Med 11:66–73, 1948
5. Andersson GBJ: Interdiscal pressure, intraabdominal pressure and myoelectric back muscle activity related to posture and loading. Clin Orthop 129:156–164, 1977
6. Andersson GBJ: Epidemiology of low back pain. In Bueger AA, Greenman PE (eds): Empirical Approach to the Validation of Spinal Manipulation. Springfield, IL, Charles C Thomas, 1985
7. Andersson GBJ, Jonsson B, Örtengren R: Myoelectric activity in individual lumbar erector spinae muscles in sitting. I: A study with surface and wire electrodes. Scand J Rehabil Med Suppl 3:91–108, 1974
8. Andersson GBJ, Örtengren R: Lumbar disc pressure and myoelectric back muscle activity during sitting. II: Studies on an office chair. Scan J Rehabil Med 6(3):115–121, 1974
9. Andersson GBJ, Örtengren R: Myoelectric back muscle activity during sitting. Scan J Rehabil Med Suppl 3:73–101, 1974
10. Andersson GBJ, Örtengren R: Lumbar disc pressure and myoelectric back muscle activity during sitting. III: Studies on a wheelchair. Scand J Rehabil Med 6:128–133, 1974
11. Andersson GBJ, Örtengren R, Herberts P: Quantitative electromyographic studies of back muscle activity related to posture and loading. Orthop Clin North Am 8:85–96, 1977
12. Andersson GBJ, Örtengren R, Nachemson A: Intradiskal pressure and myoelectric back muscle activity related to posture and loading. Clin Orthop 129:156–164, 1977
13. Andersson GBJ, Örtengren R, Nachemson A: Quantitative studies of the load on the back in different working postures. Scand J Rehabil Med 6:173–178, 1978
14. Andersson GBJ, Örtengren R, Nachemson A, et al: Lumbar disc pressure and myoelectric back muscle activity during sitting. Parts I–III. Studies on an experimental chair. Scand J Rehabil Med 6:104–127, 1974
15. Andersson GBJ, Örtengren R, Nachemson A, et al: Lumbar disc pressure and myoelectric back muscle activity during sitting. II. Studies on a car driver's seat. Scand J Rehabil Med 6(3):128–133, 1974.
16. Aprill C, Dwyer A, Bogduk N: Cervical zygapophyseal joint pain patterns. II: A clinical evaluation. Spine 15(6):458–461, 1990
17. Arkin AM: The mechanism of rotation in combination with lateral deviation in the normal spine. J Bone Joint Surg 32(A):180–188, 1950
18. Aryanpur J, Ducker TB: Differential diagnosis and management of cervical spine pain. In Tollison CD (ed): Handbook of Chronic Pain Management, pp 320–325. Baltimore, Williams & Wilkins, 1989
19. Bartelink DL: The role of abdominal pressure in relieving the pressure on the lumbar intervertebral discs. J Bone Joint Surg 39(B):718–725, 1975
20. Basmajian JV: Electromyography of iliopsoas. Anat Rec 132:127–132, 1958
21. Beaman D, Glover R, Graziano G, et al: Substance P innervation of lumbar facet joints. International Society for the Study of the Lumbar Spine, Chicago, IL, May 20–24, 1991. Abstract
22. Boas R: Facet joint injections. In Stanton-Hick M, Boas R (eds): Chronic Low Back Pain, pp 199–212. New York, Raven Press, 1982
23. Bogduk N: The innervation of the lumbar spine. Spine 8:286–293, 1983
24. Bogduk N: Lumbar dorsal ramus syndromes. In Grieve G (ed): Modern Manual Therapy of the Vertebral Column, pp 396–404. Edinburgh, Churchill Livingstone, 1986
25. Bogduk N, MacIntosh JE: The applied anatomy of the thoracolumbar fascia. Spine 9:164–170, 1984
26. Bogduk N, Marsland A: The cervical zygoapophyseal joints as a source of neck pain. Spine 13:610–617, 1988
27. Bogduk N, Twomey LT: Clinical Anatomy of the Lumbar Spine, pp 139–147. Melbourne, Churchill Livingstone, 1987
28. Bowen V, Cassidy JD: Macroscopic and microscopic anatomy of the sacroiliac joint from embryonic life until the eighth decade. Spine 6:620–628, 1980
29. Brain WR, Northfield D, Wilkinson M: The neurological manifestations of cervical spondylosis. Brain 75:187–225, 1952

30. Brasseur K, Melvin J: Myoelectric activity in deep muscles of the back. A review. Arch Phys Med Rehabil 59:546, 1978
31. Buckwalter JA, Cooper RR, Maynard JA: Elastic fiber in human intervertebral discs. J Bone Joint Surg 58(A):73–76, 1976
32. Butler DS: Clinical consequences of injury. In Butler DS: Mobilization of the Nervous System, pp 75–88. Melbourne, Churchill Livingstone, 1991
33. Cailliet R: Low Back Pain Syndrome, 4th ed. Philadelphia, FA Davis, 1988
34. Cailliet R: Tissue sites of low back pain. In Cailliet R: Low Back Pain Syndrome, 4th ed, pp 63–75. Philadelphia, FA Davis, 1988
35. Cailliet R: Pain: Mechanisms and Management. Philadelphia, FA Davis, 1993
36. Chaffin JB, Park KS: A longitudinal study of low back pain as associated with occupational lifting factors. J Am Ind Hyg Assoc, 34:513–525, 1973
37. Chamberlain WE: The symphysis pubis in the roentgen examination of the sacroiliac joint. J Bone Joint Surg 24(A):621–623, 1930
38. Cloward RB: Cervical diskography. Ann Surg 150:1052–1064, 1959
39. Colachis S, Worden R, Bechtol C, et al: Movement of the sacroiliac joint in the adult male: A preliminary report. Arch Phys Med Rehabil 44:490–498, 1963
40. Collins G, Cohen M, Naliboff B, et al: Comparative analysis of paraspinal and frontalis EMG, heart rate and skin conductance in chronic low back pain patients and normals to various postures and stress. Scand J Rehabil Med 14:39–46, 1982
41. Collis DK, Ponset IV: Long term follow-up of patients with idiopathic scoliosis not treated surgically. J Bone Joint Surg 51(A):425–455, 1969
42. Cotch MT: Biomechanics of the thoracic spine. In American Academy of Orthopedic Surgeons: Atlas of Orthotics: Biomechanical Principles and Applications. St Louis, CV Mosby, 1975
43. Cram J, Steeger J: EMG scanning in the diagnosis of chronic pain. Biofeedback Self Regul 8:229–241, 1983
44. Cuatico W, Parker JC, Papptert E, et al: An anatomical and clinical investigation of spinal meningeal nerves. Acta Neurochir 90:139–143, 1988
45. Cyriax J: Perineuritis. Br Med J 1(May):570–580, 1942
46. Cyriax J: Textbook of Orthopedic Medicine, 8th ed, vol I. London, Bailliere Tindall, 1982
47. Cyriax J: Textbook of Orthopaedic Medicine, 11th ed, vol 2. Treatment by Manipulation, Massage and Injection. London, Bailliere Tindall, 1984
48. Cyron BM, Hutton WC: The tensile strength of the capsular ligament of the apophyseal joints. Anatomy 132:145–150, 1981
49. Davis PR: Posture of the trunk during lifting of weights. Br Med J 11:87–89, 1959
50. Davis PR: The causation of herniae by weight lifting. Lancet 2:155–157, 1959
51. Davis PR: The use of intraabdominal pressure in evaluating stresses on the lumbar spine. Spine 6:90–92, 1981
52. Dory MA: Arthrography of the lumbar facet joints. Radiology 140:23–27, 1981
53. Dubuisson D: Pathophysiology of pain. In Warfield CA: Principles and Practice of Pain Management, pp 13–25. New York, McGraw-Hill, 1993
54. Edgar MA, Nundy S: Innervation of the spinal dura mater. J Neurol Neurosurg Psychiatry 29:530–534, 1966
55. Egund N, Olsson TH, Schmid H, et al: Movements of the sacroiliac joints demonstrated with roentgen stereophotogrammetry. Acta Radiol 19:833–846, 1978
56. Ehni G: Cervical Arthrosis: Disease of the Cervical Motion Segments. Chicago, Year Book Medical Publishers, 1984
57. Eie N: Load capacity of the low back. J Oslo City Hosp 16:73–78, 1966
58. Eie N, Wehn P: Measurement of the intraabdominal pressure in relation to weight bearing of the lumbo sacral spine. J Oslo City Hosp 12:205–217, 1962
59. Epstein BS: The Spine. Philadelphia: Lea & Febiger, 1962
60. Farfan HF: Mechanical Disorders of the Low Back. Philadelphia, Lea & Febiger, 1973
61. Farfan HF: Muscular mechanism of the lumbar spine and the position of power and efficiency. Orthop Clin North Am 6:135–144, 1975
62. Farfan HF, Sullivan JD: The relation of the facet orientation to intervertebral disc failure. Can J Surg 10:179, 1967
63. Fielding JW: Normal and selected abnormal motion of the cervical spine from the second cervical vertebra to the seventh cervical vertebra based on cineroentgenography. J Bone Joint Surg 46(A):1779–1781, 1964
64. Fischer FJ, Houtz SJ: Evaluation of the function of the gluteus maximus muscle: An electromyographic study. Ann Phys Med 47:182–191, 1968
65. Floyd WF: The function of the erector spinae muscles in certain movements and postures in man. J Physiol 129:184–203, 1955
66. Floyd WF, Silver PHS: Function of the erector spinae in flexion of the trunk. Lancet 1:133–134, 1951
67. Frankel V, Nordin M: Basic Biomechanics of the Skeletal System. Philadelphia, Lea & Febiger, 1980
68. Frigerio N, Stow R, Howe J: Movement of sacroiliac joint. Clin Orthop 100:370–371, 1974
69. Frymoyer JW: Back pain and sciatica. N Engl J Med 318:291–300, 1988
70. Galante JO: Tensile properties of the human lumbar annulus fibrosis. Acta Orthop Scand Suppl 100:9–96, 1967
71. Gallois J, Japoit T: Architecture interieuredes vertebre du point de vue statique et physiologique. Rev Chir Orthop (Paris) 63:689, 1925. (Cited in Steindler A (ed): Kinesiology of the Human Body. Springfield, IL, Charles C Thomas, 1958)
72. Gamble JG, Simmons SC, Freedman M: The symphysis pubis. Clin Orthop 203:261–272, 1986
73. Gibson GJ, Clark E, Pride NB: Static transdiaphragmatic pressures in normal subjects and in patients with chronic hyperinflation. Am Rev Respir Dis 124:685–689, 1981
74. Gilbertson LG, Krag MH, Pope MH: Investigation of the effect of intra-abdominal pressure on load bearing of the spine. Orthop Trans 7:313, 1983. Abstract
75. Golding JSR: Electromyography of the erector spinae in low back pain. Postgrad Med J 28:401–440, 1952
76. Gould JA: The spine. In Gould JA, Davies GJ (eds): Orthopedics and Sports Physical Therapy, 2nd ed. St Louis, CV Mosby, 1985
77. Grabel J: Electromyographic study of low back muscle tension in subjects with and without chronic low back pain. United States International University Dissertation Abstracts International (1973) 34:292–293, 1974. Doctoral thesis
78. Gracovetsky S, Farfan H, Helleur C: The abdominal mechanism. Spine 10:317–324, 1985
79. Gracovetsky S, Farfan HF, Lamy C: The mechanism of lumbar spine. Spine 6:249–262, 1981
80. Grant JCB: Grant's Atlas of Anatomy. Baltimore, Williams and Wilkins, 1972
81. Gregersen GG, Lucas DB: An in vivo study of the axial rotation of the human thoracolumbar spine. J Bone Joint Surg 49(A):247–262, 1967
82. Grew ND: Intra-abdominal pressure response to load applied to the torso in normal subjects. Spine 5:149–155, 1980
83. Grieve GP: Manipulation therapy for neck pain. Physiotherapy 65:136–146, 1979
84. Grieve GP: Common Vertebral Joint Problems, 2nd ed. New York, Churchill Livingstone, 1988
85. Grieve GP: Diagnosis. Physiother Pract 4:73–77, 1988
86. Guyton AC: Basic Human Physiology: Normal Function and Mechanisms of Disease, 2nd ed. Philadelphia, WB Saunders, 1977
87. Hall MC: The Locomotor System: Functional Anatomy. Springfield, IL, Charles C Thomas, 1965
88. Hamilton WJ (ed): Textbook of Human Anatomy, 2nd ed. St Louis, CV Mosby, 1976
89. Hemborg B, Moritz V: Intra-abdominal pressure and trunk muscle activity during lifting. II. Chronic low-back patients. Scand J Rehabil Med 17:5–13, 1985
90. Hemborg B, Moritz V, Hamberg J, et al: Intraabdominal pressure and trunk muscle activity during lifting-effect of abdominal muscle training in healthy subjects. Scand J Rehabil Med 15:183–196, 1983
91. Hemborg B, Moritz V, Hamberg J, Holmstrom E, et al: Intra-abdominal pressure and trunk muscle activity during lifting. III. Effect of abdominal muscle training in chronic low back patients. Scand J Rehabil Med 17:15–24, 1985
92. Hemborg B, Moritz V, Lowing H: Intra-abdominal pressure and trunk muscle activity during lifting. IV. The causal factors of intra-abdominal pressure rise. Scand J Rehabil Med 17:25–38, 1985
93. Hendry NG: The hydration of the nucleus pulposus and its relation to intervertebral disc derangement. J Bone Joint Surg 40(B):132–144, 1958
94. Hettinga DL: I. Normal joint structures and their reaction to injury. J Orthop Sports Phys Ther 1:10, 1979
95. Hirsch C, Ingelmark BE. Miller M: The anatomical basis for low back pain: Studies on the presence of sensory nerve endings in ligamentous, capsular and intervertebral disc structures in the human lumbar spine. Acta Orthop Scand 33:1–17, 1963
96. Hollinshead WH: Anatomy for Surgeons, 2nd ed. New York, Harper and Row, 1969
97. Hollinshead WH, Jenkins DB: Functional Anatomy of the Limbs and Back. Philadelphia, WB Saunders, 1981
98. Hoyt W, Hunt H, De Pauw M, Bard D, et al: Electromyographic assessment of chronic low back pain syndrome. J Am Osteopath Assoc 80:728–730, 1981
99. Hutton WC, Stott JRR, Cyron BM: Is spondylosis a fatigue fracture? Spine 2:202–209, 1977
100. Inman VT, Ralston HJ, Todd F: Human Walking. Baltimore, Williams and Wilkins, 1981
101. Iwasaki T, Ito H, Yamada M, et al: Electromyographic study of the lifting weights. J Jpn Phys Ther Assn 4:52–61, 1978
102. Jonsson B: The Lumbar Part of the Erector Spinae Muscle. A Technique for Electromyographic Studies of the Function of its Individual Muscles. Gîteborg, Sweden, University of Gîteborg, 1970
103. Jonsson B: Topography of the lumbar part of the erector spinae muscle: An analysis of the morphologic conditions present for insertion of EMG electrodes into individual muscles of the lumbar part of the erector spinae muscle. Z Anat Entwickl Gesch 130:177–191, 1970
104. Jonsson B: The function of individual muscles in the lumbar part of the spinae muscle. Electromyogr Clin Neurophysiol 10:5–21, 1970
105. Jonsson B: Electromyography of the lumbar part of the Erector spinae muscle. Medicine and Sport, vol 6. In Komi PV (eds): Biomechanics II, pp 185–188. Basel, S Karger, 1971
106. Jonsson B: Electromyography of the Erector spinae muscle. Medicine and Sport, Vol 8 Biomechanics III, pp 295–300, Basel, S Karger, 1973
107. Jonsson B, Synnerstad B: Electromyographic studies of muscle function in standing. A methodological study. Acta Morphol Neerl Scand VI:361–370, 1966
108. Joseph J: Man's Posture: Electromyographic Studies. Springfield, IL, Charles C Thomas, 1960
109. Kapandji IA: The Physiology of the Joints, vol 3: The Trunk and Vertebral Column. Edinburgh, Churchill Livingstone, 1974
110. Karlsson E, Jonsson B: Function of the gluteus maximus muscle. An electromyographic study. Acta Morphol Neerl Scand 6:161–169, 1965
111. Kazarian L: Dynamic response characteristic of the human vertebral column. An experimental study of human autopsy specimens. Acta Orthop Scand (Suppl) 146:1–186, 1972
112. Kazarian L: Creep characteristics of the human spinal column. Orthop Clin North Am 6:3–18, 1975
113. Keller TS, Holm SH, Hansson TH, et al: The dependence of intervertebral disc mechanical properties on physiological conditions. Spine 15:751–761, 1990
114. Kenna C, Murtagh J: Patterns of spinal pain. In Kenna C, Murtagh J: Back Pain & Spinal Manipulation, pp 1–10. Sydney, Butterworths, 1989
115. King AI, Prasad P, Ewing CL: Mechanism of spinal injury due to caudocephalad acceleration. Orthop Clin North Am 6:19–31, 1975
116. Kos J, Wolf J: Intervertebral menisci and their possible role in intervertebral blockage. Burkart SL (trans): Special Edition, Bull Orthop Sports Med, Sect APTA 1:8, 1976
117. Kraft, GL, Levinthal DH: Facet synovial impingement. Surg Gynecol Obstet 93:439–443, 1951
118. Krag MH, Wilder DG, Pope MH: Internal strain and nuclear movements of the intervertebral disc. Proceeding of International Society for Study of the Lumbar Spine, Cambridge, England, April 15, 1983
119. Krag MH: Three dimensional flexibility measurements of preload human vertebral motion segments. New Haven, Yale University School of Medicine, 1975. PhD dissertation
120. Krammer J: Treatment of the Lumbar Syndrome in Intervertebral Disk Disease. Chicago, Year Book Medical Publishers, 1981
121. Kraus H: Stress analysis. In Farfan HF (ed): Mechanical Disorders of the Low Back, pp 112–133. Philadelphia, Lea & Febiger, 1973
122. Kravitz E, Moore M, Glaros A: Paralumbar muscle activity in chronic low back pain. Arch Phys Med Rehabil 62:172–176, 1981
123. Krenz J, Troup JDG: The structure of the pars interarticularis of the lower lumbar vertebrae and its relation to the etiology of spondylosis with a report of healing frac-

ture in the neural arch of a fourth lumbar vertebra. J Bone Joint Surg 55(B):735–741, 1973

124. Kuluk RF, Belytshko TB, Schultz AB, et al: Non-linear behavior of the human intervertebral disc under axial load. J Biomech 9:377–386, 1976
125. La Rocca H: Biomechanics of the cervical spine. In American Academy of Orthopedic Surgeons: Atlas of Orthotics: Biomechanical Principles and Application. St Louis, CV Mosby, 1975
126. Lee D: Anatomy. In Lee D: The Pelvic Girdle, pp 17–38. Edinburgh, Churchill Livingstone, 1989
127. Legg SL: The effect of abdominal muscle fatigue training on the intra-abdominal pressure developed during lifting. Ergonomics 24:191–195, 1981
128. Lewis T, Kellgren JH: Observation relating to referred pain, visceromotor reflexes and other associated phenomena. Clin Sci 4:47–71, 1939
129. Lindl M: Biomechanics of the lumbar spine. In Frankel V, Nordin M: Basic Biomechanics of the Skeletal System. Philadelphia, Lea & Febiger, 1980
130. Loebl WY: Regional rotation of the spine. Rheum Rehabil 12:223, 1973
131. Lorenz M, Patwardhan A, Vanderby R: Load-bearing characteristics of lumbar facets in normal and surgically altered spinal segments. Spine 8:122–130, 1983
132. Lumsden RM, Morris JM: An in vivo study of axial rotation and immobilization at the lumbosacral joint. J Bone Joint Surg 50(A):1591–1602, 1968
133. Lysell E: Motion in the cervical spine. Acta Orthop Scand (Suppl) 123:1–61, 1969
134. MacConaill MA, Basmajian JV: Muscles and Movements. Baltimore, Williams and Wilkins, 1969
135. Maigne R: Orthopaedic Medicine. Springfield, IL, Charles C Thomas, 1976
136. Maldague B, Mathurin P, Malghem J: Facet joint arthrography in lumbar spondylosis. Radiology 140:29–36, 1981
137. Manning DP, Shannon HS: Slipping accidents causing low-back pain in a gearbox factory. Spine 6:70–72, 1981
138. McCall IW, Park WM, O'Brien JP: Induced pain referral from posterior lumbar elements in normal subjects. Spine 4:441–446, 1979
139. McGregor M, Cassidy JD: Post-operative sacroiliac syndrome. J Manipulative Physiol Ther 6:1–11, 1983
140. McNeill T, Warwick D, Andersson G, et al: Trunk and strengths in attempted flexion, extension and lateral bending in healthy subjects and patients with low-back disorders. Spine 5:527–538, 1980
141. Messerer O: Uber Elastizitat und Festigkeit der Menschlichen Knochen. Stuttgart, JG Cottasche Buchhandlung, 1880
142. Meyer GH: Der Mechanismus der Symphysis Sacroiliaca. Archiv fur Anatomie und Physiologie Leipzig 1:1–16, 1978
143. Michele AA: Iliopsoas. Springfield, IL, Charles C Thomas, 1962
144. Miles M, Sullivan WE: Lateral bending at the lumbar and lumbar sacral joints. Anat Rec 139:387–398, 1961
145. Mitchell FL: Structural Pelvic Function. Academy of Applied Osteopathy, vol 2. Chicago, Year Book Medical Publishers, 1965
146. Mitchell FL: An Evaluation and Treatment Manual of Osteopathic Muscle Energy Procedures. Valley Park, MO, Mitchell, Moran and Pruzzzo, 1979
147. Moll JMH, Wright V: Normal range of spinal mobility. An objective clinical study. Ann Rheum Dis 3:381–386, 1971
148. Mooney V: The syndromes of low back disease. Orthop Clin North Am 14:505–515, 1983
149. Mooney V: Facet joint syndrome. In Jayson MIV (ed): The Lumbar Spine and Back Pain, 3rd ed, pp 370–382. Edinburgh, Churchill Livingstone, 1987
150. Mooney V, Robertson J: The facet syndrome. Clin Orthop 115:149–156, 1976
151. Morris JM: Biomechanics of the spine. Arch Surg 107:418–423, 1973
152. Morris JM, Benner G, Lucas DB: An electromyographic study of intrinsic muscles of the back in man. J Anat 96:509–520, 1962
153. Morris JM, Lucus DB, Bresler B: Role of the trunk in stability of the spine. J Bone Joint Surg 43(A):327–351, 1961
154. Murphy RW: Nerve roots and spinal nerves in degenerative disc disease. Clin Orthop 129:46–60, 1977
155. Nachemson AL: Lumbar interdiscal pressure. Acta Orthop Scand Supp 43:9–104, 1960
156. Nachemson A: The load on lumbar disc in different positions of the body. Clin Orthop 45:107–122, 1966
157. Nachemson A: Electromyographic studies on the vertebral portion of the psoas muscle with special reference to its stabilizing function of the lumbar spine. Acta Orthop Scand 37:177–190, 1966
158. Nachemson AL: The lumbar spine: An orthopaedic challenge. Spine 1:59–71, 1976
159. Nachemson A: Disc pressure measurements. Spine 6:93–97, 1981
160. Nachemson A: Low back pain including biomechanics of the intervertebral joint complex. In Straub LR, Wilson PD (eds): Clinical Trends in Orthopaedics. New York, Theime-Stratton, 1982
161. Nachemson A, Elfstrom G: Intravital dynamics pressure measurements in lumbar discs. A study of common movements, maneuvers and exercises. Scand J Rehabil Med 2 (Suppl 1):1–40, 1970
162. Nachemson AL, Evans J: Some mechanical properties of the third lumbar inter-laminar ligament (ligamentum flavum). J Biomech 1:211–219, 1968
163. Nachemson AL, Morris JM: In vivo measurements of intradiscal pressure. Discometry, a method for the determination of pressure in the lower discs. J Bone Joint Surg 46(A):5:1077–1092, 1964
164. Nemeth G: On hip and lumbar biomechanics, A study of joint load and muscular activity. Scand J Rehabil Med Suppl 10:1–35, 1984
165. Nemeth G, Ekholm J, Arborelius UP: Hip load moments and muscular activity during lifting. Scand J Rehabil Med 16:103–111, 1984
166. Norkin CC, Levengie DK: Joint Structure and Function: A Comprehensive Analysis, 2nd ed. Philadelphia, FA Davis, 1992
167. Okada M: Electromyographic assessment of the muscular load in forward bending postures. Journal of the Faculty of Science, University of Tokyo 3:311–336, 1970
168. Okada M: An electromyographic examination of the relative muscular load in different human postures. J Hum Ergol I:75–93, 1972
169. Örtengren R, Andersson GBJ: Electromyographic studies of trunk muscles with special reference to the functional anatomy of the lumbar spine. Spine 2:44–52, 1977
170. Panjabi MM, Brand RA, White AA: Mechanical properties of the human thoracic spine as shown by three-dimensional load-displacement curves. J Bone Joint Surg 8(A):642–652, 1976

171. Panjabi MM, Goel VK, Takata K: Physiologic strains in the lumbar ligaments: An in vitro biomechanical study. Spine 7:192–203, 1983
172. Panjabi MM, Krag MM, White AA, et al: Effect of preload on load displacement curves of the lumbar spine. Orthop Clin North Am 88:181–192, 1977
173. Paris SV: Anatomy as related to function and pain. Orthop Clin North Am 14:475–487, 1983
174. Pauly JE: An electromyographic study of certain movements and exercises: I. Some deep muscles of the back. Anat Rec 155:223–234, 1966
175. Perry O: Fracture of the vertebral end-plate in the lumbar spine. Acta Orthop Scand 25 (Suppl) 25:3–101, 1957
176. Perry O: Resistance and compression of the lumbar vertebrae. In Ranninger K (ed): Encyclopedia of Medical Radiology. New York, Springer-Verlag, 1974
177. Platzer W: Color Atlas and Textbook of Human Anatomy: Locomotion System, vol 1. Chicago, Year Book Medical Publishers, 1978
178. Poland JL, Hobart DJ, Payton OD: The Musculoskeletal System. New York, Medical Examination Publishing, 1977
179. Pope MH, Lehmann TR, Frymoyer JW: Structure and function of the lumbar spine. In Pope MH, Frymoyer JW, Andersson G (eds): Occupational Low Back Pain. New York, Praeger, 1984
180. Pope MH, Rosen JD, Wider DG, et al: The relation between biomechanical and psychological factors in patients with low back pain. Spine 5:173–178, 1983
181. Porterfield JA, DeRosa C: Articulations of the lumbopelvic region. In Porterfield JA, DeRosa C: Mechanical Low Back Pain: Perspectives in Functional Anatomy, pp 83–122. Philadelphia, WB Saunders, 1991
182. Porterfield JA: The sacroiliac joint. In Gould JA, Davies GJ (eds): Orthopedics and Sports Physical Therapy. St Louis, CV Mosby, 1985
183. Portnoy H, Morin F: Electromyographic study of postural muscles in various positions and movements. Am J Physiol 186:122–126, 1956
184. Poulsen E, Jorgensen K: Back muscle strength, lifting and stooped working postures. Appl Ergon 2:133–137, 1971
185. Reichmann S: Motion of the lumbar articular processes in flexion-extension and lateral flexion of the spine. Acta Morphol Neerl Scand 8:261–272, 1970–1971
186. Resnick D, Niwayama G, Goergen TG: Degenerative disease of the sacroiliac joint. Invest Radiol 10:608–621, 1975
187. Rissanen PM: Comparisons of pathological changes in the intervertebral discs and interspinous ligaments of the lower part of the lumbar spine. Acta Orthop Scand 34:54–65, 1964
188. Roberts S, Chen PH: Global characteristics of typical human ribs. J Biomech 5:191–201, 1972
189. Rolander SD: Motion of the lumbar spine with special reference to the stabilizing effect of posterior fusion. Acta Orthop Scand (Suppl) 90:1–144, 1966
190. Rolander SD, Blair WE: Deformation and fracture of the lumbar vertebral end-plate. Orthop Clinic North Am 6:75–81, 1975
191. Rothman RH, Simeone FA: The Spine, 2nd ed, vol 1. Philadelphia, WB Saunders, 1982
192. Rothman RH, Simeone FA: The Spine, 2nd ed, vol 2. Philadelphia, WB Saunders, 1982
193. Roussos CS, Macklem PT: Diaphragmatic fatigue in man. J Appl Physiol 43(2):189–197, 1977
194. Sashin D: A critical analysis of the anatomy and pathological changes of the sacroiliac joints. J Bone Joint Surg 12:891–910, 1930
195. Schmorl G: Die Pathologische Anatomie der Wirbelsaule. Vern Dtsch Orthop Ges 21:3, 1927
196. Schultz A, Andersson G, Örtengren R, et al: Loads on the lumbar spine. J Bone Joint Surg 64(A): 713–720, 1982
197. Shah JS, Hampson WGJ, Jayson MIV: The distribution of surface strain in the cadaveric lumbar spine. J Bone Joint Surg 60(B):246–251, 1978
198. Sherman RA: Relationships between strength of low back muscle contraction and reported intensity of low back pain. Am J Phys Med 64:190–200, 1985
199. Shore LR: On osteoarthritis in the dorsal intervertebral joint. Br J Surg 22:833–849, 1935
200. Sluijter ME, Koetsvedl-Baart CC: Interruption of pain pathways in the treatment of the cervical syndrome. Anesthesia 35:302–307, 1984
201. Smidt GL, Amundsen LR, Dostal WF: Muscle strength of the trunk. J Orthop Sports Phys Ther 1:165–170, 1980
202. Soderberg GL, Barr JO: Muscular function in chronic low-back dysfunction. Spine 8:79–85, 1983
203. Solonen KA: The sacro-iliac joint in the light of anatomical, roentgenological and clinical studies. Acta Orthop Scand Suppl 26:9–127, 1957
204. Spilker RL: Mechanical behavior of a simple model of an intervertebral disk under compressive loading. J Biomech 13:895–901, 1980
205. Stillwell GK: The Law of Laplace: Some clinical applications. Mayo Clin Proc 48:863–868, 1973
206. Stoddard A: Manual of Osteopathic Technique. London, Hutchinson, 1962
207. Tauber J: An unorthodox look at backaches. J Occup Med 12:128–130, 1970
208. Tesh JH, Evans J, Shawdunn J, O'Brien JP: The mechanical interaction between the thoracolumbar fascia and the connective tissue of the posterior spine. In Bueger AA, Greenman PE (eds): Empirical Approach to the Validation of Spinal Manipulation. Springfield, IL, Charles C Thomas, 1985
209. Tkaczuk H: Tensile properties of human lumbar longitudinal ligament. Acta Orthop Scand Suppl 115:9–69, 1968
210. Troup JDG, Hood CA, Chapman AE: Measurements of the sagittal mobility of lumbar spine and hips. Ann Phys Med 9:308–321, 1976
211. Urschel HC, Razzuk MA, Wood RE, Parckn M, Paulson DL: Objective diagnosis (ulnar nerve conduction velocity) and current therapy of the thoracic outlet syndrome. Ann Thorac Surg 12:608–620, 1971
212. Warwick R, Williams P: Gray's Anatomy, 36th ed (Br). Philadelphia, JB Lippincott, 1980
213. Watanabe K: A study on the posture: The function of the human erector spinae. Jpn J Phys Educ 21:69–76, 1976
214. Weisl H: The articular surfaces of the sacro-iliac joint and their relation to the movement of the sacrum. Acta Anat 22:1–14, 1954
215. Weisl H: The movements of the sacro-iliac joint. Acta Anat 23:80–91, 1955
216. Weisman G, Pope MH, Johnson RJ: Cyclic loading in knee ligament injuries. Am J Sport Med 8:24–30, 1980

217. Weismantel A: Evaluation and treatment of sacroiliac joint problems. Bull Orthop Sect APTA 3:5–9, 1982.
218. White AA: Analysis of the mechanics of the thoracic spine in man. Acta Orthop Scand (Suppl) 127:8–105, 1969
219. White AA, Hirch C: The significance of the vertebral posterior elements in the mechanics of the thoracic spine. Clin Orthop 81:2–20, 1971
220. White AA, Panjabi MM: Clinical Biomechanics of the Spine, 2nd ed. Philadelphia, JB Lippincott, 1990
221. White AA, Southwick WO, Panjabi MM, et al: Practical biomechanics of the spine for orthopaedic surgeons. Instr Course Lect 23:62–78, 1974
222. Wilder DG, Msme, Pope MH, Frymoyer JW: The functional topography of the sacroiliac joint. Spine 5:575–579, 1980
223. Wolf SL, Basmajian JV: Assessment of paraspinal electromyographic activity in normal subjects and in chronic back pain patient using muscle biofeedback device. In Asmussen E, Gorgensen J (eds): International Series in Biomechanics, pp 319–323. Baltimore, University Paris Press, 1977
224. Wolf SL, Basmajian JV, Russe CTC, Kutna M: Normative data on low back mobility and activity levels. Am J Phys Med 58:217–229, 1979
225. Wyke BD: The neurology of joints. Ann R Coll Surg Engl 41:25–50, 1967.
226. Wyke B: Receptor systems in lumbosacral tissues in relation to the production of low back pain. In White AA, Gordon SL (eds): American Academy of Orthopaedic Surgeons Symposium on Idiopathic Low Back Pain. St Louis, CV Mosby, 1982

17
CHAPTER

The Cervical Spine

MITCHELL BLAKNEY AND DARLENE HERTLING

- **Review of Functional Anatomy**
  Osseous Structures
  Joints and Ligaments
  Muscle Groups
  Innervation
  Blood Supply
- **Joint Mechanics**
  Lower Cervical Spine (C2–T1)
  Upper Cervical Spine (Occiput–C1–C2)
  Head-Righting Mechanism
- **Examination**
  History
  Observation
  Inspection

Selective Tissue Tension
Neurological Testing
Palpation
Roentgenographical Analysis
- **Common Disorders**
  Acceleration Injury
  Cervical Instability
  Acute Disk Bulge
  Degenerative Joint Disease
- **Treatment Techniques**
  Manual Techniques—Muscles
  Manual Techniques—Joints
  Positional Traction

REVIEW OF FUNCTIONAL ANATOMY

☐ Osseous Structures

The seven vertebrae of the cervical spine can be divided into two groups, according to structure and function. The vertebrae of the *lower cervical spine* (C2–C7) are similar in structure to the vertebrae of the thoracic and lumbar spine with clearly defined vertebral bodies and spinous processes (Fig. 17-1).[11] The transverse processes are abbreviated to allow better mobility, and there is a foramen to allow passage of the vertebral artery. The lateral portions of the vertebral bodies form the joints of Luschka, which also facilitate mobility of the lower cervical spine.[11] The facet joints of the lower cervical spine are in the sagittal plane and incline forward at approximately 45°. This

forward inclination allows the facet joints to bear weight and guides the motion of the segment.

The bony structure of the *upper cervical spine* (occiput–C1–C2) is specialized to allow a great deal of mobility and to protect the medulla oblongata (Fig. 17-2*A,B*). The inferior facet of C2 has the same form and function as the facets of the lower cervical spine. The joint surfaces of the superior facet of C2 are aligned in the horizontal plane to allow approximately 90° rotation. The dens portion of C2 is a vertical pin of bone that acts as a pivot around which the atlas rotates (Fig. 17-2*C,D*).[11] The atlas is a wide, thin ring of bone with a well-developed transverse process but no spinous process. There is no intervertebral disk between the C1 and C2 because the atlas, with concave joint surfaces above and below, serves the function of the disk. The anterior portion of the transverse ligament of the atlas forms a socket for the dens.

Darlene Hertling and Randolph M. Kessler: MANAGEMENT OF COMMON
MUSCULOSKELETAL DISORDERS: Physical Therapy Principles and Methods, 3rd ed.
© 1996 Lippincott-Raven Publishers.

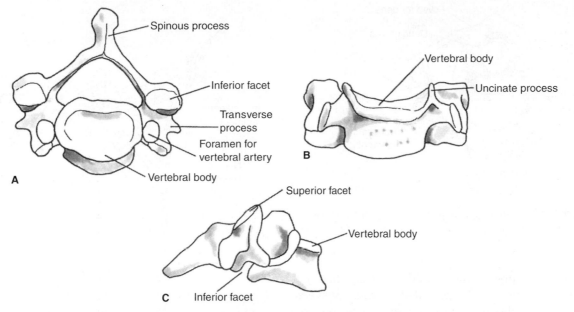

FIG. 17-1. A typical lower cervical vertebra: (**A**) inferior, (**B**) anterior, and (**C**) sagittal views.

The atlanto-occipital joint is the one true convex-on-concave joint in the spine. The superior facet surfaces of the atlas are oval, concave, and toed-in slightly. The convex condyles of the occiput are slightly larger than the joint surfaces of the atlas, making maximal congruence possible on only one side at a time, when the occiput is laterally bent on the atlas. The anterior placement of the center of rotation of the atlas causes a lateral movement to the opposite side whenever the atlas is rotated (Fig. 17-3). This can be palpated as the transverse process becoming more prominent on the side opposite rotation. When viewed from the side, the superior facet joint of C2 is rounded as the atlas rotates. It rolls down the shoulder of the side of

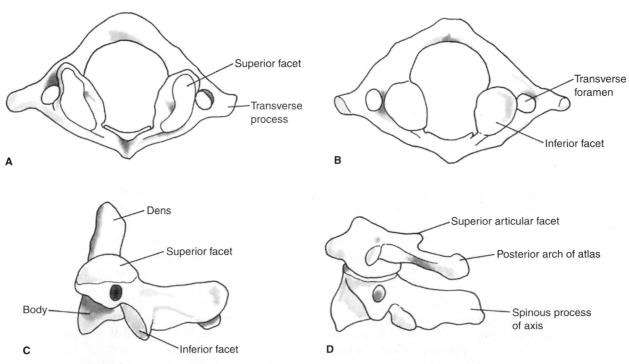

FIG. 17-2. The upper cervical spine: (**A**) superior view of atlas, (**B**) inferior view of axis, (**C**) lateral view of axis, and (**D**) lateral view of atlantoaxial articulation.

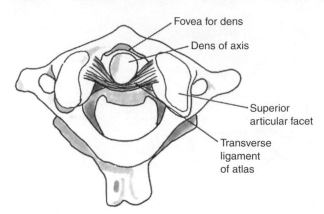

FIG. 17-3. Fovea for dens

Dens of axis

Superior articular facet

Transverse ligament of atlas

FIG. 17-3. The atlantoaxial joint from a superior view, showing the dens and the transverse ligament of the atlas.

rotation and climbs up the shoulder of the side opposite rotation. This can be palpated as the transverse process of the atlas becoming higher and farther forward on the side opposite rotation and lower and more posterior on the side of rotation.[18]

The atlanto-occipital, atlantoaxial, and, arguably, the Luschka joint surfaces are lined with articular cartilage; they have synovial membranes and, like other synovial joints, have rich proprioceptive and nociceptive innervation.[23]

☐ Joints and Ligaments

The *anterior* and *posterior longitudinal* ligaments and the *ligamentum flavum* are present in the cervical spine from C2 through C7 and perform the same functions as in the thoracic and lumbar spine (see Fig. 16-10).

The *interspinous* and *supraspinous* ligaments blend with the nuchal ligament of the cervical spine (Fig. 17-4). The *nuchal* ligament has its origins on the spinous processes of the cervical spine and its insertion on the occiput. Its function in quadruped animals is to support the head. Its function in humans is to prevent overflexion of the neck. The nuchal ligament tightens at the extreme of neck flexion. It also becomes tight, flattening out the cervical lordosis, with approximately 15° of nodding of the upper cervical spine.[18]

The *posterior longitudinal* ligament ends at C2. The tectorial membrane, which is thin and diaphanous through the rest of the spine, thickens into the *tectorial* ligament arising from C2, bypasses the atlas, and inserts on the occiput (Fig. 17-5). The tectorial ligament becomes tight with flexion of the head.

Deep to the tectorial ligament is the *cruciform* ligament, which has both vertical and transverse portions (see Fig. 17-5). The vertical portion of the cruciform ligament has its origin on C2 and has the same insertion and function as the tectorial ligament. It also by-

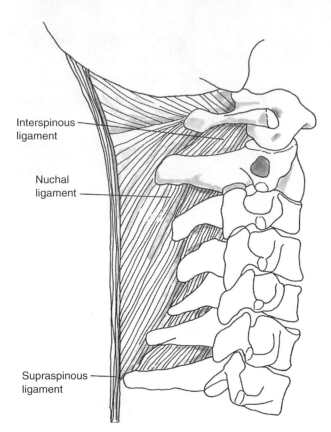

Interspinous ligament

Nuchal ligament

Supraspinous ligament

FIG. 17-4. A lateral view of the cervical spine, showing the interspinous, supraspinous, and nuchal ligaments.

passes C1. The horizontal portion of the cruciform ligament has its origin and insertion on the interior surface of the anterior ring of the atlas. It encircles the dens to reinforce the transverse ligament of the atlas (see Fig. 17-3).

The *transverse* ligament of the atlas has its origin and insertion on the interior surface of the anterior ring of the atlas. It encloses the dens and is lined with a synovial membrane and articular cartilage to provide lubrication as the atlas rotates around the dens. If the transverse ligament of the atlas and the horizontal portion of the cruciform ligament are weakened by systemic inflammatory disease or injured in an accident, there is danger of damage to the medulla oblongata by dislocation of the dens. If this is suspected, traction or mobilization of the cervical spine should be considered gravely dangerous.

The *alar* ligament is a winglike structure that has its origin on the lateral borders of the dens and its insertion on the occiput (see Fig. 17-5). It is a major portion of the stabilization system of the upper cervical spine. The configuration of the atlanto-occipital joints could allow considerable lateral flexion, which would damage the medulla oblongata. This lateral flexion is checked by the alar ligament. If the alar ligament is congenitally absent or damaged or if the dens is frac-

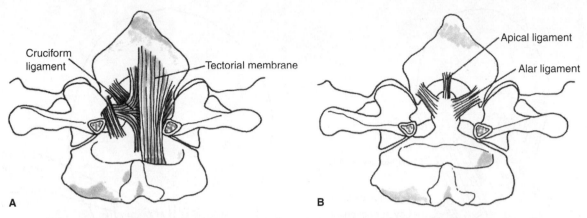

FIG. 17-5. A posterior view of the ligaments of the upper cervical spine: the more superficial tectorial and cruciform ligaments (**A**) and the deeper alar and apical ligaments (**B**). (Note: the cruciform ligament is not shown so that the deeper ligaments can be seen.)

tured or congenitally absent, mobilization or traction to the cervical spine should be considered gravely hazardous.

The *apical* ligament has its origin on the tip of the dens and inserts on the occiput (see Fig. 17-5). It becomes taut when traction is applied to the head. The joint capsule of the atlanto-occipital joint is reinforced with ligaments. The lateral placement of the atlanto-occipital joint capsules and ligaments severely limits rotation of the occiput on the atlas.

CLINICAL CONSIDERATIONS

The ligaments of the upper cervical spine may be damaged in high-velocity accidents, weakened by rheumatoid arthritis or other types of systemic inflammatory diseases, or may be congenitally absent or malformed. Before any kind of mechanical treatment is begun, the integrity of the upper cervical ligament should be tested.

The Sharp-Purser test has been described as a safe and effective method to evaluate alar ligament stability and correlates strongly (r = 0.88) with radiographic findings.[20,21] To perform this test the patient should be sitting in a relaxed position with the cervical spine in a semiflexed position. The examiner places the web space of one hand around the spinous process of the axis for fixation and then presses with the palm of the other hand on the patient's forehead dorsally. While the examiner presses dorsally with the palm, an excessive sliding motion of the head posteriorly in relation to the axis can be appreciated, which indicates atlanto-axial instability.[1,21] Symptoms exhibited when the head is in the forward-flexed position should be alleviated with posterior movement of the head.

In order to distract by traction the atlanto-occipital or atlanto-axial joint, the head must be in a neutral or slightly extended position to slacken the nuchal and posterior longitudinal ligaments.

The upper cervical spine can be thought of as an upper joint which flexes and extends and has some sidebending but no rotation, and as an inferior joint that allows approximately 90° rotation, no sidebending, and limited flexion–extension; therefore, if the lower cervical spine is locked in full flexion or sidebending, movements of the atlanto-occipital joint are tested by lateral flexion, and movements of the atlanto-axial joint are tested by rotation.[11]

☐ **Muscle Groups**

The muscles of the cervical spine can be considered in four functional groups: superficial posterior, deep posterior, superficial anterior, and deep anterior. Normal function of the cervical spine depends on proper flexibility and balance of these muscle groups.

The trapezius muscle is the largest, strongest, and most prominent of the posterior neck muscles (Fig. 17-6). It is very well developed in quadruped animals and serves to hold the head up against gravity. It inserts into the nuchal ligament and occipital ridge and extends the head and neck. In its function of maintaining the head in an erect position against the pull of gravity, the trapezius muscle works most efficiently when the head and neck are in their optimal position; that is, with the deepest part of the cervical lordosis no more than 4 to 6 cm from the apex of the thoracic kyphosis. The levator scapulae, splenius capitis, and splenius cervicis are other large superficial muscle groups that assist in extending the head and neck and holding the head up against gravity.

The multifidi and suboccipital muscles make up the deep posterior muscle group (Fig. 17-7). The multifidi have their origins on the transverse processes and in-

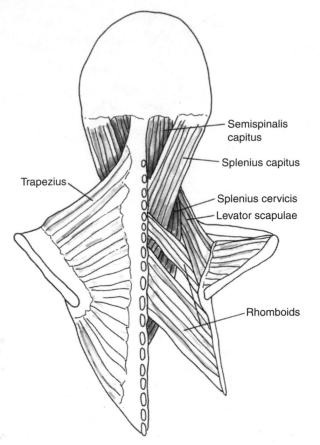

FIG. 17-6. The superficial muscles of the head, neck, and shoulders. This posterior view shows the trapezius, levator scapulae, splenius capitis, splenius cervicis, and rhomboid muscles.

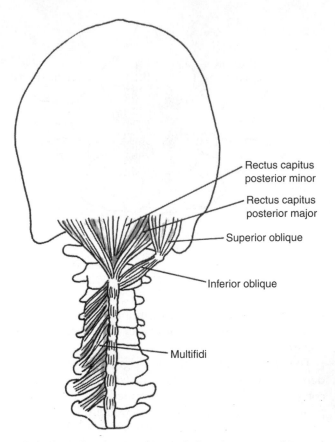

FIG. 17-7. A posterior view of the deep posterior neck muscles, showing the multifidi and suboccipital muscles.

sertions on the spinous process of the vertebra one to two segments above. When contracted together they extend the cervical spine; when contracted unilaterally they rotate the cervical spine to the opposite side and sidebend to the same side.

The sternocleidomastoid muscle is the largest and strongest of the anterior neck muscles (Fig. 17-8). From its dual origins on the sternum and clavicle, it inserts on the mastoid process, posterior to the center of gravity of the head. When both heads of the sternocleidomastoid are contracted together, they are flexors of the neck but extensors of the head. When only one side is contracted, the head and neck are laterally flexed and are rotated to the opposite side. The sternocleidomastoid muscles are very strong, and when injured or in spasm, they hold the neck and head in the head-forward, chin-out posture.

The other major neck flexors are the scalenus muscles, which have their origins on the first and second ribs and their insertions on the lateral tubercles of C2 to C7 (see Fig. 17-8). The scalenus anticus and scalenus medius are the anterior and posterior walls of the thoracic outlet. The first rib forms the bottom of the box, and the clavicle forms the top.[10] If the scalenus muscles are hypertrophied or in spasm, they may impinge on the lower roots of the brachial plexus or the subclavian artery as it passes through the thoracic outlet. Flexion of the head is accomplished by stabilization of the mandible by the muscles of mastication and a downward pull on the mandible by the strap (suprahyoid and infrahyoid) muscles (Fig. 17-9).[11]

The deep anterior neck muscles are the longus colli and longus capitis (Fig. 17-10). They are small muscles with origins and insertions on the bodies of the cervical vertebrae. In spite of their size, they are very strong and have very good leverage. Their function is to prevent anterior collapse of the cervical lordosis to resist the compressive force of the long cervical muscles. When these muscles are injured or in spasm, they exert a constant force that gradually flattens out the curve in the cervical spine.[11]

☐ **Innervation**

Sensory and sympathetic innervation of the head and neck is a complex overlapping of cervical plexus and

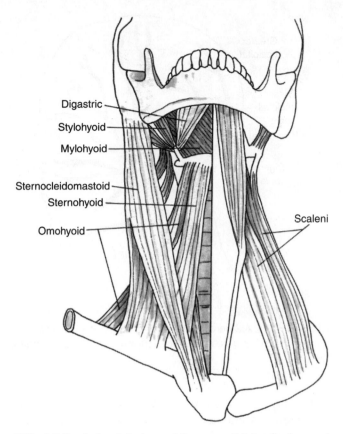

FIG. 17-8. A frontal view of the superficial anterior neck muscles, showing the sternocleidomastoid, scaleni, suprahyoid, and infrahyoid muscles.

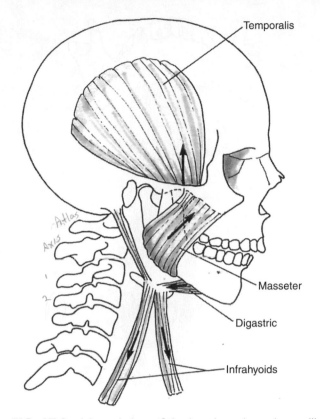

FIG. 17-9. A lateral view of the head, neck, and mandible showing the muscular forces that flex the head: the infrahyoid muscles pulling downward on the hyoid bone, the suprahyoids pulling downward on the mandible, and the muscles of mastication stabilizing the jaw.

cranial nerves, making evaluation of pain complaints difficult. Sensory and sympathetic innervation of the face come from the facial and trigeminal nerves, both of which have sensory ganglia in the medulla oblongata and have anastomoses with sensory nerves of the cervical plexus (Fig. 17-11). The posterior portion of the head and upper cervical spine is primarily innervated by the greater and lesser occipital nerves, which arise from the cervical plexus but also have twigs from the trigeminal nerve. The joint and ligamentous structures and the segmental spinal muscles of the cervical spine are innervated by the recurrent fibers of the segmental spinal nerves. The brachial plexus arises from the roots of the fifth through eighth cervical nerves and provides the sensory and motor innervation to the scapula and upper extremity.[9]

CLINICAL CONSIDERATIONS

Mechanical irritation of deep somatic structures in the cervical spine may refer pain to the face, head, upper extremity, or interscapular area.[5]

Neuritis and neuralgia of the cranial nerves, particularly V, VII, IX, and XI and also the greater and lesser occipital nerves, are common and may be mistaken for musculoskeletal pain.[2]

Peripheral entrapment of the brachial plexus is possible at the thoracic outlet, the shoulder, the elbow, and the carpal tunnel; this can produce symptoms that may be mistaken for shoulder tendinitis, elbow tendinitis, nerve root pain, or musculoskeletal pain of the neck or shoulder.

The nerve roots may be irritated by pressure from the bulging nucleus pulposus or by stenosis of the intervertebral foramen.

☐ Blood Supply

The blood vessels in the cervical region of particular interest to physical therapists are the subclavian arteries, which pass between the scalenus anticus and scalenus medius and may be compressed (see Thoracic Outlet Syndrome on page 576), and the vertebral arteries. The vertebral arteries passes upward through the lateral foramen of the cervical vertebrae. There is a redundant portion that allows full rotation of the atlas in both directions (Fig. 17-12). The vertebral arteries

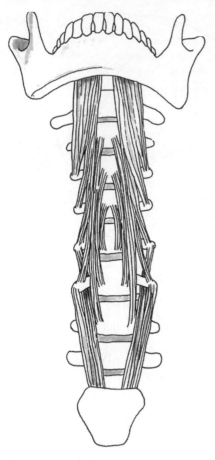

FIG. 17-10. The deep anterior neck muscles include the longus colli.

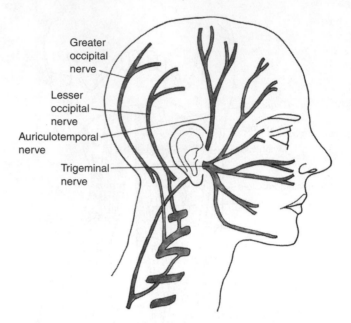

FIG. 17-11. A lateral view of the neck, head, and face showing the cervical plexus, trigeminal, and occipital nerves.

of this type of catastrophe involves an attempt to rotate the atlas and usually involves an exceptionally forceful maneuver. In many cases the patient felt violently ill, dizzy, briefly lost consciousness after manipulation, was manipulated again, and died several hours later. Because death may occur several hours after manipulation, it is possible that the number of

enter the cranium at the foramen magnum and come together to form the basilar artery.[12] The normal blood supply for the brain is through the carotid arteries if the circle of Willis is complete. If the circle of Willis is incomplete or if there is interruption of the blood supply through the carotid arteries, the vertebral arteries may form a major portion of the blood supply for the brain, particularly the brain stem and cerebellum. The vertebral arteries are at least partially occluded by extension and rotation of the cervical spine; maximum occlusion occurs with the combination of extension and rotation. Brief occlusion of the vertebral artery is not a problem in a patient who has normal carotid arteries and a normal circle of Willis; however, if there is interruption of the normal blood supply to the brain, occlusion of the vertebral artery may cause a reduction of blood flow to the brain stem and cerebellum, the symptoms of which are dizziness, nystagmus, slurring of speech, and loss of consciousness.[14]

There are many well-documented cases of coma and death secondary to vasospasm or thrombosis of the vertebral arteries caused by manipulation of the upper cervical spine.[4,12,15] The most common history

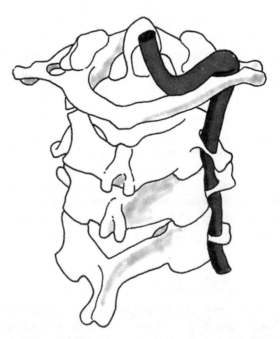

FIG. 17-12. A posterior view of the upper cervical spine, showing the vertebral artery emerging from C2 with a redundant loop that allows mobility of the atlas.

catastrophic responses to upper cervical manipulation is actually underreported.

Blood vessels in the cervical spine have no nociceptive innervation *per se,* but when overdilated, intense headaches (migraines) are perceived. Migraine headaches may be accompanied by blurring of vision from pressure of the distended cranial blood vessel on the optic nerves. They may also be accompanied by nausea and muscle spasm in the neck. The migraine headache may be distinguished from the musculoskeletal headache in that the pain is generally throbbing rather than constant, and the pattern of the headache is generally irregular and not related to trauma or activity.[2]

CLINICAL CONSIDERATIONS

Before using traction or mobilization techniques on the upper cervical spine, the vertebral arteries should be carefully tested one at a time by placing the neck in full rotation, extension, and lateral flexion to each side and holding for approximately 1 minute. The clinician should observe the patient for nystagmus, slurring of speech, blurring of vision, dizziness, or unconsciousness. Dizziness as a result of vertebral artery testing is fairly common and should be a warning sign to the practitioner to proceed very cautiously. Nystagmus, slurring of speech, or loss of consciousness should be considered contraindications to traction and mobilization of the neck, and the practitioner should take care when treating the patient to make sure that the neck is not positioned in extension or the extremes of rotation.[17]

If a patient has a history of throbbing headaches or headaches accompanied by blurring of vision and nausea, or if the history of headaches is irregular and not related to activity, the possibility of migraine headaches should be investigated before investing in a long course of physical therapy treatment.

▪ JOINT MECHANICS

☐ Lower Cervical Spine
(C2–T1)

The facet joints of the lower cervical spine are planar; at the single-joint level the only motions possible are superior and inferior glide. In inferior glide or extension the joint surfaces are maximally congruent, and the facet and joint capsules are maximally taut. Extension is the close-packed position and the position of maximal stability of the cervical spine. In full flexion the ligaments of the joint capsule are also taut, but the surfaces of the joint are barely engaged, making flexion the position of instability.[18]

CLINICAL CONSIDERATIONS

When the cervical spine is positioned in slight lordosis, there is good passive stability from the facet joints and supporting ligaments. When the cervical lordosis is lost or the cervical curve is reversed, passive stability is lost, and the segmental muscles must go into constant contraction to stabilize the spine. When there is slight lordosis in the cervical spine, the facet joints are able to bear approximately one third each of the compressive forces on the spine. When the cervical lordosis is lost, the entire compressive force is borne by the disk, causing excessive pressure and flattening.

Motion of a lower cervical segment involves movement of the vertebral bodies, which use the disk as a pivot, as well as movement of the joints of Luschka and the facet joints. Flexion of a cervical segment is superior glide of both facet joints. Extension of the cervical spine is inferior glide of both facet joints. Rotation and sidebending of the lower cervical spine are the same movements: there is inferior glide of the facet joint on the side to which the spine is rotated or sidebent, and superior glide of the facet on the side opposite rotation. Because of the 45° slope of the facet joints, the lateral tubercle on the same side moves downward and backward while that on the opposite side moves upward and forward. With either rotation or lateral flexion, there is always slight extension of the segment as well.[11]

☐ Upper Cervical Spine
(Occiput–C1–C2)

When the ring of the atlas lifts up posteriorly, there is approximately 20° of flexion–extension of the atlanto-occipital joint and approximately 15° of flexion of the atlanto-axial joint. When the atlanto-occipital joint is in extension, the ring of the atlas gets closer to the occiput and may compress the neurovascular structures in the suboccipital area. When the atlanto-occipital joint is flexed by nodding the head, the space between the atlas and occiput is maximally opened (Fig. 17-13). This can be seen clearly on mobility roentgenograms. Sidebending of the atlanto-occipital joint is always accompanied by a small conjunct rotation to the opposite side, which allows the condyle of the occiput on the side of lateral flexion to become congruent with the superior joint surface of the axis below. Lateral flexion is checked by the alar ligament, which because of its insertion on the dens, causes rotation of the axis toward the side of lateral flexion. This can be palpated as the spinous process of the axis swinging to the side opposite lateral flexion. Palpating for motion of the spinous process of the axis with sidebending of the atlanto-occipital joint is one test for integrity of the alar

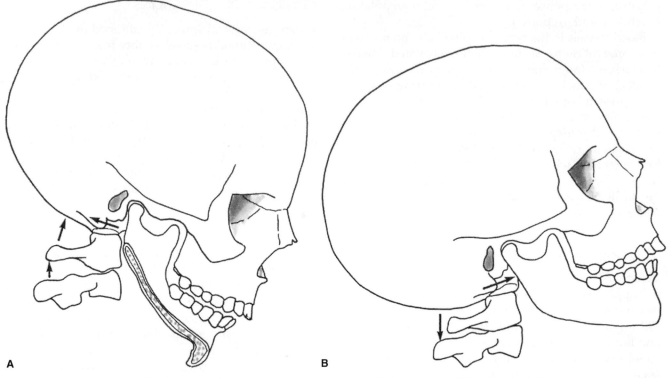

FIG. 17-13. Mobility of the upper cervical spine: (**A**) flexion and (**B**) extension. (Note: In flexion, the space between the occiput and C1 increases, and it decreases with extension.)

ligament. Rotation of the atlas around the axis always involves a swing to the side opposite rotation and an elevation of the transverse process opposite rotation as the atlas slides up the shoulder of the axis. This is accompanied by a tilting of the atlas toward the side of rotation, which may be palpated as the transverse process of the atlas moving posteriorly and inferiorly, and the transverse process on the side opposite rotation moving anteriorly and superiorly. Because the atlas has considerable mobility with relatively little ligamentous stability, it is possible for the atlas to be jammed or locked in a rotated position.

The combined movement of flexion of the head and neck involves full flexion of the atlanto-occipital joint, flexion of the atlas on the dens, and full flexion of the lower cervical segments. The combined movement of extension of the head and neck consists of extension of the atlanto-occipital joint, extension of the atlas on the axis, and extension of the lower cervical segments. As mentioned above, in the lower cervical spine there is no difference between rotation and sidebending. In the upper cervical spine, rotation of the head and neck is rotation of the atlantoaxial joint to the same side and sidebending of the atlanto-occipital joint to the opposite side. Sidebending actually involves lateral flexion of only the atlanto-occipital joint, but rotation of the atlanto-axial joint to the opposite side. Both rotation and sidebending involve slight flexion of the at-

lanto-occipital joint to compensate for extension of the lower cervical spine (Fig. 17-14).[11]

As an example, in left rotation of the head and neck, each segment of the lower cervical spine is in the combined movement of left lateral flexion and rotation, and each segment is slightly extended. The atlanto-axial joint is in full left rotation. The atlanto-occipital joint is in sidebending to the right and is slightly flexed. In left lateral flexion of the neck and cervical spine, each segment of the lower cervical spine is as in left rotation, with lateral flexion, rotation, and slight extension. The atlanto-axial joint is fully rotated to the right. The atlanto-occipital joint is in sidebending to the left and in slight flexion.

The only difference between left lateral flexion of the head and neck and left rotation of the head and neck is what happens in the upper cervical spine.

☐ Head-Righting Mechanism

The posture and righting mechanism seen in infants and lower animals are present in adult human beings as well. There is a strong tendency for the eyes to face forward and level in the horizontal plane. This means that any lateral or rotational deviation from normal posture must be compensated for in the upper cervical spine. This also means that if there is a rotational

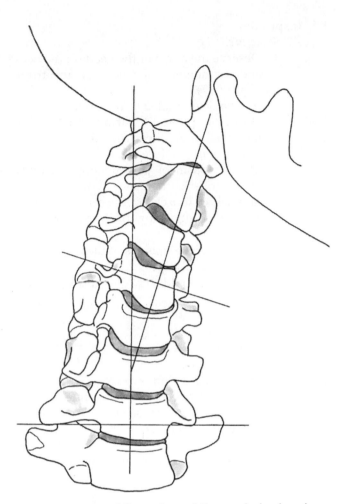

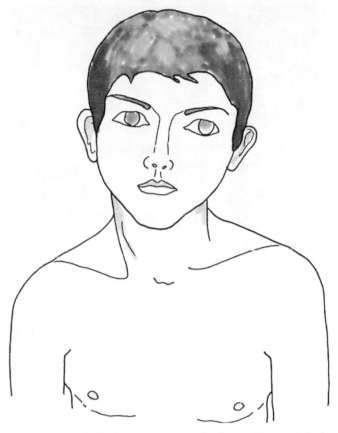

FIG. 17-15. Clinical appearance of a boy with a rotated atlas.

FIG. 17-14. An oblique view of the cervical spine showing full rotation: external rotation and lateral flexion of the lower cervical segments, rotation of the atlantoaxial joint, and flexion of the atlanto-occipital joint.

or sidebending fault in the upper cervical spine, it will impart scoliosis to the rest of the spine. For example, in an atlanto-occipital joint locked in left lateral flexion, the cervical spine will move into right sidebending to bring the eyes level, thus producing an S-shaped scoliosis in the rest of the spine. Another example would be a left leg-length discrepancy that imparts a long C-shaped scoliosis; this is compensated for by left lateral flexion at the atlanto-occipital joint to bring the eyes level (Fig. 17-15).[18]

■ **EXAMINATION**

I. **History**

In addition to the general musculoskeletal history (see Chapter 5, Assessment of Musculoskeletal Disorders and Concepts of Management), the following factors should be considered:

A. *Rule out migraines by determining if headache symptoms are as follows:*
   1. Of an intermittent irregular pattern unrelated to activity or trauma
   2. Accompanied by nausea or blurring of vision
   3. Throbbing like a pulse rather than steady
   4. Relieved by beta blockers, ergotamine, or related compounds
B. *Determine if pain is caused by neuritis or neuralgia.*[2]
   1. Unrelated to activity or trauma
   2. Superficial, stimulating in quality, or electric
   3. Follows the pattern of innervation of a cranial or peripheral nerve
C. *Evaluate upper extremity pain.* If the patient is complaining of upper extremity pain, is it in the pattern of a nerve root or peripheral entrapment?

II. **Observation**

A. *Posture*—Observe in sitting and standing.
   1. General alignment
   2. Does the head deviate from the optimal posture (4–8 cm from the apex of the tho-

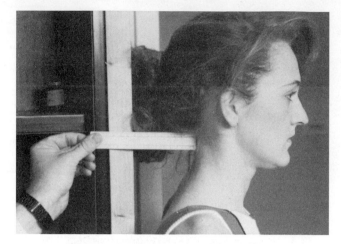

FIG. 17-16. Measurement of head posture.

racic kyphosis to the deepest point in the cervical lordosis)? (Fig. 17-16)[18]

3. When the sternocleidomastoid muscle is in its normal rest position, it angles backward slightly. If the sternocleidomastoid muscle is vertical, this indicates forward head posture and/or tightness of the sternocleidomastoid muscle.

4. Function. How willing is the patient to turn the neck when dressing, undressing, or filling out paperwork?

III. Inspection

A. *Structure*
1. Observe the angle of the head on the neck and the angle of the neck on the trunk (Fig. 17-17).
2. Are clavicles angled or horizontal?
3. Do the scapulae lie flat against the thoracic wall or are they winged?

B. *Soft tissue signs*
1. Muscle spasm or parafunctional activity of the muscles of mastication, the facial muscles, or muscles of the cervical spine
2. Segmental guarding or hypertrophy of muscle
3. Atrophy of the muscles of the neck, upper extremity, or scapula

C. *Skin*—Neck, shoulder girdle, and upper extremity regions
1. Color
2. Moisture
3. Redness or swelling
4. Scars or blemishes

IV. Selective Tissue Tension

A. *Active range of motion*—Test in sitting
1. Flexion—extension (see Fig. 17-18A,B)
2. Rotation (see Fig. 17-18C)
3. Sidebending (see Fig. 17-18D). (If sidebending is severely limited, suspect

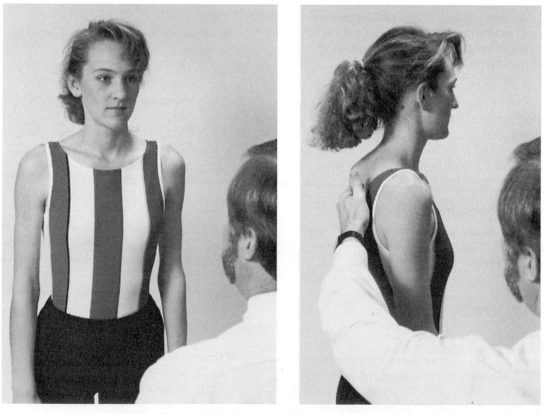

FIG. 17-17. Observation view of the head, neck, and shoulder girdle.

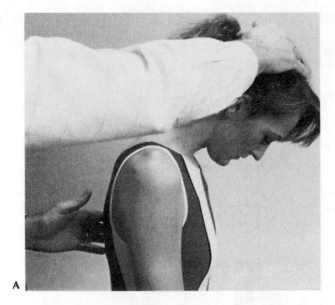

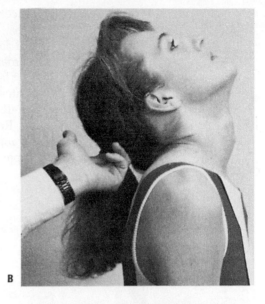

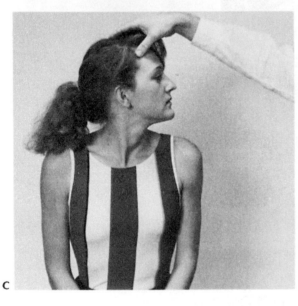

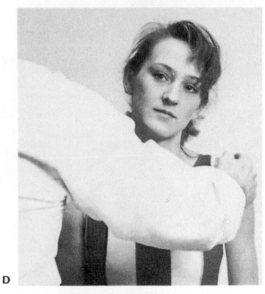

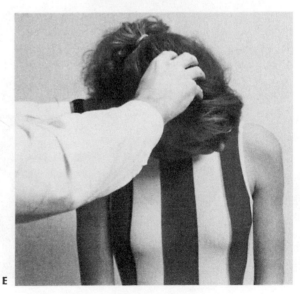

FIG. 17-18. Active movements of the cervical spine: (**A**) flexion, (**B**) extension, (**C**) rotation, (**D**) sidebending, and (**E**) atlantoaxial rotation.

capsular tightness of the lower cervical spine.)

4. Lock lower cervical spine in full lateral flexion or full flexion. Test movement of the atlanto-occipital joint by testing lateral flexion. Test movement of the atlanto-axial joint by testing rotation (see Fig. 17-18*E*).

B. *Passive range of motion*—Test supine. Repeat tests for active motion, noting the range of motion, end feel, muscle spasm, and pain.

C. *Isometrically resisted motions*

1. Gently test rotation, lateral flexion, and flexion of the cervical spine (see page 564).

2. Test rotator cuff muscles, noting pain and/or weakness (see Chapter 9, The Shoulder and Shoulder Girdle).

D. *Joint play*

1. Atlanto-occipital joint
   a. Distraction (Fig. 17-19*A*)
   b. Lateral glide (Fig. 17-19*B*)
2. Atlanto-axial joint
   a. Distraction
   b. Rotation (Fig. 17-20)
3. Lower cervical facets—Test glide by placing the web space of the thumb over the joint and gently gliding laterally (Fig. 17-21).

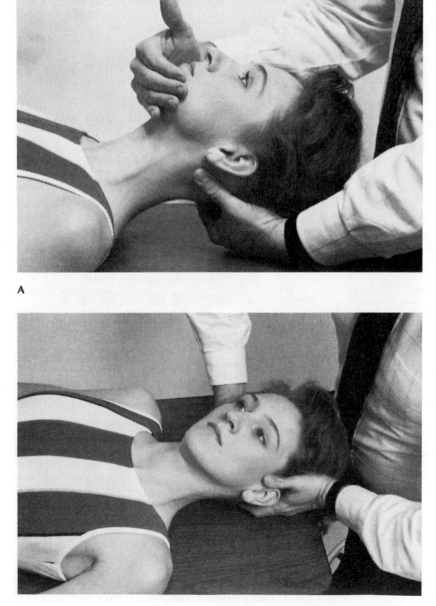

A

B

FIG. 17-19. Joint-play movements of the atlanto-occipital joint: (**A**) distraction and (**B**) lateral glide.

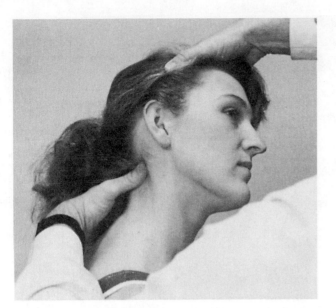

FIG. 17-20. Joint-play movements of the atlantoaxial joint rotation.

V. Neurological Testing

A. *Neurological involvement suspected:*

1. For neurological function in various sites, test the levels noted (muscle power):
   a. Abduction—C5
   b. Biceps—C6
   c. Triceps—C7
   d. Pronator teres—C7
   e. Wrist extension—C6
   f. Wrist flexion—C7
   g. Finger abduction—C8
   h. Finger adduction—T1
2. Reflex testing
   a. Biceps—C6 (Fig. 17-22*A*)
   b. Triceps—C7 (Fig. 17-22*B*)
   c. Wrist extensor—C6 (Fig. 17-22*C*)

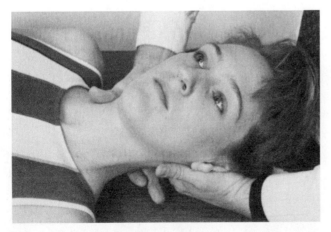

FIG. 17-21. Joint-play movements of the lower cervical facets.

3. Neural tension test (see Chapter 9, The Shoulder and Shoulder Girdle, and Fig. 9-21)

B. *Sensation*—Test sensation, particularly around the hand (Fig. 17-23). (See Chapter 18, The Cervical–Upper Limb Scan Examination.)

C. *Spurling test* (foramen compression)
   1. Place the neck in extension, lateral flexion, and rotation to one side. Watch for referred pain or neurological signs in the extremity (Fig. 17-24*A*).
   2. Apply traction to the neck and watch for improvement of referred pain and neurological symptoms (Fig. 17-24*B*).

D. *Carpal tunnel test* (see Chapter 11, The Wrist and Hand Complex) (Fig. 17-25)

E. *Tests for scalenus anticus and thoracic outlet* (Fig. 17-26).
   1. Scalenus anticus (Fig. 17-26*A*)—Apply firm pressure over the lower bellies of the scalenus muscles near their origins on the first and second ribs. Maintain pressure for at least 30 seconds. The scalenus muscles, if involved, may refer pain to the anterior chest, neck, or interscapular area, even if there is no neurovascular compression.
   2. Test for neurovascular compression (Fig. 17-26*B*)
      a. Patient—In a sitting position
      b. Operator—Stands behind and to one side
      c. Movement—Operator guides the motion of the patient's head to the extreme of rotation and into slight extension, holding this position for at least 30 seconds, palpating for pulse at the wrist, and watching for reproduction of radiating symptoms in the hand or arm.
   3. Neurovascular test with depression of the scapula (Fig. 17-26*B*). The patient and operator are in the same position as above for neurovascular compression test. In addition to rotating and extending the neck, the operator presses down on the shoulder, depressing the clavicle and closing down the thoracic outlet. Hold for 30 seconds and watch for the same signs and symptoms as above.
   4. Neurovascular test with clavicle depressed and ribs elevated. The procedure in the previous test is repeated, and the patient is asked to take a deep breath and hold for 30 seconds.

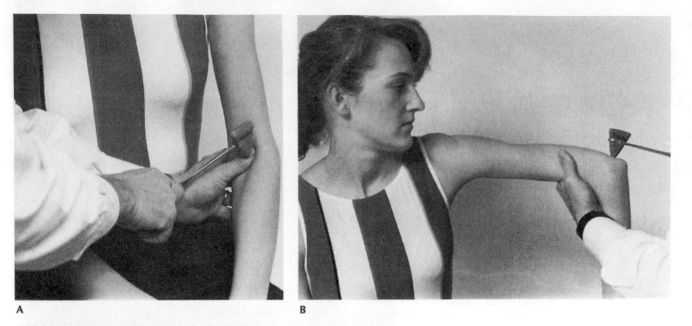

A

B

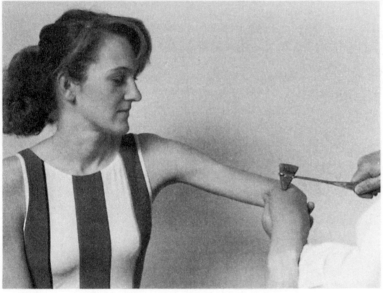

C

FIG. 17-22. Test of upper limb reflexes: (**A**) biceps, (**B**) triceps, and (**C**) brachioradialis.

5. Overhead test (Fig. 17-26C). With the patient in the same position as above, a 2- or 3-pound weight is placed in the patient's hand. With the shoulder in flexion, the patient actively flexes and extends the elbow (repeatedly). If there is compression of the subclavian artery, the muscles of the elbow will fatigue very rapidly, and the symptoms may be reproduced.

VI. Palpation

The following structures should be carefully palpated for guarding, spasm, and particularly to see if deep palpation reproduces pain referred to another area.

A. Trapezius—Palpate inferior, middle, and superior portions (Fig. 17-27A).
B. Levator scapula—Palpate particularly close to the origin.
C. Multifidi—Should be palpated segmentally from C2–C7, particularly noting segmental guarding at the C4, C5, or C6 segments (Fig. 17-27B).
D. Lesser occipital nerve (Fig. 17-28A)
E. Greater occipital nerve and suboccipital musculature (Fig. 17-28B)
F. Belly of the temporalis muscle (Fig. 17-28C)
G. Masseter muscle—Palpate bimanually with the thumb inside the mouth and fingers over

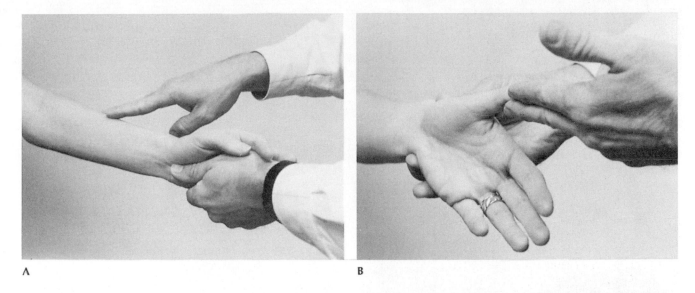

A   B

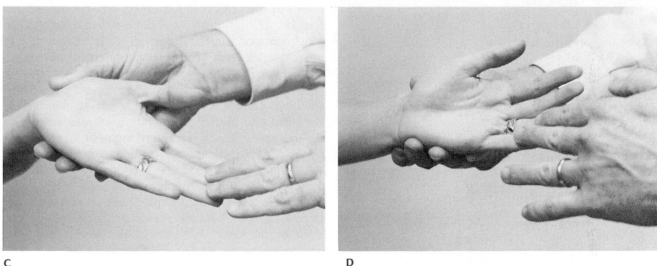

C   D

FIG. 17-23. Sensory testing of the dermatomes of the hand: (**A**) C5, (**B**) C6, (**C**) C7, and (**D**) C8 sensory areas.

the cheeks (Fig. 17-28*D*) and outside the mouth (Fig. 17-28*E*).

H. Inferior head of the lateral pterygoid muscle (Fig. 17-28*F*)

I. Medial pterygoid—Palpate at its insertion under the angle of the mandible.

J. The sternocleidomastoid muscle (Fig. 17-28*G*)

K. The thyroid cartilage and longus colli muscle (Fig. 17-28*H*)

L. The suprasternal notch and sternoclavicular joint (Fig. 17-28*I*)

M. The acromioclavicular joint (Fig. 17-28*J*)

N. The sternocleidomastoid muscle in supine (Fig. 17-29)—Stimulataneous palpation.

VII. Roentgenographical Analysis

A. Cervical curve—Normal or abnormal curvature
   1. There should be a slight lordotic curve in the cervical spine.
   2. Note a straight or kyphotic spine suggesting spasms of the longus colli or overdevelopment of the anterior neck musculature.
   3. Ankylosis or instability on mobility films

B. Lipping or spurring of the vertebral bodies or uncinate processes indicating abnormal weight-bearing or degeneration of the disk. Also note disk height (Fig. 17-30).

C. Intervertebral foramina: Look for opening on an oblique film. Note any narrowing or encroachment.

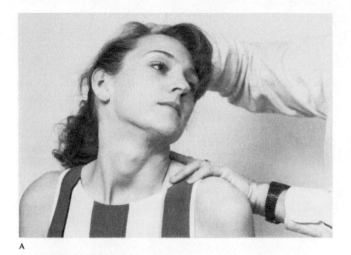

A

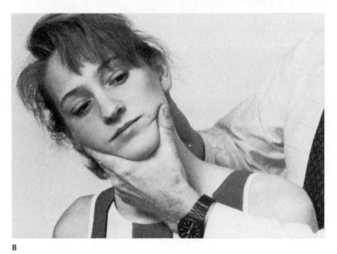

B

FIG. 17-24. Spurling test.

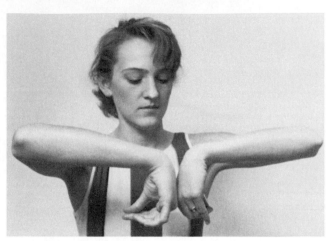

FIG. 17-25. Carpal tunnel test.

D. A 9–12 mm space between the ring of the atlas and the occiput. There should be a minimum of 9–12 mm of space visible on the x-ray film between the occipital bone and the posterior arch of the atlas. Less than 9 mm of space indicates extension of the upper cervical spine and possible compression of the neurovascular structures in the suboccipital area.

E. Through-the-mouth view for the relationship of the odontoid process to the adjacent bones.

COMMON DISORDERS

☐ Acceleration Injury

The mechanism of acceleration injury (or whiplash) is acceleration of the head and neck relative to the body. It usually results from the collision of two automo-

biles but also can result from contact sports such as football or high-velocity sports such as skiing. The most common mechanism of injury is an automobile at rest struck from behind. At the moment of impact, the trunk of the body, which is supported by the car seat, moves rapidly forward. The moment of inertia of the head creates a relative backward acceleration of the head and neck.[19] Acceleration injuries are not as dangerous as flexion injuries of the neck, in which the head is stabilized and the momentum of the body weight forces the neck into flexion, but they can be very persistent and difficult to treat.

Because there is often a question of insurance compensation, and because roentgenographical reports, even in the most severe cases, are usually negative, the question arises as to whether there actually is an injury, and if so, which structures are injured. As with low back injuries, there is a natural history to acceleration injuries; 80 percent of patients reporting symptoms following a motor vehicle accident will be better within 3 to 4 weeks.[6,8,16] If this is so, are there any factors that would allow one to predict from the physical examination who the 20 percent will be who will not improve spontaneously?

These questions have been partially answered by experimental animal research and longitudinal studies of patients injured in automobile accidents. In a study of 525 patients injured in automobile accidents, the *direction of the initial impact* was found to be an important predictor of prognosis. In this group, the 100 patients who were in cars involved in head-on collisions had no prolonged symptoms. The 200 cases where initial impact was from the side had lingering symptoms for a short period of time but no symptoms lasting more than a few months. Of the 250 patients in cars that were hit from the rear, 50 percent were still having symptoms 1 year after the accident.[13] The possibility of in-

(text continues on page 548)

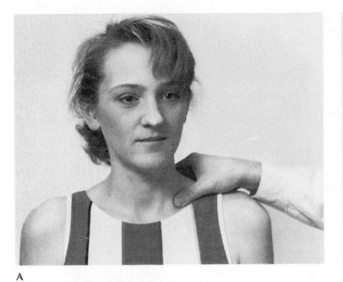

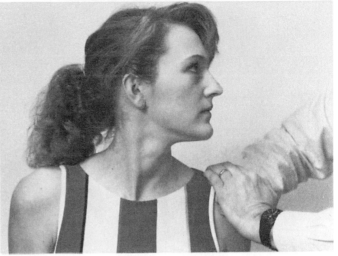

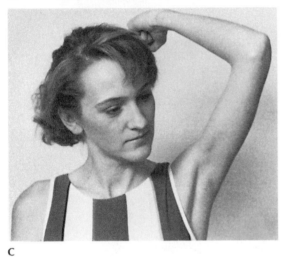

FIG. 17-26. Thoracic outlet tests: (**A**) scalenus anticus test; (**B**) neurovascular compression test with depression of the scapula; and (**C**) overhead test.

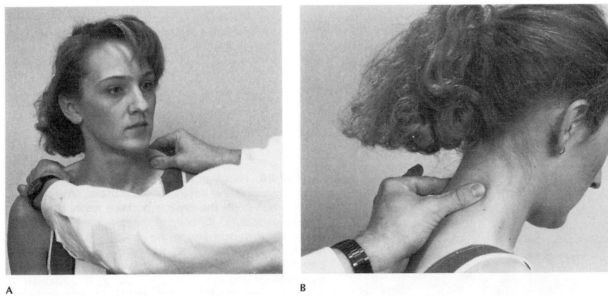

FIG. 17-27. Palpation of the (**A**) trapezius and the (**B**) multifidi muscles (segmentally).

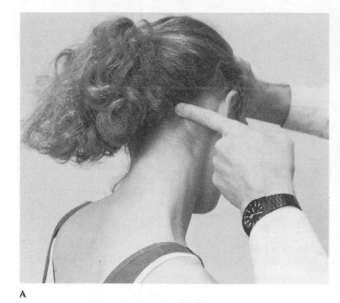

A

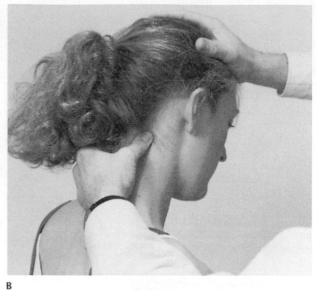

B

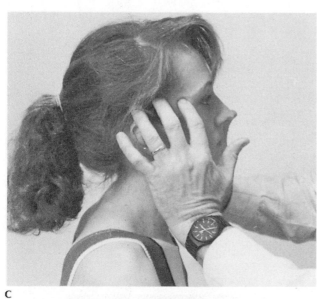

C

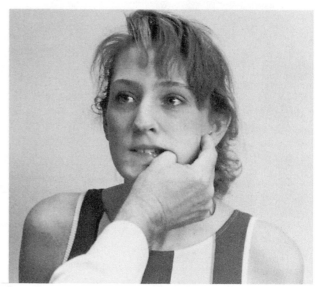

D

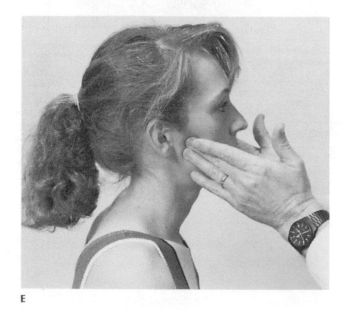

E

FIG. 17-28. Palpation of the occipital region, muscles of mastication, and the anterior neck muscles: (**A**) the lesser occipital nerve, (**B**) the greater occipital nerve and suboccipital musculature, (**C**) belly of the temporalis muscle, (**D**) the masseter muscle (inside the mouth), (**E**) the masseter muscle (superficial fibers), (**F**) the inferior head of the lateral pterygoid, (**G**) the sternocleidomastoid muscle, (**H**) the thyroid cartilage and longus colli muscle, (**I**) the suprasternal notch and sternoclavicular joint, and (**J**) the acromioclavicular joint.

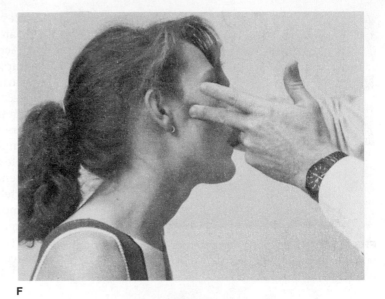

F

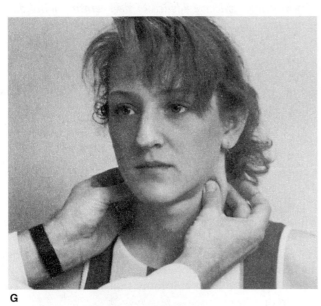

G

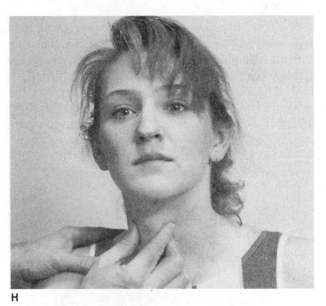

H

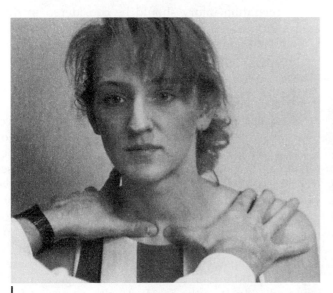

I

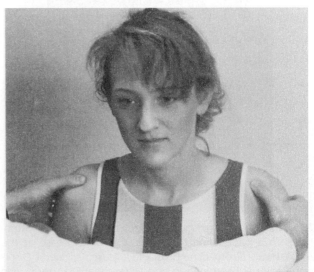

J

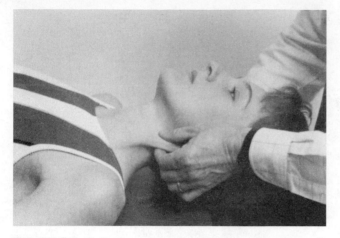

FIG. 17-29. Palpation of the sternocleidomastoid from its origin to its base. (Both sternocleidomastoids should be palpated simultaneously.)

surance compensation did not seem to be a factor in prognosis. Presumably, when the initial impact is from the front, the chin hits the chest before the cervical spine reaches its anatomical limit of motion. When the initial impact is from the side, the head hits the shoulder before the anatomical limit of range of motion is reached. When the impact is from behind, however,

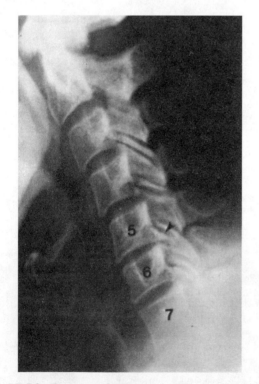

FIG. 17-30. Roetgenogram depicting posterior osteophytes in a patient with degenerative disk disease at the C5–C6 level. (From D'Ambrosia RD: Musculoskeletal Disorders: Regional Examination and Differential Diagnosis, 2nd ed, p. 256. Philadelphia, JB Lippincott, 1986.)

unless the back of the car seat is high enough, there is no anatomical stop to prevent hyperextension.

Acceleration injuries were simulated in monkeys by strapping them to car seats and dropping them backward from various heights. The animals were sacrificed and dissected at intervals afterwards. The most common injuries found were complete and partial tears of the sternocleidomastoid muscle followed by complete and partial tears of the longus colli, complete and partial tears of the anterior longitudinal ligament, and finally, separation of the disks from the vertebral bodies.[13] Five patients who had persistent symptoms from rear-end impact were found at surgery to have disks torn away from the vertebral body.[13] After anterior fusion, their symptoms were resolved, even though most of them had long since settled their insurance claims.

Two other predictors of a poor prognosis are *roentgenographical evidence of degenerative joint disease* and *neurological signs* soon after the accident.[16]

CLINICAL CONSIDERATIONS

Patients with injuries from initial impact from the rear should be followed more closely and should be considered to be at higher risk for having prolonged symptoms. Patients who have roentgenographical evidence of degenerative joint disease or neurological signs soon after the accident must also be considered at higher risk and followed more closely.

Muscle injury to the anterior neck must not be overlooked, particularly the sternocleidomastoid and deep anterior neck musculature.

Acceleration injuries should be considered legitimate trauma with potential anatomical damage sufficient to cause the symptoms that most patients complain of.

Acceleration injury should be considered in three phases: acute, subacute, and chronic. The injury should be classified according to the findings from examination, rather than the length of time since the accident.

ACUTE PHASE

The acute phase begins at the moment of the accident and may last as long as 2 to 3 weeks. The most severe injury is from a rear impact. As the head hyperextends on the trunk, the sternocleidomastoid muscle becomes tight and it is pulled or torn. With higher velocity impacts, the longus colli may be pulled or torn, the anterior longitudinal ligament may be pulled or torn, and the annulus of the disk may tear away from the vertebral body. The facet joints are hyperextended and their capsules may be strained or torn. There is generally little pain and fairly free range of motion immediately after the accident, with painful stiffness gradually developing over 24 to 48 hours. There is a possibility of fracture, traction injury to the nerve roots, contusion to the spinal cord, head injury, or tearing of the supporting ligaments of the upper cervical spine. These conditions cannot be ruled out definitively without a roentgenographical evaluation. Consultation with a physician prior to mechanical treatment is wise.

Evaluation. The patient will generally feel very little pain or stiffness immediately after the accident. As the large muscles swell and develop spasm, the patient will note onset of muscle soreness, stiffness, and swelling. The therapist may observe spasm of the sternocleidomastoid muscle, and the head will often be pulled into the head-forward posture. The skin may be red, and the muscles will be warm, rubbery, and tender to touch. Active range of motion will be quite limited with muscle spasm end feel. Passive range of motion will be greater than active. Joint play will be very difficult to assess because of muscle spasm. The sternocleidomastoid muscle will generally be warm, swollen, and in spasm. There may be palpable tears, particularly in the proximal third. There may be clearly delineated segmental spasm of the multifidi at the C4–C5 or C5–C6 level.

Treatment. The goal of treatment in the acute phase is to allow the cervical musculature to rest without becoming stiff and to progress to the subacute phase as rapidly as possible. Very little treatment is needed in the acute phase. The patient should be instructed in the use of heat or ice at home and in the use of a soft cervical collar. The patient should also be instructed in active rotation of the cervical spine within limits of pain to maintain joint range of motion. The patient should be given an explanation of the mechanics of the acceleration injury, including the information that most cases are completely healed in 4 to 5 weeks. The patient should be encouraged to be as active as possible and should be rechecked at approximately 1-week intervals.

SUBACUTE PHASE

In the subacute phase, which usually lasts 2 to 10 weeks, the larger muscles have healed and are no longer swollen or tender. General muscle guarding will be reduced, and a more detailed evaluation of the cervical spine will be possible.

Evaluation. The patient will report that the muscle pain originally experienced has gone away but has been replaced by deep, aching pain that may be referred to the head, the interscapular area, or the upper extremity. The large cervical muscles will no longer feel warm, rubbery, and swollen. There will be focal areas of intense tenderness in the sternocleidomastoid, suboccipital, multifidi, and deep anterior neck

muscles. These areas of tenderness may refer pain to the head, shoulder, or upper extremity when palpated. Active range of motion will have increased considerably. The end feel will be capsular muscle guarding. If the facet joints have been injured, there will be capsular restriction of the neck with limitation of joint play when tested. The patient should be given a complete neurological screening, which in most cases will be negative. The major muscle groups of the neck should be carefully palpated noting tenderness, guarding, spasm, or anatomical shortening. The longus colli should be carefully palpated. As the patient progresses through the subacute phase, the longus colli should become progressively less tender. Roentgenograms may show flattening of the cervical spine from spasm of the longus colli.

Treatment. The treatment goal in the subacute phase is to restore flexibility to the cervical muscle groups and facet joints, if they are involved. Mechanical treatment is most effective in the subacute phase because muscle guarding has subsided, and stretching and mobilization will be fairly comfortable, but adhesions between muscle and joint fibers will not have solidified into scars.

Physical therapists have many effective techniques for dealing with tight, painful muscles. The following principles will make treatment of the muscles of the cervical spine more effective:

1. The most likely muscle to be injured in an acceleration injury is the sternocleidomastoid muscle. In order to stretch the sternocleidomastoid, the head and neck must be put into an extreme of rotation and lateral flexion, which can be uncomfortable and can also be damaging to joints and smaller muscles. The sternocleidomastoid muscle can be easily treated by massage.

2. The sternocleidomastoid muscles will be overshortened and very strong. Any strengthening program that increases the strength of the sternocleidomastoid or anterior neck musculature will contribute to muscle imbalance.

3. The most effective treatment for the longus colli and multifidi is to restore normal resting length (slight lordosis).[18]

4. Lordosis is a dynamic position and cannot be restored passively. Strengthening of the multifidi is the best way to restore cervical lordosis and to stabilize the midcervical spine. Multifidi strengthening through isometric exercise should be started as early as possible (see Figs. 17-35 to 17-37).

5. The large posterior neck musculature should be strengthened but not stretched. These muscles need to be strong to counteract the anterior pull of the sternocleidomastoid muscle. All of the muscles of the cervical spine are accessory muscles of respira-

tion. They can be aerobically strengthened by any activity that increases heart rate above the target level. Aerobic training of muscle is very helpful in reducing lactic acid to carbon dioxide. Blood flow to muscle can be increased by a factor of one or two by massage, but by a factor of six with aerobic exercise.

In addition to muscle therapy, attention must also be directed toward the facet joints. The cervical facet joints are approximately the same size as the distal interphalangeal joint of the little finger. The capsule and ligaments are delicate, and the mechanical forces that the facet joints undergo in an acceleration injury are severe. Because the facet joints are so deep, swelling, warmth, and redness are not apparent; however, the facet joints do go through the same stages that any acutely injured joint does. Mobilization or stretching that causes an increase in swelling will be harmful to the joint, because the presence of edema contributes to scarring. It is possible that overstretching or mobilization of swollen joints may lead to ankylosis or degenerative joint disease. Based on the information that we have about peripheral joint injuries, immobilization of injured joints also contributes to scarring.

The following guidelines are useful in treating the facet joints during the subacute phase:

1. During the acute phase, the patient should be instructed in active rotation within limits of pain to be done every hour.
2. Joint mobilization in the subacute phase should not be painful to the patient or cause lingering discomfort after treatment.
3. Hypermobile areas should be identified and mobilization avoided.
4. Gross passive stretching of the head and neck should be avoided because of the possibility of overstretching hypermobile segments. Range of motion should be restored by segmental joint mobilization (see Figs. 17-38 to 17-42).

CHRONIC PHASE

The chronic phase of an acceleration injury begins when the acute healing process is over. The large muscle groups will have completely healed, but they may be shortened and fibrotic. The longus colli remains in chronic spasm and will be acutely tender to palpation. The longus colli exerts a force that gradually flattens the cervical spine and may lead eventually to cervical instability. The multifidi at the C5 or C6 segment will be in constant contraction and may feel rubbery and inflamed as a result of overwork, in an attempt to stabilize the lower cervical spine.

Evaluation. The patient will complain of symptoms which are consistent with irritation of the deep somatic structures. The pain will be deep, aching, vague,

and often referred to the head, shoulders, interscapular area, or upper extremity. It is very common to have a headache in the suboccipital area, which begins in the morning and gets gradually worse with the day's activity. The patient will have hypertrophy of the sternocleidomastoid muscles and may have parafunctional hyperactivity of the anterior neck muscles and muscles of mastication.

The patient will have a forward-head posture with protraction of the scapula and superior angulation of the clavicles. Active range of motion of the neck may be limited by as much as 50 percent. Active and passive ranges of motion will be approximately the same. When tested segmentally, the upper and midcervical spine will be limited in a capsular pattern of restriction with segmental hypermobility of the C4, C5, or C6 segments. Neurological testing will generally be negative, but there is the possibility of nerve-root irritation or thoracic outlet syndrome from shortening and hypertrophy of the scalenus muscles. On palpation there will generally be segmental guarding of the multifidus muscle at the C5 or C6 segment. There may be tenderness and spasm of the suboccipital muscles from overcontracting in a shortened position from the forward-head posture. There may be tenderness of the greater or lesser occipital nerve from mechanical compression. The muscles of mastication should be carefully palpated if tenderness is present. A temporomandibular joint evaluation should be performed (see Chapter 15, The Temporomandibular Joint). The sternocleidomastoid muscle will be hypertrophied and may have palpable fibrous nodes. The longus colli will be acutely tender, particularly at the C4 through C7 segments.

Roentgenograms may begin to show flattening or kyphosis of the cervical spine. If retropharyngeal swelling is present, it may be seen along the anterior border of the cervical spine on the lateral roentgenogram. The intervertebral foramina will be open. There may be less than 8 mm of space noted on the lateral film between the occiput and atlas, indicating chronic extension of the upper cervical spine secondary to forward-head posture. If mobility films are taken, they may show hypermobility of C4, C5, or C6.

Treatment. The treatment approach in the chronic phase must be gradual. Rapid increases in range of motion should not be expected because fibrosis of joints and muscles will respond well to gentle repetitive stretching, but attempts to overstretch will result in increased swelling and scarring. The emphasis of treatment must be to gradually restore cervical lordosis by mobilization into extension and specific segmental strengthening of the multifidus at the hypermobile segments. Normal muscle balance should also be restored by stretching the large anterior neck musculature and strengthening the posterior neck musculature.

Treatment of the acceleration injury in the chronic phase must be undertaken carefully and gradually, with a view not only to short-term symptoms but also to long-range outcome. A few precautions should be noted:

- Stretching of the posterior neck musculature, particularly by pulling the head into flexion, may give temporary reduction of muscular symptoms, but in the long run will contribute to cervical instability.
- The "chin-tuck" exercise (Fig. 17-31) may be helpful in stretching the suboccipital muscles, but it also completely flattens the curve in the cervical spine. When instructing a patient in this exercise, always give the precaution that it should be continued for no longer than 6 weeks.
- Strengthening exercises should be light, as the multifidi are very small muscles. Care should be taken in the exercise instruction to avoid strengthening of the sternocleidomastoid or anterior neck muscles.
- Vigorous rotatory mobilization or passive stretching may overstretch segments that are already hypermobile, contributing to cervical instability.

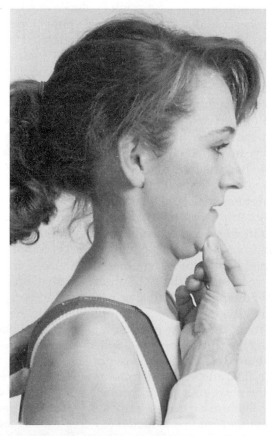

FIG. 17-31. The chin-tuck exercise.

- The patient should be encouraged to remain as active as possible, and 20 minutes of aerobic activity should be a component of every treatment program.

☐ Cervical Instability

Passive stability of the cervical spine comes from the tripod configuration of the two posterior facet joints and the anterior disk. When the cervical spine is in its normal rest position of slight lordosis, the facet joints are engaged and bear approximately one third of the vertical compressive force. Very little muscle contraction is needed to maintain stability in this position. Passive stability may be lost as a result of an injury (see Acceleration Injury, earlier) or may develop after years of poor posture or activities that involve flexion of the neck. If cervical lordosis is lost, the facet joints disengage and are no longer capable of stabilizing rotational forces. The vertical compressive forces are shifted forward onto the disk, which gradually begins to lose height. Over time the annulus of the disk stretches out and weakens, and the vertebral bodies may show lipping and traction spurs as an attempt to compensate for increased vertical compressive forces (see Degenerative Joint Disease, page 552). The multifidus muscle must be in constant contraction to prevent overrotation or overflexion. The segmental muscle will progress from constant guarding to spasm and inflammation. The annulus of the disk is weakened, and there may be acute episodes of bulging of nuclear material, either anteriorly or posteriorly. Patients with cervical instability may have chronic headaches, chronic neck pain, and chronic shoulder or interscapular pain. They also may have asymptomatic periods and acute episodes of disk bulging that happen suddenly for no apparent reason.

Evaluation. The patient may have a history of acceleration injury or an occupation that involves flexion of the neck such as office or laboratory work. The patient may have a forward-head posture but observation alone should not be relied on to determine cervical lordosis or compression of the upper cervical spine. There will generally be hypertrophy of the anterior neck and anterior chest and protraction of the scapula with elevation of the clavicles. Active and passive ranges of motion will be limited. When tested segmentally, the upper cervical spine will be restricted. There will be hypermobility of C4 or C5, usually accompanied by ankylosis of the segment below. The patient should be given a careful neurological examination. Neurological tests will generally be negative. There may be nerve irritation from peripheral entrapment or a bulging disk but rarely from bony compression. The multifidi will be in segmental guarding or spasm and may feel rubbery or acutely inflamed. The sternocleidomastoid muscles are hypertrophied and may have localized areas of fibrosis that are acutely tender. The deep anterior neck musculature, particularly the longus colli, will be in spasm and may be acutely inflamed.

Treatment. The only effective conservative treatment for cervical instability is to restore the normal lordosis to the cervical spine. This should be accomplished by mobilizing the upper and midcervical spine to restore range of motion, segmental strengthening of the multifidi to hold the lordosis, followed by restoration of the muscular balance of the cervical spine. As with chronic acceleration injuries, care must be taken when working with the neck to avoid strengthening the sternocleidomastoid or anterior neck musculature and to avoid stretching segments that are already hypermobile.

☐ Acute Disk Bulge

If the annulus of the disk is weakened, acute bulging of the disk, either anteriorly or posteriorly, may occur. If the disk bulges anteriorly, it presses on the anterior longitudinal ligament and may cause spasm of the longus colli. The patient may have difficulty swallowing or have the sensation of a sore throat. If the disk bulges posteriorly, it may press on the posterior longitudinal ligament, the spinal cord, or the nerve root.

Evaluation. Sudden onset of acute neck pain, usually noticed early in the morning, is probably from bulging of the disk. It has also been described as acute dislocation of a facet joint or entrapment of the synovial villi. The pain begins with clearly delineated, sharp neck pain and progresses during the day to generalized muscle spasm and inability to rotate the neck in one direction. The patient may present with the neck rotated and bent to one side and may be in acute distress. Active range of motion will be limited in rotation, and lateral flexion to one side and fairly free to the opposite side. Active and passive range of motion will be limited by pain and muscle spasm, with passive range of motion usually considerably greater than active. A position of comfort is usually a combination of extension and lateral flexion to the opposite side, and traction often makes the condition immediately more comfortable.

Treatment. These conditions generally resolve in a few days if left untreated, but there is an excellent treatment method described by Cyriax that will provide greatly increased comfort and range of motion for the first few days.[3] This consists of placing the neck in as much extension as possible under fairly strong manual traction. Range of motion under traction is begun first to the pain-free side. When full range of motion of the pain-free side is achieved, range of motion under traction to the painful side is begun.[3]

The patient should be instructed to avoid flexion of the neck. A soft collar will be helpful for the first few days. The patient should be reassured and encouraged to be as active as possible. When the acute symptoms subside, treatment for cervical instability should begin.

☐ Degenerative Joint Disease

Degenerative joint disease begins as capsular restriction of the facet joints without bony changes on roentgenograms and gradually progresses over months or years to the characteristic flattening, lipping, and spurring of the vertebral bodies (see Fig. 17-30) and facet joints that become clearly visible on roentgenographical studies. Degenerative joint disease must be considered a normal aging process (most older people have at least some evidence of it), but it should be considered abnormal in younger people. Degenerative joint disease may be accelerated by injury. Bony stenosis of the intervertebral foramen is possible and may cause symptoms of neck pain, shoulder pain, radiating pain in the arm, numbness in the extremity, or muscle weakness.

One of the paradoxes of degenerative joint disease is that the patient may have foraminal stenosis for many years without symptoms and then suddenly begin to have neurological signs and symptoms. After treatment with traction or passage of time, these signs or symptoms may resolve. Clearly the bony changes have not improved, so what accounts for the sudden appearance and disappearance of symptoms?

Pain from compression of nerve roots is complex. In an experimental study, ligatures were placed around nerve roots at the time of surgery so that pressure could be applied after the surgical incision had healed. When pressure was applied to the healthy nerve roots, there were no symptoms of pain or paresthesia. When pressure was applied to injured nerve roots, there was a gradual onset of anesthesia, diminished reflex, and eventually motor weakness. If, however, the nerve root was ischemic, very light pressure by the ligature produced immediate pain and paresthesia in the arm.[22,23] A model of nerve-root irritation then might be that some unusual activity, probably involving extension or sidebending of the neck, causes the nerve root to swell. With impingement of the blood supply to the nerve root, it becomes extremely sensitive. When pressure is removed by traction or proper positioning, swelling of the nerve root diminishes, and the symptoms disappear. This would also seem to explain some of the complexities of peripheral entrapments. If the nerve root has slight compression and is ischemic, the nerve would be considerably more sensitive to pressure at the shoulder, wrist, or carpal tunnel.

Evaluation. The patient will generally give a history of gradual or sudden onset of neck pain, shoulder pain, and paresthesia in the upper extremity. (It is also possible to have motor weakness, muscle atrophy, and loss of reflex without symptoms of pain.) The patient will generally have a forward-head posture, and the lower cervical spine will be kyphotic to palpation. Active rotation and lateral flexion toward the painful side will be limited by pain, as will extension. There will be capsular restriction of the lower cervical spine with possible ankylosis. The mobility of the upper cervical spine is generally quite good. The Spurling test will reproduce paresthesia in the upper extremity. There may be diminished reflex, motor weakness, anesthesia, or muscle atrophy. Roentgenograms may reveal generalized degenerative joint disease, stenosis of the intervertebral foramen, or both.

Treatment. The prognosis for treatment is much better if the symptoms are of a recent and sudden onset. Large-fiber nerves are more susceptible to pressure than small-fiber nerves, so as the pressure increases, the signs and symptoms will progress from paresthesia to reflex loss, then to motor weakness and anesthesia. A patient who has a recent, sudden onset of only paresthesia has a very good prognosis compared with a patient who has a gradual, silent onset of muscle atrophy and weakness; the latter has a relatively poor prognosis.

Many patients will respond well to a combination of cervical traction and instruction to position the head in flexion and sidebending away from the painful side (positional traction) (Fig. 17-32), with reduction of symptoms being the best indicator of proper position. Mobilization of adjacent segments may reduce some of the mechanical forces on the involved segment. The patient should also be given instruction in activities of daily living to avoid extension. These may include thoracic extension exercises to improve back bending at the C6 and C7 segments, switching from bifocal glasses (which require extension of the neck to read) to reading glasses, and general avoidance of working above the head.

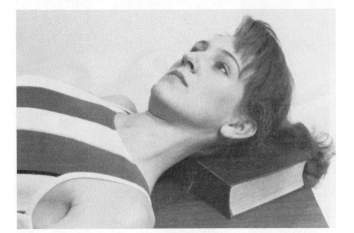

FIG. 17-32. Positional traction of the cervical spine.

▪ TREATMENT TECHNIQUES

I. **Manual Techniques—Muscles**
  A. *Bimanual massage and manual stretching of the sternocleidomastoid muscle* (see Fig. 17-29)
    Note: P—patient; O—operator; M—movement.
    P—Lies in supine position
    O—Sits at head of treatment table
    M—*Bimanual massage:* The sternocleidomastoid muscle can be grasped between the thumb and fingers and rolled and massaged between them. Begin at the insertion behind the mastoid process and cover both the sternal and clavicular heads. (**Note:** Patient may be instructed to do this as a home program.)
    Manual stretching: Grasp the belly of the muscle between the thumb and fingers, holding the head and neck in slight lateral flexion to the opposite side. Glide the hand toward the table, stretching the belly of the sternocleidomastoid muscle.
  B. *Stretching of the suboccipital muscle* (Fig. 17-33)
    P—Lies in supine position
    O—Sits at head of treatment table. The thumb, forefinger, and web space of the right hand should be along the nuchal line. The left hand should be placed lightly on the patient's forehead to make the grip firmer.
    M—3 to 4 lbs traction should be applied to the occiput. The patient's head should be in the chin-tuck position.
  C. *Scalenus stretching* (Fig. 17-34)
    P—Lies supine, with the neck in slight extension
    O—Sits at end of treatment table. If the

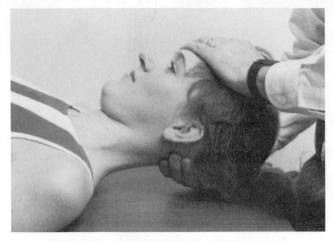

FIG. 17-33. Stretching of the suboccipital muscles.

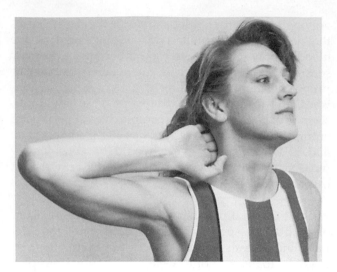

FIG. 17-35. Isometric strengthening of the multifidi.

scalenus muscles on the left are to be stretched, the operator's right hand should be cupped underneath the neck. The heel of the left hand should be on the first and second ribs to stabilize them while the muscle is stretched. (Hand position is reversed if the right scalenus is to be stretched.)

M—The neck is rotated toward the side to be stretched and laterally flexed away from the side to be stretched. Vapor coolant spray may be helpful but is not necessary.

D. *Isometric strengthening of the multifidi muscle—* This may be performed by the therapist or taught as a home program (Fig. 17-35).

P—In a sitting position

O—Stands behind and to one side. A hand is cupped behind the neck, forming a slight backward curve. Light pressure is applied to the back of the head. The patient is asked to hold. (**Note:** The pressure should be applied with one finger only to avoid the possibility of overworking the multifidus muscle.)

E. *Specific segmental strengthening of the multifidi muscle*—This may be done as a manual technique or taught as a home program (Fig. 17-36).[18]

P—In a sitting position

O—Stands behind and to one side. Two fingers are placed at the level to be strength-

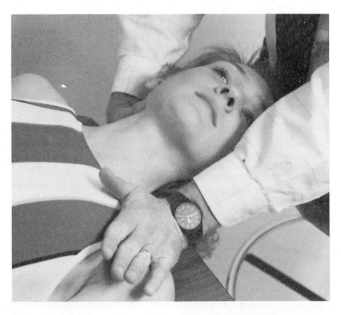

FIG. 17-34. Stretching of the scaleni muscles.

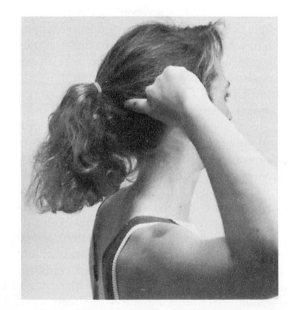

FIG. 17-36. Segmental strengthening of the multifidi.

ened. The patient is asked to extend and sidebend the neck over the fingers. The patient is asked to hold while the force is applied in the direction of flexion and sidebending to the opposite side. As progress is made, this exercise may be modified by having the operator give the command to "push" and allowing 10° or so of motion.

F. *Antigravity strengthening of the multifidi* (Fig. 17-37)

P—Lies prone, with head off the table. The top of the patient's head should be resting in the therapist's hand.

O—Sits at the head of the table with the patient's head resting in a hand, which is supported by the knee. The operator lifts the patient's head until a slight backward curve can be palpated. The operator gives the command to "hold" and allows the multifidi muscles to take some of the weight. As progress is made, the therapist should allow the patient to accept

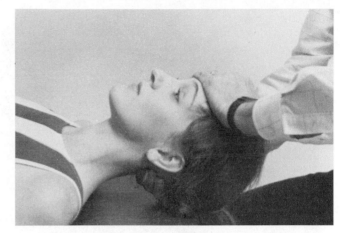

Fig. 17-38. Manual traction to the upper cervical spine.

more weight as long as the patient is strong enough to maintain a curve in the neck. (**Precaution:** If the patient's multifidus muscle is not strong enough to support the weight of the head, this exercise should not be done.)

II. Manual Techniques—Joints

A. *Manual traction to the upper cervical spine* (Fig. 17-38)

P—Lies supine, with the upper cervical spine in slight extension with slackening of the suboccipital muscles and the nuchal ligament

O—Sits at the head of the table with the thumb, web space, and index finger of the right hand along the nuchal line. The left hand is placed lightly on the patient's forehead to improve grip.

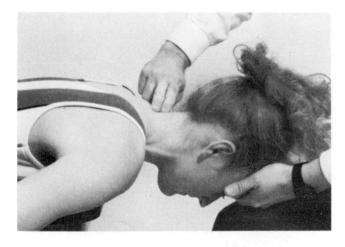

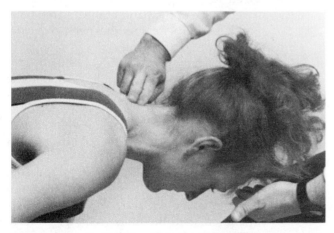

FIG. 17-37. Antigravity strengthening of the multifidi.

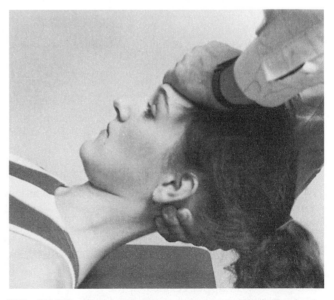

FIG. 17-39. Manual traction to the lower cervical spine.

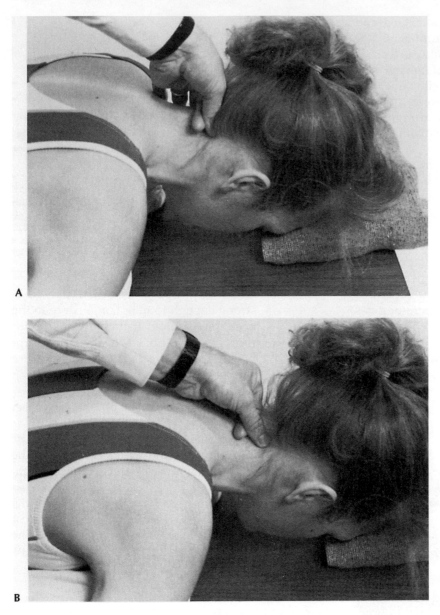

FIG. 17-40. Vertical oscillations to the joints of (**A**) the atlantoaxial, atlanto-occipital, and (**B**) the C2–C7 segments.

M—The operator applies 3 to 5 lbs of traction by leaning backward, holding the arms rigid. (**Note:** Because motion has isolated the upper cervical spine, strong traction is not necessary. Traction may be sustained or oscillated, depending on patient response.)

B. *Manual traction to the lower cervical spine* (Fig. 17-39)

P—Lies supine, with the neck supported in flexion by a pillow. The upper cervical spine is flexed, drawing the nuchal ligament tight and transferring the force to the lower cervical spine.

O—Same position as for manual traction of the upper cervical spine

M—The operator leans backward, applying 3 to 5 lbs of traction. Traction may be localized to a single segment by placing the web space of the hand at the desired level and laterally flexing the neck over the web space of the hand.

C. *Vertical oscillation extension* (Fig. 17-40)

P—Lies prone, with two pillows under the chest and a small pillow under the forehead

O—Stands next to the table, with thumb reinforced by a middle finger on the lamina of the joint to be mobilized

M—For the atlanto-axial and atlanto-occipital joints, oscillatory motion from grades I to IV should be applied in a direction perpendicular to the table (see Fig. 17-40*A*). (The atlanto-axial, atlanto-occipital, and

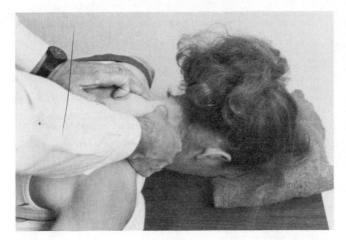

FIG. 17-41. Rotational oscillations.

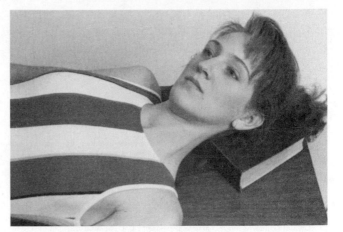

FIG. 17-43. Positional traction.

facet joints are all oriented in the horizontal plane.) For C2 to C7, the oscillation should be applied downward and forward at a 45° angle. (The lower cervical facet joints are aligned at 45° off the sagittal plane.) (Fig. 17-40*B*)

D. *Rotational oscillation* (Fig. 17-41)

P—Lies prone, with two pillows under the chest; forehead supported with a small block

O—Stands beside table, with thumb on the lateral side of the spinous process of the segment to be mobilized

M—The operator makes graded oscillating movements, from grades I to IV, in a direction to induce rotation of the segment.

E. *Lateral glide* (Fig. 17-42)

P—Lies supine

O—Sits at the head of the table, with the patient's head cupped in one hand and the web space of the other hand cupping the facet joint of the segment to be moved

M—The operator takes up the slack by sidebending the neck over the web space of the hand and applies oscillations into sidebending grades I to IV.

III. Positional Traction (Fig. 17-43)

A. *Positional traction*—This is a method of opening the intervertebral foramen by carefully positioning the head and neck.[17] Cervical traction may be applied in the positional traction position to further open the intervertebral foramen.

P—Lies supine

O—Palpates the interspinous ligament at the segment to be distracted. The patient's head is elevated using small blocks or pillows until the interspinous ligament at the desired segment becomes taut, indicating the segment has flexed. The operator then places a hand on the lateral portion of the desired segment and, taking care to keep the head flexed at the same level, laterally flexes the neck over the finger. The patient can rest indefinitely in this position.

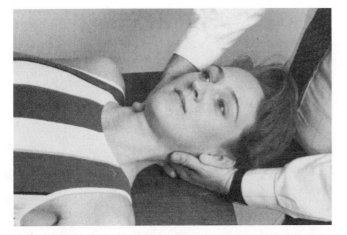

FIG. 17-42. Lateral glide.

REFERENCES

1. Aspinall W: Clinical testing for the craniovertebral hypermobility syndrome. J Orthop Sports Physiother 12:2, 1990
2. Bell W: Temperomandibular Disorders. Classification, Diagnosis, Management. Chicago, Year Book Medical Publishers, 1986
3. Cyriax J: Textbook of Orthopedic Medicine, 11th ed. Vol 2: Treatment by Manipulation, Massage, and Injection. London, Balliere Tindall, 1984
4. Davidson KC, Welford EC, Dixon GD: Traumatic vertebral artery pseudoaneurysm following chiropractic manipulation. Radiology 115:651–652, 1975
5. Feinstein B: Referred pain from paravertebral structures. In Buerger AA, Tobis JF (eds): Approaches to Validation of Manipulation Therapy. Springfield, IL, Charles C Thomas, 1977
6. Gotten N: Survey of one hundred cases of whiplash injury after settlement of litigation. JAMA 162(9):865–867, 1956
7. Greenfield GB: The joints. In Greenfield GB: Radiology of Bone Disease, 4th ed, pp 474–910. Philadelphia, JB Lippincott, 1986
8. Hohl M: Soft tissue injuries of the neck in automobile accidents: J Bone Joint Surg 56(A):1675–1682, 1974
9. Hollinshead WH: Functional Anatomy of the Limbs and Back, 5th ed. Philadelphia, WB Saunders, 1981

10. Hoppenfeld S: Physical Examination of the Spine and Extremities. New York, Appleton-Century-Crofts, 1976
11. Kapandji IA: Physiology of the Joints. Vol 3: The Trunk and Vertebral Column. New York, Churchill Livingstone, 1974
12. Krueger BR, Okazak H: Vertebrobasilar distribution infraction following chiropractic cervical manipulation. Mayo Clin Proc 55:322–332, 1980
13. Macnab I: Acceleration injuries of the cervical spine. J Bone Joint Surg 46(A):1797–1799, 1964
14. McKenzie JS, Williams JF: The dynamic behavior of the head and cervical spine during whiplash. J Biomech 4:477–490, 1971
15. Miller RG, Burton R: Stroke following chiropractic manipulation of the spine. JAMA, 229:189–190, 1974.
16. Norris SH, Watt I: The prognosis of neck injuries resulting from rear-end vehicle collisions. J Bone Joint Surg 65(B):608–611 1983
17. Paris S: S-I: Introduction to spinal evaluation and manipulation. Continuing education course, Institute of Graduate Health Sciences, Los Angeles, May 19, 1978
18. Rocabado M: Advanced upper quarter. Continuing education course, Rocabado Institute, San Francisco, December 10, 1984.
19. Severy DM, Mathewson JH, Bechtol CO: Controlled automobile rear-end collisions: An investigation of related engineering and medical phenomena. Can Serv Med J 11:727–759, 1955
20. Sharp J, Purser DW: Spontaneous atlanto-axial dislocation in ankylosing spondylitis and rheumatoid arthritis. Ann Rheum Dis 20:47–72, 1961
21. Uivlugt G, Indenbaum S: Clinical assessment of atlanto-axial instability using the Sharp-Purser test. Arthritis Rheumatol 31:918–922, 1988
22. Wyke B: Cervical articular contributions to posture and gait: Their relation to senile disequilibrium. Age Ageing 8(4):251–258, 1979
23. Wyke B: Neurology of the cervical spine joints. Physiotherapy 65(3):72–76, 1979

RECOMMENDED READING

Beeton K, Jull G: Effectiveness of manipulative physiotherapy in the management cervicogenic headache: A single case study. Physiotherapy 80:417–423, 1994
Bisbee, LA, Hartsell HD: Physiotherapy management of whiplash. Spine: State Art Rev 7: 501–516, 1993
Bogduk N: Cervical causes of headache and dizziness. In Grieve G (ed): Modern Manual Therapy, pp 289–302. Edinburgh, Churchill Livingstone, 1986
Butler D: Mobilization of the Nervous System. Edinburgh, Churchill Livingstone, 1991
Cassidy JD, Lopes AA, Yong-Hing K: The immediate effect of manipulation versus mobilization on pain and range of motion of the cervical spine: A randomized controlled trial. J Manipulative Physiol Ther 15:570–575, 1992
Dalton M, Coutts A: The effect of age on cervical posture in a normal population. In Boyling J, Palastanga N (eds): Grieve's Modern Manual Therapy of the Vertebral Column. Edinburgh, Churchill Livingstone, 1994.
Derrick L, Chesworth B: Post-motor-vehicle-accident alar ligament laxity. J Orthop Sport Phys Ther 16:6–11, 1992
Dvorak J: Soft tissue injury to the cervical spine. New possibilities of diagnosis with computed tomography. J Man Med 4:17–21, 1989
Dvorak J: The neurologic work-up in patients with cervical spine disorders. Spine 15:1017–1022, 1990
Edward BC: Manual of Combined Movements. Edinburgh, Churchill Livingstone, 1992
Gargan MF, Bannister GC: Longterm prognosis of soft-tissue injuries of the neck. J Bone Joint Surg 72(B):901–903, 1989
Greenman PE: Manual and manipulative therapy in whiplash injuries. Spine: State Art Rev 7:517–530, 1993
Grant R (ed): Physical Therapy of the Cervical and Thoracic Spine, 2nd ed. Edinburgh, Churchill Livingstone, 1994
Koe B, Bouter L, van Mameren H, et al: The effectiveness of manual therapy, physiotherapy and treatment by the general practitioner for nonspecific back and neck complaints: A randomized clinical trial. Spine 17:28–35, 1992
Labon M: Whiplash: Its evaluation and treatment. Phys Med Rehabil 4:293–307, 1990
Olesen J, Tfelt-Hansen P, Welch KMA (eds): The Headache. New York, Raven Press, 1993
Rocabado M, Iglarsh ZA: The Musculoskeletal Approach to Maxillofacial Pain. Philadelphia, JB Lippincott, 1991
Sjaastad O: Cervicogenic headache: The controversial headache. Clin Neurol Neurosurg 94(Suppl i):147–149, 1990
Sjaastad O, Freriksen TA, Pfaffenrath V: Cervicogenic headache: Diagnostic criteria. Headache 30:725–726, 1991
Sweeny T: Neck school: Cervicothoracic stabilization training. Spine: State Art Rev 5:367–378, 1992
Teasell R: The whiplash patient: A sympathetic approach. In Hachinski J (ed): Challenges in Neurology, pp 29–52. Philadelphia, FA Davis, 1992
Teasell R, McCain G: Clinical spectrum and management of whiplash injuries. In Tollison CD (ed): Painful Cervical Trauma: Diagnosis and Rehabilitative Treatment of Neuromusculoskeletal Injuries, pp 2292–2318. Baltimore, Williams & Wilkins, 1992
Vernon H, Mior S: The neck disability index: A study of reliability and validity. J Manipulative Physiol 14:409–415, 1991
Watson D, Trott P: Cervical headache: An investigation of natural head posture and upper cervical flexor muscle performance. Cephalagia 13:272–284, 1993

18

The Cervical–Upper Limb Scan Examination

DARLENE HERTLING AND RANDOLPH M. KESSLER

The limbs are derived from spinal segments: the myotomes, dermatomes, and sclerotomes. Those corresponding to C4 through T1 extend into the arms, whereas those from L2 through S2 extend into the legs. The clinical significance of this is that symptoms and signs related to pathological spinal processes are often referred to the limbs, and, conversely, symptoms from common limb lesions are often referred to the spine (or other parts of the involved extremity). In the case of deep somatic lesions, referred symptoms and signs are the rule rather than the exception. This is most significant with respect to pain, since pain is the most frequent clinical manifestation of deep somatic disorders. Thus, the patient with a cervical problem is very likely to experience scapular, shoulder, or arm pain, perhaps even more so than cervical pain. In addition, paresthesias, weakness, or sensory changes may affect the related segment in the arm or hand. Similarly, it is not unusual for patients with common extremity disorders to experience pain that is referred in a retrograde direction to the proximal aspect of the limb or the related spinal region. Indeed, patients with carpal tunnel syndrome often experience pain up the forearm and arm into the scapular region and neck.

The clinical problem encountered when dealing with the common phenomenon of referred symptoms is that information elicited from the history does not always reliably narrow the source of the problem to a particular region. When this is the case, the clinician may have trouble knowing in which area to direct the physical, or objective, examination. The situation may be compounded by the fact that many patients present with symptoms that occur as the result of summation of afferent input from two separate disorders affecting tissues innervated by the same segment. This is especially true for middle-aged and older people, since degenerative joint changes in the cervical spine are common by middle age and may cause "hyperexcitability" of the involved segments.

The purpose of performing a spinal–limb scan examination is to help identify the major area of involvement so that the physical examination can be directed accordingly. It is most useful in cases in which the history or the referring diagnosis does not provide adequate information to indicate the area to be examined. It should be used with most middle-aged or older patients presenting with chronic musculoskeletal complaints because it will often reveal disorders, other than those identified by the referral or by the history, that are the primary cause. For example, a scan examination often reveals that the patient who describes symptoms suggestive of a C6 radiculopathy actually has carpal tunnel syndrome, that the patient with carpal tunnel syndrome may have symptoms that are enhanced by lower cervical facet joint tightness, that a person with some lower cervical problem is also developing a frozen shoulder, or that someone who describes what sounds like pain referred distally into the C7 segment from the neck actually has pain referred proximally from a tennis elbow condition. Such situations are surprisingly common and can be a frequent source of error in evaluation and treatment planning unless recognized.

The tests that make up the scan examination include those that can be considered *key tests* for the common musculoskeletal lesions affecting the cervical spine and upper limb, or the lumbar spine and lower limb. Listed below are the key tests and positive findings for the common disorders for which the scan examination is intended to be sensitive.

■ COMMON DISORDERS OF THE CERVICAL SPINE, TEMPOROMANDIBULAR JOINT, AND UPPER LIMB

I. The Cervical Spine

A. *Localized cervical facet joint restriction*
  1. Typical subjective complaints include
    a. Aching in the scapular region, perhaps into the arm, usually unilaterally; occasional headaches
    b. Gradual onset with perhaps a history of cervical trauma or intermittent acute episodes of neck pain
    c. Worse at the end of the day and during periods of prolonged muscular tension such as during emotional stress and long periods of holding the head against gravity (*e.g.,* typing or reading)
    d. Patient age is usually 25 to 50 years
  2. Key objective findings
    a. Active cervical movements with passive overpressure
      i. Pain at the extremes of sidebending and rotation to the involved side
      ii. Possible pain on extension
    b. Quadrant test (passive rotation, sidebending, and extension to one side). Pain when performed toward the side of involvement.

B. *Generalized cervical degenerative changes*—Bilateral, multisegmental facet joint capsular tightness
  1. Typical subjective complaints include the following:
    a. Gradual onset of neck stiffness with associated pain into shoulder girdles and perhaps the arms. Pain and stiffness may be bilateral, although they are usually worse on one side. Frequent headaches originate from the occiput and radiate to the frontal region.
    b. History of intermittent cervical problems over many years
    c. Stiffness and headaches noted in the morning, easing somewhat during midday, with increased neck and shoulder pain by evening
    d. The patient is usually 50 years old or older.
  2. Key objective findings: Active cervical movements with passive overpressure
    a. Marked restriction of extension, moderate restriction of sidebending, mild to moderate restriction of rotations and flexion
    b. Pain at the extremes of some movements

C. *Cervical nerve root impingements* (see Chapter 17, The Cervical Spine)
  1. Typical subjective complaints include the following:
    a. Gradual or sudden onset of unilateral neck, scapular, or arm pain. Often paresthesias into fingers are described. Arm pain may be sharp or aching.
    b. Pain may be intense, relieved somewhat with recumbency, and worse with weight-bearing.
    c. The patient is usually 35 to 60 years old.
  2. Key objective findings

a. Quadrant test (foraminal compression); reproduction of *arm* pain
b. Upper limb sensory (see Figs. 5-4 and 19-7), motor, and reflex tests. Neurological deficit is confined to the involved segment.
C5—Weak shoulder abduction or external rotation
—Sensory changes over the radial aspect of the forearm
—Diminished biceps or brachioradialis jerk
C6—Weak elbow flexion or wrist extension
—Sensory changes over the thumb or index finger
—Diminished biceps or brachioradialis jerk
C7—Weak elbow pronation, extension, or wrist flexion
—Sensory changes over the index, middle, and ring fingers
—Diminished triceps jerk
C8—Weak thumb abduction, small finger abduction, or wrist ulnar deviation
—Sensory changes over the little or ring fingers
T1—Weak adduction of the extended fingers (interossei muscles)
—Sensory changes over the inner side of the forearm

II. The Temporomandibular Joint
A. *Dysfunction syndrome*
1. Typical subjective complaints include the following:
a. Often associated with an insidious onset of emotional stress or overload such as bruxism, for a long period of time.
b. The presenting complaint is usually pain, which is either in the jaw or ear but which often radiates widely into the face, temporal region, or around the neck. Jaw pain or difficulty in chewing, or worse, after meals and at end of day.
c. Early incoordination associated with clicking, popping, subluxation, and recurrent dislocation. Often reversible but may lead to limitation phase.
d. The patient is often a women, usually of 20 to 40 years.
2. Key objective findings (incoordination phase): Active motions
a. Excessive joint mobility, often characterized by excessive anterior transla-

tion during opening. Patient may be able insert three knuckles between the incisors.
b. Clicking, popping, or cracking with mandibular depression or elevation
c. Abnormality of movement: mandibular deviations (protrusively as well as laterally)
d. Tenderness and thickening around the joint with the mouth both closed and open
B. *Internal derangement such as a disk or degenerative joint disease*
1. Typical subjective complaints include the following:
a. May occur at any age, usually middle or old age, associated with the aging process and repeated minor trauma.
b. Pain is present at rest or during movements such as chewing or yawning and is often described as a deep-seated, dull aching type of pain felt in the preauricular region. There may be facial pain that is obscure in character and location.
c. Morning stiffness that subsides with jaw use
d. Jaw pain that is associated with clicking or crepitus
2. Key objective findings
a. Limitation in a capsular pattern of restriction; in unilateral conditions, contralateral excursions and opening are the most restricted.
b. Accessory movements are limited and reproduce temporomandibular joint pain.

III. The Shoulder
A. *Frozen shoulder* (adhesive capsulitis)
1. Typical subjective complaints include the following:
a. Gradual onset of shoulder pain and stiffness, noted especially when combing hair, fastening buttons, bras, *etc.*, behind the back, or reaching into the hip pocket
b. Frequently there are problems with being awakened at night when rolling onto the painful side.
c. The patient is more often a woman, usually 40 years old or older.
2. Key objective findings: Active shoulder movements with passive overpressure
a. Considerable loss of external rotation and abduction, mild to moderate loss of flexion and internal rotation

    b. Pain at the extremes of shoulder movements, especially external rotation and abduction, with a capsular or muscle-spasm end feel

B. *Shoulder tendinitis* (rotator cuff or biceps)

    1. Typical subjective complaints include the following:

        a. Gradual onset of lateral brachial pain, occasionally radiating into arm and forearm

        b. The onset may be associated with increased use of the arm, such as in athletics.

        c. Painful twinges are felt with specific movements, such as putting on a jacket and reaching behind the back.

        d. The patient is likely to be 20 to 50 years old.

    2. Key objective findings: Resisted shoulder, elbow, and forearm movements and pain on contraction of the involved muscle–tendon complex

        a. Supraspinatus: pain on resisted shoulder abduction

        b. Infraspinatus: pain on resisted external rotation

        c. Subscapularis: pain on resisted internal rotation

        d. Biceps (long head): pain on resisted elbow flexion or forearm supination

C. *Shoulder tendon rupture* (rotator cuff or biceps)

    1. Typical subjective complaints include the following:

        a. Gradual onset of inability to use the arm normally, especially above shoulder level if a rotator cuff tendon is involved. The onset may be sudden, especially in the case of a biceps rupture.

        b. History of intermittent shoulder pain over many years

        c. Possible history of repeated local corticosteroid injections

        d. Pain may or may not be a problem

        e. The patient is usually 50 years old or older

    2. Key objective findings

        a. Resisted movement tests

            i. Supraspinatus: resisted abduction is weak and painless

            ii. Infraspinatus: resisted external rotation is weak and painless

            iii. Biceps: resisted elbow flexion and forearm supination are weak and painless

        b. Observable muscular atrophy

D. *Shoulder atraumatic instability*

    1. Typical subjective complaints include the following:

        a. Presence of mechanism likely to tear the ligaments or capsule. Typically instability often begins with some minor event or series of events that leads to progressive decompensation of the glenohumeral stability mechanism.

        b. The patient may notice that the shoulder slips out and "clunks" back in with different activities. Patients with multidirectional glenohumeral instabilities may have difficulty sleeping, lifting overhead, and throwing.

        c. Pain may or may not be a problem.

        d. Patients are predominantly younger than 30 years of age.

    2. Key objective findings

        a. Diminished resistance to translation or increase joint-play motions in multiple directions as compared with normal.

        b. Duplication of the patient's symptoms with certain motions or position of the arm.

E. *Acute subdeltoid bursitis*

    1. Typical subjective complaints include the following:

        a. Gradual development of relatively intense, constant lateral brachial pain over a 48- to 72-hour period. Pain may radiate down the entire arm.

        b. Often a history of more minor, intermittent shoulder problems suggestive of preexisting tendinitis.

        c. Difficulty sleeping or using the arm at all because of intense pain.

        d. The patient is likely to be 30 to 50 years old.

    2. Key objective findings: Active shoulder movements with passive overpressure. Marked restriction of active flexion and abduction, with an empty end feel to passive overpressure. Mild-to-moderate restriction of internal and external rotation with the arm to the side.

IV. The Elbow

  A. *Elbow tendinitis*

    1. Typical subjective complaints include the following:

        a. Gradual onset of medial or lateral elbow pain that may radiate into the ulnar aspect of the forearm (medial tennis elbow) or into the dorsum of the forearm and hand and into the posterior brachial region (lateral tennis elbow)

b. Onset may be associated with some activity such as playing tennis or golf or pruning shrubs

c. Pain is aggravated by grasping activities, such as hammering or carrying a suitcase, and by prolonged fine finger activities such as knitting or sewing.

d. The patient is usually 35 to 60 years old.

2. Key objective findings

  a. Resisted wrist movements, performed with elbow extended

    i. Lateral tennis elbow (tendinitis at origin of extensor carpi radialis brevis): pain on resisted wrist extension

    ii. Medial tennis elbow (tendinitis at common flexor-pronator origin): pain on resisted wrist flexion

  b. Active wrist movements with passive overpressure, performed with elbow extended

    i. Lateral tennis elbow: pain on full wrist flexion with the elbow extended and forearm pronated

    ii. Medial tennis elbow: pain on full wrist extension with the elbow extended and forearm supinated

V. **The Wrist and Hand Complex**

A. *Carpal tunnel syndrome* (pressure on the median nerve in the carpal tunnel)

  1. Typical subjective complaints include the following:

    a. Gradual onset of paresthesias into any or all of the median nerve distribution of hand (thumb and middle three fingers). An aching sensation may be referred up the forearm and arm to the scapula and neck.

    b. Symptoms often awaken the patient at night and are aggravated by activities involving the finger flexors, such as writing, sewing, or knitting.

    c. Women are affected more often than men. The patient is usually 40 years old or older.

  2. Key objective findings: Three-jaw-chuck pinch with wrist held in sustained flexion (modification of Phalen's test). Reproduction of paresthesias into median nerve distribution of the hand (see Fig. 17-25).

B. *De Quervain's disease* (tenosynovitis of the abductor pollicis longus and extensor pollicis brevis at the wrist)

  1. Typical subjective complaints include the following:

    a. Gradual onset of pain over the radial aspect of the distal radius that may radiate distally into the thumb or proximally up the radial aspect of the forearm

    b. Pain is worse with activities involving thumb movements or wrist ulnar deviation.

    c. The patient is usually 40 years old or older.

  2. Key objective findings

    a. Resisted finger movements. Pain occurs over the radial styloid region on resisted thumb extension.

    b. Active wrist movements with passive overpressure. Pain occurs over the radial styloid region on full ulnar deviation with thumb held in patient's clenched fist.

C. *Carpal ligament sprain*

  1. Typical subjective complaints include the following:

    a. History of acute trauma, usually a fall on the dorsiflexed or palmarly flexed hand, followed by chronic wrist pain. The patient often has trouble localizing the pain to a particular aspect of the wrist.

    b. Pain is often felt only with specific activities, such as those requiring repeated wrist or weight movements or weight-bearing through the hand and wrist.

    c. The patient is usually a young or active person.

  2. Key objective findings

    a. Active wrist movements with passive overpressure

      i. Dorsal radiocarpal, dorsal lunocapitate, or capitate–third metacarpal ligament: pain on full wrist flexion

      ii. Palmar radiocarpal or palmar lunocapitate ligament: pain on full wrist extension

    b. Upper extremity weight-bearing (through dorsiflexed wrist and straight arm). Pain is noted with either dorsal or palmar ligament sprains.

▪ FORMAT OF THE CERVICAL– UPPER LIMB SCAN EXAMINATION

The patient sits at the edge of the plinth with the neck, arm, and shoulder girdles exposed. The examiner briefly inspects the upper spine, shoulder girdles, and arms for obvious muscular atrophy or deformity (see Figs. 17-15 and 17-17).

I. Cervical Tests

Problems in the cervical spine can be ruled out by applying a series of joint-clearing tests.

A. *Active cervical movements* (see Fig. 17-18). The patient is asked to perform each of the six cervical movements (flexion, extension, right and left lateral flexion, and right and left rotations), or the joints can be passively cleared by spring testing each cervical segment. If each active movement exhibits a full range of pain-free motion, then some passive overpressure is applied at the extreme of each movement.
   1. Tests for cervical joint restriction
   2. Overpressure to stress the noncontractile structures

B. *Isometrically resisted movements.* Isometrically resisted movements at mid range are performed in each direction to stress the contractile units. One hand is placed on each side of the patient's head (without covering the auditory meatus). The forearms and elbows rest over the patient's trapezial ridges to help stabilize against trunk movements. From this position the examiner resists cervical rotation and sidebending to the left and right, without allowing movement of the head.

   To resist cervical extension, the examiner places one hand over the back of the patient's head, such that the wrist lies over the patient's cervical spine and the forearm rests against the thoracic spine. The other hand reaches across the front of the patient to grasp the opposite shoulder. Extension of the patient's head and neck is resisted without allowing movement.

   Flexion is resisted by approaching the patient from behind, resting the elbows against the back of the patient's shoulders, and placing both hands over the patient's forehead.
   1. Tests the integrity of the upper cervical myotomes
   2. Tests for lesions of the cervical muscles

C. *Quadrant test.* Position the patient's head in combined rotation, sidebending, and extension to one side. With the patient's head in this position, a gentle axial compression is applied through the neck by downward pressure to the top of the head.
   1. Tests for localized capsular facet-joint tightness

   2. Tests for interforaminal nerve root impingement
D. *Neuromuscular Tests*
   1. Key sensory areas (C5–C8)—stroking test along dermatomes and sensibility to pin prick (see Fig. 17-28)
   2. Resisted isometric (myotomal) tests (C5–T1). Compare both sides (see p. 90).
   3. Neural tension tests (brachial tension or upper limb tension tests) (see Fig. 9-21)
   4. Reflexes (see Fig. 17-22)
      a. Biceps—C6 (C5)
      b. Wrist extension (brachioradialis)—C6
      c. Triceps—C7

II. Temporomandibular Joint

This joint is checked by palpation by the patient actively opening and closing the mouth, and by tests of provocation.

A. *Active opening and closing of mouth.* While the examiner is palpating the temporomandibular joints, the patient is asked to carry out active opening and closing of the mouth to demonstrate the following:
   1. Any localized swelling or tenderness
   2. Abnormal dynamics of the joint or changes in range of motion
   3. Clicking and pain during active motion or on closure

B. *Provocation tests.* If active movement exhibits a full range of pain-free motion, then provocation tests may be applied to stress the noncontractile structures of the temporomandibular joints by applying loading by forced biting or forced retrusion.

III. Acromioclavicular Joint

A. *Inspection and palpation.* Inspection may show swelling and elevation of the clavicular end of this joint due to sprain. There will be a step deformity in the presence of a third-degree sprain or dislocation. Palpation is performed for normal positioning, tenderness, and crepitation (see Fig. 17-28J).

B. *Active and passive movements.* Active ranges of depression, elevation, abduction, adduction, protraction, retraction, and circumduction are requested of the patient, followed by passive motion by the examiner through these same ranges. The joint is palpated during active motion for crepitus and abnormal excursions. The patient is instructed to horizontally adduct the arm across the chest. If horizontal flexion exhibits a full range of pain-free motion, then passive overpressure is applied at the end of range to reproduce pain.
   1. Tests for pain. If pain is elicited in any of

these movements, the patient should be asked if it is the same type of pain that brought him or her to the clinician for examination.

2. Tests for range and symmetry of motion

IV. Sternoclavicular Joint

A. *Inspection and palpation.* Synovitis is usually evident as a rounded soft-tissue swelling localized over the joint. Subluxation of the joint usually occurs in an anterosuperior direction and is best appreciated by looking down onto both joints. With anterior subluxation the clinician should be able to momentarily reduce the subluxation. On palpation there may be tenderness (see Fig. 17-28*I*).

B. *Active and passive movements.* The same seven ranges as for the acromioclavicular joint are performed.

1. Tests for pain
2. Tests for restriction of motion. The sternoclavicular joint moves with movement of the shoulder girdle, but it is not practical to measure exact range. The examiner should observe range and note symmetry.
3. Tests for crepitus and abnormal excursions during motion

V. Costosternal Joints and Ribs

A. *Inspection and palpation.* Adjacent to the sternum the examiner should palpate the sternocostal and costochondral articulations, noting any swelling or tenderness. Swelling may indicate an inflammation or subluxation of the costosternal joint (costochondritis or Tietze's syndrome). The first rib on both sides is palpated for position and tenderness. Any differences on caudal pressure are noted.

B. *Active and passive motion.* There is normally little motion of these joints. Raising and lowering the arms and breathing deeply may elicit a click and produce pain if there is a subluxation. If manual compression of the ribs causes pain, the individual joint or joints should be palpated to determine which ones have abnormal motion.

1. Tests for abnormal motion
2. Tests for pain

VI. Scapulothoracic Joint

A. *Inspection.* Inspection may reveal winging of the scapula if the long thoracic nerve has been injured.

B. *Active and passive motion.* Active motions are observed from behind: elevation, forward, sideways, horizontal abduction–adduction, external and internal rotation. Of particular importance is notation of scapular rotation for bilateral asymmetry and scapulohumeral rhythm. Passive motion testing (retraction, protraction, elevation, depression, and mediolateral rotation [in sidelying]) is included with palpation.

1. Tests for excessive or reduced movement
2. Tests for contracture
3. Tests for pain or tenderness

VII. Costovertebral and Costotransverse Joints

Palpation may reveal tenderness if there is joint involvement. Deep breathing may induce pain and refer it to the shoulder or arm.

VIII. Upper Thoracic Spine

A. *Inspection and palpation.* Inspection may reveal a sharp kyphosis at the site of an injured vertebra or a flat back or reversal of the curve in a mobile spine. Injured vertebrae will usually be tender on compression of the spinous process.

B. *Active-passive movements.* Active range of flexion, extension, rotation, and lateral bending should be observed. If active motions are full and painless, overpressure is given to clear the joint.

1. Tests for limitation and asymmetrical movement
2. Tests for pain and muscle spasm

IX. Glenohumeral Joint

A. *Active shoulder movements with passive overpressure.* The patient is asked to perform flexion of the arm (in the sagittal plane), abduction (in the frontal plane), and horizontal adduction (reaching across to behind the opposite shoulder); to touch the palm to the back of the neck and retract the elbow; and to crawl the thumb up the back as far as possible. If range of motion is full and painless, gentle passive overpressure is applied at the end point of each movement. Both arms are tested simultaneously for comparison, noting the presence of pain, muscle spasm, or loss of movement.

1. Tests for shoulder tendinitis: Typically full range of motion with pain at the extremes of elevation and movements that stretch the involved tendon. A painful arc on abduction suggests rotator cuff tendinitis.
2. Tests for capsular restriction of the glenohumeral joint: Considerable pain and restriction on external rotation and abduction, moderate restriction of flexion and internal rotation
3. Tests for acute bursitis: Marked pain and

restriction of elevation of the arm in any plane

B. *Resisted isometric shoulder movements.* The patient sits with the elbows close to the sides, the elbows bent to 90°, and the fingers pointed forward. Abduction is resisted with the arms held at about 30° abduction. External rotation and internal rotation are resisted with the elbows held tight against the sides, applying counterpressure just proximal to the wrist. All movements are resisted bilaterally and simultaneously for easy comparison of one side with the other and for most efficient stabilization against trunk movements. Maximal contractions should be encouraged. Any joint movement should be prevented and the presence of pain or weakness noted.

1. Tests for the presence of tendinitis: the contraction of the involved muscle and tendon will be strong and painful.
2. Tests for the presence of a tendon rupture: the contraction will be weak and painless.
3. Tests the integrity of the C5 and C6 myotomes.

C. *Quadrant test and locking position of the shoulder if applicable.* Compare findings with those of the opposite side (see Chapter 9, The Shoulder and Shoulder Girdle).

D. *Neurological test of reflexes, sensation, and distal muscle (C8–T1)*

X. Elbow Joint

A. *Active movements with passive overpressure.* The patient is asked to fully flex and extend both elbows together. If this exercise is full and painless, passive overpressure is applied at the extremes of each movement and the patient is observed for pain, spasm, or restricted movement. These tests may be performed with the shoulder extended, in neutral, or flexed to test for involvement of the long head of the biceps or triceps.

1. Tests for capsular restrictions: Flexion is limited to about 90° to 100°, extension is lacking by 20° to 30°.
2. Tests for extracapsular pain or restrictions
   a. Loose body—Extension is restricted; flexion is relatively free. Often there are painful twinges or crepitus noted during movement.
   b. Brachialis tightness—Extension is limited; flexion is free. Tightness is felt anteriorly by the patient on forced extension. The restriction is

unaffected by the position of the shoulder.
   c. Biceps tendinitis—Pain may be reproduced with elbow extension performed with the shoulder extended.

B. *Resisted isometric movements.* The trunk is stabilized by placing a hand over the top of the patient's shoulder and resisting isometric flexion and extension of the elbow. Pronation and supination are resisted with the elbow bent to 90°. Pain or weakness is noted.

1. Tests the integrity of the C6 and C7 myotomes (biceps [C6], triceps [C7], and pronator teres [C7])
2. Tests for biceps tendinitis: Resisted elbow flexion and forearm supination will be strong and painful.
3. Tests for biceps tendon rupture: Flexion and supination will be weak and painless.

XI. Wrist Joint

The patient's elbow is maintained in extension. The patient's arm is held snugly between the examiner's elbow and side, and the patient's forearm is cradled in the examiner's forearm and hand.

A. *Active movements with passive overpressure*

1. With the forearm pronated, the wrist is moved into full flexion and ulnar deviation. If movement is full and painless, passive overpressure is applied, once with the patient's fingers flexed, once with them relaxed. Pain or restricted motion is noted.
2. With the forearm supinated, the wrist is brought into full extension and radial deviation. If movement is full and painless, overpressure is applied, once with the fingers extended, once with them relaxed. Pain or restricted motion is noted.
   a. Tests for lateral tennis elbow: Elbow pain is reproduced on full wrist flexion and ulnar deviation with the forearm pronated and the fingers flexed.
   b. Tests for medial tennis elbow: Elbow pain is reproduced with full wrist extension with the fingers extended and forearm supinated.
   c. Tests for carpal ligament sprain: Pain on movement that stretches the involved ligament.
   d. Tests for de Quervain's tenosynovitis: Pain over the radial styloid region when the wrist is ulnarly deviated while the thumb is held flexed

e. Tests for capsular restriction of wrist movements: All wrist movements are limited.
B. *Resisted isometric wrist movements.* With the patient's arm held as described above and the patient's fist clenched, wrist flexion, extension, ulnar deviation, and radial deviation are resisted and pain or weakness is noted.
  1. Tests the C6 (extension), C7 (flexion), and C8 (ulnar deviation) myotomes
  2. Tests for tennis elbow: Pain on resisted wrist extension
  3. Tests for golfer's elbow: Pain on resisted wrist flexion
C. *Modified Phalen's test* (see Fig. 17-25). The patient is asked to perform a "three-jaw-chuck" pinch with both hands and to maintain both wrists in extreme flexion by pressing the dorsum of the hands against one another. This position is held for 30 to 60 seconds. The production of pain or paresthesias is noted.
  1. Tests for carpal tunnel syndrome: Paresthesias into the thumb or index, middle, and ring fingers are reproduced on the involved side.
  2. Tests for dorsal carpal ligament sprain: Wrist pain is reproduced on full wrist flexion.
D. *Upper extremity weight-bearing*
  1. While still seated, the patient is asked to place both hands to the side on the plinth and to attempt to raise the body off the plinth by pressing down with the hands.
  2. Tests for carpal ligament sprain: This is often the only maneuver that will reproduce the wrist pain.

XII. **The Hand**
A. *Grasp–release.* The patient is asked to squeeze two of the examiner's fingers simultaneously with both hands, as hard as possible, and then to open the hands as wide possible. Pain, weakness, or joint restriction is noted.
  1. Tests for the integrity of the T1 myotome: Weakness will be noted on grasp.
  2. Tests for tennis elbow: Strong grasp may reproduce the elbow pain because the wrist extensors must contract to stabilize.
  3. Tests for restriction of finger movement
B. *Resisted isometric abduction–adduction.* The patient attempts to keep the fingers spread apart as the examiner adducts the small finger and thumb simultaneously. Both hands are tested at the same time for comparison.

Then the examiner interlaces his fingers between the patient's extended fingers and asks the patient to adduct the fingers. Pain or weakness is noted.
  1. Tests the C8 myotome (thumb and small finger abduction) and the T1 myotome (finger adduction)
  2. Tests for de Quervain's tenosynovitis: Pain is produced with resisted thumb abduction.

XIII. **Sensory Tests**
The patient sits with the forearms resting on the thighs, palms facing upward. Using a sharp pin or pinwheel, the examiner assesses sensation by applying the stimulus to a small area on one extremity and asking the patient if it feels sharp, and then he repeats the test on the same area on the opposite extremity. Then the patient is asked if it feels the same on both sides. The key sensory areas in the hand are checked first, then various aspects of the forearms, arms, and shoulder girdles, using the procedure described above. Asymmetries and reduction of sensation are noted. For more subtle testing, a wisp of cotton or tuning fork may be used.
A. *Tests the integrity of the C4 through T1 dermatomes.* Rarely is a deficit noted proximal to the distal forearm in the case of nerve root lesions because of the extensive overlapping of dermatomes in all but the wrist and hand (see Fig. 17-23).
  C4—Trapezial ridge to tip of shoulder
  C5—Upper scapula, lateral brachial region, radial aspect of forearm
  C6—Upper scapula, lateral brachial region, radiovolar aspect of forearm, thumb, and index finger
  C7—Middle scapula, posterior brachial region, dorsum of forearm and hand, and palmar surface of index, middle, and ring fingers
  C8—Middle to lower scapula, ulnar aspect of forearm, and palmar surface of ring and little fingers
  T1—Ulnovolar aspect of forearm
B. *Tests sensory integrity of upper extremity peripheral nerves*

XIV. **Deep Tendon Reflex Tests**
The patient sits with forearms resting on thighs.
A. *Jaw jerk* (V cranial nerve; see Fig. 15-26). With the mandible in the physiological rest position, place the thumb over the mental area of the patient's chin. The examiner then taps the thumbnail with the reflex hammer; the reflex elicited will close the mouth. A

brisk reflex may be due to an upper motor neuron lesion.

B. *Biceps* (C5, C6; see Fig. 17-22*A*). As the patient maintains relaxation of the arm, the examiner places his thumb firmly over the patient's biceps tendon at the antecubital fossa and strikes the dorsum of the thumb with the reflex hammer to elicit the reflex. One should feel for tensing of the tendon and observe for contraction of the muscle and slight flexion of the elbow. Asymmetries in responses and clonic responses are noted.

C. *Triceps* (C7; see Fig. 17-22*B*). As the patient maintains relaxation of the arm, the examiner grasps the patient's upper arm (near elbow) and, while supporting the forearm at 90° elbow flexion, strikes the distal triceps tendon just above the olecranon. One should observe for triceps contraction and feel for slight elbow extension. Asymmetrical or clonic responses are noted.

D. *Brachioradialis* (C5, C6; see Fig. 17-22*C*). Alternative test: As the patient maintains relaxation of both arms, the examiner supports both forearms at about 90° elbow flexion by grasping both of the patient's thumbs in one hand (or the thumb of one hand, as illustrated). The brachioradialis tendon is struck just above the radial styloid process, slightly volarly. The brachioradialis muscle belly is observed for contraction and felt for slight elbow flexion and forearm pronation. Asymmetrical or clonic responses are noted. The integrity of the C5, C6, and C7 segments is tested.

XV. Referred and Related Tissues

A. *Thoracic outlet syndrome* (see Chapter 17, The Cervical Spine). Because the thoracic outlet syndrome induces pain in the upper quadrant, specific tests should be used to rule out its causes. If applicable, hyperabduction tests, costoclavicular tests, scalenus anticus tests, neurovascular compression tests, overhead tests, and the Adson's maneuver may be carried out. Conditions that can cause or contribute to a thoracic outlet syndrome include the following: pseudoarthrosis of the clavicle, exostosis of the first rib and cervical rib, and fascial fusion of muscles.

B. *Visceral conditions.* Pain may be referred to the upper quadrant from irritation of the diaphragm or peritoneum due to infection, the presence of free air or blood, an inflamed gallbladder, distended or inflamed stomach, or an injury to the liver or spleen.

Cardiac ischemia may also cause shoulder pain.

▧ SUMMARY OF STEPS TO CERVICAL–UPPER LIMB SCAN EXAMINATION

In order for the scan examination to be of practical use, it must be performed within a very short period of time—5 minutes or less. Otherwise, one of its primary purposes, that of saving time in the clinic, is defeated. In order to perform the scan examination within a reasonable period of time, the clinician must sequence the tests so that they are performed as efficiently as possible. In doing so, care must be taken to avoid undue haste, which might lead to poor evaluative technique and inaccurate findings. The scan examination condenses a number of tests within a short time period; in order to avoid confusion or the possibility of omitting crucial steps, the clinician must drill herself on the sequencing of steps and the rationale for each step in order to be able to use the scan examination effectively in the clinic.

The steps to the scan examination are listed below in the order that they can be most efficiently performed.

1. Active cervical movements with passive overpressure
2. Cervical resisted movements
3. Quadrant test, left and right
4. Active shoulder movements with passive overpressure
   a. Flexion
   b. Abduction
   c. Hand to opposite shoulder
   d. Hand to back of neck, wing elbow back
   e. Hand behind and up back
5. Resisted shoulder movements
   a. Abduction (C5)
   b. Internal rotation
   c. External rotation
6. Active elbow and forearm movements with passive overpressure, resisted elbow and forearm movements
   a. Flexion (C6): passive overpressure, resist flexion
   b. Neutral: resist extension (C7), resist pronation (C7) and supination
   c. Extension: passive overpressure
7. Active forearm and wrist movements with passive overpressure
   a. Combined wrist flexion and ulnar deviation with the forearm pronated and elbow extended: (1) passive overpressure with fingers

flexed; (2) passive overpressure with fingers relaxed

   b. Combined wrist extension and radial deviation with the forearm supinated and elbow extended: (1) passive overpressure with fingers extended; (2) passive overpressure with fingers relaxed

  8. Resisted wrist movements

    a. Flexion (C7)

    b. Extension (C6)

    c. Radial deviation

    d. Ulnar deviation

  9. Modified Phalen's test

 10. Active and resisted finger movements

    a. Grasp–release

    b. Finger abduction (C8)

    c. Finger adduction (T1)

 11. Upper extremity weight-bearing

 12. Sensory tests

    a. C4–T1

 13. Reflex testing

    a. Jaw jerk (V cranial nerve)

    b. Biceps (C5)

    c. Triceps (C6)

    d. Brachioradialis (C7)

RECOMMENDED READINGS

American Society for Surgery of the Hand: The Hand: Examination and Diagnosis. New York, Churchill Livingstone, 1983

Boyling J, Palastanga N (eds): Grieve's Modern Manual Therapy of the Vertebral Column. Edinburgh, Churchill Livingstone, 1994

Butler: Mobilization of the Nervous System. Melbourne, Churchill Livingstone, 1991

Corrigan B, Maitland GD: Practical Orthopaedic Medicine. London, Butterworths, 1985

Cyriax JH, Cyriax PJ: Illustrated Manual of Orthopaedic Medicine, 2nd ed. London, Butterworths, 1993

Donatelli R (ed): Physical Therapy of the Shoulder. New York, Churchill Livingstone, 1987

Dvorak J, Dvorak V: Manual Medicine: Diagnostics. New York, Thieme Medical, 1990

Evans RC: Illustrated Essentials in Orthopedic Physical Assessment. St Louis, CV Mosby, 1994

Grant R (ed): Physical Therapy of the Cervical and Thoracic Spine. New York, Churchill Livingstone, 1988

Grant R (ed): Physical Therapy of the Cervical and Thoracic Spine, 2nd ed. New York, Churchill Livingstone, 1994

Grieve GP: Mobilisation of the Spine: A Primary Handbook of Clinical Method, 5th ed. Edinburgh, Churchill Livingstone, 1991

Hartley A: Practical Joint Assessment: A Sports Medicine Manual. St Louis, Mosby Year Book, 1990

Magee DJ: Orthopedic Physical Assessment, 2nd ed. Philadelphia, WB Saunders, 1992

Maitland GD: Vertebral Manipulations, 5th ed. Boston, Butterworths, 1986

Matsen FA, Lippitt SB, Slides JA, et al: Practical Evaluation and Management of the Shoulder. Philadelphia, WB Saunders, 1994

McKenzie RA: The Cervical and Thoracic Spine: Mechanical Diagnosis and Therapy. Waikanae, New Zealand, Spinal Publications, 1990

Morrey BF: The Elbow and Its Disorders. Philadelphia, WB Saunders, 1987

Rocabado M: Diagnosis and treatment of abnormal craniomandibular mechanics. In Solbery W, Clark G (eds): Abnormal Jaw Mechanics: Diagnosis and Treatment. Chicago, Quintessence, 1984

Rocabado M: The importance of soft tissue mechanics in stability and instability of the cervical spine: A functional diagnosis for treatment planning. J Craniomandib Pract 5:130–138, 1987

Rocabado M, Iglarsh ZA: Musculoskeletal Approach to Maxillofacial Pain. Philadelphia, JB Lippincott, 1991

Rockwood CA, Matsen FA: The Shoulder, vol 1. Philadelphia, WB Saunders, 1990

Wadsworth CT: Wrist and hand examination and interpretation. J Orthop Sports Phys Ther 5:108–120, 1983

The Thoracic Spine

DARLENE HERTLING

EPIDEMIOLOGY AND PATHOPHYSIOLOGY

Few people have a normal thoracic spine, according to Grieve.[67] The diseases that commonly affect the cervical and lumbar spine also occur in the thoracic spine. Degenerative disease changes in the thoracic spine occur as frequently as they do in the cervical and lumbar spine; the peak incidence of involvement is at C7–T1 and T4–T5. However, symptoms and signs from this region are rare, due to the anatomy and biomechanics of this area of the spine.[93]

Degenerative joint disease is common in the thoracic spine, but disk lesions are rare. Thoracic involvement occurs in only about 2% of all causes of disk problems. De Palma and Rothman reported that of 1000 disk operations, only one involved the thoracic spine.[35]

According to Cyriax,[32] unlike the cervical and lumbar regions where muscle lesions are rare, the muscles of the thorax and abdomen can suffer strain, leading to posttraumatic scarring and persistent symptoms. A pectoral or intercostal muscle may be affected in this way, as may the latissimus dorsi, the rectus abdominis, or the oblique abdominals. Maigne[104] points out that involvement of the rib cage in pathologic processes is often neglected. However, costal sprain is common and is expressed by thoracic or upper lumbar pain. Most rib lesions are accompanied, if not caused by, spasms of the intercostal muscles. A sneeze or cough with a violent contraction of the muscles of the thoracic cage may leave a persistent contraction of

Darlene Hertling and Randolph M. Kessler: MANAGEMENT OF COMMON
MUSCULOSKELETAL DISORDERS: Physical Therapy Principles and Methods, 3rd ed.
© 1996 Lippincott-Raven Publishers.

one intercostal muscle, leading to approximation of two adjacent ribs, and this may persist. The effect of sustained contraction in one intercostal muscle is to elevate the lower rib (an *inspiratory-type* lesion). *Expiratory-type* lesions, in which the lower rib is held downward, occur only in the lower ribs (mainly the 11th and 12th) because of the attachment of the quadratus lumborum.

The thoracic spine is frequently the source of pain of postural origin, particularly in adolescence. McKenzie[116] suggested that although it is not a pathological entity in itself, poor posture may be a significant factor contributing to the development of Scheuermann's disease in the young and osteoporosis in the aged. Perhaps the most common disease affecting the skeletal thoracic spine is osteoporosis. In the treatment of this disorder, the value of physical therapy has gone largely unrecognized.[116]

■ FUNCTIONAL ANATOMY

The thoracic vertebrae are characterized primarily by two features: the presence of articular facets on the vertebral bodies (for articulation with the ribs) and the long, thin spinous processes that angle downward in relation to the motion segment (see Fig. 16-4). Unlike the spinous processes in the cervical and lumbar spine, where the tip of the spinous process is found directly posterior to the body of the vertebrae, the tip of the spinous process in the thoracic area lies posterior and inferior to the body of the vertebra. It therefore can be used as a lever to rotate the vertebral body, resulting in a gliding of the facet articulations that is associated with forward and backward bending in the thoracic spine.[43] The spinous processes are quite long and overlap each other, particularly in the middle to lower region (see Fig. 16-1C).

Mitchell, Moran, and Pruzzo[123] divide the thoracic vertebrae into groups of three for the purpose of examination. The spinous processes of the first three thoracic vertebrae (T1, T2, T3) project directly backward: the tip of the spinous process is on the same line as the transverse process. The spinous processes of T4 to T6 project half a vertebra below that to which they are attached. The spinous processes of T7 to T9 are located a full vertebra lower than the vertebra to which they are attached. The spinous processes of T10 to T12 return to being palpable at the same level as the vertebral body to which they are attached (Fig. 19-1).

The typical thoracic vertebra has a body roughly

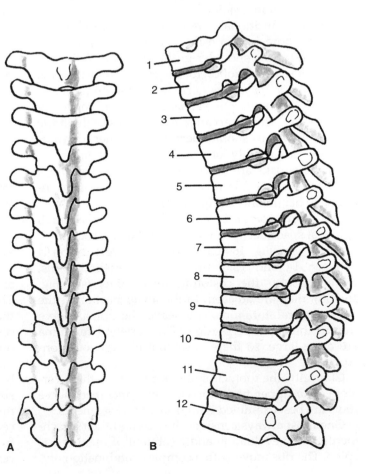

FIG. 19-1. Thoracic vertebra—"rule of 3." (Adapted from Greenman PE: *Principles of Manual Medicine,* p. 52. Balitmore, Williams & Wilkins, 1989.)

A   B

equal in its transverse and anteroposterior diameter. The apophyseal joints are vertical in orientation (at an angle of about 60° from the horizontal plane; see Fig. 16-4). The superior facet faces upward and back, and the inferior facet faces downward and forward, making them particularly well suited for rotation.

The *atypical thoracic vertebrae* (T1 and T12) are those that are transitional between the cervical and thoracic spine and the thoracic and lumbar spine. T1 has the longest transverse process in the thoracic spine. The inferior apophyseal joint surface orientation (facing) is typically thoracic, but the superior apophyseal joint is transitional from the cervical spine and may have typical cervical characteristics. T1 is also the junction for the change in the anteroposterior curve between the cervical and thoracic spine. Dysfunction of T1 profoundly affects the functional capacity of the thoracic outlet and related structures.

T12 is the location of transition to the lumbar spine. The superior apophyseal joint facing is usually typically thoracic, but the inferior apophyseal joint facing tends toward lumbar characteristics. T12 is the location for the change in the anteroposterior curve between the thoracic kyphosis and the lumbar lordosis, a location of change in mobility to two areas of the spine, and a point of frequent dysfunction.[65] T12 acts as a bridge between the lumbar-thoracic spine and is essentially a mortise joint.

T3 is the transitional zone between the cervical lordosis and thoracic kyphosis and also serves as the axis of motion for the shoulder-girdle complex. T6 is considered the axis of motion for the entire thoracic spine.

The *thoracic kyphosis* is normally a smooth posterior convexity, without severe areas of increased convexity or flattening. The observation of flat spots without the thoracic kyphosis should alert the examiner to evaluate this area carefully for vertebral dysfunction.

Thoracic disks are narrower and flatter than those in the cervical and lumbar spine. They gradually increase in height and width from superior to inferior.

The spinal canal is narrow, with only a small epidural space between the cord and its osseous environment (see Fig. 16-4C).[168] The narrowest region is between T4 and T5.[93] Besides the vertebral joints, there are also the costotransverse joints (see Fig. 16-10B): they are adjacent to the lower portion of the intervertebral foramina and leave the spinal nerve free in the superior portion. The vertebral foramina are quite large, so there is seldom any osseous constriction.

Clinically, the thoracic spine begins at the third vertebra. The upper two thoracic joints and their nerve roots are best examined with the cervical segments.[32]

One must always consider the ribs and their attachments in the evaluation and treatment of the thoracic spine. The ribs move with a complex combination of:

1. Pump-handle motions (similar to flexion and extension) (see Fig. 16-11A)
2. Bucket-handle motions (similar to abduction and adduction) (see Fig. 16-11B)
3. Caliper-like motions (analogous to internal and external rotation) (see Fig. 16-11C).

The upper ribs move mainly in a combined pump-handle/bucket-handle type of motion; middle rib motion is primarily of the bucket-handle type. The lower ribs move much like calipers. However, all ribs move with a complex combination of these motions. Ribs II, III, and IV have a somewhat greater proportion of pump-handle movement as they rise and fall with the sternum. Rib I, moving with about half pump-handle and half bucket-handle motions, is acted on in inhalation by the anterior, medial, and posterior scalene muscles. In quieter respiration they may move by the tilting manubrium, or they may not move much at all. Ribs VIII to X have a greater proportion of bucket-handle motion as they increase and decrease the transverse diameter of the chest. The floating ribs have a greater proportion of caliper-type motions.

There are three costovertebral joints for each rib. Except for ribs I and X to XII, the head of each rib articulates with two adjacent vertebrae and with one transverse process. The exceptions articulate with one vertebral body (costovertebral joint) and its transverse process. In addition, ribs I to VII articulate anteriorly with the sternum via synovial joints (see Fig. 16-10A). Rib movements are small and gliding to enable pump-handle, bucket-handle, and caliper movements to occur.

The thoracic spine is intimately related to the rib cage, and they work essentially as a single unit. Alterations in thoracic cage function alter the thoracic spine. Hence, from the respiratory/circulatory model of manual medicine, the thoracic spine assumes major importance in providing optimal functional capacity to the thoracic cage for respiration and circulation.[65] The thoracic spine takes on additional importance from the neurologic perspective because of its relation with the sympathetic division of the autonomic nervous system.

Because of the convexity of the thoracic spine, the anterior parts become subjected to considerable load. The intradiskal pressure is high in this region because the load is taken up entirely by the vertebrae and disks. Because of this, compression fractures most often appear anteriorly, and there is an invasion of disk tissue through the end-plates into the vertebral bodies.[93] Due to the continuous high intradiskal pressures, degenerative changes develop quite early in the middle and lower sections of the thoracic spine. According to Kramer,[93] disk disease with symptoms from the thoracic spine is not as common as it is in the cervical and lumbar spine. This is because:

1. The intervertebral foramina are not posterior to the disks, as is the case in the cervical and lumbar spine, but are rather on the same level as the vertebral bodies. Nerve root involvement thus requires a large prolapse of disk tissue, and this is uncommon.

2. The movements of the thoracic spine are much more restricted than those of the cervical and lumbar spine. The position of the nerve in relation to the osseous structures is fairly constant and is not subjected to a continuous change of position, as is the case in the cervical and lumbar spine.

The intercostal nerves (the anterior branches of the thoracic spinal nerves) supply the chest wall, the intercostal muscles, the costotransverse joints, the parietal pleura, and the skin. When any of these nerves becomes irritated, an intercostal neuralgia develops.

Deformities such as scoliosis and Scheuermann's disease generally develop slowly, and the nerve roots adapt to the change of position. Because of the anterior loading of the disks, dislocation of disk fragments may occur in a posterior direction, with rupture and perforation of the annulus fibrosus. The disk fragment can be as large as a cherry and will in time adhere to the dura.[12] There are also central, anterolateral, and lateral dislocations of fragments, which ultimately protrude posteriorly.[35] The region most involved is T7 to T12.[12,94,99]

COMMON LESIONS AND THEIR MANAGEMENT

Pain in the thoracic spine with referral to various parts of the chest wall and upper abdomen is common in people of all ages and can closely mimic the symptoms of visceral disease such as angina pectoris and biliary colic.[84] Cloward,[28] Maigne,[104] and Cyriax[32] have demonstrated that much of the pain experienced in the upper thoracic region to the level of T7 originates in the cervical spine.

According to Kenna and Murtagh,[84] the significant features to consider with respect to the thoracic region are:

1. People of all ages can experience thoracic problems. They are surprisingly common in young people, including children.
2. Thoracic pain is more common in patients with abnormalities such as thoracic kyphosis and Scheuermann's disease.
3. Trauma to the chest wall (including falls on the chest), such as those experienced in contact sports, commonly leads to disorders in the thoracic spine.
4. Patients recovering from open-heart surgery, when

a longitudinal sternal incision is made and the chest wall is stretched out, commonly experience thoracic pain.

5. Unlike the lumbar spine, the joints are quite superficial, and it is relatively easy to find the affected painful segment.

Mechanical causes of thoracic and rib cage dysfunction include disk lesions, facet lesions, costovertebral and costochondral lesions, and spondylosis.

Thoracic Disk Herniations

Disk lesions are relatively rare in the thoracic spine but are of concern because of their possible impingement on the spinal cord.

Disk Prolapse and Pain Patterns

Of the total number of disk problems, thoracic presentations represent 1 to 6 patients per 1000.[34] This problem appears predominantly in males, and the highest incidence is in the fifth decade. T11 and T12 are most commonly involved.

The clinical history often reveals an axial compression of the trunk, as occurs in a fall on the hindquarter or when lifting a heavy object in the forward-bent position. Localized pain corresponds to the segment involved. Coughing or increasing intrathoracic pressure increases the pain. The cord may be involved and radicular signs may develop, although the only symptom may be localized pain. Evidence of cord compression, with resultant sensory loss, upper motor neuron lesions, and bladder symptoms, is common.[99] A medial prolapse may produce cord symptoms; a disk prolapse that is more posterolateral is more likely to involve the nerve roots.

DISK BULGING AGAINST THE POSTERIOR LIGAMENT AND DURA

When a prolapsed disk exerts pressure on the posterior ligament and the dura, the result is spondylogenic referred pain, usually experienced in the upper back (if of thoracic origin) or the low back (lumbar origin). The pain, however, can be referred over a wider area. According to Cyriax,[33] as at other spinal levels, involvement of the dura mater, with a central disk protrusion, produces unilateral extrasegmal dural reference of pain. Interference with the dura mater at thoracic levels may produce posterior pain, spreading to the base of the neck or down to the midlumbar region and often pervading several dermatomal levels (Fig. 19-2). Symptoms are usually central or unilateral.

Coughing or deep breathing increases the pain.[32,33] The pain is usually dull, deep, and poorly localized.

DISK BULGING POSTEROLATERALLY AGAINST NERVE ROOT

This is a natural route because the annulus fibrosus is no longer reinforced by the posterior longitudinal ligament. According to Cyriax[33] and Cailliet,[23] if the disk exerts pressure on the dural sleeve of the nerve root only, the radicular pain is experienced along the course of the nerve root. Pain can be experienced, therefore, in any part of the dermatome of the affected nerve root.

At T1 and T2 (both rare), symptoms may be felt in the arm. Root pain of lower levels causes symptoms in the side or front of the trunk. A cervical disk lesion is the routine cause of pain felt at upper thoracic levels.[33,106] According to Cyriax,[33] discomfort below the sixth thoracic dermatome may arise from a thoracic disk lesion.

With further pressure on the nerve parenchyma, there is usually no pain. Because conduction down the nerve is affected, parenthesis or anesthesia in the dis-

tal end of the dermatome, absent or sluggish reflexes, and motor weakness results.

The most common site of prolapse is between T11 and T12. Symptoms include local back pain and radicular pain. Pain refers to the lumbar region, especially the iliac crest.

According to D'Ambrosia,[34] thoracic disk protrusion is difficult to diagnose and more often than not will have a long, puzzling history. It can be confused with ankylosing spondylitis, metastatic tumor, chronic duodenal ulcer disease, intercostal neuralgia, disk space infection, intramedullary spinal cord tumors, or neurofibromas.

☐ Minor Intervertebral Derangement Theory of Maigne

Maigne[106] proposes the existence in the involved segment of a *minor intervertebral derangement* (MID), which is usually reversed by mobilization or manipulation. It is defined as "isolated pain in one interverte-

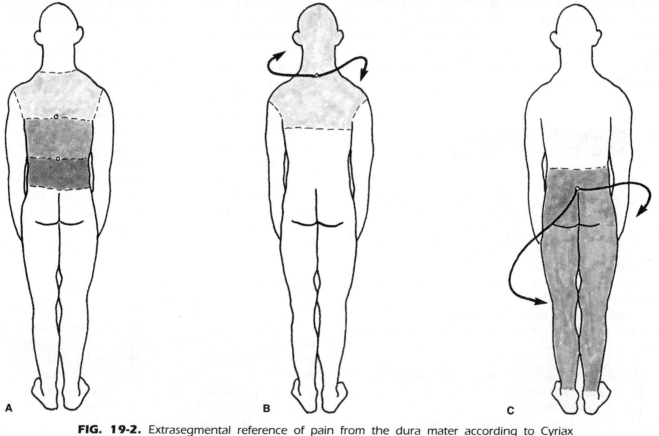

FIG. 19-2. Extrasegmental reference of pain from the dura mater according to Cyriax (1983). **(A)** Cyriax considered that thoracic dural pain could produce pain up to the base of the neck and down to the waist. **(B)** The cervical dura could refer pain to the head and midthoracic spine. **(C)** The low lumbar dural pain could spread to the legs (infrequently to the abdomen and to the mid-thoracic area). Note that the feet are excluded. (Adapted from Cyriax JH, Cyriax PJ: *Illustrated Manual of Orthopaedic Medicine,* p 245. London, Butterworths, 1993.)

bral segment, of a mild character, and due to a minor mechanical cause."[106] Most commonly, a vertebral level is found to be painful and yet has a normal static and radiological appearance.

The MID always involves one of the two apophyseal joints in the mobile segment, thus initiating nociceptive activity in the posterior primary dermatome and myotome. The overlying skin is tender to pinching and rolling, and the muscles are painful to palpation and feel cordlike.

Referral patterns based on stimulation of the apophyseal joints have recently been reported by Dreyfuss, Tibiletti, and Dreyer (Fig. 19-3).[40] This study provides preliminary confirmation that the thoracic apophyseal joints can cause both local and referred pain. Significant overlap in the referral patterns was reported.

According to Maigne,[106] the functional ability of the mobile segment depends closely on the condition of the intervertebral disk—thus, if the disk is injured, other elements of the segment will be affected. Even a minimal disk lesion can produce apophyseal joint dysfunction, which is a reflex cause of protective muscle spasm and pain in the corresponding segment with loss of function. The result is avoidance of painful pressure or movement of the involved seg-

ment. This becomes fixed, and the condition tends to become self-perpetuating.

☐ Thoracic Pain of Lower Cervical Origin

The clinical association between injury to the lower cervical region and upper thoracic pain is well known, especially with whiplash injuries. According to Maigne,[104] 70% of common thoracic pain is of lower cervical origin and is predominant in the intercellular region. These cases represent almost entirely postural thoracic pain, such as that manifested by typists and secretaries.

The examination reveals the same signs in all cases: thoracic signs with a particular localized area of tenderness called the *cervical point of the back* or the interscapular point (ISP) near T5 or T6 (2 cm from the line of the spinous process) and inferior cervical MID (C5–C6, C6–C7, or C6–T1), with the tender facet on the same side as the back pain and the thoracic signs.

An interesting sign that demonstrates the connection between cervical spine involvement and back pain is the anterior cervical doorbell or "push-button" sign.[104,107] Pressure with the thumb over the anterolateral portion of the lower cervical spine, maintained for a few seconds at the responsible vertebral level, triggers the thoracic pain. Another sign is an area of skin more or less thickened and extremely sensitive to the pinch-roll maneuver, which includes all or part of the cutaneous territory of the posterior branch of the second thoracic nerve.[106] This extends from the middle thoracic region (T5–T6) to the acromion.

In addition to these findings, a therapeutic trial of cervical mobilization is important. Disappearance of the cervical MID and ISP with diminished sensitivity in the pinch-roll maneuver of the medial thoracic zone should occur.

Pain from the lower cervical spine can also be referred to the anterior chest and mimic coronary ischemic pain. The associated autonomic nervous system disturbance can cause considerable confusion in making the diagnosis.[84]

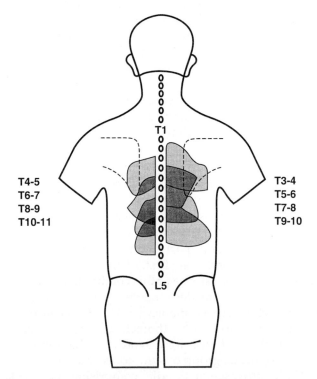

FIG. 19-3. *Referral patterns from the T3–T4 to T10–T11 thoracic apophyseal joints: a composite map from asymptomatic volunteers. (From Dreyfuss P, Tibiletti C, Dreyer SJ: Thoracic zygapophyseal joint pain patterns: A study in normal volunteers. Spine 19:807–811, 1993.)*

☐ Thoracic Pain of Thoracic Origin
(According to Maigne[106])

Thoracic pain of thoracic origin is rarer than the preceding. Postural thoracic pain resembles thoracic pain of cervical origin, but the pain is not always localized in the T5 and T6 segments. Clinical examination reveals an MID of a thoracic segment with:

1. Tenderness of the corresponding supraspinous ligament
2. Tenderness of the neighboring skin (infiltrating cellulitis) tested by the skin-rolling maneuver
3. Pain following lateral pressure on one side of the spinous process
4. Elective pain elicited by "resisted" pressure of the spinal processes in one direction.

Mobilization and a few sessions of skin-rolling massage involving the tender skin may be used if tenderness persists after the MID is corrected. Muscle re-education and postural exercises should be prescribed, and static deficiencies should be corrected.

Thoracic Hypomobility Syndromes

The most common cause of pathology arising from the apophyseal joints is capsular fibrosis. Most dysfunction is that of hypomobility. Hypermobility is uncommon, but as in the cervical spine, it is equally significant and more difficult to treat. Within their own segment, stiff apophyseal joints may result in reduction of nutrition to the disk. In neighboring segments, they may produce ligamentous and joint instability.

According to McKenzie,[116] the extension dysfunction develops in patients with both Scheuermann's disease and osteoporosis. The loss of movement that characterizes this dysfunction syndrome is caused by adaptive shortening resulting from poor postural habits over a sustained period, or from adaptive shortening as a result of derangement or trauma and the healing process. The dysfunction syndrome is presumed to be caused by a disturbance of some structure within a joint causing mechanical deformation of pain-sensitive structures.[95,116] Many patients lose mobility in extension and rotation as a result of poor postural habits. Treatment is directed at maintaining correct posture and performing extension exercises on a lifelong basis. Management of rotation dysfunction is directed at rotation exercises in sitting and extension in lying.

Mayo Clinic research in postmenopausal spinal osteoporosis has demonstrated that extension exercises performed regularly significantly reduced the number of compression fractures, and that levels of physical activity and back muscle strength may contribute to the bone mineral density of vertebral bodies.[156,157]

A primary cause of thoracic hypomobility in neurologically involved children and adults (*e.g.,* cerebral palsy, traumatic head injury, multiple sclerosis) is the lack of active thoracic extension, leading to immobility of the spine and rib cage. Common problems seen in these patients include:

1. Forward head and increased thoracic kyphosis
2. Decreased thoracolumbar mobility
3. Limited spinal extension with associated hip flexion contractures or excessive lumbar lordosis with increased thoracic kyphosis and genu recurvatum on weight-bearing
4. Hypomobility of the rib cage resulting from lack of mobility and postural and muscular imbalances
5. Altered breathing patterns, usually avoiding diaphragmatic breathing (diaphragm is restricted)
6. In the neurologically involved child, retention of the neonatal thoracolumbar kyphosis (thoracolumbar flexion) with posterior tilt of the pelvis (sacral sitting)
7. Spasticity (resulting in hyperactivity of spinal gamma motor neurons) and static postural reflexes. These are often present and interfere with voluntary movement.

Treatment aimed at reducing tone and abnormal movement patterns may be successful using various physical therapy approaches: therapeutic exercise, positioning, and modalities. Joint articulations using long-lever articulations, thoracic stretching, and soft-tissue manipulations are useful.

Developmental activities and exercises, as well as joint articulations aimed at reducing tone and restoring motions, should concentrate on trunk and proximal movements, as many patterns of hypertonus seem to arise from these key areas.[15] Trunk activities should include segmental rolling, in addition to upper and lower trunk rotation and counterrotation.[130] Activities, exercise, and articulation techniques that stress extension with trunk rotation are generally most effective. When extensor tone seems to predominate, flexion activities and articulations with trunk rotation should be considered.

Thoracic Outlet Syndrome

This condition, considered a neurovascular compression syndrome of the thoracic outlet, gained great importance in the early part of this century and was diagnosed frequently at first. Time has given less credence to the existence of this condition, to the point that many now consider it neither anatomically possible nor clinically verifiable.[26,27,143,171] According to Phillips and Grieve,[137] "thoracic outlet" is a convenient anatomical term for a syndrome that represents a heterogeneous group of symptoms and signs.

The neurovascular bundle, comprising the subclavian vasculature and the brachial plexus, may be compressed in its course through the thoracic outlet in the neck. This compression is considered the source of the syndrome's symptoms and signs. Obstruction may be caused by a number of abnormalities, including degenerative or bony disorders, trauma to the cervical spine, fibromuscular bands, vascular abnormalities, and spasms of the anterior scaleni or pectoralis minor muscle.[31,101] When soft-tissue tests do not reproduce the symptoms or signs, examination of the lower cervical and upper thoracic spine and palpation of the first rib may prove more valuable.

Cailliet[22] outlined the "compression syndromes" of the thoracic outlet as the anterior scalene syndrome, clavicocostal syndrome, pectoralis minor syndrome, scapulocostal syndrome, and pectoralis minor syndrome, emphasizing the role of hypertonic muscles. There are other diagnostic labels, such as the first rib syndrome,[32,117] myofascial thoracic outlet compression,[104] axonopathic neurogenic TOS (thoracic outlet syndrome), and "droopy shoulder" TOS.[71] According to McNair and Maitland,[117] the syndrome may be a product of the combined anomalies of the soft tissues and the bony boundaries of the outlet; hence, treatment must address both conditions.

Symptoms depend on whether the nerves, the blood vessels, or both are compressed. The nerve symptoms are paresthesia and subjective weakness or pain; the vascular symptoms are edema, discoloration, pallor, or venous congestion. Symptoms range from diffuse arm pain to a sensation of fatigue in the arm, frequently aggravated by carrying anything in the hand or doing overhead work. In axonopathic TOS, there is objective weakness and wasting of the median and ulnar nerve distribution of the hand and forearm.[22] Sensory impairment is usually of the ulnar distribution. Pain, when present, may also be in the dermatomal distribution.

Several authors[22,117,108,137] have outlined test procedures to help differentiate the most likely offending soft-tissue or bony structure (see Chapter 17, The Cervical Spine). According to Butler,[20] all tension tests should be performed (see Chapter 9, The Shoulder and Shoulder Girdle). Tension tests on the opposite arm and a slump test, both in long-sitting and in sitting, are suggested to look for any spinal canal components of adverse tension. The first and second rib joints and the apophyseal joints, especially in the lower cervical and upper thoracic spine must be examined. The acromioclavicular, glenohumeral, and possibly elbow and wrist joints need to be examined, particularly if a double or multiple crush syndrome is evident.[102,165]

Treatment options are physical therapy, strengthening exercises, re-education for postural change, and surgical decompression in patients with well-defined supernumerary bony or fibrotic abnormalities.[37,76,87,136,158]

Physical therapy is designed to restore pain-free movements at the site of the compression and then to correct any postural abnormalities present. Exercises to strengthen the shoulder muscles or to stretch any soft-tissue tightness should be done. Joint mobilizations and supportive devices to reduce symptoms on the nerve trunk or to take the downward strain off the thoracic spine occasionally are required.[32,117] Improved posture in activities of daily living should be stressed, because faulty posture remains the major culprit. Corrective actions may include bed elevation, proper use of pillows, seating and lighting, body mechanics, and training techniques to reinforce coordinated chest and abdominal breathing.[22,32,164]

☐ Upper Thoracic Spinal Syndromes

The upper thoracic spine is considered the stiffest part of the thoracic spine. Pain is usually well localized but may cause distal symptoms, probably via the autonomic nervous system.[84] A specific syndrome in this region is known as the T4 syndrome.[113] This condition is associated with a hypomobility lesion at the T4 level and has the following features:

1. Arm pain or vague discomfort in the arm associated with paresthesias that do not follow any dermatome pattern, with the hand always involved
2. Diffuse posterior head and neck pain in some patients
3. Hypomobility at one or more levels (T3–T4, T4–T5, or T5–T6); T4 is invariably involved.
4. Tenderness and stiffness, especially at T3–T4 and T4–T5.

The mechanism is unknown, but an associated disturbance of autonomic nerve control has been postulated. Predisposing factors have been attributed to unaccustomed lifting, stretching, pushing activities, or trauma (*e.g.*, a motor vehicle accident, a fall). A relaxed posture, with a forward head, accentuated thoracic kyphosis, and protracted shoulder girdle, may predispose the patient to this syndrome.

Butler[20] has explained the symptom distribution and the apparent epiphenomenon of symptomatic involvement based on the clinical observation made by many manual therapists over the past few years that patients with the symptom complex have a positive upper limb tension test and some have a positive slump test. The T4 to T9 segment of the spinal canal is a narrow zone where minimal reduction in the size of the canal will result in possible compromise of the neuraxis and the meninges.[38] With injury to surrounding joints, a site of adverse tension may be initiated. Other structures such as the thoracic sympathetic trunk and ganglia, dura mater, nerve roots, and even the preganglionic neurons in the cord may eventually be irritated.

TREATMENT

Articulations or manipulation of this involved area almost always relieve symptoms after three or four treatments, according to Corrigan and Maitland.[30] McGuckin[113] endorsed this and emphasized Klapp's quadrapedic exercises.[89,104] If the relaxed posture is considered a predisposing factor, postural correction exercises can be useful.

Butler[20] recommends using both upper limb tension tests 1 and 2 and also the slump test, with combinations of thoracic rotation and lateral flexion in evaluation and treatment if needed. A technique in which the costotransverse joint is mobilized in the slump long-sitting and thoracic rotation positions may be used. For a complete description of the evaluation process and illustrations of these valuable techniques, refer to his textbook.

☐ Midthoracic and Costovertebral Disorders

The T5 to T7 segments are the most common sites for apophyseal joint pain; the T8 to T10 segments are the most common sites for rib articulation problems (costovertebral disorders) and the most common site for referred pain mimicking visceral pain.[84]

Localized degenerative disk lesions are relatively uncommon. There is a higher incidence in people whose occupations involve repeated thoracic rotation (*e.g.,* professional golfers).[30] Nerve root involvement may occur with pain radiating around the chest wall following the line of the rib; this is sometimes associated with paresthesias or numbness over the same distribution. Pain is aggravated by movement and is often worse on lying down. Treatment is difficult: traction, some form of back support, and gentle mobilization techniques may help.

The costovertebral joint may be involved in inflammatory or degenerative joint disease. Complaints of pain in this region are common early in ankylosing spondylitis due to synovitis, and examination reveals local tenderness and reduced chest expansion. Chest measurements can also be used to assess disease progress.

Dysfunction of the costovertebral joint commonly causes localized pain about 3 to 4 cm from the midline, where the rib articulates with the transverse process and the vertebral body.[84] The costovertebral joint is frequently responsible for referred pain ranging from the midline, posterior to the lateral chest wall, and even to the anterior chest wall. Diagnosis is confirmed only when movement of the rib provokes pain at the costovertebral joint.

Degenerative changes may occur, although they are usually asymptomatic. They begin in the fourth decade, but symptoms such as tenderness and localized pain usually result only after some form of localized trauma. Nathan and associates[129] found the inferior rather than the superior joint facet to be the usual site of involvement. They also found that the joints with a single facet (1, 11, 12) have a much higher incidence of degenerative changes than the others, which have two hemifacets.

Treatment with mobilization techniques is usually successful. Local anesthetic injections are often beneficial.

☐ Lower Thoracic Spine and Thoracolumbar Junction Dysfunction

Lower thoracic and thoracolumbar junction pain is common and is the most common level for thoracic disk lesions. Pain is referred to the lumbar region, especially the iliac crest and often the buttock (see Fig. 19-8). There is sometimes pain in the inguinal or apparently in the abdominal areas and occasionally pain in the trochanteric region. The initial impression is that the symptoms are arising from the lower lumbar spine. The pain in these cases is low, lumbar, deep, or sacroiliac, or at the level of the iliac crest.

The skin over the iliac crest and upper outer buttock areas is supplied by the posterior primary rami of nerves arising from the thoracolumbar region.[106] Similarly, anterior groin pain can arise form this region as the nerve supply is from the anterior rami of spinal nerves T12 and L1. The dermatomal symptoms can be present in either the posterior or anterior branches of the dorsal rami. Consequently, with anterior abdominal symptoms, and in some cases of hip pain where the radiological examination of the hip is normal, irritation of the 12th thoracic or first lumbar nerve should be considered.

According to Maigne,[106] in these cases an iliac crest ("crestal") point is found at the gluteal level, usually 8 or 10 cm from the median line, more lateral or more medial. Pressure and friction over the iliac crest will reveal this well-localized and actually painful point. Examination of the thoracolumbar region will also reveal the signs of an MID between T10 and L2. The two most characteristic signs are pain to lateral pressure over the spinous process and posterior articular sensitivity on the same side as the crestal point.

Pain may be acute or chronic. Acute lumbago or dorsalgia of thoracolumbar junction origin or higher can be seen at all ages, but is most common in those over 40. Typically the patient does not assume an antalgic posture as in the lumbar spine with a lateral shift (lumbar scoliosis). There is, however, marked local contracture, stiffness, vertebral tenderness to pressure, and signs of an acute intervertebral disturbance, probably of diskogenic nature.[39] During attempted active motions there is severe pain on lateral flexion of the trunk and rotation to one side.[104]

Management is similar to that of the lumbar spine (see Chapter 20, The Lumbar Spine). Chronic involvement is most common. Treatment with mobilization techniques is usually successful. Therapeutic exercise is usually of little value and may frequently be irritating in this form of low back pain.

☐ Thoracic Derangement Syndrome of McKenzie

According to McKenzie,[116] derangements occur in the thoracic spine, but apart from radiating pains there is little remarkable to differentiate between them. The pain of derangement is thought to be produced by displacement or altered position of joint structures, resulting in mechanical deformation of pain-sensitive tissues. Change within the joint may prevent the joint surfaces from moving normally, resulting in altered movement patterns.

McKenzie argues that the derangement syndrome is usually caused by a mechanical disturbance of the intervertebral disk.[116] He has divided these into posterior disk and anterior disk derangements because the clinical presentations suggest that one or the other part of the disk is involved. Anterior derangement is rare in the thoracic spine, with perhaps one case having been identified.[140] The mechanism of posterior derangement may be similar to that demonstrated by Adams and Hutton.[1]

The following derangement patterns are seen in the thoracic spine, but there are many variations and not all patients fit precisely into this listing. The classification is simplified to give a clear explanation of the principles.

- Derangement 1: Central or symmetrical pain between T1 and T12; rapidly reversible
- Derangement 2: Acute kyphosis; rare, usually the result of trauma or serious pathology
- Derangement 3: Unilateral or asymmetrical pain across the thoracic region, with or without radiation around the chest wall; rapidly reversible

Diagnosis involves assessing the effect of posture and movement on the symptoms. Each problem is manifested differently, and more than one problem may be present in the same patient.

With respect to treatment, the patient with a derangement should be taught the postures and movements that will reduce the mechanical deformation of involved structures. In the thoracic spine, this typically involves static thoracic extension (in supine or prone lying) and thoracic rotation in sitting. Such exercises should be expected to reduce the severity or the extent of symptoms. The course of treatment must follow the normal physiological healing process. Full range of motion without the production of symptoms is the goal.

McKenzie[116] has also classified nonspecific thoracic spine pain into the postural and dysfunction syndrome. Described simply, postural pain appears eventually by the overstretching of normal tissue. Usually the postural syndrome is of insidious onset. Symptoms are time-dependent, and range of motion is within normal limits. The postural patient is taught how to maintain optimal alignment of spinal segments to avoid pain.

The pain of the dysfunction syndrome is thought to be caused by the stretching of adaptively shortened pain-sensitive soft tissues.[131] The pain of dysfunction is probably due to specific shortening or scarring of tissue rather than a general age-related loss of movement. The onset may be acute or insidious; symptoms may or may not be time-dependent. The patient usually complains of intermittent pain with increased pain on movement. Range of motion is limited in one or more directions. The dysfunction patient should be given exercises to elongate shortened tissues. Such exercises will be expected to produce end-range pain. The principles of treatment for this syndrome are based on the mechanism of tissue healing, and the response of soft tissue to the application of controlled forces.[3,4,50,60,135,175]

Back conditions due to mechanical deformation of soft-tissue structures do not respond to palliative treatment only. A comprehensive program, including posture and body mechanics instruction and specific individualized exercises, is vital to success. The reader should refer to McKenzie's textbook to plan a treatment program.[116] It is critical to determine the classification or syndrome.

☐ Thoracic Hypermobility Problems

Hypermobility is fairly uncommon but is as significant as hypomobility and more difficult to treat. Hypermobility of the thoracic segments usually results from postural and muscle imbalances, often at levels above restricted segment(s), or from trauma such as pulling, lifting, or reaching, resulting in ligament and capsular sprain.[110] Several signs and symptoms may alert the examiner to the presence of hypermobility and instability.

HISTORY

Typically the patient reports back pain on assuming a static position (such as sitting) and fatigue of the muscles as a result of their protective role. Movement brings temporary relief, signifying the presence of ligamentous insufficiency.[110,133] Paris[133] defines hypermobility as a range of motion somewhat in excess of that expected for that particular segment given the patient's age, body type, and activity status. Hypermobile joints are generally considered normal. However, complaints of "giving away" or "slipping out" and being able to "twist it back into position" are due to *instability*. The differences between hypermobility and instability should be detected during the physical examination.

ALIGNMENT

Efficient alignment allows for equal weight-bearing distribution throughout the spine. Functional tasks such as lifting and carrying objects reveal the position and use of the cervical, thoracic, and lumbar spine. Assess the segmental relation of these three areas and any changes that occur during functional activity.

An important objective assessment of the vertical alignment of the thoracic and lumbar spine is the *vertical compression test*.[24,152,153] This test, described by Johnson and Saliba,[77] provides kinesthetic feedback as to how weight is transferred through the spine to the base of support. With the patient standing in a comfortable, natural stance, the therapist applies vertical compression through the shoulders, feeling for any giving away or buckling in the spine (Fig. 19-4). The idea is to test the amount of "spring" the spine has under direct compression.[24] The patient should relate any increase or reproduction of symptoms. The examiner usually feels and may observe an instability at the level of dysfunction, and the patient often reports pressure or pain from the vertical compression in the same area.

Deviations such as an increased posterior angulation of the thoracic spine, increased lumbar lordosis, or anterior shear of the pelvis suggest instability and the prevention of efficient weight transfer through the spine.[54,75,133] According to Saliba and Johnson,[153] when the natural segmental relation of the three spinal curves is interrupted, the spine no longer efficiently transfers the weight to the pelvis, but concentrates the force of the vertical loading at the biomechanically altered segment. This concentration of force appears to facilitate a progressive breakdown of the

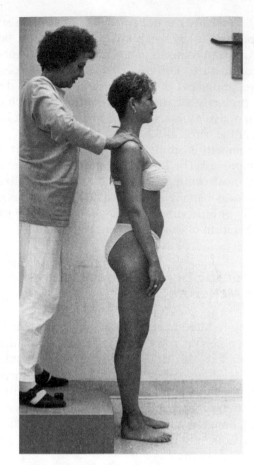

FIG. 19-4. Compression testing of the spine.

structural and neuromuscular stability at those segments.[133,147]

Wadsworth[167] describes another test for segmental vertebral instability particularly suited for the lower thoracolumbar spine. In this test the patient lies prone with the legs over the edge of the table and feet resting on the floor. If vertebral posterior-anterior glide applied by the therapist produces pain when the feet are supported by the floor and the paraspinal muscles are relaxed, but not when the legs are actively extended from the hips (bilateral hip extension) and the paraspinal muscles are contracted, the test is positive, implicating segmental instability.

During the objective examination, other signs that suggest hypermobility or instability of the lumbar spine, according to Paris,[133] and that would seem applicable to the middle and lower thoracic spine include:

1. During active forward-bending, one may observe (when standing at the patient's side) a sharply angulated segment suggesting hypermobility. If one also observes a "shake," "catch," or "hitch," then there is instability.

2. When examining the patient from behind during forward-bending, if the apophyseal joint is hypermobile, the vertebra will slide up more freely on that side, producing a sidebending to the opposite side at that level. Simultaneous uncoordinated muscle contraction or spasm suggests instability.

3. During standing, a hypertrophied band or hypertonic band of muscle may be evident. When palpated, it will show an increased tone or firmness to touch. If the tone is substantially reduced in prone lying, an instability exists, not a simpler hypermobility, according to Paris.[133]

4. Palpation for mobility using passive intervertebral motion has a satisfactory inter-rater reliability.[64] When performing these tests (forward-bending, side-bending, and rotation), the clinician may notice that movements feel "too free" or that there is a forward step or slip in forward-bending.

CONSERVATIVE TREATMENT

Treatment should be directed at decreasing the stresses on the unstable segment. The desired outcomes are to prevent worsening of instability and to reduce pain. The most harmful motion appears to be rotation, which produces both compression and shear.[54]

Physical therapy should include a program of stabilization techniques: isometric, abdominal, and back exercises, as well as localized techniques for the erector spinae muscles, with particular focus on the multifidi. The multifidi are the most influential in extension of small segments and in stabilizing the spine. Work should stress exercises done in midrange or beginning range and those directed at increasing endurance, strength, dynamic control, and sensitivity to stretch. Many of the stabilization programs for the cervical and lumbar spine are equally effective for the upper and lower thoracic spine respectively (see Chapter 17, The Cervical Spine, and Chapter 20, The Lumbar Spine). One should also include correction of neighboring hypomobility, support of the involved segment, postural re-education to reduce the strain, and diaphragmatic breathing exercises.

☐ Rib Conditions

Some painful thoracic or lumbar conditions are associated with small derangements of the costovertebral or costotransverse articulations. Typically they are due to trauma or an unguarded movement in rotation, such as turning too rapidly, or minimal motions such as reaching back to roll up the back window in a car.

There are also "anterior chondrocostal sprains," which are usually posttraumatic. According to Maigne,[104] costal sprains are common during judo, particularly at the level of the false ribs. Postural and muscle imbalances may also be a source of pain.

COSTAL SPRAINS

Most rib lesions are due to intercostal muscle spasms that diminish the normal expansion and contraction between the two ribs.[159] The most common cause is a sneeze or unexpected cough. These simple dysfunctions consist of restriction of excursion in either inhalation or exhalation and are commonly known as respiratory rib dysfunctions.[17,65] They are associated with hypertonus in the intercostal muscles above and below, and although they may not cause pain, the restriction of motion may cause a predisposition to recurrence of the spinal joint problem if not treated.

Costal sprains are expressed by thoracic or upper lumbar pain. Clinical examination does not reveal tenderness of the spine, but pain is produced by pressure on one rib only. The false ribs are usually involved.[104] The patient complains of a continuous soreness at the costovertebral angle that is aggravated by certain movements or positions. It may vary from a simple feeling of discomfort to pronounced chronic lumbar pain when the false ribs are involved.

A key test in the evaluation of costal sprain is the rib maneuver described by Maigne (see Fig. 19-27).[104] Whenever a rib lesion is suspected, the corresponding apophyseal joint must also be evaluated. Also, because ribs 1 to 7 articulate anteriorly with the sternum, the sternoclavicular and costochondral joints may also need to be assessed.

The course of costal sprain is good, with relief of pain in a few days. However, a costal sprain may become chronic, resulting in thoracic and lumbar pain, and this may be responsible for diagnostic error. Rib articulations are described later in this chapter. Mobilization is performed by articulating the rib in the nonpainful direction.[104]

HYPOMOBILITY AND HYPERMOBILITY DYSFUNCTIONS

The intercostal muscle may be irritated from a central source—that is, an intervertebral joint lesion may cause nerve irritation and muscle contraction, which leads to restricted rib mobility. This type of dysfunction is sometimes called a structural rib deformity.[17] Positional alterations become evident on palpation and may consist of alterations in *eversion* (the lower rib margin becomes more prominent) or *inversion* (reverse findings), lateral flexion, anteroposterior compression, lateral compression, and subluxation.[17,65,123,159]

FIRST RIB SYNDROME

Often considered a compression syndrome, this condition is characterized by local unilateral pain or tenderness over the supraspinous fossa and by constant referred pain, aching, or paresthesia in the C8 or T1 dermatomal distribution of the arm, forearm, or hand.[117] With involvement of the first rib only, the costotransverse joint may be subluxed superiorly by the pull of the scaleni. This is not uncommon and is often associated with dysfunction of either C7–T1 or T1–T2.[17] The vertebral joints should always be checked and treated first if they are dysfunctional. On palpation, unilateral posteroanterior pressure on the costotransverse joint and on the first rib (caudally) readily reproduce some or all of the symptoms. Functionally there may be hypertrophy or adaptive shortening of the scalenus anticus or medius muscles, with associated elevation, hypomobility, or subluxation of the first rib.

Other signs may include a forward head and protracted shoulders and restriction of the acromioclavicular and sternoclavicular joints. In addition to restricted myofascia of the scalenus anticus and medius, there may also be restriction in the pectoralis minor and major, trapezius, levator scapulae, and sternoclavicular muscles.[110]

Initially the palpation technique that elicits the symptoms is the method used for treatment. Manipulations of restricted joints, soft-tissue manipulation for tight muscles, and postural re-education are all beneficial. There is often associated cervical joint dysfunction, and this must be treated to avoid recurrence from tightness in the scalene muscles.

HYPOMOBILITY

In hypomobility dysfunctions of the ribs the patient often presents with a forward head and increased thoracic kyphosis. Pain is usually posterior at the costovertebral or costotransverse joint, with occasional reference of pain laterally into the chest wall. Diaphragmatic breathing and movements requiring rib cage excursion may be uncomfortable. Signs that may be present during evaluation include:[110]

1. An altered breathing pattern, avoiding diaphragmatic breathing
2. With an *inhalation restriction* the rib will not move upward during inspiration; with an *exhalation restriction* the rib will not descend.
3. On palpation, tenderness may be found involving

the costovertebral joint as well as an altered position of the rib.
4. Restriction of motion on testing

Treatment includes mobilization of the restricted segments, soft-tissue mobilizations, and stretching of the involved intercostal muscles, self-mobilization and stretching to increase rib cage excursion, and postural re-education.

HYPERMOBILITY

With hypermobility of the ribs, the patient complains of pain localized to the involved costal margin or costochondral area.[110] The pain is usually a dull ache but there may be sharp episodes. Pain may be intermittent, aggravated by activities involving rotation, such as twisting while bending forward. Clicking sounds may be present. Signs include:

1. Protective posture and shallow breathing
2. Tenderness to palpation of the costochondral junction
3. Excessive joint play motion or passive motion with spring tests
4. Tenderness of the costochondral junction

Treatment includes gentle stretching to the intercostal area to minimize soft-tissue changes resulting from protective postures, correction of any hypomobilities, and advice on body mechanics to decrease the strain to the area.

☐ Kyphosis

Kyphosis is most prevalent in the thoracic spine. There are four types of kyphotic deformities: localized, sharp, posterior angulation (a *gibbous*); dowager's hump, which results from postmenopausal osteoporosis; decreased pelvic inclination (20°) with a thoracolumbar or thoracic kyphosis (round back); and decreased pelvic inclination (20°) with a mobile spine (flat back).[51] The normal pelvic angle is 30° (Fig. 19-5).

Faulty posture, with excessive thoracic kyphosis and the protracted shoulder position that accompanies this, prevents the shoulder girdle joints from functioning normally. The internal rotators and serratus anterior shorten; the rhomboids and the lower trapezius lengthen. Adaptive anterior shortening of the glenohumeral capsule can result. Consequently, these patients develop restriction of movement of both shoulders as well as the upper thoracic spine.

Thoracolumbar kyphosis, due to a postural deficit, is classified as a *round back type I* or *type II*.[51] Patients with type I round back are not round-shouldered but are round-backed. Type I results from postural habits,

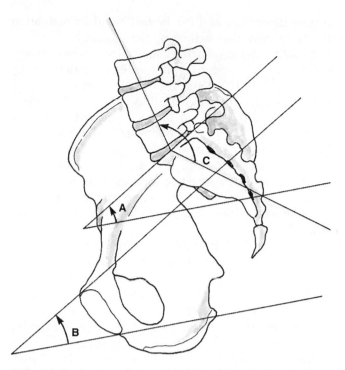

FIG. 19-5. *Angles of the pelvic joint: (**A**) sacral angle (normal = 30°); (**B**) pelvic angle (normal = 30°); (**C**) lumbosacral angle (normal = 140°). (Adapted from Magee DJ: Orthopaedic Physical Assessment, 2nd ed, p. 312. Philadelphia, WB Saunders, 1992.)*

type II from structural abnormalities. Often this is the presentation seen as a consequence of Scheuermann's disease (osteochondrosis in adolescence) and vertebra plana.[14,51] Scheuermann's disease frequently leads to an anterior wedging of the vertebra. This growth disorder affects about 10% of the population, and several vertebrae are usually affected. The most common area is between T10 and L2.[103] Regularly, with the dramatic and adverse changes of thoracic kyphosis, there is a parallel development of scoliosis.

Few conditions produce decreased kyphosis. Decrease or a reversal of the kyphosis of the interscapular thoracic spine (Pottenber's saucering) involves the T2 to T6 vertebra. The etiology of this flattened spine may be a congenital fixation of the thoracic spine.[51]

☐ Senile Kyphosis

This common condition is responsible for the round shoulders and forward carriage of the head associated with advancing age. It occurs in older patients of either sex and is associated with severe degeneration of the midthoracic intervertebral disks. The principal radiological changes involve the anterior part of these disks, with loss of disk space.[30]

Upper thoracic kyphosis (dowager's hump), with accompanying fluid retention, is common in postmenopausal women, men with heavy shoulders, and persons with poor postural sense. According to May,[110] the result is a loss of movement in the upper thoracic region, forcing hypermobility in the lower cervical spine, with tenderness and discomfort in the lower cervical spine aggravated by motion or sustained positions. Patients with dowager's hump at the cervicothoracic junction typically present with compensatory increased cervical lordosis and a forward head. They may also have an abnormally flat interscapular region, which is either very stiff or exceptionally irritable on palpation.[14] When this exists, the patient presents with various symptoms including localized upper thoracic, shoulder, cervical, and arm pain.

Senile kyphosis and upper thoracic kyphosis are usually asymptomatic, but some patients present with severe, aching pain that has been present for many years, is worse after activity, disturbs sleep, and tends to be episodic and difficult to control effectively with analgesics.[30]

Pain relief is difficult. Use of a brace, analgesics, exercise, postural control, stretching to the intercostal area, and mobilization techniques may provide temporary or partial relief of symptoms.

☐ Osteoporosis

Osteoporosis frequently is associated with senile kyphosis or upper thoracic kyphosis in postmenopausal women. As a consequence of calcium deficiency, bones weaken; in the spine this causes thinning and wedging of the vertebral bodies, placing the person at risk for fractures. Mayo Clinic research has demonstrated that extension exercises, performed regularly, significantly reduce the number of compression fractures in persons with this disorder (see Fig. 20-5A).[156,157] These studies demonstrated a significant correlation of the bone mineral density of the spine and the strength of back extensors with the patient's level of physical activity.

According to McKenzie,[116] the muscles strengthened by performing the exercises recommended by these Mayo Clinic studies are also the muscles responsible for maintaining the upright posture. Maintaining good posture may assist in the strengthening process and reduce the likelihood of small compression fractures.

Use caution when prescribing an exercise program for the patient with spinal osteoporosis. Not all types of exercise are appropriate for these patients because of the fragility of their vertebrae. Exercises that place flexion forces on the vertebrae tend to cause vertebral fractures in these patients. Isometric abdominal strengthening exercises seem more appropriate than flexion exercises.[156,157]

McKenzie[116] recommends that extension exercises should be performed from perhaps the age of 40 for the rest of the patient's life. He recommends prone extension with pillows under the abdomen and the hands clasped behind the back. The patient lifts the head, shoulders, and legs simultaneously as high as possible. This position is held for a second, then the patient relaxes. The exercise is repeated as many times as possible; repetitions are increased until at least 15 to 20 are done in each session. In patients with severe osteoporosis the Mayo Clinic recommends extension exercises in sitting to minimize pain.[157]

☐ Postural Disorders

Muscle pain may be felt without any underlying lesion of the cervical or thoracic joints and is related to postural changes. The patient is typically a woman who complains of stiffness and tenderness of the muscle groups related to the shoulder girdle and thorax. Frequently the patient has a sedentary occupation and in general lacks physical fitness. In addition to upper back pain, the patient often describes pain in the cervical and lumbar region. The pain usually worsens as the day goes on, and the patient is often conscious that it may be related to postural activities such as sitting for prolonged periods, typing, or other forms of continuous use. Writers, musicians, dentists, and computer programmers are all common victims. Pain may be aggravated by fatigue or stress or sometimes by changes in the weather.[30] This same pain pattern has been described in women with a postural sagging of the shoulder girdles or in those with large, pendulous breasts.

Treatment of these postural disorders involves simple measures such as reassurance, prophylactic advice, correction of sitting, standing, and sleeping postures, muscle-bracing exercises, and relief positions (*i.e.*, upper back stretch), Brugger's relief positions, and special chairs (*i.e.*, chairs with the seat tilted forward and a knee rest; a proper chair enforces lumbar lordosis and thus automatically achieves positional relief), as well as advice regarding problems peculiar to his or her occupation.[25] Changing posture or position is a form of exercise; proprioceptive neural circuits are directly involved.[115,138]

Numerous clinicians have written extensively on exercise programs for postural correction. The principles proposed by Kendall and coworkers[83] and Sahrmann[148–150] are most beneficial. The number of soft-tissue treatment options is almost infinite. Muscle length can be restored with stretching techniques. Stretching can be specific for certain muscles or for

certain directions, and can be facilitated by activating the antagonist, then activating the agonist.[2,52,92,155]

Assistive devices such as specialized taping procedures can be used to apply external tension (Fig. 19-6).[112,122,150] This tension can be corrective, guiding the soft tissues into a new position and thereby relieving stress on overloaded or overstretched tissues or applying a low-level stretch to restricted tissues, or by both.[122] Tension can also serve as a simple behavior reminder, regularly cuing the patient to assume a better position. Other assistive devices include posture-correction braces or a good support bra with crisscross back straps or large back and shoulder straps.[83,150]

Posture should be addressed from a static viewpoint and more importantly from a dynamic one. Most of these clients, as well as others with thoracic dysfunction, especially with thoracic osteoporosis, will benefit from movement therapies intended to correct inefficient movement patterns (*e.g.*, the Alexander technique,[5,11,25,62,78] the Feldenkrais method,[55–57,146] Aston patterning,[8,100,121,141] Klein-Vogelbach's Func-

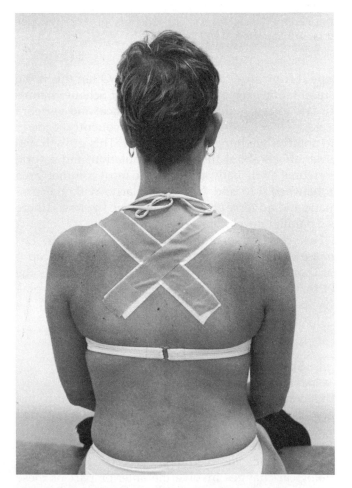

FIG. 19-6. Taping for postural correction and reeducation.

tional   Kinetics,[90,91]   and   Trager's   Mentastics,[80,163,172–174] which take the form of neuromuscular re-education).

THORACIC SPINE EVALUATION

☐ Clinical Considerations

Dysfunction of the joints of the thoracic spine is common in people with stresses and strains due to poor posture and heavy lifting. The costovertebral joints are unique to the thoracic spine. Together with the apophyseal joints, they can present with well-localized pain close to the midline or with referred pain often quite distal to the spine. The major symptoms may appear to have no relation to the thoracic spine.

Clinical features to be considered in the evaluation include the following:[84,128]

1. Pain of lower cervical origin (C4 to C7) may be referred to the upper thoracic region. The lower cervical spine must be included in the evaluation of the upper thoracic spine, because the movement of one occurs in conjunction with the other.
2. The upper thoracic spine (T1 to T4) is the stiffest part of the spine. Pain is usually well localized.
3. The midthoracic spine (T5 to T7) is the most common site for apophyseal joint pain. T8 to T10 is the most common site for rib cage articulation problems and for referred pain mimicking visceral pain.
4. Pain of the thoracolumbar region (T11 to L1) is common. Pain can be referred to the lumbar region, especially the iliac crests. T11–T12 is the most common level for thoracic disk lesions.

THORACIC DISK LESIONS

Thoracic disk lesions in this region are less common than those of the cervical and lumbar spine. The clinical history often reveals an axial compression of the trunk, as occurs in a fall on the hindquarter or lifting a heavy object in the forward-bent position. The mode of onset is various: it can be sudden, or a posterior thoracic backache can come on slowly. As at other spinal levels, the mechanism of dural pain may be present, giving rise to unilateral extrasegmental reference of pain in the presence of a central protrusion (see Fig. 19-2). Alternatively, a posterolateral displacement produces root pain referred anteriorly. At T1 and T2 symptoms may be felt in the arm; at lower levels symptoms are experienced at the side or front of the trunk (Fig. 19-7). The dermatomal pain pattern should act as a guide only, because dermatomes overlap and there are variations between patients.

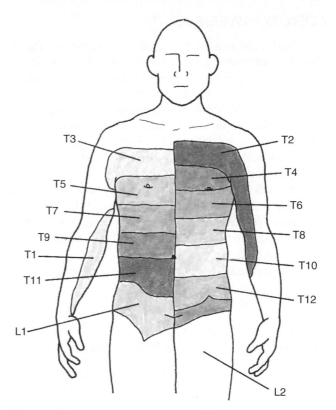

FIG. 19-7. The cutaneous dermatomes (areas) supplied by the thoracic nerve roots. (Adapted from Williams P, Warwick R [eds]: Gray's Anatomy, 36th British ed. New York, Churchill Livingstone, 1980.)

THORACIC PAIN OF LOWER CERVICAL ORIGIN

The clinical association between injury to the lower cervical region and upper thoracic pain is well known.[106] The T2 dermatome, which is in close proximity to the C4 dermatome, appears to represent the cutaneous areas of the lower cervical segments, as the posterior primary rami of C5 to C8. This is why patients present with interscapular pain following cervical spine injury. Such pain may have no connection with dysfunction of the thoracic spine, but instead represents injury to the lower cervical spine (which because of an apparent anomalous dermatome pattern refers pain to the interscapular region, usually corresponding to the T5 and T6 region). The scapula originates as part of the developing limb bud (see Chapter 1, Embryology of the Musculoskeletal System). As the limb develops, the scapula migrates to become folded back on the posterior thoracic wall. This is why the scapula, although it lies level with the thoracic segments, is innervated primarily by cervical segments. Thus, pain of cervical origin is often referred to the scapulae, as well as to the arms. The pain from the lower cervical spine can also refer to the anterior chest and mimic coronary ischemic pain.

COSTOTRANSVERSE JOINTS

So-called costotransverse joint syndrome is due to arthrosis of these joints. Symptoms develop either spontaneously or when there has been an extenuation of these joints, as after a rib fracture. According to Hohmann,[73] the clinical symptoms include pain on forced and deep breathing that radiates along the ribs, a "whooping" feeling, and a sudden lightening-like pain that makes breathing difficult and may give a feeling of constriction.

Dysfunction of this joint commonly causes localized pain about 3 to 4 cm from the midline, where the ribs articulate.[84] It may also be responsible for referred pain ranging from the midline, posterior to the lateral chest wall, and even the anterior chest wall. Diagnosis may be confirmed when movement of the rib provokes the pain at the costovertebral joint.

LOWER THORACIC SPINE AND THORACOLUMBAR JUNCTION

Dysfunction of joints in the thoracolumbar region can cause pain presenting primarily as iliac crest or buttock pain.[106] The skin over the iliac crest and upper outer buttock area is supplied by the posterior primary rami of nerves arising from the thoracolumbar junction (T12 and L1) (Fig. 19-8A,B). Similarly, anterior groin pain can arise from this region, as the nerve supply is from the anterior rami of the spinal nerves T12 and L1 (Fig. 19-8A).[106] Because dermatomal symptoms can be present in either the posterior or anterior branches of the dorsal rami, with anterior abdominal symptoms the thoracic spine must be palpated.

MUSCLE PAIN

Muscle pain may also be experienced with no underlying lesion of the cervical or thoracic joints, and this is often related to postural changes of the thoracic spine.[30] Muscle injury occurs more often in the thoracic region than the cervical or lumbar regions.[33] The strong paravertebral muscles do not appear to be a cause of chest pain, but strains of the intercostal, pectoral, and latissimus dorsi muscles, as well as the musculotendinous origins of the abdominals, can cause pain. Injuries to these muscles can be provoked by overstrains or attacks of violent coughing or sneezing.

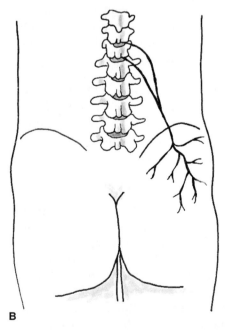

FIG. 19-8. (A) Spinal nerves T12 and L1: 1, anterior branch, 2, posterior branch, 3, lateral branch. **(B)** Cutaneous innervation of the upper portion of the gluteal area (T11–T12 to L1) according to Maigne (1980). (Adapted from Rogoff JB [ed]: Manipulation, Traction and Massage, 2nd ed, p. 100. Baltimore, Williams & Wilkins, 1980.)

OTHER CAUSES OF THORACIC PAIN

Apart from vertebral dysfunction, there are many other causes of thoracic pain. Although posterior pain is often caused by vertebral dysfunction, there are several important visceral and vascular origins of this type of pain, some of which can be life-threatening. Features of the history that indicate the pain is arising from thoracic spine dysfunction include the following:[84]

1. Visceral disorders are not influenced by thoracic movements.
2. Aggravation and relief of pain on trunk rotation: the pain may be increased by rotating toward the side of pain but is eased by rotating in the opposite direction.
3. Aggravation and relief of pain on trunk side-flexion: typically flexion away from the painful side does not hurt, but flexion toward the painful side increases the pain. A neuroma on one side of the spine will painfully limit side-flexion away from that side.
4. Aggravation of pain by coughing, sneezing, or deep inspiration tends to implicate the costovertebral joint.
5. Pain is relieved by firm pressure over the back.

☐ Subjective Examination

A general approach to history-taking and the subjective examination is described in Chapter 5, Assessment of Musculoskeletal Disorders and Concepts of Management. The concepts there and in Chapter 20, The Lumbar Spine, all apply to the evaluation of the thoracic spine. One item peculiar to this area is the effect of breathing on the symptoms. Inspiration frequently causes pain; expiration does so far less commonly.[108] The history should include the chief complaints and a pain drawing (see Fig. 20-8). As with the lumbar spine, the Oswestry function test and McGill Pain Questionnaire are helpful in trying to objectify the quality of pain and its effect on function.[111,118]

When listening to the patient's history of pain, bear in mind the cervical spine, the costochondral articulations, and the scapulothoracic movement, as well as the obvious costovertebral and intervertebral joints. When the patient's symptoms refer to the legs, arms, head, or neck, assess these areas as well. Patience and care with assessment is extremely important, particularly when symptoms have both visceral and vertebral components.

☐ Physical Examination

OBSERVATION

Observe the patient's posture, body type (*i.e.*, ectomorphic, mesomorphic, endomorphic, or mixed), gait, and ability to move freely. A good time to observe the patient's general sitting posture is during the subjective examination. The patient will automatically choose the posture that he or she habitually assumes.

FUNCTIONAL ACTIVITIES

Assess whether spinal movements are free or restricted by watching the patient get in or out of a chair. Observe the position that he or she adopts while sitting and undressing. This can be done before undertaking a more formal inspection of bony structure and alignment.

INSPECTION

With the patient standing with the back, shoulders, and legs exposed, observe features such as the level of the pelvis and any disturbance of spinal curves. View the patient from the front, back, and sides. Record specific alterations in bony structure or alignment, soft-tissue configurations, and skin status.

BONY STRUCTURE AND ALIGNMENT

Refer to the section on assessment of structural alignment in Chapter 22, The Lumbosacral–Lower Limb Scan Examination, for a complete discussion of this part of the examination with respect to the lower thoracic spine. Observe the total body posture from the head to the toes and look for any deviations. Alterations in overall spinal posture may lead to problems in the thoracic spine. Look for kyphosis and scoliosis. Younger patients in particular should be screened for scoliosis.

I. **Posterior Alignment** (the patient is viewed from behind in the standing position)
   A. *Shoulder level:* Posteriorly the spine of the scapula should be level with the T3 spinous process. The inferior angle of the scapula is level with the T7 spinous process. The medial borders of the scapulae are parallel to the spine and about 5 cm lateral to the spinous processes.[103] A common sign of scoliosis is unequal shoulder levels and apparent winging of a scapula.
   B. *Spinal posture:* Look for scoliosis and the presence of a lateral shift.

1. *Lateral shift:* This is present if the shoulders and trunk have moved laterally in relation to the pelvis. It is described in terms of the direction of the shift of the shoulders and the upper trunk—that is, if they have moved to the left it is described as a left lateral shift. When it is present and symptomatic it often indicates a derangement, usually of the lumbar spine.[46,114]

2. *Scoliosis:* In this deformity there are one or more lateral curves of the lumbar or thoracic spine (Fig. 19-9). It is gauged from the line of the spinous processes and described with respect to the convexity of the curve. Scoliosis may be structural or nonstructural and compensated (Fig. 19-9*A*) or uncompensated (see Fig. 19-9*B*). A structural scoliosis does not straighten during forward-bending or sidebending into the convexity of the spine. Because lateral bending is always accompanied by rotation, there will be a lumbar bulge or rib hump (gibbous) with forward-bending if a structural scoliosis is present (Fig. 19-9*C*). The criteria for screening, evaluation, and diagnosis and a review of nonoperative methods of treatment are covered extensively in the literature.[9,10,21,29,53,58,59,82,83,86,88,125,145,166,169,170]

   a. A *functional scoliosis* can be caused by muscle imbalance, poor posture, or a leg-length discrepancy. This type of scoliosis generally straightens on forward-bending and sidebending into the convexity, except in the presence of muscle spasm or guarding.

   b. *Acute scoliosis:* Facet joint impingement may cause an acute scoliosis in any area of the spine. This disorder involves the entrapment of soft tissue within the facet joint.[126,154] If this happens, the patient may shift to the opposite side of impingement to take the weight off the painful structure. A more common type of lateral curve is the lateral shift or protective scoliosis (see above).[114]

3. *Rib cage:* Have the patient cross the forearms in front of the body. Posteriorly, inspect for rib asymmetry and carriage of the scapulae. Palpate for rib prominence by a flat-handed sweep over the posterolateral surface of the hemithorax.

4. *Sacral base and leg length:* Inspect for the presence of segmental vertical asymmetries. See Chapter 22, The Lumbosacral–Lower Limb Scan Examination.

II. **Anterior Alignment** (the patient is viewed from the front)

   A. *Shoulders:* Common faults include dropped or elevated shoulders. Note any clavicular, sternoclavicular, or acromioclavicular joint asymmetry.

   B. *Rib cage:* Inspect for rib cage deformities such as pigeon chest (pectus carinatum), funnel chest (pectus excavatum), or barrel chest (Fig. 19-10). Note any increase or decrease in the infrasternal angle (more or less than 90°). See the section on soft-tissue inspection below.

III. **Sagittal Alignment** (the patient is viewed from the side; obvious abnormalities or asymmetries of the extremities and spine are noted)

   A. *Cervical spine:* Does the head deviate from the optimal posture (4 to 8 cm) from the apex of the thoracic kyphosis to the deepest point in the cervical lordosis? (See Fig. 17-16.)[142]

   B. *Shoulders:* The acromion process often lies anterior to the plumb line; the scapulae are abducted and are associated with excessive kyphosis and forward head. Tightness of the pectoralis major and minor, serratus anterior, and intercostal muscles is most often found.

   C. *Thoracic spine:* Note increased anteroposterior curves (*e.g.,* localized or generalized dowager's hump [osteoporosis causing excessive kyphosis in the C7 to T1 area]). Kyphosis may be generalized, with the back having a smooth, uniform contour, or it may be localized if it is due to a collapsed vertebra, as occurs in an older person with osteoporosis. In-

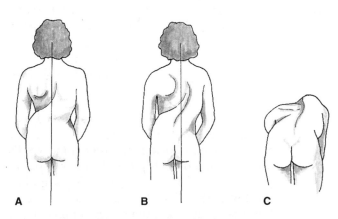

FIG. 19-9. Scoliosis: To distinguish between a compensated and an uncompensated deviation of the posture, a plumb line is dropped from the first thoracic spinal process. **A** indicates a compensated right thoracic–lumbar curve, and **B** an uncompensated right thoracic curve with a right list. (**C**) When viewed from behind, minor degrees of structural scoliosis can be detected in forward bending. A rotatory component produces a rib deformity or hump.

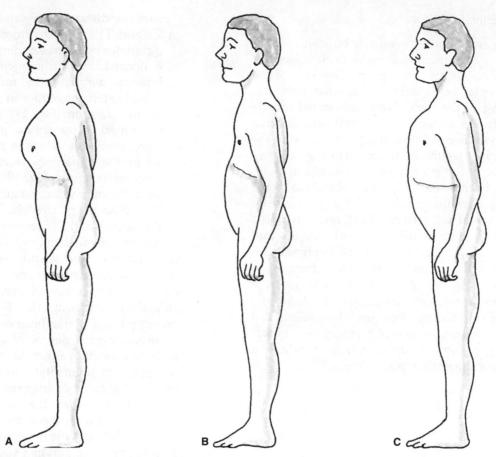

FIG. 19-10. Chest deformities: (**A**) pectus carinatum, (**B**) pectus excavatum, and (**C**) barrel chest.

creased posterior convexity (generalized kyphosis) may be due to tightness of the anterior longitudinal ligament and the upper abdominal and anterior chest muscles. Other muscle findings include stretched thoracic extensors, middle and lower trapezius, and posterior ligaments.

D. The *angle of minimum kyphosis* can be obtained by a 2-inclinometer measurement. Standing and sitting techniques, with the inclinometer at T1 and T12 and with the subject in the erect "military brace" posture, are used to obtain the angle of minimum kyphosis.[6]

E. *Chest and rib cage:* Note any depression of the anterior thorax and sternum (funnel chest), increased overall anteroposterior diameter of the rib cage (barrel chest), or projection of the sternum anteriorly and downward (pigeon chest).

F. *Lumbar spine:* Observe for an accentuated or reduced lordosis. Note whether the sacrovertebral or lumbosacral angle is normal (see Fig. 19-5).

IV. Transverse Rotary Alignment (the patient is viewed from the front and from behind. The stance width should be normal and the feet slightly [5° to 10°[pointed outward. Assess segmental rotatory alignment, working upward from the feet. See Chapter 22, The Lumbosacral–Lower Limb Scan Examination, for assessment of the lower limbs.)

A. *Anterior-superior iliac spines:* These should be positioned in a frontal plane. If the pelvis is rotated (one iliac spine is more anterior then the other) the common causes to be considered are:

1. A fixed (structural) spinal scoliosis, the rotatory component of which is transmitted the pelvis through the sacrum via the lumbar spine

2. Torsional asymmetry of the sacroiliac joints.

B. *Rib cage:* Note whether the ribs are symmetrical and whether the rib contours are normal and equal on both sides. The contours should both be positioned in a frontal plane. In scoliosis the ribs are pushed posteriorly and the thoracic cage is narrowed on the convex side of the curve; the ribs on the concave side move anteriorly.

SOFT-TISSUE INSPECTION

Note obvious asymmetries in muscle bulk and prominence of the trapezius on one side. Seek regions of muscle tightness and muscle spasm. One side of the erector spinae may be tighter than the other, with subsequent listing of the torso. Note abdominal muscle length (*i.e.*, rectus abdominis, internal and external obliques). According to Sahrmann,[150] shortness of the rectus abdominis results in anterior rib cage depression, shortness of the internal oblique results in an increase in the infrasternal angle, and shortness of the external oblique results in a decreased angle. If the internal and external obliques are short, one may find a long lumbar lordosis with paraspinal atrophy and a narrow infrasternal angle, or thoracic kyphosis with a depressed chest and a narrow infrasternal angle.

Observe the skin for any abnormality or scars. If there are scars, what were the causes? Look for any local swelling or cutaneous lesions such as café-au-lait spots, patches of hair, or areas of pigmentation, or any abnormal depressions. A tuft of hair may indicate a spina bifida occulta or diastematomyelia.[109]

SELECTIVE TISSUE TENSION: ACTIVE MOVEMENTS

I. Active Physiological Movements of the Spine

Since the lumbar and thoracic spine form part of a continuous coordinated motion pattern, they are assessed together. With all movements, determine the range, rhythm, and quality of active movement. Note any localized restriction of movement and any protective deformity, muscle guarding, or painful arc of motion. Note whether the patient's symptoms are reproduced. Not every movement listed below is needed for every patient.

First test the patient while standing. Have him or her extend and laterally flex the spine. This is followed by flexion and rotation.

II. Standing Tests

A. *Extension* (backward-bending). After observing the global range of motion from the side, kneel behind the patient and while supporting his or her pelvis ask the patient to extend again while observing the thoracic extension. Ask the patient to bend the head, shoulders, middle back, and lower back sequentially.

1. The thoracic curve should flow backward or at least straighten in a smooth, even manner. If the patient shows excessive kyphosis, this curvature will remain on extension.

2. Thoracic spine extension is normally 25° to 45°. A tape measure may be used to measure the distance between two points (the C7 and T12 spinous processes). A 2.5-cm difference between standing and extension is normal.[51,103] Inclinometry and spondylometry may also be used to measure spinal extension, either in standing or the sphinx position (Fig. 19-11).[41,63] The values found in the sphinx position may be compared with values in minimal kyphosis or the military posture (in standing). This method (see Fig. 19-11) can also be used for measuring extension of the lumbar spine by placing the inclinometer at the sacrum and T12 respectively.

B. *Lateral flexion* (sidebending): Have the patient sidebend the head, shoulders, middle back, and lower back, first to one side and then to the other. Symmetry of movement may be judged by comparing the distance from the fingertip to the fibular head on either side and by observing the degree of spinal curvature with movement in either direction. Assess the continuity of segmental movement and look for any tightness or hypermobility at a specific segment when the movement is performed. Lateral flexion is the best movement with which to test the hypomobile lesion.

1. Bilateral limitation in a young person suggests serious disease but in the elderly person may be attributed to no more than decreased mobility with the passage of time.[33]

2. With multisegmental capsular restriction, sidebending is restricted in both directions.

3. Lateral flexion is about 20° to 40°. Some observers measure lateral flexion by measuring the distance between the fingers and knee, or between the fingers and the floor. A more objective method devised by Moll (Fig. 19-12)[124] involves placing two ink marks on the skin of the lateral trunk. The upper mark is placed at a point where a horizontal line through the xiphosternum crosses the coronal line. The lower mark is drawn at the highest point on the iliac crest. The distance between the two marks is measured in centimeters using a tape measure first with the patient standing erect, and again after full lateral flexion. The new distance between the two marks is measured and subtracted from the first measurement. The remainder is taken as an index of lateral spinal mobility. Distraction on the contralateral trunk or approximation of the marks on the homolateral trunk may be used. Lateral spinal

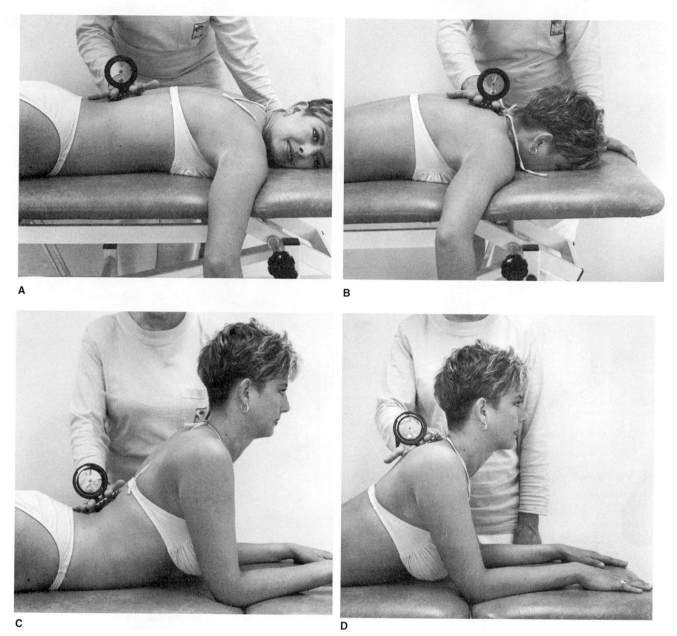

FIG. 19-11. Measuring extension of the thoracic spine in the Sphinx position. In prone (**A**), the inclinometer is placed over T12 and set at zero. (**B**) The inclinometer is then moved to T1 and the degrees of neutral kyphosis are read. The patient then assumes the Sphinx position (**C**); the inclinometer is moved to T12 and set at zero. (**D**) The inclinometer is then moved to T1 and the degrees are read on the dial. The values taken in the Sphinx position are subtracted from the values in neutral kyphosis to determine true extension motion.

movement may also be measured with an inclinometer.[6,63,98]

C. *Flexion* (forward-bending): Have the patient bend the head and cervical spine forward, then the thoracic spine, and finally the lumbar spine. Have the patient repeat the motion with the eyes closed. Assess the general and specific mobility of the spine. Ask the patient if he or she is experiencing any pain, stiffness, or other symptoms with the movement.

1. Note whether the patient drifts to the left or right instead of bending straight forward. If this is found, it indicates unilateral hypomobility of the apophyseal joint(s), unilateral muscular tightness, or a posterolateral disk protrusion. Drift can often be more readily seen when patients close their eyes, because it is natural for patients to fix their eyes to the floor and guide themselves straight down, thus overriding the tendency to drift laterally.

2. Note whether the thoracic spine shows in-

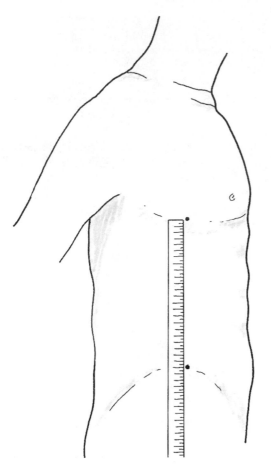

FIG. 19-12. Measuring thoracolumbar lateral flexion with a tape measure.

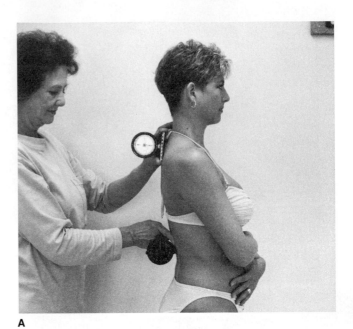

A

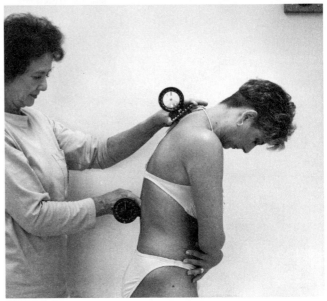

B

creased kyphosis or any evidence of a structural scoliosis. With a nonstructural scoliosis, the scoliotic curve will disappear on forward-flexion, but with a structural scoliosis it will remain.

3. Flexion may be measured with a tape measure as the distance the fingertips reach from the floor or as the distance from C7 to T12, with the patient in the erect position and then again in maximum forward-bending. However, it is more important to observe the relative movement of the spinous processes and to record any loss of range. Other objective clinical methods include the use of the spondylometer and inclinometer.[6,7,41,63] The normal range of motion is 20° to 45°. The inclinometer may also be used to assess segmental lateral flexion and flexion (Fig. 19-13) of the spine.[63]

D. *Rotation in standing:* Have the patient bend forward to 45° with the hands folded across the chest and the feet together. The patient then rotates fully to the right and left while the exam-

FIG. 19-13. Testing flexion with an inclinometer. (**A**) One inclinometer is placed in the sagittal plane at the T1 level and the other at the T12 level. Both instruments are zeroed. (**B**) The thoracic spine is flexed forward so as not to involve the lumbar spine. Both instruments' readings are recorded. The T12 value is subtracted from the T1 value to arrive at the thoracic flexion angle.

iner observes the amount of rotation and compares one side to the other. When the two-inclinometer method is used, one inclinometer is placed at the T1 level in the coronal plane and the other at the T12 level. Restrained active rotation of the thoracic spine of 20° or less is an impairment of the function of the thoracic spine in the activities of daily living.[51] Rotation in standing can also be tested in the fully erect position with or without the help of outstretched arms or folded arms. Such rotation is more likely to include detectable movement of the lower thoracic spine.

Rotation should be further tested with the patient seated and the trunk alternatively in flexion and then extension (see below).

III. Sitting Tests

Overpressure can easily be applied in this position and may be necessary to reproduce the pain. Note the range of each of these movements, whether symptoms are reproduced, any disturbance in normal synchronous rhythm, and the presence of muscle spasm.

A. *Rotation:* Rotation of the thoracic spine is the key movement that requires scrutiny on examination. According to Cyriax,[33] the movement most likely to hurt with a disk lesion is the extreme of passive rotation. In a minor protrusion this may be the only painful movement.

  1. With the patient's arms folded across the chest, active rotation can be tested in the erect or extended position. This can then be compared with the same rotation in the flexed position.

  2. In the erect position the patient can usually rotate about 60° to 70°. Pavelka[134] devised a simple objective clinical method to measure thoracolumbar rotation with a tape measure (Fig. 19-14).

  3. Rotation with passive overpressure (Fig. 19-15). Fix the patient's pelvis by stabilizing his or her knees with your own knees. Have the patient cross the arms with the hands resting on opposite shoulders and actively rotate, or the examiner may move the trunk passively toward end range (patient's arms at side). Apply gentle overpressure by placing a hand on each shoulder and applying further pressure or small oscillatory movements at the end of the painless range in each direction. Note not only the end range but also the end feel of the movement. A normal end feel is springy or elastic; an abnormal end feel is usually that of a firm, hard stop.

B. *Auxiliary tests:* If the above movements do not reproduce the patient's pain, auxiliary tests that may do so include:

  1. Performing the test movements repeatedly and at increasing speeds in erect sitting (*i.e.*, flexion, extension, and rotation)

  2. Applying sustained pressure at the limit of the range of relevant movements

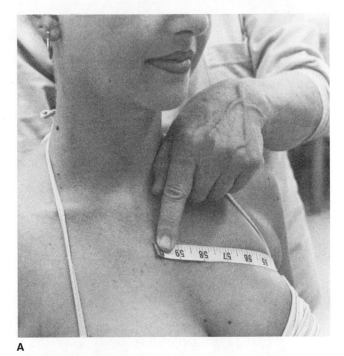

A

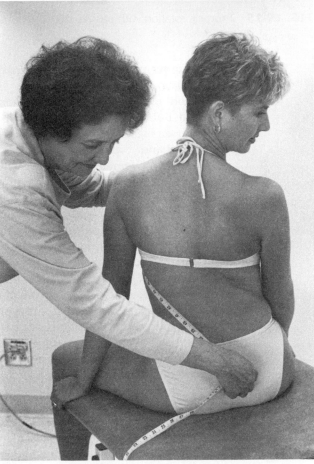

B

FIG. 19-14. Measurements of thoracolumbar rotation in sitting with a tape measure are made over the spinous process of L5 and over the jugular notch. Using a tape measure, the distance between these two points is recorded before (**A**) and after (**B**) full trunk rotation.

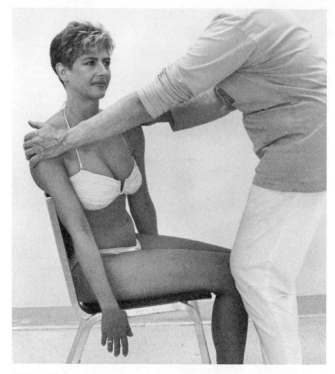

FIG. 19-15. Thoracic rotation with passive over-pressure.

3. Combined movement tests involving many sequences of combined movements, as well as combined motions with compression, can be used, but they are beyond the scope of this text (see Figs. 20-9 to 20-12). See the works of Maitland[108] and Edwards.[44,45]

4. Cervical spine movements should always be tested to exclude pain referred from the lower cervical spine. Cervical flexion may exacerbate any thoracic pain, even if pain arises from the thoracic spine.[30] It helps to keep the thoracic spine immobile to determine whether the cervical spine is responsible for the pain. One way to achieve this, according to McKenzie,[116] is to have the patient sit unsupported in the slump position while active cervical motions are carried out. If the patient's thoracic symptoms are altered in this position, they probably arise from the cervical spine.

5. With the patient sitting, examine the upper limbs in a cursory fashion to determine if they are free of symptoms. Elevating the arms extends the thoracic spine. Try to clarify the effect of neck and arm movements on the thoracic spine. Tightness of the latissimus dorsi muscles and the thoracolumbar fascia will prevent full shoulder joint flexion and flatten the lumbar lordosis.

C. *Active physiological (segmental) mobility testing:* A useful test of vertebral motion and restriction is to monitor changes in the relation of individual segments during active forward- and backward-bending (Fig. 19-16).[65,96] Standing behind the seated patient, palpate the transverse processes (with the thumbs) at individual levels while having the patient either flex forward or extend. Note the cranial/caudal displacement of the transverse processes. Asymmetry may indicate dysfunction.

IV. **Rib Motion and Thoracic Excursion**

General mobility of the ribs can be observed by watching the respiratory range anteriorly and posteriorly with the patient sitting. Note whether expansion is mainly costal or diaphragmatic and if there is a painful phase of inspiration.

A. *Evaluation of thoracic excursion during inspiration and exhalation:* Have the patient maximally inhale and exhale. Excursion of both the

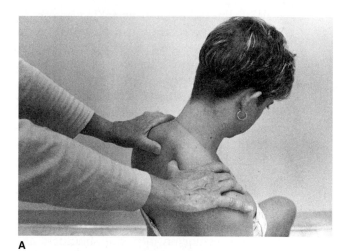

A

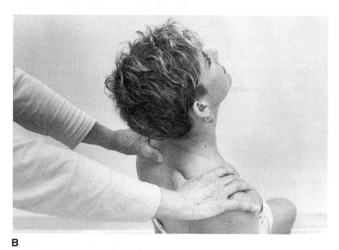

B

FIG. 19-16. Active (segmental) physiological mobility testing of (**A**) forward and (**B**) backward bending.

upper and lower halves of the thorax is evaluated by placing the thumbs along the midline of the trunk (posterior and anterior aspect) with the hands embracing the thoracic cage. Note the amount of excursion and asymmetrical movements. Possible findings include decreased thoracic excursion in the presence of various pulmonary diseases, such as ankylosing spondylitis and scoliosis, or pronounced abdominal breathing, which is almost always associated with decreased thoracic excursion.[42]

B. *Active physiological mobility testing* (specific articular mobility [individual rib motion testing during respiration])

1. With the patient prone, palpate the ribs just lateral to the tubercle and medial to the rib angle during full inspiration and expiration. Note the quantity and quality of motion. Repeat this test for each rib. Compare the sides.

2. With the patient supine, starting on the cranial aspect of the ribs at the sternocostal junction, palpate for rib excursion during full inspiration and expiration. Note the quantity and quality of motion. Repeat this test for each rib. Compare the sides and note any asymmetry.

3. With the patient supine and during full inspiration and expiration, palpate (with the index fingers) the lateral aspect of the ribs in the midaxillary line. Possible findings include decreased rib motion, either regionally or segmentally, or asymmetry, indicating possible dysfunction.

V. Chest Expansion (Costovertebral Expansion)
Rigidity of the thoracic cage is characteristic of spinal and chest disorders and of the late stages of ankylosing spondylitis. An expansion of 3 cm at T4 level is considered within the lower limits of normal.[124] The patient should be sitting with the hands on the head and the arms flexed in the sagittal plane to prevent maximum contraction of the shoulder adductors. Measure the circumference at rest and during maximum expiration and inspiration at the fourth rib level. Measurements may also be taken at the ninth rib level (three finger-widths below the xiphoid) and subcostally (level of the umbilicus). Record measurements taken at rest, during inspiration, and during expiration. Subtract the smaller figure (expiration) from the larger (inspiration). When the subcostal measurement is greater on expiration and less on inspiration, the results should be recorded as minus.

SELECTIVE TISSUE TENSION: PASSIVE MOVEMENTS

The passive movements that should be tested include the compression test of the spine,[24,153] static postures,[116] passive physiological movements including segmental palpation (feeling movement between the adjacent spinous processes or ribs), and segmental mobility (accessory movements) of the spine.

I. Compression Testing
In deviations, such as increased lordosis, posterior angulation of the thoracic spine, or anterior shear of the pelvis, or in regions of instability, efficient weight transfer through the spine is prevented. A useful objective assessment of the patient's vertical alignment and determination of a biomechanically altered segment is the vertical compression test.[24,77,152] Have the patient stand in a comfortable, natural stance. Apply vertical compression through the shoulders, feeling and observing for any give or buckling in the spine (see Fig. 19-4). Generally, patients with accentuated curvatures have an increased springiness, indicating decreased lever arms for the effects of gravity and increased stress on the myofascial structures.[24] The spines of patients with decreased curvatures do not have enough spring, leading to decreased shock attenuation. Have the patient relate any increase or reproduction of symptoms. In the presence of postural deviations, the examiner usually feels an instability at the level of the dysfunction, and the patient may report an increase in symptoms.

II. Static Postures
When thoracic pain is of postural origin, many of the auxiliary tests above will not provoke pain. In such cases, according to McKenzie,[116] the structures must be loaded for a prolonged time before deformation is sufficient to reproduce the pain. Each position is held for no more than 3 minutes, and the effects are recorded. The test postures include:

A. Static flexion in sitting (slouched with the back totally rounded). The totally flexed position is most often responsible for the production of mechanical thoracic pain.

B. Lying prone, with the lower thoracic spine fully extended and the weight supported on the hands (Fig. 19-17). The patient allows the lower thoracic spine and pelvic girdle to sag into the treatment table. This position extends the thoracic spine from about T4–T5 to L1.

C. Lying supine in extension, which extends the thoracic spine from about T1 to T4–T5. The

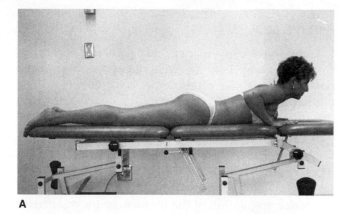

A

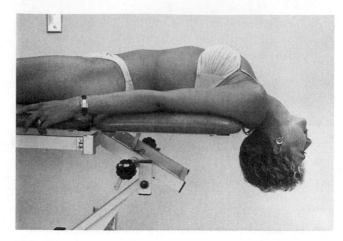

FIG. 19-18. Supine lying upper thoracic extension.

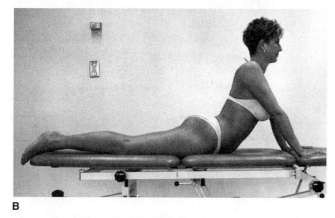

B

FIG. 19-17. Prone lying thoracolumbar extension: (**A**) starting position; (**B**) end position.

patient lies supine over the end of the table so that the head, neck, and shoulders are unsupported down to the level of T4. With the support of one hand the head is lowered until the neck and upper back are fully extended (Fig. 19-18). If the test is impossible in supine, it can be performed in prone on the elbows with cervical extension.

III. Passive Physiological Movements of the Spine
Passive motion is done with palpation to appreciate the movement of each segment. Palpate between the spinous processes and compare the movement obtained at each level. The chief movements of the T4 to T12 region are forward- and backward-bending. Sidebending and rotation are limited by the ribs. Rotation occurs mostly at the lower thoracic and upper lumbar spine.

A. C7 to T4 passive motion of flexion (forward-bending), extension (backward-bending), lateral flexion (sidebending), and rotation at individual segments. Standing at the side of the seated patient, place your middle finger over the spinous process of the vertebra being tested and the index and ring fingers between the spinous processes of the two adjacent vertebrae. Place your other hand on the patient's

head or forehead, and introduce flexion and extension (passive movement) to this area (Fig. 19-19*A,B*). Then introduce passive lateral flexion and rotation (Fig. 19-19*C,D*). With each motion component introduced, evaluate the movement by assessing its quality, paying particular attention to the coupled movements and determining whether the movement is hypermobile or hypomobile relative to the adjacent vertebrae.

Findings: Asymmetrical movement, abnormal coupling patterns, and hypomobility or hypermobility may indicate pathology. According to Dvořák,[42] pain with movement, especially in the cervicothoracic junction and during extension, may be due to a segmental somatic dysfunction—that is, impaired or altered function of related components of the somatic system, such as skeletal, arthrodial, and myofascial structures, as well as related vascular, lymphatic, and neural elements.[17]

B. T4 to T12 passive motion testing of flexion and extension. The patient sits with the fingers clasped behind the neck and the elbows together in front. Via the patient's hands or arms, introduce passive flexion and extension (Fig. 19-20) while palpating over the spinous processes as previously described. Pay attention to the gliding motion of the thoracic spinous processes in relation to each other.

Findings: The spinous processes do not separate during flexion, do not approximate during extension, or both. Two or more segments are usually involved. Typically this is due to joint dysfunction secondary to degenerative joint disease. In young people it may be related to Scheuermann's disease.

C. T4 to T12 passive motion testing of lateral flexion (sidebending). The patient sits with

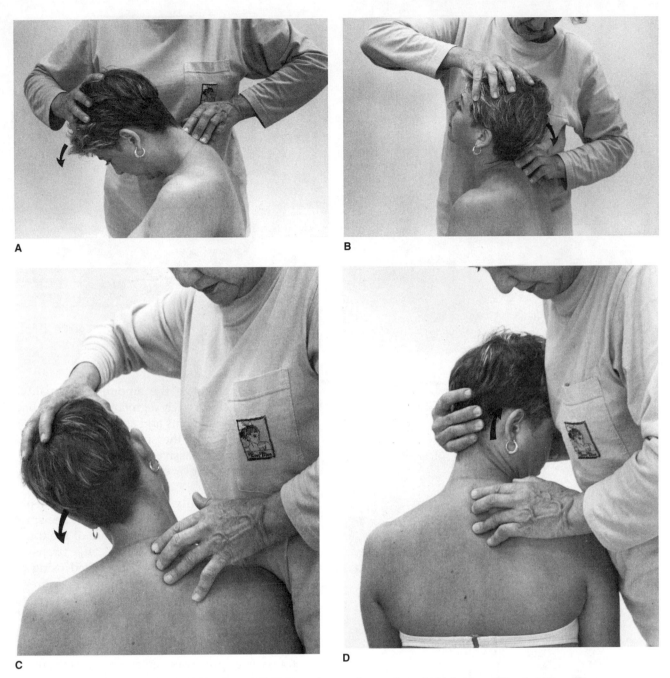

FIG. 19-19. Upper thoracic (C7–T4) passive motion testing of (**A**) flexion, (**B**) extension, (**C**) lateral bending, and (**D**) rotation.

the hands clasped behind the neck and the elbows together in front. Reach across the front of the patient and place the stabilizing hand over the patient's shoulder. Use the fingers of the monitoring hand to palpate the spinous processes (Fig. 19-21). Use your chest to introduce sidebending movement or force against the patient's shoulder girdle, against which the patient rests. During normal passive sidebending, the spinous processes rotate to the same side (toward the side of the convex-

ity of the thoracic spine).[42] Compare movement at the various levels.

Findings: A segmental dysfunction may be suspected when the spinous processes do not exhibit coupled rotation with induced lateral flexion.[42]

D. T4 to T12 motion testing of rotation. The patient sits astride the plinth with arms clasped behind the neck. Standing at the patient's side, reach across the patient from below or thread your arm through the patient's flexed

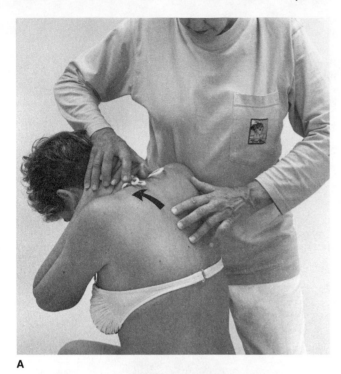

A

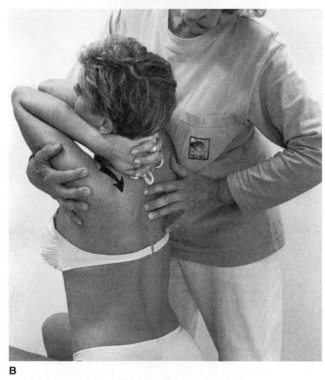

B

FIG. 19-20. Middle and lower thoracic spine (T4–T12) passive motion testing of (**A**) flexion and (**B**) extension.

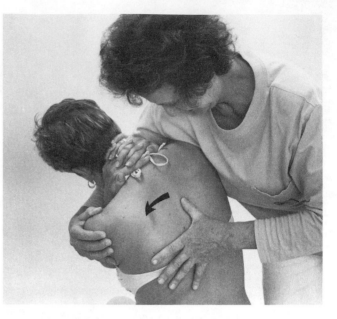

FIG. 19-21. Middle and lower thoracic spine (T4–T12) passive motion testing of lateral flexion.

19-22). Evaluate the amount and quality of movement of each segment, as well as that of adjacent segments and any pain induced.

Findings: If the spinous processes do not rotate with passive rotation, a segmental or regional joint or somatic dysfunction is suggested.

IV. **Segmental Mobility (Accessory Movements)**
These passive movements (except for the springing test) are produced by pressure of the thumbs on the spinous process and the transverse process. Spinous processes are tested using posteroanterior (central) and transverse pressures (on the side of spinous processes); these may be varied by angling the direction of the pressure toward the head or the feet, or diagonally. This is followed by posteroanterior pressures against the transverse processes, over the costotransverse junctions (unilateral), and over the ribs (unilateral).

Passive movement is the key to examination and treatment. It helps identify the site and origin of the pain and is the basis of specific mobilization techniques.

The preferred position for examining the lower thoracic spine is with the patient lying prone across the table (see Fig. 20-14), with a cushion or pillow under the abdomen to place the lower thoracic spine in neutral (resting position). A fully prone position is used for the middle and upper thoracic spine, but ideally the spine should be in slight flexion. This position can be obtained by putting a wedge under the chest or by lowering

arms and grasp the opposite shoulder. With the patient stabilized against your trunk, move your whole body to effect rotation. Use the fingers of the free hand, placed on the spinous processes as previously described, to palpate the coupled rotatory movement (Fig.

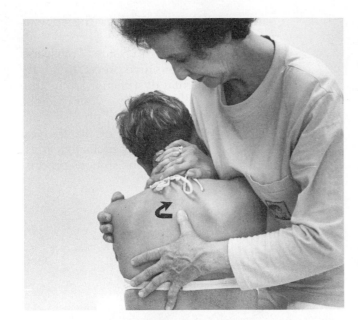

FIG. 19-22. Middle and lower thoracic (T4–T12) passive motion testing of rotation.

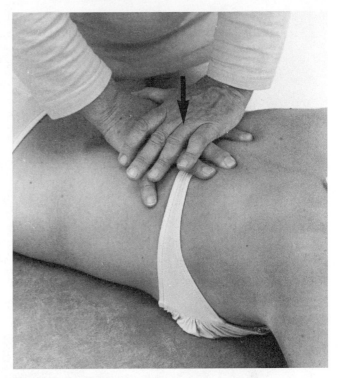

FIG. 19-23. Springing tests to the articular processes.

the top of the table. The head is supported by the palms or with a towel roll.

Throughout springing and vertebral and rib pressures, ask the patient to report when and where he or she feels pain or other symptoms; relate this information to the test being performed. Knowing that upper thoracic pain is often cervical in origin, when testing the cervicothoracic junction and upper thoracic region, central and unilateral pressures from C4 to C7 must be done before proceeding to the upper thoracic region. The upper thoracic region is examined with the patient in same position.

A. *Thoracic vertebrae (springing and vertebral pressures)*

1. Springing tests over the articular processes (transverse processes) of individual segments of the thoracic spine. First, examine for tenderness by palpating the spinous processes with the fingertips. Then perform the springing test, which examines resistance and tenderness of the deep structures of the spinal segment (*i.e.,* the disk and apophyseal joints).

Stand at the side of the table facing the head of the table (Fig. 19-23). Use the index and middle fingers of the examining hand to palpate the area over the articular processes. With the hypothenar eminence of the other hand, produce a spring-like (up and down) motion. Then place the palpating fingers over the costotransverse joint and apply a springing force.

Findings: Pain, either localized or referred, induced by this maneuver indicates segmental instability (with little or no resistance) or articular blockage with increased resistance.[42,97] Additional specific mobility tests must be used to localize the segment precisely.

2. Central posterior/anterior pressures against the spinous process. Using the tips of the thumbs applied to the spinous process, direct rhythmic pressure anteriorly (Fig. 19-24*A*). At first the pressure is applied gently in a rhythmic fashion and then more firmly to reproduce pain if it is present. Pressures over the spinous process may be inclined in a cephalic, caudal, or diagonal direction.

Findings: Dysfunction of a level is characterized by reproduction of local pain or symptoms and restriction of motion. This test may be performed several times to determine the quality of motion. Pain may be felt at any stage in the range.

3. Posterior/anterior unilateral pressure over the apophyseal joints. Move your thumbs laterally so that they rest on the transverse process of the thoracic vertebra, 2 to 3 cm from the midline to elicit symptoms from the apophyseal joints and 4 to 5 cm from the midline to provoke the costovertebral

joints (Fig. 19-24*B*). Pressure may be varied by directing it in a cephalic, caudal, medial, or lateral direction. Again, start gently with rhythmic oscillations and assess the segments immediately above, below, and on the opposite side.

Findings: Same as 2A above, but unlike central palpation this method can determine quite localized symptoms.[84] Remember that the transverse process is not neces-

sarily at the same level as the spinous process (see Fig. 19-1).

4. Transverse vertebral pressure. Transverse pressure is the definitive procedure for localizing segmental dysfunction in the thoracic spine.[84,104,106] Place your thumbs along the side of the spinous process, lying flat across the curvature of the thoracic wall (Fig. 19-24*C*). Apply oscillatory pressure along the side of the spinous process.

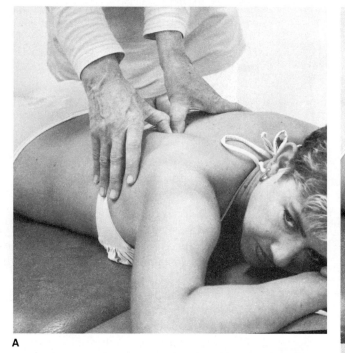

A

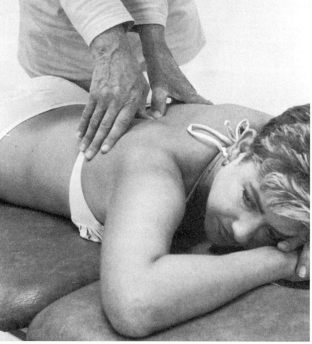

B

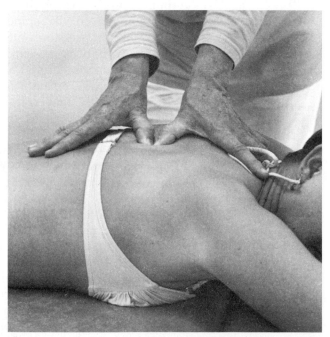

C

FIG. 19-24. Segmental testing for joint play movements. (**A**) posteroanterior central pressures, (**B**) posteroanterior unilateral pressures, and (**C**) transverse vertebral pressures.

A rotatory movement (very small in range) is being reproduced, rather than a transverse glide. When the slack is taken up, gently push the spinous process toward the opposite side. Repeat this at each level until the painful segment is located.

Findings: Same as above. The side on which the thumbs are applied to the transverse process is the side responsible for the pain. For example, if pressure from the left toward the right elicits pain, but palpation from the right is painless, the painful lesion is left-sided.

B. *Ribs and Costovertebral Joints*
Methods to elicit symptoms at the costovertebral joint include direct pressures over the costovertebral joint and springing of the ribs, thus producing an indirect stretching of the joint, and the rib maneuver described by Maigne.[104]

1. Posterior/anterior unilateral pressures over the costovertebral joints. The costovertebral joints and intercostal movements are tested by using posteroanterior pressure of the thumbs over the angle of the rib unilaterally, about 4 to 5 cm from the midline. Vary the pressure by directing it in a posterior/anterior direction or in a cranial/caudal direction to attempt to reproduce the symptoms.

    Findings: If affected, the costovertebral joint will be very sensitive to pressure because it is relatively superficial and also produces soft-tissue irritation in its vicinity.[84]

2. First rib. Palpate the first rib for position and tenderness. Palpation on the superior aspect of the first rib just anterior to the rhomboid muscle commonly shows that a dysfunctional rib is elevated in relation to the contralateral side or that it is hypomobile (Fig. 19-25). To assess mobility, passively flex the cervical spine of the supine patient, rotate it away from and laterally flex it toward the side to be examined.[65] Using the thumb of your free hand, after making contact with that rib, introduce an oscillatory or spring-like force in the caudal direction while evaluating the mobility and ease of displacement.

    Caudal pressures of the first rib with the thumbs should be repeated in prone. The bulk of the trapezius should be raised posteriorly to allow easy access to the rib angle.

    Findings: Immediate localized pain, arm

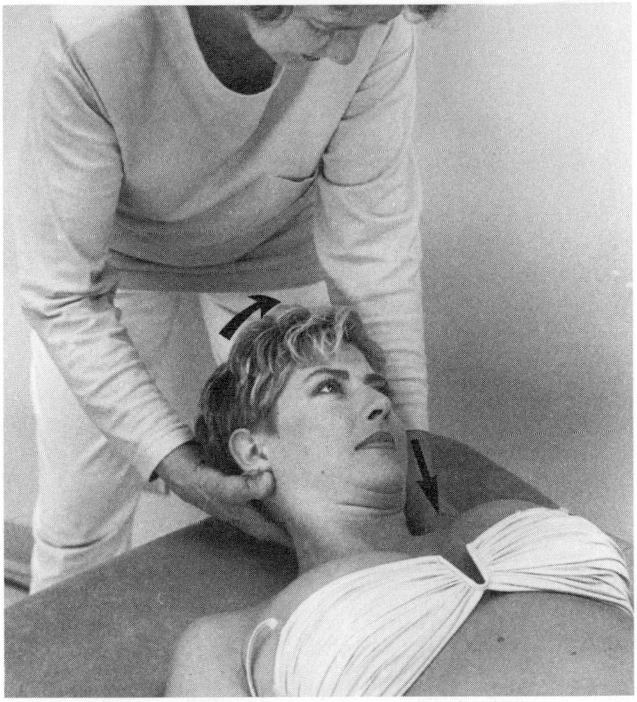

FIG. 19-25. First rib passive motion testing: Caudal glide.

pain, or both. Pain may be elicited in the cervical region as well with this maneuver, suggesting the presence of the scalenus anticus syndrome.[42,97] Hypertonicity of scalene muscles may also be noted on the ipsilateral side. There may be an absence of spring-like movement due to motion restriction.

3. Ribs III to XII—rib springing. With the patient lying prone, stand at the side or head of the table. Place your hands around the posterolateral aspect of the rib cage so that the heel of each hand rests on the angles of the ribs (Fig. 19-26). Keep your elbows fully extended as you gently spring the ribs, starting at the top of the rib cage and progressing caudally along the whole length of the thoracic spine. Note the amount and quality of movement. This general springing test is especially valuable in providing a good general impression of regional restrictions. If one rib appears hypermobile or hypomobile relative to another, it can be tested individually by applying unilateral posterior rib pressures with the ulnar border of the hand over the rib as it curves around the posterior wall.

    Findings: Provocation of the costovertebral symptoms produced by indirect stretching of the joint; absence of spring-

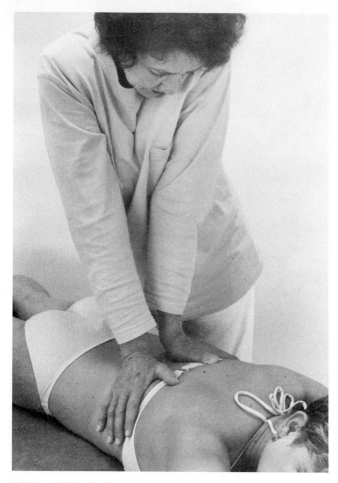

FIG. 19-26. Rib II–XII: Springing tests for joint play movements.

like movement due to dysfunction with motion restriction.

4. Rib maneuver for costal sprain.[104] With the patient sitting and the examiner standing behind, move the patient's trunk in lateral flexion to the side opposite the painful side. The arm on the painful side is raised over the head and held there while the ribs are examined. Perform a caudal glide with the tip of the thumb on the upper border of the rib (Fig. 19-27A). Apply the same maneuver with the tips of the fingers pulling upward (cranial glide) (Fig. 19-27B). With a costal sprain, one of these maneuvers will increase the pain but the other will be painless. Assessment should include anteroposterior pressures (joint play) and palpation of the ribs at their costochondral junctions. With upper thoracic dysfunction, palpate the sternoclavicular, acromioclavicular, and xiphoid joints and assess them for increase or loss of joint play. Screening tests of the sacroiliac joint should be considered when there is lower thoracic involvement, as joint abnormalities here can refer pain to areas that also receive a thoracic supply. For instance, T12 supplies the lateral aspect of the buttock.[14]

SELECTIVE TISSUE TENSION: RESISTED MOVEMENTS

Unlike the cervical and lumbar spine, the muscles of the thorax and abdomen suffer strain, so that resisted isometric testing has a significant role in the evaluation of the thoracic spine.[33] According to Cyriax,[33] the thorax should be in a neutral position and the most painful movements should be performed last. Grimsby[68] suggests performing resisted tests not only in the midrange but also in the inner and outer ranges to open or close the joint spaces; this helps determine the effect of compression on pain production. The following motions are tested.

1. *Side flexion* (standing or sitting in a chair with the feet supported). Side flexions (left and right) are resisted by the patient bending outward against the examiner's unyielding resistance. Stabilize the patient's trunk with your trunk and resist the motion with your upper limb(s), which embrace the patient's opposite shoulder. Have the patient match your resistance so that the movement is truly isometric (Fig. 19-28A).
2. *Forward flexion* (sitting in a chair with the spine in a neutral position). Stabilize the patient's knees. Prevent movement at the sternum and knees as the patient attempts to flex forward (Fig. 19-28B).
3. *Rotation* (sitting in a chair, spine in a neutral position). Stand in front of the patient and stabilize the lower limbs. Prevent movement of the pelvis by clamping the patient's knees between your knees. Resist the patient by using your hands (which are placed on the shoulders) as he or she tries to rotate right and then left (Fig. 19-28C).
4. *Extension* (prone lying). Have the patient try to extend his or her back while you offer unyielding resistance to upper thoracic extension with the cranial hand. The caudal hand stabilizes the pelvic girdle.

PALPATION

The thoracic spine is palpated for any alteration in bony alignment, muscle spasms or guarding, muscle and skin consistency, temperature alterations, swelling, and any localized tenderness that may be felt over the supraspinous ligament or the side of the interspinous ligament. Tapping sharply with the finger or a percussion hammer on the spinous processes, with the patient standing fully flexed, often elicits local tenderness over the affected level.[30]

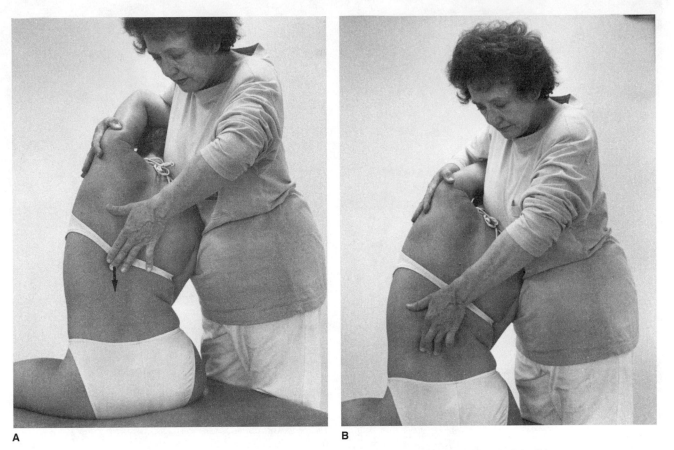

FIG. 19-27. Rib maneuver for costal sprain: (**A**) caudal glide and (**B**) cranial glide.

I. Patient in Supine Lying

A. Palpation of the costochondral articulations of the ribs often identifies one or more rib articulations that are exquisitely tender to palpation. This is frequently described as osteochondritis (Tietze's syndrome) but may be associated with dysfunction of that rib.[65,67]

B. Palpate for symmetry of ribs and intercostal spaces. A widened intercostal space above and a narrowed intercostal space below suggest a rib fault. Place the index fingers into corresponding anterior interspaces and feel for approximation or separation. In theory, a rib can be blocked both in the expiration and inspiration positions. From this it follows that the rib is more prominent if blocked in inhalation and less so if blocked in exhalation. According to Lewit,[97] it is wiser to rely on examination and comparison of mobility rather than on position. Palpate for positional alterations, such as eversion of the rib.

C. Search for the presence of tissue texture abnormality, primarily hypertonicity and tenderness of a muscle attachment to a rib.

D. When indicated, palpate the abdomen for tenderness or other signs suggestive of pathology.

II. Prone Lying (arms to the side, head to one side)

A. *General palpation*

1. Sweep the flat of the hand paravertebrally to assess the state of the skin, texture, and moisture.

2. Use the skin-rolling technique (pinch while rolling) for painful subcutaneous tissue and regions with loss of mobility—for instance, painful subcutaneous regions in the gluteal area with low back pain may originate in the thoracolumbar junction.[104,106] Normally the skin can be rolled over the spine and gluteal regions freely and painlessly.

3. Palpate the anterior aspect of the medial, lateral, and superior borders of the scapula for any tenderness or swelling. Palpate the posterior aspect of the scapula and the rotator cuff muscles as well.

B. *Segmental palpation*

1. Seek abnormalities such as thickening or undue tenderness and bony prominences.

2. Palpate the spinous processes for tender-

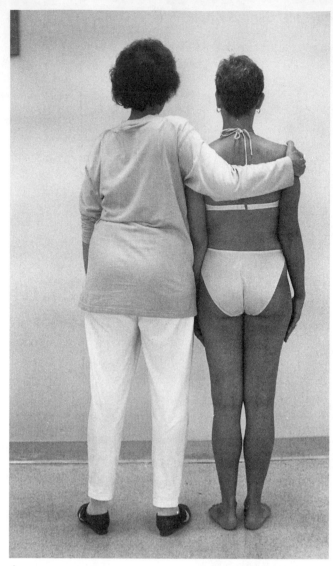

A

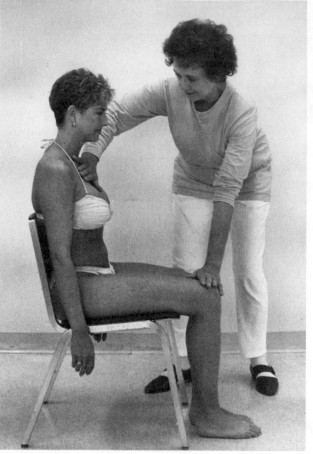

B

FIG. 19-28. Resisted isometric testing: (**A**) resisted side bending, (**B**) resisted flexion, and (**C**) resisted rotation.

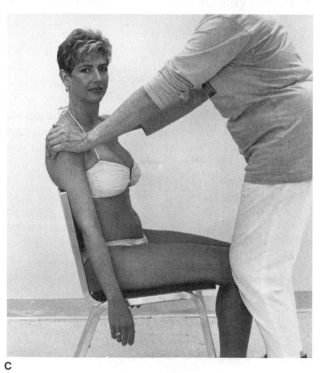

C

ness and abnormalities. By placing the fingers in the paravertebral sulcus, note any malalignment of the spinous process, as well as the prominences and depressions of the transverse process.

3. Apply pressure over the supraspinous ligament with the edge of a coin held lightly between two adjacent spinous processes. Such pressure on the normal ligament is painless; on the involved vertebral area it is usually more painful than over the others.[104,106]

4. Again, palpate the ribs and intercostal spaces for positional faults and symmetry.

5. Palpate along the iliac crest for signs such as Maigne's syndrome[105,106] (see Fig. 19-8B).

NEUROLOGICAL EXAMINATION

Occasionally patients presenting with thoracic pain complain of weakness, pain, and paresthesias in both lower limbs at rest as well as while walking. This should alert the examiner to the possibility of spinal cord involvement. If a tumor is developing, ankle clonus may be present, lower limb reflexes may be exaggerated, and the plantar reflex may be positive. Sensation and power in the lower limbs may be deficient. Neurological testing should include a full neurological assessment of the upper and lower limbs. If you suspect a problem with movement of the spinal cord, any of the tests that stretch the cord may be performed: these include the straight-leg raising test, the slump test, and others.

I. **Sensory Testing (Dermatomal and Myotomal)**
Gross sensory testing may be performed. Within the thoracic spine there is a great deal of overlap in the dermatomes (see Fig. 19-7). The dermatomes tend to follow the ribs. The absence of only one dermatome may not result in loss of sensation. Remember that sensory changes occur two segments *lower* than the location of a pathological thoracic spine condition. Like the myotomes, dermatomes of the trunk are arranged in regular bands from T2 to L1. T2, however, includes a Y-shaped area that stretches from the inner condyle of the humerus up the arm and then divides into two areas, reaching the sternum anteriorly and the vertebral border of the scapula behind.[32] T9, T10, and T11 encircle the trunk at the level of the umbilicus. T12 remains uncertain. L1 is in the region of the groin.

II. **Reflex Testing**
Although there are no deep tendon reflexes to test in conjunction with the thoracic spine, assess the lumbar reflexes because pathology in the thoracic spine can affect them. Other reflexes in this area, which depend on the integrity of the appropriate sensory and motor peripheral nerves and spinal cord segment, as well as on intact suprasegmental input to the spinal reflex center, include the so-called superficial abdominal reflexes.[144] The abdominal reflex in the upper quadrant depends on segments T7 to T9, and in the lower quadrant on segments T10 to T12. Unlike deep tendon reflexes, superficial reflexes are abolished by upper motor neuron lesions. Scratching the skin some distance away from the umbilicus in any one quadrant of the anterior abdominal wall causes contraction of the underlying abdominal muscles. The umbilicus is drawn toward the side of the contraction.

III. **Dural Mobility Testing**
If you suspect a problem with movement of the spinal cord, any of the tests that stretch the cord may be performed. These include the dural mobility test for the sciatic nerve and the femoral nerve traction test (see Chapter 20, The Lumbar Spine). The following tests may also be considered.

A. *Slump test* (see Chapter 20, The Lumbar Spine).[108] This test is used to assess the movement of the pain-sensitive structures in the vertebral canal and intervertebral foremen. According to Maitland,[108] this test should be part of the examination of the thoracic spine, but remember that this test causes pain at roughly the T8–T9 area in at least 90% of all subjects.

B. *First thoracic nerve root stretch.*[32] Have the patient abduct the arms to 90° and flex the pronated forearms to 90°. This should not alter the symptoms. The patient then fully flexes the elbow and puts the hands behind the neck. This stretches the ulnar nerve, which in turn pulls the T1 nerve root. Pain in the scapular area or arm indicates a positive test.

C. *Upper limb neural tension tests.*[20,47–49,66,81,85,108] Upper limb tension tests are recommended for all patients with symptoms in the arm, head, neck, and thoracic spine (see Chapter 9, The Shoulder and Shoulder Girdle).

IV. **Chief Physical Signs**
Physical signs that may be helpful in distinguishing the compression or interruption of neighboring spinal nerves include:[144]

A. *T1.* Intrinsic muscles of the hand are severely affected but more proximal muscles are spared. All reflexes are normal.

B. *T2 to T12.* Isolated spinal nerve lesions are difficult to detect. The distribution of pain, tenderness, muscle spasm, and careful evaluation of sensory changes are the chief factors in diagnosis. Lesions of upper thoracic nerves may abolish the sympathetic input to the upper limb and head and neck. Abdominal reflexes are absent usually only if more than one of T6 to T12 spinal nerves are blocked.

GENERAL PHYSICAL EXAMINATION

The mechanisms causing pain originating in or from the thoracic spine are numerous.[16] They occur primarily from stimulation of nociceptive endings in the periosteum, ligaments, and joints of the thoracic spine. Fracture, dislocation, arthritis variants, metabolic disorders, infection, or tumors may elicit thoracic pain. Myofascial pain frequently manifests in the thoracic spine muscles, as does pain referred from the shoulder.[23] Neuropathic pain from the thoracic cord must always be suspected, for instance from intrinsic and extramedullary spinal cord lesions.[23] About 50% of spinal cord tumors originate in the thoracic area of the cord.[139]

A general physical examination, including the abdomen and chest, may be necessary. Chest pains include those of cardiac origin and those of pulmonary etiology involving the pleura, lungs, trachea, and bronchi. The esophagus is a common site and source of chest pain.[23] Chest pain can also occur from diseases of the mediastinum, the diaphragm, the pancreas, and various visceral organs.[33,79,84,151]

It is important to be able to differentiate between chest pain due to vertebral dysfunction and that caused by myocardial ischemia.[84] Typically myocardial ischemia patients are older and present with no history of injury. The pain is described as constricting or at times burning in nature. The site of the pain and radiation is epigastric, retrosternal, parasternal, jaw, neck, inside the arm (left more common than right), and interscapular. The pain of myocardial ischemia is aggravated by exercise, heavy meals, cold, or stress; the typical elements that increase pain in dysfunction of the thoracic spine include deep inspiration, postural movement of the thorax, slumping, bending, and activities such as lifting.

OTHER STUDIES

See Chapter 20, The Lumbar Spine, for a discussion of roentgenograms and other imaging studies.

■ THORACIC SPINE TECHNIQUES

The following are representative passive movement techniques. For complete descriptions and illustrations of the great variety of mobilization and passive movements available for the thoracic spine, consult other texts.*

*See references 13,17,30,33,36,42,43,61,65–68,72,81,84,96,97,104,106, 108,110,116,117,120,123,127,132,154,159–162.

As defined earlier, *articulation* is the gradual application of passive movements in a smooth and rhythmic fashion to stretch contracted muscles, fascia, ligaments, and joint capsules. Direct techniques (on spinous or transverse processes to effect a small range of passive movement between two adjacent vertebrae) or indirect techniques (using a lever system) may be used. Indirect techniques tend to be more effective for the patient with multisegmental restriction.

An important part of treatment deals with active mobility and stability. The goal is to restore normal painless joint range of motion, including the stabilization of unstable segments, correction of muscle weakness or imbalance, restoration of soft-tissue pliability and extensibility, relief of pain and reduction of muscle spasms, postural correction, and return to normal activity.

☐ Cervicothoracic Region

FIRST AND SECOND RIB TECHNIQUES

(For simplicity, the patient is referred to as a female, the operator as a male. P—patient; O—operator; L—localization or fixation; M—movement; WB—weight-bearing; NWB—non-weight-bearing.)

  I. **Caudal Glide** (elevated first rib)—WB (Fig. 19-29)
        P—Sitting
        L—The scalene muscles may be placed on slack

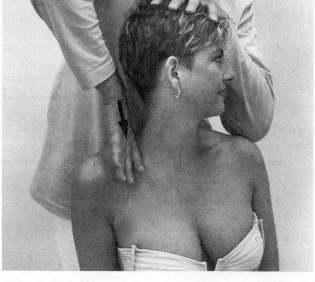

FIG. 19-29. Technique for the first rib: caudal glide (weight-bearing [WB]).

by sidebending the head to the side of restriction, or by using sufficient sidebending of the head to the side of the restriction with extension and rotation of the head and neck in the opposite direction to lock the cervical column. The examiner maintains the head position by placing the stabilizing hand on top of the head or over the vertex of the skull.

O—Stand behind the patient. With the mobilizing hand, contact the first rib posteriorly and laterally on the transverse process of the T1 vertebra with the metacarpophalangeal joint of the index finger.

M—The elbow of the mobilizing hand must be high enough so that the operator can direct downward and forward motion through the hand to the costovertebral joint. Apply mobilization pressure in an inferior, medial, anterior direction to the first rib. Time with exhalation. Follow with a stretch of the scalene muscles.

II. **Caudal Glide** (elevated first and second ribs), NWB, Supine (Fig. 19-30)

P—Supine

O—Stand at the end of the treatment table by the patient's head.

L—Place the head in sidebending to the side of the restriction to place the scaleni on slack. By adding rotation away from the restriction, one can lock the cervicothoracic spine. The fixating hand supports the cranium and cervical spine in this position.

M—Using the mobilizing hand, place the radial side of the index finger on the superior aspect of the first rib just posterior to the clavicle. With the mobilizing hand and body, move the first rib in a caudal and ventral direction.

To facilitate movement, apply pressure during exhalation. Repeat two or three times, taking up the slack with each exhalation. Follow with stretching of the scaleni muscles (see Fig. 17-34). To modify for the second rib, contact the second rib just lateral to its articulation with the sternum.

CERVICOTHORACIC SPINAL ARTICULATIONS

Oscillatory mobilizations of the thoracic spine are extensions of the segmental mobility testing, with the addition of appropriate grading (see Figs. 19-24*A*–*C*).

I. **Backward Bending or Traction,** NWB (Fig. 19-31)

P—Supine with hands behind neck (arms abducted as far as possible), hips flexed and feet resting on the table, or with the legs positioned over a wedge

O—Stand behind the patient with the arms laced between the patient's arms by going over the patient's forearm and behind the patient's back so that your fingers can reach underneath to the upper thoracic vertebrae to be mobilized.

L—Place the fingers on either side of the transverse processes on the cephalic vertebra of the segment to be treated.

M—By pulling longitudinally toward you and at

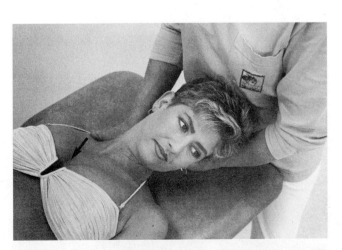

FIG. 19-30. Technique for the first and second rib: caudal glide (non–weight-bearing [NWB]).

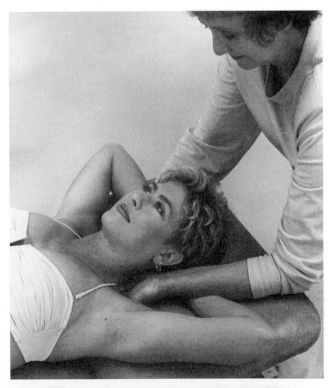

FIG. 19-31. Backward bending or traction (NWB).

the same time gently lifting up with the fingers and down with the forearms against the patient's arms, you can strongly mobilize the thoracic vertebrae into backward-bending.

Note: For traction, a combination of ordinary skin traction and of gently lifting the patient toward you can be used. Traction is effected upward and backward by using body weight and gravity to result in distraction. Do not pull with the fingers; use the body.

II. **Forward Bending/Backward Bending,** NWB (Fig. 19-32)

 P—Lying on the side, the upper arm is adducted so that the forearm rests on the table in front of the patient

 O—Facing the patient's head, the upper limb supports the patient's head and cervical spine with the hand and forearm.

 L—The caudal hand grasps the spinous process with the finger and thumb to control or localize the movement on the caudal vertebra of the segment to be treated.

 M—Support the patient's upper shoulder girdle with the trunk. The cephalic or mobilizing hand is then used to produce flexion or extension of the segment to be treated.

Note: For an alternative NWB forward-bending technique of the cervicothoracic spine, see Technique III, lower and middle thoracic spine (see

Fig. 19-38). WB techniques may also be used (see Fig. 19-19*A,B*).

III. **Sidebending and Rotation Techniques,** NWB (Fig. 19-33)

 P—Lying on the side

 O—Facing the patient, the upper limb supports the patient's head and cervical spine with the hand and forearm.

 L—The caudal hand stabilizes the segment by stabilizing the lateral aspect of the spinous process (with the finger or thumb) of the caudal vertebra of the segment to be treated to mobilize in either direction (*i.e.,* on the near side of the spinous process when mobilizing in your direction).

 M—With the caudal segment stabilized, the mobilizing hand is used to sidebend or rotate the neck to the limit of range.

Coupled movement in flexion or extension with sidebending and rotation to the same side may also be used.

IV. **Sidebending,** WB (Fig. 19-34)

 P—Sitting

 O—Stand at the side of the patient to which sidebending is to occur.

 L—With one hand, palpate on the far side of the interspace with the thumb. With the other hand on the vertex of the patient's skull, gently sidebend the head toward you until motion arrives at the level of the palpating thumb.

 M—Transverse mobilizing pressure is applied to the lateral aspect of the caudal spinous process in the direction of the restriction or the operator.

Note: This technique can be used effectively for levels C7 to T3.

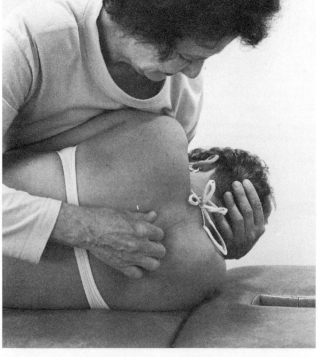

FIG. 19-32. Forward–backward bending (NWB).

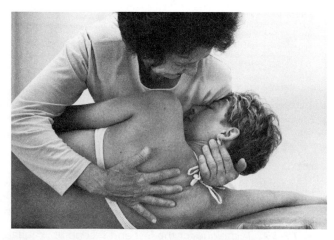

FIG. 19-33. Side bending and rotation (NWB).

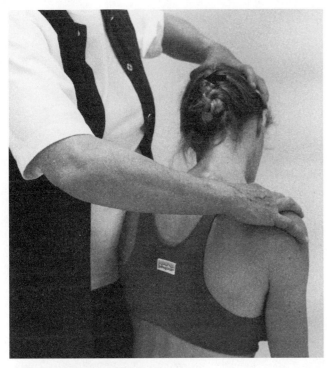

FIG. 19-34. Side bending (WB).

V. **Flexion, Sidebending, and Rotation** (active mobilization in WB; Fig. 19-35)

  P—Sitting

  O—Stand behind the patient.

  L—Contact the interspinous space of the restricted segment. The lower of the two vertebrae is fixed on the far side with the thumb. The motion barrier is localized by flexing, sidebending, and rotating the joint complex to its pathological limit.

  M—Have the patient perform a minimal isometric contraction away from the pathological barrier (*i.e.,* attempt to extend, backward-

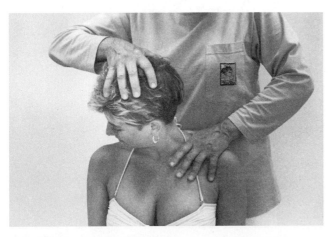

FIG. 19-35. Flexion, side bending, and rotation.

bend, and rotate away) against the resistance of your hand. Have the patient relax, then take up the slack in forward-bending and rotation in the direction of the restricted barrier. Repeat two or three times.

Note: The indication for this technique is combined motion restriction of flexion sidebending and rotation to the same side. Similar combined techniques may be used for the cervical and lower thoracic spine. Many of the techniques described earlier for cervical spine stabilization and articulations can also be effective for C7 and T1–T2, as well as the midthoracic spine techniques described below.

☐ **Thoracic Spine**
(Middle and Lower Segments)

Using segmental mobility testing (see Figs. 19-20 through 19-24) for evaluation is important in articulations of the thoracic spine. Graded oscillatory movements (from grade I to IV) should be used appropriately. Many of the segmental spinal movements described in Chapter 20, The Lumbar Spine, are appropriate for the thoracic spine (see Figs. 20-30 through 20-34). The long-lever extension (see Fig. 20-35) and rotational mobilization (see Figs. 20-36*B* and 20-38) are particularly well suited for the lower thoracic spine.

I. **Vertical Intermittent Traction**, nonspecific (Fig. 19-36)

  P—Sitting with arms folded across the chest, with hands on the shoulders or with both arms folded across the waist

  O—Stand behind the patient and cup your hands under the patient's elbows, or lace your arms under the patient's arms and secure the patient's forearms.

  M—Crouch behind the patient by bending the legs and flattening the lumbar spine. Both the therapist and the patient lean back slightly, and traction is applied upward by straightening the legs.

  Note: Some degree of localization can be obtained by using the following positions: upper thoracic—position the patient in forward-bending; midthoracic—position the patient with the back straight; entire spine—position the patient in backward bending. For a specific level, forward-bend the patient to the level with body contact or by using a wedge to fixate the cranial or caudal vertebra between your chest and the patient's body.

II. **Forward-Bending,** WB (Fig. 19-37)

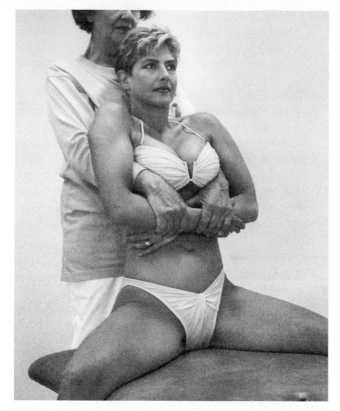

FIG. 19-36. Vertical intermittent traction: non-specific.

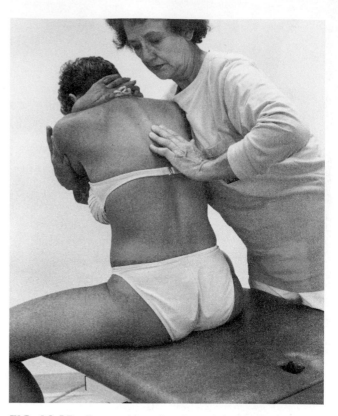

FIG. 19-37. Forward bending in weight-bearing.

P—Sitting with the hands clasped behind the neck

O—Stand at the patient's side.

L—The pad of the thumb or fingers of the stabilizing hand contacts the spinous process of the caudal vertebra of the segment to be mobilized.

M—Using the patient's elbows held close together as a lever, flex the thoracic spine to the segment to be mobilized while fixating the spinous process of the lower vertebra.

Note: If shoulder range is limited, the patient's forearms can be crossed on the chest with hands on the opposite shoulders. Position your mobilizing arm across the patient's forearms with the hand grasping the opposite shoulder. One arm controls the weight of the upper torso and imparts forward-bending while the finger or thumb of the opposite hand palpates motions between the segment, or the thumb stabilizes the spinous process to be mobilized.

III. **Forward-Bending,** NWB (Fig. 19-38)

P—Prone with the trunk over a therapy wedge or resting on the forearms, thoracic spine extended

O—Stand at the patient's side. The mobilizing hand supports the top of the patient's head or forehead.

L—With the index finger or thumb, palpate the spinous process of the caudal vertebra of the involved segment. The head is flexed down to the level with your cranial hand.

M—Counterpressure of the thumb or the heel of the hand is applied against the spinous

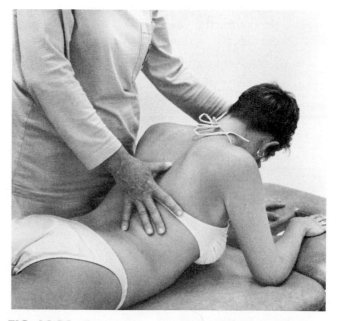

FIG. 19-38. Forward bending in non–weight-bearing.

process below the segment to be mobilized. Slow alternating movements of slight pressure and release are applied, thus mobilizing into flexion via the head. In this position the head can be used as a lever for mobilizing into extension, sidebending, or rotation as well as flexion.

Note: An alternate technique in this position is to use one hand to maintain the anterior flexion of the head while other hand exerts caudal glide (with the heel of the mobilizing hand) on the spinous process of the caudal vertebra of the involved segment.

IV. Backward-Bending, WB (Fig. 19-39)

P—Sitting with arms folded across the waist or crossed to opposite shoulders

O—Stand at the patient's side.

L—With the index finger of the dorsal hand, palpate the interspinous space of the restricted segment. Place the ventral hand on the patient's contralateral elbow or shoulder.

M—The ventral hand mobilizes the patient's thoracic spine backward into extension.

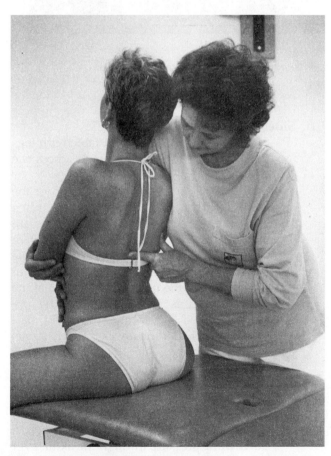

FIG. 19-39. Backward bending (WB).

V. Backward-Bending, WB (middle and lower thoracic region; Fig. 19-40A)[104]

P—Sitting, with arms flexed and supported on the operator's ventral forearm and femur of the supporting leg

O—Stand at the patient's side with one foot on a stool and the ventral forearm supporting the patient's outstretched arms.

M—The dorsal hand exerts pressure on the thoracic region to be mobilized. While accentuating this pressure, move your knee laterally, thus effecting a traction of the dorsal spine in extension. Then, as traction is released, perform a series of slow, alternating, rhythmic elastic movements.

Note: For a similar and equally effective technique for the midthoracic region (Fig. 19-40B), stand in front of the patient with the patient resting the crossed forearms on your chest or upper arms. Place your hand at either side of the region to be mobilized. To mobilize in extension, draw the patient toward you by leaning backward, then release the pull by moving forward.

VI. Backward-Bending, WB (upper thoracic spine; Fig. 19-41)

P—Sitting with the hands clasped behind the neck and the arms resting on the thorax or on the operator's arms

O—Stand in front of the patient, with your arms laced through the patient's arms with the hands in contact with the patient's thorax.

M—While palpating and monitoring the movement with the fingers, pull the patient toward you by slightly elevating the elbows and extending the trunk backward. Thus a lever is formed that acts on the upper thoracic spine, which is mobilized into extension. The pull is released by moving the trunk forward and lowering the elbows. The movement is repeated several times slowly.

Note: By pulling to the left or right, one can mobilize in combined extension and lateral flexion.

VII. Rotation, WB (Fig. 19-42)

P—Sitting astride the plinth with hands placed on opposite shoulders, clasped across the chest or behind the neck

O—Stand at the patient's side and grasp the patient's far shoulder with the ventral hand. When the alternate position is used (patient's hands behind the neck), first thread your arm through the patient's flexed arms before grasping the far shoulder.

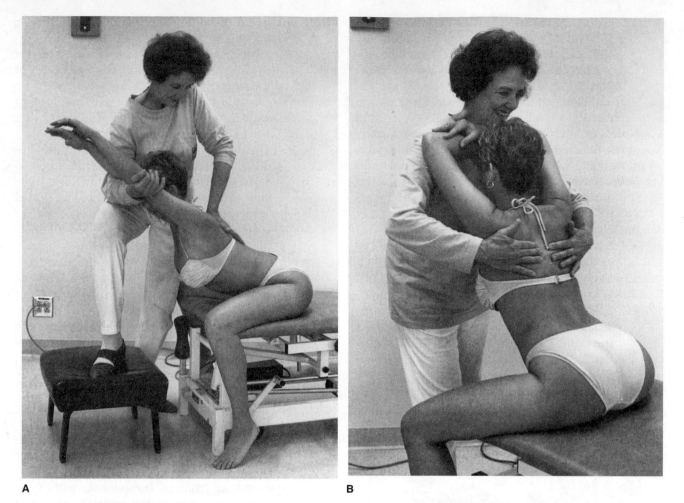

A   **B**

FIG. 19-40. Backward bending, middle and lower thoracic spine: (**A**) operator at side of patient or (**B**) in front of patient.

L—With the thumb or finger of the dorsal hand, palpate the interspinous space of the restricted segment.

M—Rotation of the spine is effected by rotating your whole body and at the same time augmenting and localizing the movement with the dorsal hand.

Note: In a variation of this technique, the restricted segment can be rotated to its pathological barrier. Steadily increase the pressure over the side of the spinous process of the inferior vertebra of the restricted spinal segment, thereby effecting passive mobilization. Active mobilization can be used by localizing the rotation to its pathological barrier, and having the patient hold the trunk still while you apply a minimal force toward the midline with the ventral hand. Coupled motions of flexion/rotation/sidebending or extension/rotation/sidebending by localizing to the segment can also be employed, using active or passive mobilization.[44,45,81,96,123]

VIII. Sidebending, WB (Fig. 19-43)

P—Sitting astride the treatment table with legs over one side and arms clasped across the chest

O—Stand at the patient's side and support the patient's arms and trunk.

L—The thumb or fingers of the dorsal hand are used to palpate laterally between the two spinous processes of the segment to be treated to ensure that movement occurs at that level. For the upper thoracic spine, the ventral hand is wound through the patient's crossed arm to grasp the contralateral shoulder. For the lower thoracic spine, the ventral hand is placed on the contralateral scapula or elbow. The patient's near shoulder is positioned under the operator's axilla.

M—The patient's trunk is sidebent by means of the operator's near axilla, which exerts a downward pressure through the axilla over the near shoulder. An upward lift is given

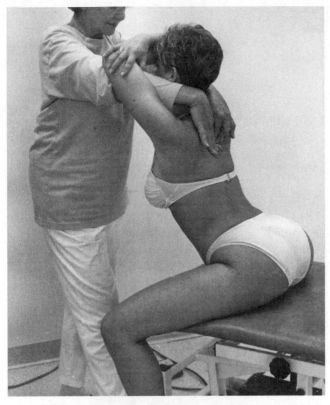

FIG. 19-41. Backward bending: upper thoracic spine.

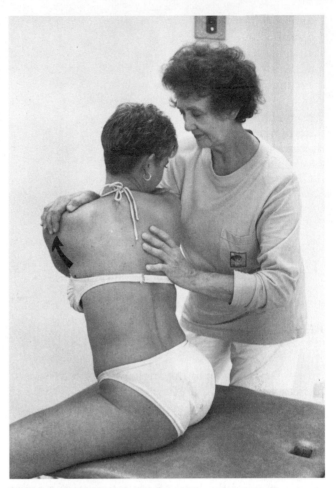

FIG. 19-42. Rotation: patient with arms across the chest.

to the patient's contralateral shoulder with the ventral hand on the far shoulder, scapula, or elbow while the dorsal hand palpates the gapping or approximation of the spinous process.

Note: The same NWB technique (see Fig. 20-39) for the lumbar spine, using the patient's thigh as a lever and applying leg abduction until motion arrives at the level of the stabilizing thumb or hand, can be used effectively for the lower thoracic spine.

☐   **The Thoracic Cage:**
     Articular Techniques of the Ribs

HYPOMOBILITY OF THE RIBS

Rib dysfunction is indicated if the rib will not move upward during inspiration (inhalation restriction); if the rib will not descend (exhalation restriction); or if there is restriction of motion or position of the rib.

MIDDLE AND LOWER RIB
CAGE TECHNIQUES
(Ribs 2 TO 12)
I. Posterior Articulation, NWB (exhalation restriction; Fig. 19-44)

P—Prone, head facing toward the side to be mobilized
O—Stand at the patient's head, take hold of the patient's arm just proximal to the elbow, and position the arm into abduction. With the opposite hand, fix each rib involved in turn with the thumb and thenar eminence at the angle of the lower rib.
M—The ribs are mobilized by stretching the arm into full abduction, achieving quite a powerful stretch of each intercostal space using the leverage of the latissimus dorsi.
Note: One can also stabilize the arm and mobilize the rib in a caudal direction by contacting the superior angle of the rib with the thumb or the heel of the hand.
II. Posterior Articulation, NWB (rib restriction when the arm cannot be used as a lever; Fig. 19-45A)
P—Prone, head facing toward the side to be mobilized. When working with the upper rib cage, the arm can be abducted or placed behind the patient's back so that the scapula is drawn away from the chest wall to allow

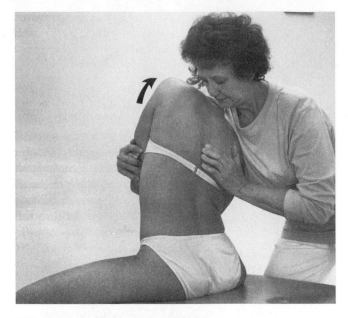

FIG. 19-43. Side bending (WB).

easy access to the angle of the rib to be mo-
bilized.
  O—Stand at the patient's head.
  M—For the upper ribs, contact the angle of the
    rib with pisiform contact and take up the
    slack in a caudal and lateral or a caudal and
    central direction. As the patient breathes out
    toward the limit of expiration, give a series
    of oscillations. For the middle and lower ribs
    the contact is with both the pisiform and the

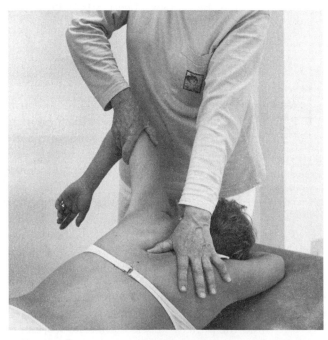

FIG. 19-44. Posterior articulations.

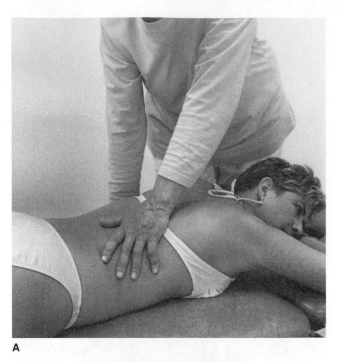

A

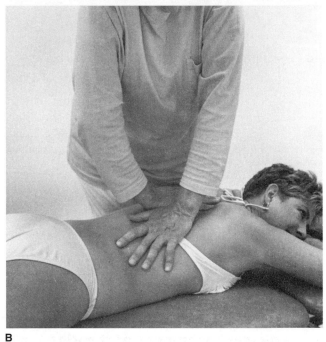

B

FIG. 19-45. Posterior articulations: (**A**) without stabilization and (**B**) with stabilization.

base of the metacarpal. Pressure is again applied in a caudal/central or caudal/lateral
direction.
  Note: The opposite rib can be stabilized with the
  other hand. The operator than stands opposite
  the side to be mobilized (Fig. 19-45*B*).
III. **Anterior Articulation** (exhalation restriction;
    Fig. 19-46)
  P—Supine

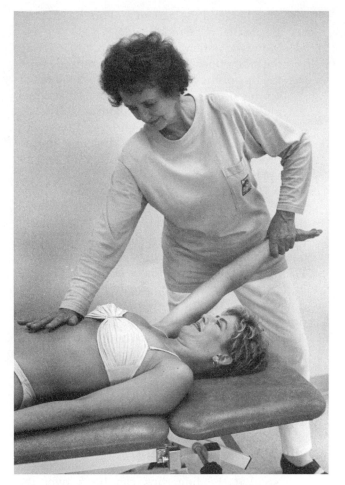

FIG. 19-46. Anterior articulations using the arm as a lever.

O—Stand on the side to be mobilized, facing the foot of the table. Grasp the forearm above the wrist with the inner hand and stretch the arm upward while fixing the anterior ends of the rib with the outer hand. The operator may use the radial border of the hand or the thumb and thenar eminence to fix the lower of the two ribs.

M—Quite a powerful stretch of the involved segments can be achieved by using the leverage of the pectoral muscles. To reinforce the stretch and separation of the ribs, muscle energy or PNF techniques may be used, or have the patient inspire deeply as you synchronize the stretch with full inspiration.

Note: Either a caudal glide may be performed with the right hand as the arm is maintained at its end range, or the right hand may maintain the caudal glide of the rib as the arm is moved into its end range.

IV. **Anterior Articulation** (exhalation restriction when the arm cannot be used as a lever; Fig. 19-47)

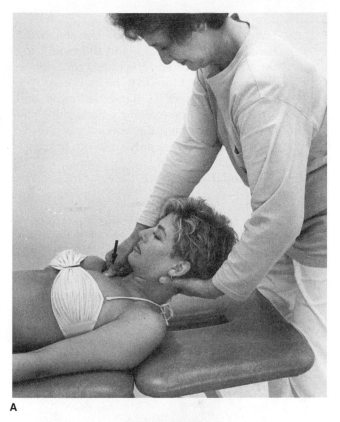

A

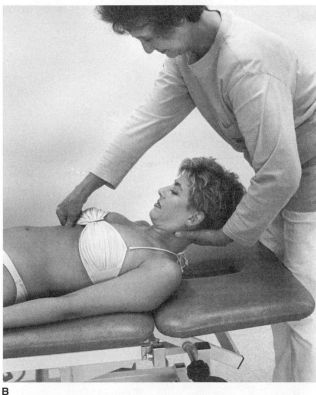

B

FIG. 19-47. Anterior articulations (alternative technique) when the arm cannot be used as a lever: (**A**) upper ribs and (**B**) lower ribs.

P—Supine with arms at side

O—Stand at the patient's head. The stabilizing hand supports the neck and the mobilizing thumb (reinforced by the hand) contacts the superior edge of the rib to be mobilized.

M—With the supporting hand, sidebend and forward-bend the patient's neck until you feel tension under the mobilizing thumb. During exhalation, apply pressure to the rib in a caudal direction.

V. Cranial/Caudal Glide, WB (lower ribs; see Fig. 19-27)[104]

P—Sitting astraddle the table

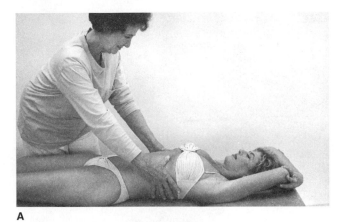

A

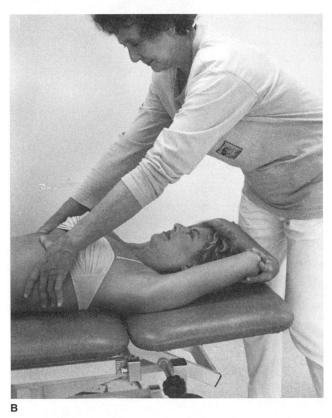

B

FIG. 19-48. Cephalic/caudal glides (NWB): (**A**) cephalic glide and (**B**) caudal glide.

O—Stand behind the patient and on the side opposite that to be mobilized.

M—Move the patient's trunk in lateral flexion to the side opposite that to be mobilized. With the tips of the fingers, hook onto the inferior border of the rib and pull upward (cranial glide) during the end of expiration. The reverse technique, caudal glide or downward pressure, can be used by directing thumb pressure to the superior border of the involved rib (see Fig. 19-27*A*).

Note: This maneuver can also be done in supine (NWB) with both arms of the patient elevated (for a bilateral technique); if a unilateral technique is used, the arm on the side to be mobilized can be maximally elevated and supported. With the thumbs on the lower border of the ribs, glide the rib(s) upward (during expiration) or downward on the upper border (during inspiration) (Fig. 19-48).

VI. Active Mobilization (inhalation restriction of the middle ribs, to raise the front of the ribs; Fig. 19-49)[96,123]

P—Supine

O—Stand on the noninvolved side (or same side). The patient's arm on the involved side is flexed as far as possible by your cephalic hand and maintained at end range. Insert your caudal hand under the patient's back so that the fingertips can hook over the inner shafts of the lower ribs. Four ribs can be treated at once. Remember that in restricted inhalation, the uppermost restricted rib is the key.

M—Have the patient inhale and bring the arm down against your unyielding resistance, if using an isometric contraction. At the same

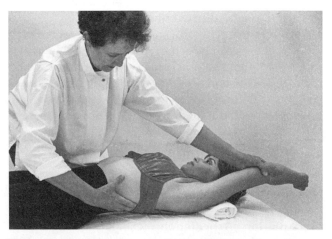

FIG. 19-49. Elevation technique using muscle energy or PNF.

time pull caudally and laterally on the angles of the ribs with the opposite hand.

Note: An isotonic contraction of the serratus anterior and pectoralis major can also be used to raise the front of the ribs while using respiration and downward pressure on the rib angles to assist. To use these muscles, the arm is elevated near its end range with the elbow bent so the forearm lies above the patient's head (or end range). While resisting at the patient's arm, have the patient inhale deeply and pull the arm down to the side as you resist the arm, and pull caudally and laterally on the angles of the ribs with the opposite hand. Have the patient relax and take up the slack. Repeat three times or more.

There are many variations of PNF or muscle energy approaches. They are extremely effective when the client can isolate movement.

VII. **Lateral Articulation** (intercostal stretch; Fig. 19-50

P—Lying on the side opposite that to be mobilized

O—Stand at the head of the table.

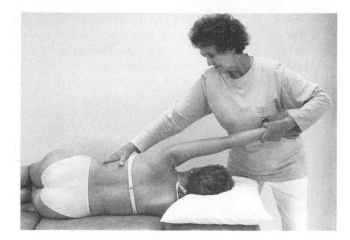

FIG. 19-50. *Lateral articulations.*

M—Place the arm at end range of abduction and stabilize it. Use the caudal hand to impart a caudal glide to each involved rib. During inhalation, resist elevation of the rib. As the patient relaxes, apply caudal pressure to the rib. Repeat two or three times.

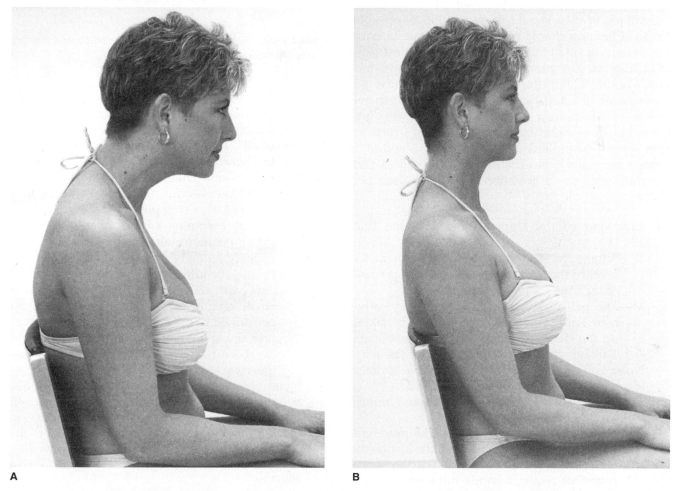

A   B

FIG. 19-51. *Extension, upper thoracic spine: (A) starting position and (B) end position.*

Note: This technique can be reversed by using the caudal hand (thumb and thenar eminence or web space) to stabilize the ribs. The cephalic arm stretches the arm into full abduction, while fixating the lower (level to be mobilized) rib in the midaxillary line with the caudal hand.

Additional treatment considerations for management of hypomobility of the ribs include stretching and soft-tissue mobilizations of involved intercostal muscles; follow-up facilitation and activities to enhance rib cage excursion; and diaphragmatic breathing exercises to increase the anteroposterior and the transverse diameters of the thoracic cavity by its influence on the ribs.

Thoracic Spine: Self-Mobilization

Self-segmental spinal mobility exercises, previously considered rather specialized, have become more widely used and discussed in the literature in the last few years.[18,19,66,69,70,74,97] Motivation for self-treatment is being encouraged, and the logical trend is to teach patients to deal with their problems themselves.

Self-mobilization should be as specific as possible. These techniques should be gentle, deliberate, coaxing movements of small range to induce, at the most, only mild distress. For painful conditions, repetitive motion working within the painless limits provides the proprioceptive input for inhibition.[119] For restricted movement, the patient should be advised to work into the painful range gradually to stretch tight structures over several days. Precise clinical diagnosis and indications are mandatory. The examples presented here correlate with the articulation techniques described above.

  I. **Extension of the Upper Thoracic Spine** (Fig. 19-51)
    P—Sitting, back supported by the chair at the level of the lower vertebra (spinous process) of the upper segment to be treated
    M—The patient shifts the head and cervicothoracic spine backward to the point of taking up the slack at the segment to be mobilized. This is repeated in a slow, rhythmic fashion.
    Note: Use a higher-back chair for upper thoracic levels and the cervical thoracic junction.
 II. **Flexion–Extension, Middle and Lower Thoracic Spine** (Fig. 19-52)
    P—Forearm and knees position. The more cranial the mobilization required, the further the elbows are placed forward. For the thoracolumbar region, a hands and knees position is assumed.

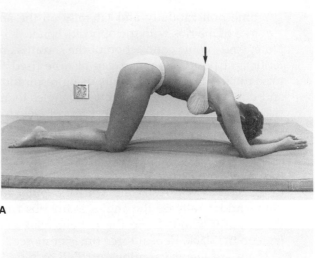

A

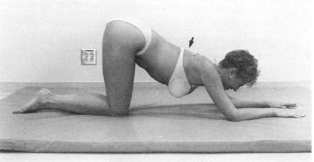

B

FIG. 19-52. Flexion–extension, middle and lower thoracic spine: (**A**) flexion and (**B**) extension.

    M—The patient actively moves the thoracic spine into flexion and extension, breathing in with flexion and out with extension.
III. **Localized Thoracic Extension, Middle and Lower Thoracic Spine** (Fig. 19-53*A*)
    P—Sitting in a chair. Fixation can be assisted with a pillow adjusted to the segmental level required. By using pillows at various heights and by assuming various erect or slumped sitting positions, almost any level of the thoracic spine can be mobilized.
    M—By back-bending to the fixation point, the patient can actively mobilize into extension. Small repetitive oscillatory movements are performed at the end range. With fixation either at a spinous process or a rib, movement can be directed at either the spinal or costovertebral joints.
    Note: This self-mobilization technique may also be performed in the supine position over a roll. The level of the axis of motion is determined by the placement of the roll (Fig. 19-53*B,C*). With this technique the upper ribs are mobilized as well.
IV. **Upper Rib/Thoracic Spine Mobilization** (Fig. 19-54)
    P—Supine with one leg supported by the flexed

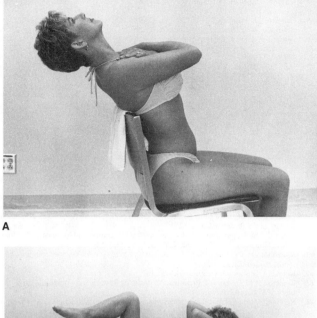

A

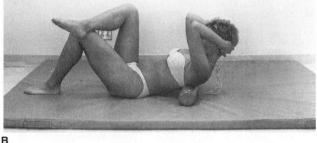

B

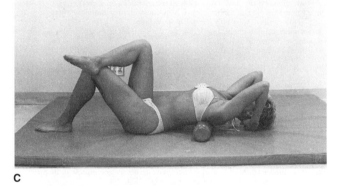

C

FIG. 19-53. Localized thoracic extension: (**A**) sitting (WB); (**B**) supine, starting position; and (**C**) end position (NWB).

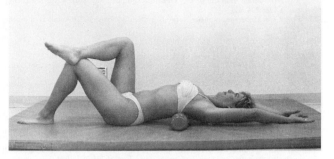

FIG. 19-54. Upper thoracic spine and rib mobilizations.

upper leg is extended with the lower leg flexed for stabilization.

M—The patient actively sidebends and reaches with the arm overhead. This technique can be used to effectively mobilize the lower ribs as well as the thoracic spine.

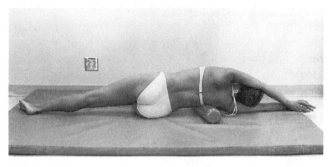

FIG. 19-55. Lower rib mobilization.

knee of the opposite side (to flatten the lumbar spine) with hands clasped behind the neck or with the arms elevated. A foam roll or firm cushion is used to provide segmental fixation at the desired level of the thoracic spine.

M—The patient performs backward-bending in time with breathing. The end position should be held as the patient exhales and relaxes.

V. Lower Rib Mobilization (Fig. 19-55)

P—Lying on the side with a hard roll positioned for fixation of the desired thoracic level. The

REFERENCES

1. Adams MA, Hutton WC: Gradual disc prolapse. Spine 10:524–531, 1985
2. Adler SS, Beckers D, Buck M: PNF in Practice: An Illustrated Guide. Berlin, Springer-Verlag, 1993
3. Akeson WH, Amiel D, LaViolette D, et al: The connective tissue response to immobility: An accelerated aging response. Exp Gerontol 3:289–301, 1968
4. Akeson WH, Amiel D, Woo S: Immobility effects of synovial joints: The pathomechanics of joint contracture. Biorheology 17:95–110, 1980
5. Alexander FM: The Use of Self. New York, Dutton, 1932
6. AMA: A Guide to the Evaluation of Permanent Impairment, 4th ed. AMA, 1993
7. Asmussen E, Heeboll-Nielsen K: Posture, mobility and strength of the back in boys 7 to 16 years old. Acta Orthop Scand 28:174–189, 1959
8. Aston J: Your ideal body: A new paradigm for movement. Physical Therapy Today, Summer 1991
9. Axelgaard J, Brown JC: Lateral electrical surface stimulation for the treatment of progressive idiopathic scoliosis. Spine 8:242–260, 1983
10. Axelgaard J, Nordwall A, Brown JC: Correction of spinal curvature by transcutaneous electrical muscle stimulation. Spine 8:463–481, 1983
11. Barlow W: The Alexander Technique. New York, Warner Books, 1980
12. Benson MDK, Byrnes DP: The clinical syndromes and surgical treatment of thoracic intervertebral disk prolapse. J Bone Joint Surg 57B:471–477, 1975
13. Blackman J, Prip K: Mobilization Techniques, 2nd ed. Edinburgh, Churchill Livingstone, 1988
14. Blair JM: Examination of the thoracic spine. In Grieves GP (ed): Modern Manual Therapy of the Vertebral Column. New York, Churchill Livingstone, 1986:534–537
15. Bobath B: The treatment of neuromuscular disorders by improving patterns of coordination. Physiotherapy 55:18–22, 1969
16. Bonica JJ, Sola AF: Chest pain caused by other disorders. In Bonica JJ (ed): The Management of Pain, 2nd ed, Vol. 2. Philadelphia, Lea & Febiger, 1990:1114–1145
17. Bourdillon JF, Day EA, Bookhut MR: Spinal Manipulation, 5th ed. Oxford, Butterworth-Heinemann, 1992
18. Buswell J: A manual of home exercises for the spinal column. Auckland, NZ, Manipulative Therapy Association, 1978

19. Buswell J: Exercises in the treatment of vertebral dsyfunction. In Grieve GP (ed): Modern Manual Therapy of the Vertebral Column. New York, Churchill Livingstone, 1986:834–838
20. Butler DS: Mobilisation of the Nervous System. Melbourne, Churchill Livingstone, 1991
21. Cailliet R: Scoliosis. Philadelphia, FA Davis, 1975
22. Cailliet R: Neck and Arm Pain, 3rd ed. Philadelphia, FA Davis, 1991
23. Cailliet R: Pain: Mechanisms and Management. Philadelphia, FA Davis, 1993
24. Cantu RI, Gordin AJ: Myofascial Manipulations: Theory and Clinical Application. Gaithersburg, MD, Aspen Publications, 1992
25. Caplan D: Back Trouble: A New Approach to Prevention and Recovery. Gainesville, Fla., Triad Publishing Co., 1987
26. Cherington M: Surgery for thoracic outlet syndrome? N Eng J Med 314:322, 1986
27. Cherington M, Happer I, Machanic B, et al: Surgery for the thoracic outlet syndrome may be hazardous for your health. Muscle Nerve 9:632–634, 1986
28. Cloward RB: Cervical diskography: A contribution to the etiology and mechanism of neck, shoulder, and arm pain. Ann Surg 150:1052–1064, 1959
29. Connolly BH, Michael BT: Early detection of scoliosis: A neurological approach using the asymmetrical tonic neck reflex. Phys Ther 64:304–307, 1984
30. Corrigan B, Maitland GD: Practical Orthopedic Medicine. Boston, Butterworths, 1983
31. Cuetter AC, Bartoszek DM: The thoracic outlet syndrome–controversies, overdiagnosis, overtreatment and recommendations for management. Muscle Nerve 12:410–419, 1989
32. Cyriax JH: Textbook of Orthopaedic Medicine, Diagnosis of Soft-Tissue Lesions, 8th ed, Vol. 1. London, Bailliere Tindall, 1982
33. Cyriax JH, Cyriax PJ: Illustrated Manual of Orthopaedic Medicine, 2nd ed. Boston, Butterworths, 1993
34. D'Ambrosia RD (ed): Musculoskeletal Disorders: Regional Examination and Differential Diagnosis, 2nd ed. Philadelphia, JB Lippincott, 1986
35. De Palma A, Rothman RH: The Intervertebral Disc. Philadelphia, WB Saunders, 1970
36. DiGiovanna EI, Sahiowitz S (eds): An Osteopathic Approach to Diagnosis and Treatment. Philadelphia, JB Lippincott, 1991
37. Dobrusin R: An osteopathic approach to conservative management of thoracic outlet syndromes. J Am Osteopath Assoc 89:1046–1057, 1989
38. Dommisse GF: The blood supply of the spinal cord: A critical vascular zone in spinal surgery. J Bone Joint Surg 56B:223–235, 1974
39. Dreyfuss P, Levernieux J: Les hernies discales dorsales. In L'actualite rheumatologique. Paris, Expansion Scientifique, 1966
40. Dreyfuss P, Tibiletti C, Dreyer SJ: Thoracic zygapophyseal joint pain patterns: A study in normal volunteers. Spine 19:807–811, 1994
41. Dunham WF: Ankylosing spondylitis: Measurement of the hip and spinal movements. Br J Phys Med 12:126–129, 1949
42. Dvořák J, Dvořák V: Manual Medicine, Diagnostics. New York, Georg Thieme Verlag, Thieme Medical Publishers, 1990
43. Edmond SL: Manipulation and Mobilization: Extremity and Spinal Techniques. St. Louis, CV Mosby, 1993
44. Edwards BC: Combined movements of the lumbar spine: Examination and clinical significance. Aust J Physiother 25:147–152, 1979
45. Edwards BC: Combined movements in the cervical spine (C2–7): Their value in examination and technique choice. Aust J Physiother 26:165–171, 1980
46. Edwardson B: Musculoskeletal Assessment: An Integrated Approach. San Diego, Singular Publishing Group, 1992
47. Elvey RL: Painful restriction of shoulder movement: A clinical observation study. In: Proceedings, Disorders of the Knee, Ankle and Shoulder. Perth, Western Australian Institute of Technology, 1979
48. Elvey RL: Treatment of arm pain associated with abnormal brachial plexus tension. Aust J Physiother 32:224–229, 1986
49. Elvey RL, Quintner JL, Thomas AN: A clinical study of RSI. Aust Fam Phys 15:1314–1322, 1986
50. Evans P: The healing process at a cellular level. Physiotherapy 66:256–259, 1980
51. Evans RC: Illustrated Essentials in Orthopedic Physical Assessment. St, Louis, CV Mosby, 1994
52. Evjenth O, Hamberg J: Muscle Stretching in Manual Therapy: A Clinical Manual, Vol. 2: The Spinal Column and the TMJ. Alfta, Sweden, Alfta Rehab Forlag, 1984
53. Farady JA: Current principles in the nonoperative management of structural adolescent scoliosis. Phys Ther 63:512–523, 1983
54. Farfan H, Gracovetsky S: The nature of instability. Spine 9:714–719, 1984
55. Feldenkrais M: Body and Mature Behavior: A Study of Anxiety, Sex, Gravity and Learning. New York, International Universities Press, 1949
56. Feldenkrais M: Awareness Through Movement—Health Exercises for Personal Growth. New York, Harper & Row, 1972
57. Feldenkrais M: The Potential Self: The Dynamics of Body and the Mind. San Francisco, Harper & Row, 1985
58. Ford DM, Bagnall KM, Clements CA, et al: Muscle spindles in the paraspinal musculature of patients with adolescent idiopathic scoliosis. Spine 13:461–465, 1988
59. Ford DM, Bagnall KM, McFadden, KD, et al: Paraspinal muscle imbalance in adolescent idiopathic scoliosis. Spine 9:373–376, 1984
60. Frank C, Akeson WH, Woo S, et al: Physiology and therapeutic value of passive joint motion. Clin Orthop 185:113–125, 1984
61. Fryette HH: Principles of Osteopathic Technique. Carmel, Calif., Academy of Applied Osteopathy, 1954
62. Gelb M: An Introduction to the Alexander Technique. New York, Henry Holt & Company, 1987
63. Gerhardt JJ: Documentation of Joint Motion: International Standard Neutral-Zero Measuring S.F.T.R. Recording and Application of Goniometers, Inclinometers and Calipers. Portland, Oregon, ISOMED Inc., 1992
64. Gonnella C, Paris S, Kutner M: Reliability in evaluating passive intervertebral motion. Phys Ther 62:437–444, 1982
65. Greenman PE: Principles of Manual Medicine. Baltimore, Williams & Wilkins, 1989
66. Grieve GP: Mobilisation of the Spine: Notes on Examination, Assessment and Clinical Method, 4th ed. Edinburgh, Churchill Livingstone, 1984
67. Grieve GP: Thoracic joint problems and simulated visceral disease. In Grieve GP (ed): Modern Manual Therapy of the Vertebral Column. New York, Churchill Livingstone, 1986:377–395
68. Grimsby O: Lumbar-Thoracic Spine. Continuing education course, Institute of Graduate Health Sciences, Nashville, Tenn., 1976
69. Gustavsen R: Fra aktiv avspenning til trening. Oslo, Norlis, 1977
70. Gustavsen R: Training Therapy: Prophylaxis and Rehabilitation. New York, Thieme, 1993
71. Hall CD: Clinical Concepts in Regional Musculoskeletal Illness. London, Grune & Stratton, 1987:227–244
72. Hartman L: Classification and application of osteopathic manipulative techniques. In Glasgow EF, Twomey LT, Scull ER, et al (eds): Aspects of Manipulative Therapy, 2nd ed. Edinburgh, Churchill Livingstone, 1985
73. Hohmann G: Orthopadische Technik Bandagen and Apparate. Stuttgart, Ihre Anzeige und ihr Bau, 1968
74. Holten O: Medisinski Treningsterapi. Oslo, Holten Institutt, 1967
75. Howes RG, Isdale IC: The loose back: An unrecognized syndrome. Rheumatol Phys Med 11:72–77, 1971
76. Jobe FW, Bradley JP: The diagnosis and nonoperative treatment of shoulder injuries in athletes. Clin Sports Med 8:419–438, 1989
77. Johnson GS, Saliba VL: Functional Orthopedics I, Course Outline. San Anselmo, CA: Institute of Physical Arts, 1984
78. Jones FP: The Alexander Technique: Body Awareness in Action. New York, Schocken Books, 1976
79. Judge RD, Zuidema GD, Fitzgerald FT: Clinical Diagnosis: A Physiologic Approach. Boston, Little, Brown & Co., 1982
80. Juhan D: The Trager approach: Psychophysical integration and Mentastics. In Drury N (ed): The Body Book. Burbank, CA, Prism Alpha, 1984
81. Kaltenborn F: The Spine: Basic Evaluation and Mobilization Techniques. Oslo, Olaf Norlis Bokhandel, 1993
82. Keim HA: Scoliosis. Clin Symp 24:1–30, 1978
83. Kendall FP, McCreary EK, Provance PG: Muscles: Testing and Function, 4th ed. Baltimore, Williams & Wilkins, 1993
84. Kenna C, Murtagh J: Back Pain and Spinal Manipulation: A Practical Guide. Boston, Butterworths, 1989
85. Kennealy M, Rubenach H, Elvey R: The upper limb tension test: The SLR test of the arm. In Grant R (ed): Physical Therapy of the Cervical and Thoracic Spine. Edinburgh, Churchill Livingstone, 1988
86. Kennelly KP, BPhty(Hons), Stokes MJ: Pattern of asymmetry of paraspinal muscle size in adolescent idiopathic scoliosis examined by real-time ultrasound imaging: A preliminary study. Spine 18:913–917, 1993
87. Kenny A, Traynor GB, Withington D, Keegan DJ: Thoracic outlet syndrome: A useful exercise treatment option. Am J Surg 165:282–284, 1993
88. Kisner C, Colby LA: Scoliosis. In Kisner C, Colby LA: Therapeutic Exercise: Foundations and Techniques, 2nd ed. Philadelphia, FA Davis, 1990:519–543
89. Klapp B: Das Klappishe Kreichverfahren. Stuttgart, B. Thieme, 1955
90. Klein-Vogelbach S: Functional Kinetics: Observing, Analyzing and Teaching Human Movement. Berlin, Springer-Verlag, 1990
91. Klein-Vogelbach S: Therapeutic Exercises in Functional Kinetics: Analysis and Instruction of Individually Adaptable Exercises. Berlin, Springer-Verlag, 1991
92. Knott M, Voss DE: Proprioceptive Neuromuscular Facilitation: Patterns and Techniques, 2nd ed. New York, Harper & Row, 1968
93. Kramer J: Intervertebral Disk Disease: Causes, Diagnosis, Treatment and Prophylaxis. Chicago, Year Book, 1981
94. Kroll F, Reiss E: Der Thoracle Bandscheibeprolaps. Dtsch Med Wschr 76:600–603, 1951
95. Laslett M: The role of physical therapy in soft-tissue rheumatism. Patient Management 15:57–68, 1986
96. Lee D, Walsh M: A Workbook of Manual Therapy Techniques for the Vertebral Column and Pelvic Girdle. Delta, B.C., Canada, Nascent Publishers, 1985
97. Lewit K: Manipulative Therapy in Rehabilitation of the Motor System, 2nd ed. Boston, Butterworths, 1991
98. Loebl WY: Measurement of spinal posture and range of spinal movement. Ann Phys Med 9:103–110, 1967
99. Love JG, Schorn VG: Thoracic-disk protrusions. JAMA 191:627–631, 1965
100. Low J: The modern body therapies, Part 4: Aston patterning. Massage Magazine 1988
101. Maachleder HI, Moll F, Verity MA: The anterior scalene muscle in thoracic outlet compression syndromes. Arch Surg 121:1141–1144, 1986
102. Mackinnon SE, Dellon AL: Surgery of the Peripheral Nerve. New York, Thieme, 1988
103. Magee DJ: Orthopedic Physical Assessment, 2nd ed. Philadelphia, WB Saunders, 1992
104. Maigne R: Orthopaedic Medicine. Springfield, Ill., Charles C. Thomas, 1972
105. Maigne R: Semeiologie clinique des derangements intervertebraux mineurs. Ann Med Phys 15:275–292, 1972
106. Maigne R: Manipulation of the spine. In Basmajian JV (ed): Manipulation, Traction and Massage. Baltimore, Williams & Wilkins, 1986
107. Maigne R, Le Corre F: Sur l'origine cervicale de certaines dorsalgies rebelles et benignes. Ann Med Phys 1:1–18, 1964
108. Maitland GD: Vertebral Manipulation, 5th ed. London, Butterworths, 1986
109. Matson DD, Wood RP, Campbell JB, et al: Diastematomyelia (congenital clefts of the spinal cord). Pediatrics 6:98–112, 1950
110. May P: Thoracic spine. In Payton OD, Difabio RP, Paris SV, et al: Manual of Physical Therapy. New York, Churchill Livingstone, 1989
111. McCarthy RE: Coping with low back pain through behavioral change. Orthop Nurs 3:30–35, 1983
112. McConnell J: McConnell patellofemoral treatment plan. Course notes, McConnell Seminars, 1990
113. McGuckin N: The T4 Syndrome. In Grieve GP (ed): Modern Manual Therapy of the Vertebral Column. Edinburgh, Churchill Livingstone, 1986:370–376
114. McKenzie RA: The Lumbar Spine: Mechanical Diagnosis and Therapy. Waikanae, New Zealand, Spinal Publications Ltd, 1981
115. McKenzie RA: Care of the Neck. Waikanae, New Zealand, Spinal Publications Ltd, 1983

116. McKenzie RA: The Cervical and Thoracic Spine: Mechanical Diagnosis and Therapy. Waikanae, New Zealand, Spinal Publications Ltd, 1990
117. McNair JFS, Maitland GD: Manipulative therapy techniques in the management of some thoracic syndromes. In Grant R (ed): Physical Therapy of the Cervical and Thoracic Spine. New York, Churchill Livingstone, 1988
118. Melzack R: The McGill pain questionnaire: Major properties and scoring methods. Pain 1:277–299, 1975
119. Melzack R, Wall PD: Pain mechanisms: A new theory. Science 150:971–979, 1965
120. Mennell JM: Back Pain. Boston, Little, Brown & Co, 1960
121. Miller B: Alternative somatic therapies. In White A, Anderson R (eds): Conservative Care of Low Back Pain. Baltimore, Williams & Wilkins, 1991:120–136
122. Miller B: Manual therapy treatment of myofascial pain and dysfunction. In Rachlin ES: Myofascial Pain and Fibromyalgia. St. Louis, CV Mosby, 1994:415–454
123. Mitchell FL, Moran PS, Pruzzo NA: An Evaluation and Treatment Manual of Osteopathic Muscle Energy Procedures. Valley Park, MO, Mitchell, Moran, and Pruzzo Associates, 1979
124. Moll JMH, Wright V: Measurement of spinal movement. In Jayson M (ed): The Lumbar Spine and Back Pain. New York, Grune & Stratton, 1981:93–112
125. Montgomery F, Willner S: Screening for idiopathic scoliosis. Acta Orthop Scand 64:456–458, 1993
126. Mooney V, Robertson J: The facet syndrome. Clin Orthop 115:149–156,1976
127. Mulligan BR: Manual Therapy: "Nags," "Snags," "Prp's," etc. Wellington, New Zealand, Plane View Services Ltd, 1989
128. Murtagh J, Findlay D, Kenna C: Low back pain. Aust Fam Physician 14:1214–1224, 1985
129. Nathan H, Weinberg H, Robin GC, Aviad I: Costovertebral joints: Anatomico-clinical observation in arthritis. Arth Rheum 7:228–240, 1964
130. O'Sullivan SB: Multiple sclerosis. In O'Sullivan SB, Schmitz (eds): Physical Rehabilitation: Assessment and Treatment. Philadelphia, FA Davis, 1988
131. Oliver MJ, Lynn JW, Lynn JM: An interpretation of the McKenzie approach to low back pain. In Twomey LT, Taylor JR (eds): Physical Therapy of the Low Back. New York, Churchill Livingstone, 1987:250–251
132. Paris SV: The Spinal Lesion. New Zealand, Degasus Press, 1965
133. Paris SV: Physical signs of instability. Spine 10:277–279, 1985
134. Pavelka K von: Rotationsmessung der wirbelsaule. A Rheumaforschg 29:366, 1970
135. Peacock E, Van Winkle: Wound Repair. Philadelphia, WB Saunders, 1976
136. Peltier LF: Surgical treatment for symptoms produced by cervical ribs and the scalene anticus muscle. Clin Orthop 207:3–13, 1986
137. Phillips H, Grieve GP: The thoracic outlet syndrome. In Grieve GP (ed): Modern Manual Therapy of the Vertebral Column. Edinburgh, Churchill Livingstone, 1986:359
138. Pickering SG: Exercises for the Autonomic Nervous System. Springfield, Ill., Charles C. Thomas, 1981
139. Rasmussen TB, Kernohan JW, Adson AW: Pathologic classification with surgical consideration of intraspinal tumors. Ann Surg 111:513–530, 1940
140. Rath WW, Rath JND, Duffy CG: A Comparison of Pain Location and Duration with Treatment Outcome and Frequency. Presented at the International McKenzie Conference, Newport Beach, CA, 1989
141. Richardson N: Aston Patterning. Phys Ther Forum 6:1–3, 1987
142. Rocabado M: Advanced Upper Quarter. Continuing education course, Racobado Institute, San Francisco, 1984
143. Roos DB: The thoracic outlet is underrated. Arch Neurol 47:327–328, 1990
144. Rosse C: Segmental innervation. In Rosse C, Clawson DK (eds): The Musculoskeletal System in Health and Disease. Philadelphia, Harper & Row, 1980:169–177
145. Ruggerone M, Austin JHM: Moire topography in scoliosis: Correlations with vertebral lateral curvature as determined by radiography. Phys Ther 66:1072–1076, 1986
146. Rywerant Y: The Feldenkrais Method: Teaching by Handling. San Francisco, Harper & Row, 1983
147. Saal JA: Rehabilitation of sports-related lumbar injuries. Phys Med Rehab: State-of-the-Art Reviews 4:613–638, 1987
148. Sahrmann S: A program for correction of muscular imbalances and mechanical imbalances. Clin Manag 3:23–28, 1983
149. Sahrmann S: Adult posturing. In Kraus S (ed): TMJ Disorders; Management of the Craniomandibular Complex. New York, Churchill Livingstone, 1988
150. Sahrmann S: Diagnosis and treatment of muscle imbalances and associated regional pain syndromes. Course notes, Seattle, 1993
151. Saibil FB, Edmeades J: Chest pain arising from extrathoracic structures. In Levene DL (ed): Chest Pain: An Integrated Diagnostic Approach. Philadelphia, Lea & Febiger, 1977:130
152. Saliba VL, Johnson GS: Back education and training. Course outline, San Anselmo, CA: The Institute of Physical Arts, 1988
153. Saliba VL, Johnson GS: Lumbar protective mechanism. In White AH, Anderson R (eds): Conservative Care of Low Back Pain. Baltimore, Williams & Wilkins, 1991
154. Saunders HD: Evaluation, Treatment and Prevention of Musculoskeletal Disorders. Minneapolis, Viking, 1985
155. Sherrington C: The Integrated Action of the Nervous System, 2nd ed. New Haven, Yale University Press, 1947
156. Sinaki M, Kenneth P, Offord MS: Physical activity in postmenopausal women: Effect on back muscle strength and bone mineral density of the spine. Arch Phys Med Rehabil 69:277–280, 1988
157. Sinaki M, Mikkelsen BA: Postmenopausal spinal osteoporosis: Flexion versus extension exercises. Arch Phys Med Rehabil 65:593–596, 1984
158. Stallworth JM, Horne JB: Diagnosis and management of thoracic outlet syndrome. Arch Surg 119:1149–1151, 1984
159. Stoddard A: Manual of Osteopathic Practice. London, Hutchinson, 1969
160. Stoddard A: Manual of Osteopathic Technique, 8th ed. London, Hutchinson, 1974
161. Stoddard A: The Back—Relief From Pain. London, Dunitz, 1979
162. Sydenham RW: Manual therapy techniques for the thoracolumbar spine. In Donatelli R, Wooden MJ (eds): Orthopedic Physical Therapy. Edinburgh, Churchill Livingstone, 1989:359–401
163. Trager M: Psychophysical integration and Mentastics. J Holistic Health 7:15–25, 1982
164. Travell JG, Simons DG: Myofascial Pain and Dysfunction: The Trigger Point Manual. Baltimore, Williams & Wilkins, 1983
165. Upton ARM, McComas AJ: The double crush in nerve entrapment syndromes. Lancet 2:359–362, 1973
166. Veldhuizen AG, Sholten PJM: Kinematics of the scoliotic spine as related to the normal spine. Spine 12:852–858, 1987
167. Wadsworth CT: Manual Examination and Treatment of the Spine and Extremities. Baltimore, Williams & Wilkins, 1988
168. Warwick R, Williams PL (eds): Gray's Anatomy, 35th British ed. Philadelphia, WB Saunders, 1973
169. Weiss HR: The effect of an exercise program on vital capacity and rib mobility in patients with idiopathic scoliosis. Spine 16:88–93, 1991
170. Weiss HR: Influence of an inpatient exercise program on scoliotic curve. Ital J Orthop Traum 18:395–406, 1993
171. Wilbourn AJ: The thoracic outlet syndrome is overdiagnosed. Arch Neurol 47:328–330, 1990
172. Witt PL: Trager psychophysical integration: An additional tool in treatment of chronic spinal pain and dysfunction. Whirlpool 9:24–26, 1986
173. Witt PL, MacKinnon J: Trager psychophysical integration: A method to improve chest mobility of patients with chronic lung disease. Phys Ther 66:214–217, 1986
174. Witt PL, Parr C: Effectiveness of Trager psychophysical integration in promoting trunk mobility in a child with cerebral palsy: A case report. Physical and Occupational Therapy in Pediatrics 8(4):75–94, 1988
175. Woo S, Matthews JV, Akeson WH, et al: Connective tissue response to immobility: Correlative study of biomechanical and biochemical measurements of normal and immobilized rabbit knees. Arthritis Rheum 18:257–264, 1975

The Lumbar Spine

DARLENE HERTLING

■ EPIDEMIOLOGY

Backache ranks high as a cause of lost working days among Americans. Second only to the common cold as a reason for outpatient visits, it represents the single most common and most expensive industrial and occupational health problem.[113] Each year about 500,000 workers in the United States sustain back injuries, leading to lost time from work and financial compensation. Health-care costs, disability payments, and lost productivity related to low back pain syndromes are estimated at some $20 billion annually. An estimated 8 million Americans suffer from chronic low back pain.[582] Each year more than 200,000 Americans undergo some sort of back surgery. About 30% of workers at some time miss work because of a back ailment; 2% to 4% actually change jobs at least once because of this problem, in addition to the ones who become disabled.[628] According to Kelsey and White, workers who are off the job more than 6 months with back pain have only a 50% chance of returning to work; this decreases to 25% after 1 year.[300]

Nachemson's 1976 report may be the most quoted paper in the field.[446] It states that 80% of citizens will suffer back pain "to some extent," men as often as women, "white collar as often as blue collar workers." About 50 in 100 workers are significantly affected each year, leading to 1400 to 2600 lost workdays per 1000 workers each year. Thus, back pain is the most expensive ailment in the 30- to 60-year-old age group.

The patient with acute low back pain presents different problems due to the self-limiting nature of the first episode: 88% will be asymptomatic in 6 weeks, 98% in 24 weeks, and 99% in 52 weeks; 97% of causes

Darlene Hertling and Randolph M. Kessler: MANAGEMENT OF COMMON MUSCULOSKELETAL DISORDERS: Physical Therapy Principles and Methods, 3rd ed. © 1996 Lippincott-Raven Publishers.

are unknown, 2% are attributed to disk problems, and 1% to apophyseal joint disorders. No more than 29% require conservative measures, 1% surgery, and the rest recover spontaneously.[326]

According to Dagi and Beary, about 80% of all back cases can be attributed to soft-tissue conditions (*i.e.*, muscle or ligament sprain, postural abnormalities, poor muscle tone, or neuromuscular disease) and 10% to intervertebral disk disease with or without radiculopathy.[113] The annual incidence of diagnosed disk prolapse is about 5% per year in 20- to 40-year-olds. These lesions occur most often at L4–L5 and L5–S1 segments. Thirty percent of all those who have back pain have a syndrome consistent with radiculopathy at some time in their life.[628] Those operated on for disk herniation are usually 30 to 39 years old, tending to confirm the theory that partly degenerated disks are the most likely to herniate in such a way as to lead to surgery.

Roentgenographic evidence of disk space narrowing or osteophytosis is found in 70% of men and 50% of women aged 55 to 64 years. Autopsy studies show that disk degeneration begins at 20 to 25 years of age.[300] With respect to facet joint disease, Kelsey and White state that disk and facet joint disease are closely but most inevitably linked.[300] About 90% of autopsies in patients older than 45 years reveal lumbar facet osteoarthrosis, and more joints are affected as age increases. Most studies have found that symptomatology is not significantly related to such findings.

The epidemiology of other specific diagnoses is not discussed thoroughly in the literature. For example, Shealy suggests that 20% of chronic unoperated back pain patients had sacroiliac joint symptoms as their major complaint, but did not further specify how this was demonstrated.[548] Travel and Simons make only scant reference to the epidemiology of myofascial pain and quote Kraft and Levinthal as stating that the affected patients were most likely aged 31 to 50 years.[320,617] A large number of soft-tissue-related anatomical or clinical syndromes (*i.e.*, iliolumbar ligament strains, piriformis syndrome, lumbodorsal fascia tears, iliac crest syndrome) are described in the literature, but few research studies or controlled tests have been conducted. Many of the more accepted terms used to describe these conditions, as Flor and Turk point out, are more descriptive than etiological or useful, especially with respect to the treatment of individual patients.[175]

Recently, a considerable amount of work has been done concerning risk factors, individual characteristics, and the natural history of low back pain. Low back pain in general, and disk herniation specifically, are influenced by many factors, including age and gender.[33,37,61,263,265,299,366,367,575,601,628] Low back pain in general is as common in females as in males,

but the pattern changes when the work situation is taken into account.[263,601,628] Magora found that 35% of women in physically heavy jobs had low back pain, compared to 19.1% of males.[366,367] Strength factors could be a reason, or a mismatch between the worker's physical strength and the job requirements.[14]

Repeated lifting of heavy loads is often considered a risk factor for back pain,[33,265–267,298,368,446] although others deny this.[265,266,404,628] Magora found sudden unexpected maximal efforts to be particularly harmful.[368] Glover, Tichauer, and Troup and associates expressed the same opinion about lifting in combination with lateral bending and twisting.[200,614,622] Magora found no relation to heavy lifting while standing, but he did find that workers who handled materials while seated and bent over had a high incidence of back pain.[366,367]

In general, postural deformities, scoliosis/kyphosis, hypo- or hyperlordosis, and leg-length discrepancy do not seem to predispose to low back pain.[38,263,265,266,370,520,575] Although there is considerable disagreement, studies of static work postures indicate an increased risk of low back pain in subjects with predominantly sitting working postures.[265,266,322,334,368] Sitting with a bent-over working posture seems to carry a significant increased risk factor. Kelsey[298] and Kelsey and Hardy[299] found that men who spend more than half their workday in a car have a threefold increased risk of disk herniation. This could be due to the combined effects of sitting and vibration.

Andersson reviewed the industrial epidemiology of the last 30 years and stated that physically heavy, static work postures, frequent bending and twisting, lifting and forceful movements, and repetitive work and vibration were vocational factors in back pain.[13] He and others noted as well that tallness provides an increased risk of injury[13,298,334,608] and that sciatica is more common in the obese.[267]

Physical fitness and conditioning have significant preventive effects on back injuries. Weak trunk muscles and decreased endurance are significant risk factors in the development of back problems.[288] Cady and associates showed that among fire-fighters, muscle strength was an accurate prognostic indicator for the development of low back pain.[69] Chaffin[82] and Keyserling and associates,[307] using pre-employment strength testing, found that the risk of back injury increases threefold when the job requirements exceed the worker's capabilities on an isometric simulation of the job.

Clinical observations led Rowe[520] and Berguist-Ullman and Larsson[33] to conclude that abdominal and spinal extensor muscle strength was decreased in patients with low back pain.[330] Many other investigators have established that patients with low back pain have lower mean trunk strength than do healthy subjects.[5,8,34,240,277,282,410,470,475,498,541] Some investigators have found the extensors to be more influenced (weaker) than the flexors,[465,541] whereas others have identified relatively greater extensor strength.[38,39,40] Biering-Sorenson found that patients with recurrent back pain had weaker trunk muscles and diminished flexibility (particularly flexion) when compared with asymptomatic persons.[39] Conversely, good isometric endurance in men appears to prevent low back problems. Very little data concerning the endurance capacity of the back muscles are found in the literature.[256,465] The most striking finding of Nicolaisen and Jorgensen in persons with early, serious low back trouble was decreased endurance capacity of the trunk extensors rather than muscle strength, when compared with normal subjects.[465]

Other factors significantly associated with low back pain include smoking and coughing.[191,601] Svensson speculated that coughing led to increased intradiskal pressure and thus to increased loading and low back pain.[601] Disk degeneration, osteoporosis, and spondylolisthesis are all associated with increased low back pain. The major risk for an episode of back pain is a previous history of back pain.[254]

Several reports give a fairly clear picture of how the patient with acute back pain fares.[16,33,133,621] Horal documented that 90% of acute symptoms resolve in the 2 months after the first episode.[263] It is often suggested that little can be done in the way of treatment to alter this course. Some evidence exists, however, that short periods of bed rest (2 days), back school, and early and comprehensive care of the patient can speed the return to work.[33,127] Thus, when the initial history and physical examination suggest limited injury or abnormality, without significant neurological deficit, an initial trial of empirically based conservative treatment and early mobilization is warranted.[127] Nachemson has summarized a variety of data suggesting that motion, rather than rest, may be beneficial in healing soft tissues and joints.[447] For the patient who appears to have a herniated disk with a motor deficit, there is a good biological rationale for recommending longer periods of bed rest (*i.e.*, reduction of intradiskal pressure).[444]

The risk that the typical patient with acute low back pain will suffer a recurrence over the next few years is about 60%.[33,620] The next attack, however, may be shorter and have a more benign course. According to Troup and associates, attacks of accident-related pain take longer to subside, both during the first attack and with recurrence.[621] Other factors influencing recurrence include sciatic pain, alcoholism, specific job situations, sociopsychological stigmata, and general insurance benefits.[450]

Social problems are greatest in chronic low back pain. Nachemson lists just as many social or psychological findings as mechanical or occupational ones in considering the correlates of back pain.[446] He mentions abnormal profiles on the Minnesota Multiphasic Personality Inventory (MMPI), the most widely used psychological test, as well as alcoholism, history of divorce, educational level, and depression as some of the factors that may affect the relation between acute injury or pain and chronic back pain. Severe mental problems are no more common in low back patients, but changes in the MMPI are seen.[14]

Many different diseases can present as low back pain. The purpose of this chapter is not to classify the numerous known causes for low back pain, but rather to deal with the more common types of back pain, including so-called "idiopathic" low back pain.[649] Other sources offer an exhaustive classification of the etiology of low back pain.[9,363,406,450,504]

Musculoskeletal disorders are of primary importance because they are the largest group of complaints most often seen by physical therapists and other health-care practitioners. However, systemic and visceral problems may mimic low back pain.[56,214,558,657] Thus, a thorough abdominal examination may direct attention away from the spine to a source of viscerogenic pain. Here, we are interested only in minor mechanical derangements; this excludes fractures, dislocations, inflammatory disorders, and tumors.

■ APPLIED ANATOMY

□ Three-Joint Segment

At any one level, the motion segment is composed of three distinct parts: the two facet (zygapophyseal) joints and the intervertebral joint (the disk) (Fig. 20-1). In a normal motion segment, these three joints are anatomically linked and mechanically balanced. With age or as a result of various pathological processes, degeneration may affect the motion segment. The segment as a whole may be somehow programmed to fail, with the chondrocytes of the disk nucleus involuting at the same time that the subchondral bone fractures; or, by attrition, each component structure may succumb to stress in turn. Narrowing of the disk space, spondylolisthesis, and transitional vertebrae tend to apply abnormal stress to the posterior structures.[156,157] Conversely, dysplasia of the lumbosacral facet structures or degenerative changes in the facet joints can cause spondylolisthesis.[462] The two major sites of pathological change—the intervertebral disks and facet joints—must not be considered independently of one another: dysfunction of one, if allowed

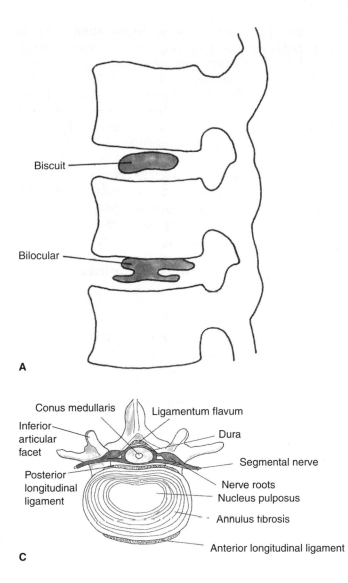

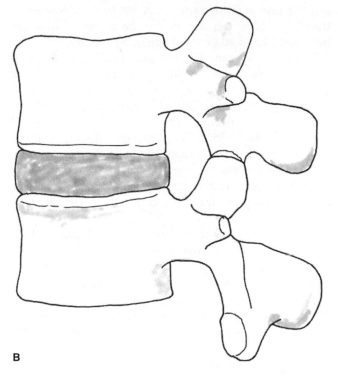

FIG. 20-1. (**A**) Some normal diskogram configurations. (**B**) A properly spaced lumbar vertebra. (**C**) Superior view of a normal intervertebral disk. (*A* adapted from Finneson BE: Low Back Pain, 2nd ed, p 104. Philadelphia, JB Lippincott, 1980.)

to progress, ultimately leads to dysfunction of the other.

The disk depends on normal movement (and therefore adequate mobility at the facet joints) for its nutrition and for an even distribution of force to the annulus over time. On the other hand, normal arthrokinematics at the facet joints depend, in part, on a healthy disk. An inelastic disk at a given level tends to alter the normal centroid of movement for the respective facet joints, a factor likely to contribute to the initiation of a degenerative cycle of events, as discussed in Chapter 3, Arthrology.[163,164,438,651]

In considering joint dysfunction of the spine, as with the peripheral joints, our conceptual model must include all the anatomical and physiological structures of the joint. Only by looking at the whole picture can we judge which tissues seem to be primarily affected in a particular disorder, as well as the probable or possible secondary effects on other joint tissues. In the spine, it is best to think more in terms of segmental dysfunction rather than joint dysfunction, because

of the intimate dependency of the paired facet joints and the intervertebral joint. Therefore, always consider that a segment includes two vertebrae with their paired facet joints, the intervening intervertebral joint with its disk, the muscles and ligaments controlling the segment, the nerves supplying the segment, the nerve tissue within the vertebral canal at the segment, and the spinal nerves leading from the segment and the tissues they innervate.[93] This is why spinal dysfunction is much more complex than peripheral joint dysfunction.

☐ Vertebrae

One of the more important aspects of the skeletal aging process is bone loss. A gradual decrease in cortical bone of 3% per decade can be expected for both sexes. In postmenopausal women, a 9% rate of decrease in cortical bone per decade has been demonstrated. Trabecular bone (see Fig. 16-6) also decreases, but the rate is more variable. A 6% to 8% decrease in trabecular bone per decade can be expected to begin between 20 and 40 years of age in both sexes.[398]

These changes modify the load-bearing capacity of the vertebrae. After age 40, the load-bearing capacity of cortical cancellous bone changes dramatically.[514] Before age 40, about 55% of load-bearing capacity is attributed to cancellous bone; after age 40, this decreases to about 35%. Bone strength decreases more rapidly than bone quantity.[29] This decrease in strength accounts for the end-plates bending away from the disk, wedge fractures of vertebral bodies, and the end-plate fractures common in osteoporotic spines.[139]

The cartilaginous end-plate of the vertebral body is the weak point of the disk (see Fig. 16-12). It is the site of failure when compressive loads become excessive. Between age 23 and 40, there is a gradual demineralization of end-plate cartilage. By age 60, only a thin layer of bone separates the disk from the vascular channels. These nutrient channels are slowly obliterated and the arterioles and venules progressively thicken.[35] Such changes can have a significant role in the pathogenesis of lumbar disk disease. Because the adult disk has no blood supply, it must rely on diffusion for nutrition.[446]

In the upper lumbar spine, degeneration seems to start early with end-plate fractures and nuclear herniations (Schmorl's nodes) related to the essentially vertical loading of those segments (Fig. 20-2)[163] Facet disease also starts first in the upper lumbar spine. In the lower lumbar spine, disk changes begin in the late teens, facet changes in the mid-20s. Both lesions typically are seen first at L5–S1, then at L4–L5. Degenerative changes of both synovial and vertebral joints seem to occur together, most often at the lumbosacral articulation.[214] Spondylitic and arthrotic changes involving the whole segment are age-related and occur in about 60% of persons over age 45.[339]

☐ **Facet (Zygapophyseal) Joints**

All the pathologic considerations presented in Chapter 3, Arthrology, apply to the posterior elements and the spinal facet joints (see Fig. 16-9). Primary inflammatory conditions affecting spinal joints are relatively rare; the two major exceptions are ankylosing spondylitis, affecting most often the young male, and rheumatoid arthritis, which primarily involves the upper cervical spine. Osteoarthrosis is probably the major joint condition affecting the spine. It most fre-

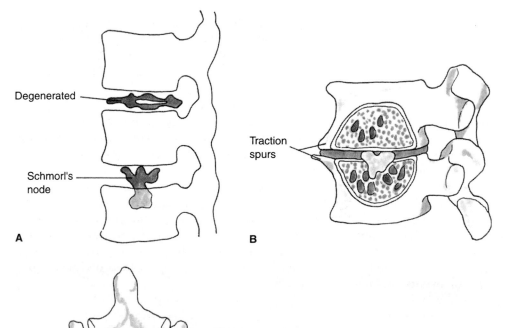

FIG. 20-2. Some abnormal diskogram configurations. (**A**) Chronic lumbar degenerative joint disease. (**B**) Narrowing of the disk and foramina and hypertrophic changes at the vertebral margins. (**B, C**) Internal disruption of the disk. (A adapted from Finneson BE: Low Back Pain, 2nd ed, p 104. Philadelphia, JB Lippincott, 1980.)

quently involves the lower cervical spine and the lower lumbar levels. In the lumbar region, degenerative changes of the facet joints are the rule rather than the exception in virtually everyone living beyond the third decade or so. This fact is attributable in part to the likelihood that the human spine has not completely adapted to the upright, weight-bearing position and to the fact that human life expectancy has been drastically extended. Normal degeneration generally progresses so gradually that only minor symptoms, if any, result. The person may develop a "stiff spine" but usually not until an age at which the normal activity level does not require much mobility anyway. Again, because the process proceeds gradually, the joint tissues gradually adapt by means of fibrosis, bony hypertrophy, or even spontaneous ankylosis; thus, little if any inflammation or pain results. For this reason it is not unusual to see very marked joint narrowing with hypertrophic bony changes on roentgenograms in a person with marked restriction of spinal mobility, even if the person denies significant back pain or dysfunction over the years.

On the other hand, some persons suffer an acceleration of the normal degenerative processes of the spinal joints. The reasons may include a genetic predisposition, such as asymmetry of facet planes in the lower lumbar spine; an occupational predisposition, such as a job involving abnormal compression of joint surfaces; or some other factor resulting in considerable alteration in normal joint mechanics, such as excessive muscle tension or sudden changes in disk mechanics. These persons eventually complain of spinal pain; the origin of their pain is the facet joint capsule, which undergoes abnormal stress from the alteration in normal mechanics. In such cases, the altered joint mechanics occur suddenly enough, or to such a degree, that the joint tissues do not have time to adapt through fibrosis and bony hypertrophy. The painful condition continues unless joint stresses sufficient to cause pain are prevented through restoration of normal mechanics and avoidance of certain activities, or until the condition runs its course—that is, over the years, the joint tissues will gradually adapt to the abnormal stresses placed on them. Symptoms are likely to appear before significant radiographic changes; conversely, roentgenographic "degenerative" changes cannot be reliably correlated with symptoms.[371]

Spinal joints, like any synovial joint, can refer pain into the relevant segments, or sclerotomes.[110,112] Pain of spinal joint origin tends to be a deep aching pain felt in an area that often does not correlate well to the skin overlying the site of the lesion; this is characteristic of pain of deep somatic origin.

Posterior element changes proceed from early degenerative joint disease with articular erosion of the facet surfaces to fibrous dysplasia, loss of normal anatomical relations of the facets, osteophyte formation (in an attempt to heal capsular injuries), synovial proliferations, and eventually hyper- or hypomobility of the joint.[164] Associated with this process are changes in the subchondral bone similar to those seen in degenerative joint disease in other joints, but in the lumbar spine there is also frequently a fatty infiltration of the joint, revealing the "abnormal widening" and the lack of mechanical function of a fully degenerated joint.

The ligamentum flavum (see Fig. 16-8) becomes less elastic and thicker, although the thickness may result from shortening secondary to lost disk height rather than the commonly implied "hypertrophy."[618] Thus, the ligament plays only a passive role in neural entrapment problems. Although the intimate association of the ligamentum flavum with the medial aspect of the facet joint capsule should retract the capsule and synovium when the capsule is slack, this system may not work well because the ligamentum flavum shortens with age and the loss of disk height.[21] Several works refer to the possibility of joint dysfunction and pain secondary to entrapment of the synovium, meniscoid bodies (or meniscoid inclusions), or capsule, or loose joint bodies, especially during re-extension after forward-flexion.[320,483,484,486]

In quick, poorly controlled movements, or, for example, in the case of a relatively lax ligamentum flavum from segmental narrowing, a meniscoid may become entrapped with a resulting pinching of the innervated portion and a pulling on the capsule to which they attach. This results in a reflex, segmental muscle spasm that tends to prevent the spontaneous release of the entrapped structure. Clinically, the patient presents with a history of a sudden onset of localized pain and "spasm," usually accompanying a combined rotation and extension movement. The pain is immediate, persistent, and associated with rather marked spinal deformity in a direction of flexion, rotation, and sidebending away from the involved side. This must be distinguished from the patient who, while bent forward, feels an immediate pain in the back, which quickly subsides for the most part, then gradually builds to a constant, intense pain over a period of 8 to 12 hours; this is invariably an acute disk protrusion.

This dysfunction concept is highly theoretical. Many believe that it is based on sound anatomical, physiological, and biomechanical principles. A review and anatomical study by Bogduk and Engel describes three types of meniscoid structures (connective tissue rim, adipose tissue pad, and fibroadipose meniscoid), which are in fact found in various percentages of lumbar facet joints.[47] A histologic study of the fibroadipose meniscoid (the only one long enough to be trapped between the articular surfaces) suggested that it is not strong enough to provide painful traction on the joint capsule in such circumstances.[47] There is a possibility of detachment of the meniscoid with resultant effusion, but that would not be relieved with manipulation, which has been considered effective in the facet joint meniscal syndrome. The authors concluded that it would be appropriate to consider other causes of "acute locked back" outside the lumbar facet joint.

Studies of intervention in the form of surgical fusion or surgical, chemical, or thermal denervation of the facets indicate that many cases of back pain may be of facet origin.[53,77,78,350,489,546] That impression is supported by the experiment of Mooney and Robertson, who produced typical sciatica, sometimes bilaterally, by facet joint injections with hypertonic saline in patients.[432]

Other proponents of the facet joint as a cause of pain have concentrated on root impingement caused by inflammatory hypertrophy of the joint margin, with resulting root compression or irritation. Vertical subluxation of the superior facet occurs with loss of disk space, leading to superior articular facet syndrome and root impingement in the intervertebral foramen by the subluxated process.[156,518]

Damage to the facet joint has always been considered secondary to disk failure. However, according to Farfan,[163,164] Grieve,[214] and others, autopsy evidence clearly shows that facet damage of varying degrees can and frequently does occur in the absence of disk failure. Helfet and Gruebel Lee maintain that lesions of the posterior element always have an effect on the disk and that disk lesions always have an effect on the posterior joints.[246]

☐ Intervertebral Disk

In a manner and at a rate not unlike those of the facet joints, human intervertebral disks (see Fig. 20-2) undergo a normal process of degeneration.[502,510] Early changes in the lumbar intervertebral disks are common as early as the second decade, when vascular channels begin to become obliterated. With the developing lumbar lordosis, the posterior lamellae of the annulus become compressed vertically and also horizontally, with an associated tendency toward posterior bulging of the annular fibers. The compaction of the posterior lamellae gives the posterior annulus the appearance of being thinner than the anterior annulus, although the number of lamellae remains the same. The nucleus remains a viscous, incompressible gel with a few collagen fibers embedded.[604]

The nucleus gradually changes from a gel to more of a viscous, fibrous structure. Associated with this process is early breakdown of mucopolysaccharide (with a net loss of chondroitin sulfate); there is a resul-

tant decrease in water-binding capacity and a slight increase in collagen content (from 15% in the first decade to about 20% in the remaining years).[67,249,457–459] The original water content decreases from 88% to about 70%.[457] Beginning at the third decade, there is a 55% decrease in the glycosaminoglycan content of the nucleus pulposus.[238] There is a gradual increase in glycoprotein (noncollagen), particularly in the cross-beta form.[361] The posterior annulus gradually becomes more weight-bearing, probably due in part to some loss in the preload condition of the nucleus and its ability to withstand vertical compression, but also because of the increasing lumbar lordosis. The posterior lamellae continue to compress posteriorly with an associated posterior bulging. The anterior annular lamellae, which have greater vertical height, remain comparatively loose but also begin bulging posteriorly. The posterolateral annulus becomes dog-eared—it tends to compact and bulge considerably in the posterolateral direction. Between the lamellae of the posterolateral annulus, clefts or gaps appear, perhaps secondary to a pressure atrophy from the combined vertical forces of weight-bearing and the horizontal pressure from the nucleus pulposus. Vascular channels have been shut off and have filled with fibrous scarring.

During the fourth decade, transformation of the nucleus from nearly a pure gel to a largely fibrous mass becomes complete. The nucleus gradually becomes less distinguishable from the surrounding annulus. A considerable portion of the nucleus, in addition to the invading collagen fibers, consists of pulpy debris left from the breakdown of the original protein-polysaccharide material. The water content continues to decrease, although the nucleus retains its volume. The cartilaginous end-plate begins to thin, and some of the scarred vascular channels tend to coalesce to form larger pits. It has been proposed that these weaker, pitted areas are often the site of Schmorl's nodes or invasion of the nucleus into the vertebral body (see Fig. 20-2A). Clefting of the posterolateral annulus continues, spreading into the posterior annulus. Some of the clefts meet, forming even larger gaps in the posterolateral annulus. A few radial tears may begin to form across adjacent lamellae, especially in the inner layers of the posterolateral annulus.

Over the next 20 years, roughly from age 40 to 60, similar processes continue. With continued loss of nuclear water content and collapse of the annular lamellae, the disk space begins to narrow. The nucleus is now a pulpy, fibrous mass that is largely adhered to adjacent vertebral bodies (see Fig. 20-2C). Clefts in the annulus continue to increase in number and distribution and to coalesce to form larger clefts. Radial tearing, especially posterolaterally, increases, often with rather large tears extending horizontally across the entire annulus, allowing the nucleus to protrude into the annular space. The annular fibers are correspondingly weaker and have lost their normal elasticity. With gradual narrowing, increased weight-bearing peripherally, and increased tension on the outer annular fibers attaching to the vertebral bodies at the periphery, the added stresses to the margins of the vertebral body result in a hypertrophic bony reaction with the development of spurs and osteophytes. These occur both anteriorly and posteriorly (see Fig. 20-2B).

After age 60, the disk space is essentially filled with a mass of relatively unorganized fibrous material connecting adjacent vertebral bodies. The area once occupied by the nucleus is virtually indistinguishable from the annular regions. The spaces are narrowed, and bony changes at the periphery of the superior and inferior vertebral bodies are considerable.

Again, this a normal process that occurs in virtually every human spine. So long as the process continues gradually over the years, the involved tissues can be expected to adapt to the altered mechanics so that although considerable changes occur, the person suffers little pain or disability. For example, although the annulus weakens considerably, the nucleus, at the same time, becomes more fibrous and loses volume and therefore exerts less pressure on the annulus, so that the annulus need not be as strong. Although the fibrosis of the disk space results in a very immobile segment, the person, at the age at which this occurs, sim-

ply does not require much spinal mobility for activities of daily living.

As with the facet joints, pathologic disk changes are those that occur prematurely or at an accelerated rate, in such a fashion that either the person or the related tissues cannot adapt to the change, resulting in pain or disability. Such pathological disk changes may result from several factors.[117,146,306,423] Hyper- or hypomobility at the related facet joints may certainly cause changes in the normal stresses to the intervertebral disk, resulting in accelerated tissue change. For instance, at a segment in which a facet on one side lacks mobility but its mate moves freely, asymmetrical movement will result in increased pressure from the nucleus on an isolated portion of the annulus. This portion of the annulus would tend to degenerate and possibly tear prematurely, resulting in a herniation or protrusion of the nucleus into the torn portion of the annulus (Fig. 20-3). If an entire segment lacks mobility, the segment above or below might tend to become hypermobile, with added stresses on the disk at the hypermobile segment. Again, the annulus at this segment may be unable to withstand the increased horizontal forces applied to it by the nucleus and may give way prematurely, allowing the nucleus to bulge into the space and applying pressure to the sensitive outer annular layers, posterior longitudinal ligament, or nerve root. Occupational factors may also play an important role. The person who must perform contin-

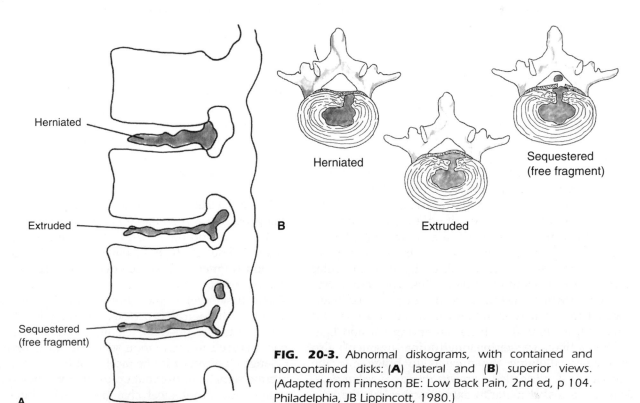

FIG. 20-3. Abnormal diskograms, with contained and noncontained disks: (**A**) lateral and (**B**) superior views. (Adapted from Finneson BE: Low Back Pain, 2nd ed, p 104. Philadelphia, JB Lippincott, 1980.)

ual forward-bending and lifting activities places heavier, more frequent horizontal stresses on the inner layers of the posterior annulus than the more sedentary person. On the other hand, the sedentary person is likely to lose normal annular elasticity and movement between annular lamellae earlier. The annulus is then less able to yield to the relatively higher demand placed on it during more strenuous activities (_e.g.,_ occasional sports participation), with an increased likelihood of tearing.

No matter what factors predispose to early disk lesions, persons aged 30 to 50 are much more susceptible to suffering an acute, symptomatic disk injury. At this age, a person usually is still quite active, has a nucleus pulposus that is of good volume, can imbibe fluid, and can exert horizontal forces on the annulus, and has an annulus that is beginning to weaken and form clefts and is therefore more likely to tear. Before this age, the annulus is strong and elastic and capable of withstanding pressures transmitted to it by the nucleus. After this period, the nucleus loses volume, narrows, and no longer can bulge posteriorly into sensitive tissues. The nucleus pulposus in the middle-aged person has been invaded by collagen tissue, which may be denser in some areas of the nucleus than in others. Because of this, the nucleus no longer exerts an even distribution of pressure on the posterior annulus; rather, areas of relatively high concentration of forces may result, again increasing the likelihood of an annular tear.

The posterolateral annulus tends to weaken first, with earlier development of clefts and tears. This is perhaps because in the lumbar region, the posterior longitudinal ligament is stronger centrally, thinning out over the posterolateral disk in its characteristic hourglass shape. The central portion of the posterior annulus is, then, better reinforced by this ligament. Also, because functional movements of the trunk tend to be diagonal rather than pure sagittal or coronal, the posterolateral annulus receives more pressure transmitted to it from the nucleus.

The person likely to experience symptoms of disk disease, then, is one in whom the inner layers of the posterior annulus tear in the presence of a nucleus pulposus that is still capable of bulging into the space left by the tear. If the tear is extensive enough, the nucleus may bulge sufficiently to cause increased pressure to the posterior longitudinal ligament or outer annular fibers, resulting in pain. This type of disk protrusion, in which the outer annulus or posterior longitudinal ligament remains intact, is called a _herniated nucleus (contained disk)._ If the outer annular and ligamentous fibers (posterior longitudinal ligament) also give way, allowing the nucleus to bulge into the neural canal, it is called a _prolapsed_ or _extruded nucleus._ When the diskal material extrudes through the pos-

terior longitudinal ligament, the condition is known as a _noncontained disk._ As long as the nuclear herniation is connected to the disk itself, a free protrusion is present. If the nuclear material has actually separated from the remaining nucleus, allowing it to be free in the neural canal, it is called a _sequestration of nuclear material_ (see Fig. 20-3). The term _disk protrusion_ is used in a general sense.

A herniation is likely to result in a deep, somatic type of pain or scleratogenous pain, which is deeply, poorly localized and perhaps referred to part or all of the relevant sclerotomal segment. Because the nucleus is still contained, the patient is likely to experience more pain in the morning after the nucleus has imbibed more fluid, because the added volume increases pressure on sensitive structures. A disk prolapse or sequestration (see Figs. 20-3 and 20-4) is more likely to impinge on nerve tissue, resulting in "neurogenic" pain and perhaps a progressive nerve root impingement syndrome, in which the symptoms change with prolonged pressure (see Chapter 4, Pain). Central prolapses, although relatively rare, may cause upper motor neuron disturbances if they occur in the cervical spine, with perhaps a plantar-flexion reflex response, lower extremity spasticity, and paresthesias into all four extremities. If the central prolapse occurs in the lumbar region, the lower sacral nerve roots may be compressed, resulting in bowel or bladder dysfunction.

☐ **Phases of Degeneration**

Generally, three conditions are considered degenerative—spondylosis, osteoarthritis, and herniated (or "slipped") disk (degenerative disk disease).[161,187,589] Alone, or more often together, they can lead to spinal stenosis and nerve root entrapment. Degenerative changes in general are the body's attempt to heal itself. Thus, the body tends to stabilize an unstable joint by immobilizing it, by the natural splintage of muscle spasms or by increasing the surface area of the joint.[139]

To define this process more clearly, Kirkaldy-Willis has proposed a reasonable system based on our current understanding of the degenerating motion segment.[308] The spectrum of degenerative change in the motion segment can be divided into three phases of deterioration.

The first level is the _early dysfunction phase_, with minor pathological processes resulting in abnormal function of the posterior element and disk. Damage has occurred in the motion segment but is reversible. Changes that occur in the facet joint during this phase are the same as those that occur in any other synovial joint. The pathological changes usually begin with

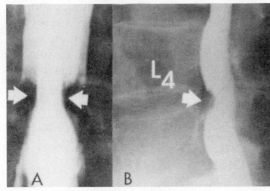

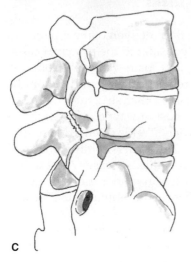

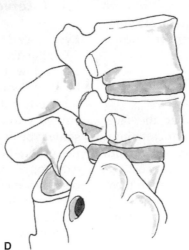

FIG. 20-4. Pathological processes of the lumbar spine. Anteroposterior (**A**) and lateral (**B**) myelogram views showing large central and bilateral disk bulge. Illustrations of (**C**) spondylosis and (**D**) spondylolisthesis. Anatomical differences between (**E**) normal and (**F**) stenotic spinal canals. (Finnesson BE: Low Back Pain, 2nd ed, p 141. Philadelphia, JB Lippincott, 1980.)

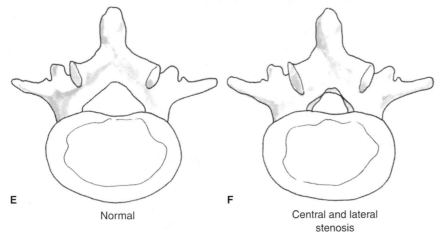

E
Normal

F
Central and lateral
stenosis

synovitis. Chronic synovitis and joint effusion can stretch a joint capsule. The inflamed synovium may in turn project folds, which can become entrapped in the joint between the cartilage surfaces and initiate cartilage damage. Most often, this early dysfunction phase involves the capsule and synovium, but it can also involve the cartilage surface or supporting bone. Disk dysfunction during this phase is less clear but probably involves the appearance of several circumferential tears in the annulus fibrosis. If these tears are in the outer layer, healing is possible because there is some

vascular supply. In the deeper layers, this is less likely because no blood supply is available. Slowly, there is progressive enlargement of the circumferential tears, which coalesce into radial tears. The nucleus begins to exhibit changes by losing proteoglycan content.

Next, an *intermediate instability phase* results in laxity of the posterior joint capsule and annulus. Permanent changes of instability may develop because of the chronicity and persistence of the dysfunction in earlier years. Restabilization of the posterior segment takes the form of subperiosteal bone formation or bone formation along ligaments and capsular fibers, resulting in perifacetal osteophytes and traction spurs.[139] Finally, the disk is anchored by peripheral osteophytes that pass around its circumference, producing a stable motion segment.

The *final stabilization phase* results in fibrosis of the posterior joints and capsule, the loss of disk material, and the formation of osteophytes.[308,644] Osteophytes form in response to abnormal motion to stabilize the affected motion segment.[463] Osteophyte formation around the three joints increases the load-bearing surface and decreases motion, resulting in a stiff, less painful motion segment.

Each of these categories defines a pattern of symptoms that may require varied treatment approaches.

☐ Incidental Complications

Although degenerative changes in either the facet joint or the disk may in themselves produce painful syndromes, the pathological interaction when both parts of the three-joint system are affected is most significant. The three-joint complex can go through these changes with very few symptoms. Pain is only a signal of impending or actual tissue damage and becomes manifest only if the tissue-failure threshold is reached. Thus, patients with minimal degenerative changes may present with chronic recurrent symptoms; others with severe roentgenographic changes present with few or no symptoms.

Each phase carries a specific set of incidental complications that may result in painful clinical syndromes. In the first phase, facet lesions may become manifest as painful facet syndrome. With increased formation of radial tears in the annulus, a disk herniation may occur, often caused by minor trauma. Disk herniations most commonly occur at the end of the dysfunction phase or the beginning of the instability phase, but may occur during the stabilization phase.[308]

During the instability phase, dynamic degenerative spondylolisthesis (see Fig. 20-4*D*) may occur when laxity predominates in the posterior restraining structures, or dynamic degenerative retrolisthesis when laxity predominates in the disk.[140] Both can produce dynamic lateral or central nerve entrapment.[501,629]

In the restabilization phase, narrowing of the central spinal canal at one level may be produced by osteophytic enlargement of the facet joints and circumferential osteophytes around the disk space, which can produce symptomatic central or lateral stenosis (see Fig. 20-4*F*). Later, the degeneration process may spread to involve several levels.

An attempt should be made to correlate this spectrum of degenerative changes and symptoms with di-

agnosis and treatment. Knowing the natural history of the disease enables the therapist to gain insight into the disease process, to make a more complete assessment, and to formulate a more rational regimen of treatment. An understanding of which forms of treatment are more likely to meet with success is important.

■ MEDICAL MODELS AND DISEASE ENTITIES

☐ Intervertebral Disks

Ever since Mixter and Barr delivered their paper in 1934, the disk has been considered the principal cause of all low back pain and pain referred from the back.[424] Because more research has been done on the intervertebral disk than any other structure, there is a tendency to attribute almost any type of backache to some type of disk disorder.[450] This often leads to tunnel vision, because many disorders, both spinal and extraspinal, may simulate disk disease. Although a disk dysfunction may result in more serious low back problems, it is rarely if ever the initial cause of low back pain.

Disk protrusion seems to be regarded by most current orthopaedists and neurosurgeons as the most probable diagnosis in cases of back pain with sciatica and evidence of nerve root involvement suggested by physical examination, electromyography, myelography, and other tests.[168,518,579,651] Cases not meeting these criteria are usually designated "mechanical" back pain; those that do meet them are treated conservatively (usually bed rest followed by flexion exercises if improved) or surgically (diskectomy or chemonucleolysis alone, unless there is added indication for fusion).

Recently, there seems to be a return to the concept that pain can arise from injured disk structures directly in cases of "annular tears."[163,308] Several classifications of clinical syndromes now include pain due to disk degeneration itself.[429,473,651] Although it was established more than 35 years ago, the concept of primary disk pain is relatively unfamiliar to clinicians because it was overshadowed by the concept of disk prolapse.[346–348,515,655] Because the peripheral third of the annulus fibrosis of every lumbar disk is innervated, the disk is a potential source of pain.[45,272] The nerve endings in the disk can be stimulated by involvement of the innervated perimeter of the annulus by the autoimmune inflammatory processes of disk degeneration, by torsional strains of the annulus, or by a bulging nucleus straining the overlying annulus. In each case, the pain is mediated by the nerves that supply the disk.

There is a wide variety of conservative and surgical means of treating intervertebral disk disorders, including immobilization, manipulation, traction, therapeutic exercises, laminectomy, spinal fusion, and chemonucleolysis, to name but a few.[72,79,107,112,159,210,255,256,283,302,344,362,403,406,472,517] A frequently mentioned disk-based treatment approach was that of Cyriax, who believed that most back pain (95%) was secondary to disk disease and herniation.[110] The diagnosis is mostly based on physical findings. According to the Cyriax approach, back pain without sciatica is secondary to the blocking effect of a disk protrusion on the motion in the involved segment; back pain with local or buttock-referred symptoms is related to dural "involvement" or irritation by a protrusion that is not affecting a specific root. Muscular pain, sacral joint pain, and buttock pain are referral patterns and are not treated except by treating the disk lesion. Back pain with sciatica or sciatica alone is secondary to root compression or irritation by a disk fragment. Treatment recommended by Cyriax is manipulation for the so-called "hard" or annular protrusions, lumbar traction for "soft" or nuclear protrusions, and epidural steroids for persistent radiculopathy.

In addition to these procedures, the maintenance of a normal or exaggerated lumbar lordosis is emphasized, especially in sitting. This is thought to prevent or reduce disk protrusion of either the soft or hard type by compressing the disk forward rather than backward. Exercise, stretching, acupressure, and massage are not used for back pain, but prolotherapy (the injection of sclerosants into connective tissue) is advocated for cases in which repeated attacks of pain are thought to indicate ligamentous laxity associated with and perhaps responsible for recurrent disk herniation. Patients are taught to avoid certain positions and stresses.

An increasingly popular conceptual system is that of McKenzie of New Zealand, who believes that the principal cause of back pain is disk disease manifested by abnormal mechanics resulting from the consequences of migration of the intact nucleus within the disk, not frank herniation.[406,407,547] Herniation is seen as a result of untreated, poorly treated, or unusually severe acute nuclear migration. A special case of nuclear migration is the "lateral shift phenomenon," a sciatic scoliosis caused by a lateral or posterior migration of the nucleus within the annulus.

The type of nucleus disk lesion is deduced through a program of prolonged or repeated stresses on the low back, attempting to reproduce painful situations. The change in the pain during such procedures as repeated extension in standing, trunk extension in lying, and lateral bending is recorded and classified according to its peripheralizing or centralizing nature. The geographic pattern of the pain response (central or near the spine as opposed to peripheral) is considered more important than its intensity. A series of positional self-mobilizations is then prescribed, based on the patterns found. Usually, these self-mobilizations are in extension. When a lateral shift is found, it is first reduced by mobilizations by the therapist (and self-mobilizations) before extension is done to prevent possible peripheralization of symptoms. More conventional spinal manipulations are recommended only for certain situations.

McKenzie also describes a postural syndrome characterized by mechanical deformation of the soft tissue as the result of prolonged postural stress that can lead to pain and a dysfunction syndrome that features pathologically involved muscles, ligaments, fascia, facet joints, and the intervertebral disk.[406] The major factor is adaptive soft-tissue shortening (fixation) of the motion segment, causing chronic mechanical deformation and loss of joint play. The precipitating causes are usually by-products of disk migration (derangement syndrome), spondylosis, or poor posture (postural syndrome). Based on the type of motion loss (flexion or extension), mobilization and home exercises are used. For example, when flexion loss is present, a static supine position is used, progressing to sustained and active lumbar stretching into flexion.

In this approach, home therapy is key to maintaining the corrective influences of therapy. McKenzie places a heavy emphasis on prevention of future attacks, usually by the use of lumbar rolls or special seating to maintain lordosis while sitting, and by instruction in body mechanics for daily activities and a daily program of exercise. McKenzie's text is valuable and must be understood in depth. We cannot cover this field adequately here, but other sources should be reviewed.[131,132,332,333,383,384,474,630,631]

☐ Facet Joints

The lumbar facet joints can be a source of both low back pain and referred pain.[44,160,400,432] Pathologically, the lumbar facet joints can be affected by a variety of disorders, but most commonly they undergo degeneration, usually secondary to some form of injury or disk disease.[44] Facet joint pain can be referred to any part of the limb, but most commonly it is the gluteal and proximal thigh or groin region.[44,160,400,432]

Some clinicians place great emphasis on the pathological processes of the facet joints in the genesis of back pain. Many manual therapists have tended to embrace views propounded by osteopaths,[442,588] orthopaedists,[44,372,373,418,419,420] and physical therapists.[289,375,376,484,485]

Mennell proposed the theory of joint play (see

Chapter 6, Introduction to Manual Therapy), a type of freedom or "slack" considered necessary for the painless function of synovial joints in the spine and extremities.[419,420] Lack of joint play reduces motion at the joint and produces secondary effects, including referred pain and the myofascial trigger point phenomenon. Treatment is by mobilization of the restricted joints and procedures to break up the cycle of epiphenomena (spray and stretch, trigger-point injections, and contract–relax programs). Manipulations are often recommended. Determination of the level of the spine to be treated is by skin rolling, observation of gross and segmental movement abnormalities, and oscillations of the vertebral spine, looking for hypersensitive levels ("facilitated segments").[317,378,485] Treatment is directed at an area of the spine that contains one or more symptomatic facet joints, in the expectation that joint mobilization will restore joint play.

Kaltenborn[289–291] and Paris[484,487] describe detailed evaluation systems for locating individual hypo- or hypermobile joints. Mobilizations are usually in the direction in which motion is blocked on examination, so that the facet motion is normalized.[485] In addition, Paris's patients are instructed in active abdominal exercises to reduce pelvic tilt and lumbar lordosis when standing and lifting. Instructions include the positioning principles of Fahrni for specific control of the spine.[159]

Maitland (a physical therapist) and Maigne (an orthopaedic surgeon) are other well-known manual therapists who operate relatively empirically, attempting to avoid the argument about underlying lesions while using mobilization techniques similar to those of the osteopaths and the "facet school."[372–376] Maitland's evaluation system is closely linked to treatment and incorporates a widely used graphic record of range of motion and its restrictions.[375] He uses gentle, graded (I to IV), oscillating motions within or at the limit of the available range of motion of the joint, concentrating on end feel and tissue characteristics (see Chapter 6, Introduction to Manual Therapy).

Maigne uses specific mobilizations and manipulation techniques. Based on the evaluation, he implements therapy based on two major rules: no painful manipulations should be performed, because they are unlikely to be successful; and mobilizations or manipulations should be done initially in the direction of greatest mobility found on the examination. The latter rule seems contradictory to other treatment systems (see Chapter 19, The Thoracic Spine).

Great importance has also been attached to the facets by clinicians who do not necessarily advocate manual therapy. Most recently, Shealy,[548] Mooney and Robertson,[432] Rothman and Simeone,[518] MacNab,[363] Fairbanks,[160] and others continue to place importance on facet pathology. Following the works by Kirkaldy-Willis and others, the role of the facet joint in radiculopathies is again becoming prominent, with a re-emergence of the facet joint syndrome theory popular between 1930 and 1945.[312]

Some authors believe that pathological processes of the facet joints occur after and perhaps because of disk degeneration; others believe they occur with disk degeneration. Asymmetry of the facet joints is well documented and has been given particular significance by Farfan and Sullivan as a contributing factor to pathological problems in the lower lumbar region.[164] These authors suggest that facet asymmetry (by producing a cam-like effect) may contribute to early degeneration of the L5–S1 intervertebral joint.[164]

☐ Segmental Intervertebral Instability

Instability is a loss of integrity of soft-tissue intersegmental control that causes potential weakness and liability to yield under stress, according to Newman.[464] Lumbar instability, where a degenerating segment is functionally incompetent because of insufficient control (whether muscle, ligament, disk, or all three), can be an intractable problem.[147,148,210,213,337,434,461,463,590] According to Grieve[210] and Paris,[488] segmental hypermobility and ligamentous or disk insufficiency are not necessarily the same thing. Paris defines hypermobility as a range of motion somewhat in excess of that expected for the particular segment, given the subject's age, body type, and activity status.[204] Simple hypermobility may be insignificant and need not result in instability. According to Paris, instability exists when, during active motion, there is a sudden aberrant motion such as a visible slip or shaking of the section.[488] Instability may be the result of postural problems, congenital defects, severe trauma, disk degeneration, traumatic ruptures of ligaments with or without fractures, unsatisfactory results following disk surgery, overtreatment by manipulation, or excessive stretching related to certain sports.[308,310] In spondylolisthesis, the spine sometimes is hypermobile. Hypermobility can also develop in areas adjacent to a hypomobile segment.

A lumbar segment is considered unstable when it exhibits abnormal movement in quality (abnormal coupling patterns) or in quantity (abnormal increased motion).[140] This instability can be asymptomatic or symptomatic, depending on the demands made on the motion segment. Instability (secondary) is seen in all ages—in the young, in spondylolisthesis or following trauma; and in middle-aged or older patients, in degenerative conditions.[246]

With disk degeneration, vertebral motion becomes irregular, allowing rocking, gliding, and rotation of the adjacent vertebrae with excessive posterior excursion of facet joints. In degenerative spondylolisthesis or retrospondylolisthesis, degenerative subluxation of the facet joint allows posterior or anterior displacement of the vertebral body. The symptoms are those of instability and spinal and intervertebral canal stenosis consequent to secondary changes. Anterior displacement of a vertebral body on the one below causes nerve root traction and compression. These patients (often elderly) may require decompression by laminectomy and stabilization by fusion.

Primary instability occurs chiefly in men in their 30s and 40s, when they are vulnerable to such strains as heavy lifting, falls, and rotational injuries.[246,434] Moran and King found "primary instability" of lumbar vertebrae to be the most common cause of low back pain.[434] This form of lumbar instability was labeled "pseudospondylolisthesis" by Jungham because there is no neural arch defect.[286,287]

The disk may not be an unstable element in spondylolisthesis or after a ligamentous rupture, despite the fact that it is always involved. In some cases, a deranged disk is part of the complex of instability; in others, it is the only unstable element.

Instability may be present in extension, flexion, lateral tilt, lateral displacement, or rotation. The main effect of rotational injuries is on the intervertebral disk itself.[246] Hyperextension strains are the most common cause of back pain resulting from segmental instability. This disruption in the normal mechanism of the joint causes a constant position of hyperextension at the posterior facet joint. In this case, there is no free play in the joint; it is held at its physiological limit constantly, so that even a slight hyperextension strain causes irritation and pain.

Dynamic roentgenograms in flexion-extension and sidebending are a simple, reliable way to determine if motion segment laxity is present.[140] The mobility examination reveals increased active and passive movement at the involved level. Some patients describe a "slipping" or catching sensation or a feeling of instability associated with movement, but this is far from being a reliable or consistent finding. The segment involved is tender to palpation.

Typically, the low back pain of patients with segmental instability is aggravated by both activity and inactivity. Prolonged sitting or standing causes aching, morning stiffness is common, and minor injury causes acute pain with diffuse radiation to the buttocks. The classic sign is lumbar insufficiency (reversal of the normal motion): when extending from the flexed position, rather than extending the upper trunk over the buttocks, the patient brings the buttocks and legs forward beneath the upper trunk in a ducking, irregular movement. Other events observed during active movement tests include pushing up from the thighs for support when returning from flexion; a tendency to maintain a lumbar lordosis during flexion; hinging or fulcruming at one or more spinal levels; a momentary catch during flexion, causing a directional change; and guarded motion performance.[471]

In the classic instability syndrome of spondylosis with a definable skeletal defect (common in adolescents), hamstring tightness (in defense of the instability) is the classical sign.[430] Transient neurological signs, such as those arising from a spondylolisthesis and causing neurogenic claudication, indicate instability.[488] For example, a runner who clinically has an unstable spondylolisthesis may develop pain and neurological deficit after 5 to 10 miles. Conservative treatment consists of postural training, muscle strengthening to improve the power of the trunk both regionally and segmentally, lumbosacral supports (corsets or braces), and prophylactic guidance and adherence to good body mechanics.

Grieve proposed a basic scheme of progressive stabilization techniques for strengthening regional and segmental muscles.[210,215,218] Abdominal exercises and dynamic abdominal bracing may also be used.[284] Exercises are selected that avoid extreme positions (flexion, extension, or rotation) liable to exacerbate the condition. For example, a potent cause of aggravation of low back pain, due to hypermobility, is that of active forced extension in the neutral starting position of prone-lying.

Mobilizations are used to relieve the pain of the hypermobile segments within the normal range of accessory movement and to mobilize stiff segments as part of the treatment for lumbar instability (i.e., where neighboring osteochondrotic segments have slowly induced hypermobility at the L5–S1 segment).[199] If the spinal extensor muscles are weak or need extra strengthening, exercises to strengthen them should avoid outer-range hyperextension movements. Therefore, the starting position should be such that the resisted movement occurs in middle range and the excursion ceases when the normal postural length of the muscle is reached (Fig. 20-5)[363] A segment held in hyperextension has no safety margin, so painful capsular lesions result.

Grimsby,[219,220] Gustavsen,[225,226] May,[388] Morgan,[435,436] Holten,[260] Johnson,[280] Saal,[521,522] Robinson,[512] White,[654] and Batson[24–26] use similar schemes of progressive stabilization for strengthening regional and segmental muscles when the joints are hypermobile or painful. Self-stabilization exercises, with the patient's active participation, and training in synergies are useful prophylaxis. The prime importance of soft tissues, particularly muscles, as opposed to the skeletal elements of joint structures is underscored by selected exercises that not only emphasize pure strength training but also improve speed and endurance.[219,260]

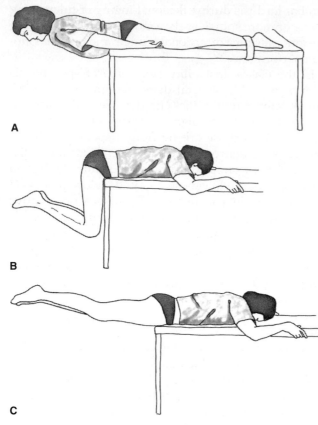

FIG. 20-5. Strengthening exercises of the low back, with the lumbar spine in a neutral position. (**A**) The trunk is stabilized by straps around the ankles; the trunk is then raised to the horizontal and sustained in this position. (**B**) Another approach is to have the patient grasp the sides of the table, (**C**) then bring one or both legs to the horizontal. In both of these exercises the patient should breathe freely.

Stabilization exercises involving the strengthening of regional and segmental muscles are shown in Figures 20-6 and 20-7. These are just a few of the exercises often necessary to complement passive movement techniques, and at times they make up the main form of treatment. When attempting to stabilize the unstable segment and to avoid further stress, there are two goals. The first is to encourage the patient to recognize and maintain functional back positions during all activities and to teach the patient to avoid postures and activities that aggravate the back dysfunction. The second goal is to improve the strength of the trunk musculature and its function specific to the task demanded and the directional intent. The trunk muscles should be able to contract (isometrically), contract and shorten (concentrically), contract and lengthen (eccentrically), stretch, and—most importantly—rest, ideally at their resting length.

Other methods of stabilization include sclerosant injections and surgical fusions. Indications for surgical intervention include lack of response to conservative

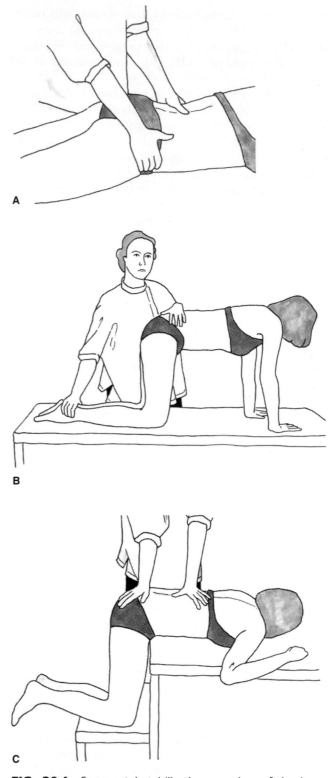

FIG. 20-6. Segmental stabilization exercises of the lower lumbar musculature. The therapist may use one hand on the lumbar region immediately above or below the involved segment. Moderate but increasing sustained pressure is applied to the patient's pelvis. (**A**) Rotation, (**B**) sidebending, and (**C**) flexion–extension techniques may be performed. Techniques may be modified to emphasize isometric, concentric, and eccentric control and to assist in stretching shortened tissue by using hold–relax techniques.

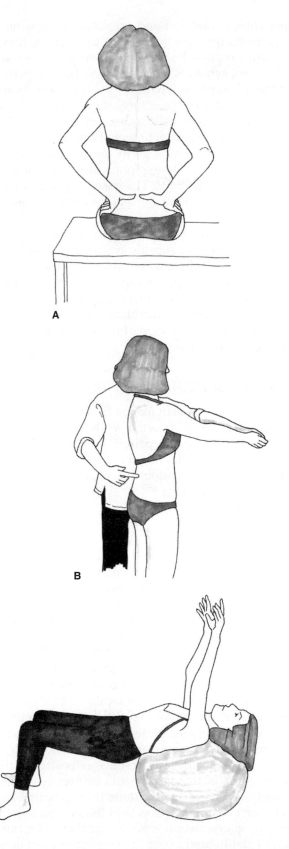

FIG. 20-7. Exercises for stabilization and strengthening. (**A**) Self-resistance may be applied using posteroanterior or lateral pressures for strengthening the segmental musculature. Regional strengthening may be achieved through (**B**) standing exercises and (**C**) assuming the bridging position while maintaining a functional back position.

measures, significant restriction of the patient's activities, and neurological findings that are progressing, or in spondylolisthesis progression of the slip itself.[52]

☐ Effects of Aging

SPINAL STENOSIS

Spinal stenosis includes narrowing of the spinal canal (see Fig. 20-4F), nerve root canals, and intervertebral foramina, all of which cause nerve root entrapment.[51] Patients with spinal stenosis experience back pain, transient motor deficits, tingling, and intermittent pain in one or both legs; this is worsened by standing or walking (neurogenic claudication) and somewhat relieved by sitting.[509] Pain of neurogenic claudication, unlike claudication of vascular origin (which disappears quickly with rest), does not ease very readily with rest and may persist for several hours.

In some patients, symptoms may be relieved by surgical correction.[89,136] Physical therapy is directed at increasing mobility (flexion–distraction mobilizations, manual stretching, exercises, or traction[530]) and improving the posture to reduce lordosis. Lordosis tends to decrease the size of the intervertebral foramen and increase the symptoms.[487]

Liyang and associates demonstrated that lumbar spinal canal capacity, specifically the dural sac, was enlarged during flexion and decreased with extension.[353] Modification of activities of daily living, achieving ideal lumbar posture through the principles of dynamic lumbar stabilization, endurance exercise, back school, stretching, and side-posture spinal manipulations (for lateral recess stenosis and central canal stenosis) are useful in the conservative management of spinal stenosis.[138,309,516]

OSTEOPOROSIS

Osteoporosis is the most common metabolic bone disease in adults.[169] Although loss of bone itself does not normally cause symptoms, associated fractures or collapse of vertebrae can cause considerable pain. The pain produced is thought to be secondary to pressure on nerve roots or on sensory fibers in the periosteum. Women are more commonly affected than men; more than half of women age 45 and older have roentgenographic evidence of osteoporosis in the lumbar spine.[270] The cause is unknown, but many theories have been proposed, including lack of estrogen and longstanding calcium deficiency.

The most prominent manifestations of osteoporosis in terms of vertebral collapse are usually localized to the thoracic and upper lumbar region, with pain referred diffusely to the low back (see Chapter 19, The Thoracic Spine).[454,543]

Treatment is concentrated on pain-reduction measures and increasing exercise and functional activities. With anterior compression fractures, active and passive exercises are emphasized. All positions and activities involving flexion should be avoided.[531]

Exercise may be an effective strategy, either by improving the peak bone mass attained in young adulthood or by reducing the rate of bone loss in later life.[476] Goals for those with established osteoporosis should include the maintenance of bone mass, strength training, increased coordination, and reduction of pain. Sinaki[559–562] has reviewed exercises that are safe and effective for osteoporotic subjects. Isometric and extension exercises are probably the most useful.[559]

KISSING LUMBAR SPINAL PROCESSES

Increased lordosis with disk collapse may lead eventually to "kissing spines" (Baastrup's syndrome).[20] This condition may develop because of degenerative changes in many segments and lordotic postural stresses. The resulting chronic impaction of the spinous processes is accompanied by ligamentous changes and interferes considerably with vertebral mechanics. The flattening of the ligamentous system and disk may create an instability of the intervertebral joint and, in some cases, hypermobility of the joint.[286] Of the lumbar movements, extension is the most limited and painful in the low back.[214] Relief is gained by bending forward or by putting the knees to the chest.

The goal of treatment is to reduce the pressure and lordosis. According to Paris, the best method is to lessen the lordosis by stretching the tight myofascia, and strengthening exercises for the abdominal muscles.[487]

☐ Other Tissues and Structures

The most common diagnoses in patients with acute low back pain of 0 to 3 months' duration are nonspecific (*e.g.*, lumbosacral or ligamentous strains, muscular sprains, lumbar dorsal syndromes); only 10% to 20% can be given a precise pathological diagnosis.[449] Many of the acute temporary painful episodes of low back pain are caused by acute muscular, ligamentous, or capsular strains.[36,95,372] Practically all anatomical structures in the region of the motion segment have been cited as a source of pain and have had their proponents in the etiological discussion. For the most part, conditions involving the soft tissues await fur-

ther clinical attention and research. There is no clear way to ascribe low back pain to fasciitis, fibrositis, myositis, ruptured or degenerative ligaments, strains or sprains, synovitis of the facet joints, or hypertrophy of the ligamentum flavum.[229,230] It is clear, however, that many of these structures do have sensory innervation and are potential sources of pain.[166,297] Hirsch and associates have documented fine and complex encapsulated nerve endings in the lumbosacral fascia, supraspinous and interspinous ligaments, and vertebral periosteum.[251,253] The facet (apophyseal) joint capsules and the outer third of the annulus are also innervated.

Most cases of uncomplicated acute low back pain can be expected to subside within 3 weeks. Management should be directed at excluding other pathological processes and providing relief of symptoms and localized therapy. Treatment may progress to graduated activity with a maintenance exercise program and education in the care of the low back in working and recreational life.

SKIN AND SUBCUTANEOUS TISSUE

In the skin and subcutaneous tissue, there are trigger points that when injected with a local anesthetic sometimes reduce the pain.[28] Lumbosacral fascia fibrositis has been diagnosed clinically, although never proved by pathoanatomical pictures, according to Nachemson and Bigos.[450]

LIGAMENTS

Ligaments have also been cited as a source of low back pain.[62,95,506,668] Ligamentous pain is thought to arise from a weakened ligament, which, when stretched, produces pain and perhaps trigger muscle guarding. Traumatic ligamentous strains include flexion strains that exceed the limits of the interspinous and supraspinous ligaments.[44,62,95,214,228,585] A typical patient with this type of lesion is a middle-aged person who complains of sudden onset (after twisting) of one-sided back pain localized to the fourth or fifth level in the lumbar spine.[441] Pain sometimes radiates down over the gluteal region. Symptoms are increased by certain movements and relieved by rest. The patient particularly resents extension of the affected level, as this movement compresses an already acutely tender and edematous interspinous ligament between the spinous process of the sacrum and that of L5. The intervertebral space is acutely tender, but flexion of the lumbar spine in the supine position gives temporary relief because the injured ligament is no longer compressed.[95]

Ligamentous strains need time to heal. During the

subacute stage, if mild mobilization and range of motion are used, normal mobility is likely to be achieved by the time complete healing has occurred. If the joint capsule or ligamentous structures are actually torn or overstretched during injury, the joints may be hypermobile (unstable) when healing is complete. Because ligamentous pain arises from weakened ligaments, it makes sense to reduce the stress on these ligaments by correct or neutral postures supported by adequate muscle action and positions. In time, the ligaments should regain some of their integrity with less movement present on examination.

MUSCLES AND MYOFASCIAL STRUCTURES

Myofascial restrictions may occur from overuse or overstrain and also accompany any other type of injury in low back pain. These restrictions limit function and may lead to adverse changes in other structures, such as the disk or facet joints.

Acute muscle strains, producing partial tears of muscle tissue attachments, typically are a young man's injury, where strong muscles are guarding a healthy spine.[247,296,363,419,420] Primary muscle disorders will probably heal no matter what care is given, but stiffness, weakness, and postural changes may occur during healing. To avoid loss of function and adaptive postural changes, the activity level and mobilization treatment should be increased as the patient progresses.

Despite the widespread use of exercises, there is little scientific information about their effectiveness in the management of acute low back pain. Kendall and Jenkins compared a variety of exercise regimens and concluded that isometric exercises were most effective.[302]

According to Wyke, myofascial pain is one of the common causes of primary backache resulting from irritation of the nociceptive system that is distributed through the muscle masses of the low back, their fascial sheaths, intramuscular septa, and the tendons that attach them to the vertebral column and pelvis.[665] Contrary to traditional opinions, inflammatory disorders of the back muscles and their related connective tissues are seldom the cause of low back pain. More often, backache of myofascial origin is the result of muscle fatigue, reflex muscle spasm, or trauma. According to Rovere[519] and Keene and Drummond,[296] the most common cause of low back pain in the athlete is overuse, with resultant strains or sprains of the paravertebral muscles and ligaments.

Several muscle pain syndromes are reported in the literature—for instance, the tenderness at motor points described by Gunn and Milbrandt,[222,223] which seem to fall within the myofascial pain and dysfunction group discussed by Travel and Simons.[617] A report by Gunn and Milbrandt and suggestions by others imply that sympathetic phenomena such as trophic changes, cutaneous and myalgic hyperalgesia, increased muscle tone, and piloerection can be seen early and late in patients with "secondary" back pain caused by some degree of injury to the dorsal root ganglion or peripheral nerve.[223,552,553] Skin, connective tissue, and muscle may share in sensory disorders, and these detectable changes may be confusing: their typical or unexpected distribution conforms more to a vasal rather than a neural topography. They are ascribed to early and reversible neuropathy rather than late and severe denervation.

Treatment of muscular back pain currently is the cause of some confusion, but major approaches include acupuncture, acupressure, spray and stretch, contract–relax techniques, soft-tissue mobilizations, dry needling, and anesthetic injections. Procaine may be the least myotoxic agent; steroids are not indicated for muscle use.[617]

Spinal disorders primarily of muscle origin are uncommon. Although muscle guarding or intrinsic muscle spasm usually accompanies spinal pain regardless of the underlying cause, there is no neurophysiological reason for a normal muscle to spontaneously go into spasm. According to Wyke, type IV joint receptors in joint capsules, fat pads, and ligaments, when subjected to sufficient irritation, provoke intense nonadapting motor unit responses simultaneously in all muscles related to the joint, as well in more remote muscles elsewhere in the body.[663]

Dysfunction may lead to nociception (noxious stimulus) that will lead to a state of prolonged involuntary holding. Prolonged muscle guarding leads to circulatory stasis and the retention of metabolites. The muscle then becomes inflamed (myositis) and localized tenderness develops. This intrinsic muscle spasm adds additional pain (see Fig. 8-4). Prolonged intrinsic muscle spasm tends to generate up and down the spine and may aggravate areas of degenerative joint and disk disease. During examination, muscle guarding and intrinsic muscle spasm may be noted during palpation or observation, and a positive weight-shift sign may be noted.

According to Nachemson and Bigos, although available data do not support the incrimination of muscle injury as a source of low back disorders, there is indirect evidence to warrant muscle rehabilitation.[450] Even if the musculature was not injured at the time of onset of low back pain symptoms, the subsequent decrease in activity would affect endurance, stamina, and fitness. They advocate aerobic exercise, which also is a means of treating depression, a common finding with at least chronic low back pain.[176,566] An increase in endorphins has been demonstrated in the CSF[17] and in the bloodstream[165] with aerobic training. Other benefits include positive effects of increased mental alertness,[142,667] sleep,[176,566] stamina,[294] improved self-image, and reversal of activity level compatible with chronic pain.[177,179]

SACROILIAC JOINT

It is impossible to discuss management of the lumbar spine without mentioning the sacroiliac joint. The pain felt at this joint is usually referred from the lumbosacral junction secondary to disk degeneration. However, subluxation (sprains) and dislocations do occur, especially before age 45. Typical presenting symptoms are pain on resistive hip abduction and weight-bearing, as well as tenderness of the symphysis pubis.

Osteopaths, followed by specialists in physical medicine and orthopaedists, have suggested that sacroiliac subluxations may be responsible for low back pain and even sciatica.[50,56,121,135,209,422,496,499,587] Involvement of this region must be ruled out when evaluating the lumbar spine. Treatment of this region and even the entire lower quadrant often must be included in the total management of lumbar spine conditions (see Chapter 21, The Sacroiliac Joint and the Lumbar–Pelvic–Hip Complex).

☐ Combined States

One of the greatest frustrations in the management of spinal pain is that the patient rarely has a single defined abnormality. The nature of degenerative or traumatic spinal disease is such that multiple joints in one or more segments can be involved, and the patient can suffer pain from each component of the disease at different times. In cases of chronic spinal pain with little improvement, the patient usually presents with more than one syndrome.

Degenerative disk disease might not produce any symptoms, but the patient can have pain from secondarily affected facet joints or can suffer from disk pain, complicating the dilemma. Any of these causes of pain can be superimposed on nerve root compression. All the elements of this lesion complex may require treatment.

Other conditions to be considered by the physician include viscerogenic pathological processes, vascular lesions, ankylosing spondylitis, Scheuermann's disease, rheumatoid arthritis of the spinal joints, extraspinal lesions, and intraspinal lesions.[603]

■ EVALUATION

An accurate history is the key component for successful treatment of the low back. The examination entails subjective questions regarding the onset of symptoms and their present status, and the physical examination, which consists of tests and measurements of the symptomatic area. Evaluation of the soft tissues and a scan examination of the lumbar spine and lower extremity are covered in Chapter 5, Assessment of Musculoskeletal Disorders and Concepts of Management, and Chapter 22, The Lumbosacral–Lower Limb Scan Examination. The scan examination of the lumbar spine and lower extremity is oriented toward detecting gross or subtle biomechanical abnormalities and determining the presence of common lumbar or lower extremity disorders.

Because of the strategic location of the lumbar spine, this structure should be included in any examination of the spine in terms of posture or in any examination of the lower extremity joints, particularly the hip and sacroiliac joints. Unless there is a definitive history of trauma, it is difficult to know to which area to direct physical examination procedures after completing the history. Thus, the lumbar spine, sacroiliac joints, and lower extremity joints should be examined sequentially.

☐ History

A general approach to history-taking is described in Chapter 5, Assessment of Musculoskeletal Disorders and Concepts of Management; the concepts presented there apply to the evaluation of the lumbar spine. History-taking of the lumbar spine is probably best done using a combination of a written questionnaire and an interview to assess reliability and to guarantee a thorough review.[268,269,578,636] All aspects of the history are important, because different conditions may be related to the patient's age, sex, occupation, and family history. Previous history of trauma, accidents, or other episodes are considered with respect to recent history. The frequency and duration of each attack and knowledge of the exact mechanism of injury is often helpful and may give clues as to which tissues may have been stressed. For example, disk lesions usually have an insidious onset caused by repeated activities related to slump sitting, lifting, and forward-bending; joint locking is often caused by a sudden, unguarded movement. Inflammatory and systemic disorders usually present with a subtle onset; sprains and strains involve aggravation or trauma.

The history should include the chief complaints and

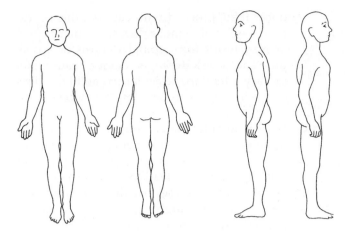

FIG. 20-8. Body chart for recording subjective and objective information.

a pain drawing. When using a body chart (Fig. 20-8), the area, type, depth, and intensity of pain are ascertained, and the areas and types of sensory disturbance are recorded. The pictorial record of information may, by reference to sclerotomes, myotomes, and dermatomes, indicate which nerve root, if any, is involved. It also helps to distinguish organic pain from psychological pain fairly well.[81,431,507,641] If pain has been present for a significant time, other tests should be used for functional overlay.[460,578,649] The Oswestry function test and the McGill Pain Questionnaire are helpful in objectifying the patient's perception of the quality of pain and its effect on function.[402,415]

Taking each symptomatic area separately, establish by questioning the severity and irritability of the symptoms, and check the level of activity necessary to bring on the pain or other symptoms. Ascertain how the patient eases the symptoms and how long this takes. Determine if there are any reliable historical clues to disease by reviewing the following points:

I. Signs and Symptoms
   A. Are there any postures or actions that specifically increase or decrease the symptoms or cause difficulty? Patients suffering from mechanical problems affecting the low back (*i.e.*, herniated disks, osteoarthritic facet joints, or spondylolisthesis) know precisely which factors aggravate and which relieve their symptoms. For example, pain arising from the facet joints is often relieved by sitting and forward-bending, but walking is likely to be painful.

   According to White, the diagnosis of annular tear is suggested by pain that is aggravated by sitting, relieved by extension, and not stimulated by standing and walking (except prolonged standing).[648]

   Classic radiculopathy causes radicular pain radiating into a specific dermatomal pattern with paresis, loss of sensation, and reflex loss. The classic history for radiculopathy resulting from disk herniation is back pain that progresses to predominantly leg pain. It is worsened by increases in intraspinal pressure such as coughing, sneezing, and sitting. Leg pain predominates over back pain and mechanical factors increase the pain.[546] Physical examination shows positive nerve-stretch signs. A dermatomal distribution of leg pain that is made worse by straight-leg raising, sitting, or supine foot dorsiflexion, neck flexion, jugular compression, and direct palpation of the popliteal nerve is characteristic of radiculopathy.

   Patients with mechanical problems do not complain of symptoms being aggravated by "everything" they do. The person who develops spontaneous low back pain initially noted at night but later presenting constantly must be investigated for organic disease (*e.g.*, tumor, abdominal or pelvic disease). The possibility of any nonmechanical pathological process may be exposed here, perhaps in the way of constant, unremitting pain that is worse at night; the patient regularly must get out of bed to find relief.

   B. Establish whether there is any diurnal or nocturnal variation. Is the pain worse in the morning or evening? As the day goes on? For example, in chronic degenerative lumbar disk disease, the history is of sudden catching pain in the back, morning stiffness that wears off to allow activity with minimal pain, and a prolonged (many hours) increase in pain after heavy use or abusive positioning. This is too much like the history given by White for facet arthropathy (transient pain reproduced with certain motions and positions, including rotation, with "catching" pains and relief in neutral) to allow a diagnosis to be made from historical information alone.[648]

   C. Which movements hurt? Which movements are stiff? Postural or static muscles tend to respond to pathological processes by tightness in the form of spasm or adaptive shortening; dynamic or phasic muscles tend to respond by atrophy.[274,275] Tightness of hamstrings or trunk erectors frequently develops in various back syndromes and similar postural defects, whereas abdominal and gluteal muscles show weakness. Janda suggests that just as we have a capsular pattern of joint restriction, so may we have a typical muscle pattern.[274]

   1. Does the patient describe a painful arc of movement on forward- or side-flexion? If so, it may indicate a disk protrusion with a nerve root riding over the bulge.[110,588] The phenomenon of a painful arc throws light on intra-articular mechanics (see Chapter 16, The Spine), in which the nucleus tends to move backward during trunk flexion (see Fig. 16-13). According to Cyriax, as trunk flexion proceeds, the movement comes to the half-flexed position when the surfaces have moved enough to reverse the tilt.[110] At this point, a mobile fragment of disk moves sharply backward, jarring the dura by pressure transmitted through the posterior longitudinal ligament. Pain may reappear at the extreme of trunk flexion if the loose part is squeezed even further backward.[110]

Pain associated with an acute injury or inflammation often presents if the joint is moved in any direction. Pain while resting suggests an inflammatory process.

2. What position does the patient sleep in? Prone-lying for a person with restricted extension compresses the posterior tissues and causes ischemia.

3. Is there a change in symptoms in rising from a sitting position? Change may indicate possible ligamentous instability. The action of changing position is painful, but when an upright position is acquired the pain is diminished.

D. Does the patient describe a slipping, popping, or clicking sensation that is associated with certain movements? Popping that cannot be repeated every time is thought to be related to the vacuum effect that is experienced if the joint surfaces are separated suddenly.[96,532] This is a normal phenomenon, and if a joint seems to pop quite easily it indicates a hypermobile joint.

II. Special Considerations for the Lumbar Spine

A. Does the patient experience tingling and numbness in the extremities or the perineal (saddle) or pelvic regions? The adult spinal cord ends at the bottom of the L1 vertebra and becomes the cauda equina. The nerve roots extend in such a way that it is rare for the disk to pinch the nerve root of the same level (except when the protrusion is more lateral). For example, a herniated disk between L4 and L5 usually compresses the fifth lumbar nerve root.

B. Has there been any change in micturition habits associated with back trouble or sphincter disturbance (particularly urinary reten-

tion)? If so, proceed with caution; this condition may involve more than the lumbar spine or may result from spinal stenosis or a disk problem. A disk derangement may cause total urinary retention, vesicular irritability, or loss of desire or awareness of the necessity to void.[364]

C. Is the patient taking any medications? Are anticoagulants or steroids being taken, or have they been taken in the past? Long-term steroid therapy can lead to osteoporosis.

D. Is there any increase in pain with coughing, deep-breathing, laughing, or the Valsalva maneuver? All of these actions increase the intrathecal pressure and suggest a pathological process pressing on the theca (wrapping of the spinal cord).[262]

E. How is the patient's general health? Is body weight stable?

F. Has the patient had a roentgenographic examination? If so, x-ray overexposure must be avoided; if not, roentgenograms may aid in the diagnosis.

G. Has the patient undergone any major surgery? If so, when was the surgery performed, what condition was being treated, and what was the site of surgery?

H. Is there any history (or family history) of rheumatoid arthritis or ankylosing spondylitis, diabetes, or vascular disease? Previous treatment for malignant disease or osteoporosis may be a clue to the current problem. Likewise, a brief systemic history might provide important information.

III. History.
The history section completes the impression of the severity, irritability, and particularly the nature of the presenting condition. Putting the history at the end of the subjective examination facilitates constructive questioning.[81]

A. *Recent history.* A good way to take a current pain history is to ask the patient to describe a typical 24-hour period. Some points in the recent history of the pain that may help to provide a clue to diagnosis include:

1. When? Sudden or gradual onset?
2. Cause, if any? If there is any obvious cause, obtain the direction, amount, and duration of any forces involved.
3. If there is no obvious cause, were there any predisposing factors?
4. Where was the pain first felt? Did it spread to the leg? Did any sensory disturbances develop?
5. How have the symptoms varied? What has been the effect of any treatment?

6. If the condition is improving or worsening, does the patient know why? Has a different activity or posture been used?

Often using a pain or symptom scale improves communication. The scale is rated from 0 to 10; 0 is no pain at all and 10 is the worst pain that the patient has ever experienced. Patients may be asked to grade their pain on a graph throughout the day. Pain that does not go below a 3 with rest may be related to a psychological problem, cancer, or a disease process originating in a location other than a degenerative spinal segment.[652]

B. *Past history.* Elicit the patient's general history, especially of any past spinal symptoms or injury. When was the first episode? Gradual or sudden? Cause? Site of pain? Any referral? Duration of first attack? What treatment was received, and what was its effect? Did the patient completely recover after the attack?

C. *From past to present.* How many episodes, and with what frequency? Local or local and referred symptoms? How long do the attacks usually last? Is treatment usually necessary? If so, what treatment is used, and what is the effect? Is the patient symptom-free between episodes?

☐ The Dilemma of Diagnosis

According to DeRosa and Porterfield[124] and others, therapists must accept the fact that it is usually impossible to identify the tissues that are causing pain. The Quebec Task Force on Spinal Disorders recognized this dilemma of diagnosis and recommended 11 classifications of activity-related spinal disorders.[580] DeRosa and Porterfield[124] have proposed a modified version of these categories that are more relevant to a scheme for manual therapy diagnosis (Table 20-1).

TABLE 20-1 SPINAL DISORDERS CLASSIFICATION

1. Back pain without radiation
2. Back pain with referral to extremity, proximally
3. Back pain with referral to extremity, distally
4. Extremity pain greater than back pain
5. Back pain with radiation and neurological signs
6. Postsurgical status (<6 months or >6 months)
7. Chronic pain syndrome

(DeRosa CP, Porterfield JA: A physical therapy model for treatment of low back pain. Phys Ther 72:261–269, 1992.)

☐ Physical Examination

OBSERVATION

Observe the patient's posture, body type (*i.e.*, ectomorphic, mesomorphic, endomorphic, or mixed), and ability to move freely. See Chapter 22, The Lumbosacral–Lower Limb Scan Examination, for common gait abnormalities and possible causes.

FUNCTIONAL ACTIVITIES

Assess whether spinal movements are free or restricted by watching the patient getting into or out of a chair and observing the position he or she adopts while sitting and while undressing. Then undertake a more formal inspection of bony structures and alignment.

INSPECTION

Have the patient stand with the back, shoulders, and legs exposed for inspection. Features such as pelvic level, disturbances of spinal curves, or other deformities may be observed; view the patient from the front, back, and sides. Record specific alterations in bony structure or alignment, soft-tissue configuration, and skin status.

I. **Bony Structure and Alignment.** See the section on assessment of structural alignment in Chapter 22, The Lumbosacral–Lower Limb Scan Examination, for a discussion of this part of the examination.

II. **Soft-Tissue Inspection**

    A. *Muscle contour.* Note obvious asymmetries in muscle bulk. The calves or hamstrings on one side may be atrophied in the presence of a chronic S1–S2 radiculopathy. Seek regions of muscle tightness and muscle spasm. Muscle spasm is noted as a tautness, particularly in the low back, where the erector spinae stands in relief. One side may be tighter than the other, with subsequent listing of the torso.

III. **Skin and Markings.** Observe the skin for any local swelling or cutaneous lesions such as café-au-lait spots, patches of hair, areas of pigmentation, or any abnormal depression. A tuft of hair may indicate a spina bifida occulta or diastematomyelia.[385]

IV. **Selective Tissue Tension Tests—Active Movements**

    A. *Active physiological movements of the spine.* With all movements, determine the range, rhythm, and quality of active movement. Watch the body contours and spinous processes carefully to observe whether the spinal joints move smoothly and evenly or whether there is any localized restriction of movement in the spinous processes between two or three vertebrae. Note disturbances of rhythm and the presence or absence of any protective deformity. Note any muscle guarding, a painful arc of motion, and whether the patient's symptoms are reproduced. The patient must actively extend the movement as far as possible. In general, facet joint restrictions are more noticeable during side-bending; conversely, restrictions caused by muscle tightness are proportionately more noticeable in forward-bending.

With the patient standing (feet a little apart and parallel), assess:

1. *Extension* (backward-bending). Kneeling behind the patient, support the patient's pelvis or shoulders for stability while observing lumbar extension. Ask the patient to sequentially bend the head, shoulders, middle back, and lower back backward. The lumbar lordosis should increase from the resting position as the patient extends. Note the movement in relation to the painful site and any deviations toward one side. Observe the point on the spine at which extension originates.
   a. In an acute spinal derangement, lumbar extension is negligible, with most of the observable backward-bending occurring at higher levels.
   b. With multisegmental capsular restriction, lumbar extension is also markedly limited due to premature close-packing of the facet joints.
   c. The spine may deviate away from the side of a localized unilateral capsular restriction.

   The normal range is about 20° to 35°. Extension is often the stiffest and most painful movement with lumbar problems. Suitable methods for measuring extension externally include the use of a kyphometer,[434] goniometer (spondylometer or hydrogoniometer),[137,182,357] inclinometer,[158,195] Flexirule,[64,615] and tape measure.[173,364,426,427] The first two methods are based on a mathematical theory of angles outlined by Loebl and are expressed in degrees.

2. *Lateral flexion* (sidebending). Have the patient sidebend the head, shoulders, middle back, and lower back, first to one side and

then to the other. Symmetry of movement may be judged by comparing the distance from the fingertip to the fibular head on either side and by observing the degree of spinal curvature with movements in either direction. Symmetry of movement, however, is significant only with respect to the starting position; if the resting position of the spine involves a right sidebending curve, then "normal" movement would be a greater degree of sidebending to the right than to the left. Also assess the continuity of segmental movement. Reproduction of pain on passive overpressure is most likely to occur when a capsular restriction exists on the side to which the movement is performed.
   a. In acute spinal derangements, such as a posterolateral disk protrusion or unilateral facet joint derangement, lumbar sidebending may be absent on one side (usually toward the involved side), especially if a functional spinal deviation exists in the erect position.
   b. With multisegmental capsular restriction, sidebending is moderately restricted in both directions. All serious diseases of the lumbar spine (*e.g.*, malignancy, ankylosing spondylitis) result in equal limitation of both left and right sidebending.[112]
   c. With localized unilateral capsular restrictions, sidebending is usually only slightly limited toward the involved side. Unilateral restrictions are often difficult to detect.

   Lateral flexion is about 15° to 20°. Suitable methods for measuring lateral flexion include the use of two Myrin goniometers, one or two inclinometers,[158,195] Flexirule,[64,615] and a tape measure, using either distraction or approximation (see Fig. 19-12).[205,425,539]

3. *Flexion* (forward-bending). Forward flexion is an important movement and the one most likely to be limited by a disk lesion. Have the patient bend the head forward, then the middle back, and finally the low back. A painful arc may be noted. Observe the level at which lumbar flexion originates. Reversal of normal spinal rhythm on attempting to regain the erect posture after forward flexion is characteristic of disk degeneration associated with a posterior joint lesion.[363] "Hitching" is sometimes seen in

patients with osteoarthritis of the facet joints; the patient first extends the lumbar spine, fixing it in lordosis, and then extends at the hips until the erect position is regained.[546] An instability problem may be present if there is a reversal of the normal pelvic rhythm, an arc or listing to one side through the range, or sharp catches of pain, or if the patient exhibits cogwheeling while he or she attempts to rise from the forward-bent position.[308,363,546]

a. If the patient has a relatively acute back problem and this movement is extremely difficult to perform—the patient may support his body weight by placing the hands on the thighs or a nearby plinth—suspect a posterior disk prolapse.

b. If the patient has a relatively acute back problem but can bend forward reasonably well, with only mild discomfort and restriction, an acute facet joint dysfunction or less severe disk prolapse might be considered. It is not unusual to see variations in lateral deviations of the spine as the patient bends forward in either instance. For example, the spine may start out deviated in the upright position and the deviations may disappear during forward-bending, or the spine may be erect on standing and deviate as forward-bending proceeds; the deviation may or may not resolve by the end point of the movement. Such patterns may occur with movement abnormalities resulting from either disk or facet joint derangements.

If a facet is limited on one side due to meniscoid locking, muscle guarding, or capsular restriction, it will not glide forward on that side. This results in a sudden shift toward the restricted side, followed by a rapid shift back.[484] Conversely, ongoing deviations with forward-bending are typically associated with disk involvement. The patient tends to shift laterally as a unit to move the protrusion away from the irritated nerve root—away from the involved side if the prolapse is lateral to the nerve root and toward the same side if the protrusion is medial to the nerve root.[305]

c. Observe the spine during forward-bending from the back, then from the side.

When viewing from behind, look for lateral deviation of the spine during movement. A deviated arc of movement is more likely to be secondary to an alteration of intervertebral disk mechanics; a deviation that exists up to the end point of movement is more likely to be the result of a unilateral or asymmetrical capsular restriction or a fixed scoliosis. If a fixed scoliosis exists, a rotary component is present; the side of the convexity appears higher than the side of the concavity in the forward-bent position.

When viewing from the side, assess the continuity of movement at the various spinal segments. The overall spinal curve should be relatively smooth; flattened areas may reflect segmental hypomobility, whereas angular areas may be associated with segmental hypermobility. These flattened areas or sharp angulation of the spinal curvature may also be identified during active sidebending and extension.

With full forward-bending of the lumbar spine, the normal lumbar lordosis should be straightened but is usually not reversed. Inadequate straightening of the lordosis may occur with localized or generalized capsular restriction. Reversal of the lumbar lordosis suggests hypermobility.

The maximum range of motion is 40° to 60°. Suitable methods for measuring flexion include the kyphometer,[137,527] the goniometer (the spondylometer or hydrogoniometer), the inclinometer, and the tape measure (including the Schober test to detect and follow the loss of spinal motions in ankylosing spondylitis). Segmental measurements of flexion of the spine (T12, L3, S1) can also be determined.[158,173,195,364,397,505,539]

4. *Lateral shift* (side-gliding). Lateral displacement of the pelvis on the thorax is an important test movement, especially for the lower lumbar spine. McKenzie described its application fully.[406] Have the patient move the pelvis and shoulder simultaneously in opposite directions while keeping the shoulders parallel to the ground. Watch for unilateral restriction or blocking. When the patient has a lateral shift, movement is restricted in the opposite direction.

While maintaining a stabilized upper thoracic area, ask the patient to allow the hips and pelvis to slide laterally in the horizontal plane to the left and right.[406]

With the patient sitting, knees together, compare the sitting posture to the standing posture. Note any changes in bony structure and alignment.

5. *Rotation.* With the arms held straight out in front and the hands together, have the patient turn toward the left and then the right. In sitting, as rotation occurs in one direction, sidebending occurs in the opposite direction. The spinous processes move in the opposite direction of rotation. Assess symmetry of movement by observing the lateral curvature of the lower spine. The same considerations apply to the assessment of rotation as discussed under sidebending. There is no significant rotation of the lumbar spine (3° to 18°), but it is a useful test for the patient with nonorganic back pain.[441] Structural stresses could include torsional and shear stresses of the disk and neural arch. The contralateral facet is compressed, and the ipsilateral joint is stretched. Suitable methods for measuring lumbar spine rotation externally include the use of a tape measure and application of the rotometer developed by Twomey and Taylor.[427,625]

B. *Chest expansion and active peripheral joint tests*
1. Measure chest expansion from normal expiration to maximal inspiration at the level of T4. An expansion of 3 cm is within the lower limits of normal.[427] Loss of chest expansion is usually a late finding in ankylosing spondylitis. Another late sign is decreased ability to extend the neck.
2. Squatting on the heels from the standing position and returning to the erect position puts the peripheral joints through a full active range of motion. The ability to squat normally reflects the state of the hip joints as well as the power of the quadriceps and gluteal muscles. A patient who complains of low back pain radiating down the anterior aspect of the thigh and who has difficulty squatting may have a midlumbar disk lesion.[546] Changes in symptoms should be noted, as well as where in the range they occur.

C. *Auxiliary tests.* In most patients with symptoms arising from the lumbar spine, the active tests described above reproduce the symptoms. If not, the following additional maneuvers may be used:
1. Passive overpressure at the end range of the active physiological motions described above. The overpressure should be applied with care because the upper body weight is already being applied by virtue of gravity.
2. Repeated motions. It may be helpful to do repeated physiological movements at various speeds.
3. Sustained pressure. This is applied for about 10 seconds with the lumbar spine first in extension and then in lateral flexion, when necessary to reproduce the pain.
4. Combined motions.[59,149–151,546] These passive movement tests are designed to position the joint under maximum stress. The combining of routine physiological movements to form test movements either opens or closes one side of the intervertebral segment. In this way, a pattern of painful movement may be found or a combination that relieves or increases symptoms. If pain is reproduced, determine whether the pain is felt in the midline or the same or opposite side, and if it radiates down the leg. Determine if the patterns are regular or irregular. These motions may be applied with and without passive overpressure.
   a. Active motions without overpressure include:
      i. Lateral flexion combined with extension to the left and right
      ii. Lateral flexion combined with flexion to the right and left
   b. Combined movements with passive overpressure. Securely stabilize and maintain the patient's pelvis. Once end range is reached, apply passive overpressure.
      i. Combined movements in flexion
         A. Combined movement of forward-flexion and right lateral flexion (Fig. 20-9). While maintaining a fully flexed position, the patient laterally flexes to the right. At the end of range, the therapist applies passive overpressure. Repeat to the left.
         B. Combined forward-flexion with rotation (Fig. 20-10). The patient bends forward in a fully flexed position. The patient's trunk is

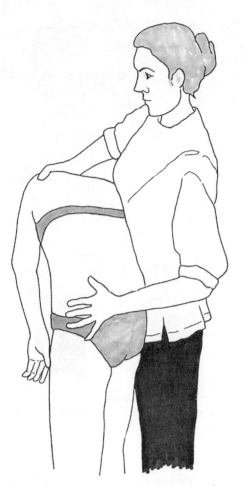

FIG. 20-9. Combined movement examination: lateral flexion in forward flexion.

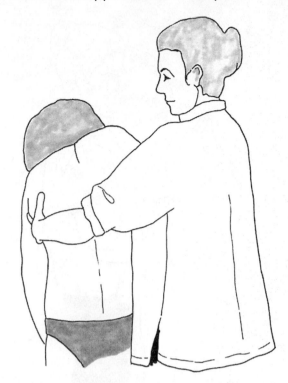

FIG. 20-10. Combined movement examination: flexion and rotation.

rotated to the right. Repeat the sequence with rotation to the left.

ii. Combined movements in extension.

  A. Extension with lateral flexion to the right (Fig. 20-11). The patient first extends, and lateral flexion is added to this position (the patient is now in a quadrant position). The examiner stands to the side (right) and places one arm across the chest so the hand grasps the patient's opposite shoulder, to which extension and lateral flexion will occur. The thumb and index finger of the examiner's opposite hand are placed over the transverse process at the level of the lumbar spine to be examined. Following active extension, coun-

terpressure is provided by the thumb while the upper arm is used to bring the patient's trunk into lateral flexion. Repeat this sequence on the left side.

  B. Extension and rotation to the right (Fig. 20-12). The examiner places one arm across the chest so the hand grasps the opposite shoulder (left). The thumb and index finger of the opposite hand are placed over the transverse process at the level of the lumbar spine to be examined. The patient is encouraged to actively extend to the limit of the range. Using the upper hand (on the patient's shoulder), the examiner guides the trunk into rotation as the thumb applies counterpressure. Repeat this sequence on the left side.

  These examining movements involve the combination of two movements. However, three movements may also be combined, and the sequence of performing movements may also

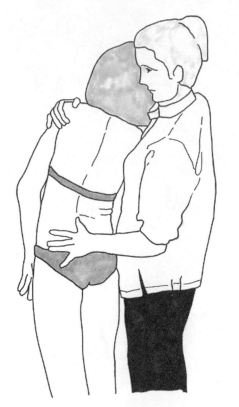

FIG. 20-11. Combined movement examination: lateral flexion in extension.

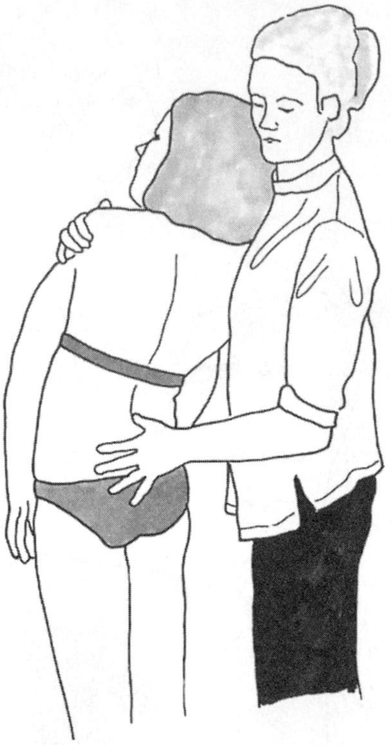

FIG. 20-12. Combined movement examination: extension and rotation.

be varied.[59,149–151,546] As a result of examining, analyzing, and treating using combined movements, a better appreciation of the mechanical presentation of spinal pathology and its application to treatment can be gained.

  5. Positive heel-drop test. Have the patient stand on tiptoes, then drop heavily onto the heels. This causes a jarring of the spine that may be sufficient to reproduce the symptoms.[546]

D. *Active segmental mobility.* With the patient standing, assess:

  1. *Upper lumbar spine lateral flexion.* Have the patient stride-stand so that motion is directed at the upper lumbar segments. With the weight transferred to the same side (right), the patient actively sidebends to the right. Repeat to the left.

  2. *L5–S1 lateral flexion.* Have the patient stride-stand with weight transferred to the opposite side (left). The patient actively sidebends to the right. Repeat to the left.

  3. *L5–S1 region.* The patient actively tilts the pelvis forward (symphysis up) and then extends it.

V. **Selective Tissue Tension—Passive Movements**
  A. *Muscle length.* See Chapter 21, The Sacroiliac Joint and the Lumbar–Pelvic–Hip Complex.
  B. *Vertical compression test.* See Chapter 19, The Thoracic Spine.
  C. *Posture correction.* Posture correction is done to determine if a return to normal posture is possible and if the symptoms are altered. This may help determine which structures are at fault and to what extent the postural deformity is involved in the current complaints. When an acute lumbar scoliosis is seen during an examination, attempt to correct it. If the scoliosis is caused by a moderate or mild disk protrusion (lateral shift), the correction procedure often causes centralization of the pain in the lumbar region but no increase in peripheral symptoms.[406] If the scoliosis is a protective scoliosis, as described by Finneson, any attempt at correction increases pain and other symptoms in the lower extremities.[167]

  The patient stands with the elbow of the arm on the side of the lumbar convexity bent to 90°. The therapist contacts the lateral aspect of the patient's thorax with the clavicular region. The arms encircle the patient and the hands interlock to contact the lateral aspect of the patient's pelvis. The sidebending deformity is very slowly reduced with a mild lateral pressure against the pelvis, toward the therapist. See Figure 20-28 for the proper positioning of the therapist and the patient.

D. *Quadrant testing.*[375] The quadrant test is a provocative test for a localized capsular restriction that may not cause an obvious restriction of motion or pain on active movement tests. The examiner stands to the patient's side and places one arm across the patient's chest to grasp the opposite shoulder. The other hand is placed over the lower back, with the thumb over the region of the mammillary process of about L2 on the side closest to the examiner. Use the upper arm to bring the patient's trunk around into sidebending, rotation, and extension, while applying counterpressure forward and inward with the other thumb. When the limit of range is reached, hold the position for 20 seconds to allow for a delayed response. This maneuver localizes a close-packed movement to the facet joint immediately superior to the examiner's thumb, therefore localizing stress to the capsule of that joint. The remaining joints, caudal to the first segment tested, are examined in the same manner in an attempt to reproduce the symptoms. The opposite side of the spine may then be tested. This test is less likely to reproduce nerve root symptoms by reducing the size of the intervertebral foramen, as it may in the cervical spine, because the lumbar intervertebral foramina are larger in diameter than the exiting nerve roots.

E. *Passive physiological movements of the spine.* Physiological movements of flexion, extension, rotation, and lateral flexion are tested by passive movements and compared with active motions.

1. *Flexion* (forward-bending). The patient lies in supine with the knees bent. Forward-bending is done by having the therapist or patient pull the knees to the chest or by approximating the patient's knees to the axillae (see Fig. 20-22). Make a general assessment of flexion; compare it with standing forward-bending. Repeated motions may be used to determine if the symptoms change.

2. *Extension* (backward-bending). Passive backward bending is checked with the patient lying prone. Have the patient press up with the arms while letting the back sag. Observe range, changes in pain (centralization or peripheralization), or other symptoms. Measure the distance of the an-

terior-superior iliac spine from the table; about 2″ is considered within normal limits.[532] Passive backward-bending (press-ups) may also be repeated several times to determine if symptoms change with repeated motion (see Fig. 20-47).

3. *Lateral flexion* (sidebending). The patient lies supine with the knees bent. The examiner holds the patient's legs together with hips and knees bent to 90°. Spinal sidebending is produced by rotating the patient's pelvis about a vertical axis, using the patient's leg as a lever (see Fig. 20-26).

4. *Rotation.* The patient lies supine with the knees bent; the thorax is stabilized by placing the arm across the rib cage. The leg furthest from the examiner is grasped behind the knee and the hip is brought to about 90° flexion. This leg is then pulled toward the operator, across the near leg. Repeat on the other side, and compare the two sides (see Fig. 20-24).

F. *Passive physiological movements with segmental palpation.* Passive motion is also done with palpation to appreciate the movement of each segment. This is achieved by palpating between the spinous processes and comparing the movement obtained at each level.

Note the end feels. Normal end feels of the lumbar spine for flexion, extension, lateral flexion, and rotation are of tissue stretch. Determine if tissue tension limits movement before the end of range. Abnormal end feel encountered may be boggy with greater than the expected movement (hypermobility), a rubbery rebound type of resistance, a fairly hard end feel (chrondro-osteophyte contact), or a block.[215] Seek abnormalities such as irritability. Does movement elicit spasm, pain, or paresthesias locally or distally?

1. *Flexion–extension.* (forward and backward bending; Fig. 20-13*A,B*). These movements may be tested by the operator flexing one or both of the patient's legs, but it is generally easier to use one leg. The patient lies on the side with the underneath leg slightly flexed at the hip and knee (a small, flat pillow under the waist keeps the lumbar spine in a neutral position). The examiner stands in front of the patient. The index or middle finger of the cranial hand rests between adjunct spinous processes, while the patient's upper leg is grasped at the knee (with the caudal hand) and passively flexed and released at the hip (extension). The movements of flexion and

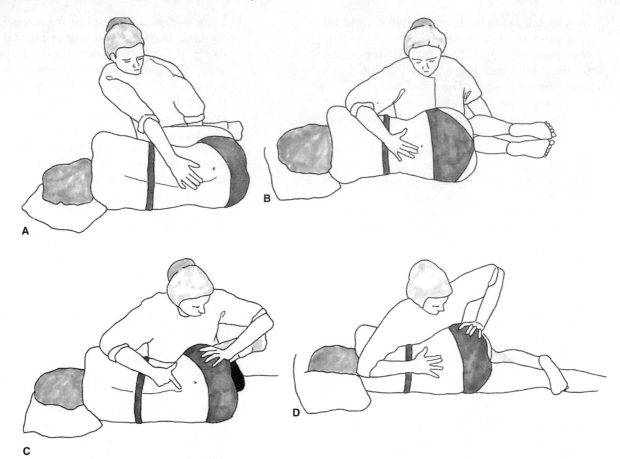

FIG. 20-13. Passive physiological testing of (**A**) flexion, (**B**) extension, (**C**) lateral flexion, and (**D**) rotation.

extension should be stretched to their limits. The amount of movement, noted as an opening and closing of the interspinous gap, is compared to other levels.

2. *Lateral flexion* (sidebending; Fig. 20-13C). The patient lies on the side with the knees and hips bent so that the lumbar spine is relaxed midway between flexion and extension. The examiner (facing the patient) applies the caudal arm around the patient's upper pelvis and under the patient's ischial tuberosity. The examiner's cranial hand palpates between the interspinous spaces of the adjacent vertebrae (the pad of the palpating finger is placed facing upward in the underside of the interspinous space). The examiner firmly grasps the patient's pelvis and upper thigh with the caudal hand, then uses a rhythmical side-sway of the trunk toward the patient's head to produce a side-flexion movement from below upward by rocking the pelvis. Movement can be appreciated either as a gapping or approximation by

the finger of the cranial hand. Repeat to the opposite side.

3. *Rotation* (see Fig. 20-13D). Although active lumbar rotation does not provide much information, testing the small range of rotation is often valuable. The positions of the examiner and patient are similar to those used for assessing lateral flexion or sidebending but with a flat pillow placed under the patient's waist to keep the lumbar spine in neutral. The examiner leans across the patient and places the cranial forearm along the lower thoracic spine, with a reinforced finger resting against adjacent spinous processes from underneath. The caudal hand is placed over the patient's greater trochanter. As the examiner stabilizes the thorax with the cranial forearm, the patient's pelvis is rocked backward and forward so the pelvis and lumbar spine rotate. Repeat on the opposite side.

Note: These three examinations can be modified and used as mobility techniques, using appropriate grades of movement based on the findings found on the evaluation.[289,485]

G. *Segmental mobility* (T10–L5). The patient is in prone-lying across the table, if necessary with a cushion under the abdomen to place the lumbar spine in neutral (resting position; Fig. 20-14). The lower legs are supported on a stool (hips and knees in 90° flexion). The correct movements are achieved by moving the joint by thumb-tip pressure or with pisiform contact against the vertebral prominences. Apply the pressure slowly and carefully so that the "feel" of movement can be recognized. This springing test may be repeated several times to determine the quality of the movement. The basic maneuvers include:

1. Posteroanterior pressure against the spinous processes (using the thumb or pisiform contact)
2. Transverse pressure against the lateral surface of the spinous process. Pressure should be applied to both sides of the spinous processes to compare the quality of movement.
3. Posteroanterior unilateral pressures over the mammillary process of the joint to be examined. The same anterior springing pressure is applied as in central pressure evaluation. Both sides are evaluated and compared. For additional information:

a. Alter the direction of posteroanterior pressure movements: cephalad (toward the head), caudally (toward the feet), and diagonally.
b. Exert counterpressure to the transverse process of the spinal process just below and over the spinous process above a tender segment to determine more precisely the location of the painful or involved segment.[372]

These procedures may elicit pain, restricted movement, or spasm. If the range of movement is limited, assess the type of resistance—caused by either a sense of tightness or muscle spasm. The direction of restriction or painful movement determines the type of mobilization therapy to be used.

H. *Passive sacroiliac and peripheral joint tests.* Painful joint conditions that may originate from the lumbosacral spine must be assessed. Pain from the spine can be referred to the hip, knee, and sacroiliac joints; pain originating in the hip or sacroiliac joint may be referred to the lumbar spine. Clearing tests of the peripheral joints include:

1. *Sacroiliac provocation/mobility tests.* These may reproduce pain from a sacroiliac disorder, and a snap might be elicited if the joint is abnormally mobile. Little or no movement should occur at this joint.

a. Posterior rotation. The patient lies on the side with the side to be tested on top. The examiner flexes the upper knee toward the patient's abdomen, then holds it flexed with the upper thigh or pelvis to free the hands. One hand is placed over the patient's anterior-superior iliac spine, the forearm directed diagonally in the posterocaudal direction with respect to the patient. The opposite hand is placed over the patient's ischial tuberosity, the forearm directed in an anterocephalad direction. The examiner then produces a force-couple movement to rotate the ilium backward on the sacrum while simultaneously moving the patient's hip and knee into more flexion with the examiner's pelvis or anterior thigh (see Fig. 20-43).
b. Anterior rotation. The patient lies prone. The examiner stands at the side to be tested. The more cephalad hand is placed over the sacrum. With the opposite hand, the examiner grasps around

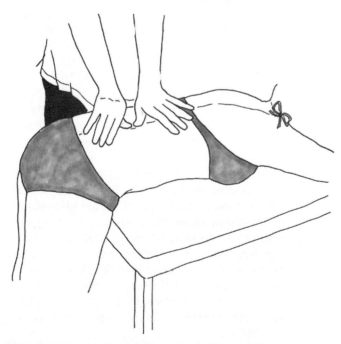

FIG. 20-14. *Position of the patient for palpation and segmental mobility testing of the lumbar spine.*

medially to the anterior aspect of the patient's knee. The examiner pushes down on the inferior aspect of the sacrum while simultaneously lifting the patient's leg into extension to move the ilium, by way of the hip joint capsule, into a forward position on the sacrum (see Fig. 20-44).

c. Tests to demonstrate sacroiliac fixation as described by Kirkaldy-Willis are often included (see Fig. 21-14).[311]

2. *Hip joint.* A test that may be used to clear the hip joint and also to assess the sacroiliac joint is the hip flexion–adduction test. This test uses the femur as a lever to stretch the posterolateral and inferior portions of the inferior capsule and to compress the superior and medial portions of the capsule. With the patient in supine, the examiner flexes the patient's knee and hip fully and then adducts the hip. As the knee is moved fully toward the patient's opposite shoulder, the examiner compresses the hip joint.

3. *Knee joint.* To clear the knee, the anterior drawer test (Lachman test) performed at 25° of knee flexion, and the valgus–varus stress test at 30° of knee flexion also may be used (see Chapter 13, The Knee).

PALPATION

This underused but important examination should be incorporated into the assessment of every patient with back pain. The aims of palpation are to detect abnormalities in bone structure (*e.g.*, spondylolisthesis), to identify the level of the lesion, and to determine the nature of the problem (*e.g.*, muscle spasm, stiffness, pain).

A useful test to assess muscle guarding in the lumbar spine is the weight-shift test.[532] With the patient standing, the examiner places the thumbs on the patient's lumbar paraspinals. The patient is then asked to shift the weight from one side to the other. Normally, the paraspinals on the side of the stance foot relax, but if muscle guarding or spasm is present, the muscle is not felt to relax.

I. **Posterior Aspect.** For further palpation of the posterior aspect of the spine, the patient is placed in a relaxed prone position. This is best achieved in the 90–90 position of the hips and knees (see Fig. 20-14). Standing behind the patient, the examiner places the fingers on the top of the iliac crests and the thumbs at the same level on the midline of the back (the level of the fourth and fifth lumbar disk interspaces). This reference point is marked and the following are palpated:

A. *Ligaments.* The supraspinous ligaments are palpated for tenderness and consistency; the supraspinous ligament is normally springy and supple. If it is thick and hardened, the segment may be hypomobile. Tenderness is usually apparent over the involved intervertebral joint. Usually, the interspinous ligament is also tender. This is found by applying exquisitely localized pressure with a key ring or the edge of a coin between the spinous processes.[372]

B. *Position of the transverse and spinous processes.* Note any alterations in the bony alignment, such as spondylolistheses and evidence of tenderness. Specific pain elicited in one segment is particularly helpful in patients with suspected instability.[450] If each spinous process is tapped sharply with a reflex hammer or fingertip, pain may be reproduced over the painful joint.

C. *Sacrum, sulcus, sacral hiatus, and coccyx.* Palpation of a the whole sacroiliac sulcus, hiatus, and coccyx should be done (see Fig. 21-10). If indicated, a rectal examination of the coccyx may be performed. The sacroiliac joint is palpated at its inferior extent in the region of the posteroinferior iliac spine. Acute unilateral tenderness is common in painful sacroiliac conditions and when well localized is a useful confirmatory sign.[209] When palpating the joint, the patient's knee is flexed to 90° and the hip is passively medially rotated while the examiner palpates the sacroiliac joint on the same side. The procedure is repeated on the opposite side.

A comprehensive examination of this joint should be regarded as an expanded section of the lumbar spine. Details of a comprehensive examination of this joint are found in other sources (see Chapter 21, The Sacroiliac Joint and Lumbar–Pelvic–Hip Complex).*

D. *Iliac crest, ischial tuberosity, and hip joint.* Beginning at the posterosuperior iliac spine, the examiner moves along the iliac crest, palpating for signs of pathological processes such as Maigne's syndrome (see Chapter 19, The Thoracic Spine).[311] Pressure and friction over the iliac crest often reveal a well-localized, acutely painful point (crestal point) at the gluteal level (8 to 10 cm from the midline). Pinching and rolling of the skin in the gluteal area will be painful, as well as lateral pressure over the spinous processes (T11–L1). According to Maigne, referred pain may be mediated by the cluneal nerves, the posterior rami of the T12 or L1 spinal nerves.[373] These nerves pass down-

---

*References 50, 96, 110–112, 156, 193, 195, 196, 311, 365, 371, 376, 422, 470, 532, 647

ward and outward on each side to supply the skin at the level of the iliac crest (see Fig. 19-8B). The referred pain is experienced at this level. Irritation of these nerves may be responsible for low back pain, pseudovisceral pain, and pseudohip pain. Because attention is usually directed to the site of referred pain, the source is frequently overlooked.[373] When Maigne's syndrome is suspected, the diagnosis is confirmed when pain is alleviated following manipulation or injections to the symptomatic posterior joints.[311]

The ischial tuberosities are palpated on both sides for any abnormalities, including the hip and greater trochanteric bursa, which sometimes mimics sciatica. It is often difficult to differentiate between hip and spine problems, because the symptoms may be similar.

E. *Muscles of the gluteal region and sciatic nerve.* Observe for apparent muscle atrophy, particularly of the gluteus maximus on one side. During palpation, one or several of the muscles often have hard, infiltrated fascicles that are sometimes cord-like and may be very sensitive to pressure. According to Maigne, the gluteal muscle pain is responsible for many instances of lumbar pain.[372] Deep petrissage gives excellent results in this type of chronic pain.[373] Palpating midway between the ischial tuberosity and the greater trochanter, the examiner may be able to palpate the sciatic nerve. Deep to the gluteal muscles, the piriformis muscle should be palpated for potential pathological processes.

F. *Skin and subcutaneous tissue.* Palpate the skin for tenderness, moisture, texture, and temperature changes. A quick wipe over the area with the back of the hand is used to register any apparent local changes in temperature or sweating. Examine any moles on the skin to determine whether they are deep or superficial. Normally, the skin can be rolled over the spine and gluteal region freely and painlessly. If there are subcutaneous pathological changes, there will be tightness and pain with skin-rolling.

II. **Anterior Aspect**

A. *Abdominal wall, iliac crest, and symphysis pubis.* Palpate the abdominal wall, iliac crest, and symphysis pubis for tenderness. Palpate the symphysis pubis bilaterally, over the superior aspect, to ensure that the two pubic bones are level and asymptomatic.

B. *Inguinal area and femoral triangle.* Probe the general area within the triangle for enlarged lymph nodes (infections), symptoms of hernia, abscess, or other pathological conditions.

C. *Arterial pulses.* Assess the arterial supply to the legs by palpating the arterial pulses in the inguinal, popliteal, and dorsalis sites.

NEUROMUSCULAR EVALUATION

The neurological part of the musculoskeletal evaluation consists of a series of tests to determine if there is segmental interference of neural conduction. The most common cause of such findings is a disk extrusion in the lumbar spine. Other causes of neurological deficits in the legs are rare but are usually more serious. Any multisegmental deficit should be viewed with some suspicion, because nerve root impingement from a disk protrusion rarely involves more than one root; the occasional exception is an L5–S1 protrusion, which may affect the L5 and S1 roots.

I. **Sensory (Dermatomal) Tests.** Subtle sensory deficits are best detected by assessing vibratory perception with a tuning fork. This is because pressure tends to affect the large, myelinated fibers that mediate vibratory and proprioceptive sensation first. Gross sensory testing may be done using a wisp of cotton or a pin.

The key sensory areas to test are in the distal part of the limb, because these are the areas where there is relatively little overlap of segmental innervation. These include L4, the medial aspect of the big toe; L5, the web space between the first and second toes; S1, below the lateral malleolus; and S2, the distal Achilles tendon region. Test these areas first, then the various aspects of the leg and thigh. If a significant deficit is detected proximal to the foot, ensure that more serious pathological processes have been ruled out.

When performing sensory tests, test a small area of one limb. Ask the patient if the expected sensation is felt (*e.g.*, vibration, touch, or pinprick). Then test the corresponding area on the opposite limb and ask the patient again if it is felt. Ask if the intensity of the stimulus felt is about the same on both sides. Proceed in this fashion for all the areas to be tested. Sensory tests are most easily done with the patient supine.

II. **Resisted Isometric Tests** (motor, myotomal tests). Because most limb muscles receive innervation from more than one segment, only subtle motor dysfunction is noted in the case of segmental deficits resulting from disk protrusions. Significant motor loss should suggest a more serious pathological process. Key muscles are tested for each segment. Large muscle groups, such as the quadriceps and calf muscles, must be tested by repetitive resistance against a load, because even in the presence of loss of segmental input to such muscles, sufficient tension may still be produced to prevent the examiner from detecting weakness by overcoming the contraction.

In general, isometric tests are used to test for any muscle weakness that may result from nerve root compressions. However, plantar-flexion of the foot cannot be adequately tested by an isometric contraction. Instead, weight-bearing ankle plantar-flexion is tested by repeated toe-raises. When testing muscles (and reflexes), look for unusual fatigue, and always compare both sides. Tests of clinical significance are listed below.

A. *Tests with patient in supine*

  1. L2—Hip flexion (iliopsoas). The patient holds the flexed hip and knee at 90° while resistance is applied just above the knee.
  2. L3—Knee extension (quadriceps). Test by repetitive one-legged half-squats in the standing position or in supine using an isometric contraction. The examiner supports the thigh with one arm underneath it, with the examiner's hand supported on top of the opposite thigh. Resistance is applied to the lower leg while the patient holds the leg just short of full extension.
  3. L4—Ankle dorsiflexion and inversion (tibialis anterior). Test bilaterally. The patient holds the feet in dorsiflexion and inversion as resistance is applied against the dorsal-medial aspect of the foot.
  4. L5—Great toe extension (extensor hallucis longus). Toe extension is tested bilaterally. The patient holds the foot and toes dorsiflexed as resistance is applied against the dorsal aspect of the great toe.
  5. L5–S1—Extension of the toes (extensor digitorum longus). The patient holds the foot and toes dorsiflexed as resistance is applied against the dorsum of the toes.
  6. S1—Ankle eversion (peroneus longus and brevis). The patient tries to keep the heels together with the feet everted as resistance is applied to the lateral borders of the feet, pushing them together.

B. *Tests with patient in prone*

  1. S2—Knee flexion (hamstrings). The hamstrings are tested bilaterally as the patient holds the knees flexed to 90° as resistance is applied behind the heels.
  2. S1—Hip extension (gluteus maximus). The patient holds the hip extended with the knee bent while the examiner applies resistance just above the knee with one hand while palpating the gluteal mass with the other hand to assess firmness.

C. *Tests with patient standing*

  1. S1—Plantar-flexion (gastrocnemius). The patient stands on one leg and plantar-flexes by rising on the toes through a full range of motion. Repeat six to ten times per side. Plantar-flexion can also be tested by having the patient walk on the toes.
  2. L3—Knee flexion (quadriceps). Unilateral half-squats; repeat six to ten times. The girth of the limbs above and below the knee is measured to document any muscle-wasting.

III. Dural Mobility Tests. The dura, nerve root sleeves, and nerve roots are sensitive to pain. Their irritants are many, as are the pathological processes that induce them. Included are disk prolapse,[55,596,626] adhesions (*e.g.,* post-traumatic or postsurgical epidural fibrosis, subarachnoid adhesions),[626,627] hypertrophic changes in the facet joints and margins of the vertebral bodies,[156,432,599] and indirect compressions from ischemic changes secondary to chronic progressive compression (*e.g.,* enlarged masses, thickening of the ligamentum flavum, apophyseal joint swelling).[375]

Dural mobility tests (sciatic nerve, straight-leg raising) may reproduce symptoms (usually pain) in the case of a disk prolapse, in which a bulging disk may approximate the anterolateral aspect of the dural sac of the cauda equina, or in the case of a disk extrusion, in which the protruded disk material may be adjacent to some part of the dural investment of a nerve root. The dura can be moved in a cephalad direction by flexing the neck, or in a caudal direction by applying tension to the femoral or sciatic nerves. The femoral nerve and its contributing nerve roots are stretched by sidelying or prone knee flexion and hip extension, the sciatic nerve and its roots by straight-leg raising. Additional tension is applied to the sciatic nerve by dorsiflexing the ankle.

A. Dural mobility tests for the sciatic nerve roots may be done sitting or supine. It is often best to perform them in both positions and to compare the results. Sitting increases the likelihood of obtaining a positive test in the case of a minor prolapse, because it is a position of relatively high intradiskal pressure. However, to judge improvement, the tests are best performed in the supine position, measuring the distance from the lateral malleolus to the plinth at which pain is produced on straight-leg raising.

A true-positive dural mobility test will reproduce back pain, hip girdle pain, leg pain, or some combination thereof, and pain should be felt somewhere between 30° and 60° of straight-leg raising. At angles less than 30°, there is very little movement of the nerve roots, and by 60° the dura will have already moved sufficiently to have reproduced pain. Also, above 60°, the reproduction of pain may be caused by movement of the spinal column as the pelvis tilts backward. Differentiate between pulling on tight hamstrings and reproduction of leg pain from dural impingement. Possible mechanical effects from movement of the spine or sacroiliac joint can be ruled out by seeing if ankle dorsiflexion further accentuates the pain produced; if so, it is likely to be a true-positive dural sign.

1. The sitting tests are done with the patient sitting at the edge of the plinth. First move one knee toward extension, noting any guarding of the movement and asking whether symptoms are reproduced. If pain is produced, hold the leg just up to the painful point and assess the effects of ankle dorsiflexion and neck flexion. Test the opposite leg similarly.

2. The supine tests are done in a similar manner by moving first one leg and then the other into flexion with the knee straight. Again, assess the effects of ankle dorsiflexion and neck flexion. Test straight-leg raising with the hip in neutral rotation and slightly adducted during straight-leg raising of the asymptomatic leg. Positive straight-leg raising of the opposite leg can be more important than ipsilateral straight-leg raising. A discussion of this sciatic traction test would be incomplete without mentioning what is called the "well leg of Fajersztan," the crossed straight-leg raising test or crossover sign, a prostrate leg raising test, Lhermitte's sign or sciatic phenomenon.[264,495,613] These tests have a high correlation with large central disk protrusions that impale on the root in its axilla.[141,264,534,575,662] The pattern of positive results yields clues as to the relation between the protrusion and the pain-sensitive structure (*e.g.*, dura or dural covering of a nerve root).

   a. If prolapsed or extruded material is anterior to the pain-sensitive tissue, ipsilateral leg raising, contralateral leg raising, and neck flexion may all hurt.

   b. If the protruded material is medial to the nerve root as it exits from the dural sac (rare), leg raising may hurt bilaterally but neck flexion may be painless.

   c. If the protrusion is lateral to the existing nerve root, ipsilateral leg raising

may reproduce symptoms, neck flexion may or may not be painful, and contralateral leg raising is painless.

Intradiskal pressure increases when the patient sits or stands, as compared with lying.[452] This may cause a discrepancy in the degree of limitation of straight-leg raising performed in the standing and lying positions, so performing tests in both positions can be valuable.[375]

3. The slump test is an excellent test for a disk lesion and dural tethering; it is performed on the patient who has low back pain with or without leg pain.[375,441] Maximum tension can be exerted on the canal structures with the patient's chin on the chest.[375] With the patient sitting erect on the table, have him or her do the following:

   a. Let the back slump through its full range of thoracic lumbar spine flexion.

   b. Having established full range of the hip and spine from T1 to the sacrum, flex the head and neck fully.

   c. Straighten first the unaffected leg and actively dorsiflex the ankle and then the affected leg.

   Note and record the pain response after each step. There are many variations of this test, including passive and sustained overpressure of the head and neck while in the slump position, releasing the neck-flexion component, raising the head to neutral, neck extension in the slump position, and performing the test in long-sitting. According to Maitland, when assessing the findings of this test, the pain response, particularly in relation to releasing the neck-flexion component, is most important.[374,375]

B. *Femoral nerve traction test.*[141] The patient lies on the unaffected side with the lower limb flexed at both the hip and knee joints to stabilize the trunk. The head is flexed slightly to increase tension on the cauda equina. The test has two components:

1. The uppermost part of the thigh is first passively extended just short of provoking lumbar spine extension to create tension in the iliopsoas, and hence traction on the upper lumbar nerve root.

2. Next, the knee is progressively flexed to increase femoral nerve tension by stretching the quadriceps femoris muscle.

In the presence of an L3 radiculitis, pain radiates down the medial thigh to the knee. When the L4 root is involved, the pain is more anterior on the thigh and extends to the midtibial portion of the leg.[141]

IV. **Reflex Tests.** Plantar responses and deep tendon reflexes are tested for any evidence of an upper motor neuron lesion.

    A. *Plantar reflex test.* With the patient's leg extended, stimulate the lateral border of the sole with a blunt object. The stroke begins on the lateral aspect of the heel and moves distally, then across the metatarsals just proximal to the toes. Plantar-flexion is a normal response; dorsiflexion (a positive Babinski response) is pathological and indicates spinal cord injury (upper motor neuron lesion).

    B. *Deep tendon reflexes.* Segmented neurological deficits may result in diminution of deep tendon reflexes on the involved side. When examining deep tendon reflexes, primarily observe for asymmetry of responses from one side to the other. Difficulty eliciting reflexes on both sides does not necessarily indicate a pathological process, so long as there is no asymmetry in response. Look for unusual fatigue. Elicit the reflex at least six times, and always compare sides.

        1. Knee jerk reflex—L3, L4
        2. Ankle jerk reflex—S1, S2
        3. Great toe reflex—L5[609]

        The medial (L5, S1) and the lateral (S1) hamstring reflexes are not routinely tested but may assist in decisions about involvement of those roots.[201]

        Superficial reflex (upper motor neuron) testing may be indicated and includes the abdominal, cremasteric, and anal reflexes.[262,365]

V. **Test for Ankle Clonus.** A test to determine if the patient has clonus may be included here. A hyperactive stretch reflex is the mechanism that supports clonus. Ankle clonus is elicited by quickly stretching the gastrocsoleus muscle group by dorsiflexing the foot and then maintaining moderate stretch to the plantar flexors. The clonus response is alternating plantar-flexion and dorsiflexion of the foot.

VI. **Balance Testing.** Balance testing is conducted to appraise the receptor integrity in the joints of the lower extremities and lumbar spine.[152,664,665] The Romberg test, "stork-standing," or digital balance boards can be used to assess balance. If a mechanical lesion of the low back is suspected, the above tests are generally sufficient. However, if neurological disease is suspected (*e.g.*, diabetic neu-

ropathy), motor performance, temperature, and proprioception should be tested as well.

GENERAL PHYSICAL EXAMINATION

A general physical examination, including the abdomen and chest, may be necessary. In cases of suspected pelvic lesions, a rectal examination is necessary. These tests help determine the severity of the back pain, the level of the lesion, the presence of nerve root pressure, and the authenticity of the pain. A history and physical examination are usually sufficient to identify most patients for whom specific therapy is required.[504] Because of the drawbacks of routine roentgenography, many authors have proposed selective studies based on clinical findings.

OTHER STUDIES

I. **Roentgenograms and Other Imaging Studies.** The examiner may review any imaging studies that have been done.[128,281,421] In addition to basic roentgenograms, other special techniques may be used.

    A. *Myelograms.* A radiopaque dye is placed within the epidural space and allowed to flow to different levels of the spinal cord. Due to its potential morbidity, this technique is usually reserved for patients with suspected spinal canal stenosis or spinal tumor, or it is used to demonstrate the level of a prolapsed disk. With disk prolapse, the column of dye should be indented or distorted with evidence of compression or shortening of the nerve root dural sheath (see Fig. 20-4*A,B*).

    B. *Diskography.* This test involves injecting a water-soluble radiopaque dye under roentgenographic control into the nucleus pulposus to reproduce signs of disk disease and to localize the level of impingement. The injection should reproduce the pain if the test is to be considered positive (see Figs. 20-1*A* and 20-2*A*).

    C. *CT scan.* Tomography, which has become a common technique, involves a computerized display that recreates a three-dimensional image of the spine.[584] It provides a noninvasive alternative to the techniques described earlier. Plane tomograms or computer isotomograms have improved the capability to outline both bony and soft tissues. CT scans are most useful in outlining structural spinal deformities such as lumbar canal stenosis, abnormalities in the facet joints, vertebral disease, and disk prolapse.[78]

    D. *Bone scanning.* This noninvasive, sensitive

technique uses chemicals labeled with isotopes such as technetium pyrophosphate, which is taken up by bone and bound to hydroxyapatite crystals. The isotope may be localized where there is a high level of activity relative to the rest of a bone. Its major role is to identify pathological changes such as stress fractures, tumors, and metabolic bone disease.

E. Other techniques include radiculography, epidural blocks, MRI, and venography.[652]

II. **Electromyography.** Electromyography may be used to localize the level of a spinal lesion with nerve root pressure.[155] Evidence of denervation may be found as early as 2 weeks after the onset of nerve damage.[96]

III. **Laboratory Tests.** A complete blood count is among the laboratory tests used to investigate spinal disease, and urinalysis should be performed routinely.

TESTS FOR NONORGANIC BACK PAIN

Several tests are useful in the differentiation of organic and nonorganic back pain (*e.g.*, that seen in patients suffering from depression, emotional disturbance, or anxiety).[96,303,518,520,525] It is difficult to assess a patient who has an organic back lesion but whose symptoms are exacerbated or prolonged by psychological factors. In these patients, the symptoms are usually out of proportion to the signs (*e.g.*, inconsistent joint findings; abnormal postures or gait). Tests include the following:

I. **Distraction Test** (leg test or flip test).[303,635,636] A positive physical finding is demonstrated in a routine manner; this finding is then checked while the patient's attention is distracted. For example, after performing the usual straight-leg raising test in supine, ask the patient to sit up, swing the legs over the end of the table, and repeat leg raising in sitting. If marked improvement is noted, the patient's response is inconsistent. Leg raising is a useful distraction test.

II. **Stimulation Tests.** These tests should not be uncomfortable: if pain is reported, a nonorganic influence is suggested.

A. Axial loading uses manual pressure through the standing patient's head. Few patients whose lumbar pain is organic will suffer discomfort on this test.[303,635,636]

B. Hip and shoulder rotation.[303] With the patient standing, examine for pain by passively rotating the patient's hips or shoulders while the feet are kept on the ground. This maneuver is usually painless for patients with organic back disorders.

C. Kneeling on a stool (Burns test).[96,303] The patient kneels on a stool or chair and is asked to bend over and try to touch the floor. Even with a severely herniated disk, most patients attempt the task to some degree. Persons with nonorganic pain often refuse on the grounds that it would cause great pain or would tend to overbalance them on the chair.

III. **Other Methods.** Other tools for assessing nonorganic physical signs include regional disturbances, which involve a divergence from the accepted neuroanatomy (*i.e.*, atypical motor and sensory disturbances), overreaction during examination (*i.e.*, disproportionate verbalization, muscle tension, and tremor), and tenderness.[637,640] Tenderness, when related to physical disease, is usually localized to a particular skeletal or neuromuscular structure. Nonorganic tenderness is nonspecific and diffuse. Further verification is possible by the use of pain drawings, as recommended by Ransford and associates (see Fig. 20-8).[507]

Several other psychopathic signs and observations have been described;[363,415,431,495,578] if found, further psychological evaluation is indicated, and the therapist must guard against potential overtreatment.[495,581,656]

Other types of investigation, such as the MMPI and other psychological tests, have been used for lumbar spine problems.* Since its development in 1940 by Hathaway and McKinley, the MMPI has become one of the most widely used personality screening tests.[241]

ACTIVITIES OF DAILY LIVING

A formal exercise obstacle course may be used to evaluate the patient's ability to perform activities of daily living.[652] Activities to be assessed include sitting, standing, walking, bending, lifting, pushing, pulling, climbing, and reaching. Endurance may be evaluated while the patient is walking or riding a stationary bicycle. Quantitative functional capacity measurements can give objective evidence of the patient's physical abilities and degree of effort, and can be useful in designing and administering an effective treatment program.[393]

COMPUTERIZED TESTS

Isokinetic forms of resisted muscle testing are the most effective and yield reliable measurements of

---

*References 27, 38, 40, 54, 63, 105, 114, 115, 122, 177, 194, 248, 316, 408, 413–415, 578, 585, 586, 623, 659

muscular strength, power (at slow and fast speeds), and endurance. These measures can be recorded in graphic form for comparison later in rehabilitation.[140] The potential value of objective measurement of spinal function has been recognized for some time, although practical and clinically useful technology has not been generally available.[38,174,444,600] The increasing understanding of disuse and deconditioning syndromes as a factor in long-term disability and recent developments in the qualification of true spinal range of motion,[394,395,397,605] trunk muscle strength,[118,329,380,451,493,567,612,613] endurance, and lifting capacity bring a new dimension to the management of low back pain.[245,313,396,467,500]

COMMON LESIONS AND MANAGEMENT

☐ Intervertebral Disk Lesions

Sciatica is caused by many intraspinal abnormalities other than disk prolapse.[4,88,208,212,258,341,494,498,568,576,577] For example, a decrease in size of the lateral bony nerve root canal can result from degenerative hypertrophy of the lumbar facets or a trefoil canal (a congenital variant in cross-sectional geometry).[18,310] Other less common causes of sciatica include congenital anomalies of the lumbar nerve roots, "hip-pocket" sciatica, the piriformis syndrome, and even viral infections.[387,583] Space does not permit a full discussion of all the causes of acute spinal dysfunction.

Despite the extensive differential diagnosis, intervertebral disk prolapse is the most common diagnosis of sciatica. Ninety-eight percent of intervertebral disk prolapse cases involve the L4–L5 or L5–S1 lumbar disk space.[576] Older patients have a relatively increased risk of disk prolapse at the L3–L4 and L2–L3 levels.[188,189]

The sensitive spinal cord has an elaborate protective mechanism, including a most pain-sensitive anterior dural sheath and the posterior longitudinal ligament. The following can occur with a prolapsed disk:

1. The disk bulges against the ligament and the dura. This produces a dull, deep, poorly localized pain in the back and over the sacroiliac region because the dura does not have specific dermatomal localization.
2. The disk bulges posterolaterally against the nerve root. This is a natural route because the annulus fibrosus is no longer reinforced by the posterior ligament. The result is sharp nerve root pain (*e.g.*, sciatica).
3. The disk ruptures and the thick gelatinous fluid of the nucleus pulposus flows around the dura and nerve roots. This is an extremely irritating substance and it causes a reaction around the nerve-sensitive tissue. It is the most likely cause of agonizing, persistent back pain. When the disk ruptures, fragments of the harder annulus fibrosus may protrude into the spinal canal; this usually requires surgical intervention.

In experiments using human volunteers by Nachemson and Morris in 1964, the intradiskal pressures in the lumbar spine were measured with a diskogram, and subsequent studies have enhanced our understanding of the intervertebral disk (Figs. 20-15 and 20-16).[446,452] Obviously, bending forward while lifting increases the pressure. The situation is aggravated by sitting, when the lumbar lordosis is reduced by leaning forward.

DISK PROLAPSE

Some clinical features associated with disk prolapse include:

1. Age—The peak age is 20 to 45 years. A prolonged work posture of lumbar flexion is a frequent factor in the history.
2. Sex—Males are more commonly affected than females by about 3:2.
3. Site—In 1000 lumbar disk operations, Armstrong found that 46.9% occurred at the lumbosacral disk, 40.4% at the L4–L5 disk, and 2.1% at the upper three disks; in 10.7% of the cases, double lesions were present.[17]

HISTORY
Back pain may occur for no apparent reason—rather, it may be caused by the cumulative effects of months or even years of forward-bending, lifting, or sitting in a slumped, forward-bent position.[83,119,123,406,466,489,573,576,649] There may be a history of attacks of back pain, sometimes associated with a sensation of back locking. Many patients tend to relate it to some minor traumatic incident or after a strain, such as bending, lifting, or twisting, which may be associated with a tearing sensation.[96]

In the early stages, the patient complains of pain, usually in the lower back but sometimes in the posterior buttocks or thigh. As a rule, leg pain indicates a larger protrusion than does back pain alone.[406] Pain may be described as a dull ache or knife-like. The onset of pain may be sudden and severe or may develop more gradually. Pain at first may be intermittent and relieved by rest, standing, lying, or changing position. Spinal pain tends to be greater on one side than the other. Bilateral spinal pain is probably secondary to a connecting branch of the sinuvertebral

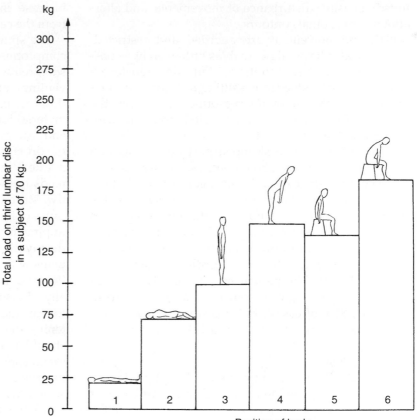

FIG. 20-15. Intradiskal pressures (relative) as they relate to body positions. (Finneson BE: Low Back Pain, 2nd ed, p. 41. Philadelphia, JB Lippincott, 1980.)

nerve, which joins the right and left portions of that nerve.[169] Pain is aggravated by straining, stooping, sneezing, coughing, car travel, and sitting. The patient also often reports that prolonged sitting causes the pain to move from the lower back into the leg. Difficulty in assuming an erect posture after lying down or sitting may also be described. Ultimately, pain usually becomes severe and may disturb sleep.

Back pain may be followed by leg pain, which is almost always unilateral and usually is severe. The back

pain may disappear when the leg pain begins. The distribution of the leg pain varies according to the nerve root involved.

CLINICAL EXAMINATION

Signs consist of varying combinations and degrees of mechanical derangement of the lumbar spinal joints and evidence of nerve root involvement. Mechanical derangement is evidenced by alterations in posture,

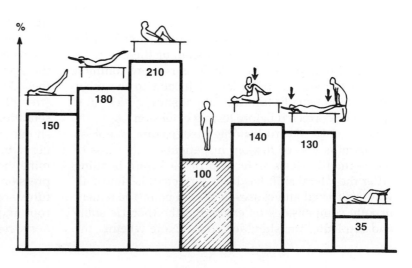

FIG. 20-16. Intradiskal pressures (relative) as they relate to activities. (Adapted from Nachemson AL: The lumbar spine: An orthopedic challenge. Spine 1:59–71, 1976.)

muscle spasms, disturbance of movements, and alterations in the spinal contours.

Gait and movement are guarded and restricted. Gait may also be antalgic, with as little weight as possible being transferred to the painful side. Transfer activities, such as rising from a sitting position and moving about on the plinth, are performed guardedly; the lumbar spine is reflexively protected from compressive loading or movement.

The patient sits in a slumped posture or insists on standing in the waiting room because of increased intradiskal pressure caused by sitting. In erect standing, patients may be unable to bear any weight on the painful leg, so they stand with the hips and knees flexed and the back held rigid. The patient may have loss of the normal lordosis and flattening of the thoracic spine and shoulder girdle retraction as well.[96,110,406,638] The patient may have a lateral shift (lumbar scoliosis) away from the side of pain (contralateral, 85% of cases), but occasionally toward the painful side (ipsilateral, 15% of cases).

INSPECTION

To evaluate active movement, the physiological movements of the spine are tested to determine their range, whether pain is reproduced, the behavior of the pain with movement, whether an arc of pain is present, and the presence of any deformity.

Lumbar forward-bending (flexion) is sometimes limited because of the severity of the pain, and the degree of its loss usually reflects the severity of the disk prolapse. The patient often tends to compensate by bending at the hips and knees and may guard the spine against excessive compression by placing the hands on the thighs. In less severe cases, where forward-bending is possible, bending may be associated with a deviated arc of movement in which the spine shifts out of and back toward the midline as movement proceeds. When tested in the standing position, flexion may cause the pain to move peripherally, especially if forward-flexion is repeated several times.[406]

Movement into lateral flexion varies. There may be full and painless range to each side, or there may be painful limitation to one side. This is more common toward the side of pain; lateral flexion to the other side is then usually full. If a lateral shift is present, it should be corrected before testing extension.

Loss of backward-bending (extension) is not as common as loss of flexion. In patients with a loss of the normal lordosis, extension or backward-bending (after the lateral shift has been corrected) is almost always restricted and causes increased pain. The patient usually compensates by extending the thoracic spine and retracting the shoulder girdle. Note whether the increase in pain centralizes or becomes peripheral from the center of the spine into the leg.

The spine is reflexively splinted in a position that compromises between minimizing intradiskal pressure, reducing tension on the dural material, and preventing impingement of the protruded materials. Lordosis is lost because the posteriorly protruded disk material forces the segment toward forward-bending, and backward-bending would tend to compromise the prolapse. Forward-bending is difficult because the marked increase in intradiskal pressure it causes tends to increase the pressure against the pain-sensitive structures.[12,444] Lateral bending is restricted because of increased intradiskal pressure and because of impingement of the protrusion when performed to the involved side. McKenzie maintains that 50% of patients with this disorder have a lateral shift because of the tendency of the nuclear gel to shift posterolaterally.[406] As the gel moves posteriorly, the patient tends to shift the body weight in an anterior direction, flattening the lumbar spine. When the patient shifts the shoulder away from the side of the nuclear movement, a lateral shift occurs.[96,162,169,305,473] Usually, the protrusion is lateral to the existing nerve root, in which case a lateral shift away from the defect minimizes the dural impingement. Less often, the bulge is located at the axilla formed by the root stemming from the dural sac. The spine is shifted toward the ipsilateral side or painful side (15% of cases). The presence of a lateral shift may be noted while the patient is standing or flexing or extending the lumbar spine. It is not rare for a patient with only unilateral pain and a contralateral list to have this change under treatment to an ipsilateral list, or vice versa.[214]

Passive movements—both physiological and accessory—are limited because of spasms, stiffness, and pain. Passive physiological restriction is usually less, because of reduced compression imposed on the spine, in a reclining position. Accessory movements are usually compromised by protective muscle guarding.

Nerve root involvement is indicated by the loss of freedom of movement of the nerve root in the spinal canal or its intervertebral foramen. True neurological signs and symptoms are produced. The patient has all the signs and symptoms previously discussed, with the addition of positive neurological signs such as strength loss, decreased muscle stretch reflexes, loss of sensation, and positive dural mobility signs. Tests should include straight-leg raising and the femoral nerve traction test. Neurological assessment to determine the nerve root involved and the degree of compression is essential. The most important clinical features are the localization of pain to an affected nerve root and the reproduction of the pain by a positive nerve root tension sign.[534]

PALPATION

The affected spinal level is usually tender to palpation in the midline or in the paravertebral area on the same side as the disk prolapse. The sciatic nerve may also be tender. If the patient has had pain for more than 1 or 2 days, the muscles may be tender from guarding and muscle spasm. Positional changes can occasionally be felt by palpating the spinous processes. For example, if the segment is locked in rotation and sidebending, the superior spinous process will not be in alignment with the adjacent inferior spinous process.

CLINICAL VARIATIONS

Many clinical variations of the pain pattern and neurological involvement are possible. The most common pain pattern is back pain followed by leg pain, but the patient may present with back pain alone, sciatic pain alone, or simultaneous back and leg pain. Pain may radiate into both legs simultaneously and consecutively. A large posterior prolapse may implicate two nerve roots on either side at the same level or at different levels.[96]

Acute nerve root compression is a severe back problem usually caused by an advanced disk protrusion. It must be handled with care. The disorder has a protracted course of 6 to 12 weeks; more than 50% of patients recover in 6 weeks.[15] Rarely is surgical treatment required, so delaying surgery is appropriate in most cases.

CONSERVATIVE TREATMENT

In the acute stage, the nonsurgical treatment of acute symptomatic disk prolapse includes bed rest, medications, epidural steroids, and minimizing the lesion by reducing intradiskal pressure. The therapist must be aware of the positions and activities that increase intradiskal pressure and must carefully instruct the patient to avoid situations that may cause the protrusion to progress (see Figs. 20-15 and 20-16).[11,12,100,101,444,447]

The optimal amount of bed rest remains to be established, but Deyo and associates observed no difference in outcome between patients with 2 days of bed rest versus those with 1 week of bed rest.[127] In patients with a demonstrated radicular compression, bed rest is efficacious, as shown in Weber's study of 2 weeks of bed rest.[642] This does not mean absolute bed rest, however, because with prolonged recumbency, the disk tends to imbibe fluid from the adjacent vertebral bodies. Activities related to feeding and personal hygiene may actually be more difficult to achieve in bed than out of bed.

Prospective, randomized trials of autotraction,[197] phenylbutazone, and indomethacin have demon-

strated that these treatment procedures diminish pain.[30]

Epidural infiltrations of cortisone and local anesthetics have been the topic of several clinical studies, and results have been variable; their utility remains controversial.[51,104,572] Epidural steroids reduced pain and increased function in one randomized study,[130] but a recent comparison of epidural steroid therapy and placebo (saline) demonstrated no differences 24 hours after the injections.

Traction can be applied by means of autotraction, inversion traction, gravity reduction, 90–90 traction, and motorized techniques, including three-dimensional lumbar traction.* Some clinical studies have compared the effects of different types of traction, but no controlled study has demonstrated their relative efficacy.[338,504,534,564,676] At least 60% of the body weight must be applied for dimensional changes in the lumbar disk to occur.[189] Claims that disk prolapse can be reduced are unproven. Autotraction, gravity axial traction, and positional traction have a short-lived benefit in acute low back pain and sciatica.[65,197,484]

When treating an acute disk protrusion with spinal traction, the treatment time should be short. The patient may feel less pain while the distractive force is applied, but as the traction is released a marked increase in pain often is experienced.[534] Such an effect is probably secondary to absorption of additional fluid by the nucleus while the traction is applied, and the development of a high intradiskal pressure as the distractive force is relaxed. This adverse reaction has not been observed if treatment times are kept under 10 minutes for intermittent traction and under 8 minutes for sustained traction.[530]

Braces and lumbar corsets remain controversial. Morris and associates[437] and Nachemson and Morris[452] have shown that when a garment such as a lumbosacral corset that compresses the abdomen is worn, intradiskal pressure is diminished by about 25%. Significant unloading of the disk occurs in both the standing and sitting positions.

The first step in any treatment program for acute low back pain should be education. The following points should be considered with respect to the reduction of intradiskal pressure:

1. Sitting (see Fig. 20-15), especially with the lumbar part of the spine in a forward-bent position, causes high intradiskal pressure.[446] Sitting with the knees and hips flexed is especially contraindicated. The patient must be taught to sit and rise to standing

---

*References 65, 66, 98, 106, 112, 125, 153, 261, 331, 338, 344, 381–383, 440, 455, 469, 479, 492, 525, 530, 532, 576, 624

without bending forward at the lumbar part of the spine. Sitting for a bowel movement may cause a marked increase in intradiskal pressure because of the Valsalva maneuver. The patient must be taught to sit leaning back, with a wide base of support, with one or both legs outstretched. Use of a raised toilet seat and of a laxative also may be advisable.

2. Most patients are more comfortable while standing than sitting, which confirms Nachemson and Morris's findings that on standing intradiskal pressure is decreased by 29%.[452] The normal lumbar curve should be maintained. If the patient is fixed in some degree of forward-bending, walking should be allowed only with the aid of crutches to reduce weight-bearing compressive forces to the disk.[517]

3. Isometric abdominal contractions and pelvic-tilt exercises that increase intradiskal pressure should not be instituted in the early acute stage.

PHYSICAL THERAPY

Oscillatory techniques may relieve pain by increasing large-fiber proprioceptive input, which in turn relieves some of the protective muscle spasm. Physical programs (*e.g.*, ultrasound, hot packs, cold packs, and diathermy) have no impact on the disease process but provide temporary pain relief.[96,446]

Perhaps the most controversial form of treatment is *manipulative therapy*, which Haldeman has divided into manipulation, mobilization, manual traction, soft-tissue massage, and point-pressure massage.[233,234] Others have evaluated multiple critical trials that have compared manipulative therapy with other treatments such as medications and sham therapy; they concluded that short-term manipulative treatment may temporarily decrease pain and improve function.[57,126,232,233,477] Although sciatica is not considered a contraindication to manipulation by its proponents, there are reports that forceful manipulations may cause new or increased neurological deficits.[116]

Total management often involves passive exercises as soon as they can be done without increasing peripheral signs and symptoms. An organized form of exercise, "the McKenzie program," has been found to be effective against both chronic and acute low back pain.[630] This program uses a series of individualized, progressive exercises to localize and ultimately to eliminate the pain. A comparative study found the McKenzie protocol twice as effective in alleviating low back pain as traction and back schools.[131,630] More than 40 different exercise regimens are available. The appropriate exercise regimen must be individualized, incorporating only those movements (done in the proper sequence and with or without the effects of gravity) that bring about symptom centralization.[131]

Typically, McKenzie advocates correction of any lateral shift and passive extension exercises to move the nucleus of the disk centrally.[406] He also advocates constant maintenance of the correction to allow healing of the annular fibers. Healing of the disk can occur.[163,186,239,252,351] The key is to reduce the bulge and then to maintain the posterior aspect of the disk in close approximation so the scar formed will protect it from further protrusion.[106,406,492] The patient must avoid positions and activities that increase the intradiskal pressure or cause a posterior force on the nucleus (*e.g.*, slump sitting, forward-bending, and flexion exercises). The restoration of full mobility is a necessary component of treatment as soon as the protrusion is stable. Passive exercises and joint mobilization are indicated if mobility is restricted. Finally, a full fitness program should be implemented.

☐ Disorders of Movement

Disorders of spinal movement may be classified as acute mechanical derangement, hypomobility, and hypermobility lesions.

ACUTE MECHANICAL DERANGEMENT

The *acute locked back*, *sudden backache*, *facet syndrome*, *facet blockage*, *subluxation or fixation*, and *acute lumbago* are all terms used to describe sudden pain in the back. This condition may be regarded as an acute form of mechanical derangement and locking of the intervertebral joint complex. Several theories have been proposed to explain its occurrence: ligamentous tears,[36,62] a primary muscle lesion,[363,593] apophyseal joint (facet) lesions (including subluxation—an overriding or shifting of the facet joint out of its normal congruous relation),[545] synovitis, an impacted synovial fringe or intra-articular structure such as a meniscoid body,[318,320] acute nuclear prolapse of the disk, acute hydrops of the disk,[87] and an annular tear.[89]

In this form of acute backache (lumbago), more than one condition can produce a typical attack.[215] The term *lumbago* is used here to describe a lumbar spinal syndrome characterized by the sudden onset of severe persistent pain, marked restriction of lumbar movements, and a sensation of locking in the back. Attacks may vary in severity from severe and incapacitating to more minor discomfort. During an attack, it is impossible to know the exact mechanism; one can only speculate.

Lumbago can occur at any age but is most common between ages 20 and 45 years.[545] The mechanism of injury is usually a sudden, unguarded movement involving backward-bending, forward-bending, sidebending, or rotation. If the attack is severe, the patient presents with an onset of sudden, intense lower lumbar pain. It may be bilateral but typically is unilateral. The pain and sensation of back locking may render the patient immobile, with the back stuck in one position. The patient may even fall down or may have had to crawl on hands and knees off a tennis court or into bed from the bathroom. Not all attacks are severe: the patient may be aware only of a mild discomfort in the low back after the triggering movement. Symptoms are initially mild but within a few hours or after having gone to bed, the patient awakens to find that he or she cannot get out of bed because of agonizing pain in the low back. Some examples of sudden back pain, which may serve as a guide when planning initial treatment, are described below.

IMPACTED SYNOVIAL MENISCOID[215]

The patient with a sudden backache caused by a presumed locking of a facet joint by an impacted synovial meniscoid is often a young person with a degree of hypermobility. Lumbar synovial joint locking typically results during some activity involving reaching up (*e.g.*, to open a window) or after a forward-flexion movement, which may have been slight (*e.g.*, picking up a piece of paper or a tennis ball), in which a hypermobile segment undergoes additional distraction.

Examination reveals:

1. Marked paraspinal muscle spasm, more prominent on one side than the other. A spinal deformity is present.
2. Physiological movements. Extension and lateral flexion toward the painful side may be nearly full, with pain near the extremes of range; lateral flexion toward the painless side is restricted early in the range and is more painful. Flexion is cautious and limited.
3. Straight-leg raising is limited by pain, with movement of the contralateral (painless) leg equally restricted. Straight-leg raising usually provokes acute discomfort in the region of the posterosuperior iliac spine.
4. Negative neurological signs.

LOCKING OF ARTHROTIC FACET JOINT[213]

A typical patient is a middle-aged or older person, with a degree of presupposed degenerative joint disease, who complains of sudden onset (after twisting) of one-sided back pain localized to the fourth or fifth level in the lumbar spine. The history is that of a simple, nonstressful daily activity such as getting out of a bathtub, bending over to tie a shoe, leaning over a bathroom sink, coughing, sneezing, or lifting a weight. Sudden pain to one side fixes the patient in a flexed posture, and a vertical position can be regained only with some difficulty. The patient may present with a kyphosis or a reversal of the normal lumbar curve.

Examination reveals:

1. Pain is unilateral; extension and lateral flexion away from the side of pain are the most painful.
2. Flexion may not appear to be limited and may be painless, but is performed with the lumbar spine fixed in lordosis. Passive overpressure may provoke localized lumbosacral pain.
3. There are no neurological signs. Straight-leg raising is usually negative; there may be localized pain at the extreme of leg raising on the painful side.

Most cases of acute mechanical derangement subside within 3 weeks; spinal mobilizations shorten that time. One mobilization technique useful in early treatment is gentle, rhythmic manual traction applied to the patient's legs. As the patient improves, other mobilization techniques may be added. Specific and nonspecific rotational manipulations are appropriate. Vertebral manipulation is probably the therapeutic modality most frequently studied in controlled trials. A few studies have shown that short-term manipulative treatment may temporarily decrease pain and improve function.[57,99,126,129,201,207,229,233,259,278,293,373,384,477,504,508]

Traction can be applied by manual, autotraction, gravity reduction, and motorized methods. It is often wise to precede mobilization or traction with ice or heat and massage to relieve the muscle guarding and spasm that may accompany acute mechanical derangement. Finally, the restoration of normal mobility of the lumbar spine, particularly in patients who have had several attacks, is facilitated by appropriate therapeutic exercise.

This condition cures itself in most cases when enough time is allowed to pass and when rest (relative) is prescribed. Nevertheless, mobilizations shorten the duration of pain, often dramatically.

HYPOMOBILITY LESIONS

LOCALIZED RESTRICTION

Facet joint capsular tightness or degenerative changes in the disk result in localized hypomobility lesions. The chronic form of a mechanical derangement, usually of the intervertebral joint complex, is the result of prolonged immobilization secondary to injury or poor posture. Often there is a history of acute low back dysfunction. The onset of pain may be gradual or sudden; the patient may relate it to bending, twisting, or trauma. Pain varies in degree from minor to severe and is usually described as a dull aching in the lumbosacral region or referred into the buttocks, leg, or abdomen. Symptoms are aggravated by long periods of standing, walking, or activity involving prolonged or repetitive lumbar extension. Symptoms are worse in the evening than in the morning.

When evaluating a patient, it is often difficult, if not impossible, to determine if pain is coming from the disk or the facet joints. Determining the mechanism of aggravation and analyzing the most painful position may give reliable clues. If extension (standing and walking) is the most aggravating, the facets are probably involved. If the pain is diskogenic in nature, it may be because of mechanical irritation or inflammation of the outer wall of the annulus.[532] In this case, flexion (sitting and forward-bending) is the most painful movement or is the mechanism of aggravation.

Consider the following points and tests in evaluating the patient:

1. Possible subtle predisposing biomechanical factors, such as leg-length discrepancy
2. Physiological motions may appear normal but usually show some evidence of restricted motion only in certain directions (*e.g.*, minor restriction of sidebending to the involved side; deviation of the spine toward the involved side on forward-bending and away from the involved side on extension). When motions are restricted, they should also reproduce the patient's pain. The normal, rhythmic pattern of lumbar movement may also be disturbed. This is best appreciated by standing behind the patient to observe spinal movement.
3. There is usually loss of the normal passive joint-play movements that reproduce the pain. However, because degenerative joint or disk disease can develop because of hypermobility or instability of the joint, accessory movements are sometimes excessive. Pain may occur within the limited range, but most often it occurs at the limits of the range. The examination consists of direct pressure over the spinous process, lateral pressure over the spinous process, pressure over the facet joints, and pressure over the interspinous and supraspinous ligaments. Pain may be referred and is usually unilateral.
4. Special tests may be indicated if the above tests fail to reproduce symptoms. The quadrant test or combined movements are used in attempt to reproduce the symptoms at the appropriate level. Examination using combined movements and recognition of regular (or irregular) patterns of movement can be most helpful in the selection of treatment techniques.[149]
5. The involved level is tender to palpation. Often, a thickened supraspinous ligament can be palpated.
6. Roentgenograms should be normal for the patient's age.

Manipulations, segmental distraction techniques, and mobilizations (including muscle energy techniques and combined movements) are the manual treatments of choice. On the whole, mobilization techniques are most effective because of the variety of joint responses that can be facilitated.[327] A vast array of mobilization techniques can be used.

With hypermobility, localized stabilization techniques should be used instead. Sometimes both mobilization and stabilization techniques are indicated. Mobilizing exercises are indicated if the condition has been present for a long time. Based on the evaluation, the home program should include localized segmental self-mobilization or stabilization techniques (see Figs. 20-6 and 20-7). Prolonged rest and use of supports are contraindicated, because they tend to increase the restrictions.

MULTISEGMENTAL BILATERAL CAPSULAR RESTRICTION

Degenerative joint or disk disease, osteoarthritis, lumbar spondylosis, and facet arthritis are included in this category. Various terms, including spondylosis, are used to describe the osteoarthritic changes in the spine that may lead to back pain, which is more common in middle-aged or older persons. Although degenerative joint or disk disease is a natural process of aging and is often asymptomatic, symptoms sometimes develop as the result of hypomobility and repeated trauma. (Hypermobility can also contribute to the development of degenerative joint or disk disease.) Patients with symptomatic degenerative joint disease often have difficulty bending because of stiffness and aching in the low back. On stooping over a wash basin, they usually lean on one arm to support the body weight. After simple loosening-up exercises or a hot shower, the discomfort eases tremendously. As the condition progresses, the patient tends to get worse as the day goes on, but at times the pain may be more pronounced after a night of rest and then ease as the patient becomes more mobile. Patients also may note discomfort with increasing sports activities and may even cut down on sports as they become aware that pain and stiffness tend to be more pronounced the following day.

A striking symptom relates to many patients' avocations or occupational activities—they do not like to hold their backs in a flexed position.[545] Homemakers, carpenters, plumbers, and others who must frequently work in a stooped position find their symptoms increased. They do not like standing for lengthy periods because this increases the lumbar lordosis. Aching is relieved if one foot is placed on a stool or step while standing. If facet arthrosis is more advanced, turning over in bed becomes increasingly difficult because of movement imposed on the facet joints.

Because degenerative changes involve both the anterior and posterior portions of the intervertebral joint complex, it is impossible to determine the exact mechanism of symptom production. The most likely basis for attacks of mechanical derangement is recurrent episodes of synovitis in the facet joints after overuse, such as excessive bending (as in gardening), stressful unaccustomed activity, or abrasive positioning with resultant strain of the joints. After several hours of heavy use, pain develops that can last for hours. Pain is typically at the lower lumbar midline but may radiate out to the groin or buttock. Degenerative joint or disk disease may also occur with neurological complications (*i.e.*, lateral spinal stenosis). Pain may be experienced in one or both legs, and three mechanisms may be involved: pain may be referred with stimulation of the sinuvertebral nerve; sciatica may result from nerve root pressure, or leg pain may be caused by the pressure of a spinal canal stenosis.[96]

Consider the following in evaluating a patient:

1. Activities that aggravate and relieve symptoms. Some loss of normal lordosis may be noted. The pain may increase if the patient tries to sit up straight or slumps. Symptoms are decreased with the back in a neutral or functional position. Pain is increased when upright (standing and walking). One test that Seimons found positive in almost all of these patients is to have the patient stand semi-stooped and to maintain this position for 1 to 2 minutes.[545] This increases the tension in the disks and also strains the capsular ligaments of the facet joints.
2. Physiological movements. Early on, spinal motions may appear normal. Most of the discomfort and stiffness occurs early in the day and may have subsided by the time of the assessment. With advanced chronic degeneration, restriction of active and passive motions occurs in a generalized capsular pattern: marked restriction and equal limitation of side flexion, and moderate restriction of rotation, forward-bending, and backward-bending.
3. Moderate to marked restriction of all accessory motions may be noted.
4. The neurological findings in uncomplicated degenerative disease are normal. Patients who complain of pain on coughing, sneezing, jarring movements, or turning over in bed often have a positive heel-drop test.
5. Degenerative changes are observed on roentgenograms, affecting the disk and facet joints. The severity of pain is out of proportion to the roentgenographic findings.[545]

With advanced degenerative joint or disk disease, movements are stiff in all directions, so treatment requires several techniques in different directions, including intermittent variable lumbar traction, mobi-

lization, and a program of exercises. There may also be attacks of mechanical derangement. First, settle any localized single joint signs superimposed on an otherwise stiff spine by local treatment, as these will be worsened by a generalized regimen. The facet joints are more vulnerable to facet impingement, sprains, and inflammation when degenerative joint disease is present.

Nonsteroidal anti-inflammatory drugs are used in patients with more severe degrees of degenerative joint disease in an attempt to reduce any associated synovitis.[441]

Passive movements (*i.e.*, flexion, extension, and sidebending) play a major role in the management of patients with multisegmental involvement. Starting in the direction opposite that of pain aggravation, exercises are progressed to include motions in all directions. Manual and mechanical lumbar traction and spinal mobilization techniques increase mobility and relieve pain. Use joint mobilization and exercise cautiously in the presence of nerve root irritation, because they may increase symptoms. Postural training and carefully instituted isometric exercises to strengthen the abdominal and back muscles may be indicated. Patients may be overweight, and their type of work may aggravate the disorder. The overweight patient should be encouraged to lose weight and to exercise by walking or swimming within the limits of pain. Brisk walking (in patients who are bothered by standing) often relieves pain.

☐ Chronic Low Back Pain

After 3 months of low back pain, only 5% to 10% of patients have persisting symptoms,[189,450] but these patients account for 85% of the costs in terms of compensation and loss of work related to low back pain.[190,574] In these patients, the presence of a treatable active disease has been carefully eliminated. Pain has become the patient's preoccupation, limiting daily activity.[504] It is important to reach a definitive diagnosis if possible, and to rule out any of the causes for back pain for which specific treatment exists. No study demonstrates a specific method of treatment for chronic idiopathic low back pain.[450]

The differential diagnosis of chronic low back pain includes all the conditions previously discussed, which may be overlooked or neglected during the acute and subacute phases. The additional diagnostic possibilities include various degenerative conditions, spondyloarthropathies, and ill-defined syndromes of fibrositis. Some psychologists[177] maintain that this pain represents a behavior reaction, whereas neurophysiologists lean toward the hypothesis that nervous structures irritated for a prolonged period generate new mechanisms of pain generation. Chronic pain has also been described as a variant of depression. In a study of patients with chronic low back pain, a structured diagnosis was possible in 50%; no diagnosis could be determined in the remainder.[497]

Included in this diagnostic category are degenerative spondylolisthesis[628] and degenerative lumbar stenosis,[18,310,311] affecting either the central canal or the lateral recesses, or consisting of isolated disk resorption.[102] Also included are several degenerative conditions with less certain criteria, such as facet syndromes,[432] disk-disruption syndrome,[103] segmental instability,[192,210,312,434,448,592] idiopathic vertebral sclerosis,[650] diffuse idiopathic skeletal hyperostosis,[192] inflammatory spondyloarthropathy,[73] myofascial syndromes,* fibrositis,[2,74,254,319,356,569–571,616,617,660,661] and primary fibromyalgia.[74,76,292,616,661,669,670,672–674]

According to Maigne, in many cases of chronic distal lumbago and sciatica, a cellulomyalgic syndrome is often present, revealed by the presence of myalgic cordlike structures in the muscles of the external iliac fossa (*i.e.*, the gluteus medius, tensor fasciae latae, gluteus maximus, or piriformis).[372] In the syndromes of sciatica, in addition to the muscles of the iliac fossa, the distal portion of the biceps femoris, the lateral gastrocnemius (S1), and the anterior lateral aspect of the leg (L5) may be involved. With joint manipulation, tenderness often disappears, but in some cases pain remains. In addition to procaine injections of trigger points, treatment by slow, deep massage and long, continued stretching can be helpful.

EVALUATION

A definitive diagnosis requires a careful history to identify the distribution of back and leg pain as well as such aggravators of pain as poor posture, mechanical loads, and walking.[145] The physical examination should include observation of gait, trunk mobility, deformities, leg-length inequalities, and assessment of coordination, endurance, and function. The examination should also include a careful search for neurosensory and motor loss and signs of nerve root tension. The neurological examination may be confusing and show no anatomical sensory losses in patients with spinal stenosis.[206] In addition to a detailed neuromuscular examination, abdominal and vascular evaluations should be included, particularly in the elderly and those with symptoms suggesting neurogenic claudication. The degenerative conditions that may be causing the pain can be classified according to the

*References 19, 32, 75, 170, 171, 202, 231, 257, 379, 399, 480, 550, 554–557, 572, 617, 643, 660, 661, 671

clinical history, roentgenographic findings, diagnostic blocks, and imaging studies. Psychological testing should be used to determine the patient's psychological status and to explore the relations between pain behavior and reinforcing consequences.

The results of a physical examination in such patients are often nonspecific, except for demonstration of restricted motion and muscle spasm. However, many degenerative conditions can be strongly suggested by roentgenographic studies. When segmental instability is suspected, flexion and extension films may demonstrate abnormal displacements.[192,308,434] If nerve root symptoms or claudication is present, myelography is the most sensitive study for identifying the level of neural encroachment, followed by CT scanning. CT and MRI are rapidly surpassing myelography as the imaging technique of choice in most patients with radiculopathies. Electromyography may also be used to provide additional confirmation of the levels of nerve root involvement.[154] In patients with suspected facet syndrome, a CT scan may reveal degeneration, but a definitive diagnosis is based on the relief of symptoms by the injection of local anesthetics into the affected joints.[160,428,431] In patients with suspected internal disruption, diskography may be diagnostic, particularly when combined with CT scanning, but this remains controversial.

TREATMENT CONSIDERATIONS

Most patients with chronic low back pain can be treated with anti-inflammatory medications and exercise programs.[189] As in other nonmalignant chronic pain syndromes, narcotic analgesics are avoided. Alternative therapeutic modalities have been used, including biofeedback, acupuncture, transcutaneous nerve stimulation, implanted neurostimulators, and ablative neurosurgical procedures.[416] These methods have varying degrees of success; all have methodological problems.[126] For selected patients, trigger-point injections may be beneficial.[509]

SOFT-TISSUE MOBILIZATION TECHNIQUES, MASSAGE, AND RELAXATION

Soft-tissue techniques, with the specific purpose of improving the vascularity and extensibility of the soft tissues, are another approach to pain management. Massage and myofascial release types of soft-tissue mobilization are being used now more than ever before.[23,31,85,111,143,144,324,325,373,412,439,481,482,588,639,646]

These techniques are beneficial, although research has been lacking in this area for hundreds of years.[214,215] Their effectiveness is attributed in part to increased circulation to the area, release of muscle spasm, stretching of abnormal fibrous tissue (connective tissue), increased proprioception, and extensibility of the soft tissues. An increase in extensibility may also allow a secondary increase in circulation.[91] Acupressure massage presumably produces some of the same beneficial effects as acupuncture and acupuncture-like transcutaneous electrical nerve stimulation.[86,606,666] Rocking-chair therapy and mechanical vibration are other forms of sensory stimulation that reportedly relieve both chronic and acute pain.[108,236,237,358–360,417,478,664] Relaxation techniques can affect the pain cycle by eliciting relaxation, increasing circulation, and decreasing pain (see Chapter 8, Relaxation and Related Techniques). Stress and tension influence strongly the perception of pain and pain tolerance.

ANTERIOR ELEMENT PAIN

Anterior element pain is pain that is made worse by sustained flexion of the lumbar spine.[551] Characteristically, anterior element pain is made worse by sitting and is relieved by standing. Patients assume the hyperlordotic posture to relieve pain. Fracture of the vertebral body and prolapsed intervertebral disks produce anterior element symptoms. In young patients, in whom anterior element pain is the most common presentation, extension exercises and press-ups are more likely to produce remission than flexion exercises.[302] This is borne out by the tendency of many flexion exercises to increase intradiskal pressure; extension exercises unload the disk.[271] Therefore, the hyperextension principles advocated by Cyriax[110] and McKenzie[406,407] are logical for patients with anterior element pain.[333] Lesions resulting in chronic anterior pain are obscure; it is tempting to assume that anterior element pain is diskogenic in origin, but there is no evidence for this. Unlike the acute group, patients with chronic anterior element pain may respond to manipulative techniques.[332,551]

POSTERIOR ELEMENT PAIN

In posterior element pain, pain is worsened by increasing the lumbar lordosis, standing, and walking. It is eased by maintained forward-flexion, sitting, and hip flexion (with or without the knees extended). Patients with structural or postural hyperlordosis, facet arthropathy, or foraminal stenosis show features of posterior element pain.[537,551] Pain from extension and rotation is usually of facet origin.[652] Flexion treatment frequently improves facet disease, spondylolysis, flexion dysfunction, and certain types of derangement.[131,132,406,652] Hyperextension exercises may make the condition worse.[302]

MOVEMENT-RELATED PAIN

Patients with movement-related pain are most comfortable at rest; pain is precipitated only by activity or jarring. Heavy manual work, repeated twisting, fast walking or running (especially on hard surfaces), and traveling in cars over rough ground all precipitate pain. Movement-related pain occurs in association with traumatic fracture/dislocations, in symptomatic spondylolysis or spondylolisthesis, and as a result of chronic degenerative segmental instability. Diagnosis may be confirmed by obtaining lateral flexion and extension roentgenograms of the lumbar spine and noting abnormal translational movements. A basic scheme of progressive stabilization by strengthening regional and segmental muscles isometrically should be considered.[210,211,218] According to Grieve, mature patients and those in most pain may need to start abdominal exercises with their knees bent, and progress more slowly.[218] Sidelying stabilization techniques and dynamic abdominal bracing also may be used.[304] Home exercises must be efficiently monitored, and the patient must be taught to avoid aggravating postures and activities.[538]

MECHANICAL PAIN WITHOUT POSTURAL OR MOVEMENT EXACERBATIONS (Static-Sensitive)

Patients with static-sensitive low back pain cannot maintain any one position (other than lying) for a normal length of time and obtain relief by changing position and moving. Many of these patients appear to have discrete structural disease, such as scoliosis.[58]

ALTERED PATTERN OF MUSCLE RECRUITMENT

Janda has delineated the altered patterns of muscle recruitment in chronic low back pain (see Table 21-1).[274–277,284–285] One of the most common is the overuse and early recruitment of the low back muscles.[411] Another common pattern associated with low back pain is overuse of the hip flexors (psoas) and weakness of the abdominals. Often the the gluteal muscles must be retrained and the overuse of lumbar extension inhibited, a common maladaptive pattern.

Numerous clinicians have written on exercise programs for the treatment of muscle imbalances and programs for postural correction, with or without mechanical or manual resistance or assistance.*

SPINAL BRACING

Several lumbar supports have been advocated. Spinal bracing seems justified in patients with osteoporotic compression fractures, spondylolisthesis, or segmental instability, and in some patients with spinal stenosis, although no controlled studies have demonstrated its efficacy. About 80% to 90% of patients wearing a simple support find it of benefit.[450] It

---

*References 48, 71, 134, 193, 217, 218, 224, 226, 227, 240, 301, 349, 433, 490, 491, 521–524, 526, 598

prevents excessive motion and reminds the wearer not to exaggerate the lumbar load.

EDUCATIONAL PROGRAMS

Educational programs are an essential part of the care of patients with chronic low back pain.* All patients must be educated in how to live with their discomfort. Advice regarding everyday activities must be individualized; in many instances this is the most important aspect of treatment. Educational programs are more effective than flexion exercises, although some studies have questioned the effectiveness of low back schools. Historical surveys have demonstrated that only 40% of patients disabled for 6 months can be successfully rehabilitated; at 1 year, the figure drops to 20%; and 2 years after injury, the chances for rehabilitation are virtually nil. We cannot cover the various intervention programs here, so the reader is directed to the references in each section.

FUNCTIONAL TRAINING

These structured programs include the identification of routine daily living and work postures and activities, and advice on re-education exercises and instructions.[504] Mayer and associates have devised a functional program that emphasizes restoration of muscle strength and aerobic capacity, vocational assessment, and short-term psychological intervention, with careful qualification of progress.[390,392] A year after this 3-week intervention, 85% of patients had returned to work.

BACK SCHOOLS

These structured intervention programs are aimed at groups of patients and include general information on the spine, recommended posture and physical activities, preventive measures, and exercises for the back.[3,33,172,181,235,243,314,330,349,352,386,405,652,658,675] The main objective is to transmit information on anatomy and disorders of the spine and to teach the principles underlying healthy posture, daily activities, and sports. The content of the programs varies considerably. Overall patient satisfaction with back schools is 75% to 96%. According to White, 70% to 90% of patients find their pain is at an acceptable level after attending back school.[652] One American program forms the basis of White's book on back schools. This book entails a hospital back school for acute back pain and incorporates education with progressive remobilization. White includes McKenzie's protocol and techniques in his school.

Acute back schools and education can often keep patients out of the hospital and return many of them to a normal life in just days.[652] Back schools in the home and at work, and an athletic back school for chronic patients have also been described.

Work-hardening or work-capacity training is the "Super Bowl" of back schools. A high rate of recurrent low back injury and poor work tolerance may be due to underlying pathological processes and incomplete rehabilitation before return to work. With the work-endurance program, there has been a significant improvement in work tolerance and a decreased rate of recurrent injury.[335,336,342,343,392,653]

SPECIALIZED CENTERS

Exercises and therapeutic activities may be prescribed, directed, and supervised by a health professional.[193,260,304,405,435,436] Generally, exercises are done in a specialized center for a limited time only, mainly to instruct the patient, and then are continued at home by the patient. Sometimes specific rehabilitation demands prolonged therapy in a specialized environment.

Most of these programs emphasize the functional position of the spine, defined by Morgan and Vollowitz as "the optimal position in which the spine functions."[436] These positions vary depending on the physical condition of the spine and the stresses it must withstand. There is no one position for all functional tasks, and the best functional position varies from person to person. It is often near the midrange of all available movement. The functional position should not be confused with the theoretical "neutral" position of the spine.

The spinal control method (stabilization) is a form of body mechanics that trains and uses any or all of the muscles associated with body alignment to place a given spinal segment in its functional balanced position and hold it there while other joints and muscle groups accomplish a specific task. Thus, the involved spinal segment is stabilized to whatever degree is necessary to allow pain-free activity.[436]

PAIN CLINICS

Pain clinics focus on behavioral adaptation to help patients withstand and control their condition.[401,504] This form of intervention is recommended to evaluate the factors that modify the patient's perception of pain and to support the patient. Improved understanding of the relation between pain and activity has resulted in a change in management from a negative philosophy of treatment for pain to more active restoration of function. Fordyce and colleagues[179] and other behavioral psychologists have investigated the relation between chronic pain and physical activity, and suggest that pain behaviors are influenced and modified by their consequences.[178,180,349,549]

---

*References 73, 80, 92, 109, 159, 172, 184, 242, 243, 314, 322, 323, 336, 342, 363, 390, 392, 404, 405, 531, 533, 540, 545, 592, 594, 595, 597, 632, 634, 652

ERGONOMICS

Knowledge of the patient's work environment and a functional evaluation can help ensure a better balance between job assignments and capabilities.[504] For chronic conditions, ergonomic interventions are an integral component of therapy. Ergonomists seek to create a harmonious balance between workers and their equipment, work patterns, and the working environment, both at work and at home. Manual handling and lifting has received more attention from ergonomists[83,84,120,190,191,368,369,602] than virtually any other topic. Since Brackett first identified the possible dangers of lifting a heavy load from the ground with the back in a fully flexed position,[53] ergonomists have sought to identify safer lifting techniques and load limits.[119,242–244,444,445,593,595]

Another aspect of back pain that has interested ergonomists is work postures, particularly the seated work posture. Several epidemiological studies point to the relation between sitting and back pain, and clinicians use the increase of pain in sitting as a diagnostic indicator.[298,299] Many authors—as early as Staffel in 1884[581]—have made recommendations about seating design.[49,60,242,377,632] The importance of the design of the back rest was underlined by Akerblom in 1948.[6,295] More recently, Andersson and associates measured changes in intradiskal pressure at the L3–L4 disk in different sitting positions and for different configurations of the back rest and lumbar support.[10–12] To reduce intradiskal pressure, they recommended a positive lumbar support maintaining the lumbar spine in lordosis.

Reports about seating and driving positions have demonstrated a confusing lack of agreement. Until recently, concepts of correct design have been based more on aesthetics, ethics, and wishful thinking than on science, but that is beginning to change. The chair is a principal adjunct in industrialized labor, and seating design must be integrated into the whole of the work space and also the job design. It is hoped that car manufacturers will propose alternative seating designs to substantially reduce stresses on the spine.

EXERCISE

Currently, aerobic exercise is a popular form of treatment. The bases for these exercise programs have been extensively reviewed with respect to their effects on disk nutrition, pain modulation, and spinal mechanics.[116,271,449] Knowledge of the body's endogenous chemical pain-modulating capability, the endorphin system, continues to increase.[7,453,544,610,667] Activity in large muscle groups yields an increased amount of endorphins in both the bloodstream and the CSF.[7,165] This, in turn, lessens the pain sensitivity.[389,453,544,667] Johansson and associates[279] demonstrated in 10 patients with chronic back pain a significantly lower amount of endorphins in the CSF, a finding recently corroborated by Pug and coworkers.[503] Aerobic exercise also relieves depression,[176,566] a common finding with at least chronic low back pain. Other benefits include increased mental alertness,[142,667] sleep,[176,566] and stamina,[294] improved self-image, and an increase in the activity level compatible with chronic pain.[177,566]

Walking and jogging on soft, even ground are recommended. Indoor cross-country skiing machines are preferable to stationary bikes, and water aerobics are preferable to swimming.

Experts agree that some exercise is useful, and its role has been summarized by Jackson and Brown.[271] High levels of physical fitness reduce the risk of further injury and speed rehabilitation. The more physically fit a person is, the more pain he or she can tolerate.[94,183,544] However, there is little agreement about what form the exercise should take. Any exercises selected must be based on a thorough clinical evaluation.[271]

■ TREATMENT TECHNIQUES

The following are examples of spinal movement techniques and should be useful in treating properly selected patients when applied according to the above guidelines. For complete descriptions and illustrations of the great variety of mobilizations and passive movements available, other texts should be consulted.[112,216,289,309,372,373,375,406,418–420,422,484] Although some of McKenzie's techniques are briefly described here, refer to his textbook to plan a treatment program.[383] Determination of the tissue type involved is critical.

Assessment continues throughout the treatment period, and the patient's response guides the next step in treatment. For example, the aim to make a hypomobile joint able to sustain a grade IV movement (a small-amplitude movement, conducted at the very end of the range of motion without pain) is not always possible or advisable. If the symptoms have been relieved, it is often better not to attempt to influence joint limitations that are clearly the result of adaptive shortening. *Do not overtreat;* when signs and symptoms are cleared, stop. Passive movement treatments should be adapted according to presenting signs and symptoms; as these change, so should the treatment.

For mobilization to be effective, a sense of "feel" of movement is required. The movements occurring are often not seen but sensed.[96]

Many passive movements have been described for the lumbar spine, but only a few of the more common techniques are presented here.

☐ **Active Treatment**

The term *active* is used here to define treatment in which the patient independently performs activity or in which the patient may assist.[512] These treatments include unloading activities, self-mobilization, stabilization, and conditioning exercises.

UNLOADING

The concept of unloading is an integral part of the Norwegian spinal treatment technique called *medical exercise training*.[260] This type of unloading may occur by assisting with the upper extremities while performing lower extremity activities, such as squats or step-up activities (Fig. 20-17), by exercising on an incline board, or by using inversion traction (hanging from the lower extremities) while strengthening the trunk muscles (Fig. 20-18).[70,71] It improves the body's

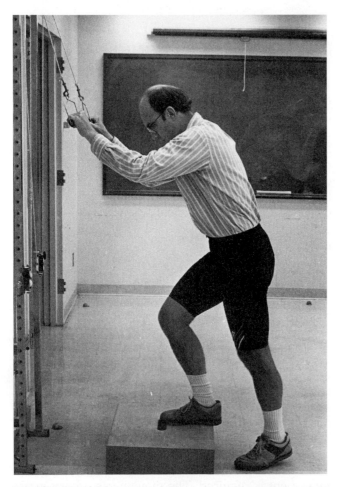

FIG. 20-17. Unloading a patient (so-called minus weight exercise), performed by utilizing a wall pulley with weights to assist with stair climbing. This exercise might be used with patients who can bear only partial weight on one limb.

ability to control and stabilize in a position with reduced body weight and decreases the nociceptive input, while allowing the affected tissues to adapt at a tolerable level.

Unloading or "de-weighting" the spine with the use of manual (see Figs. 20-40 through 20-42),[102,216,354,355] positional (see Fig. 20-45), suspended, or gravity traction is often used to bring temporary pain relief when an irritable tissue (*i.e.*, nerve root) is provoked by an exercise program or activities of daily living. These mild forms of traction should not be confused with other forms of traction in which a body part's gravitational weight is exceeded by the distraction force. Self-traction (Fig. 20-19),[535,536] autotraction (including the gymnastic table for home use),[41,197–199,218,309,344,345,354,355,443,455,456] positional traction,[456,484] Cottrell 90-90 traction,[97,98] inversion traction,[70,71,185,196,328,529] and the development of various forms of gravity traction,[66,203,479,528,611] in which gravity is applied to the body, are useful home traction methods for the lumbar spine. The principle of gravity traction is that the weight of the upper or lower body stretches all the tissues of the low back—the muscles, fascia, ligaments, and possibly the disk.[70,71,536] Traction may exert some of its beneficial effects by stretching the mechanoreceptors of the apophyseal joints, disk, and ligaments.[607]

One of the more common methods of unloading the spine is through hydrotherapy.[1,42,90,409,563,618,645] Although a fair amount has been written regarding the benefits of water exercises for people with orthopaedic problems of the spine and extremities, Cirullo[90] was one of the first to address specific low back diagnoses. A land-based program is integrated with an aquatic program of basic lumbar stabilization training. Before engaging in multiple stabilization training activities, full understanding of what lumbopelvic motion is at both ends of the available range, training in cocontraction techniques, and demonstration of the concept of midrange or pelvic neutral[521] is stressed. As with land programs, early emphasis is placed on lengthening the "guy wires" of the spine (iliopsoas, quadriceps, hamstrings, and hip rotators) if needed, and strengthening the key stabilizing muscles (abdominals and latissimus dorsi).[521] All four abdominals are strengthened separately at first, and then together for more advanced work. The program also includes strengthening of the gluteus maximus, spinal extensors, and multifidi. Also included is a general program for cervicothoracic stabilization training.

Unloading is recommended for most spinal dysfunction patients with radicular syndromes, disk derangement, hypomobility, strains, sprains, and degenerative disk disease. Unloading with activity offers great benefits because it allows patients to engage in activity at a reduced percentage of body weight.

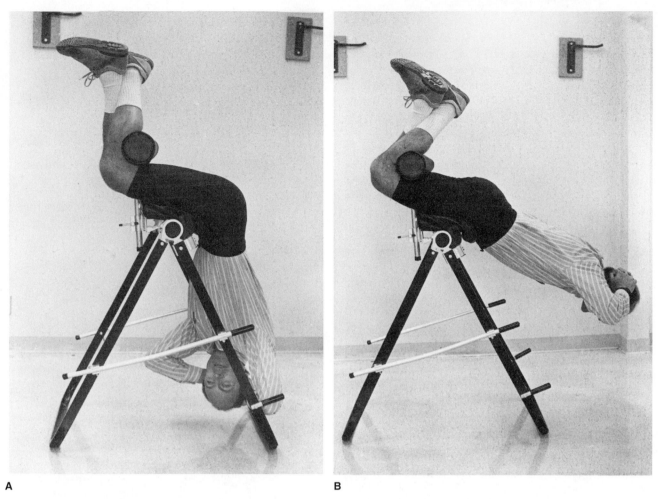

FIG. 20-18. An inversion machine: (**A**) gravity-assisted traction and (**B**) gravity-assisted traction with active exercise (extension).

A

B

SELF-MOBILIZATION EXERCISES

The purpose of self-mobilization exercises is to increase joint mobility at hypomobile segments. Specificity of motion may be accomplished through ligamentous or facet-locking techniques, by the use of the patient's hands, or by a device (*e.g.*, a roll or the back of the chair) to allow motion to occur at a particular segment without creating unwanted extension at other areas (see Fig. 19-53).

Based on the Holten's medicine training theory,[260] hypermobile joints should be trained with endurance exercises (30 repetitions, 60% of 1 resistance maximum [RM]) initially to provide an increase in tissue capillarization and to promote an increase in mobility and control through low-intensity repetitive movements.[226] This is followed by training for strength and endurance (15 to 30 repetitions, 60% to 75% of 1 RM) in the outer range of motion; this allows an increase in strength to maintain the gained range of motion. Finally, the patient should be trained with 8 to 12 repetitions at 80% or more of their 1 RM for pure strength. Such training is designed to provide optimal stimulus

for the regeneration of tissue (see Chapter 2, Properties of Dense Connective Tissue and Wound Healing) as well as pain modulation (see Fig. 9-26).

SELF-STABILIZATION EXERCISES

Hypermobile joints should be trained initially with many repetitions, at low speed, and with minimal resistance at the beginning or midrange.[219] This is followed by increasing (isometric) contractions in the inner range of motion to facilitate increased sensitivity to stretch, particularly of the deep rotators such as the multifidi (see Fig. 20-7). Finally, the patient is trained with submaximal resistance (isometric contractions) in any range except the outer range.

Stabilization training uses exercises specifically designed to provide a "muscle corset,"[521] limiting undesirable motions and allowing healing to occur. Saal[521] described the anatomical basis for this method of control, stating that the "abdominal mechanism, which couples the midline ligaments as well as the dorsolumbar fascia, combined with a slight reduction in

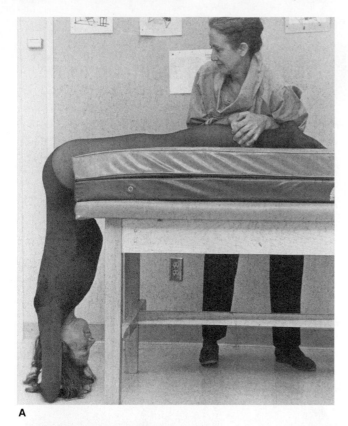

A

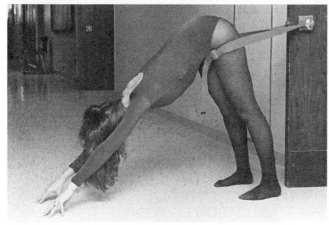

B

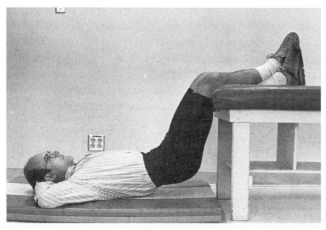

C

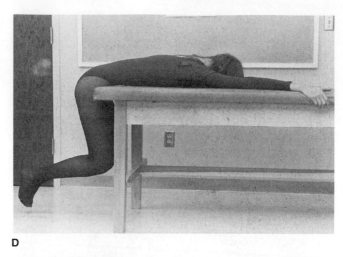

D

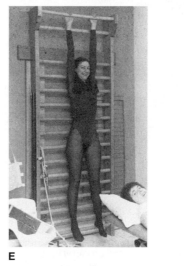

E

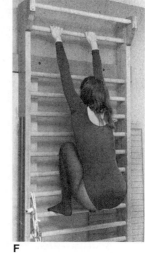

F

FIG. 20-19. Self tractions. Traction methods include (**A**) torso hang over a table or (**B**) via a belt around the pelvis; (**C**) leg hang over a table in supine or (**D**) prone position; and (**E**) arm hang in either an extended or (**F**) flexed position.

lumbar lordosis, can eliminate shear stresses to the lumbar intervertebral segments." He argued that the coupled action of this musculature, together with the latissimus dorsi, allows a muscle "fusion" for spinal protection. Spinal extensors, particularly the multifidi, are essential for balancing the stress to the intervertebral segments.

Contrary to some beliefs, spinal stabilization is not about maintaining a static position but rather about maintaining a controlled range of motion that varies with the position and with the activity. As Morgan[435] stated, the "functional position" is the most stable and asymptomatic position of the spine for the task at hand.

CONSIDERATIONS

Joint structures and the optimal stimulus for regeneration that should be considered include:

1. **Vertebrae:** The optimal stimulus for regeneration of bone is biomechanical energy in the line of stress (longitudinal axis of bone). This biomechanical energy is transmitted to the bone through intermittent compression and distraction by way of antigravity muscle contraction and through the forces of gravity and body weight in upright postures (see Chapter 3, Arthrology). Exercises involving repeated high-force movements in weight-bearing positions produce greater bone densities.[591]
2. **Zygapophyseal joints:** The optimal stimulus for regeneration of articular cartilage is intermittent compression and decompression and gliding, which can be achieved through specific active movements of the lumbar spine while avoiding static loading.[221]
3. **Ligaments:** Joint immobilization results in reduced synthesis of proteoglycan and plasticity of ligaments over time. Ligamentous laxity tends to be prominent in the lumbar spine secondary to chronic improper postural loading or traumatic ligamentous strain.[511] When ligaments are torn or overstretched, they may remain lax, in which case neutral postures and muscle stabilization is required. According to Grimsby,[221] ligaments respond well to modified tension in the line of stress. This modified tension may be applied to the ligaments through selected exercises designed to target the specific ligament. Tension to the posterior longitudinal, interspinous, and supraspinous ligaments, for example, may be applied by flexion of the lumbar spine at the end range (see Fig. 20-22), either by the therapist or the patient.
4. **The disk:** The annulus, like ligaments, contains mainly of type I collagen fibers, which are highly organized and resist tension. The nucleus pulposus contains mainly type II collagen fibers, which respond to pressure. The nucleus pulposus has a greater concentration of water and proteoglycans than the annulus. The exercise of choice for stimulating disk repair is lumbar rotation. Modified tension in the line of stress stimulates protein synthesis of type I collagen of the annulus; intermittent compression and distraction promotes regeneration of type II collagen and proteoglycans.[511] Rotations can be performed either in non-weight-bearing (supine or prone; Fig. 20-20) or in weight-bearing (Fig. 20-21), with or without weights. Pain is theoretically reduced by producing mechanoreceptor activity. Strengthening and segmental coordination of the deep rotators may also be improved. In sitting, because of the ability to produce end-range stretch, this may be useful in restoring function.

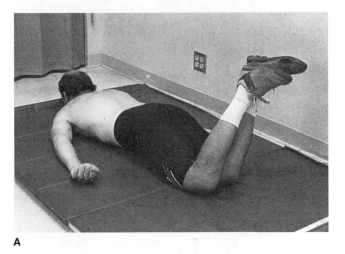

A

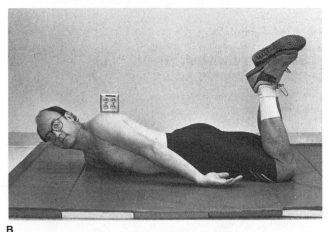

B

FIG. 20-20. Prone rotations (**A**) performed caudad-to-cephalad with knee flexion. The patient is instructed to slowly lift the pelvis and anterior thigh with the rotator muscles. (**B**) Cephalad-to-caudad. The patient is instructed to roll slowly while lifting one shoulder and stabilizing the pelvis.

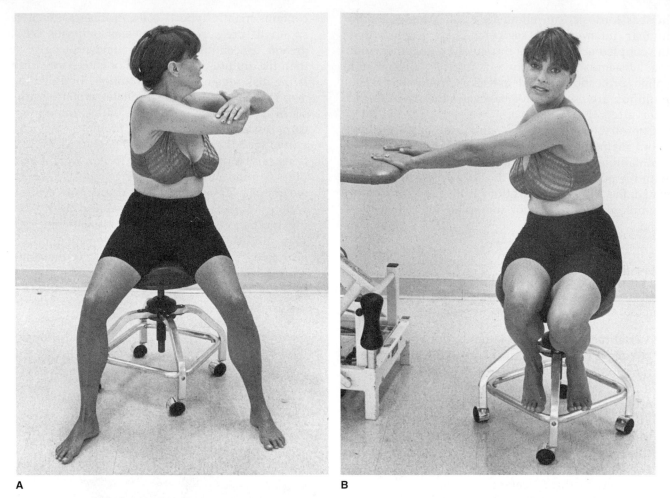

A   B

FIG. 20-21. Sitting rotations: (**A**) cephalad-to-caudad with active upper trunk rotation performed with a neutral lumbar spine and a fixed pelvis, and (**B**) caudad-to-cephalad performed with a fixed upper torso. The patient is rotating the pelvis (while sitting on a swivel stool).

5. **Muscles:** Phasic muscles, such as the erector spinae, act as movers of the spine; tonic muscles, such as the multifidi, act as stabilizers. The lumbar multifidus, considered be particularly important for stability,[340] is also particularly prone to atrophy.[250] The optimal stimulus for the regeneration of tonic fibers is high-repetition, low-resistance exercise to improve capillarization to the muscle. Because tonic muscles atrophy first, muscle endurance exercises should be performed initially, followed by strengthening exercises.[221] The optimal stimulus for regeneration of phasic fibers is low-repetition, high-resistance exercise without increasing speed.[511]

Based on Holten's medicine training theory, muscle endurance is enhanced by performing about 30 repetitions at 60% of one resistance maximal (1 RM).[226,260] Pure strength is achieved by performing 8 to 12 or fewer repetitions at 80% to 100% of 1 RM. For a combination of strength and endurance, Holten proposed performing 20 to 25 repetitions at 70% of 1 RM.

GENERAL CONDITIONING

A conditioning program initially focuses on mobility, followed by progressive resistive exercise training for strength, including both resistive and repetitive low-load exercises. Endurance is then improved through aerobic exercise, followed by protocols to improve whole-body coordination and agility.[391] For the athlete, plyometrics is useful in late-stage rehabilitation and functional precompetitive testing after injury (see Chap. 12, The Hip).[468] Although plyometric activity is primarily used for lower limb training, it is also important in training the upper limb and trunk. Throwing and catching from a bent-knee position is an example.

☐ Joint Mobilization Techniques

NONSPECIFIC SPINAL MOBILIZATIONS

(**Note:** P—patient, O—operator, M—movement)

I. **Flexion** (Fig. 20-22)

P—Supine with knees bent

O—Grasps across the anterior aspect of both proximal tibias and approximates the patient's knees to the axillae

M—Traction may be used by passing the left arm behind the knees and the right arm in front of the thighs. The hands are interlocked; by lifting and pulling with the arms, the knees are flexed toward the chest. Some traction is carried out along the line of the femurs by lifting the pelvis with the left arm as the knees are flexed.

Global stretching into flexion is used for patients with a generally tight back (particularly with loss of flexion), or for apprehensive patients beginning a home stretching program. Large-amplitude oscillations can increase general mobility, stimulate joint motion, or reduce active muscle guarding. Gentle, small-amplitude oscillations can relieve pain.

II. **Extension** (Fig. 20-23)

P—Lies prone

O—Grasps across the anterior aspect of the patient's distal femurs

M—The spine is extended by extending the patient's legs and hip girdle.

This technique is used as in flexion above and to prepare the patient for more specific techniques. Sometimes this method is better tolerated than specific, more vigorous techniques.

III. **Rotation** (Fig. 20-24)

P—Supine with knees bent

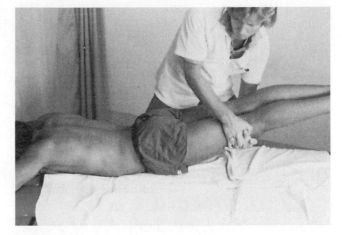

FIG. 20-23. Nonspecific long-lever extension mobilization of the lumbar spine.

O—Stabilizes the patient's thorax by placing an arm across the lower rib cage. The leg further from the operator is grasped at the knee and the hip is brought to about 90° flexion.

M—This leg is then pulled toward the operator, across the near leg. Maintain some knee and hip flexion of the near leg to prevent overextension of the spine.

IV. **Rotation** (Fig. 20-25)

P—Sidelying, hips and knees slightly flexed. This movement is localized to one area by the positioning of the patient's pelvis and thorax. For the lower lumbar spine, rotation is used with the spine toward flexion; for the upper lumbar spine, rotation is used with the spine in minimal extension

O—Stands behind patient. Simultaneously rotate the patient's top shoulder toward and the hip away until all slack is taken up.

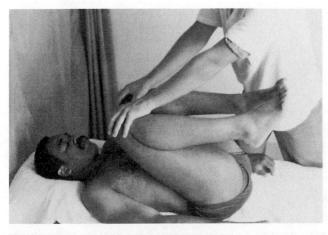

FIG. 20-22. Nonspecific long-lever flexion mobilization of the lumbar spine.

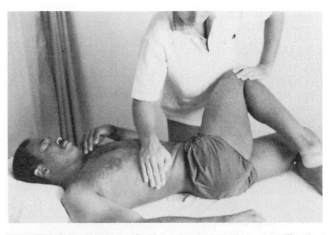

FIG. 20-24. Nonspecific long-lever rotation mobilization of the lumbar spine.

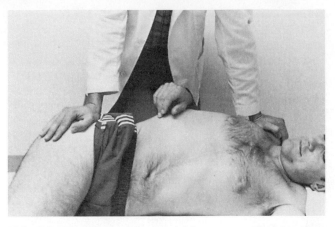

FIG. 20-25. *Alternative method for nonspecific long-lever rotational mobilization of the lumbar spine.*

Then, positioned directly over the patient with both elbows straight, apply firm pressure down and cranially against the shoulder, and down and caudally against the greater trochanter, taking up additional slack.

M—An oscillation movement is produced by the therapist's caudal hand, which rotates the pelvis while the cranial hand stabilizes the thorax (grade III). Additional stretch or thrust (given through the shoulder and hip) may be performed (grade IV).

This is a useful technique for unilateral back or leg pain. Gentle, small-amplitude oscillations can relieve pain, and large-amplitude oscillations can increase general mobility or reduce active guarding.

V. Lateral Flexion (sidebending; Fig. 20-26)
 P—Supine with knees bent
 O—Holds the patient's legs together with the hips and knees bent to 90°

M—Spinal sidebending is produced by rotating the patient's pelvis about a vertical axis, using the patient's legs as a lever.

VI. Lateral Flexion (sidebending; Fig. 20-27)
 P—Lies on the side toward which sidebending is to occur. A small, soft roll may be placed under the lumbar spine to create a greater excursion of movement. The hips and knees are comfortably flexed.
 O—Contacts the lateral aspects of the patient's hip girdle and shoulder girdle with the forearms. The fingertips contact the far sides of the spinous processes.
 M—Movement is produced by pressing outward, then down, with the forearms and pulling up on the spinous processes. Additional leverage is gained by caudal pressure of the operator's chest on the patient's top hip and thigh.

This technique is useful for global stretching and pain relief. Its potential for separating vertebral bodies and opening intervertebral foramina may be valuable in relieving nerve root entrapment.

VII. Correction of Acute Lateral Deviation (Fig. 20-28)
 P—Standing, with the elbow bent to 90° and resting on the side to which the thorax deviates (Fig. 20-28*A*)
 O—Contacts the patient's thorax and arm with the shoulder or chest. The operator's arms encircle the patient and the hands interlock to contact the lateral aspect of the patient's pelvis.
 M—The lateral deviation is *slowly* (may take several minutes or attempts) reduced with simultaneous pressure against the thorax and the hips. Small-amplitude oscillations

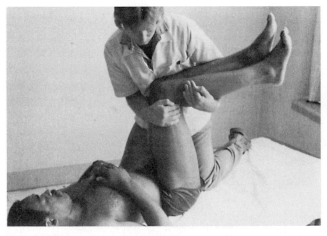

FIG. 20-26. *Nonspecific long-lever lateral flexion mobilization of the lumbar spine.*

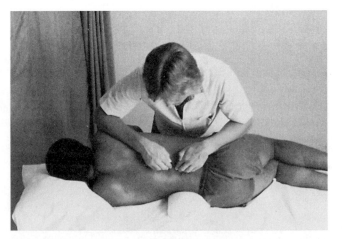

FIG. 20-27. *Alternative method for nonspecific long-lever lateral flexion mobilization of the lumbar spine.*

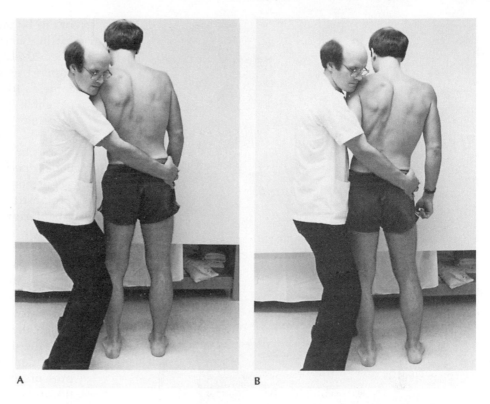

FIG. 20-28. Correction pressure to the patient's trunk for lateral deviation: (**A**) the initial contact and (**B**) with slight "overcorrection" at the end.

may be superimposed on slow pressure, for patient comfort. The original deviation should be slightly overcorrected (Fig. 20-28*B*).

Note: The patient may be taught to perform this maneuver at home (see Fig. 20-48). In performing this technique, original or more central back discomfort is acceptable; more distal pain is not. This technique is useful for acute disk prolapse and is more successful if radicular signs or symptoms are not present.[403,406] This procedure is usually followed by the next technique.

VIII. **Correction of Flexion Deformity in Standing** (Fig. 20-29)

   P—Standing, as relaxed as possible

   O—Contacts the low lumbar spine with the thenar eminence of one hand (if the level at which the blockage occurs can be identified, the thenar eminence should contact the spinous process *below* that level). The opposite arm reaches across the front of the patient's thorax to grasp the shoulder on the opposite side.

   M—Extension is slowly and gradually produced with a mild forward pressure of the contacting hand, while the thorax is gently moved backward.

Note: The patient may be taught to perform this maneuver at home (see Fig. 20-46).

SEGMENTAL SPINAL MOVEMENTS

I. **Posteroanterior Central Vertebral Pressure** (Fig. 20-30)

   P—Prone. The spine may be positioned in the desired degree of extension by placing a

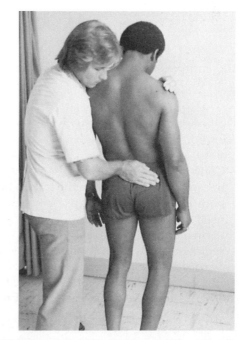

FIG. 20-29. Correction pressure to the patient's trunk for flexion deformity.

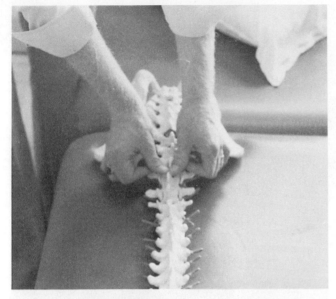

A

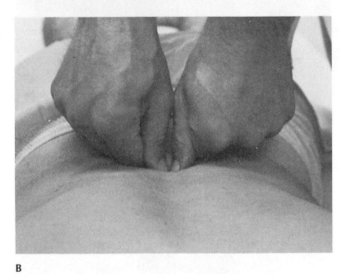

B

FIG. 20-30. Posteroanterior central vertebral pressure on the spinous process.

pillow under the abdomen (for more flexion) or the chest or thighs (for more extension).

O—Contacts the spinous process of the vertebra to be mobilized with the thumb pads of both hands. The fingertips or knuckles are used to stabilize the hand-hold by placing them along the spine on both sides.

M—Segmental movement is localized by downward pressure through the arms, forearms, and thumbs. Graded oscillations are used.

II. **Posteroanterior Central Vertebral Pressure** (Fig. 20-31)

P—Prone; may be positioned as described in the previous technique.

O—Contacts the spinous process of the verte-

bra to be mobilized with the ulnar border of the hand closest to the patient's head (Fig. 20-31*A*). The other hand is used for support, as shown in Figure 20-31*B*.

M—Same as for the previous technique. If the patient is positioned in flexion, overpressure may be applied cranially into more flexion.

This is a technique of choice for pain reduction or gentle, specific mobilization, for stretching stiff segments, and for helping patients with disk prolapse to achieve greater extension.

III. **Posteroanterior Unilateral Vertebral Pressure** (Fig. 20-32)

P—Prone, with the spine positioned in the desired degree of initial extension

O—Places both thumb pads over the mammillary process of the joint to be mobilized; these are roughly level with the spaces between the spinous processes and perhaps 1″ to the side.

M—Movement is produced with a downward pressure in an oscillatory manner through the arms, forearms, and thumbs, in a direction perpendicular to the contour of the spine.

IV. **Transverse Vertebral Pressures** (rotational gliding; Fig. 20-33)

P—Prone

O—The thumbs are applied against the side of the spinous process at the painful level or the level to be mobilized.

M—The thumbs apply a rhythmic oscillatory force directed toward the opposite side (the painful side or the side of restriction). It is often useful to overlap the thumbs to generate reinforcement.

This technique achieves a rotational mobilization by means of localized direct pressure to the side of the spinous process of the affected vertebral level. Its greatest value is in conditions in which the symptoms have a unilateral distribution.

Note: Isometric exercises for strengthening the segmental muscles related to a hypermobile joint may be performed in a similar fashion to the preceding segmental spinal movements (see Figs. 20-30 to 20-33). The patient is taught to prevent displacement of the spinous or mammillary process at the level of the hypermobile segment. The direction of the applied sustained pressures may be altered (diagonally, transversely, posteroanteriorly, caudally, and cephalad) to recruit the appropriate muscles. Progression is made by increasing the pressure being sustained and the duration of the hold.

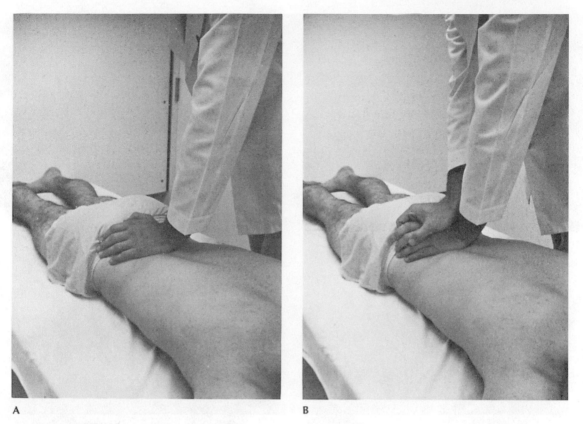

FIG. 20-31. Alternative method for posteroanterior central vertebral pressure on the spinous processes, with (**A**) ulnar border contact and (**B**) support of the other hand.

V. Flexion (Fig. 20-34*A*)
P—Sidelying, with the hips and knees comfortably flexed, arms resting in front of the body
O—Rest the patient's upper arm across the lateral aspect of the thorax. Grasp the lower arm at the distal humerus, gaining a pur-

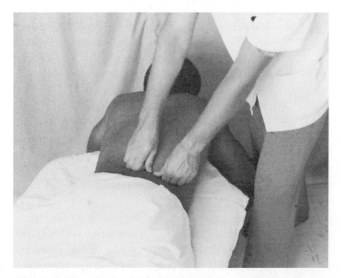

FIG. 20-32. Posteroanterior unilateral vertebral pressure.

chase on the humeral epicondyles. Pull the shoulder forward until the restricted segment is localized and engaged by rotating the thoracic and lumbar vertebrae above the restricted segment (slack is taken up to the restricted segment). The hip is flexed to prevent further motion in that joint. The patient's lower leg rests against the operator's body.
—The operator's cranial forearm stabilizes along the patient's upper shoulder and rib cage with the fingers placed on the transverse processes or the spinous process of the cranial vertebra of the targeted segment to provide fixation.
—The caudal arm and forearm encircle the sacrum, and the fingers are placed on the spinous or transverse processes of the caudal vertebra of the targeted segment.
M—Flexion is introduced by the operator's caudal hand and body moving as a unit, stabilizing with the cranial hand. The pelvis is moved in a caudal–ventral direction.
This technique involves locking the cranial segments in extension and rotation. If this position is not tolerated well, locking from above (via rotation) may be achieved by rotating the thoracic

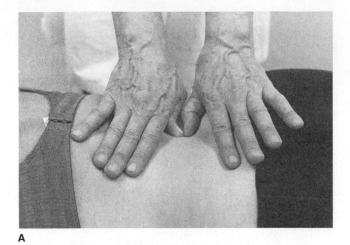

A

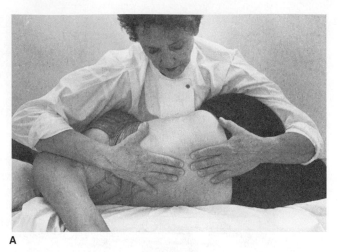

A

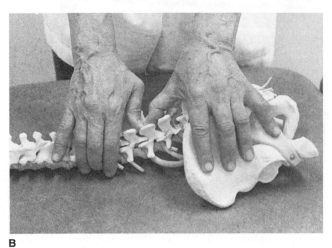

B

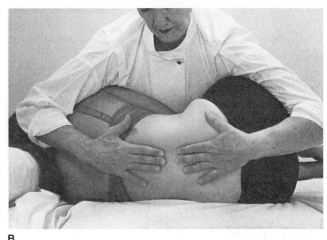

B

FIG. 20-33. Transverse vertebral pressures: (**A**) transverse directed rotational gliding using the thumbs; (**B**) position of the thumbs on the spinous processes for transverse gliding.

FIG. 20-34. (**A**) Segmental flexion mobilization and (**B**) alternative method for flexion mobilization.

and lumbar spine forward (Fig. 20-34*B*). Active mobilization (muscle energy or post-isometric relaxation techniques) is often effective. The operator introduces traction to the spinous process of the caudal segment, thereby effecting passive mobilization and flexing the spinal segments. The hips are concurrently flexed as well.

—The restricted segment is brought up to the pathological barrier. Isometric extension is effected away from the barrier during inhalation. During the relaxation phase, the segment is mobilized beyond the pathological barrier while the patient exhales.

VI. Extension (Fig. 20-35)

P—Prone

O—The ulnar border of the cranial hand contacts the spinous process of the segment to be mobilized (Fig. 20-35*A*). The other hand grasps firmly around the patient's near thigh, just above the knee, and raises (extends) that leg until motion occurs at the

desired segment. Alternatively, the thumb pad contacts the mammillary process on the near side for unilateral extension (Fig. 20-35*B*).

M—Movement is produced by pressing down on the spinous process or mammillary process, or extending the leg.

Because of the long lever arm (the patient's leg), a significant amount of force can be applied with this technique, so it is a technique of choice for patients with chronic lumbar stiffness. It may be too vigorous for patients with more acute disorders and should be used with caution.

VII. Rotation (Fig. 20-36)

P—Prone

O—Grasp across to the opposite anterosuperior iliac spine with the more caudal hand. Contact the far side of the spine over the mammillary process of the upper vertebra of the segment to be mobilized with the

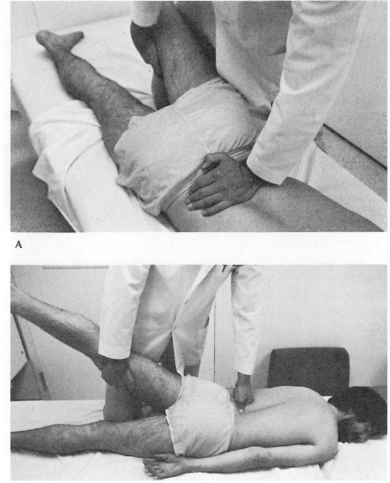

FIG. 20-35. Long-lever extension mobilization of the lumbar spine with (**A**) ulnar border contact or (**B**) thumb contact with the stabilizing hand.

ulnar border or the pisiform of the opposite hand (Fig. 20-36A). Alternatively, the thumb or pisiform can contact near the side of the spinous process of the upper vertebra of the segment to be mobilized (Fig. 20-36B).

M—Movement is performed by simultaneously lifting the pelvis and pressing down with the contacting hand. This produces rotation (of the spine) away from the side of the pelvis contacted.

This is an effective stretching (grade IV) and pain-reducing (grades I to III) technique and is also useful for disk prolapse (without neurological deficit), usually with the painful side toward the operator.

VIII. **Rotation** (Fig. 20-37)

P—Prone, knees flexed to 90°

O—The cranial hand contacts the upper vertebra of the segment to be mobilized at the far side (mammillary process), using pisiform contact. The other hand grasps the patient's ankles and lowers them until movement just occurs at the desired segment (Fig. 20-37A). Alternatively, contact is made on the near side of the spinous process of the upper vertebra with the pisiform or thumb (Fig. 20-37B).

M—Movement is produced by lowering the ankles or pressing down and laterally with the contacting hand.

IX. **Rotation** (Fig. 20-38)

P—Lying on the side opposite that to which movement will occur. The hips and knees are comfortably flexed, the head and neck slightly flexed, and the arms at rest in front of the patient.

O—Flexes the upper hip, keeping the knee level with the plinth, until movement just occurs at the segment below that to be moved (palpate motion with the middle finger). Position the dorsum of the patient's foot behind the opposite knee or thigh. Rest the patient's upper arm across the lat-

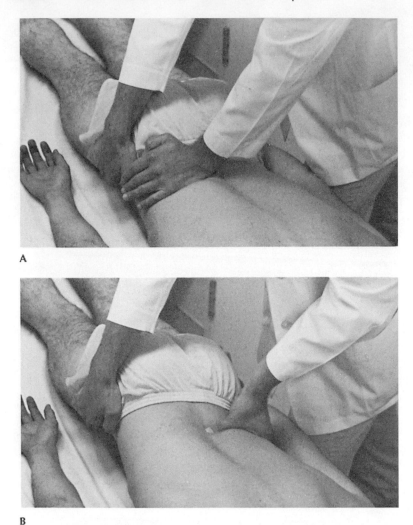

A

B

FIG. 20-36. Rotational mobilization using (**A**) ulnar border or (**B**) thumb contact with the lumbar spine.

eral aspect of the thorax. Grasp the lower arm at the distal humerus, gaining a purchase on the humeral epicondyles. The third finger of the opposite hand palpates between the spinous processes at the level above that to be moved. The patient relaxes and the spine is rotated until movement just occurs at the segment palpated by pulling out on the patient's arm.

—The forearm is placed across the posterolateral aspect of the patient's pelvis, the opposite forearm across the deltopectoral groove. The middle finger of the caudal hand hooks underneath to the opposite side of the spinous process of the more caudal vertebra of the segment to be moved. The opposite middle finger or thumb contacts the near side of the spinous process of the more cranial vertebra.

—Slack is taken up in the shoulder girdle by pushing down and away with the forearm, and in the hip girdle by pulling down and toward the operator.

M—Movement is produced by pulling up on the caudal spinous process while continuing to move the pelvic girdle (as above), and simultaneously pushing down on the cranial spinous process while moving the shoulder girdle (as above). Use body weight to complete end-range distraction. Oscillations can also be used.

Note: Sometimes a gentle thrust is performed at the end point of movement, or a contract–relax technique may be used to facilitate maximum range of motion.

X. **Sidebending** (Fig. 20-39)

P—Prone

O—The cranial hand makes thumb or pisiform contact at the near side of the upper spinous process of the segment to be mobilized. The other hand grasps the patient's near thigh just above the knee. The patient's leg

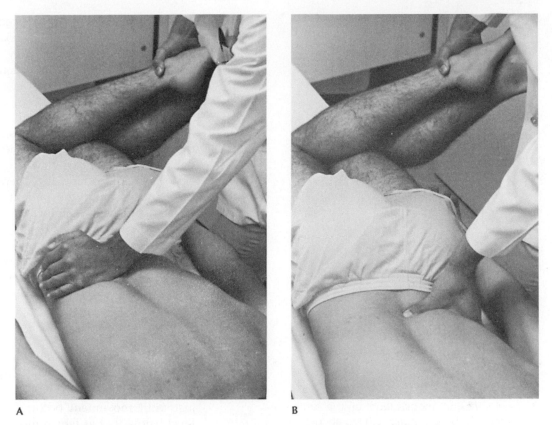

A   B

FIG. 20-37. Alternative method for rotational mobilization using (**A**) pisiform contact on the far side or (**B**) thumb contact on the near side of the lumbar spine.

is abducted, which sidebends the lumbar spine, until motion reaches the desired level.

M—Overpressure is applied at the spine through the thumb or at the leg (into more abduction).

Because of the long lever arm, significant force can be used, so this is a technique of choice for patients with chronic joint stiffness.

XI. Traction (Fig. 20-40)

P—Supine, knees and hips flexed

O—Sits or stands at the patient's feet, securing them with the buttocks or thighs. Grasps behind the patient's knees.

M—The operator leans backward, exerting a longitudinal movement through his arms and the patient's legs to the patient's spine. Movement can be graded, depending on pa-

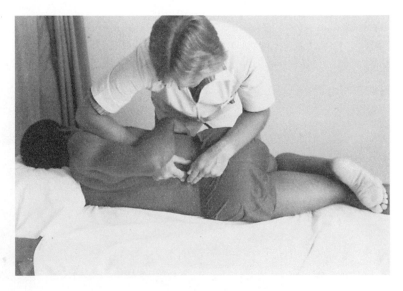

FIG. 20-38. Alternative method for rotational mobilization of the lumbar spine.

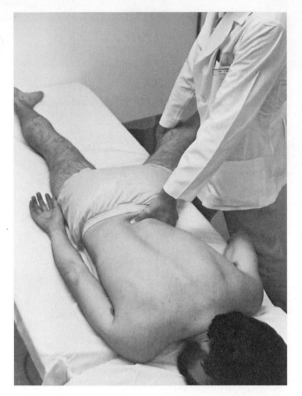

FIG. 20-39. Lateral flexion mobilization of the lumbar spine with transverse vertebral pressure and leg abduction.

tient tolerance and desired result. This technique provides gentle traction to relieve pressure on the disk and also comfortable stimulation and movement to pain segments that may not tolerate more vigorous techniques. Belt traction may be used.[440] The belt is placed around the patient's upper calves, with a pad interposed for comfort. The clasped loop of the adjustable belt is placed around the therapist's upper back.

By leaning the trunk in the desired direction, lumbar traction is applied. A foam or nonslip plastic pad (Dysem) may be placed under the patient's trunk and next to the skin to prevent slipping.

XII. **Traction** (Fig. 20-41)
  P—Supine, at the end of the plinth
  O—Assumes a walk-standing position at the foot of the table, facing the patient. The patient's crossed legs are placed over the operator's shoulder, and the operator clasps the hands around the patient's proximal thighs, keeping the elbows in tight to the chest.
  M—The patient's hips are drawn toward the operator, thus distracting the spine, when the operator's body is simultaneously rocked backward and the trunk is tucked (flexed).

XIII. **Unilateral Traction** (Fig. 20-42)
  P—Supine or prone
  O—Grasps the distal tibia on the side to be distracted, gaining a purchase on the malleoli. The patient's leg is flexed and adducted just until movement occurs at the spinal level below that at which movement is desired.
  M—Movement is produced by a longitudinal pull through the leg, leaning backward with body weight. Countermovement is provided against the sole of the patient's opposite foot with the anterior aspect of the operator's thigh. The opposite leg may be placed in a hook position (hip and knee flexed, feet flat on the plinth) or held in the Thomas position, to flatten out the lumbar spine.

XIV. **Sacroiliac Backward Rotation** (Fig. 20-43)

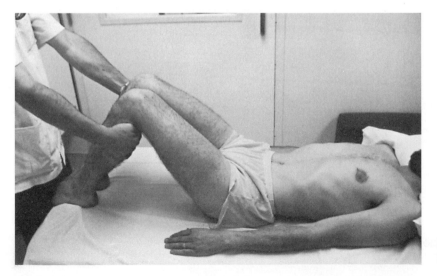

FIG. 20-40. Traction mobilization of the lumbar spine, using the legs.

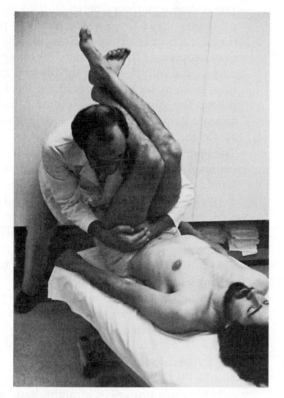

FIG. 20-41. *Alternative method for traction mobilization of the lumbar spine, using the hips.*

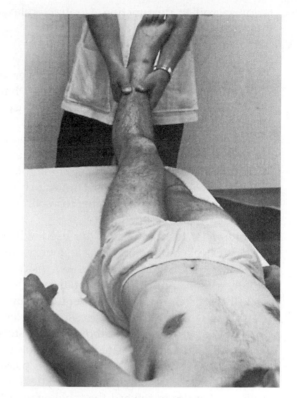

FIG. 20-42. *Unilateral traction mobilization of the lumbar spine, using the leg.*

P—Lying on the side opposite the joint to be moved

O—Flexes the patient's hip and knee as far as possible and holds the leg in that position by contacting the anterior aspect of the leg around the operator's waist. The patient's other leg is extended, and the dorsum of the foot is secured at the far edge of the plinth. The operator's more cranial hand contacts the patient's anterosuperior iliac

spine, and the opposite hand contacts the ischial tuberosity. The forearms are parallel to each other in a direction to create a force-couple around the joint axis.

M—Movement is produced by a force-couple, pushing the anterosuperior iliac spine backward and the ischial tuberosity forward. Further pressure is placed against the patient's leg with the operator's abdomen.

This is an effective technique for correcting an-

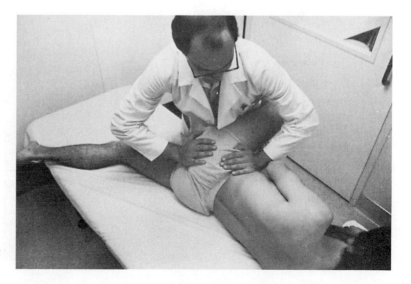

FIG. 20-43. *Posterior rotation of the innominate on the sacrum.*

terior sacroiliac dysfunction. Contract–relax or muscle-energy techniques may be used.

XV. Sacroiliac Anterior Rotation (Fig. 20-44)

P—Prone

O—Places the cranial hand directly over the patient's sacrum. The opposite hand reaches around to grasp the anterior aspect of the distal thigh of the near leg.

M—Movement is produced by simultaneously pressing on the distal sacrum with the heel of the hand and lifting the leg, thus rotating the proximal ilium forward (anteriorly).

This is an effective technique for correcting posterior sacroiliac dysfunction.

Note: This technique may be used with an isometric relaxation or muscle-energy technique.[50,422] The leg is elevated in extension and usually slight abduction and rotation to loose-pack the sacroiliac joint (the operator monitors the sulcus with the fingers). Pressure is exerted on the iliac crest slightly above the posterior iliac spine. The leg is elevated in extension until the restrictive barrier at the limit of passive range of motion is engaged. The patient then pulls the leg down toward the table against the resistance of the therapist's hand. The patient relaxes and additional slack in the joint motion is taken up until a new restrictive barrier is engaged. This process is repeated three or four times.

XVI. Positional Distraction (Fig. 20-45)

P—Sitting on the side of the plinth, with a soft roll placed at the side, between the pelvic crest and the chest wall (Fig. 20-45*A*)

M—The patient is carefully assisted into the sidelying position; sidebending occurs due to the roll. The patient's hips and knees are slightly flexed for comfort (Fig. 20-45*B*).

—The operator palpates between the spinous processes at the level where maximal positional traction is desired. Grasping the patient's top knee, the operator slides it up the edge of the plinth, flexing the hip and spine until movement just occurs at the level palpated. The dorsum of the patient's foot is secured behind the other knee or thigh (Fig. 20-45*C*).

—The operator then palpates at the next highest level, with the third finger of the other hand. The opposite hand grasps the patient's distal humerus and pulls up and out, rotating the upper spine, until motion just occurs at the level palpated (Fig. 20-45*D*).

—The patient's arm is placed across the chest. This position is maintained as long as tolerated (usually 5 to 25 minutes).

This technique is used primarily to relieve pressure on the lumbar nerve root in patients with radicular signs and symptoms.

I. Standing Extension (Fig. 20-46)

A. *General*—Place hands on hips, thumbs forward. Keeping the knees straight, bend back over the hips, extending the lumbar spine. Keep the cervical spine neutral.

B. *Specific*—Place hands on hips, thumbs making contact with the lower spinous process of the segment to be mobilized. Extend the lumbar spine, maintaining pressure with the thumbs and localizing the force at the desired level (Fig. 20-46*A*).

C. *Unilateral*—As above, with single general or specific contact (thumb just lateral to the spinous process) only. Bend back and to the side of hand contact (Fig. 20-46*B*).

(text continues on page 689)

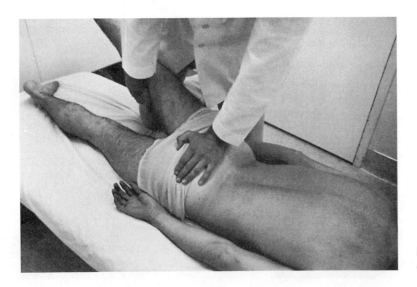

FIG. 20-44. Anterior rotation of the innominate on the sacrum.

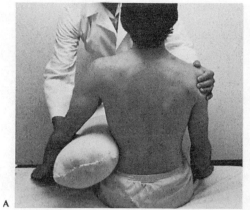
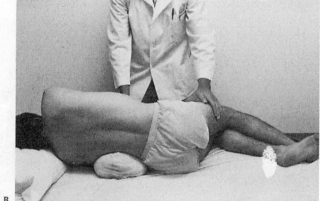
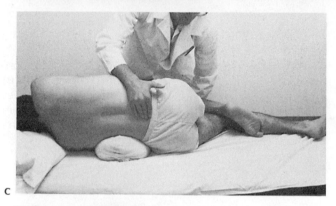
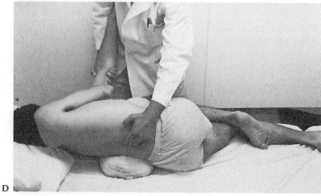
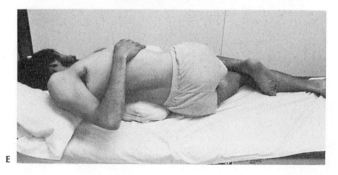

FIG. 20-45. Positional distraction technique. Beginning with the patient (**A**) sitting on the side of the plinth, (**B**) assist him into sidelying. While palpating the level where maximal positional traction is desired, the hip and spine are flexed (**C**), the upper spine is rotated (**D**), and the position is maintained (**E**).

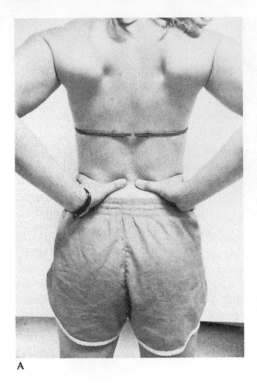

A

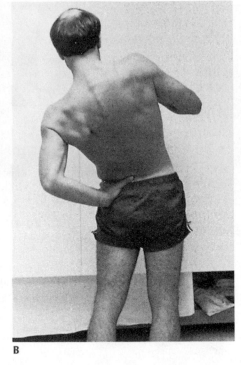

B

FIG. 20-46. Self-mobilization: (**A**) specific bilateral and (**B**) unilateral extension techniques for localized acute back pain with some loss of normal lumbar lordosis.

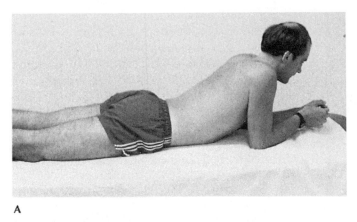

A

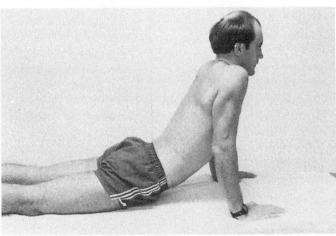

B

FIG. 20-47. (**A**) Prolonged and (**B**) intermittent prone extension.

II. Prone Extension (Fig. 20-47)

   A. *Prolonged*—Lie prone with elbows and shoulders flexed about 90°, cervical spine neutral. Relax the back and abdomen, allowing the spine to stretch into extension (see Fig. 20-40*A*).

   B. *Intermittent*—Lie prone with hands at shoulder level. Push the shoulders up until motion is halted by stiffness or discomfort. The back and abdomen remain completely relaxed (see Fig. 20-40*B*).

   Prolonged or intermittent, vigorous stretching into extension is used to relieve stiffness, or to allow the patient with acute disk prolapse to achieve desired extension.

III. Self-Correction of Lateral Deviations (Fig. 20-48)[405]

   A. Standing, the hands contact the protruding hip and chest (lateral chest wall to the same side as trunk deviation, and the pelvic crest on the opposite side). Hand pressure slowly forces the spine into straight, then slightly overcorrected, position (Fig. 20-48*A*).

   B. Alternatively, the elbow to the side of deviation is held at 90° against the lateral chest wall. Contact the wall with that arm and shoulder. Slowly move hips toward the wall, eventually assuming a slightly overcorrected position (Fig. 20-48*B*).

IV. Sidebending (Fig. 20-49)

   A. Standing, arms behind neck. Positioning of the lower extremities is critical to localize motion to the targeted segment and to prevent sagging of the pelvis. By moving the legs apart or abducting the ipsilateral leg to the level of the targeted segment, active mobilization can be localized to the hypomobile segment while avoiding hypermobile segments that may be present distal to the segment.

   B. The patient actively sidebends the upper trunk.

   Note: Combined motions may be done (*i.e.,* extension, right sidebending and left rotation).

☐ Neural Tension Techniques

According to Grieve,[216] the development of neural tension techniques of the lumbar spine has been encouraged by the success of including hamstring stretching techniques in the treatment plan,[22,273] progressive stretching of nonirritable (presumed) lumbar root adhesions,[216] and the slump test.[68,375,619]

Localized segmental changes should generally be treated first when tethering lesions are suspected. If this does not relieve the so-called canal signs, neural

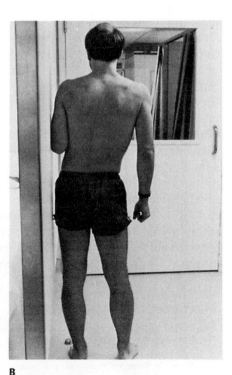

FIG. 20-48. Self-correction of lateral deviation using (**A**) hand pressure and (**B**) wall contact. (Note: In both *A* and *B*, a left lateral deviation has been slightly overcorrected so that the patient is shown in a slight right lateral deviation.)

A   B

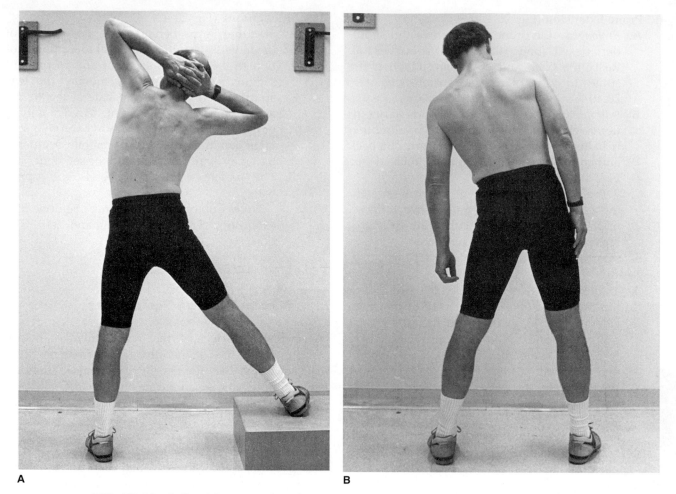

FIG. 20-49. *Self-mobilization—sidebending using the lower limbs for localization: (**A**) ipsilateral leg abduction and (**B**) legs apart.*

tension techniques should be considered. Any of the slump tests may be used in treatment as a mobilization technique. Physical therapists have prescribed straight-leg raising stretches for many years not only to stretch the hamstrings but also, in some situations, to stretch the sciatic nerve. Butler[68] recommends that to turn a hamstring stretch into a nervous system stretch, it should be done with the hip in medial rotation; this allows better access to the neural tissue. Several variations of straight-leg raising techniques and prone knee bends to stretch the upper part of the femoral nerve are described in the literature.[68,375] Neural tension techniques are beyond the scope of this text, but manipulative and clinical reasoning courses are available that include the concepts and practice of mobilization of the nervous system.

REFERENCES

1. Abboudi SY: The aquatic solution. Rehabil Management 6:77–79, 1993
2. Abel OJR, Siebert WJ: Fibrositis. J Missouri Med Assoc 36:43–437, 1939
3. Aberg J: Evaluation of an advanced back pain rehabilitation program. Spine 7:317–318, 1982
4. Adams MA, Hutton WC: Gradual disc prolapse. Spine 10:524–531, 1985
5. Addison R, Schultz A: Trunk strength in patients seeking hospitalization for chronic low back disorders. Spine 5:539–544, 1980
6. Akerblom B: Standing and Sitting Posture with Special Reference to the Construction of Chairs. Thesis. Stockholm, Nordiska Bockhandeln, 1948
7. Almay BG, Johansson F, Von Knorring L, et al: Endorphins in chronic pain: I. Differences in CSF endorphin levels between organic and psychogenic pain syndromes. Pain 5:153–162, 1978
8. Alston W, Carlson KE, Feldman DJ, et al: A quantitative study of muscle factors in chronic low back syndrome. J Am Geriatr Soc 14(10):1041–1047, 1966
9. American Academy of Orthopaedic Surgeons: A Glossary on Spinal Terminology. Chicago, American Academy of Orthopaedic Surgeons, 1981
10. Andersson BJ, Murphys RW, Ortengren R, et al: The influence of back-rest inclination and lumbar support on lumbar lordosis. Spine 4:52–58, 1979
11. Andersson BJ, Ortengren R, Nachemson A, et al: Lumbar disc pressure and myoelectric back muscle activity during sitting: 1. Studies on an experimental chair. Scand J Rehabil Med 6:104–114, 1974
12. Andersson BJ, Ortengren R, Nachemson A, et al: The sitting posture: An electromyographic and discometric study. Orthop Clin North Am 6:105–120, 1975
13. Andersson GBJ: Epidemiologic aspects on low back pain in industry. Spine 6:53–60, 1981
14. Andersson GBJ, Pope MH: The patient. In Pope MH, Frymoyer JW, Andersson G (eds): Occupational Low Back Pain. New York, Praeger, 1984:137–156
15. Andersson GBJ, Sevensson HO, Oden A: The intensity of work recovery in low back pain. Spine 8:880–884, 1983
16. Andersson JAD: Back pain and occupation. In Jayson M (ed): The Lumbar Spine and Back Pain. London, Pittman Medical, 1980:57–82
17. Armstrong JR: Lumbar Disc Lesions. London, Livingstone, 1967
18. Arnoldi CC, Brodsky AE, Cauchoix J, et al: Lumbar spinal stenosis and nerve root entrapment syndromes: Definitions and classification. Clin Orthop 115:4–5, 1976
19. Awad EA: Interstitial myofibrositis: Hypothesis of mechanism. Arch Phys Med Rehabil 54:449–453, 1975
20. Baarstrup C: On the spinous processes of the lumbar vertebrae and soft tissues between them and on pathological changes in that region. Acta Radiol 14:52, 1933
21. Badgley CE: The articular facets in relation to low-back pain and sciatica radiation. J Bone Joint Surg 23:481–496, 1941
22. Baer WS: Sacroiliac strain. Bull Johns Hopkins Hosp 28:159, 1917
23. Bajelus D: Hellerwork: The ultimate. International Journal of Alternative & Complementary Medicine 1 2:26–38, 1994

24. Batson G: Balancing mobility with stability for dynamic spine function: Part I. Mobility. Kinesiology for Dance 9(3):8–10, 1987
25. Batson G: Balancing mobility with stability for dynamic spine function: Part II. Stability. Kinesiology for Dance 9(4):12–15, 1987
26. Batson G: Balancing mobility with stability for dynamic spine function: Part III. Strengthening the trunk. Kinesiology for Dance 10(1):12–16, 1987
27. Beals RK, Hickman NW: Industrial injuries of the back and extremities. J Bone Joint Surg 54A:1593–1611, 1972
28. Becker DP, Gluck H, Nulsen FE, et al: An inquiry into neurophysiological basis for pain. J Neurosurg 30.1–13, 1969
29. Bell GH, Dunbar O, Beck SJ, et al: Variation in strength of vertebrae with age and their relation to osteoporosis. Calcif Tissue Res 1:75–86, 1967
30. Bell GR, Rothman RH: The conservative treatment of sciatica. Spine 9:54–56, 1984
31. Benjamin BE: Are You Tense? The Benjamin System of Muscular Therapy: Tension Relief Through Deep Massage and Body Care. New York, Pantheon Books, 1978
32. Bennet RM: Fibrositis: Misnomer for a common rheumatic disorder. West J Med 134:405–413, 1981
33. Berguist-Ullman M, Larsson U: Acute low back pain in industry: A controlled prospective study with specific reference to therapy and vocational factors. Acta Orthop Scand [Suppl] 170:1–117, 1977
34. Berkson M, Schultz A, Nachemson A, et al: Voluntary strengths of male adults with acute low back syndromes. Clin Orthop 129:84–95, 1977
35. Bernick S, Cailliet R: Vertebral end-plate changes with aging of human vertebrae. Spine 7:97–102, 1982
36. Bianco AJ: Low back pain and sciatica: Diagnosis/indications for treatment. J Bone Joint Surg 50A:170–181, 1968
37. Biering-Sorensen F: Low back trouble in a general population of 30-, 40-, 50- and 60-year-old men and women: Study design, representativeness and basic results. Dan Med Bull 29(6):289–299, 1982
38. Biering-Sorensen F: A prospective study of low back pain in a general population: I. Occurrence, recurrence and aetiology. Scand J Rehabil Med 15(2):71–78, 1983
39. Biering-Sorensen F: Physical measurement as risk indication for low back trouble over a 1-year period. Spine 9:106–118, 1984
40. Biering-Sorensen F, Hilden J: Reproducibility of the history of low-back trouble. Spine 9:280–286, 1984
41. Bihaung O: Autotraksjon for ischialgipasienter: En kontrolleert sammenlikning mellon effekten av Autotraksjon-B og isometriske ad modum Hume Kendell OG Jenkins. Fysioterapeuten 45:377–379, 1978
42. Blades K: Hydrotherapy in orthopedics. In Champion MR (ed): Adult Hydrotherapy. London, Heinemann, 1990
43. Blumett AE, Modesti LM: Psychological predictions of success or failure of surgical intervention for intractable back pain. In Bonica JJ, Albefessard D (eds): Advances in Pain Research and Therapy, Vol. I. New York, Raven Press, 1976:323–326
44. Bogduk N: Lumbar dorsal ramus syndrome. Med J Aust 2:537–541, 1980
45. Bogduk N: The innervation of the lumbar spine. Spine 8:286–293, 1983
46. Bogduk N: Lumbar dorsal ramus syndrome. In Grieve GP (ed): Modern Manual Therapy of the Vertebral Column. New York, Churchill Livingstone, 1986
47. Bogduk N, Engel R: The menisci of the lumbar zygoapophyseal joints. Spine 9:454–460, 1984
48. Bookhout MR: Examination and treatment of muscle imbalances. In Bourdillon JF, Day EA, Bookhout MR (eds): Spinal Manipulation, 5th ed. Oxford, Butterworth Heinemann, 1992:313–333
49. Boothby B: Seating by design. Physiotherapy 70:44–47, 1984
50. Bourdillon JF, Day EA, Bookhout MR: Spinal Manipulations, 5th ed. Oxford, Butterworth Heinemann, 1992
51. Bourne IHJ: Treatment of chronic back pain comparing corticosteroid-lignocaine injections with lignocaine alone. Practitioner 228:333–338, 1984
52. Boxall D, Bradford DS, Winter RB, et al: Management of severe spondylolisthesis in children and adolescents. J Bone Joint Surg 61A:479–495, 1979
53. Brackett EG: Low back strain with particular reference to industrial accident. JAMA 83:1068–1075, 1924
54. Bradley LA, Prokop CK, Margolis R, et al: Multivariate analyses of the MMPI profiles of low back pain patients. J Behav Med I(3):235–272, 1978
55. Braunarski DT: Clinical trails of spinal manipulations: A critical appraisal and review of the literature. J Manip Physiol Ther 7:243–249, 1984
56. Breig A, Troup JDG: Biomechanical consideration in straight leg-raising test. Spine 4:242–250, 1979
57. Brewerton DA: The doctor's role in diagnosis and prescribing vertebral manipulations. In Maitland GD (ed): Vertebral Manipulations, 5th ed. London, Butterworths, 1986:14–17
58. Brinckmann P: Injury of the annulus fibrosus and disc protrusions: An in vitro investigation on human lumbar disc. Spine 11:149–153, 1986
59. Brown L: An introduction to the treatment and examination of the spine by combined movements. Physiotherapy 74:347–353, 1988
60. Brunswic M: Ergonomics of seat design. Physiotherapy 70:40–43, 1984
61. Buckle PW, Kember PA, Wood AD, et al: Factors influencing occupational back pain in Bedfordshire. Spine 5:254–258, 1980
62. Burnell A: Injection techniques in low back pain. In Twomey LT (ed): Symposium: Low Back Pain. Perth, Western Australia Institute of Technology, 1974:111
63. Buros OK: Eighth Mental Measurements. Lincoln, University of Nebraska Press, Year Book, 1978
64. Burton AK: Regional lumbar sagittal mobility: Measurement by flexicurves. Clin Biomech 1:20–26, 1986
65. Burton CV: Conservative management of low back pain. Postgrad Med 70(5):168–183, 1981
66. Burton CV, Nida G: Gravity Lumbar Reduction Therapy; Rehabilitation Publication No. 731. Minneapolis, Sister Kenny Institute, 1976
67. Bush HD, Horton WG, Smare DL, et al: Fluid content of the nucleus pulposus as a factor in the disk syndrome. Br Med J 2:831–832, 1956
68. Butler DS: Mobilization of the Nervous System. Melbourne, Churchill Livingstone, 1991
69. Cady LD, Bischoff DP, O'Connell ER, et al: Strength and fitness and subsequent back injuries in firefighters. J Occup Med 21:269–272, 1979
70. Cailliet R: Low Back Pain Syndrome, 4th ed. Philadelphia, FA Davis, 1988
71. Cailliet R: Soft Tissue Pain and Disability, 2nd ed. Philadelphia, FA Davis, 1988
72. Cairns D, Thomas L, Mooney V, et al: A comprehensive treatment approach to chronic low back pain. Pain 2:301–308, 1976
73. Calin A, Porta J, Fries JF, Schurman DJ: Clinical history as a screening test for ankylosing spondylitis. JAMA 237:2613–2614, 1977
74. Campbell SM, Clark S, Tindall EA, et al: Clinical characteristics of fibrositis: I. A "blinded" controlled study of symptoms and points. Arthritis Rheum 26:817–824, 1983
75. Caro XJ: Immunofluorescent studies of skin in primary fibrositis syndrome. Am J Med [Suppl 3A] 81:43–48, 1986
76. Caro XJ, Wolfe F, Johnston WH, et al: Controlled and blinded study of immunoreactant deposition at dermal/epidermal junction of patients with primary fibrositis syndrome. J Rheumatol 13:1086–1092, 1986
77. Carrera GF: Lumbar facet arthrography and injection in low back pain. Wisc Med J 78:35–37, 1979
78. Carrera GF, Haughton VM, Syversten A, Williams AL: Computerized tomography of the lumbar facet joints. Radiology 134:145–148, 1980
79. Carvin PJ, Jennings RB, Stern IJ: Enzymatic digestion of the nucleus pulposus: A review of experimental studies with chymopapain. Orthop Clin 8:27–35, 1977
80. Chadwick PR: Advising patients on back care. Physiotherapy 65:277–278, 1979
81. Chadwick PR: Examination, assessment and treatment of the lumbar spine. Physiotherapy 70:2–7, 1984
82. Chaffin DB: Human strength capacity and low back pain. J Occup Med 16:248–253, 1974
83. Chaffin DB: Manual materials handling: The case of overexertion injury and illness in industry. J Environ Pathol Toxicol 2:31–36, 1979
84. Chaffin DB, Herrin GD, Keyserling WM: Pre-employment strength testing—An updated position. J Occup Med 20:403–408, 1978
85. Chamberlain GJ: Cyriax's friction massage: A review. J Orthop Sports Phys Ther 4:16–22, 1982
86. Chan PC: Finger Acupressure. Los Angeles, Price/Stern/Sloan, 1982
87. Charnley J: Orthopaedic signs in the diagnosis of disc protrusion with specific reference to straight leg-raising test. Lancet 1:186–192, 1951
88. Chrisman DO, Mittnacht A, Snook GA: A study of the results following rotatory manipulation in the lumbar intervertebral disc syndrome. J Bone Joint Surg 46A:517–524, 1964
89. Ciric I, Milhael MA, Tarkington JA, et al: The lateral recess syndrome: A variant of spinal stenosis. J Neurosurg 53:433–443, 1980
90. Cirullo JA: Aquatic physical therapy approaches for the spine. Orthop Phys Ther Clin North Am 3:179–208, 1994
91. Clelland J, Savinar E, Shepard KF: The role of the physical therapist in chronic pain management. In Burrows GD, Elton D, Stanley GV (eds): Handbook of Chronic Pain Management. New York, Elsevier, 1987:243–258
92. Clements L, Dixon M: A model role of occupational therapy in back education. Can J Occup Ther 46:161–163, 1979
93. Cloward RB: The clinical significance of the sinuvertebral nerve of the cervical spine in relation to the cervical disc syndrome. J Neurol Neurosurg Psychiatry 23:321–326, 1960
94. Colt EWD, Wardlaw SL, Frantz AG: The effect of running on plasma B-endorphin. Life Sci 28:1637–1640, 1981
95. Coplans CW: The conservative treatment of low back pain. In Helfet AJ, Gruebel LDM (eds): Disorders of the Lumbar Spine. Philadelphia, JB Lippincott, 1978:135–183
96. Corrigan B, Maitland GD: Practical Orthopaedic Medicine. Boston, Butterworths, 1985
97. Cottrell GW: 90/90 traction in the treatment of low back pain. Orthop Trans/J Bone Joint Surg 4:80, 1981
98. Cottrell GW: New, conservative and exceptionally effective treatment for low back pain. Compr Ther 11:59–65, 1985
99. Coulehan JL: Chiropractic and the clinical art. Soc Sci Med 21:383–390, 1985
100. Coventry MB, Ghormley RK, Kernohan JW: The intervertebral disc: Its microscopic anatomy and pathology: 2. Changes in the intervertebral disc concomitant with age. J Bone Joint Surg 27:233–247, 1945
101. Coventry MB, Ghormley RK, Kernohan JW: The intervertebral disc: Its microscopic anatomy and pathology: 3. Pathological changes in the intervertebral disc. J Bone Joint Surg 27:460–474, 1945
102. Crock HV: Isolated lumbar disk resorption as a cause of nerve root canal stenosis. Clin Orthop 115:109–115, 1976
103. Crock HV: Internal disc disruption: A challenge to disc prolapse 50 years on. Spine 11:650–653, 1986
104. Cuckler JM, Bernini PA, Wiesel SW, Booth RE Jr, Rothman RH, Pickes GT: The use of epidural steroids in the treatment of lumbar radicular pain: A prospective, randomized, double-blind study. J Bone Joint Surg 67A:63–66, 1985
105. Cummings GS, Routon JL: Validity of unassisted pain drawings by patients with chronic pain [abstract]. Phys Ther 5:668, 1985
106. Cyriax J: Treatment of lumbar disk lesions. Br Med J 2:1434–1438, 1950
107. Cyriax J: Conservative treatment of lumbar disc lesions. Physiotherapy 50:300–303, 1964
108. Cyriax J: Deep friction. Physiotherapy 63:60–61, 1977
109. Cyriax J: The Slipped Disc. New York, Charles Scribner's Sons, 1980
110. Cyriax J: Textbook of Orthopaedic Medicine, 8th ed, Vol. I: Diagnosis of Soft-Tissue Lesions. London, Bailliere-Tindall, 1982
111. Cyriax JC, Coldham M: Textbook of Orthopaedic Medicine, 11th ed, Vol. 2: Treatment by Manipulation, Massage and Injection. Philadelphia, Bailliere-Tindall, 1984
112. Cyriax J, Cyriax P: Illustrated Manual of Orthopedic Medicine. Boston, Butterworths, 1983
113. Dagi FT, Beary JF: Low back pain. In Beary JF (ed): Rheumatology and Outpatient Orthopedic Disorders: Diagnosis and Therapy, 2nd ed. Boston, Little, Brown, 1987:97–103
114. Dahlstrom WG, Welsh GS, Dahlstrom LE: MMPI Handbook, Vol. 1. Minneapolis, University of Minnesota Press, 1975
115. Dahlstrom WG, Welsh GS, Dahlstrom LE: MMPI Handbook, Vol. 2. Minneapolis, University of Minnesota Press, 1975
116. Dan NG, Saccason PA: Serious complications of lumbar spine manipulations. Med J Aust 2:672–673, 1983
117. Davidson EA, Woodhall B: Biochemical alterations in herniated intervertebral disks. J Biol Chem 234:2951–2954, 1959

118. Davies G, Gould J: Trunk testing using a prototype Cybex II isokinetic stabilization system. J Orthop Sports Phys Ther 3:164–170, 1982
119. Davis P: Reducing the risk of industrial bad backs. Occup Health Safety 48:45–47, 1979
120. Dehlin O, Lindberg B: Lifting burden for a nursing aide during patient care in a geriatric ward. Scand J Rehabil Med 7:65–72, 1975
121. Delmas A: Fonction sacro-iliaque et statique du corps. Rev Rhuna 17:475–481, 1950
122. Dennis MD, Greene RL, Farr SP, et al: The Minnesota Multiphasic Personality Inventory: General guidelines to its use and interpretation in orthopaedics. Clin Orthop 150:125–130, 1980
123. DePalma A, Rothman RH: The Intervertebral Disc. Philadelphia, WB Saunders, 1970
124. DeRosa CP, Porterfield JA: A physical therapy model for the treatment of low back pain. Phys Ther 72:261–269, 1992
125. deVries HA, Cailliet R: Vagotonic effect of inversion therapy upon resting neuromuscular tension. Am J Phys Med 64(3):119–129, 1984
126. Deyo RA: Conservative therapy for low back pain: Distinguishing useful from useless therapy. JAMA 250:1057–1062, 1983
127. Deyo RA, Diehl A, Rosenthal M: How many days of bed rest for acute low back pain? N Engl J Med 315:1065–1070, 1986
128. Deyo RA, Diehl AK: Lumbar spine films in primary care: Current use and the effects of selective ordering criteria. J Gen Intern Med 1:20–25, 1986
129. DiFabio RP: Clinical assessment of manipulation and mobilization of the lumbar spine: A critical review of the literature. Phys Ther 66:51–54, 1986
130. Dike TFW, Burry HC, Grahame R: Extradural corticosteroid injection in management of lumbar nerve root compression. Br Med J 2:635–637, 1973
131. Dimaggio A, Mooney V: Conservative care of low back pain: What works? J Musculoskel Med 4(4).27–34, 1987
132. Dimaggio A, Mooney V: The McKenzie program: Exercise effective against back pain. J Musculoskel Med 4(12):63–74, 1987
133. Dixon ASJ: Progress and problems in back pain research. Rheumat Rehabil 12(4):165–175, 1973
134. Dominguez RH, Gajda R: Total Body Training. New York, Warner Books, 1982
135. Dontigny RL: Function and pathomechanics of the sacroiliac joint: A review. Phys Ther 65:35–44, 1985
136. Dorwart RH, Volger JB III, Helms CA: Spinal stenosis. Radiol Clin North Am 21:301–325, 1983
137. Dunham WF: Ankylosing spondylitis measurement of hip and spine movements. Br J Phys Med 12:126, 1949
138. DuPriest CM: Nonoperative management of lumbar spinal stenosis. J Manip Physiol Ther 16:411–414, 1993
139. Dupuis PR: The natural history of degenerative changes in the lumbar spine. In Watkins RG, Collis JS (eds): Principles and Techniques in Spine Surgery. Rockville, MD, Aspen, 1987
140. Dupuis PR, Yong-Ling K, Cassidy JD, et al: Radiologic diagnosis of degenerative lumbar spinal instability. Spine 10:262–276, 1985
141. Dyck P: Sciatic pain. In Watkins C (ed): Lumbar Discectomy and Laminectomy. Rockville, MD, Aspen, 1987
142. Eastmond CJ, Woodrow JC: The HLA system and the arthropathies associated with psoriasis. Ann Rheum Dis 36:112, 1977
143. Ebner M: Connective tissue massage. Physiotherapy 64:208–212, 1978
144. Ebner M: Connective Tissue Manipulations, Therapy and Therapeutic Application. Malabar, FL, Robert Kreiger, 1985
145. Echternach JL: Evaluation of pain in the clinical environment. In Echternach JL (ed): Pain. New York, Churchill Livingstone, 1987:39–72
146. Eckert C, Decker A: Pathological studies of intervertebral discs. J Bone Joint Surg 29:447–454, 1947
147. Edgar MA: Backache. Br J Hosp Med 32:290–301, 1984
148. Edgar MA, Park WM: Induced pain patterns on passive straight leg-raising in lower disc protrusion. J Bone Joint Surg 56B:658–667, 1974
149. Edwards BC: Combined movements of the lumbar spine: Examination and significance. Aust J Physiother 25:147–152, 1979
150. Edwards BC: Combined movements in the lumbar spine: Examination and treatment. In Grieve GP (ed): Modern Manual Therapy of the Vertebral Column. New York, Churchill Livingstone, 1986:561–566
151. Edwards BC: Clinical assessment: The use of combined movements in assessment and treatment. In Twomey LT, Taylor JR (eds): Physiotherapy of the Low Back. New York, Churchill Livingstone, 1987:81–109
152. Eggart JS, Leigh D, Vergamini G: Preseason athletic physical evaluations. In Gould JA, Davies GJ (eds): Orthopaedic and Sports Physical Therapy. St. Louis, CV Mosby, 1985:605–642
153. Eggertz AM: Autotraction, a nonsurgical treatment of low back pain and sciatica. In Grieve GP (ed): Modern Manual Therapy of the Vertebral Column. New York, Churchill Livingstone, 1986:796–804
154. Ehard R, Blowling R: The recognition and management of the pelvic component of low back and sciatic pain. Presented at the Annual Meeting of the American Physical Therapy Association (Orthopaedic Section), Miami, 1967
155. Eisen A, Hoirch M: The electrodiagnostic evaluation of spinal root lesions. Spine 8:98–106, 1983
156. Epstein JA, Epstein BS, Lavine LS, et al: Lumbar nerve root compression at the intervertebral foramina caused by arthritis of the posterior facets. J Neurosurg 39:362–369, 1973
157. Epstein JA, Epstein BS, Lavine LS, et al: Surgical treatment of nerve root compression caused by scoliosis of the lumbar spine. J Neurosurg 41:449–454, 1974
158. Evans RC: The lumbar spine. In Evans RC (ed): Illustrated Essentials in Orthopedic Physical Assessment. St. Louis, Mosby, 1994:249–343
159. Fahrni WH: Conservative treatment of lumbar disc degeneration: Our primary responsibility. Orthop Clin North Am 6:93–103, 1975
160. Fairbanks JCT, Park WN, Mc Call JW, et al: Apophyseal injection of local anesthetic as a diagnostic aid in primary low back syndromes. Spine 6:598–605, 1981
161. Fajersztajn J: Ueber das gekreuzte ischiasphanomen. Wien Klin Wochenschr 14:41–47, 1901
162. Falconer MA, McGeorge M, Begg AC: Observation on the cause and mechanism of symptom production and low back pain. J Neurosurg Psychiatry 11:13–26, 1948
163. Farfan HF: Mechanical Disorders of the Low Back. Philadelphia, Lea & Febiger, 1973
164. Farfan HF, Sullivan JD: The relation of facet orientation to intervertebral disc failure. Can Surg 10:179–185, 1967
165. Farrell PA, Gates WK, Maksud MG: Plasma beta-endorphin/beta-lipotropin immunoreactivity increases after treadmill exercise in man [abstr]. Med Sci Sports 13(2):134, 1981
166. Feinstein B, Langton J, Jameson R: Experiments on pain referred from deep skeletal structures. J Bone Joint Surg 36A:981–997, 1954
167. Finneson B: Low Back Pain. Philadelphia, JB Lippincott, 1973
168. Finneson BE: A lumbar disc surgery predictive score-card: A retrospective evaluation. Spine 4:141–144, 1979
169. Finneson BE: Low Back Pain, 2nd ed. Philadelphia, JB Lippincott, 1980
170. Fischer AA: Documentation of myofascial trigger points. Arch Phys Med Rehabil 69:286–291, 1988
171. Fischer AA, Chang CH: Temperature and pressure threshold measurements in trigger points. Thermology 1:212–215, 1986
172. Fisk J, Dimonte P, Courington S: Back schools. Clin Orthop 179:18–23, 1983
173. Fitzgerald KG, Wynveen KJ, Rhealt W, et al: Objective assessment with establishment of normal values for lumbar spinal range of movement. Phys Ther 63:1776–1781, 1982
174. Flint M: Effect of increasing back and abdominal strength on low-back pain. Res Q 29:160–171, 1955
175. Flor H, Turk DC: Etiological theories and treatments for chronic back pain: Somatic models and interventions. Pain 19:105–121, 1984
176. Folkins CH, Sime WE: Physical fitness training and mental health. Am Psychol 36(4):373–389, 1981
177. Fordyce WE: Behavioral Methods for Chronic Back Pain and Illness. St. Louis, CV Mosby, 1976
178. Fordyce WE, Fowler RS, Lehmann JF, et al: Some implications of learning in problems of chronic pain. J Chron Dis 21:179–190, 1968
179. Fordyce WE, Mc Mahon R, Rainwater G, et al: Pain compliant/exercise performance relationship in chronic pain. Pain 10:311–321, 1981
180. Fordyce WE, Shelton JL, Dundore DE: The modification of avoidance learning pain behaviors. J Behav Med 5.405–414, 1982
181. Forssell MZ: The back school. Spine 6:104–106, 1981
182. Fox RF, Van Breemer J: Chronic Rheumatism: Causation and Treatment. London, Churchill, 1934
183. Fraioli F, Moretti C, Paulucci D, et al: Physical exercise stimulates marked concomitant release of B-endorphins and adrenocorticotrophic hormones (ACTH) in peripheral blood in man. Experientia 36:987–989, 1980
184. Fredrickson BE, Trief PM, Van Beveren P, et al: Rehabilitation of the patient with chronic back pain. Spine 13:351–353, 1987
185. Friberg RR, Weinreb RN: Ocular manifestation of gravity inversion. JAMA 253:1755–1757, 1985
186. Friberg S, Hirsch C: Anatomical and clinical studies on lumbar disc degeneration. Acta Orthop Scand 19:222–242, 1949
187. Fries JF, Mitchell DM: Joint pain or arthritis. JAMA 233:199–204, 1976
188. Frymoyer JW: Basics for all [abstr]. Challenge of the Lumbar Spine: Ninth Annual Meeting, New York City, 1987
189. Frymoyer JW: Back pain and sciatica. N Engl J Med 318:291–300, 1988
190. Frymoyer JW, Pope MH, Clements JH, et al: Risk factors in low back pain: An epidemiological survey. J Bone Joint Surg 65A:213–218, 1983
191. Frymoyer JW, Pope MH, Clostanza MC, Rosen JC, et al: Epidemiologic studies of low-back pain. Spine 5:419–423, 1980
192. Frymoyer JW, Selby DK: Segmental instability: Rationale for treatment. Spine 10:280–286, 1985
193. Garrett R: Back strength and fitness programme using Norsk and sequence training. Physiotherapy 73:573–575, 1987
194. Gatchel RJ, Mayer TG, Capra P, et al: Qualification of lumbar function: VI. The use of psychological measures in guiding physical functional restoration. Spine 11:36–42, 1986
195. Gerhardt JJ: Documentation of Joint Motion. International Standard Neutral-Zero Measuring SFTR. Recording and Application of Goniometers, Inclinometers and Calipers. Portland, Isomed Inc., 1992
196. Gianakopoulos G, Waylonis GW, Grant PA, et al: Inversion devices: Their role in producing lumbar distraction. Arch Phys Med Rehabil 66:100–102, 1985
197. Gillstrom P, Ehrnberg A: Long-term results of autotraction in the treatment of lumbago and sciatica: An attempt to correlate clinical results with objective parameters. Arch Orthop Trauma Surg 104:294–298, 1985
198. Gillstrom P, Ehrnberg A, Hinmarsh T: Autotraction in lumbar disk herniation: A myelographic study before and after treatment. Arch Orthop Trauma Surg 104:207–210, 1985
199. Gillstrom P, Ehrnberg A, Hinmarsh T: Computed tomography examination of the influence of autotraction on herniation of the lumbar disc. Arch Orthop Trauma Surg 104:289–293, 1985
200. Glover JR: Back pain and hyperaesthesia. Lancet 1:1165–1169, 1960
201. Godfrey CM, Morgan PR, Schatzker J: A randomized trial of manipulations for low back pain in a medical setting. Spine 9:301–304, 1984
202. Goldenberg DL: Psychologic studies in fibrositis. Am J Med (suppl 3A) 81:67–81, 1986
203. Goldish GD: Lumbar traction. In Tollison CD, Kriefel ML (eds): Interdisciplinary Rehabilitation of Low Back Pain. Baltimore, Williams & Wilkins, 1989:305–321
204. Gonnella C, Paris S, Kutner M: Reliability in evaluating passive intervertebral motion. Phys Ther 62:437–444, 1982
205. Gorman HO, Gwendolen J: Thoracic kyphosis and mobility: The effect of age. Physiotherapy Practice 3:154–162, 1987
206. Grabias S: The treatment of spinal stenosis. J Bone Joint Surg 60A:308–313, 1980
207. Greenland S, Reisbord LS, Haldeman S, et al: Controlled clinical trials of manipulation: A review and proposal. J Occup Med 22:670–676, 1980
208. Grieve GP: Sciatica and the straight leg-raising test in manipulative treatment. Physiotherapy 58:337–346, 1970
209. Grieve GP: The sacroiliac joint. Physiotherapy 62:384–400, 1976
210. Grieve GP: Lumbar instability. Physiotherapy 68:2–9, 1982
211. Grieve GP: Lumbar instability. In Grieve GP (ed): Modern Manual Therapy of the Vertebral Column. New York, Churchill Livingstone, 1986:416–441
212. Grieve GP: Diagnosis. Physiotherapy Practice 4:73–77, 1988
213. Grieve GP: Pathological changes—Combined regional. In Grieve GP (ed): Common Vertebral Joint Problems, 2nd ed. New York, Churchill Livingstone, 1988:249–298
214. Grieve GP: Clinical features. In Grieve GP (ed): Common Vertebral Joint Problems, 2nd ed. New York, Churchill Livingstone, 1988:299–353
215. Grieve GP: Common patterns of clinical presentation. In Grieve GP (ed): Common Vertebral Joint Problems, 2nd ed. New York, Churchill Livingstone, 1988:355–458

216. Grieve GP: Passive movements. In Grieve GP (ed): Mobilisation of the Spine: A Primary Handbook of Clinical Methods, 5th ed. Edinburgh, Churchill Livingstone, 1991:177–285
217. Grieve GP: Manually assisted or manually resisted movements. In Grieve GP (ed): Mobilisation of the Spine: A Primary Handbook of Clinical Methods, 5th ed. Edinburgh, Churchill Livingstone, 1991:305–318
218. Grieve GP: Active movements. In Grieve GP (ed): Mobilisation of the Spine: A Primary Handbook of Clinical Methods, 5th ed. Edinburgh, Churchill Livingstone, 1991:319–358
219. Grimsby O: Advanced Course: Lumbar– Thoracic Spine. Continuing Education Course, Institute of Graduate Health Sciences, Nashville, TN, 1976
220. Grimsby O: Advanced Extremity Mobilizations. Continuing Education Course, Sorlandet Institute, Portland, OR, 1979
221. Grimsby O: Fundamentals of Manual Therapy: A Course Workbook, 3rd ed. Norway, Sorlandet Fusikalske Institutt, 1981
222. Gunn CC, Milbrandt WE: Tenderness at motor points: A diagnostic and prognostic aid for low back injury. J Bone Joint Surg 58A:815–825, 1976
223. Gunn CC, Milbrandt WE: Early and subtle signs in low back sprain. Spine 3:267–281, 1978
224. Gunnari H, Evjenth O, Brady MM: Sequence Exercise. Oslo, Breyers Forlag, 1983
225. Gustavsen R: Fra aktiv avspenning. Oslo, Olaf Norlis Bokhandel, 1977
226. Gustavsen R, Streeck R: Training Therapy: Prophylaxis and Rehabilitation, 2nd ed. Stutgart, Georg Thieme Verlag, 1993
227. Guymer AJ: Proprioceptive neuromuscular facilitation for vertebral joint conditions. In Grieve GP (ed): Modern Manual Therapy of the Vertebral Column. New York, Churchill Livingstone, 1986:622–634
228. Hackett GS: Referred pain from low back ligament disabilities. AMA Archives of Surgery 73:878–883, 1956
229. Hadler NM: Legal ramifications of the medical definition of back disease. Ann Intern Med 89:992–999, 1978
230. Hadler NM: A critical reappraisal of the fibrositis concept. Am J Med 81A:26–30, 1986
231. Hadler NM: Regional back pain. N Engl J Med 315:1090–1092, 1986
232. Hadler NM: A benefit of spinal manipulations as adjunctive therapy for acute low back pain: A stratified controlled trail. Spine 12:703–706, 1987
233. Haldeman S: Spinal manipulative therapy as a status report. Clin Orthop 179:62–70, 1983
234. Haldeman S: Soft-Tissue Techniques. Challenge of the Lumbar Spine, Ninth Annual Meeting, New York, 1987
235. Hall H, Iceton JA: Back school: An overview with specific reference to the Canadian Back Education Units. Clin Orthop 179:10–17, 1983
236. Hansson P, Ekblom A: Acute pain relieved by vibratory stimulation [letter]. Br Dent J 151:213, 1981
237. Hansson P, Ekblom A: Transcutaneous electrical nerve stimulation (TENS) as compared to placebo: TENS for the relief of acute orofacial pain. Pain 15:157–165, 1983
238. Happey T, Pearson CH, Palframan J, et al: Proteoglycans and glycoproteins associated with collagen in the human intervertebral disc. Z Klin Chem 9:79, 1971
239. Harris RI, MacNab I: Structural changes in the lumbar intervertebral disc: Their relationship to low back pain and sciatica. J Bone Joint Surg 36B:304–322, 1954
240. Hasue M, Fujiwara M, Kikuchi S: A new method of quantitative measurement of abdominal and back muscle strength. Spine 5(2):143–148, 1980
241. Hathaway SR, McKinley JC: A multiphasic personality schedule (Minnesota): I. Construction of the schedule. J Psychol 10:249, 1940
242. Hayne CR: Ergonomics and back pain. Physiotherapy 70:9–13, 1984
243. Hayne CR: Back schools and total care programs. Physiotherapy 70:14–17, 1984
244. Hayne CR: Prophylaxis and ergonomic considerations. In Grieve GP (ed): Modern Manual Therapy of the Vertebral Column. New York, Churchill Livingstone, 1986:860–872
245. Hazard RG, Reid S, Fenwick J, et al: Isokinetic trunk and lifting strength measurements: Variability as an indicator of effort. Spine 13:54–57, 1988
246. Helfet AJ, Gruebel Lee DM: Disorders of the Lumbar Spine. Philadelphia, JB Lippincott, 1978
247. Henderson I: Low back pain and sciatica: Evaluation and surgical management. Aust Fam Phys 14:1149–1159, 1985
248. Hendler N: Psychological tests for chronic pain. In Hendler N: Diagnosis and Nonsurgical Management of Chronic Pain. New York, Raven Press, 1981:101–120
249. Hendry NGS: The hydration of the nucleus pulposus and its relation to intervertebral disc derangement. J Bone Joint Surg 40B:132–144, 1958
250. Hides JA, Stokes MJ, Saide M, et al: Evidence of lumbar multifidus muscle-wasting ipsilateral to symptoms in patients with acute/subacute low back pain. Spine 19:165–172, 1993
251. Hirsch C: Studies on the mechanism of low back pain. Acta Orthop Scand 20:261–273, 1951
252. Hirsch C: The reaction of the intervertebral discs to compressive forces. J Bone Joint Surg 37A:1188–1196, 1955
253. Hirsch C, Ingelmark BE, Miller M: The anatomical basis for low back pain: Studies on the presence of sensory nerve endings in ligamentous, capsular and intervertebral disc structures in the human lumbar spine. Acta Orthop Scand 33:1–17, 1963
254. Hirsch C, Jonsson B, Lewin T: Low-back symptoms in a Swedish female population. Clin Orthop 63:171–176, 1969
255. Hirsch C, Nachemson A: The reliability of lumbar disc surgery. Clin Orthop 29:189–195, 1963
256. Hirschberg GG: Treating lumbar disc lesions by prolonged continuous reduction of intradiscal pressure. Tex Med 70:58–68, 1974
257. Hirschberg GG, Froetscher L, Naem F: Iliolumbar syndrome as a common cause of low back pain: Diagnosis and prognosis. Arch Phys Med Rehabil 60:415–419, 1979
258. Hitselberger WE, Witten RM: Abnormal myelograms in asymptomatic patients. J Neurosurg 28:204–206, 1968
259. Hoehler FK, Tobin JS, Buerger AA: Spinal manipulations for low back pain. JAMA 245:1835–1838, 1981
260. Holten O: Medisinsk Trenigsterapi Trykk. Fugseth and Lorentzen, Medical Training Course, Salt Lake City, 1984
261. Hood LB, Chrisman D: Intermittent pelvic traction in the treatment of the ruptured disc. Phys Ther 48:21–30, 1968
262. Hoppenfeld S: Physical Examination of the Spine and Extremities. New York, Appleton-Century-Crofts, 1976
263. Horal J: The clinical appearance of low back pain disorders in the city of Goteborg, Sweden: Comparison of incapacitated probands and matched controls. Acta Orthop Scand (suppl 118):1–109, 1969
264. Hudgins WR: The crossed straight leg-raising test. N Engl J Med 297:1127, 1977
265. Hult L: The Munfors investigation: A study of the frequency and causes of the stiffneck brachalgia and lumbago-sciatica syndromes as well as observation on certain signs and symptoms from the dorsal spine and the joints of the extremities in industrial and forest workers. Acta Orthop Scand (suppl 16):1–76, 1954
266. Hult L: Cervical, dorsal and lumbar spinal syndromes: A field investigation of a nonselected material of 1200 workers in different occupations with special reference to disc degeneration and so-called muscular rheumatism. Acta Orthop Scand (suppl 17):1–102, 1954
267. Ikata T: Statistical and dynamic studies of lesions due to overloading spine. Shikoku Acta Med 40:262–286, 1965
268. Ingham JG: A method of observing symptoms and attitudes. Br J Soc Clin Psychol 4:131–140, 1965
269. Ingham JG: Quantitative evaluation of subjective symptoms. Proc R Soc Med 62:492–494, 1969
270. Iskrant AP, Smith RW: Osteoporosis in women 45 years and over related to subsequent fracture. Public Health Rep 84:33–38, 1969
271. Jackson CP, Brown MD: Is there a role for exercise in the treatment of patients with low back pain? Clin Orthop 179:39–45, 1983
272. Jackson HC, Winkelmann RK, Bichel WH: Nerve endings in ligamentous, capsular and intervertebral disc structures in the human lumbar spine. J Bone Joint Surg 48A:1272–1281, 1966
273. Jackson RH: Chronic sacroiliac sprain with attendant sciatica. Am J Surg 24:456–477, 1934
274. Janda V: Muscles, central nervous motor regulation and back problems. In Korr I (ed): The Neurobiologic Mechanisms in Manipulative Therapy. London, Plenum Press, 1978:27–42
275. Janda V: Muscle Function Testing. Boston, Butterworths, 1983
276. Janda V: Muscle weakness and inhibition (pseudoparesis) in back pain syndromes. In Grieve GP (ed): Modern Manual Therapy of the Vertebral Column. New York, Churchill Livingstone, 1986:197–201
277. Janda V, Schmid HJA: Muscles as a pathogenic factor in back pain. Proceedings, 4th Conference of International Federation of Orthopaedic Manipulative Therapists, Christchurch, New Zealand, 1980
278. Jayson MIV, Sim-Williams H, Young S, et al: Mobilization and manipulations for low back pain. Spine 6:409–416, 1981
279. Johansson F, Almay BG, von Knorring L, et al: Predictors for the outcome of treatment with high-frequency transcutaneous electrical nerve stimulation in patients with chronic pain. Pain 9:55–61, 1980
280. Johnson G: Functional Orthopaedics II: Advanced Techniques of Soft-Tissue Mobilizations for Evaluation and Treatment of the Extremities and Trunk. Continuing Education Course, San Francisco, 1985
281. Jones MD: Basic Diagnostic Radiology. St. Louis, CV Mosby, 1969
282. Jorgensen K: Back muscle strength and body weight as limiting factors for work in the standing slightly stooped position. Scand J Rehabil Med 2:149–153, 1970
283. Judovich B, Nobel GP: Lumbar traction therapy: A study of resistive forces. Am J Surg 93:108–114, 1957
284. Jull GA: Examination of the lumbar spine. In Grieve GP (ed): Modern Manual Therapy of the Vertebral Column. New York, Churchill Livingstone, 1986:547–560
285. Jull GA, Janda V: Muscles and motor control in low back pain: Assessment and management. In Twomey LT, Taylor JR (eds): Physical Therapy of the Low Back. New York, Churchill Livingstone, 1987:253–278
286. Jungham H: Spondylolisthesen ohne Spalt im Zwischengelenkstuck (pseudospondylolisthesen). Arch Orthop Unfall-chir, 29:118–123, 1930
287. Jungham H: Die wirbelsaule in der Arbeitmedizin. Wirbel saule Forch Praxis 79:1–395 Teil II, 1979
288. Kahanovitz N, Nordin M, Verderame R, et al: Normal trunk muscle strength and endurance in women and the effect of exercises and electrical stimulation: Part 2. Comparative analysis of electrical stimulation and exercise to increase trunk muscle strength and endurance. Spine 12(2):112–118, 1987
289. Kaltenborn FM: Test Segment: Moblis Columbia Vertebris. Oslo, Freddy Kaltenborn, 1975
290. Kaltenborn FM: Manual Therapy for the Extremity Joints. Oslo, Olaf Norlis Bokhandel, 1976
291. Kaltenborn FM: Manual Mobilizations of the Extremity Joints: Vol II. Advanced Treatment Techniques. Oslo, Olaf Norlis Bokhandel, 1986
292. Kalyan-Raman UP, Kalyan-Raman K, Yunus MB, et al: Muscle pathology in primary fibromyalgia syndrome: Light microscopic, histochemical and ultrastructural study. J Rheumatol 11:808–813, 1984
293. Kane RL, Craig L, Olsen D, et al: Manipulating the patient: A comparison of the effectiveness of physician and chiropractor care. Lancet 1:1333–1336, 1974
294. Kavanagh T: Exercise: The modern panacea. Ir Med J 72:24–27, 1979
295. Keegan JJ: Alterations to the lumbar curve related to posture and seating. J Bone Joint Surg 35:589—603, 1953
296. Keene JS, Drummond DS: Mechanical back pain in the athlete. Compr Ther 11:7–14, 1985
297. Kellgren JH: On the distribution of pain arising from deep somatic structures with charts of segmental pain areas. Clin Sci 4:35, 1939
298. Kelsey JL: An epidemiological study of the relationship between occupations and acute herniated lumbar intervertebral discs. Int J Epidemiol 4:1997–204, 1975
299. Kelsey JL, Hardy RJ: Driving a motor vehicle as a risk factor for acute herniated lumbar intervertebral disc. Am J Epidemiol 102:63–67, 1975
300. Kelsey JL, White AA: Epidemiology and impact of low-back pain. Spine 5:133–142, 1980
301. Kendall FP, Mc Creary EK, Provance PG: Muscles: Testing and Function, 4th ed. Baltimore, Williams & Wilkins, 1993
302. Kendall PH, Jenkins JM: Exercises for backache: A double-blind controlled study. Physiotherapy 54:154–157, 1968
303. Kenna O, Murtagh A: The physical examination of the back. Aust Fam Physician 14:1244–1256, 1985
304. Kennedy B: An Australian programme for management of back problems. Physiotherapy 66:108–111, 1980
305. Kessler RM: Acute symptomatic disc prolapse: Clinical manifestations and therapeutic considerations. Phys Ther 59:978–987, 1979

306. Keyes DC, Compere EL: The normal and pathological physiology of the nucleus pulposus of the intervertebral disc. J Bone Joint Surg 14:897–938, 1932
307. Keyserling WM, Herrin GD, Chaffin DB: Isometric strength testing as a means of controlling medical incidents on strenuous jobs. J Occup Med 22:332–336, 1980
308. Kirkaldy-Willis WH: The three phases of the spectrum of degenerative disease. In Kirkaldy-Willis WH (ed): Managing Low Back Pain. New York, Churchill Livingstone, 1983:75–90
309. Kirkaldy-Willis WH: Manipulation. In Kirkaldy-Willis WH (ed): Managing Low Back Pain. New York, Churchill Livingstone, 1983:175–183
310. Kirkaldy-Willis WH: The relationship of structural pathology to the nerve root. Spine 9:49–52, 1984
311. Kirkaldy-Willis WH (ed): Managing Low Back Pain, 2nd ed. New York, Churchill Livingstone, 1988
312. Kirkaldy-Willis WH, Wedge JH, Yong-Hing K, et al: Lumbar spinal nerve entrapment. Clin Orthop 169:171–178, 1982
313. Kishino ND, Mayer TG, Gatchel J, McCrate Parrish M, et al: Qualification of lumbar function IV: Isometric and isotonic lifting simulation in normal subjects and low-back dysfunction patients. Spine 10:921–927, 1985
314. Klaber Moffett JA, Chase SM, Portek I, et al: A controlled prospective study to evaluate the effectiveness of a back school in low back pain. Spine 11:120–122, 1986
315. Knott M, Voss DE: Proprioceptive Neuromuscular Facilitation, 2nd ed. New York, Harper & Row, 1968
316. Kopala B, Matassarin-Jacobs E: Sensory-perceptual pain assessment. In Bellack J, Banford PA (eds): Nursing Assessment: A Multidimensional Approach. Belmont, CA, Wadsworth, 1984
317. Korr IM: Proprioceptive and somatic dysfunction. J Am Osteopath Assoc 74: 123–135, 1975
318. Kos J, Wolf J: Intervertebral menisci and their possible role in intervertebral blockage. Bulletin of the Orthopedic Section, American Physical Therapy Association 1:8, 1976
319. Kraft GL, Johnson EW, LaBan MM: Fibrositis syndrome. Arch Phys Med Rehabil 49:155–162, 1968
320. Kraft GL, Levinthal DH: Facet synovial impingement. Surg Gynecol Obstet 93:439–443, 1951
321. Kramer J: Intervertebral Disc Disease. Chicago, Year Book Medical Publishers, 1987
322. Kroemer KHE, Robinette JC: Ergonomics in the design of office furniture. Industr Med Surg 38:115–125, 1969
323. Kvien TK, Nilsen H, Vik P: Education and self-care of patients with low back pain. Scand J Rheumatol 10:318–320, 1981
324. La Freniere JG: The Low-Back Patient: Procedures for Treatment by Physical Therapy. New York, Masson, 1979
325. La Freniere JG: La Freniere Body Techniques. Chicago, Year Book Medical Publishers, 1984
326. Lageard P, Robinson M: Back pain: Current concepts and recent advances. Physiotherapy 72:105, 1986
327. Lamb DW: A review of manual therapy for spinal pain with reference to the lumbar spine. In Grieve GP (ed): Modern Manual Therapy of the Vertebral Column. New York, Churchill Livingstone, 1986:605–621
328. Lancourt JE: Traction technique for low back pain. J Musculoskel Med 3:44–50, 1986
329. Langrana N, Lee C, Alexander H, et al: Quantitative assessment of back strength using isokinetic testing. Spine 9:287–290, 1984
330. Lankhorst GL, Vanderstadt RJ, Vogelaar JW, et al: The effect of the Swedish back school in chronic idiopathic low back pain. Scand J Rehabil Med 15:141–145, 1983
331. Larsson V, Choler V, Lidstrom A, et al: Autotraction for treatment of lumbago-sciatica. Acta Orthop Scand 51:791–798, 1980
332. Laslett M: The role of physical therapy in soft tissue rheumatism. Patient Management 15:57–68, 1986
333. Laslett M: Use of manipulative therapy for mechanical pain of spinal origin. Orthop Rev 16:65–73, 1987
334. Lawrence JS: Rheumatism in coal miners: Part III. Occupational factors. Br J Industr Med 12:249–261, 1955
335. Lee CL: Work hardening: Return to work and work hardening [abstr]. Challenge of the Lumbar Spine: 9th annual meeting, New York, 1987
336. Lee SLK, Wesers B, McInnis S, et al: Analysing risk factors for preventive back education approaches: A review. Physiother Can 40:88–98, 1988
337. Lettin AWF: Diagnosis and treatment of lumbar instability. J Bone Joint Surg 49B:520–529, 1967
338. Levernieux J: Traction Vertebrale. Paris, Expansion Scientifique, 1960
339. Lewin T: Osteoarthrosis in lumbar synovial joints. Gottesborg, Orstadius Bokryckeri Aktiebolag, 1964
340. Lewin T, Moffett B, Viidik A: The morphology of the lumbar synovial intervertebral joints. Acta Morph Neder Scand 4:299–319, 1962
341. Leyshon A, Kirwan E, Wynn-Parry GB: Is it nerve root pain? J Bone Joint Surg 62B:119, 1980
342. Lichter R: Work hardening: Simulated job training using work performances for worker rehabilitation and testing [abstr]. Challenge of the Lumbar Spine: 9th annual meeting, New York, 1987
343. Lichter RL, Hewson JK, Radke S, et al: Treatment of chronic low-back pain. Clin Orthop 190:115–123, 1984
344. Lind G: Autotraction: Treatment of Low Back Pain and Sciatica. Thesis, University of Kinkopinj, 1974
345. Lind GAM: Autotraction treatment of low back pain and sciatica. Scand J Rehabil Med 2:37–42, 1974
346. Lindblom K: Technique and results in myelography and disc puncture. Acta Radiol 34:321–330, 1950
347. Lindblom K: Technique and result of diagnostic disc puncture and injection (discography) in the lumbar region. Acta Orthop Scand 20:316–326, 1951
348. Lindblom K: Intervertebral disc degeneration considered as a pressure atrophy. J Bone Joint Surg 39A:933–945, 1957
349. Linton SJ: The relationship between activity and chronic pain. Pain 21:289–294, 1985
350. Lippit AB: The facet joint and its role in spine pain management with facet joint injections. Spine 9:746–750, 1984
351. Lipson SJ, Muir H: Proteoglycans in experimental intervertebral disc degeneration. Spine 6:194–210, 1981
352. Liston CB: Back schools and ergonomics. In Twomey LT, Taylor JR (eds): Physical Therapy of the Low Back. New York, Churchill Livingstone, 1987:279–303
353. Liyang D, Yinkan X, Wenming Z, et al: The effect of flexion–extension motion of the lumbar spine on the capacity of the spinal canal. Spine 14:523–525, 1989
354. Ljunggren AE, Eldevik P: Autotraction in lumbar disk herniation with CT examination before and after treatment, showing no change in appearance of the herniated tissue. J Oslo Hosp 36:87–91, 1986
355. Ljunggren AE, Weber H, Larson S: Autotraction versus manual traction in patients with prolapsed lumbar intervertebral disks. Scand J Rehabil Med 16:117–124, 1984
356. Llewellyn RLJ, Jones AB: Fibrositis. London, Heinemann, 1915
357. Loebl WY: Measurement of spinal posture and range of spinal movement. Ann Phys Med 7:103–110, 1967
358. Lundeberg T: Vibratory stimulation for alleviation of chronic pain. Acta Physiol Scand [Suppl] 523:8–51, 1983
359. Lundeberg T: Long-term results of vibratory stimulation as a pain-relieving measure for chronic pain. Pain 20:13–23, 1984
360. Lundeberg T, Nordemar R, Ottoson D: Pain alleviation by vibratory stimulation. Pain 20:25–44, 1984
361. Lyon HE, Jones FE, Quinn FE, et al: Changes in the protein-polysaccharide fraction of the nucleus pulposus from human intervertebral disc with age and disc herniation. J Lab Clin Med 68:930, 1966
362. MacNab I: Chemonucleolysis. Clin Neurosurg 20:183–191, 1973
363. MacNab I: Backache, 2nd ed. Baltimore, Williams & Wilkins, 1990
364. MacRae IF, Wright V: Measurement of back movement. Ann Rheum Dis 28:584–589, 1969
365. Magee DJ: Orthopedic Physical Assessment, 2nd ed. Philadelphia, WB Saunders, 1992
366. Magora A: Investigation of the relation between low back pain and occupation: Age, sex, community, education and other factors. Industr Med Surg 39:465–471, 1970
367. Magora A: Investigation of the relation between low back pain and occupation: 2. Work history. Industr Med Surg 39:504–510, 1970
368. Magora A: Investigation of the relation between low back pain and occupation: 3. Physical requirements: Sitting, standing and weight-lifting. Industr Med Surg 41:5–9, 1972
369. Magora A: Investigation of the relation between low back pain and occupation: 4. Physical requirements: Bending, rotation, reaching, and sudden maximal effort. Scand J Rehabil Med 5:186–190, 1973
370. Magora A: Investigation of the relation between low back pain and occupation: 7. Neurologic and orthopedic conditions. Scand Rehabil Med 7(4):146–151, 1975
371. Magora A, Schwartz A: Relation between the low back pain syndrome and X-ray findings: I. Degenerative osteoarthritis. Scand J Rehabil Med 8:115–125, 1976
372. Maigne R: Orthopaedic Medicine. Springfield, IL, Charles C. Thomas, 1976
373. Maigne R: Manipulation of the spine. In Rogoff JB (ed): Manipulations, Traction and Massage, 2nd ed. Baltimore, Williams & Wilkins, 1980:59–120
374. Maitland GD: Movement of pain-sensitive structures in the vertebral canal in a group of physiotherapy students. S Afr J Physiother 36:4–12, 1980
375. Maitland GD: Vertebral Manipulation, 5th ed. Boston, Butterworths, 1986
376. Maitland GD: The Maitland concept: Assessment, examination and treatment by passive movements. In Twomey LT, Taylor JR (eds): Physical Therapy of the Low Back. New York, Churchill Livingstone, 1987:135–156
377. Mandal AC: The correct height of school furniture. Physiotherapy 70:48–53, 1984
378. Mannheimer JS, Lampe GN: Clinical Transcutaneous Electrical Nerve Stimulation. Philadelphia, FA Davis, 1984
379. Masi AT, Muhammad B, Yunus MD: Concepts of illness in populations as applied to fibromyalgia syndromes. Am J Med [Suppl 3A]81:19–25, 1986
380. Matheson L, Ogden L: Work Tolerance Screening. Trabues Canyon, CA, Rehabilitation Institute of Southern California, 1983
381. Mathews J: Dynamic discography: A study of lumbar traction. Ann Phys Med 9:275–279, 1968
382. Mathews J: The effects of spinal traction. Physiotherapy 58:64–66, 1972
383. Mathews JA, Hickling J: Lumbar traction: A double-blind controlled study for sciatica. Rheumatol Rehabil 14:222–225, 1975
384. Mathews JA, Mills SB, Jenkins VM, et al: Back pain and sciatica: Controlled trials of manipulation, traction, sclerosant and epidural injections. Br J Rheumatol 26:416–423, 1987
385. Matson DD, Woods RP, Campbell JB, et al: Diastematomyelia (congenital clefts of the spinal cord). Pediatrics 6:98–112, 1950
386. Mattmiller AW: The California back school. Physiotherapy 66:118–121, 1986
387. Maxwell TD: The piriformis muscle and its relation to the long-legged syndrome. J Can Chiro Assoc 51:10–24, 1978
388. May P: Exercise and training for spinal patients: Part A. Movement awareness and stabilization training. In Basmajian JV, Nyberg R (eds): Rational Manual Therapies. Baltimore, Williams & Wilkins, 1993:347–359
389. Mayer DJ, Price DD: CNS mechanisms of analgesia. Pain 2:379–404, 1976
390. Mayer H, Mayer TG: Functional restoration: New concepts in spinal rehabilitation. In Kirkaldy-Willis (ed): Managing Low Back Pain. New York, Churchill Livingstone, 1988
391. Mayer TG: Rehabilitation of the patient with spinal pain. Orthop Clin North Am 14:623–637, 1983
392. Mayer TG, Gatchel RJ: Functional Restoration for Spinal Disorders: The Sports Medicine Approach. Philadelphia, Lea & Febiger, 1988
393. Mayer TG, Gatchel RJ, Kishino N, et al: Objective assessment of spine function following industrial injury: A prospective study with comparison and 1-year follow-up. Spine 10:482–493, 1985
394. Mayer TG, Kishino N, Kedy J, et al: Using physical measurements to assess low back pain. J Musculoskel Med 2:44–51, 1985
395. Mayer TG, Smith SS, Keeley J, Mooney V: Qualification of lumbar function: II. Sagittal plane trunk strength in chronic low-back pain patients. Spine 10:765–772, 1985
396. Mayer TG, Smith SS, Tencer A, et al: Measurement of Isometric and Multispeed Isokinetic Strength of Lumbar Spine Musculature Using a Prototype Cybex Testing Device on Normal Subjects and Patients with Chronic Low Back Pain. Proceedings of the International Society for Study of the Lumbar Spine, Montreal, 1983
397. Mayer TG, Tencer AF, Kristoferson S, et al: Use of noninvasive techniques for qualification of spinal range-of-motion in normal subjects and chronic low-back dysfunction patients. Spine 9:588–595, 1984
398. Mazess RB: On aging bone loss. Clin Orthop 165:237–252, 1983
399. McCain GA: Role of physical fitness training in the fibrositis/fibromyalgia syndrome. Am J Med [Suppl 3A]81:73–77, 1986

400. McCall IW, Park WM, O'Brien JP: Induced pain referral from posterior lumbar elements in normal subjects. Spine 4:441–448, 1979
401. McCarthy RE: Coping with low back pain through behavioral change. Orthop Nurs 3:30–35, 1983
402. McKenna O, Murtagh A: The physical examination of the back. Aust Fam Physician 14:1244–1256, 1985
403. McKenzie RA: Manual correction of sciatic scoliosis. NZ Med J 76(484):194–199, 1972
404. McKenzie RA: Prophylaxis in recurrent low back pain. NZ Med J 89:22–23, 1979
405. McKenzie RA: Treat Your Own Back. Waikanae, New Zealand, Spinal Publications Ltd, 1980
406. McKenzie RA: The Lumbar Spine: Mechanical Diagnosis and Therapy. Waikanae, New Zealand, Spinal Publications Ltd, 1981
407. McKenzie RA: Mechanical diagnosis and therapy for low back pain: Toward a better understanding. In Twomey LT, Taylor JR (eds): Physical Therapy of the Low Back. New York, Churchill Livingstone, 1987:157–174
408. McKinley JC, Hathaway SR: The identification and measurement of the neuroses in medical practice. JAMA 23:161–167, 1943
409. McNeal RL: Aquatic therapy for patients with rheumatic disease. Rheum Dis Clin North Am 16:915–929, 1990
410. McNeill T, Warwick D, Andersson G, et al: Trunk strengths in attempted flexion, extension and lateral bending in healthy subjects and patients with low back disorders. Spine 5:529–538, 1980
411. McQuarrie A: Physical therapy. In Kirkaldy-Willis WH (ed): Managing Low Back Pain. New York, Churchill Livingstone, 1988:345–354
412. Meagher J, Boughton P: Sports Massage. New York, Doubleday, 1980
413. Meikle JCE: The Minnesota Multiphasic Personality Inventory (MMPI) and back pain. Clin Rehabil 1:143–145, 1987
414. Melzack R: The Puzzle of Pain. New York, Basic Books Inc, 1973
415. Melzack R: The McGill pain questionnaire: Major properties and scoring methods. Pain 1:277–299, 1975
416. Melzack R, Vetere P, Finch L: TENS for low back pain. Phys Ther 63:489–493, 1983
417. Melzack R, Wall PD: The Challenge of Pain. New York, Basic Books Inc, 1983
418. Mennell JB: The Science and Art of Joint Manipulation, Vol. 2. London, Churchill, 1952
419. Mennell JMCM: Back Pain. Boston, Little, Brown & Co, 1960
420. Mennell JMCM: Joint Pain. Boston, Little, Brown & Co, 1960
421. Miller WT: Introduction to Clinical Radiology. New York, Macmillan, 1982
422. Mitchell FL: An Evaluation and Treatment Manual of Osteopathic Muscle Energy Procedures, 1st ed. Valley Park, MO, Mitchell Moran Pruzzo, 1979
423. Mitchell PEG, Hendry MGC, Billewicz WZ: The chemical background of intervertebral disc prolapse. J Bone Joint Surg 43B:141–151, 1961
424. Mixter WJ, Barr JS: Rupture of the intervertebral disc with involvement of the spinal canal. N Engl J Med 211:210–215, 1934
425. Moll JMH, Liyanange SP, Wright V: An objective clinical method to measure lateral spine flexion. Rheum Phys Med 11:225–239, 1972
426. Moll JMH, Liyanange SP, Wright V: An objective clinical method to measure spinal extension. Rheum Phys Med 11:293–312, 1972
427. Moll JMH, Wright V: Measurement of spinal movement. In Jayson M (ed): The Lumbar Spine and Back Pain. New York, Grune & Stratton, 1981:93–112
428. Mooney V: Alternative approaches for the patient beyond the help of surgery. Orthop Clin 6:331–334, 1975
429. Mooney V: The syndromes of low back disease. Orthop Clin North Am 14:505–515, 1983
430. Mooney V: Evaluation and guidelines for nonoperative care of the low back. In Stauffer SE (ed): American Academy of Orthopaedic Surgeons—Instructional Course Lectures. St. Louis, CV Mosby, 1985
431. Mooney V, Cairns D, Robertson JA: A system for evaluating and treating chronic back disability. West J Med 124:370–376, 1976
432. Mooney V, Robertson J: The facet syndrome. Clin Orthop 115:149–156, 1976
433. Moore M: Endorphins and exercise: A puzzling relationship. Phys Sports Med 10:111–114, 1982
434. Moran FP, King T: Primary instability of the lumbar vertebrae as a common cause of low back pain. J Bone Joint Surg 39B:6–22, 1957
435. Morgan D: Concepts in functional training and postural stabilization for low-back-injured. Topics in Acute Care and Trauma Rehabilitation: Part II. Clinical Applications. Aspen, CO, Aspen Publishers Inc, 1988
436. Morgan D, Vollowitz E: Training the Patient with Low Back Dysfunction. Folsom Physical Therapy Education Division, Folsom, CA, 1988
437. Morris JM, Lucus DB, Besler B: The role of the trunk in the stability of the spine. J Bone Joint Surg 43A:327–351, 1961
438. Morris JM, Markoff KL: Biomechanics of the lumbar spine. In American Academy of Orthopaedic Surgeons: Atlas of Orthotics. St. Louis, CV Mosby, 1975:312–331
439. Mottice M, Goldberg D, Bennr EK, et al: Soft-Tissue Mobilization. Monroe Falls, Ohio, JEMD Publications, 1986
440. Mulligan BR: Belt techniques. In Grieve GP (ed): Modern Manual Therapy of the Vertebral Column. New York, Churchill Livingstone, 1986
441. Murtagh J, Findlay D, Kenna C: Low back pain. Aust Fam Physician 14:1214–1224, 1985
442. Murtagh JE, McKenna OJ: Muscle energy therapy. Aust Fam Physician 15:756–765, 1987
443. Myrin SO: Bedomining av Ryggpatienter. Stockholm, LIC Rehab, 1978
444. Nachemson AL: The load on lumbar discs in different positions of the body. Clin Orthop 45:107–122, 1966
445. Nachemson AL: Towards a better understanding of low back pain: A review of the mechanics of the lumbar disc. Rheum Rehabil 14:129–143, 1975
446. Nachemson AL: The lumbar spine: An orthopedic challenge. Spine 1:59–71, 1976
447. Nachemson AL: Work for all: For those with low back pain as well. Clin Orthop 179:77–85, 1983
448. Nachemson AL: Lumbar instability: A critical update and symposium summary. Spine 10:290–291, 1985
449. Nachemson AL: Recent advances in the treatment of low back pain. Intern Orthop 9:1–10, 1985
450. Nachemson A, Bigos SJ: The low back. In Cruess RL, Rennie WRJ (eds): Adult Orthopedics, Vol. 2. New York, Churchill Livingstone, 1984:843–938
451. Nachemson A, Lindh M: Measurement of abdominal and back muscle strength with and without low back pain. Scand J Rehabil Med 1:60–65, 1965
452. Nachemson A, Morris JM: In vivo measurement of intradiskal pressures. J Bone Joint Surg 46A:1077–1092, 1964
453. Nagi SZ, Riley LE, Newby LG: A social epidemiology of back pain in a general population. J Chronic Dis 26:769–779, 1973
454. Nassim R, Burrows HJ (eds): Modern Trends in Diseases of Vertebral Column. London, Butterworths, 1959
455. Natchev E: A Manual on Autotraction Treatment for Low Back Pain. Stockholm, E Natchev, 1984
456. Natchev E, Valentino V: Low back pain and disc hernia observation during autotraction treatment. Manual Med 1:39–42, 1984
457. Naylor A: The biophysical and biochemical aspects of intervertebral disc herniation and degeneration. Ann R Coll Surg 31:91–114, 1962
458. Naylor A: Intervertebral disc prolapse and degeneration. Spine 1:108–114, 1976
459. Naylor A, Happey F, MacRae T: The collagenous changes in the intervertebral disc with age and their effect on its elasticity. Br Med J 2:570–573, 1954
460. Nelson MA, Allen P, Clamp SE, et al: Reliability and reproducibility of clinical findings in low back pain. Spine 4:97–101, 1979
461. Newman PH: "Sprung back." J Bone Joint Surg 34B:30–37, 1952
462. Newman PH: The etiology of spondylolisthesis. J Bone Joint Surg 45B:39–59, 1963
463. Newman PH: The spine, the wood and the trees. Proc R Soc Med 61:35–41, 1968
464. Newman PH: Surgical treatment for derangement of the lumbar spine. J Bone Joint Surg 55B:7–19, 1973
465. Nicolaisen T, Jorgensen K: Trunk strength, back muscle endurance and low-back trouble. Scand J Rehabil Med 17:121–127, 1985
466. Norby E: Epidemiology and diagnosis in low back injury. Occup Health Safety 50:38–42, 1981
467. Nordin M, Kahanovitz N, Verderame R, et al: Normal trunk muscle strength and endurance in women and the effect of exercise and electrical stimulation, Part I: Normal endurance and trunk muscle strength in 101 women. Spine 12(2):105–111, 1987
468. Norris CM: Physical training and injury. In Norris CM (ed): Sports Injuries: Diagnosis and Management for Physiotherapists. Oxford, Butterworths-Heinemann, 1993:89–116
469. Nosse LJ: Inverted spinal traction. Arch Phys Med Rehabil 59:367–370, 1978
470. Nummi J, Jarvinen T, Stambej U, et al: Diminished dynamic performance capacity of back and abdominal muscles in concrete-reinforcement workers. Scand J Work Environ Health 4(Suppl 1):39–46, 1985
471. Nyberg R: Clinical assessment of the low back: Active movement and palpation testing. In Basmajian JV, Nyberg R (eds): Rational Manual Therapies. Baltimore, Williams & Wilkins, 1993:97–140
472. O'Brian JP: The role of fusion for chronic low back pain. Orthop Clin North Am 14:639–647, 1983
473. O'Connell JEA: Protrusion of lumbar intervertebral discs: A clinical review based on 500 cases treated by excision of the protrusion. J Bone Joint Surg 33B:8–30, 1951
474. Oliver JO, Lynn JW, Lynn JM: An interpretation of the McKenzie approach to low back pain. In Twomey LT, Taylor JR (eds): Physical Therapy of the Low Back. New York, Churchill Livingstone, 1987:225–251
475. Onishi N, Nomara H: Low back pain in relation to physical work capacity and local tenderness. J Human Ergo 2:119–132, 1973
476. Orwell ES: The influence of exercise on osteoporosis and skeletal health. In Goldberg L, Elliot DL (eds): Exercise for Prevention and Treatment of Illness. Philadelphia, FA Davis, 1994:228–244
477. Ottenbacker K, Defabio RP: Efficacy of spinal manipulations/mobilization therapy: A meta-analysis. Spine 10:833–837, 1985
478. Ottoson D, Ekblom A, Hansson P: Vibratory stimulation for the relief of pain of dental origin. Pain 10:37–45, 1981
479. Oudenhoven RC: Gravitational lumbar traction. Arch Phys Med Rehabil 59:510–512, 1978
480. Pace JB, Nagle D: Piriformis syndrome. West J Med 124:435–439, 1976
481. Palastanga N: The use of transverse frictions of the soft tissue. In Grieve GP (ed): Modern Manual Therapy of the Vertebral Column. New York, Churchill Livingstone, 1986:819–826
482. Palastanga N: Connective tissue massage. In Grieve GP (ed): Modern Manual Therapy of the Vertebral Column. New York, Churchill Livingstone, 1986:827–833
483. Paris SV: The theory and technique of specific spinal manipulations. NZ Med J 62:320–321, 1963
484. Paris SV: The Spinal Lesion. New Zealand, Pegasus Press, 1965
485. Paris SV: Mobilization of the spine. Phys Ther 59:988–995, 1979
486. Paris SV: Anatomy as related to function and pain. Orthop Clin North Am 14:475–489, 1983
487. Paris SV: Clinical decision: Orthopaedic physical therapy. In Wolf SL (ed): Clinical Decision-Making in Physical Therapy. Philadelphia, FA Davis, 1985:215–254
488. Paris SV: Physical signs of instability. Spine 10:277–279, 1985
489. Park WM: Radiological investigation of the intervertebral disc. In Jayson MIV (ed): The Lumbar Spine and Back Pain, 2nd ed. Kent, England, Pittman, 1980:185–230
490. Parker I: Beyond conventional exercise. Forum July 24:4–7, 1992
491. Parker I: Integrated Feldenkrais for Stabilization Approach to Exercise: The Connecting Link Between the Neurological and Musculoskeletal System. Continuing education course. Seattle, 1993
492. Parson W, Cummings J: Mechanical traction in the lumbar disc syndrome. Can Med Assoc J 77:7–11, 1957
493. Pederson OF, Peterson R, Staffeldt ES: Back pain and isometric back muscle strength of workers in a Danish factory. Scand J Rehabil Med 7(3): 125–128, 1975
494. Peltier LF: The classic back strain and sciatica. Clin Orthop 219(6):4–6, 1987
495. Pheasant HC: Sources of failure in laminectomies. Orthop Clin North Am 6:319–329, 1975
496. Piedalla P: Problemes sacroiliaques. Home Sain II. Bordeaux, Biere, 1952
497. Pope MH: Rosen JD, Wilder DG, et al: The relation between biomechanical and psychological factors in patients with low back pain. Spine 5:173–178, 1980
498. Porter RW, Hibbert C, Evans C: The natural history of the root entrapment syndrome. Spine 9:418–421, 1984
499. Porterfield JA: The sacro-iliac joint. In Gould JA, Davies GJ (eds): Orthopaedic and Sports Physical Therapy. St. Louis, CV Mosby, 1985:550–580
500. Porterfield JA, Mostardi RA, King S, et al: Simulated lift testing using computerized isokinetics. Spine 12:683–687, 1987
501. Posner I, White AA, Edwards WT, et al: A biomechanical analysis of the clinical stability of the lumbar and lumbosacral spine. Spine 7:374–389, 1982

502. Pritzker KPH: Aging and degeneration in the lumbar intervertebral discs. Orthop Clin North Am 8:65–75, 1977
503. Pug MM, Laorden ML, Miralles FS, et al: Endorphin levels in cerebrospinal fluid of patients with postoperative and chronic pain. Anesthesiology 57:1–4, 1982
504. Quebec Task Force on Spinal Disorders: Report. Spine [Suppl] 12:S1–S54, 1987
505. Rae PS, Waddell B, Verner RM: A simple technique for measuring lumbar flexion. J Roy Coll Surg Edinb 29:281–284, 1984
506. Ramani PS, Perry RH, Tomlinson BE: Role of ligamentum flavum in the symptomatology of prolapsed lumbar intervertebral disc. J Neurol Neurosurg Psychiatry 38:550–557, 1975
507. Ransford AO, Cairns D, Mooney V: The pain drawing as an aid to the psychologic evaluation of patients with low back pain. Spine 1:127–134, 1976
508. Rasmussen GG: Manipulation in the treatment of low back pain: A randomized clinical trial [abstr]. Man Med 1:8–21, 1979
509. Reuler JB: Low back pain. West J Med 143:259–265, 1985
510. Ritchie JH, Faharni WH: Age changes in intervertebral discs. Can J Surg 13:65–71, 1970
511. Ritzy S, Lorren T, Simpson S, et al: Rehabilitation of degenerative disease of the spine. In Hochschuler SH, Colter HB, Guyer RD (eds): Rehabilitation of the Spine: Science and Practice. St. Louis, CV Mosby, 1993:457–481
512. Robinson R: The new back school prescription: Stabilization training: Part I. Occupational Medicine: State of the Art Review. Philadelphia, Hanley & Belfus, 1992:17–31
513. Rockey PH, Tomkins RK, Wood RW: The usefulness of X-ray examination in the evaluation of patients with back pain. J Fam Pract 7:455–465, 1978
514. Rockoff SD, Sweet E, Bluestein J: The relative contribution of trabecular and cortical bone to the strength of human lumbar vertebrae. Calcif Tissue Res 3:163–175, 1969
515. Roofe PG: Innervation of annulus fibrosis and posterior longitudinal ligaments: Fourth and fifth lumbar level. Arch Neurol Psych 44:100–103, 1940
516. Rosomoff HL, Rosomoff RS: Nonsurgical aggressive treatment of lumbar spinal stenosis. Spine: State of the Art Review 1:383–400, 1987
517. Rothman RH: Indications for lumbar fusion. Clin Neurosurg 20:215–219, 1973
518. Rothman RH, Simeone FA: The Spine. Philadelphia, WB Saunders, 1982
519. Rovere GD: Low back pain in athletes. Phys Sports Med 15:105–117, 1987
520. Rowe ML: Low back pain in industry: A position paper. J Occup Med 11(4):161–169, 1969
521. Saal JA: Rehabilitation of sports-related lumbar spine injuries. In Saal JA (ed): Physical Medicine and Rehabilitation: State of the Art Reviews. Philadelphia, Hanley & Belfus, 1987:613–637
522. Saal JA: The new back school prescription: Stabilization training: Part II. Occupational Medicine: State of the Art Review. Philadelphia, Hanley & Belfus, 1992:33–42
523. Sahrmann S: A program for correction of muscular imbalance and mechanical imbalance. Clin Manag 3:23–28, 1983
524. Sahrmann S: Diagnosis and Treatment of Muscle Imbalances and Regional Pain Syndromes, Level II course notes. Seattle, 1993
525. Salib R: Gravity lumbar reduction traction—The results for documented lumbar disc herniation. Presented at the meeting of the Society for the Study of the Lumbar Spine, Sydney, Australia, 1985
526. Saliba VL, Johnson G: Lumbar protective mechanism. In White AH, Anderson R (eds): Conservative Care of Low Back Pain. Baltimore, Williams & Wilkins, 1991:112–119
527. Salisbury PJ, Porter RW: Measurement of lumbar sagittal mobility: A comparison of methods. Spine 12(2):190–193, 1987
528. Sallade J: Variation on Robin McKenzie's technique for correction of lateral shift. J Orthop Sports Phys Ther 8:417–420, 1987
529. Sanborn GE, Friberg TE, Allen R: Optic nerve dysfunction during gravity inversion: Visual field abnormalities. Arch Ophthalmol 105:774–776, 1987
530. Saunders DH: Use of spinal traction in the treatment of neck and back conditions. Clin Orthop 179:31–37, 1983
531. Saunders DH: Educational back care programs. In Saunders DH (ed): Evaluation, Treatment and Prevention of Musculoskeletal Disorders. Minneapolis, Viking Press, 1985:297–324
532. Saunders DH: Evaluation, Treatment and Prevention of Musculoskeletal Disorders. Minneapolis, Viking Press, 1985
533. Sawyer WM: The role of the physical therapist before and after lumbar spine surgery. Orthop Clin North Am 14:649–659, 1983
534. Scham SM, Taylor TKF: Tension signs in lumbar disc prolapse. Clin Orthop 75:195–204, 1971
535. Schatz MP: Living with your lower back. Yoga Journal July/August: 316–345, 1984
536. Schatz MP: Back Care Basics. Berkeley, Rodmell Press, 1992
537. Schatzker J, Pennal GF: Spinal stenosis, a cause of cauda equina compression. J Bone Joint Surg 50B:606–608, 1968
538. Schmorl G, Jungham H: The Human Spine in Health and Disease, 2nd ed. New York, Grune & Stratton, 1971
539. Schned ES: Ankylosing spondylitis. In Beary JF, Christian CL, Johanson MA (eds): Manual of Rheumatology and Outpatient Orthopedic Disorders: Diagnosis and Therapy. Boston, Little, Brown & Co., 1987
540. Schuchmann JA: Low back pain: A comprehensive approach. Compr Ther 14:14–18, 1987
541. Schultz A, Andersson G, Ortengren R, et al: Loads on the lumbar spine: Validation and biomechanical analysis by measurements of intradiscal pressures and myoelectric signals. J Bone Joint Surg 64B:713–720, 1982
542. Scott J, Huskisson EC: Graphic representation of pain. Pain 2:175–184, 1976
543. Scott ME: Spinal osteoporosis in the aged. Aust Fam Phys 3:281, 1974
544. Scott V, Gijsbers K: Pain perception in competitive swimmers. Br Med J 283:91–93, 1981
545. Seimons LP: Low Back Pain: Clinical Diagnosis and Management. Norwalk, CT, Appleton-Century-Crofts, 1983
546. Selby DK, Paris SV: Anatomy of facet joints and its correlation with low back pain. Contemp Orthop 31:1097–1103, 1981
547. Shah JS: Structure, morphology and mechanics of the lumbar spine. In Jayson M (ed): The Lumbar Spine and Low Back Pain. London, Pittman Medical, 1980:359–406
548. Shealy CN: Facet denervation in the management of back and sciatic pain. Clin Orthop 115:159–164, 1976
549. Shealy CN, Shealy M: Behavioral techniques in control of pain: A case for health maintenance vs. disease treatment. In Weisenberg M, Tursky B (eds): Pain: New Perspectives in Therapy and Research. New York, Plenum Press, 1976:21–34
550. Sheon RP: Regional myofascial pain and the fibrositis syndrome (fibromyalgia). Compr Ther 12(a):42–52, 1986
551. Sikorski JM: A rationalized approach to physiotherapy for low-back pain. Spine 10:571–579, 1985
552. Simons DC. Muscle pain syndromes: Part I. Am J Phys Med 54:289–311, 1975
553. Simons DG: Muscle pain syndromes: Part II. Am J Phys Med 55:15–42, 1976
554. Simons DG, Travell JG: Myofascial origins of low back pain: 1. Principles of diagnosis and treatment. Postgrad Med 73:66–77, 1983
555. Simons DG, Travell JG: Myofascial origins of low back pain: 2. Torso muscles. Postgrad Med 73:81–92, 1983
556. Simons DG, Travell JG: Myofascial origins of low back pain: 3. Pelvic and lower extremity muscles. Postgrad Med 73:99–108, 1983
557. Simons DG, Travell JG: Myofascial pain syndromes. In Wall PD, Melzack R (eds): Textbook of Pain. New York, Churchill Livingstone, 1984:263–276
558. Sims FH, Dahlin DC: Primary bone tumors simulating lumbar disc syndrome. Spine 2:65–74, 1977
559. Sinaki M: Postmenopausal spinal osteoporosis: Physical therapy and rehabilitation principles. Mayo Clin Proc 57:699–703, 1982
560. Sinaki M: Beneficial musculoskeletal effects of physical activity in the older woman. Geriatr Med Today 8:53–72, 1989
561. Sinaki M: Osteoporosis. In Delisa JA, Gans BM, Currie DM, et al (eds): Rehabilitation Medicine: Principles and Practice, 2nd ed. Philadelphia, JB Lippincott, 1993:1018–1035
562. Sinaki M, Mikkelsen BA: Postmenopausal spinal osteoporosis: Flexion versus extension exercises. Arch Phys Med Rehabil 65:593–703, 1984
563. Skinner AT, Thompson AM (eds): Duffield's Exercise in Water. London, Bailliere Tindall, 1983
564. Smidt G: Inversion traction: Effects on spinal column, heart rate and blood pressure [abstr]. Presented at the meeting of the International Society for the Study of the Lumbar Spine, Sydney, Australia, 1985
565. Smidt GL, Blanpied PR, Anderson MA, et al: Comparison of clinical and objective methods of assessing trunk muscle strength: An experimental approach. Spine 12:1020–1024, 1987
566. Smith AE: Physical activity: A tool in promoting mental health. J Psychiatr Nurs 11:24–25, 1979
567. Smith SS, TG Mayer, Gatchel RJ, et al: Qualification of lumbar function: I. Isometric and multispeed isokinetic trunk strength measures in sagittal and axial planes in normal subjects. Spine 10:757–764, 1985
568. Smyth MJ, Wright V: Sciatica and intervertebral disc: An experimental study. J Bone Joint Surg 40A:1401–1418, 1958
569. Smythe HA: Nonarticular rheumatism and the fibrositis syndrome. In Hollander JL, McCarty DJ (eds): Arthritis and Allied Conditions, 8th ed. Philadelphia, Lea & Febiger, 1972:874–884
570. Smythe HA: Nonarticular rheumatism and psychogenic musculoskeletal syndromes. In McCarty DJ (ed): Arthritis and Allied Conditions: Textbook of Rheumatology, 9th ed. Philadelphia, Lea & Febiger, 1979:1083–1094
571. Smythe HA: Referred pain and tender points. Am J Med (Suppl. 3A) 81:90–98, 1986
572. Snoek W, Weber H, Jorgensen B: Double-blind evaluation of extradural methylprednisolone for herniated lumbar disc. Acta Orthop Scand 48:635–641, 1977
573. Snook SH: The design of manual handling tasks. Ergonomics 21:963–641, 1978
574. Snook SH: Low back pain in industry. In White AA, Gordon SL (eds): American Academy of Orthopaedic Surgeons Symposium on Idiopathic Low Back Pain. St. Louis, CV Mosby, 1982:23–48
575. Sorensen KH: Scheuermann's Juvenile Kyphosis. Thesis. Copenhagen, Munksgaard, 1964
576. Spangfort EV: The lumbar disc herniation: A computer-aided analysis of 2504 operations. Acta Orthop Scand (Suppl 142):1–95, 1972
577. Spencer DL, Irwin GS, Millar JAA: Anatomy and significance of fixation of the lumbosacral nerve roots in sciatica. Spine 8:672–679, 1983
578. Spengler DM, Freeman CW: Patient selection for lumbar discectomy: An objective approach. Spine 4:129–134, 1979
579. Spengler DM, Freeman CW: Low Back Pain: Assessment and Management. New York, Grune & Stratton, 1982
580. Spitzer WO: Quebec task force on spinal disorders: Scientific approach to the assessment and management of activity-related spinal disorders. Spine 12:S1–S58, 1987
581. Staffel F: Zur Hygiene des Sitzens. Gesundheitspflege 3:403–421, 1983
582. Steindler A, Luck JV: Differential diagnosis of pain low in the back. JAMA 110:106–112, 1938
583. Steiner C, Staubs C, Ganon M, et al: Piriformis syndrome: Pathogenesis, diagnosis, and treatment. J Am Osteopathic Assoc 87:318–323, 1987
584. Steinmetz ND: MRI of the Lumbar Spine: A Practical Approach to Image Interpretation. Thorofare, NJ, Slack, 1987
585. Sternbach RA: Pain Patients: Traits and Treatment. New York, Academic Press, 1974
586. Stewart ML: Measurement of clinical pain. In Jacox AK (ed): Pain: A Source Book for Nurses and Other Health Professionals. Boston, Little, Brown & Co., 1977
587. Stoddard A: Conditions of the sacro-iliac joints and their treatment. Physiotherapy 44(4):97, 1958
588. Stoddard A: Manual of Osteopathic Technique. London, Hutchinson, 1959
589. Stoddard A: Cervical spondylosis and cervical osteoarthritis. Man Med 2:31, 1970
590. Stokes IAF, Frymoyer JM, Lunn RA: Segmental motion and segmental instability [abstr]. Orthop Trans 10:517–518, 1986
591. Stone MH: Implications of connective tissue and bone alterations resulting from resistance exercise training. Med Sci Sports Exerc 20(suppl):162–168, 1988
592. Strachan A: Back care in industry. Physiotherapy 65:249–251, 1949
593. Strange FG: Debunking the disc. Proc R Soc Med 9:952–956, 1966
594. Stubbs DA, Buckle PW, Hudson MP, et al: Back pain in the nursing profession: I. Epidemiology and pilot methodology. Ergonomics 26:755–765, 1983
595. Stubbs DA, Buckle PW, Hudson MP, et al: Back pain in the nursing profession: II. The effectiveness of training. Ergonomics 26:767–779, 1983
596. Sugiura K, Yoshida T, Mimatsu T: A study of tension signs in lumbar disc hernia. Intl Orthop 3:225–228, 1979
597. Sullivan PE, Markos PD: Therapeutic exercise for the patient with low back disor-

ders. In Sullivan PE, Markos PD (eds): Clinical Procedures in Therapeutic Exercise. Los Altos, CA, Appleton & Lange, 1987:211–218

598. Sullivan PE, Markos PD, Minor MAD: Low back. In Sullivan PE, Markos PD, Minor MAD (eds): Approach to Therapeutic Exercise: Theory and Clinical Application. Reston, VA, Reston Pub. Co., 1982:333–351

599. Sunderland S: The anatomy of the intervertebral foramen and mechanism of compression and stretch of nerve roots. In Haldeman S (ed): Modern Developments in Principles and Practice of Chiropractic. New York, Appleton-Century-Crofts, 1980:297–299

600. Suzuki N, Endo S: A quantitative study of trunk muscle strength and fatigability in low-back syndrome. Spine 8:69–74, 1983

601. Svensson HL, Andersson GBJ: Low back pain in 40- to 47-year-old men: I. Frequency of occurrence and impact on medical services. Scand J Rehabil Med 14(2):47–53, 1982

602. Svensson HL, Andersson GBJ: Low back pain in 40- to 47-year-old men. Spine 8:272–276, 1983

603. Svensson HL, Vedin A, Wihelmsson C, et al: Low back pain in relation to other diseases and cardiovascular risk factors. Spine 8(3):277–285, 1983

604. Sylven B: On the biology of nucleus pulposus. Acta Orthop Scand 20:275–279, 1951

605. Tanigawa M: Comparison of the hold/relax procedure and passive mobilization in increasing muscle length. Phys Ther 52:725–735, 1972

606. Tappan FM: Healing Massage Techniques: Holistic, Classic and Emerging Methods. Norwalk, CT, Appleton & Lange, 1988

607. Tasuma T, Makina E, Saito S, et al: Histological development of intervertebral disc herniation. J Bone Joint Surg 68A:1066–1072, 1986

608. Tauber J: An unorthodox look at backaches. J Occup Med 12:128–130, 1970

609. Taylor TKF, Weiner M: Great-toe extensor reflexes in the diagnosis of lumbar disc disorder. Br Med J 2:487, 1969

610. Terenius L: Endorphins and pain. Front Horm Res 8:162–171, 1981

611. Thery Y, Bonjean P, Calen S, et al: Anatomical and roentgenological basis for the study of lumbar spine with the body in suspended position. Anat Clin 7:161–169, 1985

612. Thompson NN, Gould JA, Davies GJ, et al: Descriptive measures of isokinetic trunk testing. J Orthop Sports Phys Ther 7:43–49,1985

613. Thorsteinsson A, Nilsson J: Trunk muscle strength during constant and velocity movements. Scand J Rehabil Med 14:61–68, 1982

614. Tichauer ER: The Biomedical Basis of Ergonomics: Anatomy Applied to the Design of the Work Station. New York, Wiley Inter-Sciences, 1978

615. Tillotson LM, Burton AK: Noninvasive measurement of lumbar sagittal mobility, an assessment by Flexicurves technique. Spine 16:29–33, 1991

616. Traut FF: Fibrositis. J Am Geriatr Soc 16:531–538, 1968

617. Travel JG, Simons DG: Myofascial Pain and Dysfunction: The Trigger Point Manual. Baltimore, William & Wilkins, 1983

618. Triggs M: Orthopedic aquatic therapy. Clinical Management 11:30–31, 1991

619. Trott PH, Grant R, Maitland GD: Manipulative therapy for the low lumbar spine: Technique, selection, and application to some syndromes. In Twomey LT, Taylor JR (eds): Physical Therapy of the Low Back. New York, Churchill Livingstone, 1987:199–224

620. Troup JDG: Causes, prediction and prevention of back pain at work. Scand J Work Environ Health 10:419–428, 1984

621. Troup JDG, Martin JW, Lloyd DCEF: Back pain in industry: A prospective survey. Spine 6:61–69, 1981

622. Troup JDG, Roantree WB, Archibald RM: Survey of cases of lumbar spinal disability: A methodological study. Medical Officers' Broadsheet, National Coal Board, 1970

623. Tursky B: The development of a pain perception profile: A psychophysical approach. In Weisenberg M, Tursky B (eds): Pain: New Perspectives in Therapy and Research. New York, Plenum Press, 1976:171–194

624. Twomey LT: Sustained lumbar traction: An experimental study of long spine segments. Spine 10(2):167–169, 1985

625. Twomey LT, Taylor JR: A description of two new instruments measuring the ranges of sagittal and horizontal plane motions in the lumbar region. Aust J Physiother 31:106–112, 1985

626. Urban LM: The straight-leg raising test: A review. J Orthop Sports Phys Ther 2:117–133, 1981

627. Urban LM: The straight-leg raising test: A review. In Grieve GP (ed): Modern Manual Therapy of the Vertebral Column. New York, Churchill Livingstone, 1986:567–575

628. Valkenberg HA, Haanen HCM: The epidemiology of low back pain. In White AA, Gordon SL (eds): American Academy of Orthopaedic Surgeons, Symposium on Idiopathic Low Back Pain. St. Louis, CV Mosby, 1982:9–22

629. Van Akkerveeken PF, O'Brien JP, Park WM: Experimentally induced hypermobility in the lumbar spine. Spine 4:236–241, 1979

630. Vanharanta H, Videman T, Mooney V: McKenzie exercise, back traction and back school in lumbar syndrome [abstr]. Orthop Trans. 10:533, 1986

631. Van Wijmen PM: The management of recurrent low back pain. In Grieve GP (ed): Modern Manual Therapy of the Vertebral Column. New York, Churchill Livingstone, 1986:756–776

632. Vollowitz E: Furniture prescription for the conservative management of low back pain. In Topics in Acute Care and Trauma Rehabilitation, Industrial Back Injury, Part II: Clinical Applications. Aspen, CO, Aspen Publications, 1988

633. Voss DE, Ionta MK, Myer BJ: Proprioceptive Neuromuscular Facilitation, 3rd ed. Philadelphia, Harper & Row, 1985

634. Waddell G: A new clinical model for treatment of low back pain. Spine 12:632–644, 1987

635. Waddell G, Main CJ, Morris EW, et al: Normality and reliability in the clinical assessment of backache. Br Med J 284:1519–1523, 1982

636. Waddell G, Main CJ, Morris EW, et al: Chronic low back pain, psychological distress and illness behavior. Spine 9:209–213, 1984

637. Waddell G, McCulloch JA, Kummel EG, et al: Nonorganic physical signs in low back pain. Spine 5:117–125, 1980

638. Waitz E: The lateral bending sign. Spine 6:388–397, 1981

639. Walker JM: Deep transverse frictions in ligament healing. J Orthop Sports Phys Ther 6:89–94, 1984

640. Walters A: Psychogenic regional pain alias hysterical pain. Brain 84:1–18, 1961

641. Watkins R, O'Brien J, Drauglis R, et al: Comparison of preoperative and postoperative MMPI data in chronic back patients. Spine 11:385–390, 1986

642. Weber H: Lumbar disc herniation: A controlled prospective study with 10 years of observation. Spine 8:131–140, 1983

643. Weber H, Ljunggren AI, Walker L: Traction therapy in patients with herniated lumbar intervertebral disc. J Oslo City Hosp 34:61–70, 1984

644. Wedge JH: The natural history of spinal degeneration. In Kirkaldy-Willis WH (ed): Managing Low Back Pain. New York, Churchill Livingstone, 1983:3–8

645. Weider DL: Jumping in with both feet: Water therapy in sports. Rehabil Management June/July:135, 1993

646. Weintraube A: Soft-tissue mobilization of the lumbar spine. In Grieve GP (ed): Modern Manual Therapy of the Vertebral Column. New York, Churchill Livingstone, 1986:750–755

647. Wells PE: The examination of the pelvic joints. In Grieve GP (ed): Modern Manual Therapy of the Vertebral Column. New York, Churchill Livingstone, 1986:590–602

648. White AA: Injection technique for the diagnosis and treatment of low back pain. Orthop Clin North Am 14:553–567, 1983

649. White AA, Gordon SL: Synopsis workshop on idiopathic low-back pain. Spine 7:141–149, 1982

650. White AA, McBride ME, Wiltse LL, et al: The management of patients with back pain and idiopathic vertebral sclerosis. Spine 11:607–616, 1986

651. White AA, Panjabi MM: Clinical Biomechanics of the Spine, 2nd ed. Philadelphia, JB Lippincott, 1990

652. White AH: Back Schools and Other Conservative Approaches to Low Back Pain. St. Louis, CV Mosby, 1983

653. White AH: Work hardening: General conditioning [abstr 91]. Challenge of the Lumbar Spine: 9th annual meeting, New York, 1987

654. White AH: Stabilization of the lumbar spine. In White AH, Anderson R (ed): Conservative Care of Low Back Pain. Baltimore, Williams & Wilkins, 1991:106–111

655. Wiberg G: Back pain in relation to the nerve supply of the intervertebral disc. Acta Orthop Scand 19:211–221, 1949

656. Wiesel SW, Bernini P, Rothman RM, et al: Effectiveness of epidural steroids in the treatment of sciatica: A double-blind clinical trial. Presented at the meeting of the International Society for the Study of the Lumbar Spine, Toronto, 1982

657. Wilkinson M: A neurological perspective. Rheum Rehabil 14:162–163, 1975

658. Williams SJ: The back school. Physiotherapy 63:90, 1977

659. Wiltse LL, Rocchio PD: Preoperative psychological tests as predictors of the success of chemonucleolysis in treatment of low back pain. J Bone Joint Surg 57A:478–483, 1975

660. Wolfe F: The clinical syndrome of fibrositis. Am J Med (Suppl 3A)81:99–104, 1986

661. Wolfe F, Hawley DJ, Cathey MA, et al: Fibrositis: Symptom frequency and criteria for diagnosis: Evaluation of 291 rheumatic disease patients and 58 normal individuals. J Rheumatol 12:1159–1163, 1985

662. Woodhall B, Hayes GJ: The well leg-raising test of Fajersztajn in the diagnosis of ruptured intervertebral disc. J Bone Joint Surg 32A:786–792, 1950

663. Wyke B: The neurological basis of thoracic spinal pain. Rheumatol Phys Med 10:356–367, 1970

664. Wyke B: Articular neurology and manipulative therapy. In Idezak RM (ed): Aspects of Manipulative Therapy. Carlton, Victoria, Australia, Lincoln Institute of Health Sciences, 1980

665. Wyke B: The neurology of low back pain. In Jayson MIV (ed): The Lumbar Spine and Back Pain, 2nd ed. London, Pittman Medical, 1980:265–340

666. Yao J: Acutherapy: Acupuncture, TENS and Acupressure. Libertyville, IL, Acutherapy Postgraduate, 1984

667. Young RJ: The effect of regular exercise on cognitive functioning and personality. Br J Sports Med 3:110–117, 1979

668. Young-Hing K, Reilly J, Kirkaldy-Willis WH: The ligamentum flavum. Spine 1:226–234, 1976

669. Yunus MB: Primary fibromyalgia syndrome: Current concepts. Compr Ther 10:21–28, 1984

670. Yunus MB, Kalgan-Raman UP, Kalyan-Raman K: Primary fibromyalgia syndrome and myofascial pain syndrome: Clinical features and muscle pathology. Arch Phys Med Rehabil 69:451–454, 1988

671. Yunus MB, Kalgan-Raman UP, Kalyan-Raman K, et al: Pathologic changes in muscle in primary fibromyalgia syndrome. Am J Med 81(suppl 3a):38–42, 1986

672. Yunus MB, Masi AT: Association of primary fibromyalgia syndrome with stress-related syndrome. Clin Res 33:923A, 1985

673. Yunus MB, Masi AT, Aldag JC: Criteria studies of primary fibromyalgia syndrome. Arthritis Rheum 30(Suppl):S50, 1987

674. Yunus MB, Masi AT, Calabro JJ, et al: Primary fibromyalgia (fibrositis)—Clinical study of 50 patients with matched normal controls. Semin Arthritis Rheum 11:151–171, 1981

675. Zachrisson-Fossell M, Forssell M: The back school. Spine 6:104–106, 1981

676. Zylbergold RS, Piper MC: Cervical spine disorders: A comparison of three types of traction. Spine 10:867–871, 1985

The Sacroiliac Joint and the Lumbar–Pelvic–Hip Complex

DARLENE HERTLING

- ■ **Functional Anatomy**
  Arthrokinematics and Osteokinematics
  Myokinematics
- ■ **Common Lesions and Management**
  Hypomobility Lesions
  Hypermobility Lesions
  Degenerative Changes
  Osteitis Condensans Ilii
  Inflammatory Disease and Infections

- ■ **Specific Sacroiliac Examination**
  History
  Lumbar–Pelvic–Hip Complex Evaluation
  Specific Sacroiliac Evaluation
- ■ **Pelvic Girdle Treatment**
  Hypermobility
  Passive Movements
  Nonspecific Techniques
  Innominate Dysfunction Techniques
  Sacral Dysfunction Techniques

The sacroiliac joint (SIJ) is probably the most controversial in the human body. In the early years of this century, disorders of the SIJ were considered responsible for a large percentage of patients presenting with low back pain.[16] It was not until the 1930s, when the role of the nucleus pulposus became an established entity in low back pain, that the SIJ tended to be overlooked. There is a constant debate regarding the type and amount of movement and the location of the axes. Medical students are often taught that the SIJ is immobile and therefore cannot be a cause of low back pain. More recently attention has been paid to the SIJ and its involvement in low back pain.[6,8,16,21,23,29,34,35,40,51,101,107,111,153,156,177,193,208]

FUNCTIONAL ANATOMY

☐ Arthrokinematics and Osteokinematics

When discussing the pelvic girdle, we must always consider the interrelatedness of the lumbar–pelvic–hip complex (Fig. 21-1). We can think of the lum-bopelvic complex as consisting of the fourth and fifth lumbar joints (four apophyseal joints), the sacrum (two synovial joints), the two hip joints, and the pubic symphysis (amphiarthrodial joint). This complex should always be considered as a mechanical unit; do not attempt to isolate it. Involvement of any one structure affects the positioning and movement of the others. The sacrum is mechanically associated with the spine, whereas the innominate is aligned with and affected by movement of the femur. Any frontal plane asymmetry, leg-length discrepancy, or loss of motion in one joint of the complex that might alter the forces (from the spine above or the lower limbs below) can affect the lumbar–pelvic–hip complex, resulting in abnormal mechanical stresses and symptoms of overuse.[57,153] For example, fusion of the lower lumbar vertebrae can cause a compensatory increase in motion at the SIJ.[71] Cibulka and Delitto[22] compared two different treatments for hip joint pain in runners who had primary hip and SIJ dysfunction and found that a manipulative technique designed to reduce SIJ dysfunction effectively reduced hip pain. They concluded that the therapist should evaluate the SIJ in patients with hip pain.

Darlene Hertling and Randolph M. Kessler: MANAGEMENT OF COMMON MUSCULOSKELETAL DISORDERS: Physical Therapy Principles and Methods, 3rd ed. © 1996 Lippincott-Raven Publishers.

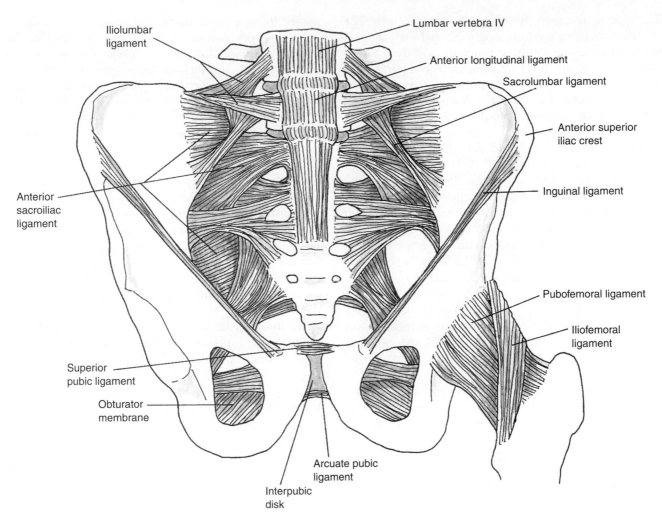

FIG. 21-1. The lumbar–pelvic–hip complex.

By establishing the relation among these functional components of the kinetic chain, the clinician can better evaluate the patient and formulate more effective treatment programs. Keep in mind the possible effect and influences of other components of the kinetic chain, such as the foot, ankle, and knee, to complete the picture of dysfunction.

The center of activity in the human body for static weight-bearing, normal biomechanics, and posture is the lumbopelvic region. Kendall and colleagues[96,97] regard the position of the pelvis as the keynote in postural alignment. The two SIJs form an integral part of this region. During ambulation the SIJs decrease the effort of ambulation and absorb shear forces to protect the disks and to decrease the effects of impact-loading on the femoral heads.[42]

The pelvis (meaning basin) is a bony ring formed by the two innominate bones, the sacrum, and the cavity of this arrangement. It is interposed between the fifth lumbar vertebra and the femoral heads (see Fig. 21-1). The ancient phallic worshipers named the base of the spine the *sacred bone*. The sacrum is the seat of the

transverse center of gravity, the keystone of the pelvis, and the foundation for the spine. The most important mechanical function of the pelvic girdle is to transmit the weight of the head, upper limbs, and trunk to the lower limbs and to transmit in the opposite direction the contact forces from the ground, through the leg, up into the trunk.[95] When trunk and ground forces exceed the normal physiological adaptive capacity of its tissues, a chronic painful condition can result.[30,122,128]

The pelvis also plays a role in energy absorption.[128] Weight is transmitted to the sacrum via the lumbosacral junction (fifth lumbar vertebra and lumbosacral disk to the first sacral segment), distributed equally along the alae of the sacrum, and transmitted through the SIJs to the acetabulum and hence to the lower limbs. The force of the body weight tends to separate the sacrum from the ilia and tends to push the first sacral segment into flexion (nutation).

The SIJ is a synovial joint formed between the medial surface of the ilium and the lateral aspect of the upper sacral vertebrae. The articular surface on the iliac side of the joint, however, is fibrocartilage. The cartilage covering the opposing joint surface (sacral) is hyaline cartilage 1.7 to five times thicker than the fibrocartilage of the iliac component.[3,15] The surfaces of the sacroiliac articulation exhibit irregular elevations and depressions that fit into one another, restrict movement, and contribute to the strength of the joint.

The SIJ changes as we age. In early childhood the joint surfaces are smooth and flat: gliding motions are possible in all directions.[15,88,115,174,199,200] After puberty the joint surfaces change their configuration, and motion is restricted to anteroposterior movement of the sacrum on the ilium or the ilium on the sacrum (flexion or rotation and extension or counterrotation).[139] Most investigators describe a decrease in motion with age.[3,15,147,166,173,174,194] Sturesson and colleagues,[184] however, noted no decrease in mobility in a sample of persons aged 19 to 45 years, and reported 0.08 mm of translation. In the elderly, the joint cavity is at least partly obliterated by fibrous adhesions and synovitis (osseous union may occur). Mobility is lower in males than females, and the joint usually becomes ankylosed in elderly men.[67,201]

The articular surface of the sacrum is shaped like a letter L lying on its side, with its upper, more vertical, limb being shorter than its lower, more horizontal limb (Fig. 21-2).[2,15,201] The sacral surface is slightly concave, the iliac surface convex.[3,15] The size, shape, roughness, and complexity of the articular surfaces vary greatly among individuals; this contributes to the unique stability of the joint.[39,181]

Besides the bony architecture, SIJ stability depends primarily on the anterior and posterior ligaments (see Fig. 16-20). The stronger posterior ligaments are nec-

essary to provide stability and prevent the tendency for the upper sacrum to be driven forward during weight-bearing. All adjacent muscles (*i.e.,* the quadratus lumborum, gluteus maximus, gluteus minimus, iliacus, latissimus dorsi, and piriformis) have fibrous expansions that blend with the anterior and posterior SIJ ligaments and contribute to the strength of the joint capsule and ligaments, and thus to the joint's stability.[196]

In addition there are the accessory ligaments. The most important is the *iliolumbar ligament*, which extends from the transverse process of the fifth lumbar vertebra (although it can reach as far superiorly as the fourth lumbar vertebra) to the posterior iliac crest (see Fig. 21-1). The multidirectional aspect of the iliolumbar bands of this ligament allows the ligament to check various motions of the L5 vertebra on the sacrum and is important in squaring the L5 vertebra on the sacrum. This ligament is frequently painful when there is true sacroiliac dysfunction.

The pelvis can move in all three body planes: in the sagittal plane during forward- and backward-bending, in the coronal plane during sidebending (lateral flexion), and in the axial plane during twisting of the trunk. During these movements, motion also occurs within the pelvis. Experiments using several different techniques (*i.e.,* gross examination, roentgenography, tomography) to demonstrate sacroiliac movement have been described.* Although there has been considerable controversy and speculation about the role and type of movements that occur in this joint, there seems no doubt that the normal range of SIJ movement (although only a few millimeters) is important.[71] Recent studies seem to have confirmed the rotatory movement described by Brooke,[17] but it is generally considered minimal.[166,181] Motion is often described as a nodding type of movement of the sacrum, in that the sacral promontory can move forward and backward between the iliac bones. Flexion or *nutation* involves movement of the anterior tip of the sacral promontory anteriorly and inferiorly while the coccyx moves posteriorly in relation to the ilium (Fig. 21-3*A*). Extension or *counternutation* refers to the opposite movement: the anterior tip of the sacral promontory moves posteriorly and superiorly while the coccyx moves anteriorly in relation to the ilium (Fig. 21-3*B*).[95] The arthrokinematics of the sacrum during rotation have not been studied, although several theories have been proposed.[56,123,132,157]

When a human stands erect, the line of gravity is posterior to the acetabula, causing a posterior rotation of the innominate bones around the acetabula. At heel-strike there is a posterior rotational force on the

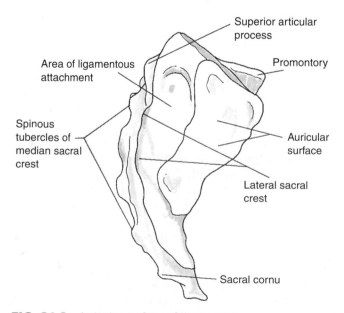

FIG. 21-2. *Articular surface of the sacrum.*

Superior articular process

Promontory

Area of ligamentous attachment

Spinous tubercles of median sacral crest

Auricular surface

Lateral sacral crest

Sacral cornu

---

*See references 13,17,19,23,26,28,41,44,48,59,64,69,70,95,103,106,112, 120,130,131,142,151,152,160,166,172,184,190,192,210,205,206.

innominate (Fig. 21-4).[133,183] As the lower extremity proceeds through the stance phase and approaches push-off, a resultant anterior rotational force creates a flexion force on the sacrum around a horizontal axis. Most agree that the axis occurs at the intersection of the cranial and caudal portions of the sacroiliac articular surfaces. However, Lavignolle and colleagues[106] calculated that the horizontal axis of the SIJ was just posterior to the pubic symphysis.

Farabeuf[206] described sacral flexion about an extra-articular axis lying posterior to the center of the articular facet and coinciding with the interosseous ligament. Bonnaire[206] argued that the axis was intra-articular at the convergence of the facetal limbs, allowing pure spin, with the sacral base turning anteriorly during flexion. Weisl[201] rejected the idea of a transverse axis and theorized pure linear motion, with sacral flexion being a straight displacement of the sacrum along the caudal facet anterosuperiorly. Wilder and associates[206] used topography and theoretical modeling with best-fit axes of rotation for each contour to calculate the optimal axes of rotation. They concluded that motion did not occur exclusively around axes proposed by Weisl, Bonnaire, or

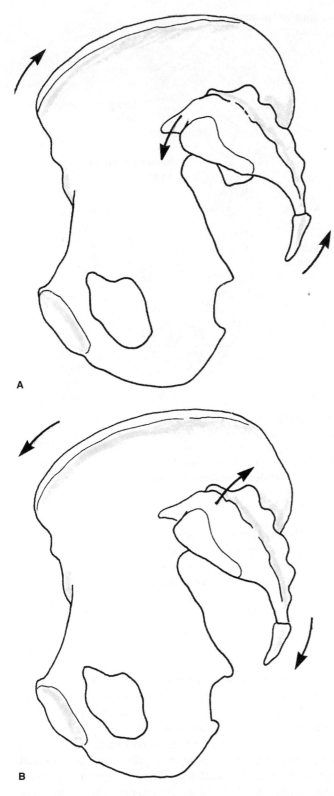

FIG. 21-3. Nutation (**A**) and counternutation (**B**) of the sacrum.

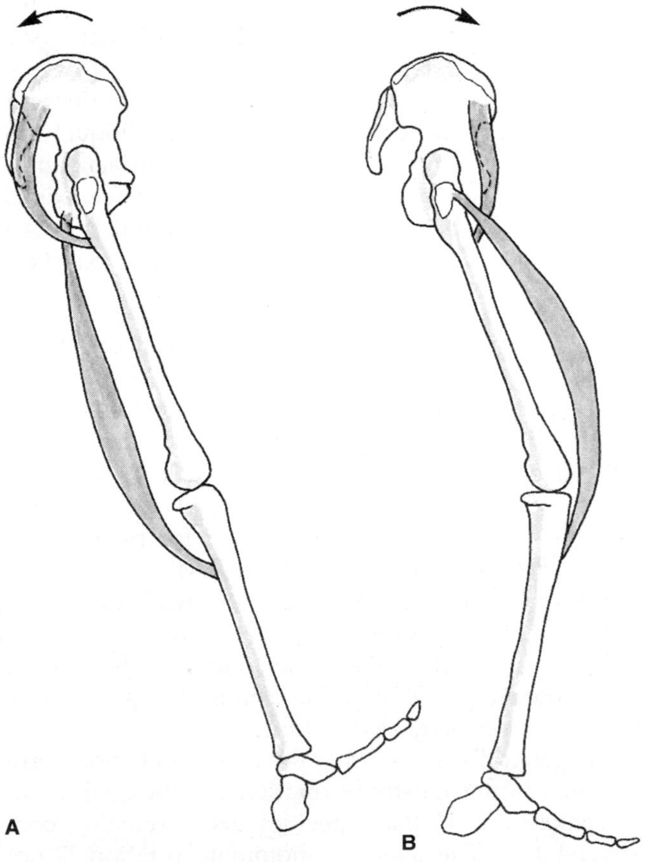

FIG. 21-4. Relative forces during early stance phase (**A**) and swing phase of gait (**B**).

Farabeuf, or in optimized axes in the median or frontal planes. They argued that translation motion occurred about a "rough axis" if some separation of the surfaces was present.

Osteopathic theory demands at least three transverse and two diagonal axes to accommodate sacroiliac and iliosacral motions and sacral torsion. It is likely that all of these axes are operative during some phase of motion, depending on the load being carried through the articulations and the age and stage of degeneration of the joint. The following axes and movements have been described by Mitchell and associates:[132,133]

1. *Superior transverse axis* (runs through the second sacral segment). This is often referred to as the respiratory axis. This axis is actually a fulcrum formed by the attachments of the posterior sacroiliac ligaments and the thoracodorsal fascia. As one inhales, the sacrum counternutates; as one exhales, the sacrum nutates (Fig. 21-5A).
2. *Middle transverse axis* (located at the second sacral body). This is the principal axis of normal sacroiliac flexion and extension (nutation/counternutation; Fig. 21-5A).
3. *Inferior transverse axis* (runs transversely through the inferior pole of the sacral articulations). This is the principal axis of normal iliosacral motion (anterior and posterior rotation of the innominates; see Fig. 21-5A).
4. *Right and left oblique axes* (run from the superior end of the articular surface of the sacrum obliquely to the opposite inferior lateral angle). Iliosacral motion occurring about the inferior transverse axis is consorted with rotation at the pubis and through the sacrum at the contralateral oblique axis (see Fig. 21-5B).

In osteopathic medicine, the SIJ is often described as two joints: the iliosacral and the SIJ.[208] The term *iliosacral* implies the innominates moving on the sacrum; conversely, the term *sacroiliac* implies the sacrum moving within the innominates. Functionally these designations hold true because they are based on the recruitment of motion and transmission of forces from the spine or lower limbs through the pelvis, although it is one and the same joint. The sacrum is mechanically associated with the spine, whereas the ilium is aligned with and affected by the lower limbs. As the lumbar spine goes, so goes the sacrum; similarly, as the lower extremity goes, so goes the ilium.[155]

It is generally agreed that the innominate bones are capable of anteroposterior rotation, but the quantity of movement and the specific axes remain controversial.[191] The axis of innominate rotation is not thought to lie in the coronal plane but rather is thought to run obliquely in the posterolateral direc-

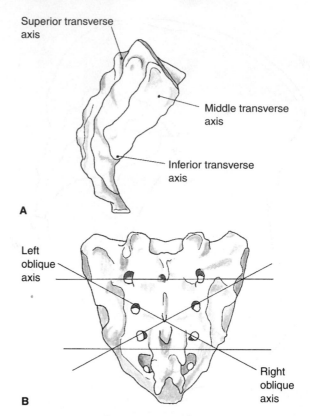

FIG. 21-5. Principal axes (about which motion of the sacrum and/or innominate bones moves) that have been proposed (Mitchell 1965, 1968). (Adapted from Saunders D: Evaluation, Treatment and Prevention of Musculoskeletal Disorder. Minneapolis, Viking Press, 1985).

tion. The craniocaudal orientation of this axis varies during anteroposterior rotation. Anterior translation (arthrokinematic) of the innominate bone (6 to 8 mm) conjoined with both anterior and posterior rotation (osteokinematic) has been confirmed, although the quantity of this translation is disputed (0.5 to 1.6 mm).[106,184]

During spinal flexion or standing up from lying down, the sacral promontory moves ventrally so that the anteroposterior diameter of the pelvic inlet is reduced and the apex of the sacrum moves dorsally. At the same time, a movement occurs in the iliac bones, in which the iliac crests and the posterior superior iliac spines (PSIS) become approximated, and the anterior superior iliac spines (ASIS) and the ischial tuberosities move apart (Fig. 21-6).[95] Flexion increases tension in the iliolumbar ligaments, the short posterior SIJ ligament, the interosseous ligaments, and the sacrotuberous ligaments, which then dynamically return the SIJs to their normal resting position.[42] In studies of functional movements, motion of the sacrum has been found to peak in the act of rising from a supine to a standing or long-sitting position.[26,28,170,184]

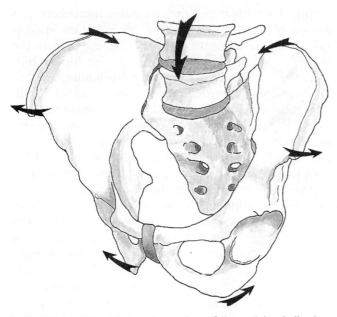

FIG. 21-6. Osteokinematic motion of the pelvic girdle during trunk flexion.

Alternatively, on spinal extension or on lying down, opposite movements occur so that the base of the sacrum moves dorsally and the apex of the sacrum moves ventrally, increasing the anteroposterior diameter of the pelvic inlet. At the same time the iliac crests and the PSIS separate and the ASIS and the ischial tuberosities approximate (Fig. 21-7).[95] Tension is increased mostly in the anterior sacroiliac ligaments, causing a relative unloading of the posterior ligaments.[40]

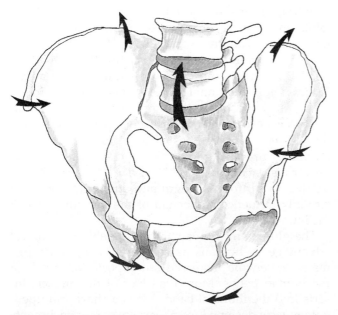

FIG. 21-7. Osteokinematic motion of the pelvic girdle during trunk extension.

Other movements of the ilia on the sacrum are possible, but do not normally occur except in dysfunctional states. These uncommon movements are described as up/down slips and in/out flares of the ilia.[40,56,68,109,133,142,202,208] Sacroiliac dysfunction is also termed *subluxation* or *posterior* or, more frequently, *anterior fixed innominate*. There are numerous tests for SIJ dysfunction, basically of two types: palpation of bony landmarks with or without measurement, and pain provocation tests.[29,40,70,71,109,196]

The symphysis pubis, a cartilaginous joint, and the sacrococcygeal joint (usually a fused line symphysis) should not be overlooked as a source of symptoms or dysfunction.[32,111] Many forces act on the symphysis pubis, especially those exerted by the muscles of the lower extremity. The symphysis pubis permits limited mobility and can be affected by excessive mobility in the SIJs. Stability of this articulation is vital to both the kinetic and kinematic functions of the pelvic girdle.

Several investigators have reported the presence of "supernumerary articular facets"[173] or "axial"[37] or accessory SIJs that may contribute to, or be responsible for, sacroiliac dysfunction.[2,37,49,77,78,189] According to Walker,[195] the fact that higher frequencies are observed in adult samples with increasing age, with no reports in fetuses or children, supports the theory that the accessory SIJs may be acquired as a result of the stress of weight-bearing.

☐ **Myokinematics**

Specific balanced muscle groups are fundamental to balancing the pelvis and lumbar spine. There are 35 muscles that attach directly to the sacrum or innominate bones and function with the ligaments and fascia to produce synchronous motion of the trunk and lower extremities.[109] Decreases in the length or strength of these muscles, caused by adaptive shortening or neuromuscular imbalances, can alter normal pelvic mechanics. Several authors have stressed that soft-tissue evaluation is the crucial factor in the diagnosis of lumbar spine and sacroiliac dysfunction.

Certain muscles respond in a typical way to a given situation, whether this be pain, impaired afferent input from the joint, or impairment in central motor regulation.[92,94,149] The tendency for muscles to respond is not random, and typical patterns of muscle reactions can be identified. The two regions where muscle imbalance is more evident or in which it starts to develop, according to Jull and Janda,[94] are the shoulder/neck complex and the pelvic/hip complex (pelvic crossed syndrome). The *pelvic crossed syndrome* is characterized by the imbalance between shortened and tight hip flexors and lumbar erector spinae and weakened gluteal and abdominal muscles. This results in anteversion of the pelvis, hyperlordosis of the lumbar spine, and slight flexion of the hip, which affects not only the efficiency of the static postural base but also dynamics such as gait.[149] In dysfunction, tonic muscles tend to shorten and hypertrophy; phasic muscles tend to become weak and atrophy.[90–94] The clinical significance is that it is essential to stretch or lengthen the tight, short tonic muscle groups before trying to re-educate the weak, dysfunctional phasic muscle groups. The main muscles and muscle groups of the pelvic/hip complex that illustrate the characteristic differences between tonic and phasic muscles are listed in Table 21-1.

According to Chapman and Nihls,[20] elsewhere in the body multijoint muscles affect the joints they traverse, and the pelvis is no exception. Pelvic articulations may also be affected by the transarticular and swing component of the muscle forces, as well as osteokinematics affecting tension, compression, and shear.

Consider the *quadratus lumborum*, a multijoint muscle. The quadratus lumborum has three portions (iliocostal, iliotransverse, costotransverse) that produce lateral guy-wire forces to the lumbar spine. Working with such structures as the iliolumbar ligament and the deep portion of the erector spinae muscles, the quadratus lumborum helps maintain the stability of the lumbar spine. Bilateral contraction may produce an anterior flexion of the sacrum through its attachments onto the base and ala. By the law of approximation, contraction of this muscle brings bony attachments together. This could produce a lateral tilt of the pelvic girdle and maintain a cranial displacement of the ipsilateral ilium on the sacrum.[20]

According to Travell and Simons,[187] the quadratus lumborum is one of the most commonly overlooked muscular sources of low back pain. Mechanical perpetuation of quadratus lumborum trigger points may depend on skeletal asymmetries, particularly inequality in leg length, or a small hemipelvis. Many authors have identified the quadratus lumborum as a source of back pain.[66,75,138,178,180,207] More specifically, they have identified it as referring pain to the sacroiliac region,[94,98,161,175,179,186] to the hip or buttock,[65,175,179,186] and to the greater trochanter.[175,186]

The abdominal muscles are also longitudinal, multijoint muscles. The abdominal muscles, including the two obliques, the transversus abdominis and the rectus abdominis, insert on the superior aspect of the pelvic girdle and are joined by the quadratus lumborum, the lumbodorsal fascia, and the erector spinae. A key point with respect to the abdominal muscles is their contribution to the stability of the symphysis pubis.[95,198] They retain the viscera and act in respiration and maintenance of the lumbosacral angle. The abdominal wall contributes to the attenuation of trunk and ground forces as they converge into the lumbopelvic region.[185] A weak abdominal wall promotes a forward pelvic tilt (increases the lumbosacral angle), creating an anterior migration of the center of gravity. To counter the anterior migration and maintain postural equilibrium, the person must increase the extension of the lumbar spine with a posterior movement of the weight line.[153]

The first sacral segment, which is inclined slightly anteriorly and inferiorly, forms an angle with the horizontal called the *lumbosacral angle* (see Fig. 19-5). The size of the angle varies with the position of the pelvis and affects the lumbar curvature. An increase in this angle increases the anterior convexity of the lumbar curve and increases the amount of shear stress at the lumbosacral joint.[139] The greater the sacral angle, the greater the shear forces and, therefore, the greater the weight carried by the soft tissues and articular processes, as opposed to the sacrum itself.[113] Added weight-bearing must be taken on by the apophyseal joints and may become an important source of both low back pain and referred pain.[9,52,112,121,134,148]

Lower extremity rotation is directly related to pelvic inclination and thus to the lumbosacral angle. External hip rotation facilitates posterior pelvic tilt and so may decrease the lumbosacral angle. One of the external rotators, the piriformis, primarily a tonic muscle, is considered responsible for restricting SIJ motion or producing local pain and symptoms of the piriformis syndrome.[18,81,132,137,143,144,175,182,188] Imbalance in piriformis length and strength appears to strongly influence movement of the sacrum between the innominates.[68]

The gluteus maximus has considerable mechanical advantage in humans as compared with other primates, given the increased anteroposterior depth of the human pelvis. More than half of this muscle inserts into the iliotibial band.[54] It is a short, multipennate muscle designed for power. Its bony attachments are close to both hip joints and SIJs, so its action in-

TABLE 21-1 FUNCTIONAL DIVISION OF MUSCLE GROUPS

Muscles Prone to Tightness	Muscles Prone to Weakness
Erector spinae	Gluteus maximus
Quadratus lumborum	Gluteus medius
Rectus femoris	Gluteus minimus
Iliopsoas	Rectus abdominis
Tensor fasciae latae	Vastus medialis
Piriformis	Vastus lateralis
Short hip adductors	
Hamstrings	

volves a large transarticular force. It can posteriorly rotate the ilium. Because the gluteus maximus, medius, and minimus are phasic muscles, in a weakened and dysfunctional state they reduce the dynamic stability of the pelvic girdle, thus predisposing to recurrent articular strains of the lumbosacral junction and the SIJ.[109] Weakness of the gluteus medius results in limited hip abduction and loss of lateral stabilization of the ilium.

The hamstrings (multijoint muscles), with their distal attachments further from the pelvic joint, help reduce the lumbosacral angle, and with unilateral action there is the potential for posterior torsion of one ilium.[20] Along with the deep rotators of the hip and the gluteus maximus, the force of these posterior thigh muscles is readily transmitted to the pelvis when the femur or foot becomes fixed and a closed kinetic chain is established.

The multifidus, along with the rotatores (transversospinalis group), is considered primarily a tonic or postural muscle and stabilizes the lumbar spine (see Fig. 16-17B).[176] The extensive attachment of the multifidus muscle to the dorsal surface of the sacrum makes it a major mass filling the deep sulcus formed by the overlapping ilium and sacrum. The attachment of the multifidus to the spinous processes results in an effective lever arm for extension of the lumbovertebral segments.[9] A unilateral contraction may produce a posterior rotation of the vertebrae on that side. A bilateral contraction may produce a posterior force on the pelvis through its attachments with the erector spinae, the posterior-superior iliac spine, and the posterior sacroiliac ligaments. Contraction also exerts a compressive force between each lumbar vertebra and between L5 and the sacrum. Stability of the lumbar spine increases when compressive forces are placed on it. Also, because of its greater tonic or stabilizing function, functional training of the multifidus may offer treatment for segmental instability. Evidence of lumbar multifidus muscle-wasting ipsilateral to symptoms in patients with acute and subacute low back pain indicate that wasting may be due to inhibition from perceived pain via a long-loop reflex pathway.[85]

The psoas, a longitudinal, multijoint muscle, does not directly attach to either the innominate bone or the sacrum but does have a significant biomechanical influence due to its potential to increase lumbar lordosis and produce hip flexion. Thoracolumbar lordosis effects a compensatory change in the lumbosacral angle and can produce a unilateral anterior iliac torsion and anterior movement of the sacrum on that side. Simultaneously, it may produce a torsion of the sacrum on the opposite side.[208] The force of the multifidus muscle is opposite that of the psoas muscle, and they may function together to "square" the vertebral unit in the sagittal plane.[153]

Other muscles to consider are:

1. The tensor fasciae latae, sartorius, and rectus femoris (multijoint) muscles can act as potential anterior rotators of the ipsilateral innominate.
2. The muscles of the adductor group have a direct effect on superior and inferior motion of the pubic rami. The short adductors and obturator externus, functioning as a unit, could produce a distracting force at the pubic ramus. Tightness or weakness of the adductors may influence hip position, which in turn influences the SIJ.
3. The pelvic floor muscles play an important supporting role. If the lumbosacral angle is increased, the stretched urogenital diaphragm becomes inefficient in its action.[20] Imbalance is highly significant in patients with rectal, gynecological, and urological problems.68

Always consider the influence of the thoracolumbar fascia, which represents not only fascial tissue but also the fused aponeurosis of several muscles (see Fig. 16-14A and Chap. 16, The Spine).[86] It serves as an attachment for the transversus abdominis, the internal oblique, and the latissimus dorsi muscles. The thoracolumbar fascia can influence and be influenced by the lumbar spine and pelvic positions and their surrounding muscles. Motions of the pelvis directly influence the thoracolumbar fascia: anterior pelvic movements tighten it and posterior pelvic movements loosen it.

■ COMMON LESIONS AND MANAGEMENT

SIJ pain is normally described as a dull ache and is characteristically experienced over the back of the SIJ and buttock.[29] It may also refer to the groin, over the greater trochanter, down the back of the thigh to the knee, and occasionally down the lateral or posterior calf to the ankle, foot, and toes.[100] Pain may also be referred to the lower abdomen; pain is then felt in the iliac fossa and is usually associated with a localized area of deep tenderness over the iliacus muscle known as Baer's sacroiliac point.[29,126] This point is located about 2″ from the umbilicus on an imaginary line drawn from the anterosuperior iliac spine to the umbilicus. Because the pelvis is a bony ring, pain may also be experienced anteriorly over the pubic symphysis or the adductor tendon origin.[29]

Clinical signs of sacroiliac dysfunction are pain and local tenderness, with increased pain on position changes such as ascending or descending stairs or slopes or rising from sitting or lying to standing. Pain may also increase with prolonged postures in standing or sitting. Pain may be initially transient but becomes deep and boring. Typically there is early-morning stiffness that eases after a period of weight-bearing.

Abnormal or asymmetrical forces reaching the lumbar or hip area are ultimately translated to the pelvis and render the weight-bearing joints vulnerable to injury.[51] Mechanical lesions may be due to hypomobility (with or without pain), hypermobility (with or without pain), or normal mobility with pain of the SIJ.[29,109]

☐ Hypomobility Lesions

Hypomobility lesions usually occur in young people and may be associated with movements that place a rotational stress on the SIJ, such as ballet or golfing.[29] It may also develop following pregnancy or trauma. It can also occur insidiously and may be associated with certain structural faults such as asymmetrical development of the pelvis or unequal leg length. Pain may result from sustained contraction of the muscle overlying the joint[99] or from a muscle-pain disorder.[187] This hypertonicity may accompany dysfunction of the SIJ or the lumbar spine.

Disparity in leg lengths, functional or structural, and pelvic muscle length asymmetry are considered prime factors in detecting sacroiliac dysfunction.[24,71] According to Grieve,[71] the pelvis can become stuck or blocked at the SIJ, not necessarily in a position of torsion but sometimes so in people with unequal leg length. Bourdillon and Day[14] wrote, "In patients with leg inequality there is a natural tendency for the pelvis to adopt the twisted position which most nearly levels the anterior-superior surface of the sacrum." When there is frontal plane asymmetry or a leg-length discrepancy, the pelvis must drop a distance equal to the amount of the discrepancy with every step. Ground forces reach the lumbopelvic tissues in an abnormal, asymmetrical manner, resulting in comparatively more compression forces applied to the shorter side and more shear forces to the opposite sacroiliac side. The tilted position of the sacrum also results in alteration at the hip (see Chap. 12, The Hip), lumbar spine, and knee. The most serious complication is osteoarthritis of the hip on the longer side.[62,63] With respect to the lumbar spine, there is sidebending motion away from the short side, with compressive forces placed on the concave side and tensile forces on the convex side.[155] Osteophytes may develop on the lumbar vertebrae on the side of the concavity produced by leg-length inequality.[57,58,61,136] Giles and Taylor[61] illustrated wedging of the lumbar vertebrae in a manner that would represent the conversion of a functional scoliosis to a fixed scoliosis.

Conversely, when innominate torsion is present (in the absence of structural leg-length discrepancy), this gives an appearance of unequal leg length, when measured from the anterosuperior spines or by noting the relation of the medial malleoli bilaterally when using a functional sit-up test.[133,154,167,193,208] Fisk[55] illustrated how anterior rotation of an innominate bone elevates the side of the sacrum. Thus, compensatory anterior rotation of the innominate is associated with a short lower limb, compensatory posterior rotation with a long lower limb. One would expect this functional compensation to become increasingly fixed over time.[188] Denslow and associates[36] also noted the likelihood of a compensatory horizontal rotation of the pelvis toward the longer side. Studies have also shown a relation between the SIJ and limited hip mobility[45,105] and between low back pain and asymmetrical hip rotation.[21,50,53,125]

☐ Hypermobility Lesions

Hypermobility lesions, like those in which hypomobility is the causative factor, are rare and occur in one of two situations.[29] According to Corrigan and Maitland,[29] the first situation is secondary to instability of the symphysis pubis, which occurs predominantly in athletes.[82] This condition may be complicated by a mechanical lesion of the lumbar spine or one or both SIJs, and may be associated with an osteitis condensans ilii. The second occurs in young females, usually during or soon after pregnancy. Ligaments may remain lax for 6 to 12 weeks after delivery or longer. Occasionally the symphysis may become a truly mobile joint, with pelvic instability as a result.[169] Movement abnormalities of the sacroiliac, the pubic joints, and the lumbar spine may be a cause of persistent postpartum pain.

Sacroiliac pain appears to be an accepted problem during pregnancy. Berg and colleagues[6] found that of 862 women who experienced low back pain during pregnancy, 79 could not continue work because of very severe low back pain. The most common cause was dysfunction of the SIJs. Under the influence of the hormone relaxin, there is a physiological pelvic girdle relaxation that may produce symptoms.[184] Dietricks and Kogstad[38] have suggested the terms *physiological pelvic girdle relaxation* for normal ligament relaxation during pregnancy and *symptom-giving pelvic girdle relaxation* for that which results in pain or pelvic instability. When pain in one or more pelvic joints is experienced outside pregnancy and the puerperium, the authors propose the term *pelvic joint syndrome*.[195] This term reflects their findings that pain, and not mechanical dysfunction, was the common symptom. There is clinical and radiological evidence to support the presence of increased SIJ mobility near the end of pregnancy.[79,104,114,124]

Simple mobilizing techniques localized to the SIJ structures are very effective after careful exclusion of problems from the intervertebral joints.[71] Use of sacroiliac belts appears to be justified in theory, but outcome data are not yet available.[109,153,196]

☐ Degenerative Changes

Degenerative changes are increasingly common with advancing age and may occur secondary to disorders in which movement is decreased.[29] SIJ degeneration is often associated with chronic neurological conditions such as paraplegia and hemiplegia. Degenerative changes are also associated with chronic structural abnormalities such as leg-length discrepancies, scoliosis, or pelvic asymmetries, or hip disease (osteoarthritis).[194,195] In patients with unilateral hip disease degenerative changes are usually found in the contralateral SIJ.[29]

Degenerative changes first involve the iliac surface, where the cartilage is thinner than on the sacral surface. The cartilage changes are similar to those in peripheral joints with, ultimately, a fibrous ankylosis of the joint cavity.[158,159] Vleeming and associates[190,191] consider the noninflammatory fibrous or chondroid ankylosis and radiologically visible hyaline cartilage-covered ridges to be physiological, not pathological, a response to joint stress and an adaptation for greater stability.

☐ Osteitis Condensans Ilii

Osteitis condensans ilii (a noninflammatory condition) is characterized by a condensation of bone on the iliac side of the SIJ. Its nature is uncertain but it probably represents a bony reaction to unequal stress in this joint. It is usually bilateral and occurs mostly in young adults, more commonly in postpartum women. It disappears with menopause, and is important medically as it mimics inflammatory disease.[196] Treatment consists of reassurance, analgesics, correction of any postural problems present, and if necessary the use of a sacroiliac belt.[29]

☐ Inflammatory Disease and Infections

Other conditions to be considered in the differential diagnosis include infections and metabolic conditions. Infections usually involve only one SIJ and may be a staphylococcal or tubercular infection, a sexually ac-

quired infection, or one due to intravenous drug abuse, among many other sources.[196] Inflammatory sacroiliitis conditions are either infectious or seronegative spondyloarthropathies. Of the latter, the major ones are ankylosing spondylitis, Rieter's syndrome, and psoriasis.[196] Ankylosing spondylitis is usually bilateral and symmetrical; involvement of the SIJs is the hallmark.

■ LUMBAR–PELVIC–HIP COMPLEX EVALUATION

☐ History

A general approach to history-taking is described in Chapter 5, Assessment of Musculoskeletal Disorders and Concepts of Management; the concepts there as well as in Chapter 12, The Hip, and Chapter 20, The Lumbar Spine, all apply to the evaluation of the lumbo–pelvic–hip complex.

In the history, certain traumatic incidents might point to involvement of the joints of the pelvis, such as a fall on the buttock, an unexpected heel-strike, a golf swing, or abnormal stresses occurring in such activities as punting a football. Chronic pain commencing after giving birth or starting oral contraceptives is another consideration. Most patients present with the typical history of acute or chronic back pain.

The history of the patient with SIJ pain typically includes:

1. Unilateral pain, most often local to the joint (sulcus) itself, but possibly referring down the leg (usually posterolaterally and not below the knee) because of innervation from the L2 through S2 segments. It may occasionally refer into the hip, groin, or abdomen.
2. The absence of lumbar articular signs or symptoms (although patients may have lesions at both areas)
3. Pain aggravated by walking, rolling over in bed, and climbing stairs, especially when leading with the involved side
4. Increased pain with prolonged postures or with standing or sitting on the affected side ("twisted-sitting" posture)
5. Morning stiffness that eases after a short period of weight-bearing.

Additional considerations are whether the patient has a past history of conditions that can involve the SIJ, such as ankylosing spondylitis,[65,170] Reiter's disease,[5,60] or rheumatoid arthritis.[145]

Finally, this area is a common site for secondary malignant deposits or Paget's disease (osteitis deformans). Paget's disease is characteristically aggravated by exercise and is more severe during sleep.[33,84]

☐ Specific Sacroiliac Evaluation

When assessing patients with sacroiliac pain, remember that pain felt in this area may be referred from either the lower lumbar spine or the hip joint. The SIJ should not be examined comprehensively until after the lumbar spine and hip joint examinations, including neurological tests. The goal of assessment is to determine what force(s) reproduce the patient's symptoms.

OBSERVATION

Observe the patient's posture, body type, and ability to move freely. Refer to Chapter 22, The Lumbosacral–Lower Limb Scan Examination, for a discussion of common gait abnormalities and possible causes.

GAIT

Careful observation of the patient's gait pattern can be informative, as formal bipedal striding requires optimal lumbo–pelvic–hip function. Sacroiliac dysfunction may originate from a leg-length discrepancy and the accompanying excessive increase or decrease in lordosis. A painful SIJ may cause reflex inhibition of the gluteus medius, leading to a Trendelenburg gait or lurch.[117] The patient may sidebend the trunk away from the painful side or walk with difficulty.

POSTURE

Postural asymmetry does not necessarily indicate pelvic girdle dysfunction, but pelvic girdle dysfunction is often reflected via postural asymmetry. Observe the patient's standing posture, sitting posture (sitting on a stool or bench without back support), and long-sitting. In the coronal and sagittal planes, observe the head, shoulder alignment, spinal curves, and level of the pelvis. In particular, carefully observe the distribution of body weight through the lower quadrant. In weight-bearing, note whether the patient stands with equal weight on both feet or has a lateral pelvic tilt, suggesting an apparent or real leg-length discrepancy. Patients tend to bear weight on the unaffected side in standing and sitting and to step up with the unaffected side. Note the posture of the feet (pronation/supination) and the knees (hyperextension, varus, valgus). Variations in the resting position of these joints can be the result of compensation for a longstanding leg-length discrepancy. The lower limbs are also an important link in the transference of ground forces to the pelvis. In anterior dysfunction of the innominate, the lower limb may be medially ro-

tated. With spasm of the piriformis muscle, the limb may be laterally rotated on the affected side.

In integrating the myofascial system, look for muscle asymmetry, connective tissue asymmetry, and increased muscle activity that may correlate with abnormal structural deviations. For example, muscle asymmetry may be a result of prolonged shortening or lengthening of a muscle group due to pelvic obliquity or a leg-length discrepancy. Although asymmetry is important, remember that the human body is by nature's design asymmetrical; the critical factor in determining whether the asymmetry is significant is its correlation to other relevant evaluation findings.

INSPECTION

BONY STRUCTURE AND ALIGNMENT

Refer to the section on assessment of structural alignment in Chapter 22, The Lumbosacral–Lower Limb Scan Examination, for a complete discussion of this part of the examination.

I. In the standing position, compare the levels of the posterior-superior iliac spines (PSIS), the iliac crests, and the anterior-superior spines iliac (ASIS). The most common finding is the posterior innominate in which the PSIS is lower than the opposite side. The reverse is found with the anterior innominate.
   A. Palpate the summit of the greater trochanter for levelness as an indicator of apparent or structural leg-length discrepancy. See Chapter 12, The Hip, for measurement of functional leg length.
   B. The depth caliper/meter stick method may be used clinically for detecting pelvic movement (Fig. 21-8).[1] Measurement of PSIS displacement is used. By this method Alviso and colleagues[1] determined an average total pelvic tilt range of 14.3°, with a standard deviation of 5.2°. Anterior pelvic tilt averaged 7.9°; posterior tilt range of motion was an average of 6.5°.
II. In sitting (erect on a level surface), repeat palpation of the bony landmarks of the innominate. Determine if lateral pelvic tilt is still present or if the previous lateral tilt in standing is now eradicated.
III. In hyperflexion (sitting, feet supported, knees at a right angle and apart, sufficient to allow the shoulders to come between them and the lumbar spine to be fully flexed), determine the position of the sacrum for possible sacral dysfunction (Fig. 21-9). To determine the position of the sacrum, compare the posteroanterior relation of the sacral base or the depth of the two sacral sulci and the inferior lateral angles (Fig. 21-10).[14,109]

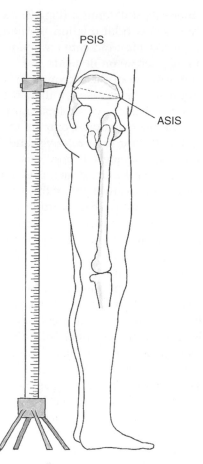

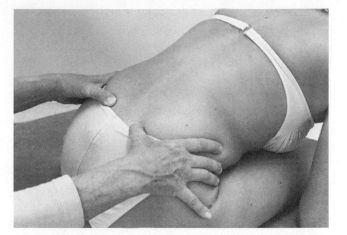

FIG. 21-9. Positional testing in hyperflexion of the lumbosacral junction.

FIG. 21-8. Measurement of pelvic inclination: measuring the distance from the PSIS to the floor. (Adapted from Basmajian JV, Nyberg R: Rational Manual Therapies, p 103. Baltimore, Williams & Wilkins, 1993.)

ligament. Note any tissue texture abnormality (see Fig. 16-20B).

As these positional findings may be manifested only in one position of the vertebral column, it is necessary to evaluate in neutral (prone) and finally in hyperextension.[109] For other types of sacral torsion lesions, refer to the works of Bourdillon,[14] Greenman,[68] Lee,[109] Mitchell,[132,133] and Woerman.[208]

IV. With the patient in supine and the crook position, have him or her lift the buttock and drop it down to the mat or treatment table, or do it for the patient. Bring the knees to the chest and slowly bring the legs down with the knees extended.

   A. Check the iliac crests for asymmetry. With the

A. The level of the sacral base is often called the *depth of the sacral sulcus*.[68] The sacral base can be described as anterior or posterior if it is not level against the coronal plane; if one sacral base is more anterior than the other, the sacral sulcus is said to be deep on that side. Using the thumbs, palpate the sacral depth (dorsal ventral distance) between the PSIS and the base of the sacrum, medially from the caudal aspect of the PSIS bilaterally.

B. The *inferior lateral angle* is the transverse process of S5 and is found by placing one finger in the sacral hiatus and the index and middle fingers of the other hand on either side at the same level about 2 cm away (see Fig. 21-10).[14] An anterior right sacral base or a deep (anterior) sacral sulcus, together with a left inferior lateral angle, suggests a left rotated sacrum.[109,141] This is the most common sacral torsion dysfunction. When palpating the inferior lateral angle, one is also palpating the superior attachment of the sacrotuberous

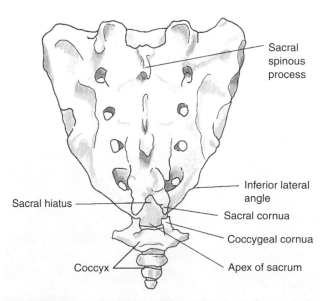

FIG. 21-10. The posterior aspect of the sacrum: anatomical landmarks used in palpation of the posterior aspect of the sacrum.

radial border of the index fingers, palpate the highest point of the iliac crest bilaterally. Compare the craniocaudal relation of the two sides.

B. Check the set of the pelvis. Determine whether either ilium is inflared (one ilium ASIS is closer to the midline than the opposite ASIS) or outflared (one ilium ASIS is further from the midline than the opposite ASIS). Use an imaginary line from the tip of the xyphoid to the pubis; ignore the navel, which is often off to one side. Over time an inflared or outflared ilium will lead to muscle imbalance.

C. Palpate bilaterally the caudal aspect of the ASIS. Check for rotation (craniocaudal relation) and the anterior-posterior relation (deep or higher).

D. Determine whether both pubic bones are level at the symphysis pubis. Test for levelness (craniocaudal position) by placing the thumbs on the superior aspect of each pubic bone and comparing the height (Fig. 21-11). This can be correlated with anterior or posterior dysfunction and the relation of the ASIS. In posterior dysfunction, one would expect the pubic bone also to be higher.

E. Assess leg-length equality (non-weight-bearing). See Chapter 12, The Hip.

V. In prone, determine:

A. Whether the ischial tuberosities are level (superoinferior position). Using the thumbs, palpate the most caudal aspect of the ischial tuberosity bilaterally (Fig. 21-12). Compare the craniocaudal relation. If one tuberosity is higher, it may indicate an *upslip* of the ilium on the sacrum on that side.[208]

B. The position of the sacrum (see above). If one sacral sulcus is deeper than the other, this could indicate a possible sacral torsion or an innominate rotation. Compare the inferior lateral angles for their relative caudad/cephalad and anteroposterior positions. If the angles are level and a deep sacral sulcus is found, it suggests a dysfunction of the innominates.[208]

VI. In the press-up or backward-bending position (prone on elbows with the patient's chin resting in the hands and the lumbar spine in hyperextension), determine the position of the sacrum by palpating the position of the:

A. Sacral sulci, to determine if there has been a change in the relative depth of the sacral sulci from that noted in the neutral prone position. In sacroiliac dysfunction, the side that is blocked will remain shallow and the side that is free to move will go deeper.[68,208]

B. The inferior lateral angles, to determine if there has been a change in their position. If the angle opposite the deep sacral sulcus becomes more posterior in this position, it suggests a forward sacral torsion. If the angle is more inferior on the same side as the deep sacral sulcus, it suggests a unilateral sacral flexion.[208]

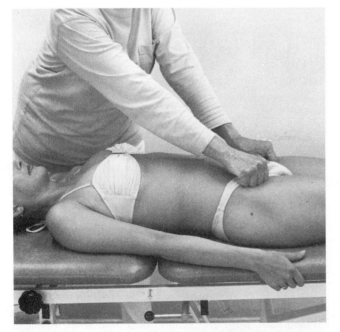

FIG. 21-11. *Determining the level of the pubic tubercles.*

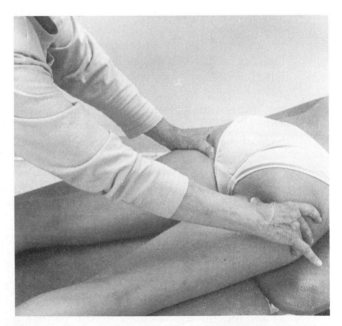

FIG. 21-12. *Determining the position of the ischial tuberosities.*

SOFT-TISSUE INSPECTION AND MUSCLE CONTOUR

With the patient standing, it is not unusual to observe a loss of bulk of the gluteal muscles of one side co-existing with sacroiliac dysfunction. View the abdominal outline and the lumbar region from the side. A weak protruding abdominal wall and a marked lumbar lordosis may be a source of stress falling on the pelvic joints.

With the patient prone, look for pelvic asymmetry and flattening of the buttock. Decreased tone in the glutei of the affected side may cause the hip to fall into more medial rotation compared to the opposite side.[203] Note a swollen appearance over either joint.

SELECTIVE TISSUE-TENSION TESTS

ACTIVE MOVEMENTS

See Chapter 22, The Lumbosacral–Lower Limb Scan Examination, for a complete discussion of this part of the examination. Perform active physiological movements of the spine and peripheral joints of the lower extremity. Note the quantity and quality of motion achieved. Look for loss of movement or hypermobility, the patient's willingness to move, and the presence and location of evoked symptoms.

I. **Forward-Flexion** (standing and seated)

   A. *Lumbosacral junction* (flexion)

     While palpating the transverse processes of the L5 vertebra, determine if any abnormal coupling (*i.e.*, two or more types of motion occurring simultaneously, such as rotation or sideflexion) manifests with flexion or extension. The transverse processes of the L5 vertebra should travel an equal distance in a superior direction. Monitor the lower thoracic and lumbar spine for segmental dysrhythmia or a compensatory scoliotic curvature.

   B. *Pelvic girdle*

     Active physiological mobility testing of the pelvis is a useful preliminary test of pelvic girdle function, as asymmetry of motion is present in all unilateral hypomobility disorders.[14,68,109,133,202]

   C. *Standing flexion test*

     1. Palpate the inferior slope of the PSIS bilaterally (following the excursion of motion), as the patient actively forward-bends, for any innominate distortion (Fig. 21-13A). The posterior-superior iliac spines should travel an equal distance in a superior direction.

     2. Repeat while palpating the sacral base or inferior lateral angles for sacral distortion (Fig. 21-13B). The angles of the sacrum

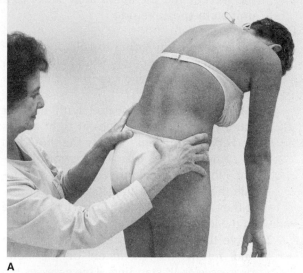

FIG. 21-13. Active physiological mobility tests: (**A**) forward bending of innominate bones and (**B**) forward bending of the sacrum.

should travel an equal distance in a superior direction without deviating in the anteroposterior plane. The test for innominate excursion is positive on the side in which the PSIS appears to move more cephalically and ventrally.[68] It is thought that the downward and backward glide of the two limbs of the SIJ has been lost, so the sacrum and the innominate move as a unit on the positive side.

D. *Seated flexion test*

Repeat the test in sitting to rule out extrinsic influences on the pelvis from below, such as leg-length discrepancy or the effect of a tight hamstring.

1. Position the patient seated with the feet flat on the floor and knees at right angles and apart, sufficient to allow the shoulders to come between them in forward-bending. Note the spinal movements and correlate them with standing forward-bending. If they have changed, the problem may be in the lower extremity.

2. Have the patient repeat forward-bending and follow the excursion of the bony processes as in standing. This assesses the movement of the sacrum with the ilium stabilized. If the PSIS moves in the same manner as in standing (more cephalically and ventrally on one side), it suggests a sacroiliac problem (as opposed to iliosacral).[202]

II. Lateral Bending (standing)

Note the ability of the pelvic girdle to translate laterally to the opposite side without deviation. See Chapter 16, The Spine, for the specific osteokinematics required during this test.

III. Auxiliary Tests

In most patients with symptoms arising from the SIJ, the active tests described above are sufficient to reproduce the patient's symptoms. If not, consider applying passive overpressure at the end range of the active physiological motions described above or using repeated motions, sustained pressure, and combined motions of the active physiological motions of the spine as well as combined motions with overpressure (see Chap. 20, The Lumbar Spine). When applying passive overpressure, consider if the overpressure is increasing compressive or tensile forces to the area.

IV. Hip Mobility (weight-bearing flexion)

Have the patient perform a bilateral or unilateral squat. Functionally, the dynamic stabilization of the hip joint and its ability to bear full weight during flexion and standing is of paramount importance.

V. Sacroiliac Fixation Tests[101,102]

Several tests have been devised to demonstrate sacroiliac fixation. This signifies ipsilateral locking, in which the sacrum and ilium move as a whole due to muscular contraction that prevents motion of the sacrum on the ilium (intrapelvic torsion). These tests include the one-legged stork test,[14,68] the ipsilateral kinetic test,[56,109,110] Gillet's test,[208] and Piedallu's sign.[69,150,168]

A. With the patient standing and using one hand for support on a table or back of a chair, palpate the inferior aspect of the PSIS with one thumb while using the other to palpate the median sacral crest directly parallel (spinous process of S2). Have the patient flex the ipsilateral femur at the hip joint and knee to 90°. Observe the displacement of the PSIS relative to the sacrum (Fig. 21-14*A–C*). This test examines the ability of the innominate bone to laterally flex and laterally rotate, as well as the ability of the sacrum to rotate.[109]

B. In a similar manner, place one thumb over the last sacral spinous process and other thumb over the ischial tuberosity. Have the patient repeat hip flexion as above, and observe the displacement of the thumb on the ischial tuberosity (Fig. 21-14*D–F*). Repeat both tests on the opposite side and compare the results.

C. A third test is required to examine the ability of the innominate bone to extend and medially rotate.[109] With the patient prone, palpate the PSIS with one thumb while the other palpates the median sacral crest directly opposite. Have the patient extend the ipsilateral femur at the hip joint. Note the superolateral displacement of the PSIS relative to the sacrum.

PASSIVE MOVEMENTS

I. Lumbosacral Junction (L5 vertebra and the sacral base)

Osteokinematic tests of physiological mobility and arthrokinematic tests of accessory motion should be performed as described in Chapter 20, The Lumbar Spine.

II. Pelvic Girdle: Osteokinematic Tests of Physiological Mobility

A. *Pelvic rock test* (Fig. 21-15). The pelvic rock test involves getting a sense of the mobility of the joint and the end feel for the relative ease or resistance to passive overpressure for each innominate. With the subject in supine, place the palms on the ASIS and gently glide and then spring or shear the innominates alternately in a medial anteroposterior direction (in the plane of the joint). While maintaining light pressure on the opposite side, press more firmly on first one side and then the other to detect resilience. A harder end feel on one side indicates a probable restriction of movement on that side.

B. *Flexion–extension of the innominate bone* (Fig.

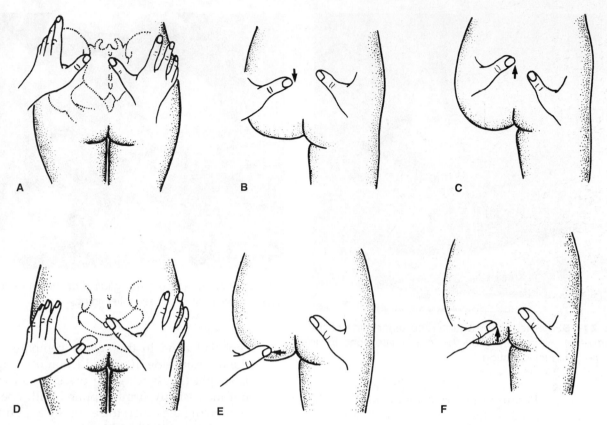

FIG. 21-14. Test for sacroiliac joint fixation. The patient is examined in standing and is instructed to flex the hip and knee to 90° during each test. To test the upper part of joint (left side): (**A**) Place one thumb over the spinous process of S2 and the other hand over the PSIS. (**B**) In the normal joint the thumb will move caudally. (**C**) In the abnormally fixed joint the thumb will move cephalad. To assess the lower part of the joint: (**D**) Place one thumb over the last sacral spinous process and the other thumb over the ischial tuberosity. (**E**) In the normal joint the thumb will move laterally. (**F**) In the abnormally fixed joint the thumb will remain stationary. (From Kirkalday-Willis WH [ed]: Managing Low Back Pain, 2nd ed, p 137. New York, Churchill Livingstone, 1988.)

21-16). With the patient sidelying, hips and knees comfortably flexed, contact the ASIS with one hand while the other contacts the ipsilateral ischial tuberosity. The innominate bone is passively flexed and extended (posteriorly and anteriorly rotated) on the sacrum; note the quantity of motion.

III. Pelvic Girdle: Arthrokinematic Tests of Accessory Joint Mobility

   A. *Anteroposterior iliac glide* (Fig. 21-17).[46,203] With the patient lying prone, palpate the sacral base with the fingertips of the cranial hand, placing them over the joint in question (over the short posterior sacral ligaments). The ilium, held by hooking the fingers under the ASIS with the caudal hand, is gently and repeatedly lifted in an anteroposterior direction. If the amplitude of movement is too large it will merely rotate the lumbar spine

and override the small but detectable joint play. The palpating fingers register the relative displacement between the iliac bone and the sacrum, which should be about 2 to 3 mm.[46]

ARTHROKINEMATIC TESTS OF STABILITY

Movement of the SIJ is produced by a series of passive movements designed to stress the joint or ligaments and to reproduce the patient's pain. That numerous tests have been devised is proof of their inadequacy. The stress tests also stress other structures, so false-positive and false-negative results are common.[29]

   I. **Sacral   Apex   Pressure   Test   or   Tripod Test**[29,46,71,203]

   The patient lies prone. Apply vertical pressure to the sacrum with the heel of the caudal hand. Rock the sacrum by repetitive pressure to

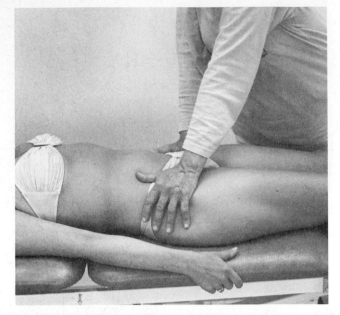

FIG. 21-15. Pelvic rock test (anteroposterior glide of the innominate). Alternately glide the innominate bone in an anterior–posterior direction.

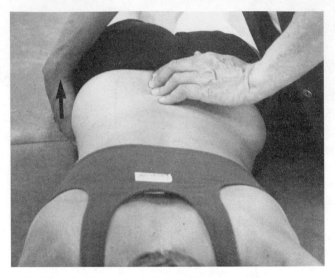

FIG. 21-17. Anteroposterior gliding of the innominate to detect movement of the sacroiliac joint.

its apex. Because the three-point contact, of the pubis and the anterior ends of the ilium, with the surface of the treatment table will stabilize the pelvis, repetitive downward pressures on the sacral apex will induce a small degree of movement of the sacrum on the ilium. This may be detected with the palpating fingers of the

cephalad hand in the sulcus; compare it with the opposite side. If reproduction of symptoms is sought (stress test), the pressure is carefully but increasingly firmly applied with one hand reinforcing the other; the arms are kept fully extended (Fig. 21-18). This produces a shearing movement across the SIJs as well as movement of the lumbosacral joint. The hand may incline medially or laterally, or in a cephalad or caudad direction to amplify the findings.

Note: In manual therapy practice, testing procedures are often used as subsequent treatment techniques. The sacral apex pressure test is a good example. As a technique it is considered a sacral counternutation manipulation to increase

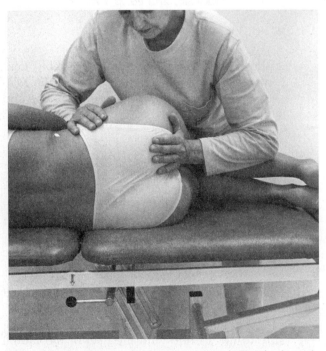

FIG. 21-16. Passive flexion/extension (posterior/anterior rotation) of the innominate bone.

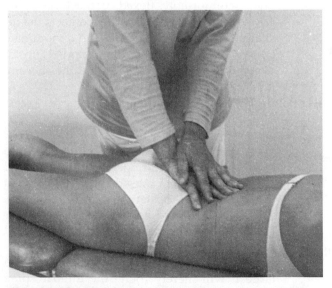

FIG. 21-18. Sacral apex pressure test.

joint play and range of motion into sacral counternutation or to reduce a sacral nutation positional fault. Bilateral sacral flexion dysfunction may be thought of as a failure to return from a fully nutated position; bilateral sacral extension dysfunction may be thought of as a failure to return from the fully counternutated position.

II. **Posteroanterior and Transverse Oscillatory Pressure** (Fig. 21-19)[120,203]

Unlike pressures applied to the spinal joints to explore the characteristics of accessory motion, these pressures, when applied to the sacroiliac region, are used to determine if they provoke or relieve the patient's symptoms. Such pressures may also be used as treatment. Thumb pressures are directed over the sacrum and adjacent ilium in an attempt to reproduce the patient's symptoms.

This useful routine was suggested by Wells.[203] With the patient in prone, first direct posteroanterior thumb pressures centrally on each sacral spinous process in turn. Next, direct posteroanterior oscillatory pressures unilaterally at each sacral level and over each PSIS (Fig. 21-19*A*). Finally, apply transverse pressures directed laterally just medial to the PSIS (Fig. 21-19*B*).

III. **Longitudinal Stress of the Sacrum** (craniocaudal and caudocranial pressures or caudocephalic shearing procedures; Fig. 21-20)[29,71,72,203]

To test these two motions, the patient is placed in the prone position. Place the heel of one hand near the apex of the sacrum and apply pressure in a cephalad direction while the heel of the other hand stabilizes the posterior third of the iliac crest. Next, apply pressure near the base of the sacrum in a caudad direction while the ilium is stabilized at the ischial tuberosity.

Note: These tests may be useful as gentle treatment techniques, applied to areas of pain noted when used as tests of sacroiliac strain.

IV. **Prone Gapping Test** (Fig. 21-21)[72,203]

This test can be done only if the hip is normal

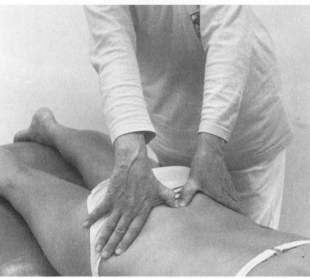

A

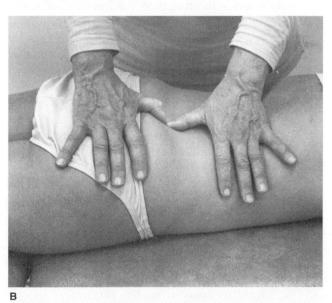

B

FIG. 21-19. Oscillatory pressures: (**A**) posteroanterior pressures applied unilaterally at each sacral level and (**B**) transverse pressures applied to the posterior superior iliac spine.

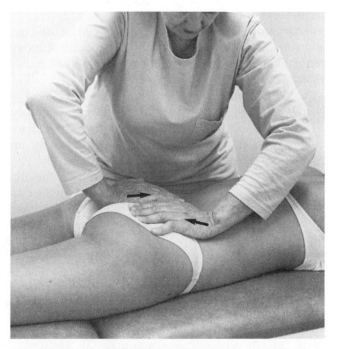

FIG. 21-20. Longitudinal stress applied to the sacrum (in a caudad direction) and the ilium (in a cephalad direction).

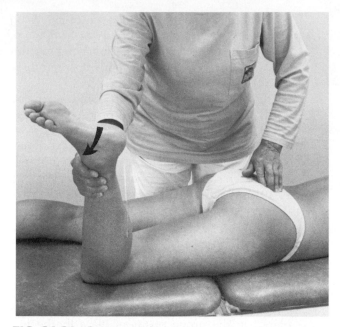

FIG. 21-21. Prone gapping test.

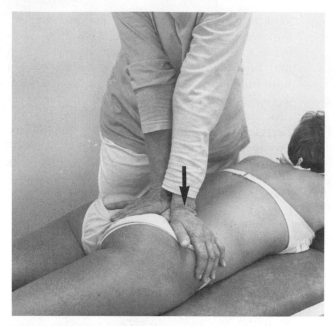

FIG. 21-22. Torsional stress test.

and full internal rotation is painless. With the patient prone, stabilize the pelvis with your thigh or abdomen while palpating the sacroiliac sulcus with the cranial hand. The patient's far knee is flexed to 90° and the hip placed in end range medial rotation while small-range oscillatory stresses are placed on the hip by the caudal hand and forearm. A small amount of sacroiliac gapping can be appreciated by the palpating fingers. Repeat the test on the opposite side, comparing the degree of opening and the quality of movement.

Note: This test is another that can be used as a treatment procedure.[69] Gentle repetitive movements can be very precisely graded when used as a treatment procedure.

V. **Torsional Stress** (Fig. 21-22)[203]

With the patient in the prone position, stabilize the sacrum at its apex with the caudad hand while the cephalad hand simultaneously applies vertical downward pressure over the PSIS on the far side. According to Wells,[203] this maneuver is particularly informative when examining a chronically hypomobile and nonirritable joint problem. Repeated oscillatory pressures reveal a markedly unyielding response in this case.

Note: This evaluation procedure can also be used either as an effective mobilization or manipulation technique for posterior dysfunction of the innominate.[71]

VI. **Compression–Distraction Tests** (transverse anterior stress test and gapping test; Fig. 21-23)[29,87,117,167,208]

Compression–distraction tests are used to ascertain a serious pathology, the presence of hypermobility, and to stress the ligaments and joint. The subject lies supine while the examiner applies crossed-arm pressure to the anterior-superior iliac spines with the heels of the hands (Fig. 21-23A). The slack is taken up and a posterolateral spring is given. This action compresses the SIJs posteriorly and gaps them anteriorly, stressing the anterior sacroiliac ligaments and the transverse pubic ligament. Then move the hands to the lateral iliac wings and compress the pelvis toward the midline of the body (Fig. 21-23B). Doing so compresses the anterior and distracts the posterior SIJs and ligaments. Some authors suggest applying a slow, steady force through the pelvic girdle (maintained for 20 seconds) rather than a spring-like force.[109]

VII. **Isometric Contraction of Hip Abductors and Adductors** (Fig. 21-24)[29,56]

A. *Hip abduction* (Fig. 21-24A)

The patient is supine with knees bent, feet flat on the treatment table, hips slightly abducted. The pelvis is in a neutral position. Place each hand on the lateral aspect of each of the patient's knees. Have the patient resist a force provided by the examiner into hip abduction, thus distracting the iliac joint surfaces away from the sacrum as the abductors contract and pull on their attachment to the iliac crest.

B. *Hip adduction* (Fig. 21-24B)

With the patient in the same position as

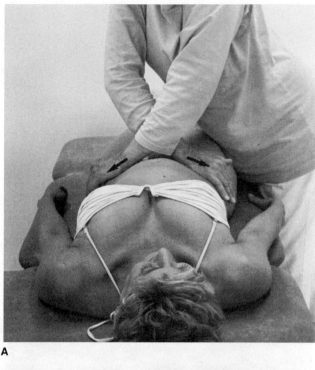

A

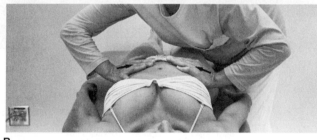

B

FIG. 21-23. Compression–distraction test using the crossed hand method (**A**) and (**B**) from the lateral aspect of the innominate.

above, the adductors of the hip are isometrically contracted by attempting to maximally adduct the hip joints against the examiner's hands, thereby recruiting the patient's short adductors. Adduction stresses the symphysis pubis because these short muscles cross the inferior aspect of the pubic articulation in a cruciate manner; when recruited, they strongly bring the joint into a balanced level position.[56] A slight popping noise is often elicited; this is felt to bring the joint strongly into a level position.[56,133]

After this test, the fixation and positioning tests are re-evaluated. If no change has occurred, a sacroiliac or iliosacral dysfunction is the probable cause.

Pain experienced over the SIJ on resisted abduction (in the absence of hip joint disease) in sidelying (positional test with the

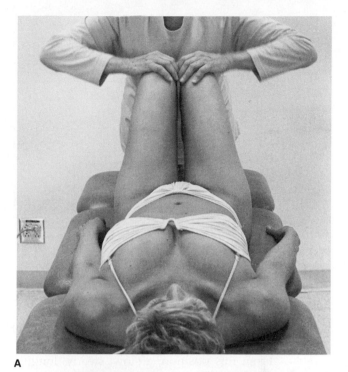

A

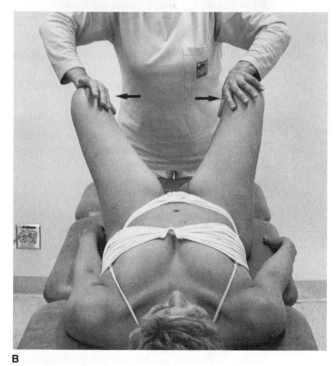

B

FIG. 21-24. Isometric contractions: (**A**) Hip abduction and (**B**) hip adduction.

knee extended) is highly suggestive of an SIJ lesion. According to Macnab,[116] when the gluteus maximus contracts to abduct the hip, it pulls the ilium away from the sacrum.

VIII. Sacrotuberous Ligament Stress Test (Fig. 21-25)[108,109,117,153]

With the patient in a supine position, the

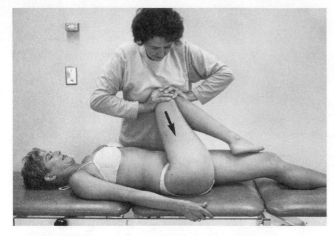

FIG. 21-25. Sacrotuberous ligament stress test.

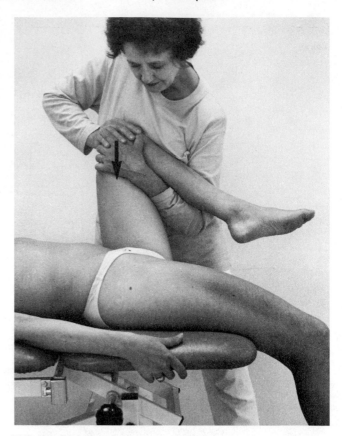

FIG. 21-26. Femoral shear test.

contralateral hip and knee are fully flexed and then adducted. The innominate bone is flexed and medially rotated until tension of the sacrotuberous ligament is perceived. From this position, a slow, steady, longitudinal (axial-loading) force is applied with both hands through the femur in an obliquely lateral direction to stress the posterior sacroiliac ligament further. The force is maintained for 20 seconds; note if local pain is provoked.[109] Another example of using the femur as a lever is to rock the SIJ by flexion and adduction of the hip, moving the knee toward the patient's opposite shoulder.[117] A long axis force is then applied down through the femur until all the tissues have become taut, and then a small adduction force is imparted through the shaft of the femur, which compresses the anterior aspect of the SIJ and results in a significant gapping at the posterior aspect.[153] These tests may induce ligamentous stretch pain, possibly indicating a functionally shortened or stressed (overloaded) posterior sacroiliac ligament.[46]

IX. Femoral Shear Test (Fig. 21-26)[117,153]

With the patient in the supine position, the leg is flexed, abducted, and laterally rotated until the thigh is at about 45°, so as to line up the force with the plane of the ipsilateral SIJ. Apply a graded force through the long axis of the femur, causing an anterior-to-posterior shear to the SIJ.

Note: There are many other tests commonly used to stress the SIJ, including the Patrick or Fabere test,[46,83,87,208] the Gaenslen test,[83,87,117] Gillet's (sacral fixation) test,[208] the flamingo test or single-leg stand,[107,117]

Yeoman's test,[25,117,168] and Goldthwait's test.[25,117,168]

TESTS TO DETERMINE FUNCTIONAL LEG-LENGTH DIFFERENCE

I. Supine-to-Sit Test (long-sitting test)[3,4,46,151,167,193,208]

This test is used to assess the ability of the SIJs to move in response to external forces that passively rotate the innominates (Fig. 21-27). To ensure a neutral alignment of the pelvis on the table, the patient performs a bridging technique, which consists of flexing the knees to place the feet flat on the table, extending the hips to lift the buttocks from the surface, and then relaxing to allow the buttocks to return to the table. With the subject in the supine position, compare the positions of the medial malleoli using the borders of the thumbs. Have the patient sit with the knees extended and recheck the malleoli for symmetry. Caudad positioning of one malleolus may indicate posterior rotation of the ilium. If the standing flexion test is positive on the same side, then this test is considered positive. Conversely, a cephalad malleolus indicates an anteriorly rotated ilium. This phenomenon (short to long or equal to long) is

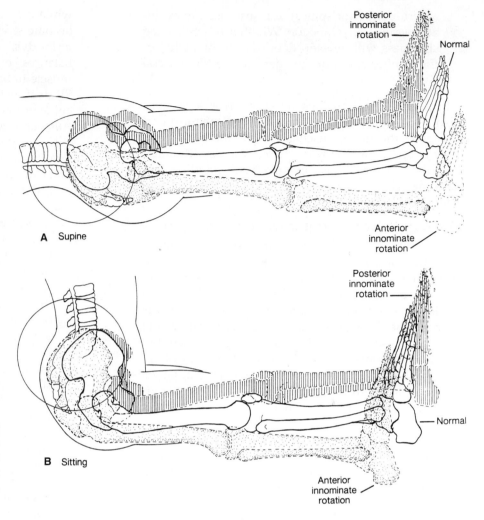

FIG. 21-27. Supine-to-sit test. Leg length reversal: supine (**A**) versus sitting (**B**). (From Wadsworth CT [ed]: Manual Examination and Treatment of the Spine and Extremities, p 82. Baltimore, Williams & Wilkins, 1988.)

thought to occur because in the posterior innominate, posterior rotation of the innominate moves the acetabulum in a superior direction and carries the leg along with it; the opposite occurs in anterior rotation. A difference of less than 2 cm is probably not clinically significant.[46]

Note: A study by Bemis and Daniel[4] suggests that this test is an accurate method of predicting iliosacral dysfunction. As with other tests, however, it should not be used alone but in conjunction with other confirmational data for accurate diagnosis.

II. **Wilson/Barlow Test of Pelvic Motion Symmetry**[133,167,208]

The patient lies supine and flexes the knees and hips. Grasp the ankles with the thumbs under the medial malleoli. To equalize the patient's position on the table, have the patient then lift the buttocks from the table, then return to the resting position. Next, passively extend the patient's legs toward yourself, maintaining good alignment. Compare the positions of the malleoli using the borders of

the thumbs. A difference in leg length should agree with the standing sacral base test. This test is also used as an alternative test for the standing and seated flexion tests. Additional steps include:

A. Passive flexion of one leg on the abdomen and then abduction, external rotation, and extension of the leg. Then compare the malleoli for levelness. The leg should appear longer.

B. Flexion of the same leg on the abdomen, internal rotation, and then extension. The leg should appear shorter. Failure of the leg to shorten or lengthen may indicate pelvic dysfunction.

III. **Testing for Leg Length** (prone)[68,132]

The patient is prone with the dorsum of the foot free at the edge of the table. Both legs are pulled toward the operator to ensure good alignment. Palpate the medial malleoli to determine any differences in length. This test is used to evaluate the position of the sacrum between the two innominates (which are triangulated on the examination table by the symphysis pubis and the two anterior-superior spines). It is also used to evaluate sacroiliac dysfunction. Whether functional leg shortness will develop depends on the ability of the lumbar curvature to adapt to the tilted sacral base.

In all these examinations, observer error is possible. Also, these non-weight-bearing tests for the most part disregard the neuromuscular control of movement. Gravity-eliminated body mechanics are very different from the body mechanics in antigravity standing, and standing assessment is thought to yield more clinically relevant information.

MYOKINEMATIC TESTS FOR MUSCLE FUNCTION

The complete lumbar and hip regions should be evaluated or screened because sacroiliac dysfunction occurs in combination with tissue injury to other lumbopelvic tissues. The pelvic girdle is the link between the lower limbs and the spine. Ligaments and fascia connect the lumbar spine, pelvis, and femur and should be tested when this area is being assessed. Important ligaments and fascia include the thoracolumbar (lumbodorsal) fascia, iliolumbar ligament, lateral fascia of the thigh, sacroiliac ligament, sacrotuberous ligament, sacrospinous ligament, and iliotibial band. The ligamentous structures (iliofemoral, ischiofemoral, and pubofemoral ligaments) and the hip joint's fibrous capsule also influence the lower limb kinetic chain. Restrictions, contractures, or laxity of the capsule can result in hip and lower quadrant mechanical dysfunction.

If the pelvis is not symmetrically balanced, then muscle imbalances occur, and with time some muscles will develop tightness while their antagonists will develop stretch weakness. Several muscles link the lumbar spine, sacrum, pelvis, and lower limbs into one kinetic chain, so any muscle imbalance or injury can influence the whole kinetic chain. A common finding in the examination of sacroiliac dysfunction is decreased passive range of motion on the side of the lesion. Hip capsule tightness or muscle shortness creates a biomechanical alteration that makes the SIJ vulnerable to overuse and sprain from what would otherwise be activities within normal tolerance.

I. **Sagittal Plane Alignment**
   A. *Anterior or posterior rotation dysfunction*

   If a unilateral posterior innominate rotation exists, the gluteus maximus, hamstrings, and adductor magnus on that side tend to become shortened and tight while the hip flexors, sartorius, and remaining adductors become stretched and weak on the affected side.[83] Conversely, if unilateral anterior rotation dysfunction exists, the hip flexors, adductors, and tensor fasciae latae become tight on that side

while the hamstrings, glutei, and abdominals become stretched and weak. Anterior or posterior dysfunction can cause these muscle imbalances, or these rotations can result from muscle imbalances. These rotations can cause SIJ dysfunction and eventual hip and lumbar spine problems.

B. *Anterior or posterior tilt*

   Excessive anterior or posterior tilt of the whole pelvis can lead to muscle imbalances and can also subject the SIJ, the lumbar spine, and the hip joint to abnormal forces and loads.

   1. If there is an anterior pelvic tilt, the lumbar spine moves into excessive lordosis and the lumbosacral angle increases. The hip flexors (chiefly the iliopsoas) and erector spinae shorten and become tight, and the abdominals, glutei, and hamstrings become stretched and weakened.[83] The anterior longitudinal ligaments in the lumbar spine and the sacrotuberous, sacroiliac, and sacrospinous ligaments are stretched.[146] There is increased compression of the lumbar spine posteriorly on the vertebrae and the articulating facets.[97]

   2. If there is a posterior pelvic tilt, the lumbar spine moves into a flat posture, characterized by a decreased lumbosacral angle. In the flat-back posture (rigid), the lumbar paraspinals become lengthened, and perhaps the hip flexors, while the hamstrings and adductor magnus become tight.[83] There is compression of the lumbar vertebrae anteriorly, stretching of the hip capsule,[146] and stress to the posterior longitudinal ligament. Kendall and associates[97] describe the flexible flat-back posture in which the low back muscles are usually normal and the abdominal muscles, especially the lower abdominals, tend to be stronger than normal. The hip extensors are usually strong and the hamstrings are short.

II. **Frontal Plane Alignment**

   A unilateral change in limb length in the closed kinetic chain position in the presence of tight muscles can alter mechanics and cause pain anywhere in the body.[197] If the leg is longer, the ilium on that side is higher, which causes imbalances of forces through the SIJ, hip joint, pubic symphysis, sacrum, lumbar spine, and whole lower limb.[83] Altered weight-bearing forces also go through the opposite side. On the long side the quadratus lumborum, iliocostalis lumborum, iliopsoas, obliques, and rectus abdominis become tight, while the hamstrings, adductors, rectus femoris, sartorius, and tensor fasciae latae become stretched and weak.[83] The opposite muscle imbalances occur on the side of the shorter leg. Subjects with leg-length differences are generally weaker on the short side.[11,197]

Any alteration of the joints or muscles in the lower extremity can result in a functional leg-length difference—that is, a foot with pronation that produces a shortening effect, or the knee in recurvatum with a weak quadriceps and gastrocnemius, which generally has a lengthening effect.[197] Anterior rotation dysfunction (ASIS low) causes a functional lengthening; posterior rotation causes a functional shortening. It is easy to miss a small right/left difference if the patient is evaluated only in a non-weight-bearing position.

With lateral pelvic tilt (a sideways tilt of the pelvis from neutral position, often associated with handedness pattern), the posterior lateral trunk muscles and thoracolumbar fascia are tighter on the high side of the pelvis, and the leg abductors and tensor fasciae latae are tighter on the low side of the pelvis.[97]

III. Transverse Plane Alignment[83]

A. On the outflare side, the adductors, obliques, and sartorius become tight; the gluteus medius, minimus, and tensor fasciae latae become stretched and weak.

B. On the inflare side, the gluteus medius, minimus, and tensor fasciae latae become tight; the adductors, obliques, and sartorius become stretched and weak. These muscle imbalances twist the pelvic girdle and cause excessive rotational forces through the lumbar spine and the whole lower limb on the involved side. The hip joint becomes rotated and the symphysis pubis, SIJ, or lumbar spine may develop dysfunction.

IV. Examination Of Lower Quadrant Muscle Length

If the regional tests of osseous and articular mobility fail to reveal the etiology of the dysfunction, the following tests of myokinematic function may help determine the cause. Some key muscles that have already been addressed include the quadratus lumborum, the abdominal muscles, the gluteus maximus, and the piriformis. Relative to the pelvic girdle, the postural muscles that tend to tighten should be assessed for their extensibility and influence on the mobility of the lumbo–pelvic–hip complex.[90–92] The postural muscles include:

A. *Erector spinae and quadratus lumborum*

Tightness of the erector spinae and quadratus lumborum is revealed in the seated for- ward-bending position. Note the quantity of the available motion, the symmetry or asymmetry of the paravertebral muscles, and the presence or absence of a multisegmental spinal curve at the limit of range. Multisegmental rotoscoliosis may indicate unilateral tightness of the erector spinae or the quadratus lumborum.[109]

An insight into quadratus lumborum tightness can be gained by positioning the patient in a half-sidelying position (Fig. 21-28).[91] Note any changes in the shape of the lumbar curve. Normally there is a smooth, symmetrical lateral curve; when the quadratus lumborum is tight, the lumbar spine remains straight or the curve reverses itself. Simultaneously, abnormal tension can be felt on deep palpation.

B. *Hamstrings*

The hamstring muscles may be assessed in the conventional straight-leg raise in supine with the knee extended. Monitor any subsequent flexion of the innominate bone via the anterior aspect of the iliac crest. A straight-leg raise with the hip in external rotation and abduction tests the length of the medial hamstrings. A straight-leg raise with the hip in internal rotation and adduction tests the length of the lateral hamstrings.[12]

The knee extension test in the sitting position offers a significant insight into restrictive hamstring length, in the presence of excessive flexibility of the lumbar spine rather than the hip extensors (flexion syndrome according to Sahrmann).[165] Typical findings in this syndrome are short abdominal muscles and associated paraspinal atrophy (multifidi).[165] While sitting in 90° of hip flexion with the lumbar spine neutral, have the patient extend the knee. Monitor the lumbar spine and pelvic

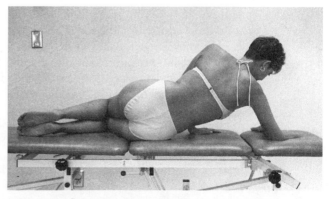

FIG. 21-28. Muscle length test of the quadratus lumborum.

girdle to assess the motion of the lumbar spine during knee extension. The patient should be able to extend the knees within 10° of complete extension without lumbar flexion or rotation and without eliciting pain.[165]

C. *Iliopsoas, rectus femoris, tensor fasciae latae, and the adductors*

With the patient lying at the end of the firm treatment table, one leg is flexed toward the chest and maintained in this position by the examiner or by the patient holding onto the knee, allowing the pelvis to tilt back and the lumbar spine to assume a flattened or neutral position. Monitor the low back position. If the knee is pulled too far forward and the back is allowed to assume a kyphotic position, the result is that the one-joint hip flexors, which may be normal in length, will appear short. The flexed leg may be supported against the examiner's trunk (Fig. 21-29A). The leg to be tested must hang free of the table.

1. Initially observe the position of the leg to assess the length of the iliopsoas and the relative length of the rectus femoris. A tight iliopsoas muscle will restrict extension of the femur; a tight rectus will restrict knee flexion. End feel is noted and passive overpressure is applied to hip extension and knee flexion.

2. If the anterior band of the tensor fasciae latae is tight, full femoral extension and knee flexion will occur; however, knee flexion will be possible only in conjunction with lateral tibial torsion.[109] If tibial rotation is passively blocked during the test, knee flexion will be restricted. Passive overpressure should also be applied to adductions. Hip adduction of less than 15° to 20° indicates tightness of the tensor fasciae and iliotibial band.[94] There will be an associated increased deepening on the outside of the thigh over the iliotibial tract.

3. To isolate the two-joint hip adductors from the one-joint adductors, the leg is abducted with the knee in extension (Fig. 21-29B) and the test is repeated with the knee flexed to 90°. A decreased range of abduction with the knee straight is a sign of shortness of the long adductors (two-joint adductors); a decreased range and compensatory flexion of the hip joint are signs of shortness of the one-joint thigh adductors.[91]

D. *Piriformis*

The patient lies supine with the hip flexed to 90° on the side where the muscle is being

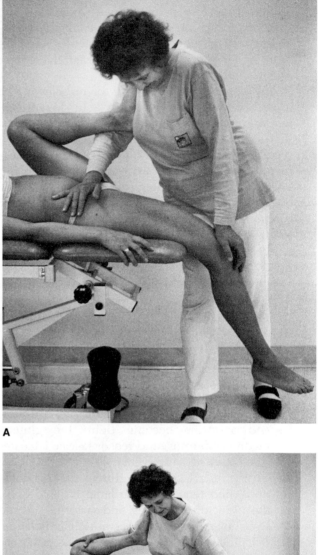

A

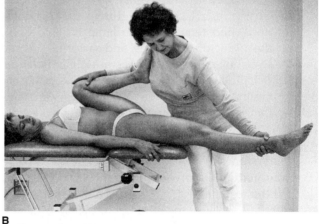

B

FIG. 21-29. Muscle length: iliopsoas, rectus femoris, tensor fascia latae, and short adductors.

examined. At this point, the piriformis muscle acts as a pure abductor of the femur. Before 60° it also laterally rotates the femur, but after 60° it medially rotates the femur.[109] Adduct the patient's hip and at the same time provide an axial force to the femur to prevent the pelvis from lifting off the table. If there is shortening of the piriformis, adduction and medial rotation are decreased and may be accompanied by stretch pain. This test does not differentiate between shortening of the piriformis muscle and a painful iliolumbar ligament. According to Janda,[91] palpation of the piriformis usually gives better results than the stretch test.

V. Examination Of Lower Quadrant Movement Patterns and Muscle Strength

If indicated, myokinetic testing is completed with a detailed examination of the contractile tissue function of all the muscles attaching to the lumbo–pelvic–hip complex. This may involve resisted isometrics for the presence of pain. Relative to the pelvic girdle, the phasic muscles that tend to weaken (the abdominals, gluteus maximus, medius, and minimus) should be specifically assessed for strength. Also observe for sequencing, quality, and coordination of muscle activity during movement.

A. *Pelvic tilt/heel slide* (abdominals; Fig. 21-30)[12,80]

With the patient lying supine with the hip joints flexed to at least 60° and the soles of the feet flat on the table, have the patient flatten the lumbar spine by doing a posterior pelvic tilt. With the back remaining flat, have the patient slide one foot along the table; if this is performed easily, have him or her slide both feet. This test assesses the ability of the lower abdominals (external obliques) to maintain a posterior tilt while the iliopsoas muscles are activated.

B. *Hip extension* (gluteus maximus)[12,91,94]

The patient is prone with the knees extended. Three muscle groups are principally involved when the patient extends the leg actively: the gluteus maximus and hamstrings, acting as prime movers, and the erector spinae, which stabilize the lumbar spine and pelvis. The correct order of patterning is ipsilateral hamstrings first, then gluteus maximus, contralateral erector spinae, and ipsilateral erector spinae. Signs of altered patterning may include the following:

1. The hamstrings and erector spinae are readily activated during the contraction, with delayed or minimal contraction of the gluteus maximus. This action may be strong enough to produce active hip extension, with little weakness noted on manual muscle testing.

2. The poorest pattern occurs when the erector spinae initiate the movement, and the activity of the gluteus maximus is again delayed or weak. Little hip extension occurs and the leg lift is achieved through forward pelvic tilt and hyperextension of the lumbar spine.

According to Bookhout,[12] chronic hamstring tightness may be a response to the substitution pattern for gluteus maximus weakness and will continue unless this muscle imbalance is corrected.

C. *Hip abduction* (gluteus medius and minimus)[91,94]

The patient lies on the side with the lower leg flexed and the upper leg extended. When abducting the leg, the gluteus medius and minimus and the tensor fasciae latae act as prime movers, while the quadratus lumborum stabilizes the pelvis. Signs of an altered pattern of movement can be observed (as well as palpated) when:

1. The patient's leg laterally rotates during upward movement, indicating that the tensor fasciae latae has initiated and even dominated the movement performance.

2. The patient compensates for weakness of the glutei by allowing flexion and lateral rotation, indicating substitution of hip flexors and iliopsoas activity for true abduction movement.

3. The quadratus lumborum acts not only to stabilize the pelvis but also to initiate the movement through lateral pelvic tilt. This pattern of movement can cause excessive stress to the lumbosacral segments and lumbar spine during walking.

PALPATION

For bony palpation and position see the section on bony structure and alignment above. The SIJ can be palpated in one locality only—at its inferior extent in the region of the posterior-inferior iliac spine. Acute unilateral tenderness and thickening are common in

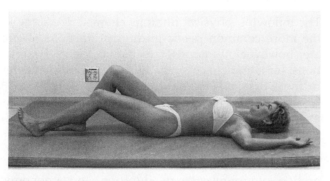

FIG. 21-30. Pelvic tilt/heel slide test for the ability of the lower abdominal to maintain a posterior pelvic tilt.

painful sacroiliac conditions, and when well localized serve as a useful confirmatory sign.[69] Tenderness here often represents a referred area of tenderness from disorders of the lower lumbar spine.

Soft-tissue palpation in prone should include the skin, subcutaneous tissues (using a skin-rolling test), gluteus maximus and medius, piriformis, and erector spinae. The lateral aspect of the erector spinae muscle is the anatomical location of the lateral raphe. At the inferior aspect of the raphe, corresponding to the level of the iliac crest, is an important connective tissue junction where the thoracolumbar fascia, the lateral aspect of the iliocostalis lumborum tendon, the deep erector spinae muscle, the lateral third of the iliolumbar ligament, and the quadratus lumborum converge to attach to the iliac crest.[153] This region is frequently tender to palpation. Palpation of ligamentous structures should include the following:

1. The iliolumbar ligaments lie deep and in a small space. The fibers arising from L4 are accessible to palpation. From a laterosuperior direction, the origin at the transverse process is palpated, whereas the insertion is palpated mediosuperiorly at the iliac crest, if accessible (see Fig. 16-20*B*).[46]
2. The posterior sacroiliac ligament may be palpated at its insertion inferiorly and slightly medially in the direction of the PSIS and through the gluteal mass (which may also be tender) (see Fig. 16-20*B*). In longstanding disorders of the SIJ, thickening overlying the posterior sacroiliac ligament may be found.
3. According to Greive,[69] changes in tension and elasticity of the sacrotuberous ligament are surprisingly easy to feel through the gluteal mass (Fig. 21-31). Using the index finger or thumb, proceed from the inferior aspect of the ischial tuberosity medially, then superiorly and posterolaterally to the superior attachment on the inferior lateral angle. A contrast in tension can be detected between the left and right ligaments by applying simultaneous pressure across the ligaments with both hands. The test is positive if one sacrotuberous ligament is more lax or tense than the normal or opposite side.[68] If the sacrum is dysfunctional in a position that places the ligament in tension, it will be tense and usually tender.
4. Anteriorly, palpate the abdominal wall, inguinal area, femoral triangle, and Baer's sacroiliac point for tenderness, muscle spasms, or other signs that may indicate the source of pathology.

NEUROLOGICAL TESTING

Neurological testing at this point has been completed as part of the earlier lumbar spine and hip examina-

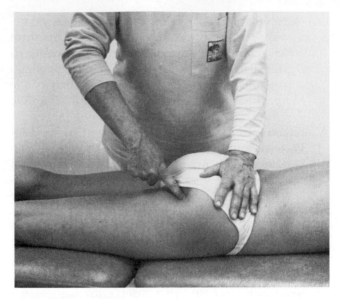

FIG. 21-31. *Palpation of the sacrotuberous ligament.*

tion, which should always precede the SIJ examination. A sacroiliac condition can co-exist in the presence of lumbosacral nerve root or cauda equina involvement. Patients with sacroiliac problems may report paresthesias in the absence of neurological signs; these appear to simulate lumbosacral involvement.[209]

RADIOGRAPHIC EVALUATION

SIJ dysfunction is diagnosed by clinical examination; radiographs rarely add any useful information but do help exclude other conditions, such as early ankylosing spondylitis.[7,100] The presence of degenerative changes usually bears no correlation with symptoms because 24.5% of patients over age 50 have abnormal-appearing SIJs on plain radiographs.[27,89,100,140,163] Radionuclide scanning of the SIJ is the procedure of choice for demonstrating infection, inflammation, stress fracture, or neoplasm involving the SIJ.[7]

CORRELATION OF FINDINGS

The following physical findings characterize some of the more common pelvic girdle dysfunctions. There are, however, numerous rare pelvic girdle dysfunctions; for complete coverage of these conditions, refer to the works of Bookhout,[12] Bourdillon and Day,[14] Greenman,[68] Mitchell,[132] Nyberg,[141] and Woerman.[208] In all dysfunctions of the pelvic girdle, correction of habitual postural stresses and sitting postures should receive primary attention. Shoe-lifts or a buttock-lift when sitting may be needed. Functional integration, neuromuscular re-education, and ergonomic measures should be emphasized.

I. Signs and Symptoms of Innominate Lesions

With respect to the pelvis, displacement of the innominate on the sacrum determines the direction of the dysfunction. The following positive findings are the most common innominate dysfunctions:

A. *Anterior dysfunction* (anterior innominate rotation)

When unilateral anterior dysfunction is present, the PSIS is higher and anterior on the affected side compared with the contralateral side when standing—that is, the ASIS is lower and more posterior. This indicates a posterior torsion (counternutation) of the sacrum on that side.[119,133] The lower limb on that side is usually medially rotated. Traumatically, anterior rotation dysfunction occurs most frequently in any forced anterior diagonal pattern, such as a golf or baseball swing, or in a posterior horizontal thrust of the femur (dashboard injury).[208]

1. In the supine-to-sit test in supine, an anterior dysfunction can cause the leg to appear longer than the contralateral limb because it brings the acetabulum closer to the plane of the table and reduces the angulation at the hip. In sitting, with unilateral anterior dysfunction, the leg may appear shorter because the acetabulum moves posteriorly relative to the SIJ (see Fig. 21-27).

2. On the involved side, the PSIS moves first and farther superiorly during the standing trunk flexion test, and the sulci are shallow.

3. Muscle findings include weak abdominals, weak gluteus maximus and medius, and tight hip flexors (particularly the iliotibial band) on the involved side.[129,141]

4. Treatment considerations:
   a. Joint mobilizations: Posterior innominate rotation (see Figs. 20-43, 21-16, and 21-35)
   b. Soft-tissue mobilization (myofascial release) techniques and stretching of tight hip flexors (particularly the psoas and tensor fasciae latae)
   c. Muscle retraining and strengthening of gluteus maximus, gluteus medius, and abdominals
   d. Greater success has been achieved by stretching shortened muscles before trying to strengthen a weakened muscle group.[90]

B. *Posterior dysfunction* (posterior innominate rotation)

Just the opposite will occur in posterior dysfunction of the innominate. This torsion may result in a spinal scoliosis and an altered functional leg length (shorter on the involved side). The posterior dysfunctions are usually the result of falling on an ischial tuberosity, lifting when forward-flexed with the knees straight, repeated or prolonged standing on one leg, vertical thrusting onto an extended leg, or sustaining hyperflexion and abduction of the hips.[117]

1. In standing, the ASIS is higher and the PSIS is lower on that side; this indicates an anterior rotation of the sacrum (nutation).[119] In the standing flexion test, the PSIS on the involved side moves first or farther superiorly. In the supine-to-sit test, the malleolus moves short to long (see Fig. 21-27). The sulcus is deep on the involved side.

2. Muscle findings include hamstring and adductor magnus tightness, tightness or tenderness of the tensor fasciae latae or piriformis, and gluteus medius weakness.

3. Treatment considerations:
   a. Joint mobilizations: Anterior iliac rotation (see Figs. 20-44 and 21-16)
   b. Increase non-weight-bearing rest time if unstable (consider a pelvic corset or belt if necessary).[141]
   c. Soft-tissue mobilization (myofascial release) and stretching of hamstrings and piriformis (occasionally the tensor fasciae latae, according to Mennell)[129]
   d. Retraining and strengthening of the gluteus medius and other muscles that may be weak (hip flexor and sartorius).

C. *Upslips* (superior innominate shear)

Vertical shear lesions of an entire innominate occur more frequently than originally thought.[68] Upslips are usually the result of jumping or falling suddenly on an extended leg.[142]

1. In standing, with unilateral anterior or posterior dsyfunction, there are differences in the relation of the ASIS and PSIS. With a unilateral upslip of the innominate, the ASIS and PSIS are higher than the ASIS and PSIS on the opposite side.[133,208]

2. The quadratus lumborum may be in muscle spasm; there may be a tight hip adductor on that side.

3. Treatment considerations:
   a. Joint mobilization: Inferior glide of the innominate joint (see Fig. 21-37) and longitudinal distraction of the lower limb (see Fig. 21-38)
   b. On the involved side, soft-tissue inhibition and myofascial release to the quad-

ratus lumborum; soft-tissue mobilization and stretch to tight hip flexors

II. **Signs of a Sacral Lesion**

A. *Sacral torsion* (left-on-left anterior torsion)

The left-on-left forward torsion is the most common sacroiliac lesion.[68,142,208] The primary axis of dysfunction is the left oblique axis. A left-on-left sacral torsion signifies flexion movement at the right sacral base and inferior movement of the left side of the sacrum. As a result, the sacrum is positioned in left rotation and left sidebending.[141] Usually there is a history of a pelvic twist injury.

1. The right sacral sulcus is deep; the left is shallow. The inferior angle is inferior and posterior on the left. Lumbar lordosis is usually increased, with a convex scoliosis on the right.[68] In prone, the left malleolus is short.

2. The piriformis, tensor fasciae latae, and posterior sacroiliac ligaments are tender on the right. The gluteus medius is usually weak (especially on the right) and the left piriformis tight.

3. Treatment considerations:
   a. Distraction of the pubic symphysis (isometric contraction of hip adductors and abductors; see Fig. 21-24) and sacral sidebending and rotation techniques
   b. If unstable, increase non-weight-bearing rest time; consider use of a pelvic belt or corset.[142]
   c. Soft-tissue mobilization (myofascial release) or stretching to piriformis and hip flexors
   d. Muscle retraining and strengthening of glutei and abdominals.

B. *Unilateral Sacral Flexion*

A unilateral sacral flexion exists when the sacrum rotates in one direction and sidebends. It may be thought of as failure of one side of the sacrum to counternutate from a fully nutated position.[208] Some of the findings for a right unilateral sacral flexion are the following:

1. The seated flexion test is positive: the blocked side (right) moves first. In prone the medial malleolus is long on the right. On the right side, the base of the sacrum (sulcus) is anterior and the inferior angle is posterior.

2. The left tensor fasciae latae is tight. Increased right piriformis and psoas tone and tenderness over the right sacroiliac ligaments are usually found.

3. Treatment considerations: Same as for sacral torsion.

■ PELVIC GIRDLE TREATMENT

The role of mobilization is limited to passive mobility, but the most important part of treatment deals with active mobility and patient self-treatment or mobilization on an ongoing basis outside the clinical setting. Joint mobilization (or stabilization) is just part of the treatment of chronic dysfunction in one or both SIJs, which is most often associated with dysfunction of the hip and lumbosacral joints. Treatment will not bring the expected relief of symptoms unless soft-tissue dysfunctions are addressed in addition to the loss of muscle strength and flexibility. Active mobilization and corrective exercises play an integral role; passive mobilization is useless if it is not followed by active specific mobilization. When patients with hypermobility are treated symptomatically, the dysfunction will reappear, leading to repeated symptoms. Recurrence can be prevented only by stabilizing the hypermobile joint or vertebral segment.

Education, in the form of ergonomic counseling, is the most important aspect of treatment. Habitual working stresses and sitting postures should be corrected.

Treatment of the pelvic girdle follows the same guidelines as for other areas of the body. Acutely, when pain is present, rest becomes an important consideration. Ice, massage, or other modalities at the disposal of the therapist may be helpful to deal effectively with the pain. Heel-lifts may be a valuable adjunct while tissue heals if they are used under the foot of the short side to minimize ground forces.[57,155] Pelvic traction may be helpful in the presence of a neurological deficit and may help correct compromised sacroiliac dysfunction by pulling the innominates caudally on the sacrum.[40]

At the appropriate time, nondestructive passive and active movements should be started to stimulate the tissue to adapt to the proper lines of stress, to modulate pain, and to provide proprioceptive input. Patient education and a return to normal function are important. Exercises should proceed with the goal of normalizing stresses by balancing muscle length and strength and ground and trunk forces.

Stabilization programs advocated for the lumbar spine[74,135,162,164,204] are also useful for problems of the SIJs. When performing stabilization exercises, the hip joints are flexed by moving the pelvis together with the lumbar spine. According to individual needs, the lumbar spine is flexed or extended by the pelvis, based on a pain-free position of the spine and pelvis. The position and range of motion are dictated by optimal positioning for the activity at hand.

☐ Hypermobility

The obvious method of treatment is rest. Passive stabilization for SIJ hypermobility may involve sacroiliac supports or belts, as advocated by Cyriax,[31] Grieve,[71] Macnab,[116] Mennell,[127] and Porterfield and DeRosa,[155] or taping. A sacroiliac belt is often used pre- and postpartum and after trauma; it is especially helpful for women just before delivery. The belt is worn when the patient is most active and is removed when sitting or lying. During the initial phase after trauma, a support is used to help stabilize the area, to enhance soft-tissue healing and minimize re-injury. The patient must be instructed thoroughly about the nature of the condition and how to prevent recurrence. Doran and Newell[43] found that the response to a corrective corset was slow, but the long-term effects were as good as those of other treatment. The support should be put on after a correction has been made to help prevent recurrence.[40]

A loose joint can become overridden and stuck so that it may appear hypomobile. Grieve,[69] in a study on lumbopelvic rhythm during simple knee-raising, found that some patients present a paradox: the joint does not move in the moving phase and is hypomobile in the stance phase.

Sometimes sclerotherapy is used. This consists of injecting the lax ligaments with an irritant substance such as dextrose. This causes an inflammatory reaction in the ligament, with resultant fibrosis and gradual shortening of the fibers.[76] According to Grieve,[70] although this is a destructive approach, it does relieve the pain and can be repeated if necessary.

Hypermobility in any joint is the result of overstretching the elastic tissue in the ligaments and the joint capsule. Normal tone in ligaments depends on the natural stimulus of intermittent gentle stretching. Therefore, controlled gentle joint mobilization techniques are useful in reducing pain and serve as a natural stimulus to the elastic tissue.

Mobilization techniques are also valuable in hypomobility, but here the aim is to provide as much stretching as possible short of causing pain. Treatment may include soft-tissue mobilizations and muscle-stretching techniques, mobilization (grade I to IV) appropriate to the degree of pain and irritability, correction of pelvic posture and muscle imbalance, support for mild laxity, and use of a heel-lift or a buttock-lift when sitting. General measures such as correction of habitual working stresses and sitting postures, weight reduction, or a change of job or athletic interest are sometimes advisable.

☐ Passive Movements

Many passive movements have been described for the pelvic girdle, but only a few of the more common ones are presented here.* The technique chosen is usually the one that reproduces the patient's pain. However, according to Maigne[118] and others, therapeutic passive movements are best applied in a direction that is painless, and therefore *opposite* to the painful movement on testing. When irritability is dominant, gently graded persuasive movements to the patient's tolerance, in the direction of the painful stress, may be just as successful.

Several of the evaluation maneuvers are useful as treatment techniques for pelvic dysfunction. The following maneuvers were described and illustrated in the section on passive movement above.

I. **Osteokinematic Tests of Physiological Mobility**
   A. *Pelvic rock test*—Anterior/posterior glide of the innominate (see Fig. 21-15). When used as a technique in the presence of asymmetrical dysfunction (*i.e.*, when gliding the innominate bones in an anteroposterior direction in the plane of the sacroiliac articular surfaces), emphasis is placed on the more hypomobile innominate.
   B. *Flexion–extension of the innominate* (see Fig. 21-16). According to Maitland,[120] the test movement that reproduces the pain should be used first as a treatment technique. At the onset it should be performed using a grade that produces only minimal discomfort.

II. **Arthrokinetic Tests of Stability**
   A. *Posteroanterior and transverse pressures around the SIJ* (see Fig. 21-19). If such pressures consistently yield a response to the same pressure and direction at certain points, they may be used not only for assessment but also for treatment.[120,203]
   B. *Prone gapping test* (see Fig. 21-21). This technique can be used as regional mobilization with a gentle gapping and gliding for the SIJ, with the near ilium stabilized. It can also be used to stretch the piriformis passively or to improve its extensibility by hold–relax or isometric techniques.[72]
   C. *Torsional stress of the SIJ* (see Fig. 21-22). This

*See references 14, 23, 29, 40, 47, 51, 56, 71–73, 108–110, 119, 120, 133, 141, 148, 154, 155, 171–183, 202, 203, 208.

technique can be used as a downward, outward, and caudal mobilization of the innominate while the sacrum is stabilized, or as an outward manipulation of the SIJ.[71,72]

D. *Compression/distraction tests of the innominates* (see Fig. 21-23). These techniques can be used to reduce a positional fault (pubic compression) or to promote motions (pubic distraction) at the pubic symphysis.[141]

Note: Other evaluation maneuvers useful in treatment techniques (not described below) include the sacral apex pressure test (see Fig. 21-28) and the longitudinal stress test of the sacrum (see Fig. 21-20).

Nonspecific Techniques

(P, patient; O, operator; M, movement)

I. **Pelvic Shift**—forward and backward, sitting (Fig. 21-32)

P—Sitting on the treatment table or bolster, or straddling a large therapy roll, with the legs abducted. Arms may be positioned on the operator's head or shoulders to facilitate upper thoracic flexion with lumbar spine extension.

O—Sit on the floor or on a mat or stool in front of the patient.

M—With your hands on the posterior aspect of the pelvic girdle, shift the pelvis forward and backward into its end range or barrier.

Note: This a useful technique for general mobilization of the pelvic girdle as well as for increasing the extensibility of the inferior hip joint capsule. It is particularly valuable in the management of pelvic dysfunction in the neurologically involved adult and child. Active pelvic shift is an excellent lead-up exercise in preparation for standing and walking.

II. **Distraction of Pubic Symphysis and SIJ: Muscle Energy**[14,47,133,154,208]

A. *Distraction of SIJ pubic symphysis* (see Fig. 21-24A)

P—Supine with knees bent, feet resting on the table, knees together

O—Stand at the end of the table facing the patient.

M—With your hands on either side of the patient's knees to resist abduction, have the patient try to spread the legs apart (abduct the legs). This is done with a maximum isometric contraction for 7 to 10 seconds. After relaxation, repeat this procedure but with the legs abducted 30°

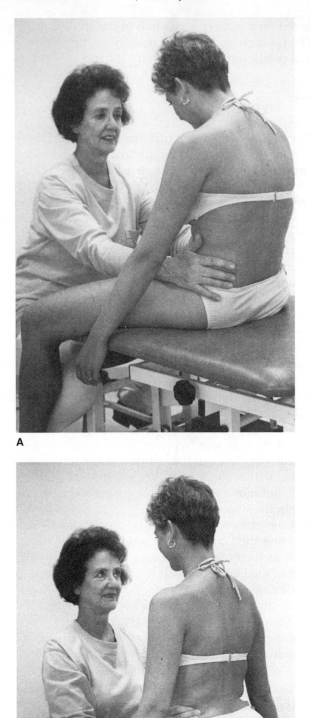

FIG. 21-32. Pelvic shift forward (**A**) and backward (**B**).

to 45°. Repeat three times and proceed to the next phase (below).

The resisted force provided by the operator into hip abduction results in distraction of the iliac joint surfaces away from the sacrum, because the abductors contract and pull on their attachments to the iliac crest.[47]

  B. *Distraction of pubic symphysis* (see Fig. 21-24*B*)

  P—Same position as above

  O—Same position as above

  M—Place the hands on the medial aspect of the patient's knees to resist adduction, or use the forearm as a brace between the knees to keep them apart. Have the patient try to bring the knees together as you oppose the adduction motion, thus distracting the pubic symphysis joint surfaces away from one another as the adductors contract and pull on their attachments to the pubic rami. After a maximum isometric hold for 7 to 10 seconds, have the patient relax. Repeat several times. Retest and repeat if indicated.

  Note: These two techniques can be used separately or in combination. Often by releasing the pubis or changing the forces in the pelvis, the sacrum is likely to correct its position as well as a left-on-left sacral torsion.[154]

III. Self-Mobilization of the SIJ (Fig. 21-33)[74,111]

  With this technique, sidebending and rotation of the lower lumbar spine are mobilized as well.

  P—Kneeling on a table, close to the edge, with the trunk supported on the hands (elbows extended) or on the elbows. One leg is shifted to hang the flexed knee over the edge of the table, with the foot supported over the heel of the other leg.

  M—The patient relaxes so the pelvis slopes obliquely down from the ilium. The slack is taken up at the SIJ of the supported side on the table. Once the patient senses tension in the joint, very small downward vertical springing motions are performed with the knee over the edge of the table, thus mobilizing the SIJ on the supported side.

□   **Innominate Dysfunction Techniques**

I. Forward Rotation (prone position)

  This is a basic technique for a posterior innominate rotation dysfunction (see Fig. 20-44). Signs on the involved side include an inferior and posterior PSIS, a superior and anterior ASIS, a positive standing flexion test, and an apparent short leg in the supine position. Hypermobility or re-

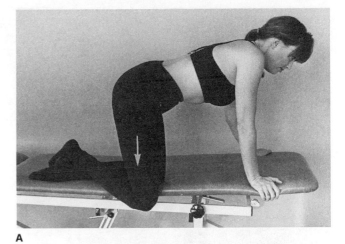

A

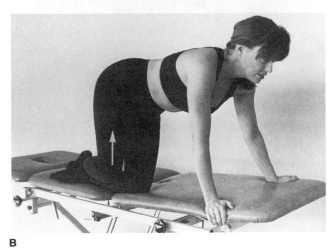

B

FIG. 21-33. *Self-mobilization of the sacroiliac joint:* (**A**) *starting position and* (**B**) *end position.*

striction in innominate anterior rotation is apparent. The hip and pelvic girdle muscles should be checked for asymmetry.

II. Forward Rotation (supine position; Fig. 21-34)

  For posterior innominate rotation dysfunction, signs on the involved side are the same as above.

  P—Supine, with the leg on the side to be mobilized extended over the edge of the table

  O—Stand opposite the side to be mobilized. The patient or operator flexes and stabilizes the opposite leg.

  M—Place the caudal hand over the thigh and use it to push the hip into further extension; the cephalic hand can be applied to the patient's PSIS, pushing upward to increase the forward rotation of the innominate on the sacrum.

Note: This technique can be modified to use muscle correction, which can place an anterior rotatory moment on the innominate (muscle energy) using the iliopsoas as the desired force.[155,208] Have the patient push the freely hanging leg up

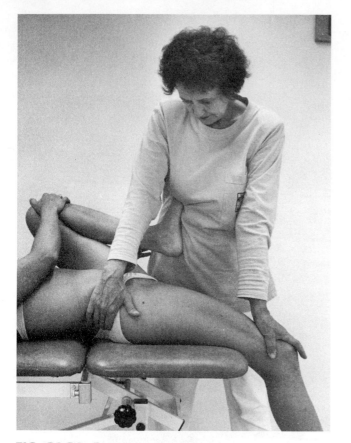

FIG. 21-34. Forward rotation for posterior iliac dysfunction.

against your hand with a submaximal force while you give unyielding resistance to the contraction for 7 to 10 seconds. This procedure is repeated three or four times or until all the slack is taken up.

The patient can be instructed in the unilateral knee-to-chest technique for home use. The patient draws the opposite knee of the posterior innominate to the chest and fixes it with the arms while maintaining the hip of the involved side in complete extension.

Management for posterior innominate rotation dysfunction should include soft-tissue inhibition and stretching to the involved muscles (hamstrings and piriformis); promotion of hip extension activities, such as prone press-ups or pushing the head and shoulders up while the pelvis remains on the floor or table; functional integration and strengthening of involved muscles (gluteus medius, hip rotators); and functional activity requiring this range (*i.e.,* coming-to-sit over the hip joint). Rolling and assuming the half-kneeling position are other activities that can improve sacroiliac mobility while gaining functional strength.

III. Backward Rotation

This is the basic technique for anterior innominate dysfunction (see Fig. 20-43). Signs on the involved side include an superior and anterior PSIS, an inferior and posterior ASIS, a positive flexion test, an apparent long leg in the supine position, and innominate posterior rotation. The hip and pelvic girdle muscles should be checked for symmetry.

Note: The same maneuver can be used to produce anterior rotation (for a posterior innominate rotation dysfunction), but the operator produces a force-couple pushing the ASIS forward and the ischial tuberosity backward. Contract–relax or muscle-energy techniques may be used effectively in either of these techniques.

IV. Backward Rotation (supine position, as in the forward rotation technique above; Fig. 21-35)

This technique is useful for anterior innominate rotation dysfunction. The cephalic hand cups the ASIS in the palm while the caudal hand grasps the ischial tuberosity. Transfer your weight toward the patient's head; this results in a backward rotation of the innominate on the sacrum.

Muscle correction (muscle energy) of this posi-

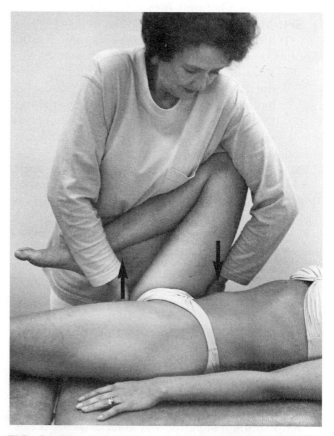

FIG. 21-35. Backward rotation for anterior iliac dysfunction.

tional fault uses muscles that can rotate the innominate in a posterior direction, mainly the gluteus maximus.[47,208] Have the patient resist a force provided by your trunk (or against the patient's own hands, which fixate the knee) with a sustained submaximal contraction for 7 to 10 seconds. This is repeated three or four times, not allowing the hip to move into extension, only flexion.

This treatment may be given to the patient to do as a home program in sitting, supine (Fig. 21-36A), or standing.[40,41] In standing, the patient places the foot on a table or bench, leans toward the knee, and stretches it into the axilla (Fig. 21-36B). DonTigny[40] recommends repeating this exercise several times a day, and always making a correction when going to bed to relieve the strain on the involved ligaments. These techniques are powerful rotators of the innominate and can be overdone unless specific guidelines are given.[208]

Management for anterior iliac rotation dysfunction should include soft-tissue mobilization techniques for the psoas; strengthening of the abdominal and gluteal muscles; and exercise and functional activities to promote hip flexion, abduction, and external rotation.

V. Iliac Upslip (inferior glide; Fig. 21-37)

An upslip is a superior subluxation of the innominate on the sacrum at the SIJ. The dysfunction is primarily articular with secondary muscle imbalances (as opposed to anterior and posterior innominate rotations, which primarily result from muscle imbalances that secondarily restrict SIJ motion).[56] Possible muscle findings include quadratus lumborum spasm and tight hip adductors. Causes include jumping or falling suddenly on an extended leg or, more commonly, from a fall on the ischial tuberosity.[56,141] Signs on the involved side include superior positioning of the ASIS, PSIS, iliac crest, pubic tubercle, and ischial tuberosity. Inferior glide of the ilium is restricted.

P—Prone

O—Stand to the involved side at the head.

M—The outer hand contacts the superior aspect of the iliac crest and applies an inferior and slightly medial force in the plane of the joint.

VI. Innominate Upslip (distraction)

Simple longitudinal distraction of one lower limb tends to induce a combined downward and forward movement of the innominate on that side.[69] Distraction may be applied in either supine or prone.

A. *Distraction in supine* (Fig. 21-38A)

P—Supine with both legs extended

O—Stand at the foot of the table and grasp the patient's ankle on one side just proximal to

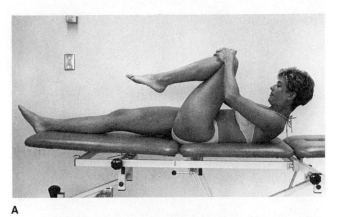

A

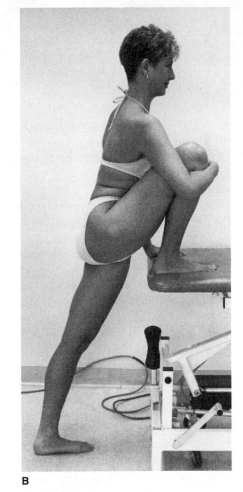

B

FIG. 21-36. *Self-mobilization of the sacroiliac joint:* (**A**) *posterior rotation in supine and* (**B**) *posterior rotation in standing.*

the malleolus. A belt may be used around the patient's trunk, or you may support the opposite foot with your thigh to stabilize the patient.

M—Apply a gentle, caudal distraction force through the lower leg until the exact position of the leg that will localize the force to the SIJ is attained. Distraction is then applied by

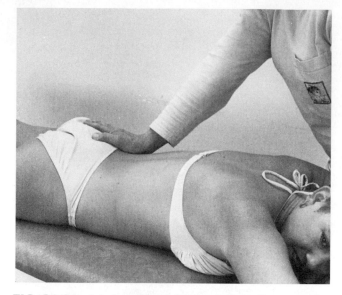

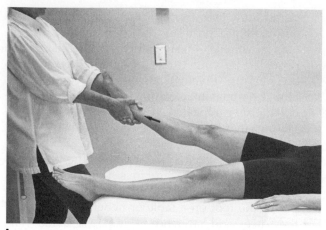

A

FIG. 21-37. Inferior glide of the innominate for an upslip.

pulling the leg, leaning backward with the trunk, and twisting the pelvis, while pushing against the other (outstretched) leg with the thigh.

B. *Distraction in prone* (Fig. 21-38B)

The signs are the same as in the iliac upslip, except that the PSIS is inferior and the ASIS is superior (iliac upslip with posterior rotation). This procedure can be performed in the prone position (Fig. 21-38B). The signs are the same as in the iliac upslip, except that the innominate is also in anterior rotation so that the PSIS is superior and the ASIS inferior on the involved side (iliac upslip with an anterior rotation). Distraction can also be performed in prone with the leg in a neutral position and the knee extended or bent to 90°. In this case the mobilizing hand applies distraction via the uppermost region of the calf; this increases the tension of the rectus femoris.

Management of an upslip should include soft-tissue inhibition and stretch to the quadratus lumborum and hip adductor muscles.

☐ Sacral Dysfunction Techniques

I. Sacral Nutation Technique (Fig. 21-39)

This is used to reduce a sacral counternutation positional fault, commonly caused by a postural flat back, or flexed sitting or standing postures. Signs include lumbar spine hyperflexion, shallow (posterior) sacral sulci, deep (anterior) inferior lateral angles, less prominent PSIS, sacral flexion restriction, and L5 to S1 (and possibly generalized) restriction in lumbar extension.

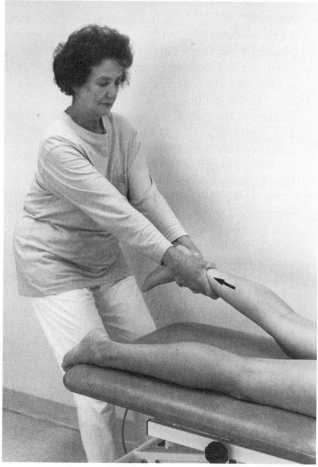

B

FIG. 21-38. Distraction in (**A**) supine and (**B**) in prone for an innominate upslip.

P—Prone with a pillow under the abdomen and the legs externally rotated

O—Stand at the level of the pelvis on the involved side, facing the foot of the table.

M—The base of the inner hand contacts the sacral base, with the arm directed at a right angle to the base. The mobilizing hand glides the cra-

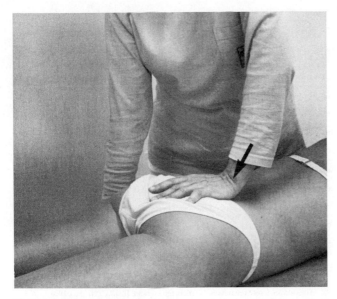

FIG. 21-39. Sacral nutation.

(posterior) inferior lateral angles, increased piriformis and psoas tone, sacral flexion hypermobility or sacral extension restriction,[141] and possibly tenderness and tightness bilaterally in the tensor fasciae latae.[208]

P—Prone with the legs internally rotated

O—To one side of the pelvis, facing the head

M—With thenar or ulnar contact of the inner hand on the sacral apex, apply a posterior/anterior force on the apex of the sacrum when the sacrum is felt to extend.

Management of sacral flexion dysfunction includes promotion of lumbar flexion activities and postures; soft-tissue mobilization and stretch for tight structures (piriformis, psoas, and possibly the tensor fasciae latae); and strengthening of the gluteus medius and maximus, as well as the abdominal muscles.

nial surface of the sacrum ventrally, directing the sacrum into nutation. Incline the pressure toward the patient's feet.

Management of sacral extension dysfunction includes postural re-education to avoid flexed sitting and standing positions; functional activities to promote lumbar extension mobility; and possibly a home exercise program of prone press-ups.

II. Sacral Counternutation Technique (Fig. 21-40)

This is used for sacral nutation dysfunction, commonly caused by an increase in the lumbosacral angle due to structure or poor abdominal tone combined with lumbar spine hyperextension and a weak gluteus medius and maximus.[141] Signs include deep (anterior) sacral sulci and shallow

SUMMARY

Dysfunctions of the pelvic girdle are often complex and not easily understood. All of the areas—the lumbar spine, pelvis, and hips—are anatomically and functionally related, and all should be examined in detail so that treatment can be applied based on these findings. The treatment goal is to normalize stresses in the lumbar–pelvic–hip complex by balancing muscle length and strength, ground and trunk forces, and afferent/efferent neuropathways. The myokinetics and arthrokinetics of the region are in their infancy as far as research is concerned; investigations have shown that motion exists at the SIJ, but it is variable and limited. Restoring pelvic girdle function within the walking cycle is a major therapeutic goal from the biomechanical, postural, and structural point of view.

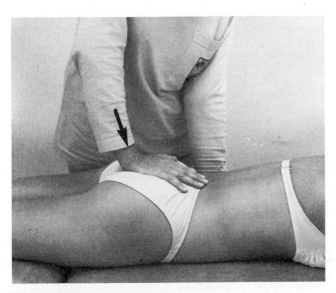

FIG. 21-40. Sacral counternutation.

REFERENCES

1. Alviso DJ, Dong GT, Lentell GL: Intertester reliability for measuring pelvic tilt in standing. Phys Ther 68:1347–1351, 1988
2. Bakland O, Hansen JH: The axial SIJ. Anat Clin 6:29–36, 1984
3. Beal MC: The sacroiliac problem: Review of anatomy, mechanics and diagnosis. J Am Osteopath Assoc 81:667–679, 1982
4. Bemis T, Daniel M: Validation of the long-sit test on subjects with iliosacral dysfunction. J Orthop Sports Phys Ther 8:336–345, 1987
5. Benson DR: The back: Thoracic and lumbar spine. In D'Ambrosia RD (ed): Musculoskeletal Disorders: Regional Examination and Differential Diagnosis, 2nd ed. Philadelphia, JB Lippincott, 1986:287–366
6. Berg G, Hammer M, Moller-Nielsen J, et al: Low back pain during pregnancy. Obstet Gynecol 71:71–75, 1979
7. Bernard TN, Cassidy JD: The SIJ syndrome: Pathophysiology, diagnosis and management. In Frymoyer JW (ed): The Adult Spine: Principles and Practice. New York, Raven Press, 1991:2107–2130
8. Bernard TN, Kirkalday-Willis WH. Recognizing specific characteristics of nonspecific low back pain. Clin Orthop 217:266–280, 1987
9. Bogduk N: Lumbar dorsal ramus syndrome. Med J Aust 2:537–541, 1980
10. Bogduk N, Twomey LT: Clinical Anatomy of the Lumbar Spine. London, Churchill Livingstone, 1987
11. Boltz S, Davies GJ: Leg-length differences and correlation with total leg strength. J Orthop Sports Phys Ther 6:123–129, 1984
12. Bookhout MR: Examination and treatment of muscle imbalances. In Bourdillon JF, Day EA, Bookhout MR (eds): Spinal Manipulation, 5th ed. Oxford, Butterworth-Heinemann, 1992:313–333

13. Borel U, Fernstrom I: The movements of the SIJs and their importance to changes on pelvic dimensions during parturition. Acta Obstet Gynecol Scand 36:42–57, 1957
14. Bourdillon JF, Day EA: Spinal Manipulation, 5th ed. Oxford, Butterworth-Heinemann, 1992
15. Bowen V, Cassidy JD: Macroscopic and microscopic anatomy of the SIJ from embryonic life until the eighth decade. Spine 6:620–627, 1981
16. Broadhurst NA: Sacroiliac dysfunction as a cause of low back pain. Aust Fam Phys 18:623–628, 1989
17. Brooke R: The SIJ. J Anat 58:299–305, 1924
18. Cailliet R: Miscellaneous low back conditions relating to pain. In Cailliet R (ed): Low Back Pain Syndrome, 4th ed. Philadelphia, FA Davis, 1988:252–270
19. Chamberlin WE: The symphysis pubis in the roentgen examination of the SIJ. J Bone Joint Surg 23A:621–625, 1930
20. Chapman L, Nihls M: Myokinematics of the pelvis. Proceedings of the 5th Conference of International Federations of Orthopaedic Manipulative Therapists. Vancouver, British Columbia, 1984
21. Cibulka M: The treatment of the SIJ component to low back pain. Phys Ther 72:917–922, 1992
22. Cibulka M, Delitto A: A comparison of two different methods to treat hip pain in runners. J Orthop Sports Phys Ther 17(4):172–176, 1993
23. Cibulka MT, Delitto A, Koldehoff RM: Changes in innominate tilt after manipulation of the SIJ in patients with low back pain: An experimental study. Phys Ther 68:1359–1363, 1988
24. Cibulka MT, Koldehoff RM: Leg-length disparity and its effect on SIJ dysfunction. Clinical Management 6(5):10–11, 1986
25. Cipriano JJ: Photographic Manual of Regional Orthopedic Tests. Baltimore, Williams & Wilkins, 1985
26. Clayson SJ, Newton IM, Debeucc DF, et al: Evaluation of mobility of hip and lumbar vertebrae in normal young women. Arch Phys Med Rehabil 43:1–8, 1962
27. Cohen AS, McNeill JM, Calkins E, et al: The "normal" SIJ: Analysis of 88 sacroiliac roentgenograms. Am J Roent Radium Ther 100:559–563, 1967
28. Colachis SD, Warden RE, Bechtol CO: Movement of the SIJ in the adult male: A preliminary report. Arch Phys Med Rehabil 44:490–498, 1963
29. Corrigan B, Maitland GD: Practical Orthopaedic Medicine. London, Butterworths, 1983:324–331
30. Coventry MB, Tapper EM: Pelvic instability. J Bone Joint Surg 54A:83–101, 1972
31. Cyriax JH: Textbook of Orthopaedic Medicine: Diagnosis of Soft-Tissue Lesions, 8th ed, Vol. 1. London, Bailliere Tindall, 1982
32. Cyriax JH, Coldham M: Textbook of Orthopaedic Medicine: Treatment by Manipulation, Massage, and Injection, 11th ed, Vol. 2. Philadelphia, Bailliere Tindall, 1984
33. D'Ambrosia RD: The hip. In D'Ambrosia RD (ed): Musculoskeletal Disorders: Regional Examination and Differential Diagnosis, 2nd ed. Philadelphia, JB Lippincott, 1986:447–490
34. Daly JM, Frame PS, Rapoza PA: Sacroiliac subluxation: A common, treatable cause of low-back pain in pregnancy. Fam Prac Res J 11:149–159, 1991
35. Davis P, Lentle BC: Evidence of sacroiliac disease a common cause of low backache in women. Lancet 2:496–497, 1978
36. Denslow JS, Chance JA, Gardner DL, et al: Mechanical stresses in the human lumbar spine and pelvis. J Am Osteopath Assoc 61:705–712, 1962
37. Derry DE: Note on accessory articular facets between the sacrum and ilium, and their significance. J Anat Physiol 45:202–211, 1911
38. Dietricks E, Kogstad O: "Pelvic girdle relaxation"—Suggested new nomenclature. Scand J Rheumatol [Suppl 88] 20:3, 1991
39. Dijkstra PF, Vleeming A, Stoeckart R: Complex motion tomography of the SIJ: An anatomical and roentgenological study. Rofo Forstschr Geb Rontgenstr Neuen Bildgeh Verfahr 150:635–642, 1989
40. DonTigny RL: Functions and pathomechanics of the SIJ: A review. Phys Ther 65:35–44, 1985
41. DonTigny RL: Dialogue on SIJ [letter to the editor]. Phys Ther 69:164–165, 1989
42. DonTigny RL: Pathomechanics and treatment of SIJ dysfunction. In International Federation of Orthopaedic Manipulative Therapists, 5th International Conference, Vail, 1992
43. Doran DMI, Newell DJ: Manipulation in treatment of low back pain: A multicentre study. Br Med J 2:161–164, 1975
44. Drerup B, Hierholzer E: Movement of the human pelvis and displacement of related anatomical landmarks on the body surface. J Biomechanics 20:971–977, 1987
45. Dunn EJ, Bryon DM, Nugent JT, et al: Pyogenic infections of the hip joint. Clin Orthop 118:113–117, 1976
46. Dvořák J, Dvořák V: Manual Medicine: Diagnostics, 2nd ed. Stuttgart, Georg Thieme Verlag/Thieme Med. Pub., 1990
47. Edmond SL: Manipulation and Mobilization: Extremity and Spinal Techniques. St. Louis, Mosby, 1993
48. Egund N, Olsson TH, Schmid H: Movement in the SIJs demonstrated with roentgen stereophotogrammetry. Acta Radiol (Stockh) 19:833–846, 1978
49. Ehara S, El-Koury GY, Bergman RA: The accessory SIJ: A common anatomic variant. AJR 150:857–859, 1988
50. Ellison JB, Rose SJ, Sahrmann SA: Patterns of hip rotation range of motion: Comparison between healthy subjects and patients with low back pain. Phys Ther 70:537–541, 1990
51. Erhard R, Bowling R: The recognition and management of the pelvic components of low back pain and sciatic pain. Bulletin of the Orthopaedics Section, APTA, 2:4–15, 1977
52. Fairbanks JCT, Park WN, McCall JW, et al: Apophyseal injection of local anesthetic as a diagnostic aid in primary low back syndromes. Spine 6:598–605, 1981
53. Fairbanks JCT, Pysant PB, Van Poortvliet JA, et al: Influence of anthropometric factors and joint laxity in the incidence of adolescent back pain. Spine 9:461–464, 1984
54. Farfan C: The biomechanical advantage of lordosis and hip extension for upright activity. Spine 3:336–342, 1977
55. Fisk JW: Medical Treatment of Neck and Back Pain. Springfield, Ill., Charles C. Thomas, 1987
56. Fowler C: Muscle energy techniques for pelvic dysfunction. In Grieve GP (ed): Modern Manual Therapy of the Vertebral Column. Edinburgh, Churchill Livingstone, 1986
57. Friberg O: Clinical symptoms and biomechanics of lumbar spine hip joint in leg-length inequality. Spine 8:643–650, 1983
58. Friberg O: The statics of postural pelvic tilt scoliosis: A radiographic study on 288 consecutive chronic LBP patients. Clin Biomechanics 2:211–219, 1987
59. Frigerio NA, Stowe RR, Howe JW: Movement of the SIJ. Clin Orthop 100:370–377, 1974
60. Gibofsky A: Reiter syndrome. In Beary JF, Christian CL, Johanson NA (eds): Manual of Rheumatology and Outpatient Orthopedic Disorders: Diagnosis and Therapy, 2nd ed. Boston, Little, Brown and Co., 1987
61. Giles LGF, Taylor JR: Lumbar spine structural changes associated with leg-length inequality. Spine 7:159–162, 1982
62. Goften JP: Studies in osteoarthritis of the hip: Part IV. Biomechanics and clinical considerations. Can Med Assoc J 104:1007–1011, 1971
63. Goften JP, Trureman GE: Studies in osteoarthritis of the hip: Part II. Osteoarthritis of the hip and leg-length disparity. Can Med Assoc J 104:791–799, 1971
64. Goldthwait JE: The pelvic articulations: A consideration of their anatomic, physiologic, obstetric and general surgical importance. JAMA 49:768–774, 1907
65. Good MB: Diagnosis and treatment of sciatic pain. Lancet 2:597–598, 1942
66. Good MB: What is "fibrositis"? Rheumatism 5:117–123, 1949
67. Gray H: SIJ pain, Part II. Mobility and axes of rotation. Int Clin 11:65–76, 1938
68. Greenman PE: Principles of Manual Medicine. Baltimore, Williams & Wilkins, 1989
69. Grieve E: Lumbopelvic rhythm and mechanical dysfunction of the SIJ. Physiotherapy 67:171–173, 1981
70. Grieve EFM. Mechanical dysfunction of the SIJ. Int Rehabil Med 5:46–52, 1983
71. Grieve GP: The SIJ. Physiotherapy 62:384–400, 1976
72. Grieve GP: Mobilization of the Spine: Notes on Examination, Assessment and Clinical Method, 4th ed. Edinburgh, Churchill Livingstone, 1984
73. Grieve GP: Common Vertebral Problems. Edinburgh, Churchill Livingstone, 1988
74. Gustavsen R, Streeck R: Training Therapy: Prophylaxis and Rehabilitation, 2nd ed. Stuttgart, Georg Thieme Verlag, 1993
75. Gutstein-Good M: Idiopathic myalgia simulating visceral and other diseases. Lancet 2:326–328, 1940
76. Hackett GS: Joint Ligament Relaxation. Springfield, Ill., C.C. Thomas, 1956
77. Hadley LA: Accessory sacroiliac articulations with arthritic changes. Radiology 55:403–409, 1950
78. Hadley LA: Accessory sacroiliac articulations. J Bone Joint Surg 34A:149–155, 1952
79. Hagen R: Pelvic girdle relaxation from an orthopaedic point of view. Acta Orthop Scand 45:550–563, 1974
80. Hall C: Diagnosis and Treatment of Movement System Imbalances and Musculoskeletal Pain as Taught by Shirley Sahrmann. Continuing education course, Seattle, 1993
81. Hallin RP: Sciatic pain and the piriformis muscle. Postgrad Med 74:69–72, 1983
82. Harris NH, Murry RO: Lesions of the symphysis pubis in athletes. Br Med J 4:211–214, 1974
83. Hartley A: Practical Joint Assessment: A Sports Medicine Manual. St. Louis, Mosby Year Book, 1990
84. Healy JH: Paget Disease of Bone. In Beary JF, Christian CL, Johanson NA (eds): Manual of Rheumatology and Outpatient Orthopedic Disorders: Diagnosis and Therapy, 2nd ed. Boston, Little, Brown and Co., 1987
85. Hides JA, Stokes MJ, Saide M, et al: Evidence of lumbar multifidus muscle wasting ipsilateral to symptoms in patients with acute/subacute low back pain. Spine 19:165–172, 1994
86. Hollinshead WH, Jenkins DB: Functional Anatomy of the Limbs and Back. Philadelphia, WB Saunders, 1981
87. Hoppenfeld S: Physical Examination of the Spine and Extremities. New York, Appleton-Century-Crofts, 1976
88. Ishimino T: Histopathological study of the aging process in the human SIJ [in Japanese]. Nippon Seikeigeka Gakkai Zasshi 63;1070–1084, 1989
89. Jajic I, Jajic Z: The prevalence of osteoarthrosis of the SIJs in an urban population. Clin Rheumatol 6(1):39–41, 1987
90. Janda V: Muscles, central nervous motor regulation and back problems. In Korr I (ed): The Neurobiologic Mechanisms in Manipulative Therapy. London. Plenum Press, 1978:27–42
91. Janda V: Muscle Function Testing. Boston, Butterworths, 1983
92. Janda V: Muscle weakness and inhibition (pseudoparesis) in back pain syndromes. In Greive GP (ed): Modern Manual Therapy of the Vertebral Column. New York, Churchill Livingstone, 1986:197–201
93. Janda V, Schmid H: Muscles as a pathogenic factor in back pain. Proceedings, 4th Conference of International Federation of Orthopaedic Manipulative Therapist. Christchurch, New Zealand, 1980
94. Jull GA, Janda V: Muscles and motor control in low back pain: Assessment and management. In Twomey LT, Taylor JR (eds): Physical Therapy of the Low Back. New York, Churchill Livingstone, 1987:253–278
95. Kapandji IA: Physiology of the Joints, 2nd ed, Vol. III. The Trunk and the Vertebral Column. Edinburgh, Churchill Livingstone, 1974
96. Kendall HO, Kendall FP, Boynton DA: Posture and Pain. Baltimore: Williams & Wilkins, 1952; Reprinted Melbourne, Fla., Robert E. Kreiger, 1971
97. Kendall HO, McCreary EK, Provance PG: Muscle Testing and Function, 4th ed. Baltimore, Williams & Wilkins 1993
98. Kidd R: Pain localization with the innominate upslip dysfunction. Man Med 3:103–105, 1988
99. Kirkaldy-Willis WH (ed): Managing Low Back Pain, 2nd ed. New York, Churchill Livingstone, 1988
100. Kirkaldy-Willis WH: The site and nature of the lesion. In Kirkaldy-Willis WH (ed): Managing Low Back Pain, 2nd ed. New York, Churchill Livingstone, 1988:133–154
101. Kirkaldy-Willis WH, Hill RJ: A more precise diagnosis for low back pain. Spine 4:102–109, 1979
102. Kirkaldy-Willis WH, Wedge JH, Yong-Hing K, et al: Pathology and pathogenesis of lumbar spondylosis and stenosis. Spine 3:319–128, 1978
103. Kissling R, Brunner C, Jacob HA: Mobility of the SIJ in vitro [in German]. Y Orthop 128:282–288, 1990
104. Kogstad D, Birnstad N: Pelvic girdle relaxation: Pathogenesis, etiology, definition, epidemiology [in Norwegian]. Tidssk Nor Laegeforen 110:2209–2211, 1990 [English abstract]
105. LaBan MM, Meerschaert JR, Taylor RS, et al: Symphyseal and sacroiliac pain associated with pubic symphysis instability. Arch Phys Med Rehabil 59:470–472, 1978

106. Lavignolle B, Vital JM, Senegas J, et al: An approach to the functional anatomy of the SIJs in vivo. Anat Clin 5:169–176, 1983
107. Leblanc KE: Sacroiliac sprain: An overlooked cause of back pain. Am Fam Physician 46:1459–1463, 1992
108. Lee D: Principles and practice of muscle energy and functional techniques. In Grieve GP (ed): Modern Manual Therapy of the Vertebral Column. Edinburgh, Churchill Livingstone, 1986
109. Lee D: The Pelvic Girdle: An Approach to the Examination and Treatment of the Lumbopelvic region. Edinburgh, Churchill Livingstone, 1989
110. Lee DG, Walsh MC: A Workbook of Manual Therapy Techniques for the Vertebral Column and Pelvic Girdle. Delta, British Columbia, Nascent, 1986
111. **Lewit K: Manipulative Therapy in Rehabilitation of the Locomotor System, 2nd ed. Oxford, Butterworth-Heinemann, 1991**
112. Lumsden RM, Morris JM: An in vivo study of axial rotation and immobilization at the lumbosacral joint. J Bone Joint Surg 50A:1591–1602, 1968
113. Lundgren B: Osteokinematics of the pelvis. Proceedings of the International Federation of Orthopedic Manipulative Therapists, 5th International Conference, Vancouver, 1984
114. Lynch FW: The pelvic articulations during pregnancy, labor and puerperium: An x-ray study. Surg Gynecol Obstet 30:575–580, 1920
115. MacDonald GR, Hunt TE: SIJs: Observations on the gross and histological changes in the various age groups. Can Med Assoc J 66:157–162, 1952
116. Macnab I: Lesions of the SIJs. In Macnab I, McCulloch J: Backache, 2nd ed. Baltimore, Williams & Wilkins, 1990
117. Magee DJ: Orthopedic Physical Assessment. Philadelphia, WB Saunders, 1992
118. Maigne R: The concept of painless and opposite motion in spinal manipulations. Am J Phys Med 44:55–69, 1965
119. Maigne R: Orthopedic Medicine. Springfield, Ill., Charles C. Thomas, 1972
120. Maitland GD: Vertebral Manipulations, 5th ed. London, Butterworths, 1986
121. McCall IW, Park WM, O'Brien JP: Induced pain referral from posterior lumbar elements in normal subjects. Spine 4:441–448, 1979
122. McKenzie RA: Mechanical diagnosis and therapy of the lumbar spine. Waikanae, New Zealand, Spinal Publications, 1981
123. Meadows J: Pelvic arthrokinematics. Proceedings of the International Federation of Orthopaedic Manipulative Therapists, 5th International Conference, Vancouver, 1985
124. Meisenbach RO: Sacroiliac relaxation: With analysis of 84 cases. Surg Gynecol Obstet 12:411–434, 1911
125. Mellin G: Correlations of hip mobility with degree of back pain and lumbar spinal mobility in chronic low-back pain patients. Spine 13:668–670, 1990
126. Mennell JB: Physical Treatment, Movement, Manipulation, and Massage. Philadelphia, Blakiston, 1947
127. Mennell JB: The Science and Art of Joint Manipulation, Vols. 1 and 2. London, Churchill, 1952
128. Mennell JB: The Science and Art of Joint Manipulation, Vol. 2: The Spinal Column. London, Churchill, 1962
129. Mennell J McM: Back Pain. Boston, Little, Brown & Co., 1960
130. Mennell J McM: Diagnosis and Treatment Using Manipulative Techniques: Joint Pain. Boston, Little, Brown & Co., 1964
131. Miller JAA, Schultz AB, Andersson GBJ: Load-displacement behavior of SIJs. J Orthop Res 5:92–101, 1987
132. Mitchell F: Structural Pelvic Function. Carmel, CA: Academy of Applied Osteopathy, 1965
133. Mitchell FL, Moran PS, Pruzzo NA: An Evaluation and Treatment Manual of Osteopathic Muscle Energy Procedures. Valley Park, MO, Mitchell, Moran and Pruzzo Associates, 1979
134. Mooney V, Robertson J: The face syndrome. Clin Orthop 115:149–156, 1976
135. Morgan D: Concepts in functional training and postural stabilization for low-back-injured. Top Acute Care Trauma Rehabil 2:8–17, 1988
136. Morscher E: Etiology and pathophysiology of leg-length discrepancies. Propr Orthop Surg 1:9–19, 1977
137. Namey TC, An HS: Emergency diagnosis and management of sciatica: Differentiating the nondiskogenic causes. Emerg Med Rep 6:101–109, 1985
138. Nielsen AJ: Spray and stretch for myofascial pain. Phys Ther 58:567–569, 1978
139. Norkin CC, Levangie PK: Joint Structure and Function, 2nd ed. Philadelphia, FA Davis, 1992
140. Norman GF: Sacroiliac disease and its relationship to lower abdominal pain. Am J Surg 116:54–56, 1968
141. Nyberg R: Pelvic girdle. In Donatelli R, Wooden MJ (eds): Orthopaedic Physical Therapy. New York, Churchill Livingstone, 1989
142. Nyberg R: Clinical studies of sacroiliac movement. In International Federation of Orthopedic Manipulative Therapists, 5th International Conference, Vail, 1992
143. Pace JB, Nagle D: Piriformis syndrome. West J Med 124:435–439, 1976
144. Pace JB: Commonly overlooked pain syndromes responsive to simple therapy. Postgrad Med 58:107–113, 1975
145. Paget S, Bryan W: Reiter syndrome. In Beary JF, Christian CL, Johanson NA (eds): Manual of Rheumatology and Outpatient Orthopedic Disorders: Diagnosis and Therapy, 2nd ed. Boston, Little, Brown & Co., 1987
146. Palmer LM, Epler M: Clinical Assessment in Physical Therapy. Philadelphia, JB Lippincott, 1990
147. Paquin JD, Rest M, Marie PJ, et al: Biochemical and morphologic studies of cartilage from the adult human SIJ. Arthritis Rheum 26:887–895, 1983
148. Paris SV: The Spinal Lesion. New Zealand, Degasus Press, 1965
149. Phillips M: Myokinetic of the pelvis. Proceedings, 5th Conference of International Federation of Orthopaedic Manipulative Therapists, Vancouver, 1984
150. Piedallu P: Problemes Sacro-iliaque. Bordeaux Biere, Homme Sain No. 2, 1952
151. Pierrynowski MR, Schroeder BC, Garrity CB, et al: Three-dimensional sacroiliac motion during locomotion in asymptomatic male and female subjects. In Cotton CE, Lamontagne M, Roberson DGE, Stothart JP (eds): Proceedings of the 5th Biennial Conference and Human Locomotion Symposium of the Canadian Society for Biomechanics, London, Ontario, 1988
152. Pitkin HD, Pheasant HC: Sacro-arthrogenetic telalgia. J Bone Joint Surg 18A:365–374, 1936
153. Porterfield JA, DeRosa CP: Mechanical Low Back Pain: Perspectives in Functional Anatomy. Philadelphia, WB Saunders, 1991
154. Porterfield JA: The SIJ. In Gould J (ed): Orthopaedic and Sports Physical Therapy. St. Louis, CV Mosby, 1985
155. Porterfield JA, DeRosa CP: The SIJ. In Gould J (ed): Orthopaedic and Sports Physical Therapy, 2nd ed. St. Louis, CV Mosby, 1990
156. Potter NA, Rothstein JM. Intertester reliability for selected clinical tests of the SIJ. Phys Ther 65:1671–1675, 1985
157. Pratt WA: The lumbopelvic torsion syndrome. J Am Osteopath Ass 51(7):335–343, 1952
158. Resnick D, Niwayama G, Georgen TG: Degenerative disease of the SIJ. Invest Radiol 10:608–621, 1975
159. Resnick D, Niwayama G, Georgen TG: Clinical, radiographic and pathologic abnormalities in calcium, pyrophosphate dihydrate deposition disease (CPPD): An analysis of 85 patients. Radiology 122:1–15, 1977
160. Reynolds HH: Three-dimensional kinematics in the pelvic girdle. J Am Osteopath Assoc 80:277–280, 1980
161. Reynolds MD: Myofascial trigger point syndromes in the practice of rheumatology. Arch Phys Med Rehabil 62:111–114, 1981
162. Robinson R: The new back school prescription: Stabilization training, part I. Occupational Medicine: State of the Art Reviews 7:17–31, 1992
163. Ryan LM, Carrera GF, Lightfoot RW, et al: The radiographic diagnosis of sacroiliitis—A comparison of different views with computed tomograms of the SIJ. Arthritis Rheum 26:760–763, 1983
164. Saal JA: The new back school prescription: Stabilization training, part II. Occupational Medicine: State of the Art Reviews 7:33–42, 1992
165. Sahrmann S: Diagnosis and Treatment of Muscle Imbalances and Associated Regional Pain Syndromes, Level II course notes. Seattle, 1993
166. Sashin O: A critical analysis of the anatomy and the pathological changes of the SI joints. J Bone Joint Surg 12A:891–910, 1930
167. Saunders HD: Evaluation, Treatment and Prevention of Musculoskeletal Disorders, 2nd ed. Minneapolis, H. Duane Saunders, 1985
168. Schafer RC: Clinical Biomechanics, Musculoskeletal Action and Reactions. Baltimore, Williams & Wilkins, 1987
169. Schmorl G, Junghanns H: The Human Spine in Health and Disease. New York, Grune & Stratton, 1971
170. Schned ES: Ankylosing spondylitis. In Beary JF, Christian CL, Johanson NA (eds): Manual of Rheumatology and Outpatient Orthopedics: Diagnosis and Therapy, 2nd ed. Boston, Little, Brown & Co., 1987:133–141
171. Schneider W, Dvořák J, Dvořák T: Manual Medicine Therapy. New York, Georg Thieme Verlag Stuttgart/Thieme Med Pub., 1988
172. Scholten PJM, Schultz AB, Luchico CW, et al: Motions and loads within the human pelvis: A biomechanical model study. J Orthop Res 6:840–850, 1988
173. Schunke GB: The anatomy and development of the sacroiliac joint in man. Anat Rec 72:313–331, 1938
174. Schunke GB: The anatomy and the development of the SIJ and their relation to the movements of the sacrum. Acta Anat 23:80–91, 1955
175. Simons DG, Travell JG: Myofascial origins of low back pain, torso muscles. Postgrad Med 73:81–92, 1983
176. Sirca A, Kostevc V: The fibre type composition of the thoracic and lumbar paravertebral muscles in man. J Anat 141:131–137, 1985
177. Snaith ML, Galvin SEJ, Short MD: The value of quantitative radioisotope scanning in the differential diagnosis of low back pain and sacroiliac disease. J Rheumatol 9:435–440, 1982
178. Sola AE: Trigger point therapy. In Roberts JR, Hedges WB (eds): Clinical Procedures in Emergency Medicine. Philadelphia, WB Saunders, 1985:674–686
179. Sola AE, Kuitert JH: Quadratus lumborum myofasciitis. Northwest Med 53:1003–1005, 1954
180. Sola AE, Williams RL: Myofascial pain syndromes. Neurology 6:91–95, 1956
181. Solonen VA: The SIJ in the light of anatomical roentgenological and clinical studies. Acta Orthop Scand Suppl 27:1–127, 1957
182. Stein JM, Warfield CA: Two entrapment neuropathies. Hosp Pract:100A–100P, 1983
183. Stoddard A: Manual of Osteopathic Technique. London, Hutchinson and Co., 1959
184. Sturesson B, Selvik G, Uden A: Movement of the SIJs: A roentgen stereophotogrammetric analysis. Spine 14(2):162–165, 1989
185. Tesh KM, Dunn JS, Evans JH: The abdominal muscles and vertebral stability. Spine 12:501–508, 1987
186. Travell JG: The quadratus lumborum muscle: An overlooked cause of low back pain. Arch Phys Med Rehabil 57:566, 1976
187. Travell JG, Simons DG: Quadratus lumborum muscle. In Travell JG, Simons DG (eds): Myofascial Pain and Dysfunction: The Trigger Point Manual, Vol. 2. Baltimore, Williams & Wilkins, 1992:28–88
188. Travell JG, Simons DG: Piriformis and other short lateral rotators. In Travell JG, Simons DG (eds): Myofascial Pain and Dysfunction: The Trigger Point Manual, Vol. 2. Baltimore, Williams & Wilkins, 1992:186–213
189. Trotter M: A common anatomical variation in the sacroiliac region. J Bone Joint Surg 22:293–299, 1940
190. Vleeming A, Stoeckart R, Snijder CJ, et al: The SIJ—Anatomical, biomechanical and radiological aspects. Man Med 5:100–102, 1990
191. Vleeming A, Stoeckart R, Volkers ACW, Snijder CJ: Relation between form and function in the sacroiliac, part I: Clinical anatomical aspects. Spine 13(2):133–135, 1990
192. Vukicevic S, Plitz W, Vukicevic D, et al: Holographic study of the stresses in the normal pelvis with particular reference to the movement of the sacrum. In Huiskes R, Van Campen D, Dewijn J (eds): Biomechanics: Principles and Applications. Dordrecht, The Netherlands, Marinus Nijhoff, W Junk Pub., 1982:223–239
193. Wadsworth CT: Manual Examination and Treatment of the Spine and Extremities. Baltimore, Williams & Wilkins, 1988
194. Walker JM: Age-related differences in the human SIJ—A histological study: Implications for therapy. J Orthop Sports Phys Ther 7:325–331, 1986
195. Walker JM: Pathology of the SIJ. In Proceedings, International Federation of Orthopaedic Manipulative Therapists 5th International Conference, Vail, 1992
196. Walker JM: The SIJ: A critical review. Phys Ther 72:903–916, 1992
197. Wallace LA: Limb-length difference and back pain. In Grieve GP (ed): Modern Manual Therapy of the Vertebral Column. Edinburgh, Churchill Livingstone, 1986
198. Warwick R, Williams P: Gray's Anatomy, 36th ed. Philadelphia, JB Lippincott, 1980
199. Weisl H: The relation of movement to structure in the SIJ. Thesis, University of Manchester, 1953

200. Weisl H: The articular surfaces of the SIJ and their relation to movement of the sacrum. Acta Anat (Basel) 22:10–14, 1954
201. Weisl H: The movements of the SIJ. Acta Anat 23(1):80–91, 1955
202. Weismantel A: Evaluation and treatment of SIJ problems. Bull Orthop Section, Am Phys Ther Assoc 3(1):5–9, 1978
203. Wells PE: The examination of the pelvic joints. In Grieve GP (ed): Modern Manual Therapy of Vertebral Column. Edinburgh, Churchill Livingstone, 1986
204. White A: Stabilization of the lumbar spine. In White A, Anderson R (eds): Conservative Care of Low Back Pain. Baltimore, Williams & Wilkins, 1991
205. Wicks T: Motion in the SIJ scanned with ultrasonography. Proceedings of the International Federation of Orthopedic Manipulative Therapists, 5th International Conference, Vancouver, 1984
206. Wilder DG, Pope MH, Frymoyer JW: The functional topography of the SIJ. Spine 5:575–579, 1980
207. Winter Z: Referred pain in fibrositis. Med Rec 157:34–37, 1944
208. Woerman AL: Evaluation and treatment of dysfunction in the lumbo-pelvic-hip complex. In Donatelli R, Wooden MJ (eds): Orthopaedic Physical Therapy. New York, Churchill Livingstone, 1989:403–483
209. Young HH: Non-neurological lesions simulating protruded intervertebral disc. JAMA 148:1101–1105, 1952

RECOMMENDED READINGS

Fortin JD, Dwyer MD, West S, et al: SIJ: Pain referral maps upon applying a new injection/arthrography technique, part I: Asymptomatic volunteers. Spine 19:1475–1482, 1994
Fortin JD, Aprill CN, Ponthieux B, et al: SIJ: Pain referral maps upon applying a new injection/arthrography technique. part II: Clinical evaluation. Spine 19:1483–1489, 1994

The Lumbosacral–Lower Limb Scan Examination

DARLENE HERTLING AND RANDOLPH M. KESSLER

A common problem in the clinical examination of patients presenting with chronic, insidious musculoskeletal problems of the low back and lower extremities is not knowing in which area to direct physical examination procedures after completing the history portion of the examination. The reason is twofold:

1. Chronic musculoskeletal disorders affecting the low back and the various regions of the lower limbs often present with similar pain patterns.
2. Biomechanical disorders affecting the back and various lower extremity regions often coexist.

The former is a result of the common phenomenon of referred pain that is characteristic of most common musculoskeletal disorders; localized pain arising from deep somatic tissues is usually perceived in an area not corresponding well to the exact pathological site. Thus, patients with "low-back pain" usually feel discomfort primarily in the upper buttock or sacroiliac region, patients with trochanteric bursitis often have significant pain in the posterior hip and lateral thigh areas, and those with chondromalacia patellae frequently feel pain over the medial aspect of the distal thigh and upper leg. Also, as the severity of the pathological process increases, there is greater likelihood

that pain may be perceived throughout a distribution corresponding to any or all of the relevant sclerotome. Thus, if a relatively acute disorder affects a tissue innervated primarily by the L5 segment, the patient may feel pain in any or all of those regions also innervated by L5.

A typical example would be the patient with moderate to advanced degenerative hip disease who invariably experiences pain in the groin, which spreads into the anterior thigh and to the knee—the L3 sclerotome. This occurs because the anterior aspect of the hip joint capsule, from which the pain primarily arises, is innervated largely by the L3 segment. Similarly, the patient with involvement of the L3 segment of the spine from, for example, the facet joint or disk, may feel pain that spreads in the same distribution as that described for hip joint disease. It may not be obvious from subjective information alone whether the hip, the low back, or both are involved. Likewise, it is often difficult to determine on the basis of subjective information alone whether a patient has trochanteric bursitis, an L5 spinal disorder, or both. The trochanteric region is innervated primarily by L5, and pain arising in conjunction with trochanteric bursitis is often felt down the lateral aspect of the thigh and

Darlene Hertling and Randolph M. Kessler: MANAGEMENT OF COMMON MUSCULOSKELETAL DISORDERS: Physical Therapy Principles and Methods, 3rd ed.
© 1996 Lippincott-Raven Publishers.

dorsum of the leg (the L5 sclerotome), as may be the case with pain originating at the L5 spinal level.

Another classic example of localization of pain to distant regions of a relevant sclerotome occurs in the child with a hip joint disorder, such as a slipped capital femoral epiphysis, who feels pain primarily in the knee; both the hip and the knee joints are innervated largely by L3. Because delocalization and reference of pain are common phenomena, the subjective account of pain distribution does not provide a reliable indication of the true site of the pathological process. Additional objective information is often required.

The prevalence of coexistent disorders or abnormalities of the low back and lower extremity regions is largely a result of the biomechanical interdependency of the weight-bearing joints in the closed kinetic chain. Normal attenuation of the energy introduced to the weight-bearing joints by the vertical displacement of the center of gravity requires that the overall displacement of the center of gravity be minimized, which, in turn, requires normal movement of the weight-bearing joints during stance phase of gait. Loss of critical movement at any of the weight-bearing joints will cause increased energy input to the entire weight-bearing skeleton from the force of the body weight acting over a greater distance, with the result being added vertical compressive loading during stance phase. Similarly, energy input to the weight-bearing joints in a horizontal plane is normally attenuated by joint movements. With the foot fixed to the ground, in order for the body to be normally moved through space in the presence of reduced critical movement at any joint, compensation is required at some other joint. Such an alteration in function is likely to result in added stresses to the compensating joint. Thus, the patient with loss of hip extension tends to walk with greater extension of the lower lumbar joints, and the person with loss of ankle dorsiflexion undergoes greater-than-normal extension movements at the knee. Since the close-packed positions of the spine and knee are extension, these abnormalities are likely to cause increased subchondral compressive stresses and increased capsular tensile stresses to the knee and spinal joints.

Less obvious are the results of abnormalities in transverse rotation of the weight-bearing joints during stance phase of gait. From heel-strike to foot-flat the pelvis, thigh, and leg normally undergo internal rotatory movements, the distal segments more so than their supra-adjacent neighbors. The segments of the leg similarly undergo external rotation during foot-flat to toe-off. Since the foot is relatively fixed to the ground, however, it does not rotate. This means that the ankle–foot complex must absorb the rotatory movements imposed from above; internal rotation is absorbed by pronation of the foot, and external rotation is transmitted to the foot as a supinatory movement. One should observe the result of rotating the leg over the foot that is fixed to the ground; internal rotation causes the calcaneus to shift into valgus position and the medial arch to lower (pronation of the hindfoot), whereas external rotation brings the heel into varus position and raises the arch (supination of the hindfoot). It should also be noted that internal rotation of the thigh with the knee slightly bent causes an increased valgus angulation at the knee. This is of practical significance because the knee remains slightly bent during all phases of the gait cycle.

Again, because attenuation of the forces of the body weight moving over the fixed foot requires a normal contribution of movement from all weight-bearing joints, abnormalities of function at any one joint may affect the function of one or more of the others in the chain. A common example occurs in the person with increased femoral antetorsion, who tends to walk with excessive internal rotation during stance phase of gait. This results in abnormal valgus angulation at the knee and increased foot pronation. The former may predispose to patellar tracking problems, while the latter may lead to a variety of problems, including plantar fasciitis, heel spurs, hallux valgus, metatarsalgia, and fatigue of the intrinsic foot musculature (see Chapter 14, The Lower Leg, Ankle, and Foot). On the other hand, a primary problem of abnormal foot pronation may lead to excessive internal rotatory and valgus stresses to the knee and increased internal rotation of the hip during gait. It should be clear that the best approach to management of pathological lesions resulting from such biomechanical derangements would be one that takes into consideration primary etiological factors. This often requires that evaluating procedures be directed to areas other than simply the primary region of involvement.

The above considerations should help emphasize the need to evaluate all of the weight-bearing joint regions in many, if not most, chronic musculoskeletal disorders affecting the low back or lower limb. A further factor to consider in this regard is the common phenomenon of summation of otherwise subliminal afferent input from coexistent minor disorders involving tissues innervated by the same or adjacent spinal segments. A common example is the person who stresses the joint capsules of the low back excessively throughout the day and who also has some low-grade inflammation of the trochanteric bursa. Noxious input from both areas may summate at the dorsal horn of the spinal cord and other central neural connections, to cause more low-back pain as well as more lateral thigh pain than would be present if either disorder existed by itself. In this particular example, the clinician must differentiate between the possibility of one lesion referring pain into another part of the relevant segment and two distinct pathological processes within the same segment. This cannot be determined without evaluating both the low-back and the hip regions. Pain arising from the summation of input from different sites of the same segment will, of course, be more likely to occur in the patient with multisegmental restrictions of motion of the lower spine, since with daily activities the soft tissues (joint capsules and ligaments) of the spine will be stressed more, causing an increase in afferent input to the relevant spinal levels. In such cases, the threshold of pain arising from minor disorders affecting tissue in the lower limbs innervated by the corresponding spinal segments is probably reduced. Any back pain is likely to be enhanced by such segmentally related pathological processes. Most persons, by middle age or later, develop some lower-lumbar facet-joint capsular restriction secondary to disk narrowing or other causes. Thus, middle-aged or older persons with chronic low-back or lower-limb pain should always be examined for coexistent segmental disorders that may be contributing to the amount of pain the person experiences.

In summary, the low back–lower extremity scan examination may be used to:

- Determine the area of involvement in cases in which relatively vague subjective information fails to suggest the site of the pathological process. This is not an uncommon occurrence and is related to the fact that pain of deep somatic origin may be referred to any or all of the relevant sclerotome.
- Examine for the presence of some distant biomechanical derangement that may be related, in cause or effect, to the patient's primary physical lesion that causes his pain.
- Rule out the possibility of some segmentally related disorder that may, by the mechanism of summation of segmentally related afferent input, contribute to the patient's pain perception.

The scan examination is oriented, then, toward detecting gross or subtle biomechanical abnormalities and toward determining the presence of common lumbar or lower extremity musculoskeletal disorders. Essential to the detection of significant biomechanical derangements are careful assessment of function (gait analysis), evaluation of bony structure and alignment, and examination of joint mobility. These examination procedures are combined with the key objective tests for the common chronic disorders affecting the lower back and lower limbs, to constitute the lumbosacral–lower limb scan examination. A discussion of the common pathological processes and their primary clinical manifestations will facilitate understanding and interpretation of the examination procedures involved in the scan examination.

COMMON LESIONS OF THE LUMBOSACRAL REGION AND LOWER LIMBS AND THEIR PRIMARY CLINICAL MANIFESTATIONS

The Lumbosacral Region

I. **Acute (severe) Posterolateral Disk Prolapse** (outer annulus or posterior longitudinal ligament still intact)
   A. *Subjective complaints*
      1. Sudden onset of unilateral lumbosacral pain, often with gradual buildup of pain intensity. Occasionally the patient denies a sudden onset and notes first experiencing pain on rising in the morning. There may be some aching in the leg.
      2. Worse with sitting and on rising after a long period of recumbency; somewhat relieved with recumbency
   B. *Key objective signs*
      1. Functional lumbar deformity, with a loss of lordosis and usually a lumbar scoliosis with the convexity to the involved side
      2. Marked, painful restriction of spinal movement, especially forward and backward bending
      3. Positive dural mobility tests

II. **Acute Facet Joint Derangement**
   A. *Subjective complaints*
      1. Sudden onset of lumbosacral pain and deformity; little or no leg discomfort
      2. Pain is aggravated by being up and about and relieved by sitting or recumbency.
   B. *Key objective findings*
      1. Marked lumbar deformity; loss of lordosis and lumbar scoliosis with convexity to side of involvement
      2. Lumbar extension and sidebending to the side of involvement are painfully restricted. Forward bending and contralateral sidebending are slightly restricted.
      3. Negative dural signs

III. **Localized, Unilateral, Facet-Joint Capsular Tightness**
   A. *Subjective complaints*
      1. Often a history of past episodes of acute low-back dysfunction
      2. Aching in the lumbosacral region, aggravated by long periods of standing, walk-

ing, or activities involving prolonged or repetitive lumbar extension; also worse with increased muscular tension, such as during periods of emotional stress, and worse in the evening than in the morning.

B. *Key objective findings*

1. Possible subtle predisposing biomechanical factors such as a leg-length disparity
2. Possible minor restriction of sidebending to the involved side and deviation of spine toward the involved side on forward bending and away from the involved side on extension
3. Discomfort on quadrant tests when localized to the involved segment

IV. **Multisegmental Bilateral Capsular Restriction of Lumbar Facet Joints—Degenerative Joint Disease**

A. *Subjective complaints*

1. The patient is middle-aged or older.
2. Often there is a long history of intermittent back problems.
3. Aching across the lower back and hip girdle is made worse with long periods of standing or walking. The back is stiff in the morning, somewhat better at midday, and aching again by evening. Some intermittent aching in one or both legs may occur.

B. *Key objective findings*

1. Some loss of the normal lumbar lordosis
2. Restriction of spinal motion in a generalized capsular pattern of limitation: marked restriction of spinal extension, moderate restriction of sidebending bilaterally, and mild to moderate restriction of rotations and forward bending

V. **Lower Lumbar Disk Extrusion with Nerve Root Impingement**

A. *Subjective complaints*

1. Sudden or gradual onset of lumbosacral pain and unilateral leg pain. The patient may describe an onset suggestive of an acute posterolateral prolapse (see earlier) with progressive loss of back pain and increase in leg pain.
2. The leg pain may be relatively sharp and is usually felt down the posterolateral thigh and into the anterolateral or posterior aspect of the lower leg. The leg pain may be aggravated by sitting or by being up and about and is relatively relieved by rest.

B. *Key objective findings*

1. Mild to moderate loss of lumbar movement, usually toward extension and in

movements toward the side of involvement; it occasionally occurs away from the involved side.

2. Mild segmental neurological deficit
3. Positive dural mobility signs

VI. **Acute Sacroiliac Dysfunction**

A. *Subjective complaints*

1. Sudden onset of unilateral sacroiliac pain, often associated with some twisting motion
2. Occasional spread of pain to the posterior thigh
3. Pain is usually aggravated by activities involving combined hip and spine extension, such as standing erect (posterior torsional displacement). Less often it is aggravated by combined hip and spine flexion, such as sitting (anterior torsional displacement).

B. *Key objective findings*

1. Posterior torsional displacement (most common)

   a. Tendency to stand with the hip, knee, and low back slightly flexed on the involved side. If so, the knee landmarks and the greater trochanter will be lower on the involved side than on the uninvolved side. The posterior-superior iliac spine and iliac crest will also be lower on the involved side, more so than the knee landmarks and trochanter. The anterior-superior iliac spine will not be as low on the involved side as the knee and trochanteric landmarks. The pelvis will be shifted away from the involved side.

      If the patient stands with the legs straight, all of the landmarks up to and including the trochanters will be level. The posterior-superior iliac spine and iliac crest will be lower on the involved side than on the uninvolved side, but the anterior-superior iliac spine will be higher. The pelvis will appear to be rotated forward on the involved side.

   b. The anterior rotation test will be quite painful; the posterior rotation test will be less painful.

   c. Contralateral straight-leg raising may cause some pain, which is relieved when the involved leg is raised.

2. Anterior torsional displacement (rare)

   a. Tendency to stand with the hip and knee in more extension on the involved side than on the uninvolved side. The pelvis may be shifted toward and inclined away from the involved side. If the patient stands in this manner, the knee landmarks and trochanter will be lower on the uninvolved side. The posterior-superior iliac spine and iliac crest will also be lower on the uninvolved side, more so than the knee landmarks and trochanter. The anterior-superior iliac spine will not be as low on the uninvolved side as the other landmarks.

If the patient can stand erect, the trochanters and landmarks below will be level. The posterior-superior iliac spine and iliac crest will be higher on the involved side; the anterior-superior iliac spine will be lower on the involved side.

   b. Posterior rotation test will be quite painful; anterior rotation test will be less painful.
   c. Ipsilateral straight-leg raising test may cause some pain, which is relieved when the opposite leg is raised.

VII. Chronic Sacroiliac Hypermobility
   A. *Subjective complaints*
      1. History suggestive of intermittent acute sacroiliac dysfunction with gradual progression to more chronic sacroiliac and posterior thigh pain. Development may be associated with past pregnancy.
      2. Pain is aggravated by prolonged or repetitive activities involving
         a. Combined hip and spine extension or hip extension with contralateral hip flexion
         b. Combined hip and spine flexion or hip flexion with contralateral hip extension
   B. *Key objective findings*
      1. Possible signs of sacroiliac asymmetry on assessment of structural alignment (see earlier under Acute Sacroiliac Dysfunction)
      2. Pain or crepitus on one or more sacroiliac stress tests

☐ **The Hip**

I. Degenerative Joint Disease
   A. *Subjective complaints*
      1. Gradual, progressive onset of hip pain and dysfunction

      2. Pain is felt first and most in the groin region. With progression, pain may spread to the anterior thigh, posterior hip, and lateral hip regions.
      3. Pain is first noticed after long periods of weight-bearing activities. Later, pain and stiffness are noted on rising in the morning, easing somewhat by midday, and then increased again by evening.
   B. *Key objective findings*
      1. Tendency to stand with hip and knee flexed and lumbar spine hyperextended; pelvis is shifted toward the involved side
      2. Gait abnormality characterized by tendency to incline the trunk toward the involved side during stance phase
      3. Painful limitation of hip motions in a capsular pattern of restriction; marked limitation of internal rotation and abduction; moderate restriction of flexion and extension; mild to moderate restriction of abduction and external rotation

II. Trochanteric Bursitis
   A. *Subjective complaints*
      1. Insidious onset of lateral hip pain, often spreading into the lateral thigh, aggravated most by climbing stairs or, occasionally, by sitting with the involved leg crossed over the uninvolved leg
      2. Occasionally an acute onset is described, associated with a "snap" felt in the hip region (the iliotibial band snapping over the greater trochanter).
   B. *Key objective findings*
      1. Pain on resisted hip abduction
      2. Pain on approximation of the knee on the involved side to the opposite axilla
      3. Possible pain on stretch of the iliotibial band
      4. Possible pain on full passive hip abduction

III. Iliopectineal Bursitis
   A. *Subjective complaint:* Gradual, usually nontraumatic, onset of anterior hip pain, made worse by activities involving extreme or repetitive hip extension
   B. *Key objective findings*
      1. Pain on resisted hip flexion
      2. Pain on full passive hip extension
      3. Possible pain on full hip flexion

☐ **The Knee**

I. Acute Medial Ligamentous Injury
   A. *Subjective complaints*
      1. Sudden onset of knee pain, usually associ-

ated with some athletic activity. There may or may not have been some external force acting on the knee at the time of injury in the case of a partial tear.

2. Gradual buildup of swelling over several hours in the case of a partial tear; there is little swelling in the case of a complete rupture.

3. The patient often attempts to continue the activity in which he was engaged in the case of a complete rupture, but much less so in the case of a partial tear.

B. *Key objective findings*
1. Antalgic, toe-touch gait in the acute phase of a partial tear; less severe gait disturbance or no gait disturbance in a complete rupture
2. Effusion with limitation of motion in a capsular pattern in the case of a partial tear; little swelling and relatively free range of motion if a complete rupture
3. Pain and spasm on valgus and external rotary stress if a partial tear; painless hypermobility in the case of a complete rupture

II. **Acute Meniscus Tear**
A. *Subjective complaint:* Essentially the same as for a partial ligamentous tear. The patient is very hesitant to continue to engage in the activity.
B. *Key objective findings*
1. The same as for a partial ligament tear except no pain on stress tests
2. Point tenderness over the anteromedial joint line
3. Disproportionate loss of extension (*e.g.,* locked knee) if a mechanical block to movement is created by a displaced piece of the meniscus

III. **Lateral Patellar Tracking Dysfunction** (chondromalacia patellae)
A. *Subjective complaints*
1. Gradual onset of medial knee pain aggravated especially by descending stairs and sitting for long periods of time
2. The onset may be associated with an increase in some activity involving repeated loaded knee extension
B. *Key objective findings*
1. There may be some predisposing structural factor such as anteversion of the hip, genu valgum, a small patella, a high-riding patella, or a diminution in the prominence of the anterior aspect of the lateral femoral condyle.
2. There may be some atrophy of the vastus medialis.

3. Lateral glide of the patella may cause some medial discomfort.
4. Palpation of the medial aspect of the back side of patella may cause discomfort.
5. Femoropatellar crepitus may be noted on weight-bearing knee flexion–extension.

IV. **Chronic Coronary Ligament Sprain** (adhesion)
A. *Subjective complaint:* Sudden medial knee pain associated with some weight-bearing twisting movement, followed by persistent aching or twinging of pain over the medial knee region. There is usually no significant disability.
B. *Key objective findings*
1. Point tenderness over the anteromedial joint line
2. Pain on passive external rotation of the tibia on the femur; no pain on valgus stress

V. **Tendinitis—Biceps, Iliotibial, or Pes Anserinus**
A. *Subjective complaint:* Gradual onset of pain, almost always associated with long-distance running or some other athletic activity. The pain is lateral for biceps or iliotibial tendinitis and medial for pes anserinus tendinitis. There is little that reproduces the pain except the activity that caused the problem.
B. *Key objective findings*
1. Pain on resisted knee flexion and external tibial rotation in the case of biceps tendinitis
2. Pain on resisted knee extension and external tibial rotation in the case of iliotibial tendinitis
3. Pain on resisted knee flexion and internal rotation for pes anserinus tendinitis
4. Pain on straight-leg raising for biceps tendinitis
5. Point tenderness over the site of the lesion, usually at the tenoperiosteal junction
6. Pain on iliotibial band extensibility test for iliotibial tendinitis

☐ The Lower Leg, Ankle, and Foot

I. **Overuse Syndromes of the Leg**
A. *Subjective complaints*
1. The term *shin splint* is often used as a blanket description of any persistent pain occurring between the knee and ankle usually associated with some increased athletic activity, such as jumping or running on a hard surface.
2. When overuse is a contributing factor, there will be a characteristic history of gradual onset of pain that may be accentu-

ated by excessive pronation or supination. Pain is aggravated by activity and relieved by rest.

B. *Key objective findings*
1. There may be some predisposing structural factors such as excessive pronation or supination, tibial varum, or the coxa varum–genu valgum combination.
2. Pain and tenderness over the involved soft tissue (tendinitis or compartment syndromes) or in an area devoid of muscles such as the tibial shaft (tibial stress reaction and stress fracture)
3. Pain is increased by stressing the involved muscles (compartment syndromes and tendinitis) actively or with manual resistance.
4. In tibial stress reaction, percussion of the tibia increases the pain. Tuning fork vibration may or may not be positive.

II. **Acute Ankle Sprain**
A. *Subjective complaints*
1. Sudden onset of lateral ankle pain, associated with plantar flexion–inversion strain, usually during some athletic activity. Continued participation in the activity, at the time of injury, is usually not possible.
2. Gradual development of lateral ankle swelling over te subsequent several hours with continued difficulty in weight-bearing

B. *Key objective signs*
1. Obvious limp associated with traumatic arthritis of the ankle mortise joint (see Table 22-1)
2. Swelling and often marked ecchymosis over the lateral aspect of the ankle
3. Pain is reproduced on
   a. Plantar flexion–inversion stress
   b. Anterior glide of the talus in the mortise

III. **Chronic Recurrent Ankle Sprains**
A. *Subjective complaint:* History of acute ankle sprain (see earlier) followed by one or more episodes of the ankle giving way during activities involving jumping or quick lateral movements. Pain, swelling, and dysfunction associated with subsequent episodes are usually not as severe as that occurring with the original injury.
B. *Key objective findings:* These are variable, depending on the causative factors. Consider the following possible causes and the related clinical manifestations.
1. True structural instability (rare)—Hypermobility of anterior glide of the talus in the mortise

2. Residual ligamentous adhesion—Hypomobility or pain on anterior glide of the talus in the mortise
3. Alteration in proprioceptive neuromuscular protective response—Poor balance reactions on one-legged standing

IV. **Achilles Tendinitis and Bursitis**
A. *Subjective complaint:* Usually a gradual onset of posterior ankle pain that may be associated with some increase in activity level. The pain is made worse when wearing lower-heeled shoes and is improved with wearing higher heels.
B. *Key objective findings*
1. Pain on strong resisted or repetitive resisted ankle plantar flexion
2. Pain on extreme hindfoot dorsiflexion
3. Tenderness to palpation over the distal Achilles region

V. **Medial Metatarsalgia**
A. *Subjective complaint:* Pain over the first two metatarsal heads after long periods of weight-bearing. The onset is usually insidious, occasionally associated with a change in foot wear.
B. *Key objective findings*
1. Pressure metatarsalgia
   a. Often associated with a pronated or pronating foot
   b. The first metatarsal may be abnormally short.
   c. The medial metatarsal heads may be tender to deep palpation.
2. Tension metatarsalgia (from increased tension on the distal insertion of the plantar fascia)
   a. Usually associated with a pronating foot
   b. The pain may be reproduced by everting the hindfoot while supinating the forefoot and dorsiflexing the toes.

VI. **Plantar Fasciitis**
A. *Subjective complaints*
1. Pain and tenderness localized to plantar aspect of foot. Pain may be localized to the heel or may present as a burning pain over the arch.
2. Pain is made worse by activity, such as climbing stairs, walking, or running, and relieved by rest.
B. *Key objective findings*
1. There may be some predisposing factors such as a high-arched cavus foot, a tight plantar fascia or Achilles tendon, weak peronei or chronic irritation from excessive

pronation, or a variety of malalignment faults.

2. Localized tenderness at the plantar fascial attachment into the calcaneus, just distal to this attachment and over the medial band of the plantar fascia. A tight plantar band can be palpated.

3. Pain may be increased on actively and passively dorsiflexing the foot, especially if the big toe is also dorsiflexed.

■ THE SCAN EXAMINATION TESTS

□ Gait Analysis

The reader should refer to Tables 22-1 and 22-2 for an overview of the primary gait abnormalities associated with various common lumbar or lower limb disorders or structural deviations. These tables emphasize the biomechanical interplay among the weight-bearing regions. A careful assessment of gait is an essential component of the evaluation of chronic low back and lower limb disorders, since it is, of course, the most important functional requirement of these regions and also because many biomechanical abnormalities will not be evident on other parts of the examination.

When evaluating chronic disorders, most of which are the result of stress overloads, it is important to realize which functional abnormalities are present and to appreciate that these are not always manifested as obvious static deviations or deformities. For example, a person's foot may undergo excessive pronation while walking but the foot may not necessarily appear "pronated" on assessment of bony structure and alignment during standing. Experience in gait analysis is invaluable in understanding the pathomechanics and, in some instances, the etiologies of many common chronic disorders. For this reason it also leads to greater sophistication in devising and implementing treatment strategies, since many chronic disorders are temporarily relieved by "symptomatic" treatment but will inevitably recur unless the underlying causes are addressed.

Tables 22-1 and 22-2 are organized to serve as a guide to the clinical assessment of gait abnormalities associated with the common disorders affecting the low back and lower limbs. After having documented the salient features of some abnormal gait pattern, the clinician may consult the tables to estimate what the underlying physical dysfunction may be and to see what the common causes are. This information should then be correlated with findings from the remainder of the physical examination.

□ Assessment of Structural Alignment

Static alterations in skeletal alignment are significant if they are relatively pronounced or if they are acquired. In either case, they affect a considerable reduction in the stresses that may be imposed on related tissues without pain or degenerative changes. Congenital skeletal deviations, as long as they fall within relatively normal limits, are usually insignificant under normal activity levels, since the related tissues automatically adapt to the various stresses they must withstand as the musculoskeletal system develops. However, such "normal" deviations may make the patient more susceptible to certain stress-overload disorders under conditions of increased activity, such as recreational or competitive athletics. To avoid omitting crucial assessments, the examination of structural alignment may be organized into the following three components: (1) frontal alignment, (2) sagittal alignment, and (3) transverse (rotary) alignment.

The patient's unstructured stance is noted. In this habitual stance the patient may be compensating for a number of postural asymmetries. It may be easier to detect these problems if the stance is structured by asking the patient to stand with the feet hip-width apart and the feet pointed slightly (about 5° to 10°) outward. The primary assessments of each position are carried out with the patient in relaxed standing position, with the low back and lower extremities well exposed. The patient is instructed to look straight ahead and to keep arms to the side.

TESTS IN STANDING

I. Frontal Alignment—Patient viewed from behind

   A. *Horizontal asymmetry* is best detected by use of a plumb bob. The plumb bob is hung so that it barely clears the ground; the patient is positioned as close as possible to the plumb line, without touching it, and with the plumb bob bisecting the heels.

   1. It should be noted, first, whether the plumb line bisects the legs, pelvis, and lower spine. If there is a lateral shift of the pelvis with respect to the plumb line, consider the following possibilities:

      a. A shorter leg on the side of the shift; this will be checked for later during assessment of vertical symmetry.

      b. Tight hip abductors (almost always the iliotibial band) on the side opposite the shift. This is often associated with a valgus deviation of the knee on the tight side. Iliotibial band extensibility should be checked later.

TABLE 22-1   EFFECTS OF COMMON PATHOLOGICAL CONDITIONS ON GAIT: SAGITTAL PLANE (PATIENT VIEWED FROM THE SIDE)

	PAINFUL OR RESTRICTED ANKLE PLANTAR FLEXION	PAINFUL OR RESTRICTED ANKLE DORSIFLEXION	PAINFUL OR RESTRICTED KNEE EXTENSION	PAINFUL OR RESTRICTED HIP EXTENSION	PAINFUL OR RESTRICTED LOW-BACK EXTENSION
Nature of Gait Disturbance					
	1. Capsular restriction (e.g., post-immobilization) 2. Traumatic arthritis (e.g., post-ankle sprain)	1. Capsular restriction (e.g., postimmobilization) 2. Heel-cord tightness (e.g., post-immobilization) 3. Traumatic arthritis (e.g., post-ankle sprain)	1. Capsular restriction (e.g., DJD or postimmobilization) 2. Traumatic arthritis (e.g., post-sprain) 3. Locked knee (e.g., bucket-handle meniscus tear)	1. Capsular restriction (e.g., DJD) 2. Iliopectineal bursitis	1. Multisegmental capsular restriction (e.g., DJD) 2. Posterior disk prolapse 3. Acute facet joint dysfunction
Pattern of Gait Disturbance					
Loss of heel-strike a. Toe-touch gait			X (if painful or locked)		
b. Flatfooted gait	X		X (if stiff)		
Loss of plantar flexion following heel-strike with accelerated stance phase	X		X (if stiff)		
Loss of dorsiflexion during foot-flat stage of stance → premature heel-rise, exaggerated hip and knee flexion during early swing phase		X	X (if stiff)		
Loss of push-off and heel-rise	X		X	X	
Shortened stance phase on involved side	X	X	X	X	X (stance shortened bilaterally)
Tendency toward increased knee extension during stance		X (if stiff)			
Trunk lurch forward during stance		X	X	X (if painful)	
Knee held in increased flexion during stance	X (early and late stance)		X	X	X
Loss of hip extension during stance		X	X	X	X
Loss of low-back extension during stance; trunk held in forward position				X (if painful)	X
Tendency toward increased low-back extension during stance				X (if stiff)	

DJD = Degenerative joint disease.

TABLE 22-2 EFFECTS OF COMMON PATHOLOGICAL CONDITIONS ON GAIT: FRONTAL PLANE AND TRANSVERSE PLANES (PATIENT VIEWED FROM THE FRONT OR BACK)

	PRONATION DEFORMITY OR FUNCTIONAL PRONATION DEVIATION OF HINDFOOT	PAINFUL OR RESTRICTED ANKLE OR KNEE FLEXION OR EXTENSION	VARUS DEFORMITY OR VALGUS DEFORMITY DEVIATION OF KNEE	VARUS DEFORMITY OR DEVIATION OF KNEE	EXTERNAL TIBIAL TORSION
Nature of Gait Disturbance					
	1. Congenital hypermobility of foot (flexible deformity) 2. Tarsal coalition (fixed deformity) 3. Increased femoral anteversion (functional) 4. Genu valgum (functional) 5. Loss of hindfoot dorsiflexion (e.g., tight heel cord)	See Table 22-1	1. DJD of lateral knee (deformity) 2. Increased femoral antetorsion (function → structural) 3. Increased foot pronation (functional) 4. Tight iliotibial band (functional)	1. DJD of medial knee (deformity) 2. Increased femoral retrotorsion (functional)	1. Congenital (structural) 2. Acquired compensation for femoral antetorsion
Pattern of Gait Disturbance					
Toeing inward					
Lowered navicular (flatfoot)	X				
Valgus deviation of heel	X		X		
Toeing outward		X			X (uncompensated)
Patella facing outward during swing phase				X (if 2° retroversion)	
Patella facing inward during swing phase					
Patella facing inward during stance	X		X (if 2° anteversion)		X (if compensated)
Patella facing outward during stance					
Pelvis rotates excessively externally (contralateral side forward) during stance					
Pelvis shifted ipsilaterally					
Pelvis shifted contralaterally					
Trunk inclined ipsilaterally during stance					
Trunk inclined contralaterally during stance					(continued)

DJD = Degenerative joint disease.

TABLE 22-2   CONTINUED

INTERNAL TIBIAL TORSION	INCREASED FEMORAL ANTEVERSION OR FUNCTIONAL INTERNAL ROTATORY DEVIATION OF FEMUR	INCREASED FEMORAL RETROVERSION OR FUNCTIONAL EXTERNAL ROTATORY DEVIATION OF FEMUR	PAINFUL OR RESTRICTED HIP ABDUCTION AND INTERNAL ROTATION	RESTRICTED HIP ADDUCTION	PAINFUL OR RESTRICTED LUMBAR LATERAL DEVIATION
		Nature of Gait Disturbance			
1. Congenital (structural) 2. Acquired compensation for femoral retrotorsion	1. Congenital (structural) 2. Increased foot pronation (functional) 3. External ti6bial torsion (compensatory)	1. Congenital (structural) 2. Internal tibial torsion (compensatory)	Capsular restriction (e.g., hip DJD)	Tight iliotibial band	1. Posterolateral disk protrusion 2. Acute facet joint dysfunction (unilateral)
		Pattern of Gait Disturbance			
X (uncompensated)	X (uncompensated)				
	X (if compensated for by external torsion)				
	X (if compensated for by external torsion)				
		X (uncompensated)	X		
		X			
	X				
	X				
X (uncompensated)		X			
	X				
			X		
				X	
			X		X (rare)
					X

c. Loss of hip abduction on the side of the shift. The most common cause is a capsular restriction secondary to degenerative hip disease. Hip range of motion should be assessed later to determine if a capsular pattern of restriction exists.

2. Note obvious valgus/varus deviations or asymmetries of the knee
   a. Bilateral genu valgum (knock knees) is often associated with femoral antetorsion, foot pronation, or both.
   b. Unilateral genu valgum is often associated with iliotibial band tightness, lateral compartment degenerative joint disease of the knee, unilateral femoral antetorsion, or unilateral foot pronation.
   c. Bilateral genu varum (bowed legs) is often associated with femoral retrotorsion.
   d. Unilateral genu varum is often associated with medial degenerative knee disease or unilateral femoral retrotorsion.
   e. Tibial varum or valgum should be differentiated from genu varum or valgum.
   f. Calcaneal valgum is usually associated with foot pronation, genu valgum, femoral antetorsion, or some combination thereof. It is evidenced by inward bowing of the Achilles tendon.
   g. Calcaneal varum may be present with foot supination, femoral retrotorsion, genu varum, or some combination and is seen as outward bowing of the Achilles tendon.

3. Note obvious asymmetries in muscle bulk. The calves or hamstrings on one side may be atrophied in the presence of a chronic S1 or S2 radiculopathy.

4. Note lateral spinal curvatures. A lumbar scoliosis may be associated with
   a. A lateral pelvic inclination. The lumbar convexity will be toward the side on which the pelvis is lower.
   b. A lateral pelvic shift. The convexity will be on the side toward which the pelvis is shifted.
   c. Acute spinal derangements (disk prolapse or facet joint dysfunction). The lumbar convexity is usually toward the side of the problem, except in some prolapses in which protruding disk material is medial to the sensitive structure (*e.g.,* the nerve root).
   d. Asymmetrical lumber degenerative changes, with asymmetrical disk narrowing and facet joint tightness. The convexity is usually away from the side of the degeneration.
   e. A structural thoracolumbar scoliosis. The patient is asked to bend forward to observe for a fixed rotary component, typical of structural curves. The lumbar convexity is usually to the left, with a left rotary component; the thoracic convexity is to the right, with a right rotary component (see Fig. 19-9C). These curves, unless severe, are generally asymptomatic.

B. *Sacral base and leg length.* The presence of segmental vertical asymmetries (leg-length disparities) is best determined by comparing the heights of the key bony landmarks listed below. This is usually done by palpating similar prominences or contours with the same finger of both hands, then assessing the relative heights of the palpating fingers. For each of the landmarks, it is not so important that the examiner feel some precise point as it is that she feel the same prominence or contour with both palpating fingers.

1. Medial malleoli. The most common cause of one being lower than the other is a foot that is more pronated on the lower side. The examiner should check transverse alignment later and correlate this with the position of the calcaneus, since with foot pronation the calcaneus will tend to be in a valgus position.

2. Fibular heads and popliteal folds. If the malleoli are level and these are not level, disparity in tibial length should be suspected. One should inquire about a previous fracture or other possible causative factors.

3. Greater trochanters. If the ankle and knee landmarks are level but the trochanters are not level, the shaft of one femur is probably shortened, barring severe degenerative changes of the knee. Again, one should inquire about previous fractures.

4. Posterior-superior iliac spines. If the ankle and knee landmarks as well as the trochanters are level, but the posterior-superior iliac spines are not, the following are possible: (1) torsional asymmetry in the sacroiliac joints, (2) valgus–varus asymmetry in the proximal femur, and (3) advanced degenerative changes of one hip joint.

a. The most common torsional displacement at the sacroiliac joint is a backward torsion of the ilium on the sacrum, in which the posterior-superior iliac spine on the involved side is lower than the one on the opposite side; however, the anterior-superior iliac spine on the involved side is higher. In this case, one should check the relative heights of the anterior-superior iliac spines.

b. In the case of femoral valgus or varus asymmetry, both the posterior-superior and the anterior-superior iliac spines are higher on the side that is in relative valgus position. Nélaton's line may be used to confirm the existence of valgus–varus asymmetry. The position of the greater trochanter is assessed with respect to a line formed from the anterior-superior iliac spine to the ischial tuberosity; with a valgus femur the trochanter will fall more inferiorly with respect to Nélaton's line compared with a varus femur. It should be realized that valgus angulation of the femur is usually associated with increased antetorsion and a relatively mobile hip joint, whereas a varus femur is usually associated with retrotorsion and a more stable hip joint.

c. Advanced degenerative changes of a hip joint, sufficient to cause noticeable lowering of the pelvis on the involved side, will invariably be associated with a capsular restriction of motion at the hip. Internal rotation and abduction are markedly restricted, flexion and extension are moderately restricted, and adduction and external rotation are somewhat limited.

5. Iliac crests. If these are not level, the cause of asymmetry should be looked for at some lower segment (see earlier). **Note:** Asymmetry in the height of landmarks at any level should result in a corresponding asymmetry of all landmarks situated more superiorly. If not, combined segmental asymmetries must be suspected (one asymmetry compensating for, or adding to, another).

II. **Sagittal Alignment**—Patient viewed from the side

Obvious abnormalities or asymmetries in flexion–extension positioning of the lower extremity joints and spine are noted. It should be realized that a fairly broad range of "normal" variation exists in sagittal alignment. For some persons, it is normal to stand with the ankles, hips, and knees slightly flexed and the spinal curves somewhat flattened. For others it might be normal to stand with the lower extremity joints well extended and with more accentuation of the spinal curves. Any "deviation" must be considered in light of other findings. Asymmetries can be considered to be more reliably significant.

A. *Hip, pelvic, and lumbar region.* In general, the front of the pelvis and thigh are in a straight line. All the muscles that control the pelvis are balanced so the angle of the top of the sacrum to a horizontal line does not exceed 50° (30° optimal) (see Fig. 19-5). The buttocks do not look prominent but slope slightly downward. Common faults include:

1. The low back arches forward too much (lordosis). The pelvis tilts forward excessively and the front of the thigh forms an angle with the pelvis when this tilt is present. The anterior-superior iliac spines lie anterior to the pubic symphysis. The amount of lordotic curve is determined not only by the slope of the sacrum but the wedge shape of L5 and the wedge shape of the L5–S1, intervertebral disk, the surrounding musculature, and the stabilizing lumbar ligament.

2. The normal forward curve in the low back has straightened out (flat back). The symphysis pubis lies anterior to the anterior superior iliac spines. The lumbosacral angle is decreased and hip extension is characteristic.

3. The entire pelvic segment shifts anteriorly resulting in hip extension, and shift of the thoracic segment posteriorly results in flexion of the thorax on the upper lumbar spine (swayback posture).[5] A compensatory increased thoracic kyphosis and forward head placement is also seen. This results in an increased lordosis in the lower lumbar region and increased kyphosis in the lower thoracic region.

4. The most common unilateral finding of the pelvis is posterior iliac torsion: the posterior superior spine is lower than the opposite side. The reverse is found with anterior iliac torsion.

B. *Knees and Legs.* Looking at the knees from the side, the knees are straight, (*i.e.*, neither bent forward nor locked backward). The plumb line passes slightly anterior to the midline of the knee creating an extension moment. Abnormal considerations include

1. Abnormal hyperextension (genu recurvatum). The knee is hyperextended and the gravitational stress lies far forward of the joint. Abnormal hyperextension of the knees is often seen with an anterior pelvic tilt and the resulting excessive lumbar lordosis. Abnormal extension is often the result of restricted ankle dorsiflexion, as from a tight heel cord or capsular ankle restriction. A less common and more serious cause of severe "back" knee is neuropathic arthropathy such as may occur with tertiary syphilis.

2. Abnormal flexion (flexed knees or antecurvatum). The plumb lines falls posterior to the joint axis. Abnormal flexion of the knees occurs with a greater variety of disorders, including the following:

   a. Restricted ankle plantar flexion (rare), the most common cause of which is capsular restriction following immobilization

   b. An internal derangement, such as a bucket-handle meniscus tear, causing a mechanical block to knee extension

   c. An acute spinal derangement, such as a disk herniation or facet joint lesion

   d. Multisegmental capsular restriction, which occurs with significant degenerative changes (*e.g.*, ankylosing spondylosis)[3]

C. *Ankles.* The plumb line lies slightly anterior to the lateral malleolus aligned with the tuberosity of the fifth metatarsal. In the forward posture (anterior deviation of the body), the plumb line is posterior to the body; body weight is carried on the metatarsal heads of the feet.[5,6] The ankles are in dorsiflexion because of the forward inclination of the leg and overstretched posterior musculature. The posterior muscles of the trunk and lower extremities tend to remain in a state of constant contraction.

III. **Transverse Rotary Alignment**—Patient viewed from the front

The stance width should be normal and the feet slightly (5° to 10°) pointed outward. Obvious foot deformities, such as hallux valgus, should be noted. Hallux valgus is often associated with abnormal foot pronation, which, in turn, often occurs in conjunction with transverse rotary abnormalities of more proximal segments. Assessment of segmental rotary alignment is performed, working upward from the feet, by examining the positioning and symmetry of the following landmarks:

A. *Navicular tubercles.* The positions of the navicular tubercles are assessed compared with a line from the medial malleolus to the point where the first metatarsal contacts the ground. The tubercle should fall just on, or below, this line. The person with a static (*i.e.*, resting) pronation deviation of the foot will have a navicular tubercle that falls well below the line. This is a true flatfoot and will invariably be associated with a valgus heel. Abnormality in bony alignment must be confirmed, since many persons have considerable bulk of the medial soft tissues of the foot, which gives the foot a flattened appearance. When a true flatfoot is detected, one must determine whether it is structural (fixed) or functional (mobile). To do so, the patient is asked to raise up on the balls of the feet or to attempt to externally rotate the legs over the stationary foot; in both cases, the arch will be seen to rise significantly if the pronated position of the foot is functional. The common cause of a structurally pronated foot is tarsal coalition. The common causes of a mobile flatfoot are congenital ligamentous laxity and femoral anteversion. It must be appreciated that a person who does not have static pronation deviation of the foot, as evidenced on examination of structural alignment, may still have a problem from abnormal foot pronation during gait. On the other hand, a person with a static pronation deviation of the foot does not necessarily have a pronation problem, especially if the deviation has existed since childhood. The tissues of the foot will have adapted to the increased pronatory stresses during development.

B. *Intermalleolar line.* A line passing through the tips of the medial and lateral malleoli should make an angle, opening laterally, of about 25° with the frontal plane when the knee axis is situated in the frontal plane (*i.e.*, when the patellae are facing straight forward).

   Note: Twenty-five degrees corresponds to the lateral malleolus being about 4 cm posterior to the medial malleolus when the intermalleolar distance is 10 cm, or about 3.5 cm posterior for a 9-cm intermalleolar width, or about 3 cm posterior for an 8-cm width.

   1. If the angle is excessive, the examiner must suspect increased external tibial torsion or increased femoral antetorsion. It is not unusual for these to coexist, the two having a mutual compensatory effect to cancel abnormal toeing inward (from femoral antetorsion) or toeing outward (from external

tibial torsion). Compensation would occur during development. The presence of femoral antetorsion is best determined clinically by femoral torsion tests (Craig's test or Ryder's method) and by assessing hip rotational range of motion in the prone position. The hip with medial femoral torsion is a very mobile hip that appears to have an increase in internal rotation at the expense of a loss of external rotation.

2. Similarly, if the angle the intermalleolar line makes with the frontal plane is diminished when the patellae face straight forward, there may be an increase in femoral retrotorsion or abnormal internal tibial torsion. A hip with lateral femoral torsion is a less mobile hip that will appear to have a loss of internal rotation, with external rotation perhaps somewhat increased.

C. *Patellae.* With the feet pointed slightly outward the patellae should face straight forward.

1. If the patellae face inward, the examiner should suspect increased femoral antetorsion, increased external tibial torsion, or both (see earlier).

2. If the patellae face outward when the feet are in a normal position, the cause may be femoral retrotorsion, internal tibial torsion, or both (see earlier).

D. *Anterior-superior iliac spines.* These should be positioned in a frontal plane. If the pelvis is rotated (one iliac spine more anterior than the other), there are two common causes to be considered:

1. A fixed (structural) spinal scoliosis, the rotary component of which is transmitted to the pelvis through the sacrum by way of the lumbar spine

2. Torsional asymmetry of the sacroiliac joints. The pelvis will appear to be rotated forward on the side on which the ilium is in more anterior torsion with respect to the sacrum.

IV. **Vertical compression test (see Fig. 19-4).**[1,8] The concept behind compressive testing is to test the amount of "spring" that the spine has when a direct compression force is applied. Spines of patients with decreased curvatures (decreased lordosis or axially extended spines) will not have enough spring, which leads to decreased shock attenuation.[1] Deviations such as an increased lumbar lordosis, posterior angulation of the thoracic spine, or regions of instability preventing sufficient weight transfer through the spine may be revealed during this test.[2,4,7]

V. **Tests in Sitting.** Observe posture with the patient seated with the back unsupported and feet on the ground. Note any changes in posture. As in the standing position, this observation is carried out for frontal, sagittal, and transverse rotatory alignment. Note any changes in the spinal curvatures. If scoliosis is observed when the client is standing and disappears in sitting, then the asymmetry is caused by the lower limbs and is therefore functional.

□ **Regional Tests**

I. **Lumbosacral Tests**

A. With the patient standing, the examiner demonstrates the movement to be performed as verbal instructions are given. The examiner is looking for the patient's willingness to do the movements and for limitation of motion and its possible causes, such as pain, stiffness, or spasm. When viewing from behind, the movements are observed for asymmetry and for the levels affected. The examiner can determine if any deviations are painful or painless when corrected. When viewing the patient from the side, the examiner should assess the continuity of movement at the various spinal segments and look for reversal of the lumbar lordosis. The most painful movements should be done last. The following active movements are carried out in the lumbosacral spine:

1. Extension (backward bending): When viewing from behind stabilize the crest of the pelvis. The pelvis should not tilt nor should the hips extend. Areas of the spine that appear to bend easier (hypermobile) and areas that seem restricted (hypomobility) should be noted.

2. Lateral flexion (sidebending) (left and right): Normally the lumbar curve should form a smooth curve on side flexion and there should be no obvious angulations. If angulation does occur, it may indicate hypomobility or hypermobility at one level of the lumbar spine. A localized capsular restriction will limit sidebending slightly towards the involved side, but a multisegmental capsular restriction can cause restriction to both sides.

3. Flexion (forward bending): The examiner must ensure that the movement is occurring in the lumbar spine and not in the hips. It should be determined if iliosacral

movement is blocked or hypomobile during palpation.

4. Active return from forward bending: The lumbosacral rhythm should be a smooth transition during lumbar reversal and pelvic return.

5. Active flexion (forward bending) in sitting position: Observe for sacroiliac motion.

6. Lateral shift (side glide): Observe unilateral restriction.

7. Rotation (patient seated, knees together, with the arms folded or held in 90° flexion and hands together) (left and right). Observe for asymmetry.

B. *Active auxiliary tests.* If the patient's symptoms have not been reproduced the following additional maneuvers may be conducted (patient standing):

1. Passive overpressure at end range of active physiological spinal motions

2. Repeated physiological motions at various speeds

3. Sustained pressure at end range of extension and lateral flexion

4. Active combined motions without overpressure (left and right)
   a. Flexion (forward bending) with rotation
   b. Lateral flexion with flexion (forward bending)

5. Passive combined motions with passive overpressure (left and right)
   a. Flexion (forward bending) and lateral flexion
   b. Flexion (forward bending) with rotation
   c. Extension (backward bending) with lateral flexion
   d. Extension with rotation

C. *Active segmental mobility.* With the patient in stride-standing position, the examiner can assess the following:

1. Upper lumbar spine—lateral flexion

2. L5–S1—lateral flexion

3. Active pelvic tilt (L5–S1—whether painful or painless)

D. *Passive movements*

1. Whether posture correction is painful or painless

2. Quadrant test (patient standing)—passive auxiliary test for segmental involvement

3. Passive physiological movements (non-weight-bearing).
   a. Flexion (forward bending)
   b. Extension (backward bending)

c. Lateral flexion (sidebending—left and right)
d. Rotation (left and right)

4. Passive physiological movements with segmental palpation. Note type of end feel and seek abnormalities.
   a. Flexion–extension (forward and backward bending)
   b. Lateral flexion (sidebending—left and right)
   c. Rotation (left and right)

5. Segmental mobility
   a. Posteroanterior central pressures—T10–L5
   b. Transverse pressures—T10–L5
   c. Posteroanterior unilateral pressures—T10–L5

   For the fullest information, one should alter the direction of posteroanterior pressure; counterpressures are exerted to the spinous process of the segment above and below, and posteroanterior pressures may be applied diagonally in caudal and cephalad directions—T10–L5.

E. *Passive movements of the sacroiliac and peripheral joints*

1. Sacroiliac auxiliary (provocation) and mobility tests
   a. Posterior rotation test
   b. Anterior rotation test

2. Hip joint: Hip flexion–adduction test

3. Knee joint
   a. Anterior drawer (Lachman) test
   b. Valgus–varus stress test at 30° knee flexion

F. *Neuromuscular tests*

1. Key sensory areas (L4–S2)—stroking test and sensibility to pin prick, if applicable

2. Resisted isometric (myotomal) tests (L2–S2). Compare both sides.

3. Dural mobility testing
   a. Straight-leg raising (sciatic nerve)—sitting and supine, with and without cervical spine flexion
   b. Slump test (sciatic nerve)
   c. Femoral nerve traction test

4. Reflexes
   a. Knee jerk (L3) and plantar response
   b. Ankle jerk (S1)
   c. Great toe jerk (L5)
   d. Posterior tibial reflex (L5)
   e. Test for ankle clonus

II. **Pelvic Joint and Sacroiliac Joint Tests**
   A. *Active movements.* Active movements of the

spine puts a stress on the sacroiliac joints as well as the lumbar and lumbosacral joints. Forward flexion movement while standing tests the movement of the ilium on the sacrum. The hip movements are also affected by sacroiliac lesions.

1. Standing and sitting active trunk flexion tests for possible locking of the ilium on the sacrum or restriction
2. Sacroiliac fixation test (active hip flexion) for fixation or restriction

B. *Passive movements.* Special tests:
1. Posterior rotation test
2. Anterior rotation test
3. Anterior ligament distraction test
4. Posterior ligament distraction test

C. *Functional leg difference due to pelvis imbalance*— Supine-to-sit test

III. Hip Tests

A. *Active movements.* The emphasis is on assessing functional activities involving the use of the hip. If the patient is able to do active flexion (knee to chest), extension in standing, and abduction and rotation in non-weight-bearing with little difficulty, the examiner may use a series of functional tests to see if increased intensity of activity produces pain or other symptoms (*e.g.,* squatting, going up and down stairs, running, and jumping).

B. *Passive movements.* Passive movements should be performed to determine the end feel and the degree of passive range of motion.
1. Perform passive hip flexion–extension, abduction–adduction, internal-external rotation, and combined flexion, adduction, and rotation.
2. If indicated, the assessment of muscle lengths is included: the Thomas test to detect a hip flexion contracture, Ely's test for the iliopsoas and rectus femoris, knee extension with the hip in 90°, straight-leg raising for hamstrings, and the Ober test for the iliotibial band.

C. *Resisted isometric movements*
1. Resisted hip flexion–extension, adduction, and internal-external rotation are tested isometrically in the supine position to determine which muscles may be at fault or for the presence of a possible bursitis. Resisted hip flexion is also done as a test for the integrity of the L2 myotome.
2. Resisted hip abduction is tested with the patient in the prone position for the presence of possible trochanteric bursitis or gluteus medius tendinitis.

IV. Knee Tests

A. *Active movements.* Flexion–extension can be assessed at the same time as hip flexion and extension and, in a weight-bearing situation, while testing the L3 myotome.
1. During weight-bearing movements, the examiner should palpate at the femoropatellar joint and at the femorotibial joint for crepitus that may indicate degenerative changes. Snapping and popping during movement is common, but a continuous grinding, suggestive of sand in the joint, is more significant.
2. During non-weight-bearing, the knee is assessed for loss of dynamic tibial function and for any evidence of quadriceps lag. These tests allow the examiner to detect subtle abnormalities that may predispose to chronic knee pain and perhaps progressive degeneration. These patients often respond well to manual therapy techniques.
3. Functional tests. If the preceding tests are performed with little difficulty, the examiner may put the patient through a series of functional tests to see if these activities reproduce the patient's symptoms or pain.

B. *Passive physiological movement with passive overpressure.* More information may be derived by testing passive ranges of extension, flexion, and axial rotation in cardinal planes and combined motions.

C. *Patellar glide.* The patella is moved passively, posteriorly, medially, and laterally. At the extremes of medial movement, the underside of the medial patella is palpated for tenderness.

D. *Resisted isometric movements*
1. Internal-external rotation with the knee bent. Resisted internal rotation will reproduce pain from pes anserinus; resisted external rotation may reproduce pain from iliotibial band tendinitis.
2. Knee flexion (also tests for the S2 myotome). This may reproduce pain from pes anserinus tendinitis or biceps tendinitis.
3. Knee extension (L3). Pain may be reproduced in patellar tendinitis.

V. Ankle and Foot Tests

A. *Active motion and passive movements*
1. Flexion–extension. The patient lies prone with the feet over the edge of the table. With the foot in subtalar neutral, active and passive dorsiflexion are assessed and then repeated with the knee bent to 90°. Pain from Achilles tendinitis may be reproduced at the extremes of dorsiflexion.

Pain from an anterior talofibular ligament sprain or adhesion may be reproduced on plantar flexion–inversion with passive overpressure.

2. Hindfoot inversion–eversion. With the patient sitting, the range of passive calcaneal inversion–eversion is assessed.

3. Forefoot supination–pronation. With the subtalar joint maintained with the calcaneus in subtalar neutral, the examiner should maximally supinate (untwist) and pronate (twist) the forefoot. With the foot held untwisted, the toes are moved into sustained dorsiflexion. Untwisting of the foot may reproduce pain from a calcaneocuboid ligament sprain; sustained toe dorsiflexion may reproduce pain from plantar fasciitis or calcaneal periostitis, since this stretches the plantar fascia.

4. Anterior glide of the talus in the mortise. Hypermobility will be present in the case of chronic anterior talofibular ligament rupture. Pain will be reproduced from a talofibular ligament sprain or adhesion.

5. Functional tests. If the patient is able to do the preceding activities with little difficulty, functional tests may be performed to see whether these activities reproduce the symptoms or pain (*e.g.,* standing and walking on the toes, standing on one foot at a time, running, and jumping). These activities should be selected and geared to the individual patient.

B. *Resisted isometrics.* With the patient in the supine position, the presence of pain and weakness is assessed. Movements tested isometrically include the following:

1. Knee flexion (S2)
2. Tibialis anterior (L4) (dorsiflexion–inversion)
3. Tibialis posterior (L5) (plantar flexion–inversion)
4. Peroneus tertius (dorsiflexion–eversion)
5. Peroneus longus and brevis (S1) (plantar flexion–eversion)
6. Toe flexion–extension: extensor digitorum (L5–S1) and hallucis longis (L5)

CLINICAL IMPLEMENTATION OF THE LUMBOSACRAL– LOWER LIMB SCAN EXAMINATION

Gait analysis and a comprehensive assessment of structural alignment should be included in the assess-

ment of virtually all chronic disorders of the low back and lower extremities. It is rare, however, to include all of the regional tests discussed during any one examination; tests are chosen as indicated by subjective information and findings on gait analysis and inspection of structural alignment. The clinician must be prepared to judge which tests might be relevant in a particular case—a judgment that is facilitated by experience.

In order for the scan examination to be of practical use in a busy clinical setting, the clinician must be able to perform the examination within a reasonable period of time, for example, 15 minutes or less. This requires knowledge of which tests are to be performed, understanding of the rationale for each test, skill in appropriately carrying out each test, and ability to interpret the results.

Clinically, the tests of the scan examination must be carried out according to the patient's position in order to minimize time requirements and to prevent omission of crucial tests. The following is a summary of the tests included in a complete lumbosacral–lower limb scan examination, according to the position of the patient. This format should be followed in the clinical implementation of the scan examination.

I. **Standing**
   A. *Gait analysis*
      1. Sagittal
      2. Frontal
      3. Transverse
      4. Equilibrium. The patient stands on one leg with the eyes closed. Check stabilization efficiency of each hip.
   B. *Inspection of structural alignment and soft tissue*
      1. Frontal—from behind
      2. Sagittal—from the side
      3. Transverse (rotatory)—from the front
      4. Posture correction
      5. Vertical compression
   C. *Functional tests*
      1. Active lumbar (physiological) movements
         a. Extension (backward bending)
         b. Lateral flexion (sidebending)
         c. Flexion (forward bending)
         d. Lateral shift (side gliding)
      2. Active lumbar segmental movements
         a. Upper lumbar
         b. L5–S1
         c. Active pelvic tilt
      3. Active peripheral joint movements
         a. Hip flexion–extension
         b. Standing unilateral half squats (L3)
         c. Standing unilateral toe raises (S1–S2)
      4. Auxiliary tests (if indicated) to clear joints.
II. **Sitting**

A. *Alignment*
   1. Sitting posture compared to standing
   2. Position of the patellae
   3. Rotatory position of the tibia
B. *Function*
   1. Active lumbar spine rotation
   2. Resisted isometrics—hip flexion (L2)
   3. Tibial rotatory mechanics
   4. Dural mobility
C. *Resisted isometrics*
   1. Resisted hip flexion (L2)
   2. Resisted knee extension (L3)

III. **Supine**
   A. *Functional tests*
      1. Active lumbar movements: Effect on symptoms
         a. Flexion
         b. Repeated flexion
      2. Passive tests—Hip, knee, ankle, and foot ranges compared with other limbs, with assessment of end feel and overpressure if applicable. Regions of muscle tightness are sought: hamstrings, hip adductors, and gastroc-soleus.
         a. Hip and knee flexion–extension range
         b. Hip adduction–abduction range
         c. Knee internal-external rotation
         d. Patellar glide, medially and laterally
         e. Ankle dorsiflexion–plantar flexion
         f. Hindfoot inversion–eversion and forefoot twisting and untwisting; dorsiflex toes when untwisted
   B. *Resisted isometrics*
      1. Resisted hip abduction
      2. Resisted dorsiflexion (L4)–plantar flexion—Tibialis posterior (L5)
      3. Resisted large toe extension (L5)
   C. *Sensation*—Include vibratory perception, stroking test, and sensibility to pin prick, if applicable
   D. *Dural mobility*
   E. *Reflexes*
      1. Knee jerk (L3–L4)
      2. Great toe jerk (L5)
      3. Test for ankle clonus
      4. Plantar response

IV. **Sidelying—Function**
   A. *Passive physiological movements with segmental palpation*—Lumbar spine
      1. Flexion–extension (forward-backward bending)
      2. Lateral flexion (sidebending)
      3. Rotation
   B. *Sacroiliac posterior rotation*
   C. *Iliotibial band extensibility*

V. **Prone**

A. *Active movements: Effect on symptoms*
   1. Lumbar spine extension
   2. Lumbar spine—Repeated extension
   3. Lateral shift—Correction
B. *Passive movements: Effect on symptoms*
   1. Sacroiliac anterior rotation
   2. Hip internal-external rotation range of motion and femoral torsion tests
   3. Lumbar spine
      a. Sidebending
      b. Rotation
C. *Accessory movements*
      a. Sacral springing
      b. Posteroanterior gliding and rotation—lumbar spine
D. *Resisted isometrics*
   1. Resisted hip extension (S1)
   2. Resisted knee rotations
   3. Resisted knee flexion
      a. Assess strength—S1, S2, myotomes
      b. Assess irritability—biceps or pes anserinus tendonitis
E. Reflexes—Ankle jerk (S1, S2)

REFERENCES

1. Cantu RI, Grodin AJ: Myofascial Manipulation: Theory and Clinical Application. Gaithersburg, MD, Aspen, 1992
2. Farfan H, Gracovetsky S: The nature of instability. Spine 9:714–719, 1984
3. Hartley A: Practical Joint Assessment: A Sports Medicine Manual. St Louis, Mosby Year Book, 1990
4. Howes RG, Isdale IC: The loose back: An unrecognized syndrome. Rheumatol Phys Med 11:72–77, 1971
5. Kendall FP, McCreary EK, Provance PG: Muscles: Testing and Function, 4th ed. Baltimore, Williams & Wilkins, 1993
6. Palmer ML, Epler M: Clinical Assessment Procedures in Physical Therapy. Philadelphia, JB Lippincott, 1990
7. Paris SV: Physical signs of instability. Spine 10:277–279, 1985
8. Saliba VL, Johnson G: Lumbar protective mechanism. In White A, Anderson R (eds): Conservative Care of Low Back Pain, pp 112–119. Baltimore, Williams & Wilkins, 1991

RECOMMENDED READINGS

Boyling J, Palastanga N (eds): Grieve's Modern Manual Therapy of the Vertebral Column. Edinburgh, Churchill Livingstone, 1994.
Butler D: Mobilisation of the Nervous System. Melbourne, Churchill Livingstone, 1991
Corrigan B, Maitland GD: Practical Orthopaedic Medicine. London, Butterworths, 1985
Cyriax JF, Cyriax PJ: Illustrated Manual of Orthopaedic Medicine, 2nd ed. Boston, Butterworths, 1993
Dvořák J, Dvořák V: Manual Medicine: Diagnostics. New York, Thieme Medical, 1990
Edwards BC: Combined movements in the lumbar spine: Their use in examination and treatment. In Grieve GP (ed): Modern Manual Therapy of the Vertebral Column, pp 561–566. New York, Churchill Livingstone, 1986
Edwards BC: Clinical assessment: The use of combined movements in assessment and treatment. In Twomey LT, Taylor JR (eds): Physiotherapy of the Low Back, pp 175–198. New York, Churchill Livingstone, 1987
Evans RC: Illustrated Essentials in Orthopedic Physical Assessment. St Louis, CV Mosby, 1994
Finneson BE: Low Back Pain. Philadelphia, JB Lippincott, 1981
Greenfield BH: Rehabilitation of the Knee: A Problem Solving Approach. Philadelphia, FA Davis, 1993
Greenman PE: Principles of Manual Medicine. Baltimore, Williams & Wilkins, 1989
Grieve P: Mobilisation of the Spine: A Primary Handbook of Clinical Methods, 5th ed. Edinburgh, Churchill Livingstone, 1991
Hunt GC: Examination of lower extremity dysfunction. In Gould JA, Davies GJ (eds): Orthopedics and Sports Physical Therapy. St Louis, CV Mosby, 1990
Hunt GC (ed): Physical Therapy of the Foot and Ankle. New York, Churchill Livingstone, 1988
Jahss MH (ed): Disorders of the Foot. Philadelphia, WB Saunders, 1982
Kaltenborn FM: The Spine: Basic Evaluation and Mobilization Techniques, 2nd ed. Oslo, Olaf Norlis Bokhandel, 1993
Kenna C, Murtagh J: Back Pain & Spinal Manipulation. Sydney, Butterworths, 1989

Lee D: The Pelvic Girdle. Edinburgh, Churchill Livingstone, 1989

Magee DJ: Orthopedic Physical Assessment, 2nd ed. Philadelphia, WB Saunders, 1992

Maigne R: Orthopedic Medicine. Springfield, IL, Charles C Thomas, 1976

Maitland GD: Vertebral Manipulations, 5th ed. Boston, Butterworths, 1986

Markolf KL: Quantitative examination for anterior cruciate laxity. In Jackson DW, Drez D (eds): The Anterior Cruciate Deficient Knee: New Concepts in Ligament Repair. St Louis, CV Mosby, 1987

McKenzie R: The Lumbar Spine: Mechanical Diagnosis and Therapy. Waikanae, New Zealand, Spinal Publications, 1981

Nicholas JA, Hershmann EB (eds): The Lower Extremity and Spine in Sports Medicine. St Louis, CV Mosby, 1986

Pauloa LE: Knee and leg: Soft tissue trauma. In American Academy of Orthopaedic Surgeons: Orthopaedic Knowledge Update 2, 1987

Porterfield JA, DeRosa C: Mechanical Low Back Pain: Perspectives in Functional Anatomy. Philadelphia, WB Saunders, 1991

Root ML, Orien WP, Weed JH: Biomechanical Examination of the Foot and Ankle, vol I. Los Angeles, Clinical Biomechanics Corp, 1971

Sonzogni JJ: Physical assessment of the injured knee. Emergency Med (April):74–92, 1988

Wells PE: The examination of the pelvic joints. In Grieve GP (ed): Modern Manual Therapy of the Vertebral Column, pp 590–602. Edinburgh, Churchill Livingstone, 1986

Woermann AL: Evaluation and treatment of dysfunction in the lumbar-pelvic-hip complex. In Donateli R, Wooden (eds): Orthopaedic Physical Therapy, pp 403–483. New York, Churchill Livingstone, 1989

Component Motions, Close-Packed Positions, Loose-Packed Positions, Rest Positions, and Capsular Patterns

Component motions are the motions in the joint complex or related joints that accompany, and are necessary for, full active range of motion. An example of a component motion is inferior glide of the head of the humerus into the lower portion of the glenoid fossa during active movement of the shoulder.

The most stable position of a joint is called the *close-packed position.*[5] In this position the tension on the articular capsule and ligaments is maximal, with the joint surfaces often temporarily locked together. The locking together is frequently performed by a screw-home component. The close-packed configuration usually occurs at a position that is the extreme of the most habitual position of the joint. For example, the close-packed position for the wrist joint is full extension. The other extreme position of the joint that is less

commonly assumed is also very congruent and is called the *potential close-packed position.*[1,15,21,29]

In the close-packed position, the joint capsule and major ligaments are twisted, causing the joint surfaces to become firmly approximated. This is a direct result either of the conjunct rotation that necessarily accompanies a diadochal movement into this position, or of the spin that accompanies an impure swing into the position. Movement into or out of a close-packed position is never accomplished by a pure chordate swing alone. Habitual movements of daily activities usually involve motions that move a joint closer to or farther from a close-packed position. An example would be the motions at the hip when walking.

Consider the relation between the close-packed position at a particular joint and the capsular pattern of restriction, as described by Cyriax,[5] at the same joint. The more intimate the anatomical and functional relation between the joint capsule and major supporting ligaments, the more likely it is that the close-packed position will be the most restricted position of the joint in a capsular pattern of restriction. Thus, in the hip and shoulder joints, in which the major ligaments blend with the joint capsule, movements into the close-packed position are the first to be lost with a capsular pattern of restriction. In the knee, however, in which the ligaments are easily distinguished from the capsule, flexion may be the most limited in a capsular restriction, whereas extension constitutes the close-packed position.

In any position of the joint other than the close-packed position, the articular surfaces are noncongruent, and some part of the joint capsule is lax. In these positions the joint is *loose-packed*. Often there is enough laxity in midrange to allow distraction of the joint surfaces by an externally applied force. The laxity of the capsule in the loose-packed position allows for the elements of spin, glide, and roll, which are present in most joint movements in various degrees. The *resting position* is the maximum loose-packed position and is the ideal position for evaluation and early treatment procedures used in restoring joint play. The resting position is also the position in which the joint capsule has its greatest capacity and where the joint is under the least stress. Accessory movement must be determined (this is traditionally part of the joint mobilization examination) if the therapist is to restore the normal roll/glide action that occurs during joint movements: joint-play and component motions.

■ TEMPOROMANDIBULAR JOINT

Both temporomandibular joints (TMJs) are involved in every jaw movement, forming a bicondylar arrangement.

☐ Component Motions

OPENING OF THE MOUTH

1. The head of the mandible first rotates around a horizontal axis (rolls dorsally) in relation to the disk (lower compartment).
2. This movement is then combined with gliding of the head anteriorly (and somewhat downward) in contact with the lower surface of the disk.
3. At the same time, the disk glides anteriorly (and somewhat downward) toward the articular eminence of the glenoid fossa (upper compartment). The forward gliding of the disk ceases when the fi-

broelastic tissue attaching to the temporal bone posteriorly has been stretched to its limits.
4. Thereafter, there is some further hinging and gliding anteriorly of the head of the mandible until it articulates with the most anterior part of the disk and the mouth is fully opened.

Closing of the Mouth. The movements are reversed.

Protrusion. The disks glide anteriorly in the upper compartment (simultaneously on both sides). Both condyles glide anteriorly and slightly downward but do not rotate.

Retraction. The movements are reversed.

Lateral Movements. Anterior gliding occurs in one joint while rotation around a cranial/caudal axis occurs in the other joint. One condyle glides downward, forward, and inward, while the other condyle in the fossa rotates and glides ipsilaterally. When the jaw is moved from side to side (as in chewing), a movement involving a shuttling of the condylar disk assembly occurs in the concave parts of the fossa.

☐ Resting Position

The mouth is slightly open. The teeth of the mandible and maxilla are not in contact but are slightly apart.

☐ Close-Packed Position

Unlike other joints, both TMJs become nearly close-packed with full occlusion of the dental arches.[11] It remains questionable whether these joints have a truly close-packed position, as the restraining capsule and ligaments are not maximally tightened during the maximum occlusion of the dental arches.[16]

Normally there is 3 to 4 mm of movement from the position of rest to the position of centric relation.[11] According to Rocabado,[24] the TMJ has two close-packed positions: maximal retrusion, where the condyles cannot go further back and the ligaments are tight, and the maximal anterior position of the condyles with maximal mouth opening (potential close-packed position).[24]

☐ Potential Close-Packed Position

This is full or maximal opening. The ligaments, in particular the temporomandibular ligament and capsular constraints of the craniomandibular articulation, seem particularly tightened during maximum opening.[14]

☐ Capsular Pattern of Restriction

In bilateral restriction, lateral movements are most restricted; opening of the mouth and protrusion are limited; closing of the mouth is most free. In unilateral capsular restrictions, contralateral excursions are most restricted. In mouth opening, the mandible deviates toward the restricted side.

▩ UPPER LIMB

☐ Glenohumeral Joint

COMPONENT MOTIONS

FLEXION (ELEVATION IN THE SAGITTAL PLANE)

1. At full elevation of the humerus, whether accomplished through coronal abduction or sagittal flexion, the humerus always ends up back in the plane of the scapula, as if it had been elevated through a pure swing (*i.e.*, at an angle midway between the sagittal and coronal planes). Because sagittal flexion is an impure swing, the humerus tends to undergo a lateral conjunct rotation on its path to full elevation. If this occurred, however, the humerus would end up with the medial condyle pointed backward, rather than forward, with the capsule of the glenohumeral joint completely twisted. This essentially would involve a premature close-packing that would prevent full elevation. To avoid this, the humerus must rotate medially on its long axis during the complete arc of sagittal flexion. The rotation occurs because the anterior aspect of the joint capsule pulls tight on flexion while the posterior capsule remains relatively lax.
2. Downward (inferior) glide of the head of the humerus on the glenoid.

ABDUCTION

1. Lateral rotation of the humerus on its long axis to counter the medial conjunct rotation that tends to occur during this impure swing (see above). In this case, the posterior capsule pulls tight during abduction, effecting a lateral rotation of the humerus.
2. Inferior glide of the humeral head on the glenoid
   External Rotation—Anterior glide of the head of the humerus
   Internal Rotation—Posterior glide of the head of the humerus
   Horizontal Adduction—Posterior glide of the humeral head
   Horizontal Abduction—Anterior glide of the humeral head

RESTING POSITION

Semiabduction: 55° to 70° abduction, 30° horizontal adduction, neutral rotation

CLOSE-PACKED POSITION

Maximum abduction and external rotation are combined.

CAPSULAR PATTERN OF RESTRICTION

External rotation is most limited; abduction, quite limited; internal rotation and flexion, somewhat limited (relatively free).

☐ Acromioclavicular Joint

COMPONENT MOTIONS

1. Allows widening and narrowing of the angle (looking from above) between the clavicle and the scapula. Narrowing occurs during protraction; widening occurs during retraction (about 10° total). This occurs about a vertical axis.
2. Allows rotation of the scapula upward, such that the inferior angle of the scapula moves away from the midline; or downward, such that it moves toward the midline. This occurs about a horizontal axis lying in the sagittal plane. Actually, very little acromioclavicular joint motion is involved in this rotation of the scapula. About 30° occurs with elevation of the clavicle at the sternoclavicular joint, but much of the remaining 30° occurs because of axial rotation of the clavicle; because the clavicle is S-shaped anteroposteriorly, an axial rotation converts the S to a superoinferior attitude, the distal end pointing more or less upward. This occurs as a result of tightening of the coracoclavicular ligaments as the scapula begins to rotate upward (the coracoid rotating downward).
3. Allows rotation of the scapula such that the inferior angle swings anteriorly and posteriorly. As the scapula moves upward and forward on the thorax, the inferior angle swings posteriorly. This occurs about an axis lying horizontally in the frontal plane and probably is accompanied by considerable length rotation at the sternoclavicular joint as well.

RESTING POSITION

Arm rests by the side in the normal physiological position.

CLOSE-PACKED POSITION

Upward rotation of the scapula relative to the clavicle is combined with narrowing of the angle between the scapula and clavicle as seen from above. This occurs during elevation of the arm (arm abducted 90°) and during horizontal adduction (see Fig. 9-3).

CAPSULAR PATTERN

Primarily there is pain into the close-packed position, such as when horizontally adducting the arm, and limitation of full extension.

☐ Sternoclavicular Joint

COMPONENT MOTIONS

1. Allows length rotation of the clavicle, as discussed above; about 50° total. This occurs during elevation of the arm and somewhat during protraction and retraction.
2. Allows upward and downward swing of the clavicle, such as during shoulder shrugging or elevation of the arm. This occurs about an axis passing through the costoclavicular ligament, so that with elevation the clavicular articular surface slides inferiorly on the sternum and, with depression, superiorly; about 30° total.
3. Allows forward and backward swing of the clavicle, such as with protraction and retraction. This occurs about an axis lying somewhat medial to the joint, so that the clavicular articular surface slides forward on protraction; about 45° to 60° total.

RESTING POSITION

Arm rests by the side in the normal physiological position.

CLOSE-PACKED POSITION

Arm abducted to 90°.

CAPSULAR PATTERN

Pain occurs at the extremes of motion. To emphasize the interplay of all joints involved with shoulder movements, we will review here the components of shoulder abduction in the frontal plane, one of the more complex shoulder movements.

With the arm at the side in the resting position, the glenoid faces almost equally anteriorly and laterally. The humerus rests in the plane of the scapula, or in alignment with the glenoid, such that the medial humeral condyle points about 45° inward and backward (see Fig. 9-2).

During the first 30° or so of abduction, the effects on the scapula are variable, but during this time it becomes set or fixed against the thoracic wall in preparation for movement. From 30° to full elevation, for every 15° of movement about 10° occurs at the glenohumeral joint and 5° at the scapulothoracic joint. The scapula must rotate upward as well as forward around the chest wall. The early part of this movement occurs as a result of elevation at the sternoclavicular joint, as well as movement at the acromioclavicular joint, such that its angle narrows (looking from above) and the scapula rotates slightly upward on the clavicle. This close-packs the acromioclavicular joint but also draws the coracoclavicular ligaments tight, because of the downward movement of the coracoid relative to the clavicle. Thus, between, say, 90° and 120°, motion stops at the acromioclavicular joint. Further elevation from scapular rotation is possible only because the coracoclavicular ligaments pull the clavicle into long-axis rotation.

The S-shape of the clavicle becomes oriented superoinferiorly such that the distal end of the clavicle points somewhat upward, allowing the acromioclavicular joint to maintain apposition as the scapula continues to rotate upward. This clavicular rotation occurs, of course, at the sternoclavicular joint.

Because the convex humeral head is moving in relation to the concave glenoid cavity to allow upward swing of the humerus, it must glide inferiorly in the glenoid. The humerus must move out of the plane of the scapula to be elevated in the frontal plane; it must undergo an impure swing. As with any impure swing, a conjunct rotation occurs, in this case a medial rotation. However, the posterior and inferior capsular fibers cannot allow this amount of rotation, so for the humerus to come back into the plane of the scapula on full elevation, it must rotate laterally on its long axis. This lateral rotation is necessary for clearance of the greater tuberosity under the acromial arch.

The clinically important considerations are that elevation is impossible without appropriate sternoclavicular and acromioclavicular movements, especially rotation of the clavicle on its long axis, without inferior glide of the humeral head, and without lateral rotation of the humerus on its long axis.

Furthermore, we must consider the motions occurring in the thoracic and lower cervical spines on shoulder movement. For example, bilateral elevation of the arms requires considerable thoracic extension; the person with a significant thoracic kyphosis will not be able to perform this movement throughout the full range. On unilateral elevation, the upper thoracic spine must sidebend toward, and the lower thoracic spine must sidebend away from, the side of motion.

Elbow

COMPONENT MOTIONS

EXTENSION
1. Superior glide of ulna on trochlea
2. Pronation of ulna relative to humerus
3. Abduction of ulna relative to humerus
4. Distal movement of radius on ulna
5. Pronation (inward rotation) of radius relative to humerus

FLEXION
1. Inferior glide of ulna on trochlea
2. Supination of ulna relative to humerus
3. Adduction of ulna relative to humerus
4. Proximal movement of radius on ulna
5. Supination (outward rotation) of radius on humerus

HUMEROULNAR JOINT

RESTING POSITION
Semiflexion: 70° flexion, 10° supination

CLOSE-PACKED POSITION
Full extension and supination

CAPSULAR PATTERN
More limitation of flexion than extension. Pronation and supination are limited only if condition is severe.

HUMERORADIAL JOINT

RESTING POSITION
Full extension and supination

CLOSE-PACKED POSITION
90° flexion, 5° supination

CAPSULAR PATTERN
Flexion and extension are most restricted; supination and pronation are limited only if condition is severe.

Forearm

COMPONENT MOTIONS

PRONATION–SUPINATION

Proximal Radioulnar Joint and Radiohumeral Joint. This movement is essentially one of pure spin of the head of the radius on the capitellum and, therefore, one of roll and slide of the radius in the radial notch of the ulna and annular ligament.

Distal Radioulnar Joint. Here the radius is said to ro-

tate around the head of the ulna, being largely a sliding movement. However, functionally the ulna also tends to move backward and laterally during pronation and forward and medially during supination. Therefore, component movements during pronation are as follows:

1. Palmar glide of radius on ulna
2. Inward rotation of radius on ulna (looking palmarly)
3. Dorsal glide of ulna on radius
4. Outward rotation of ulna on radius (looking palmarly)
5. Abduction of ulna on humerus

The reverse would naturally occur on supination.

PROXIMAL RADIOULNAR JOINT

RESTING POSITION
70° flexion, 35° supination

CLOSE-PACKED POSITION
Supination, full extension

CAPSULAR PATTERN
Pronation = supination

DISTAL RADIOULNAR JOINT

RESTING POSITION
10° supination, 90° flexion

CLOSE-PACKED POSITION
5° supination

CAPSULAR PATTERN
Involvement of the distal radioulnar joint produces little limitation of movement, but there is pain at the extremes of pronation and supination. Pronation = supination.

Wrist

COMPONENT MOTIONS

RADIOCARPAL JOINT

PALMAR FLEXION
1. Dorsal movement of proximal carpals (scaphoid and lunate) on radius and disk
2. Distraction of radiocarpal joint

DORSIFLEXION
1. Palmar movement of proximal carpals on radius (the scaphoid also spins—supinates—on the radius at full wrist dorsiflexion)

2. Approximation of scaphoid and lunate to radius and disk

RADIAL DEVIATION
1. Approximation of scaphoid to radius
2. Ulnar slide of proximal carpals on radius (this movement is quite limited and is somewhat increased by the tendency for the scaphoid to extend [slide palmarly and supinate] on the radius)

ULNAR DEVIATION
1. Distraction of scaphoid from radius
2. Radial slide of proximal carpals on radius

ULNOMENISCOTRIQUETRAL JOINT

The ulnomeniscotriquetral joint is primarily involved with pronation and supination of the forearm. During pronation and supination, the disk moves with the radius and carpals and must therefore sweep around the distal end of the ulna. During flexion and extension, the disk stays with the radius and ulna and movement occurs between the disk and the carpals. In this situation the disk acts as an ulnar extension of the distal radial joint surface to become, functionally, part of the radiocarpal joint.

During wrist radial deviation, there is considerable distraction of the triquetrum and pisiform from the ulna, with approximation on ulnar deviation.

RADIOCARPAL AND ULNOMENISCOTRIQUETRAL JOINTS

RESTING POSITION
Neutral with slight ulnar deviation

CLOSE-PACKED POSITION
Full extension

POTENTIAL CLOSE-PACKED POSITION[1,20,29]
Full flexion

CAPSULAR PATTERN
Limitation is equal in all directions.

MIDCARPAL JOINT

COMPONENT MOTIONS

PALMAR FLEXION
1. Dorsal slide of hamate and capitate on triquetrum and lunate
2. Palmar slide of trapezoid on scaphoid

Dorsiflexion. From full flexion to neutral, the reverse of the above occurs. At neutral, the hamate, capitate, and trapezoid become close-packed on the scaphoid, and these four bones tend to move together in a palmar slide and supinatory spin on the radius, lunate,

and triquetrum. The scaphoid acts as a proximal carpal from neutral into palmar flexion and as a distal carpal from neutral into full dorsiflexion. Also note the supination and radial deviation that tend to occur on extreme dorsiflexion of the wrist.

Radial Deviation. There is some ulnar slide of the hamate and capitate on the triquetrum and lunate, with considerable distraction of the base of the hamate from the lunate. The trapezoid slides radially on the scaphoid.

Ulnar Deviation. This is the reverse of radial deviation. The entire carpus might be divided into four functional units: (1) hamate, capitate, and trapezoid, always acting as distal carpals; (2) scaphoid, acting as proximal carpal into flexion and distal carpal into extension; (3) triquetrum and lunate, always acting as proximal carpals; and (4) trapezium, acting primarily in its articulation with the first metacarpal of the thumb, playing little part in movements at the wrist.

RESTING POSITION
Semiflexion: near neutral with slight ulnar deviation

CLOSE-PACKED POSITION
Of the wrist as a whole, extension (dorsiflexion) with radial deviation

CAPSULAR PATTERN
Equal limitation of palmar flexion and dorsiflexion

☐ Hand

"INTERMETACARPAL JOINTS"

Although these are not true synovial joints, movement does occur between the heads of the metacarpals on grasp and release.

Grasp. The metacarpals form an arch through the following movements:

1. Palmar movement of second relative to third, fourth relative to third, and fifth relative to fourth metacarpal head
2. Supination of fourth and fifth metacarpals; perhaps slight pronation of the second

Release. The arch is flattened through the reverse of the above movements.

COMPONENT MOTIONS

METACARPOPHALANGEAL JOINTS

FLEXION
1. Palmar glide of base of phalanx on head of metacarpal

2. Supination of phalanx on metacarpal, especially with grasp or pinch
3. Ulnar deviation of phalanx on metacarpal, especially with grasp or pinch
4. Approximation of phalanx and metacarpal

Extension. Reverse of flexion

Radial Deviation. Radial slide of base of phalanx on head of metacarpal

Ulnar Deviation. Ulnar slide of base of phalanx on head of metacarpal

COMPONENT MOTIONS
INTERPHALANGEAL JOINTS

FLEXION
1. Palmar glide of base of more distal phalanx on head of more proximal phalanx
2. Distraction of distal phalanx on proximal phalanx
3. Supination of distal phalanx on more proximal phalanx (more at distal interphalangeal than proximal interphalangeal joint)
4. Radial deviation of distal phalanx on more proximal phalanx

Extension. Reverse of flexion

COMPONENT MOTIONS
TRAPEZIOMETACARPAL JOINT

This is a sellar joint, with the trapezium concave in the plane of the palm and convex perpendicularly.

Extension. With radial deviation, there is ulnar slide of the base of the first metacarpal on the trapezium. A slight amount of lateral rotation (supination) occurs.

Flexion. Opposite of extension

Abduction. With motion away from the plane of the palm, there is palmar slide of the base of the first metacarpal.

Adduction. Dorsal slide of the base of the metacarpal

Opposition. This is a combined movement with considerable conjunct rotation as a consequence of the impure swing. It is easily visible by the rather marked medial rotation that occurs, allowing the thumb pad to oppose the pads of the fingers. It is typical for relatively more conjunct rotation to occur at a sellar joint such as this or at the interphalangeal joints or humer-oulnar joint than at ovoid joints.

RESTING POSITION
1. First carpometacarpal: Neutral position

2. Carpometacarpal (2–5): Midway between flexion and extension, with slight ulnar deviation
3. Metacarpophalangeal (2–5): Semiflexion and slight ulnar deviation
4. Metacarpophalangeal (1): Semiflexion
5. Proximal interphalangeal (1–5): 10° flexion
6. Distal interphalangeal (1–5): 30° flexion

CLOSE-PACKED POSITION

1. Most intercarpal joints: Full extension
2. Trapeziometacarpal: Full opposition
3. Metacarpophalangeal (2–5): Full flexion
4. Metacarpophalangeal (1): Full extension
5. Interphalangeal joints: Full extension

CAPSULAR PATTERNS

1. Trapeziometacarpal joint: Abduction and extension limited, flexion free
2. Carpometacarpal (2–5): Equal in all directions
3. Metacarpophalangeal joint: More restricted in flexion than extension
4. Interphalangeal joints: Flexion greater than extension

■ LOWER LIMB

☐ Sacroiliac and Pubic Symphysis[7]

RESTING POSITION
Not described

CLOSE-PACKED POSITION
Not described

CAPSULAR PATTERNS
For both joints, pain when joints are stressed.

☐ Hip

COMPONENT MOTIONS

Flexion. Posterior and inferior glide of femoral head in acetabulum

Abduction. Inferior glide of femoral head in acetabulum

External Rotation. Anterior glide of femoral head

Internal Rotation. Posterior glide of femoral head

RESTING POSITION

The hip is flexed to about 30°, abducted to about 30°, and slightly externally rotated.[12]

CLOSE-PACKED POSITION

Ligamentous: Internal rotation with extension with abduction

POTENTIAL CLOSE-PACKED POSITION

Bony: The hip is flexed to about 90°, abducted and externally rotated slightly.

CAPSULAR PATTERN

Internal rotation and abduction are most restricted; flexion and extension are restricted; external rotation is relatively free.

☐ Knee

COMPONENT MOTIONS

FLEXION
1. Medial rotation of tibia on femur during first 15° to 20° flexion from full extension
2. Posterior glide of tibia on femur
3. Inferior movement of patella
4. Inferior movement of fibula

Extension. Reverse of flexion

Analysis of Knee Motion. The knee primarily moves about a single axis that lies horizontally in the frontal plane. If the tibia moves on a stationary femur, roll and slide occur in the same direction. If the femur moves on a fixed tibia, roll and slide occur in opposite directions. Toward the last 10° to 20° extension, almost a pure roll occurs, the rolling phase being somewhat longer on the lateral side. Moving into flexion, the rolling motion between the joint surfaces gradually becomes more and more a sliding motion. Thus, the articular contact point on the femur gradually moves backward (while moving into flexion); the articular contact point on the tibia moves backward during the first phase of flexion, then gradually narrows to a point (in the case of the femur moving on the tibia).

A length rotation also occurs between the femur and tibia during flexion and extension at this joint. This rotation is a necessary part of normal joint kinematics and may be lost in certain pathological conditions, such as a torn meniscus or adhered capsule. Considering the case of the femur moving on the tibia during the last, say, 30° extension, the femur must rotate inward for close-packing and full extension to occur. There are many explanations for this phenomenon. Most include the fact that because the lateral femoral condyle is smaller, it reaches its close-packed congruent position in extension before the medial condyle does. For the medial condyle to continue movement, it must slide backward around an axis passing somewhere through the lateral femoral condyle. The resultant rotation of the lateral condyle forces the anterior segment of the lateral meniscus forward over the convex lateral tibia condyle such that the lateral femoral condyle is no longer congruent and may continue into somewhat more extension. Of course, this all happens simultaneously and continues until the knee becomes locked in its close-packed position of full extension (about 5° hyperextension). In this position, the cruciates are pulled tight and twisted so as to prevent internal rotation of the tibia on the femur. The collaterals also become twisted relative to each other (the medial ligament passes downward and forward, the lateral ligament passes downward and backward) so as to prevent outward rotation of the tibia on the femur. Both sets of ligaments prevent further extension, with help from the soft tissues posteriorly.

RESTING POSITION

About 25° knee flexion[15]

CLOSE-PACKED POSITION

Full extension with lateral rotation

CAPSULAR PATTERN

Flexion is most restricted; extension is somewhat restricted.

☐ Proximal Tibiofibular Joint

RESTING POSITION

25° knee flexion, 10° plantar-flexion[7]

CLOSE-PACKED POSITION

Not described

CAPSULAR PATTERN

Pain when joint stressed

☐ Distal Tibiofibular Joint

RESTING POSITION

10° plantar-flexion, 5° inversion[7]

CLOSE-PACKED POSITION

None; not a synovial joint

CAPSULAR PATTERN OF RESTRICTION

None; not a synovial joint

☐ Talocrural

COMPONENT MOTIONS

Dorsiflexion. Backward glide of talus on tibia; spreading of distal tibiofibular joint

Plantar-Flexion. Reverse of dorsiflexion

RESTING POSITION

The foot is in about 10° plantar-flexion and midway between maximal inversion and eversion.[12]

CLOSE-PACKED POSITION

Full dorsiflexion

CAPSULAR PATTERN

Dorsiflexion and plantar-flexion are both limited, plantar-flexion slightly more so unless the heel cord is tight.

☐ Subtalar Joint

COMPONENT MOTIONS

The subtalar joint is essentially bicondylar. The posterior facet of the talus on the calcaneus is a concave-on-convex surface; the combined anterior and medial facet forms a convex-on-concave joint. On eversion of the calcaneus on the talus, the posterior joint surface of the calcaneus must glide medially, while the anterior and medial facets must glide laterally.

RESTING POSITION

The foot is midway between maximal inversion and eversion with 10° plantar flexion.

CLOSE-PACKED POSITION

Full inversion

CAPSULAR PATTERN

Inversion (varus) is very restricted; eversion (valgus) is free.

☐ Midtarsal Joints: Talonavicular and Calcaneocuboid

RESTING POSITION

10° plantar-flexion, midway between supination and pronation

CLOSE-PACKED POSITION

Full supination

CAPSULAR PATTERN

Supination greater than pronation (limited dorsiflexion, plantar flexion, adduction, and medial rotation)

☐ Tarsometatarsal

RESTING POSITION

Midway between supination and pronation

CLOSE-PACKED POSITION

Full supination

CAPSULAR PATTERN

Not described

☐ Metatarsophalangeal

RESTING POSITION

Neutral (extension 10°)

CLOSE-PACKED POSITION

Full extension

CAPSULAR PATTERN

For the first metatarsophalangeal joint, extension is greater than flexion; for metatarsophalangeal joints 2 through 5, variable, tends toward extension greater than flexion.

☐ Interphalangeal Joints

RESTING POSITION

Slight flexion

CLOSE-PACKED POSITION

Full extension

CAPSULAR PATTERN

Tends toward extension restrictions

☐ Orientation of Joint Axes

In the embryo the lower limb started out abducted and externally rotated so that the sole of the foot faced forward. During development, the leg must rotate medially and adduct. As a result, the femoral condyles are rotated inward (about 10° in the adult) in relation to the neck of the femur, and the shaft of the femur is adducted (forming an angle of about 125° in the adult) with respect to the femoral neck. The shaft of the tibia is rotated about 25° outwardly so the axis of the ankle mortise is 25° outwardly rotated, relative

to the knee. The axis of the subtalar joint runs about 20° from back and out to front and in.

■ SPINE

In three-dimensional space, the spine has six components (degrees of freedom) of the vertebral segments.[28] A vertebral body can move in six different ways (Fig. A-1):

1. Forward and backward in the sagittal plane (anterior and posterior translation)
2. Forward and backward tilting on a frontal axis (*i.e.*, flexion and extension)
3. Laterally, in the frontal plane by a slight translation or gliding motion (*i.e.*, lateral translation)
4. Lateral tilting or rotation around a sagittal axis (movement in the frontal plane) or sidebending
5. Rotation in the horizontal plane, around a vertical axis

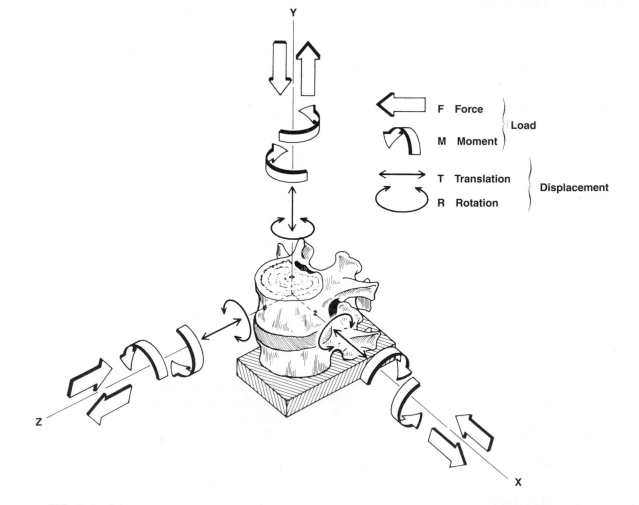

FIG. A-1. *Scheme to illustrate the six degrees of freedom of vertebral segments. (White AA, Panjabi MM: Clinical Biomechanics of the Spine, 2nd ed, p 132. Philadelphia, JB Lippincott, 1990.)*

6. Compression or distraction in the longitudinal axis of the spine

A vertebra may rotate or translate along any of these axes or move in various combinations of these motions (longitudinal, vertical, and sagittal). Pure movement in any of these three principal planes very seldom occurs. The facet joints act to guide and limit these motions; the plane of the facet joints determines the direction and amount of motion at each segment. The torsional stiffness of the spine is largely determined by the design of the facet joints.

☐ Cervical Spine

LOWER CERVICAL SPINE (C2–T2)

The only pure motions that exist in the cervical spine from C2 through C7 are that of flexion and extension in the sagittal plane, because lateral flexion and rotation are combined motions. The site of maximum motion in flexion and extension occurs between C4 and C6. In the combined movements of lateral flexion and rotation, the spinous processes of the vertebral bodies move toward the convexity of the curve, or opposite to rotation of the vertebral body. The direction of physiological rotation combined with lateral flexion appears to be the same regardless of whether the cervical spine is in flexion or extension. When we laterally bend to one side, we automatically get some physiological rotation to that side; when we rotate to one side, we automatically get some lateral flexion to the same side. According to Brown,[4] there are two degrees of coupled axial rotation for every three degrees of lateral bending. Between C2 and C7 there is a gradual cephalocaudal decrease in the amount of axial rotation that is associated.

Although movement rapidly diminishes from above downward, lateral flexion is accompanied by rotation to the same side at the cervicothoracic region (C6–T3).

RESTING POSITION

Slight forward flexion

CLOSE-PACKED POSITION

Full backward bending

CAPSULAR PATTERN

Lateral flexion and rotation are equally limited and greater limitation than extension.

OCCIPITO-ATLANTO-AXIAL COMPLEX (OCCIPUT–C1–C2)

The atlanto-occipital joint permits primarily a nodding motion of the head (*i.e.*, flexion and extension in the sagittal plane around a coronal axis).[2,16] Although there is dispute as to whether any rotation occurs between the occiput and the atlas, a small amount of rotation may be felt between the mastoid process and the transverse process on passive testing. During lateral flexion, the occiput moves in a direction opposite to that in which the head is laterally flexed.[3]

Motion at the atlanto-axial joint includes flexion, extension, lateral flexion, and rotation. About 50% of the total rotation of the cervical region occurs at the median atlanto-axial joint before rotation in the rest of cervical spine. When the atlas pivots around the dens at the median atlanto-axial joint, the skull and atlas move as one unit. The lateral atlanto-axial joint serves to guide the rotation, which is about 45°.

RESTING POSITION
Midway between flexion and extension

CLOSE-PACKED POSITION
Not described

CAPSULAR PATTERN
Atlanto-occipital joint: Forward-bending greater than backward-bending; atlanto-axial joint: Restriction with rotation

☐ Thoracic Spine

Motion in the upper thoracic spine most likely mimics the cervical spine, with sidebending and rotation coupled to the same side.[13,27,28] Motion in the midthoracic spine is variable and inconsistent among individuals.[13,28] In the lower thoracic spine (as in the lumbar spine) sidebending is accompanied by rotation to the same side only in flexion.[13] In the neutral and extended position, sidebending is accompanied by rotation to the opposite side.[13]

Vertebral rotation in the thoracic spine produces associated movement of the corresponding ribs. The rib on the side to which the vertebra is rotated moves in a dorsal direction, and the rib on the opposite side to which the vertebra is rotated moves in a ventral direction.[7] If a positional fault of the thoracic spine is detected, an associated positional fault of the ribs should also be investigated.

RESTING POSITION

Not described

CLOSE-PACKED POSITION

Full backward-bending

CAPSULAR PATTERN

Side flexion and rotation are equally limited; backward-bending is quite limited.

☐ Lumbar Spine

The lumbar region is the pivot point for most general movements of the trunk, with movements of the lower lumbar spine being the most free. The large lumbar intervertebral disks potentially allow free flexion, extension, and lateral flexion. However, these motions are limited in the lumbar spine, and the direction of the movement is controlled by the orientation of the facet joints. Because of the shape of the facets, rotation in the lumbar spine is minimal and is accomplished only by a shearing force.

The lumbar region shows certain cross-coupling of spinal motions. Two types of motion may occur at the same time, and frequently three motions simultaneously occur during normal physiological movements.[8,9,12,18,24]

Forward-bending (flexion) and backward-bending (extension) may be considered relatively pure movements to a degree. Some coupling has been proposed but has not been clearly delineated.[17,22,25,27,28] Both flexion and extension reduce the range of sidebending and rotation. Flexion sometimes slightly reverses the lumbar curve from the L3 segment upward.

As with the thoracic spine, much controversy exists in the literature as to the nature of coupling. Due to facet joint orientation, relatively less sidebending and rotation occur at the lower lumbar segments than at the upper lumbar joints.[23,28] In the three upper segments (as in the thoracic spine), sidebending and rotation to the opposite side are thought to be coupled weakly.[17,22,23,28] The L4–L5, a transitional segment, appears to exhibit inconsistent behavior but is thought to result in sidebending and rotation to the same side.[23]

Stoddard[26] stated that the direction of axial rotation varies depending on whether the lateral flexion was performed with the lumbar spine in flexion or extension. He suggests that the axial rotation is to the same side when lateral flexion is performed in flexion and to the opposite side when lateral flexion is performed in extension. Fryette[10] stated that axial rotation occurs to the same side if the segments are in full flexion or extension with the facets engaged; in neutral, without locking of the facets (erect standing), rotation is to the opposite side as sidebending. According to Edwards,[8]

the direction of axial rotation is in the opposite direction to which the lumbar spine is laterally flexed, regardless of whether the spine is in flexion or extension. Although these combined movement tendencies require further investigation, they offer a useful objective examination tool.

RESTING POSITION

According to MacConaill,[19] flexed spinal joints are loose-packed and movement is limited by soft-tissue contact. The anti-close-packed position is extreme flexion with minimal convexity of the lumbar portion of the column and minimal kinking of the lumbosacral junction.

CLOSE-PACKED POSITION

The close-packed position is that of full extension. In this position there is maximum forward convexity of the lumbar and cervical portions of the column and maximum kinking of the lumbosacral junction. At the thoracolumbar junction region, a mortise effect is produced on full extension by engagement of the articular facets. This is one of the few articular mechanisms in the body where a practically solid lock occurs at the extreme of movement.[6]

CAPSULAR PATTERN

Bilateral Pattern of Restriction. As in many synovial joints, movements toward the close-packed position are the most restricted and the earliest restricted in cases of capsular tightness. Thus, the capsular patterns of restriction in bilateral facet joint involvement are marked. There is marked and equal limitation of lateral flexion and rotation and limitation of flexion and extension (extension > flexion).

Unilateral Pattern of Restriction. In general, motion loss is most noticeable in sidebending opposite to and in rotation to the involved side. Thus, if the right facet is restricted, there will be:

1. Considerable limitation of sidebending left and rotation to the right
2. Moderate restriction of forward-bending (swings to the right)
3. Mild to slight restriction of sidebending right and rotation to the left

REFERENCES

1. Barnett C, Davies D, MacConaill MA: Synovial Joints—Their Structures and Mechanics. Springfield, IL, Charles C. Thomas, 1961
2. Basmajian BE: Primary Anatomy, 7th ed. Baltimore, Williams & Wilkins, 1976
3. Braakman R, Penning L: Injuries of the Cervical Spine. Amsterdam, Excerpta Medica, 1971

4. Brown L: An introduction to the treatment and examination of the spine by combined movements. Physiotherapy 77:347–353, 1988

5. Cyriax J: Textbook of Orthopedic Medicine, Vol. 1: Diagnosis of Soft-Tissue Lesions, 5th ed. Baltimore, Williams & Wilkins, 1969

6. Davis PR: The thoracolumbar mortise joint. J Anat 89:370, 1955

7. Edmonds S: Manipulation and Mobilization: Extremity and Spinal Techniques. St. Louis, Mosby, 1993

8. Edwards BC: Clinical assessment: The use of combined movements in assessment and treatment. In Twomey LT, Taylor JR (eds): Physical Therapy of the Low Back. New York, Churchill Livingstone, 1987

9. Farfan HF: Muscular mechanisms of the lumbar spine and the positions of power and efficiency. Orthop Clin North Am 6(1):135, 1975

10. Fryette HH: The Principles of Osteopathic Technique. Carmel, CA, Academy of Applied Osteopathy, 1954

11. Graber TM: Overbite: The dentist's challenge. J Am Dent Assoc 79:1135–1139, 1969

12. Gregerson GC, Lucas DB: An in vivo study of the axial rotation of the human thoracolumbar spine. J Bone Joint Surg 49A:247–262, 1967

13. Grieve GP: Vertebral movement. In Grieve GP (ed): Mobilisation of the Spine, A Primary Handbook of Clinical Method, 5th ed. Edinburgh, Churchill Livingstone, 1991:9–19

14. Hesse JR, Hansson JR: Factors influencing joint mobility in general and in particular respect of craniomandibular articulation: A literature review. J Craniomandibular Disord 2:19–28, 1988

15. Kaltenborn F: Manual Therapy for the Extremity Joints. Oslo, Olaf Norlis Bokhandel, 1986

16. Kent BA: Anatomy of the trunk: A review, Part I. Phys Ther 54:722–744, 1976

17. Kulak RF, Schultz AB, Belytschko T, et al: Biomechanical characteristics of vertebral motion segments and intervertebral discs. Orthop Clin North Am 6:121–133, 1975

18. Loebl WY: Regional rotation of the lumbar spine. Rheumatol Rehabil 12:223, 1973

19. MacConaill MA: Joint movement. Physiotherapy 50:359, 1964

20. MacConaill MA, Basmajian JV: Muscles and Movements: A Basis for Human Kinesiology, 2nd ed. Hunting, NY, RE Krieger Pub., 1977

21. Osborn JW: The disc of the human temporomandibular joint: Design, function and dysfunction. J Oral Rehabil 12:279, 1985

22. Panjabi M, Yamamoto I, Oxland T, et al: How does posture affect coupling in the lumbar spine? Spine 14:1002–1011, 1989

23. Pearcy MU, Tibrewal SB: Axial rotation and lateral bending in the normal lumbar spine measured by three-dimensional radiography. Spine 9:582–587, 1983

24. Rocabado M: Arthrokinematics of the temporomandibular joints. Dent Clin North Am 27:573–594, 1983

25. Rolander SD: Motion of the lumbar spine with special reference to the stabilising effect of posterior fusion: An experimental study on autopsy specimens. Acta Orthop Scand [Supp] 90:1–144, 1966

26. Stoddard A: Manual of Osteopathic Technique. London, Hutchinson, 1962

27. Veldhuizen AG, Scholten PJM: Kinematics of the scoliotic spine. Spine 12:852–858, 1987

28. White AA, Panjabi MM: Clinical Biomechanics of the Spine, 2nd ed. Philadelphia, JB Lippincott, 1990

29. Williams P, Warwick R, Dysom M (eds): Gray's Anatomy, 37th British ed. Philadelphia, JB Lippincott, 198

Modified Low-Dye Strapping

■ **Rationale for Use**

■ **Materials**

■ **Procedure**

Low-dye strapping or taping is used primarily to reduce strain on the plantar fascia and medial arch structures to help control excessive pronation.[1,2,5] It has been found to be a useful adjunct in common "overuse syndromes" that present with excessive or prolonged pronation, such as medial arch strain, plantar fasciitis (particularly in the early stages), and posterior tibial tendinitis (shin splints). At this time, much of the information regarding adhesive strapping is empirical. The ability of the low-dye taping method to modify forces on the medial arch during weight-bearing has been clearly demonstrated by Scranton and co-workers.[7] This method is felt to medialize heel strike forces and diminish duration of forces under the midfoot, as well as medialize the anterior forefoot forces resulting in diminished strain on the medial plantar fascia and plantar-tarsal ligaments.[7] In effect, external and mechanical support to the arch is provided. This taping procedure should be meticulously applied and may be used with or without heelcups and orthoses during activity. It is especially useful in controlling pronation in dancers and gymnasts who cannot wear orthoses. Light elastic tape is preferable in activities such as gymnastics, whereas heavier tape can be used in most other activities and sports. Tape should be placed directly on the skin for maximum support, but even with underwrap, proper taping will provide additional stabilization even after strenuous activity.[3,4] Low-dye strapping should be avoided in metatarsal stress fractures and metatarsalgia, since this type of taping can shift the forces anteriorly to the forefoot more rapidly, producing increased forefoot stress which may aggravate these conditions.[6]

I. **Rationale for Use**
   A. To stabilize the head of the first metatarsal by plantar flexion
   B. To decrease pain
   C. To determine need for an orthotic
II. **Materials**
   A. Moleskin strapping
   B. Tape adherent (*e.g.,* Tuf-skin)
   C. Tape—1 or $1\frac{1}{2}$ inch
III. **Procedure**
   A. Preparation
      1. Shave, clean, and thoroughly dry the forefoot.
      2. Apply tape adherent to dorsal, plantar, and medial aspect of forefoot.
      3. Place small piece of adhesive moleskin below the first and fifth metatarsal heads to reduce abrasion on these areas.
      4. Cut a 2-inch-wide adhesive moleskin strip to size of foot, measuring from the first to fifth metatarsal head. Cut a 3- $\times$ $\frac{1}{2}$-inch

Darlene Hertling and Randolph M. Kessler: MANAGEMENT OF COMMON MUSCULOSKELETAL DISORDERS: Physical Therapy Principles and Methods, 3rd ed. © 1996 Lippincott-Raven Publishers.

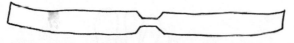

FIG. B-1. *Preparation of adhesive moleskin tape.*

angled piece from both sides of mid-portion of the moleskin (Fig. B-1).[8]

B. Tape application

1. An anchor strip of 1-inch adhesive tape is applied loosely on the dorsal and plantar aspects of the foot just proximal to the metatarsal heads (Fig. B-2).

2. Peel away the backing of the moleskin strip. Place one end on the head of the fifth metatarsal and secure it along the lateral aspect of the foot. Continue around the posterior aspect of the calcaneus (Fig. B-3).

3. Ensure that the foot is in subtalar neutral position (see Fig. 14-27). Stabilize the lateral four rays by placing your hand on the lateral aspect of the foot with your thumb on the plantar aspect of the foot. Plantar flex the first ray before securing the rest of the moleskin to the head of the first metatarsal (Fig. B-4).

   Note: If tape is used in place of the adhesive moleskin, second and third strips are placed around the foot, partially overlapping each other.

4. With 1-inch adhesive tape, strap the longitudinal arch with the "scissor" method or figure-of-eight. Half a figure-of-eight is performed by starting at the base of the great toe, angling across the longitudinal arch around the heel, and returning to the base of the great toe. The other half is reversed, using the base of the little toe as the starting position (Fig. B-5). The steps are repeated once or twice.

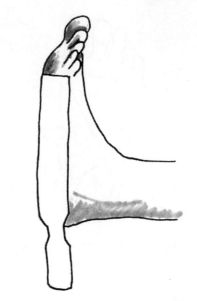

FIG. B-3. *Application of moleskin strip around calcaneus and lateral sides of foot.*

5. A closing anchor is placed on the dorsum of the foot over the original anchor. Additional anchor strips may be placed on the plantar aspect of the foot with horizontal strips applied from one side of the moleskin to the other, along the entire length of the foot. These horizontal strips are placed by pulling gently medially, from the heel to the ball of the foot (Fig. B-6).

Care must be taken to account for the expansion of the foot on weight-bearing. When the strapping is correctly applied, the great toe will be plantar flexed at the metatarsophalangeal joint and the medial longitudinal arch will be heightened and well maintained. A felt pad or a post under the medial aspect of the forefoot can be incorporated in the taping if a large defor-

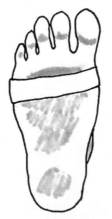

FIG. B-2. *Application of anchor strip to metatarsal heads.*

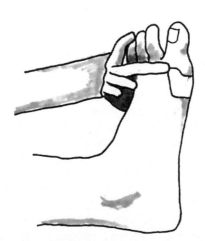

FIG. B-4. *Positioning of foot in subtalar neutral and securing rest of moleskin to metatarsal head.*

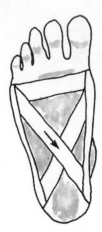

FIG. B-5. *Scissor applications of figures-of-eight from base of little toe.*

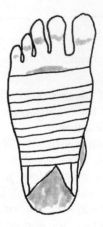

FIG. B-6. *Anchoring horizontal strips, dorsoplantar surface of foot.*

mity is present. The patient should be advised to keep the strapping dry. When weight-bearing, shoes should be worn to help prolong the life of the strapping. The foot and extremity posture should be reevaluated in stance and gait.

REFERENCES

1. Appenzeller O, Atkinson R: Sports Medicine. Fitness, Training Injuries, 3rd ed, pp 467–480. Baltimore, Urban and Schwarzenberg, 1988
2. Duggar GE: Plantar fascitis and heel spurs. In McGlawry ED (ed): Reconstructive Surgery of the Foot and Leg, pp 67–73. New York, Intercontinental Medical Book, 1974
3. Glick J, Gordon R, Nishimoto D: The prevention and treatment of ankle injuries. Am J Sports Med 4:136–141, 1976
4. Laughman RK, Carr TA, Chao EY, et al: Three-dimensional kinematics of the taped ankle before and after exercise. Am J Sports Med 8:425–531, 1980
5. Newell SG, Miller SJ: Conservative treatment of plantar fascial strain. Phys Sports Med 5:68–73, 1977
6. Scranton P: Metatarsalgia. Diagnosis and treatment. J Bone Joint Surg 62(A):723–732, 1980
7. Scranton PE, Pedegana LR, Whitesel JP: Gait analysis: Alterations in support phase forces using supportive devices. Am J Sports Med 10:6–11, 1982
8. Whitesel J, Newell SG: Modified low-dye strapping. Phys Sports Med 10:280–281, 1980

RECOMMENDED READINGS

Bruggeman A, Bruggeman JH: Modifications in the treatment program of the inversion sprain of the ankle. Int J Sports Med 5:42–44, 1984
Kosmahl EM, Kosmahl HE: Painful plantar heel, plantar fascitis, and calcaneal spur: Etiology and treatment. J Sports Med 9:17–24, 1987
Marshall P: The rehabilitation of over-use foot injuries in athletes and dancers. Clin Sports Med 7:175–191, 1988
Reed DC: Heel pain and problems of the hindfoot. In Reid DC: Sports Injury: Assessment and Rehabilitation, pp 185–214. New York, Churchill Livingstone, 1992
Roy S, Irvin R: Sports Medicine: Prevention, Evaluation, Management and Rehabilitation, pp 55–77. Englewood Cliffs, NJ, Prentice-Hall, 1983

INDEX